MW00979663

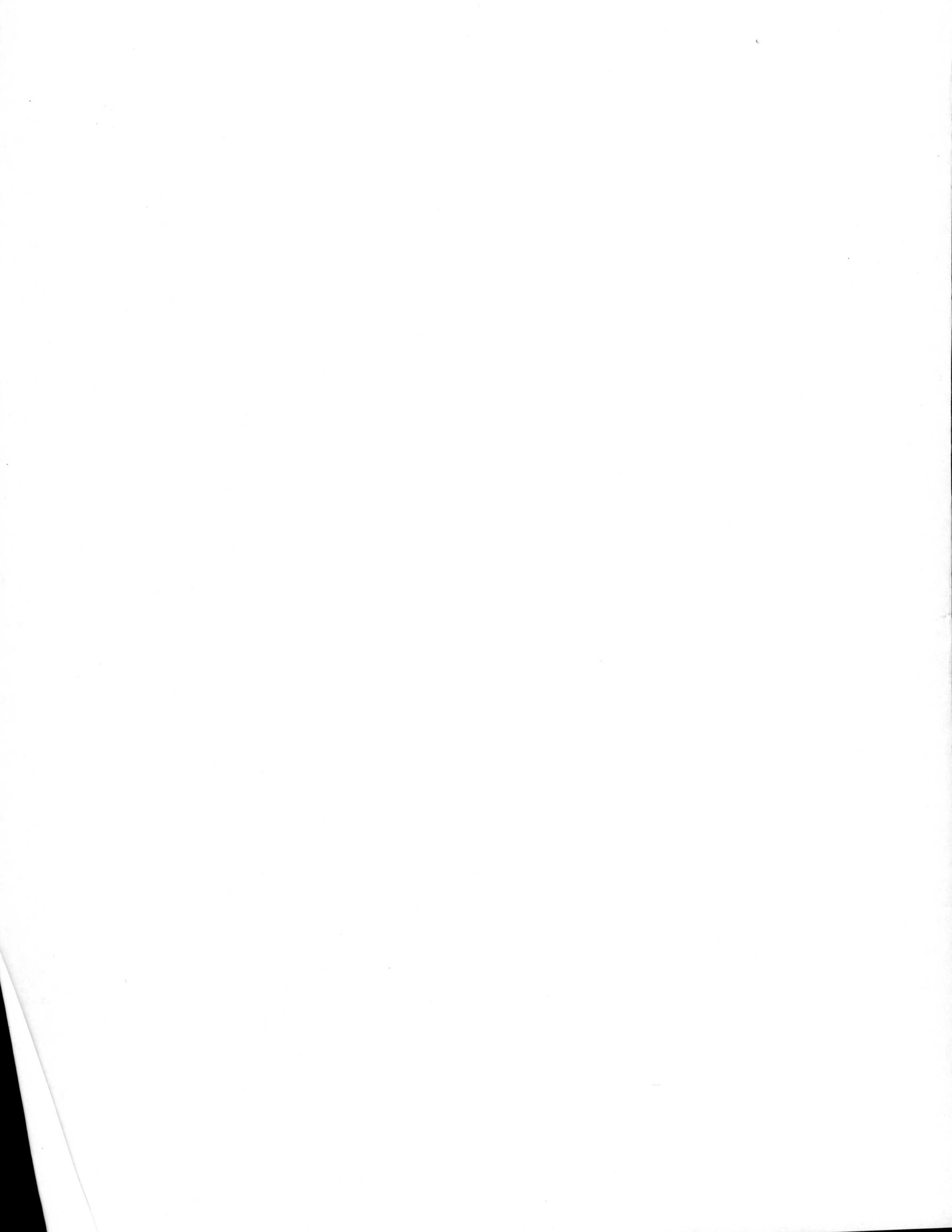

FRACTURES OF THE PELVIS AND ACETABULUM

THIRD EDITION

FRACTURES OF THE PELVIS AND ACETABULUM

THIRD EDITION

Editor-in-Chief

MARVIN TILE, M.D., M.Sc. (MED), F.R.C.S.(C)

Professor of Surgery
University of Toronto
Chairman
Sunnybrook Foundation
Sunnybrook Health Science Centre
Toronto, Ontario, Canada

Section Editors

DAVID L. HELFET, M.D.

Professor of Surgery (Orthopaedics)
Weill Medical College of Cornell University
Chief
Department of Combined Orthopaedic Trauma
Hospital for Special Surgery
New York, New York

JAMES F. KELLAM, M.D., F.R.C.S.(C)

Vice Chairman
Department of Orthopaedic Surgery
Director
Department of Orthopaedic Trauma
Carolinas Medical Center
Charlotte, North Carolina

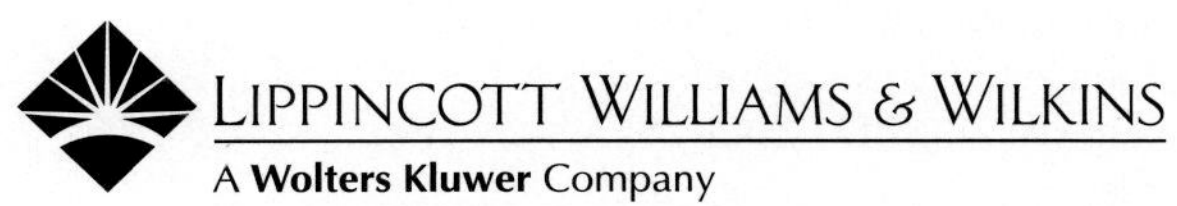

A **Wolters Kluwer** Company
Philadelphia • Baltimore • New York • London
Buenos Aires • Hong Kong • Sydney • Tokyo

Acquisitions Editor: *Robert Hurley*
Developmental Editor: *Michelle LaPlante*
Production Editor: *Deirdre Marino*
Manufacturing Manager: *Colin Warnock*
Cover Designer: *Christine Jenny*
Compositor: *Maryland Composition Company, Inc.*
Printer: *Edwards Brothers*

530 Walnut Street
Philadelphia, PA 19106 USA
LWW.com

Printed in the USA

Library of Congress Cataloging-in-Publication Data

Fractures of the pelvis and acetabulum / Marvin Tile, editor-in-chief; section editors, David L. Helfet, James F. Kellam.—3rd ed.
p. ; cm.
Rev. ed. of: Fractures of the pelvis and acetabulum / Marvin Tile. 2nd. ed. 1995.
Includes bibliographical references and index.
ISBN 0-7817-3213-1
1. Pelvic bones—Fractures. 2. Acetabulum (Anatomy)—Fractures. I. Tile, Marvin. II. Helfet, David. III. Kellam, James. IV. Tile, Marvin. Fractures of the pelvis and acetabulum.
[DNLM: 1. Pelvic Bones—injuries. 2. Acetabulum—injuries. 3. Fracture Fixation. 4. Fractures. WE 750 F798 2003]
RD549.F73 2003
617.1′58—dc21

2002043395

Care has been taken to confirm the accuracy of the information presented and to describe generally accepted practices. However, the authors, editors, and publisher are not responsible for errors or omissions or for any consequences from application of the information in this book and make no warranty, expressed or implied, with respect to the currency, completeness, or accuracy of the contents of the publication. Application of this information in a particular situation remains the professional responsibility of the practitioner.

The authors, editors, and publisher have exerted every effort to ensure that drug selection and dosage set forth in this text are in accordance with current recommendations and practice at the time of publication. However, in view of ongoing research, changes in government regulations, and the constant flow of information relating to drug therapy and drug reactions, the reader is urged to check the package insert for each drug for any change in indications and dosage and for added warnings and precautions. This is particularly important when the recommended agent is a new or infrequently employed drug.

Some drugs and medical devices presented in this publication have Food and Drug Administration (FDA) clearance for limited use in restricted research settings. It is the responsibility of the health care provider to ascertain the FDA status of each drug or device planned for use in their clinical practice.

10 9 7 6 5 4 3 2 1

To my wife and companion, Esther, for her continuing encouragement and support.

To my family, Gary, Rosemary, Katy, Sari, and Noah Tile; Stephen, Christine, David, Rachel, and Abby Tile; Steve, Deborah, Ian, and Annie Cass; and Andrew Tile and his partner Candy Ramberansingh, for their devotion and understanding, and for bringing balance and joy to my life.

To my assistant, Shirley Fitzgerald, for her selflessness, diligence, loyalty, and friendship in bringing all three editions of this text to fruition.

—Marvin Tile, M.D.

To my wife, Molly, and children, Kelly and Arthur John (A.J.) for their continued love, support and understanding.

—David L. Helfet, M.D.

To my family: Lynda, Lindsay, Stephanie, and Patrick.

—James F. Kellam, M.D.

CONTENTS

CONTRIBUTING AUTHORS

Jorge E. Alonso, M.D. Associate Professor, Department of Orthopaedic Surgery, Assistant Chief of Staff, University of Alabama at Birmingham, Birmingham, Alabama

David E. Aspirinio, M.D. Acting Chairman, Department of Orthopaedic Surgery, Westchester Medical Center, Hawthorne, New York

Jorge Barla, M.D. Orthopaedic Trauma Fellow, University of Calgary, Calgary, Alberta, Canada

Craig S. Bartlett, M.D. Assistant Clinical Professor, Department of Orthopaedics and Rehabilitation, McClure Musculoskeletal Research Center, University of Vermont College of Medicine, Burlington, Vermont

Martin Beck, M.D. Associate Professor Department of Orthopaedic Surgery, University of Bern, Inselspital, Bern, Switzerland

Martin D. Bircher, M.D. Ashtead Hospital, The Warren Ashtead, Surrey, United Kingdom

Cory Borkhoff, M.D. Associate Professor, Department of Orthopaedic Surgery, Cleveland Clinic Florida, Weston, Florida

Holly K. Brown, M.D. Associate Professor, Department of Orthopaedic Surgery, Cleveland Clinic Florida, Weston, Florida

Carol E. Copeland, M.D. Assistant Professor, Department of Orthopaedics, University of Maryland at Baltimore; and Attending Orthopaedic Traumatologist, Department of Orthopaedics, R. Adams Cowley Shock Trauma Center, Baltimore, Maryland

S. de Lange, M.D. Department of Orthopaedics, The Hague Medical Center, The Hague, The Netherlands

Victor A. De Ridder, M.D. Department of Traumatology, St. Franciscus Hospital, Rotterdam, The Netherlands

Kenneth A. Egol, M.D. Assistant Professor, Department of Orthopaedic Surgery, New York University School of Medicine, New York, New York

Thomas J. Ellis, M.D. Assistant Professor, Department of Orthopaedics and Rehabilitation, Oregon Health Science University, Portland, Oregon

Wolfgang K. Ertel, M.D. Professor and Surgeon-in-Chief, Trauma Center Berlin-Brandenburg, Department of Trauma and Reconstructive Surgery, Benjamin Franklin Medical Center, Free University of Berlin, Berlin, Germany

Axel Gänsslen, M.D. Department of Trauma, Hand and Reconstructive Surgery, University Hospital, Homburg/Saar, Hannover, Germany

Reinhold Ganz, M.D. Professor and Chairman, Department of Orthopaedic Surgery, Inselspital University of Bern, Bern, Switzerland

Emanuel Gautier, M.D. Co-Chief, Department of Orthopaedic Surgery, Hôpital Cantonal, Fribourg, Fribourg, Switzerland

William H. Geerts, M.D. Associate Professor, Department of Medicine, Sunnybrook & Women's College Health Sciences Centre, University of Toronto, Toronto, Canada

John Gorczyca, M.D. Associate Professor, Department of Orthopaedic Surgery, University of Rochester Medical Center, Rochester, New York

John H. Healey, M.D. Chief, Orthopaedic Service, Memorial Sloan Kettering Hospital, New York, New York

Trevor Hearn, B.Sc. Ph.D. Professor of Orthopaedic Research, Department of Surgery, Flinders University School of Medicine, Adelaide, South Australia

David L. Helfet, M.D. Professor of Surgery (Orthopaedics), Weill Medical College of Cornell University; and Chief, Department of Combined Orthopaedic Trauma, Hospital for Special Surgery, New York, New York

Eero Hirvensalo, M.D. Department of Orthopaedic and Traumatology, Helsinki University Central Hospital, Helsinki, Finland

Richard M. Jay, M.D. Associate Professor, Department of Medicine, Sunnybrook & Women's College Health Sciences Centre, University of Toronto, Toronto, Ontario, Canada

Matthew L. Jimenez, M.D. Assistant Professor, Advocate Lutheran General Hospital; and Department of Orthopaedic Surgery, University of Chicago, Illinois Bone and Joint Institute, Des Plaines, Illinois

Eric E. Johnson, M.D. Professor, Department of Orthopaedic Surgery, University of California—Los Angeles Medical Center, Los Angeles, California

David M. Kahler, M.D. Associate Professor, Director of Orthopaedic Trauma, University of Virginia Health System, Charlottesville, Virginia

James F. Kellam, M.D., F.R.C.S.(C) Vice Chairman, Department of Orthopaedic Surgery, Director, Department of Orthopaedic Trauma, Carolinas Medical Center, Charlotte, North Carolina

Kenneth J. Koval, M.D. Professor, Department of Orthopedics, New York University School of Medicine; and Chief, Fracture Service, Department of Orthopaedics, Hospital for Joint Diseases, New York, New York

Hans J. Kreder, M.D., M.P.H. Assistant Professor, Sunnybrook Health Science Center, University of Toronto, Toronto, Ontario, Canada

Jeffrey W. Mast, M.D. Northern Nevada Medical Center, Sparks, Nevada

Joel M. Matta, M.D. Clinical Professor, Good Samaritan Hospital, Los Angeles, California

Keith A. Mayo, M.D. Clinical Professor of Orthopaedics, University of Washington, Seattle, Washington; and Director, Department of Orthopaedic Trauma, Tacoma General Hospital, Tacoma, Washington

Alexander McLaren, M.D. Clinical Assistant Professor, University of Arizona College of Medicine; and Private Practice, Orthopaedic Surgery, Phoenix, Arizona

Dana C. Mears, M.D. Attending Surgeon, Department of Orthopaedic Surgery, University of Pittsburgh Medical Center; and Shadyside Hospital, Greater Pittsburgh Orthopaedic Associates, Pittsburgh, Pennsylvania

Douglas Mintz, M.D. Assistant Professor of Radiology, Weill Medical College of Cornell University; Assistant Attending Radiologist, New York Presbyterian Hospital; and Chief, Division of Computed Tomography, Hospital for Special Surgery, New York, New York

Berton R. Moed, M.D. Professor and Chairman, Department of Orthopaedic Surgery, St. Louis University, St. Louis, Missouri

John A. Ogden, M.D. Clinical Professor of Orthopaedics, Emory University School of Medicine; and Chairman, Department of Orthopaedics, Atlanta Medical Center, Atlanta, Georgia

Steven A. Olson, M.D. Professor, Department of Surgery, Duke University; and Chief, Orthopaedic Trauma, Division of Orthopaedic Surgery, Duke University Medical Center, Durham, North Carolina

Thomas J. Perlewitz, M.D. Resident, Department of Orthopaedic Surgery, Medical College of Wisconsin, Milwaukee, Wisconsin

Timothy Pohlemann, M.D. Unfallchirurgie, Med Hochsch, Hannover, Germany

James N. Powell, M.D. Associate Clinical Professor, University of Calgary; Department of Surgery, Foothills Hospital, Calgary, Alberta, Canada

Jeffrey Richmond, M.D. Private Practice, Orthopaedic Associates of Manhasset, Manhasset, New York

Pol M. Rommens, M.D., Ph.D. Chief, Department of Trauma Surgery, University Hospitals of the Johannes Gutenberg University of Mainz; and Professor, Johannes Gutenberg University of Mainz, Mainz, Germany

Joel Rubenstein, M.D., F.R.C.P. (C) Associate Professor, Department of Medical Imaging, University of Toronto; and Radiologist, Department of Medical Imaging, Sunnybrook Health Science Center, Toronto, Ontario, Canada

Gregory J. Schmeling, M.D. Associate Professor, Department of Orthopaedic Surgery, Medical College of Wisconsin; and Director of Orthopaedic Trauma, Department of Orthopaedic Surgery, Medical College of Wisconsin Affiliated Hospitals, Milwaukee, Wisconsin

Klaus A. Siebenrock, M.D. Staff Surgeon, Department of Orthopaedic Surgery, University of Bern, Inselspital, Bern, Switzerland

Adam J. Starr, M.D. Assistant Professor, Department of Orthopedic Surgery, University of Texas Southwestern Medical Center; and Staff, Parkland Memorial Hospital, Dallas, Texas

David J.G. Stephen, M.D. Assistant Professor, Department of Orthopaedics, Sunnybrook and Women's College Health Science Center, Toronto, Ontario, Canada

Michael D. Stover, M.D. Assistant Professor, Department of Orthopaedic Surgery, Loyola University Medical Center, Maywood, Illinois

Michael A. Terry, M.D. Senior Clinical Associate, Department of Orthopaedic Surgery, Weill Medical College of Cornell University; and Chief Resident, Department of Orthopaedic Surgery, Hospital for Special Surgery, New York, New York

Marvin Tile, M.D., M.Sc. (Med), F.R.C.S.(C) Professor of Surgery, University of Toronto; and Chairman, Sunnybrook Foundation, Sunnybrook Health Science Centre, Toronto, Ontario, Canada

Harald Tscherne, M.D. Director Emeritus, Department of Trauma, Hannover Medical School, Hannover, Germany

John H. Velyvis, M.D. Resident, Department of Orthopaedic Surgery, Albany Medical Center, Albany, New York

Mark S. Vrahas, M.D. Associate Professor, Department of Orthopaedics, Brigham and Woman's Hospital; and Chief, Partners Orthopaedics Trauma Service, Boston, Massachusetts

FOREWORD

The primary task of the fracture surgeon (despite what he is called) is the management of the injured patient, not merely the treatment of the broken bones. This emphasis on the whole patient is nowhere more vital (literally) than with pelvic fractures, whose diagnosis is so daunting and whose complications are so dangerous. Consequently, those who deal with them need wide experience in many fields—from shock, hemorrhage, and electrolyte problems, to injuries of the urogenital tract and bowel. A tall order—and that is only the beginning.

What about the bones themselves? The patient with a severe pelvic fracture is liable to say (if he can speak at all) "I feel as if I'm falling to pieces"—a shrewd self-diagnosis. Our task is to ensure that the patient ends up feeling whole again. At one time this meant letting nature slowly mend the broken bones, while we did our best to preserve joint function. Today there is another option—fixing the fragments surgically. To achieve this satisfactorily, the surgeon must first solve the three-dimensional jigsaw puzzle, by identifying each piece with precision, reassembling the fragments accurately, and fixing them securely—working all the while in what amounts to a surgical minefield.

No wonder the surgeon needs a map of the battle area and a campaign plan. And that is just what Dr. Tile has provided. He has laid out a pattern for systemically examining and critically assessing the patient for understanding the complex injuries and formulating a rational plan of treatment, not only of the bony and articular trauma, but also of the accompanying soft tissue and visceral damage. Most of us who work in this field have acquired much information but, although our sources are often both knowledgeable and authoritative, we tend to end up with a muddled mass of facts and ideas, injunctions, and prohibitions. Dr. Tile, through the alchemy of his experience and wisdom, has transmuted this murky mixture, making it clear and sparkling. He has not made pelvic injuries simple—how could they be? He has made them comprehensible.

With so many diverse disciplines involved, a leader is essential as a unifying influence to coordinate the efforts of the team and define the priorities of treatment. Who better than an orthopaedic surgeon, especially one of Professor Tile's caliber? We owe him a great debt for this book.

—Alan Graham Apley

PREFACE TO THE FIRST EDITION

"Knowledge comes, but wisdom lingers"
Alfred, Lord Tennyson

Severe injuries to the pelvic ring and to the acetabulum are occurring more frequently due to the "high-velocity" trauma so prevalent in our society. In the past decade, many advances have been made in the general management of the polytraumatized patient, thus improving the mortality rate of these patients. Also, advances in the management of major musculoskeletal trauma have considerably reduced the late morbidity associated with extremity injuries. These newer principles, methods, and implants developed for the management of musculoskeletal trauma, including techniques of both external and internal fixation, must also be applied to pelvic and acetabular injuries in order to reduce their morbidity. The first section of this book is devoted to disruption of the pelvic ring, the second section to fractures of the acetabulum.

The forces necessary to disrupt a pelvic ring in a young individual are massive, therefore, injury to the associated organs are common and often life threatening. The first order of priority for the trauma surgeon is *saving the patient's life.* Especially important in pelvic trauma is retroperitoneal hemorrhage, which may be massive and fatal. An algorithm designed by Dr. Robert Y. McMurtry will guide the reader through an orderly decision-making process and should help to control that important complication. Dr. Eric Saibil has contributed a section in the general management chapter on the use of therapeutic arteriography with clots of Gelfoam or other materials to control massive pelvic bleeding.

Often in the rush to save the patient's life, the fracture is ignored; however, the fracture should not be relegated to the bottom of the priority list to be dealt with later, when it has been determined that the patient may survive. That argument is faulty on two counts: first, early and suitable management of the fracture may contribute in a major way to the survival of the patient, and second, if care of the fracture is delayed inordinately, it may be impossible to achieve satisfactory long-term results. In this decade, it should be almost axiomatic that *"what is good for the fracture is good for the patient."* Stabilization of a major fracture in a polytraumatized patient will allow early, pain-free mobilization of the patient to the upright position for proper ventilation. Therefore, *treatment of the fracture should progress concomitantly with treatment of the associated injuries.*

The aim of fracture care is the early return of the patient to full function. For pelvic ring disruption, after careful assessment of the injury, logical management will depend upon the type of fracture. The reader may follow this management protocol in algorithm form. Stabilization of a massive, unstable pelvic ring disruption should not only help the patient's early posttrauma course, but also reduce the late complications of pain, nonunion, and malunion. The biomechanics of pelvic stabilization are outlined in detail, as well as their indications. Although I have included a chapter on internal fixation of the pelvic ring, I advise extreme caution at this time in proceeding with that treatment option. It should be reserved for those centers with particular expertise in this area, otherwise the complications may be excessive.

For fractures of the acetabulum the consequences of poor management are even greater. As in all major weight-bearing joints, fractures into the hip require anatomical reduction and early motion to ensure excellent long-term function. If this cannot be achieved by closed means, then open reduction and stable fixation are indicated, especially in young patients. The suggested treatment protocol will attempt to bridge the controversy between the proponents of closed and open methods; in effect, there would be no controversy, only a progression of logical thought. The classification suggested in Section 2 is based on related *fracture personality types:* anterior, posterior, and transverse. The methods of open reduction will be predicated on an accurate clinical and radiographic assessment, including CT scanning. Many of the common pitfalls of open reduction and internal fixation will be addressed.

In this book I have attempted to bridge the gap between the general surgical management of the associated injuries and the management of the musculoskeletal injuries by *simultaneous treatment* of both, and also the gap between the proponents of closed and open methods of management of both the pelvic ring and acetabular fracture. Treatment of these severe injuries should not *be either closed or open but, if closed fails—then open.* That form of logical decision making should be similar for all trauma care. We must individualize our care of the injured to achieve our ultimate goal—the early return of the injured patient to full function.

To paraphrase the opening quotation by Tennyson: we may learn new knowledge, but the application of that knowledge, namely sound surgical judgment, is the *lingering wisdom.*

Marvin Tile
Toronto

PREFACE

When the first edition of *Fractures of the Pelvis and Acetabulum* was published in 1984, the field of pelvic and acetabular surgery was in the adolescent phase, thanks to the previous decades' pioneering work by Pennal with the pelvic ring and Judet and Letournel with the acetabulum. By the second edition in 1995, the field had come of age, and with this third edition in 2003, it has become a full subspecialty of orthopedic traumatology.

Many changes have occurred to reflect the "conventional wisdom" of today—our diagnostic ability has been greatly enhanced, and the principles of treatment of the patient with pelvic or acetabular injury widely accepted. The field continues its rapid change, and in this new edition, we have highlighted the areas of likely change, mainly toward techniques of minimally invasive surgery.

In this edition, the book has been completely reorganized into three sections, each with its own section editor:

Section 1: General Aspects of the Pelvic Ring and Acetabulum, Marvin Tile
Section 2: Disruption of the Pelvic Ring, James F. Kellam
Section 3: Fractures of the Acetabulum, David L. Helfet

I am grateful to my co-editors for their hard work in bringing the work to fruition.

Many chapters have been completely rewritten and many new ones added, both by ourselves and by many new authors who have joined our venture, making this the most inclusive and comprehensive text on pelvic and acetabular trauma to be published to date.

The general orthopedic surgeon will find the third edition of *Fractures of the Pelvis and Acetabulum* invaluable, especially those chapters dealing with the emergency care of the polytraumatized patient with a pelvic injury, and those on decision-making in the emergency situation, even if just to direct the surgeon as to when to refer the patient to a pelvic trauma center.

For the specialist surgeon with a particular interest in pelvic and acetabular trauma, it will serve as a complete reference text for all aspects of these difficult fractures. We have greatly expanded the technical chapters, especially those on the acetabulum.

Finally, we have included a CD-ROM, with complete case documentation, of both pelvic ring and acetabular fractures.

As in the preface to the first edition, I quote Tennyson: *"knowledge grows, but wisdom lingers."* The continuing body of knowledge must be tempered with the lingering wisdom of sound clinical judgment.

Marvin Tile
Toronto

ACKNOWLEDGMENTS

In addition to those acknowledged in the first edition, I am indebted to the following individuals for their support, dedication, and hard work in bringing this third edition to completion:

To my co-editors, David Helfet and Jim Kellam, for their role in the reorganization of this edition, as well as their work as Section Editors.

To my co-authors, who contributed in the second edition and as well as the third: Jim Powell, Trevor Hearn, Joel Rubenstein, David Aspirinio, and Gregory Schmeling, for their dedication and expertise.

To the new authors who have joined our team, for their valuable contributions, we are very grateful.

These include, in Section I: General Aspects of the Pelvic Ring and Acetabulum—Martin Bircher for revision of the chapter on anatomy of the acetabulum; Trevor Hearn and Mark Vrahas for biomechanics of the pelvic injury; Steve Olson for a rewrite of acetabular injury biomechanics; Jorge Alonso for a rewrite of the pathoanatomy of the injuries; Wolfgang Ertel, who wrote a new chapter on the general management of the polytrauma patient with a pelvic injury; and Bill Geerts and Richard Jay, who contributed a new chapter on deep vein thrombosis in pelvic trauma.

In the Section II: Disruption of the Pelvic Ring—John Gorcyca and Trevor Hearn for a complete rewrite of biomechanics of pelvic fixation; Pol Rommens for a rewrite of external fixation; Roy Moed for addition of a section to the chapter on internal fixation; Tim Pohlemann, Axel Gänsslen, and Harald Tscherne for a complete rewrite on sacral fractures; Jorge Barla for open fractures; Carol Copeland, who wrote a new chapter on the obstetrical and genitourinary aspects of pelvic injury in women; Ken Egol and Ken Koval for a new chapter on insufficiency fractures; John Ogden, who contributed a rewrite of pelvic and acetabular trauma in the pediatric patient; Michael Stover and Joel Matta on malunion and nonunion; and Hans Kreder for a new chapter on outcomes in the pelvic ring patient.

In Section 3: Fractures of the Acetabulum—Douglas Mintz added to the assessment chapter; Steve Olson to decision making, nonoperative care; Martin Beck, Emanuel Gautier, Thomas Ellis, Reinhold Ganz, Klaus Siebenrock, and especially Craig Bartlett, for the rewrite of the internal fixation chapter; David Kahler and Adam Starr for new chapters on minimally invasive techniques; Jeff Mast for his major contribution on reduction and fixation techniques; Eero Hirvensalo, Victor De Ritter, S. de Lange, and Michael Terry, for contributions on techniques; David Stephen on a rewrite of the A-type fractures; Keith Mayo on a rewrite of the C-type both-column fracture; Thomas Perlewitz for adding to the complication chapter; Eric Johnson, who contributed a new chapter on malunion and nonunion; Dana Mears and John Velyvis, for new chapter on early total hip arthroplasty; Matt Jiminez for late total hip arthroplasty; Holly Brown and John Healey for a new contribution on the pathologic fracture; and Martin Bircher for outcomes of acetabular surgery.

To Trevor Hearn, former head of the Biomechanics Laboratory at Sunnybrook Health Science Centre for his contributions in the understanding of pelvic biomechanics, and to the AO Foundation and the Maurice Müller Foundation for their help with funding the laboratory.

To the team at Lippincott Williams & Wilkins—especially to Bob Hurley, Acquisitions Editor, for his help in getting this edition off the ground; Michelle LaPlante, Senior Developmental Editor, for her persistence, help, and expertise in putting together the final edit of the third edition; and Deirdre Marino, Supervising Production Editor, for seeing the project to completion.

To Cory Borkhoff, my research assistant and keeper of the Pelvic and Acetabular data bank at Sunnybrook & Women's Health Science Centre for her help with case illustrations throughout the text and the Pelvic CD-ROM; and to Dustin Dalgorf and Damian Chellaturai, our student research assistants, for helping with the case illustrations. I wish them every success in their future endeavors.

To Rena Frantzis, who made a tremendous effort on our behalf with her expertise and persistence, and to Craig Klinger, for his help in assembling the CD-ROM.

To Angela Moser and Andrew Trenholm, for their help with the text and the CD-ROM.

To Shirley Fitzgerald, who has helped so much with the previous editions, for continuing her loyalty and devotion in this third edition by reading, editing, and communicating with the editors; I am again indebted to you, more than you can imagine.

Marvin Tile

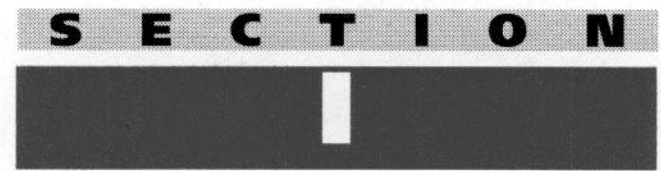

GENERAL ASPECTS OF THE PELVIC RING AND ACETABULUM

1

INTRODUCTION AND NATURAL HISTORY OF THE PELVIC RING

MARVIN TILE

INTRODUCTION

There has been an explosion of knowledge in this field since the publication of the first edition. The management of pelvic and acetabular trauma has become a subspecialty within orthopedic traumatology. Whereas three decades ago there was a limited knowledge of the injury types, early attempts at a classification, and a conservative approach to the management of the unstable pelvic ring injury; today the injury patterns are understood, there is agreement on a classification, and operative stabilization has become the treatment of choice in optimal circumstances based on sound biomechanical principles. Has this led to better outcomes for our patients? The answer is both yes and no. Yes, because we can now manage the patient to restore stability to the pelvic ring and prevent the severe deformities that were so frequent in the past; and no, because mortality and morbidity remain high, resulting from the biological effect of the injury itself, as shown in subsequent chapters.

The early major literature on pelvic fractures concentrated on the early visceral complications and made only oblique reference to late skeletal complications. At that time little attention was paid in the literature to the long-term effects of pelvic fractures on the musculoskeletal system.

There was a general feeling among practicing surgeons that most survivors of pelvic trauma did well, suffering few major late problems. However, the literature in general failed to compare similar cases; that is, there was a tendency to compare apples and oranges rather than oranges and oranges (Fig. 1-1). Most of the articles used different pelvic classifications. There was little standardization.

Today, it appears that there is more agreement in the literature on classification and natural history. The Tile classification, based on the general format of the AO/ASIF group published in the *Journal of Bone and Joint Surgery* (1), and subsequently modified (see Chapter 12), is now more widely accepted. Subsequent articles in the literature have added to our knowledge of the natural history of the disrupted pelvic ring (2,3). This new knowledge underscores the fact that not all pelvic disruptions are alike, just as all ankle fractures are not alike. The stable types of pelvic disruption generally have a good prognosis, whereas without thoughtful orthopedic management the unstable types have a much poorer prognosis.

HISTORICAL LITERATURE REVIEW

Early authors on this subject, namely Westerborn and Wilenius, suggested that sacroiliac pain was a common sequela of pelvic fractures (4,5).

Holdsworth reported on 50 pelvic fractures and helped elucidate the mechanism of injury (6). He identified retroperitoneal bleeding as the major cause of four of the six fatalities. Patients were treated nonoperatively with slings and traction, and the long-term effects were measured by the capacity of the patient to work. It became evident that the patients fell into two groups: those with a sacroiliac dislocation and those with a posterior fracture of the ilium or sacrum. Of the 27 patients with a sacroiliac dislocation, only 12 were later able to do heavy work, but 15 had pain and were unable to work. The pain usually was located in the sacroiliac area and was often severe. Of the 15 patients with a posterior fracture, only two had pain and 13 were working at heavy jobs. Many of the patients also complained of pain in the symphysis pubis, but this had usually subsided within

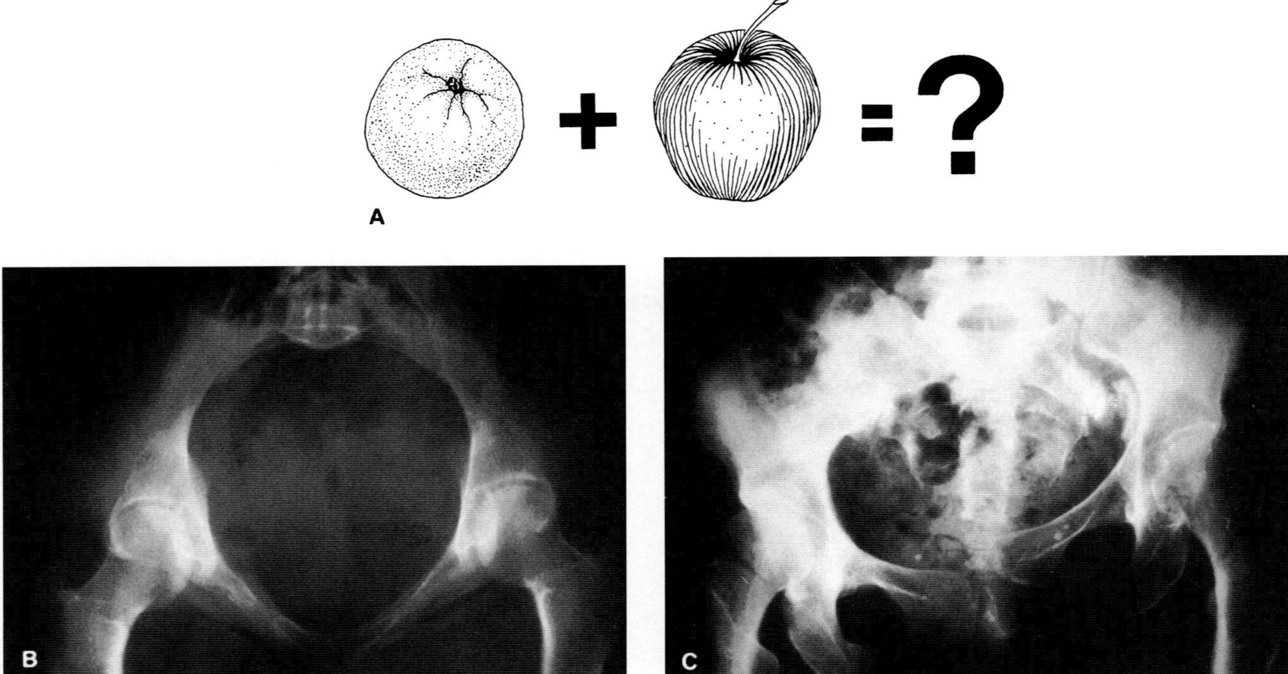

FIGURE 1-1. Comparing the relatively undisplaced pelvic ring fracture *(B)* to the very marked pelvic disruption associated with a sacroiliac fracture dislocation, nonunion, and lumbosacral plexus nerve palsy *(C)* is like comparing an orange to an apple *(A)*.

2 years of injury. Although Holdsworth stated, "Restoration of the anatomical position of any fracture is easy to assess and may or may not be important, but function is all important" (6), a careful study of his results indicates a close correlation between anatomic reduction and function. The large number of poor results in the group of patients with sacroiliac dislocation, as compared with the good results in the fracture group, suggests an unstable malreduced joint. Using modern techniques of computed tomography (CT), a sacroiliac joint that appears reasonably well reduced on the plain radiographs, is, in fact, malreduced (Fig. 1-2). Chronic pain is a common sequela.

Peltier, reporting on 186 patients with pelvic disruption, classified the cases into those that affect the weight-bearing area of the pelvis and those that do not (7). This classification identified the importance of the posterior weight-bearing sacroiliac area to the stability of the pelvic ring, because this area transfers body weight from the axial skeleton to the extremities. The rates of mortality and morbidity resulting from fractures in the weight-bearing posterior area were significantly higher than those in the non–weight-bearing area. However, in this report, little mention was made of the long-term problems associated with the musculoskeletal injury.

Raf studied 101 patients in Stockholm, Sweden who had "unstable Malgaigne" fractures (8). Of the 65 cases available for review, most patients were treated by a combination of skeletal traction for the posterior cephalad displacement and pelvic slings for the anterior disruption. Moderate or severe discomfort was reported by 22 of 65 patients (33%). The outcome was more favorable in cases in which the posterior fracture passed through the ilium. When the fracture was through the sacrum or the sacroiliac joint, 25 of 48 (52%), of the patients had persistent low back or leg pain. Pelvic tilt was present in 25 of 65 (38%) and limp in 21 of 65 patients (32%). Other complications, such as impotence, altered bowel or bladder function, and permanent nerve damage, were also common in patients with sacral fractures.

Dunn and Morris (9), using Pennal's classification based on the force patterns that cause the injury, reported on 115 of 149 cases of pelvic disruption. In the "stable group," they reported one nonunion and one nerve injury. Three deaths and many associated injuries occurred in the "unstable group." Minimal reference was made to late morbidity, although four of 31 patients (13%) with unstable fractures had disabling sacroiliac pain.

Huittinen and Slatis reported on the largest series to that date, 407 consecutive cases (10): 82% were caused by high-energy trauma and 62% had major associated injuries. The cases were divided into stable and unstable types, depending on the disruption of the posterior weight-bearing arch of the pelvis. The stable group included "isolated" pubic fractures and isolated rim fractures, whereas the unstable group included crushed pelvic, double vertical fractures (Malgaigne fracture), and fractures of the acetabulum. The overall mortality rate was 5.5%, and the genitourinary complication rate was 21%. The unstable fractures, including the double vertical fracture, had the highest number of early and late complications.

In further publications (11), Slatis and Huittinen described the late sequelae of 65 patients with double vertical (unstable) fractures of the pelvis. Of these patients, 71% had associated injuries, whereas 6.7% died of a variety of causes. The late morbidity associated with injury depended on the quality of healing of the posterior lesion. The major disabling factors in these patients were impaired gait resulting from malunion or pelvic obliquity; back or buttock pain, usually arising from the sacroiliac joint; and the sequelae of permanent neurologic damage. In general, patients with a posterior fracture of the ilium or sacrum had less pain than those with a sacroiliac dislocation; however, the highest number of nerve injuries occurred in patients with a sacral fracture. Of the 65 patients with an unstable double vertical fracture, 21 (32%) had significant gait abnormalities and 11 (17%) had pain.

In a later series (12), Slatis and Karaharju compared the results of that series with a further one on 22 patients whose unstable pelvic ring disruptions were treated with a trapezoidal external frame. In the latter group, only two patients had gait abnormalities and only one had pain. They concluded that the use of external skeletal fixation for unstable pelvic ring fractures reduces the incidence of late musculoskeletal complications.

Looser and Crombie reported 100 cases of severe pelvic trauma with a mortality rate of 18% and morbidity of 50% (13). Again, they emphasized that the patients with posterior sacroiliac disruption had the highest incidence of complications; however, they made no mention of late musculoskeletal symptoms. Reynolds and coworkers reported 273 cases with 18.6% mortality. Of 51 deaths, 33 were caused by severe hemorrhage (14). Again, no comment was made on the long-term effects of the musculoskeletal injury. Holm reported on 59 pelvic fractures, of which 16 were unstable (15). All were treated with traction techniques. Two of these patients (12.5%) had residual pain that required work modifications. One case of nonunion was also added to the literature.

Trunkey and associates (16), in a series of 173 patients treated at the San Francisco General Hospital, divided pelvic fractures into three groups based on the degree of soft tissue injury: Type 1, pelvic crush; Type 2, unstable; Type 3, stable. The crush fractures and unstable fractures had a high early complication rate of 43%, but no mention was made of late musculoskeletal complications.

Monahan and Taylor reviewed 29 patients at the Radcliffe Infirmary (Oxford, England) (17). Of the total, 57% had associated skeletal injuries, and 44.8% died of their injuries. Pain, a common complaint at review, occurred in the lumbar area in all patients, in the sacroiliac area in 15, in the pubis in three, and in the sciatic nerve area in one. Two of 15 patients complained of severe sacroiliac pain, the rest of dull, achy pain. Also, they reported a high incidence of permanent neurologic sequelae (e.g., paresthesia, numbness, and weakness) in the 37.2% of patients who had a nerve le-

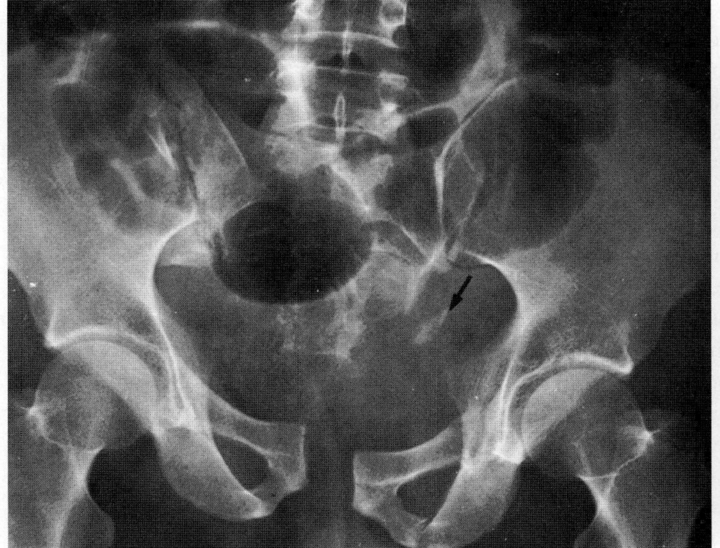
A

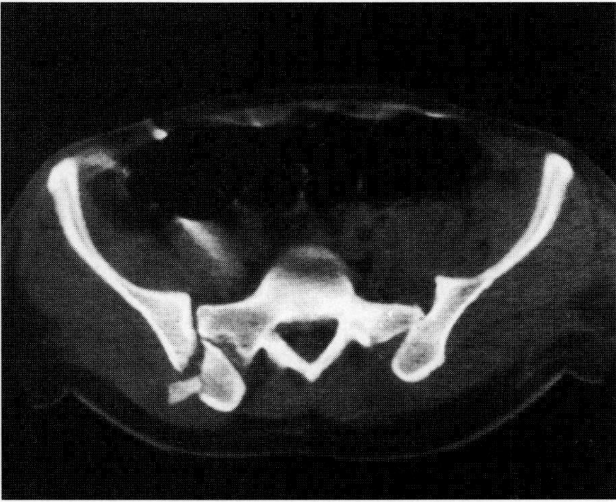
B

FIGURE 1-2. Radiograph *(A)* and computed tomography (CT) scan *(B)* of a 33-year-old patient following a motor vehicle accident. The radiograph shows disruption of the symphysis pubis, fracture dislocation of the right sacroiliac joint, and a questionable lesion of the left sacroiliac joint. Note the avulsion fracture of the sacral end of the sacrospinous ligament, indicating a left disrupted hemipelvis. The dislocated left sacroiliac joint is clearly identified on the CT scan, although it was only suspected on the plain radiograph. Chronic sacroiliac pain is a common sequela of the unreduced sacroiliac joint.

sion. Six patients had scoliosis, five a detectable deformity, and four minimal leg length discrepancy. Twenty-five patients returned to their original occupation, and three were permanently disabled.

Riska and coworkers, using external skeletal fixation with a single-bar anterior frame, reported that 43 of 51 patients were pain free, five had sacroiliac pain, and three diffuse pain (18). Five deaths (10%) were reported in this series.

Melton and associates, in an attempt to elucidate epidemiologic features of pelvic fractures, investigated the incidence of all pelvic fractures in Rochester, MN, for a 10-year period, 1968 to 1977 (3). During that period, 198 Rochester residents suffered 204 pelvic fractures. The overall incidence was 37 per 100,000 persons, substantially higher than previous population-based studies indicated. Not surprisingly, they found the incidence increased markedly with age in both sexes, but was much greater in women at all ages after 35 years, reaching a maximum incidence of 446.3 per 100,000 persons in women aged 85 years or older. In this older age group with osteoporosis, relatively minor trauma was responsible for virtually all of the fractures, whereas the incidence was also increased in the under-35 age group, most markedly in men. Severe trauma was implicated in 94 cases. In this group, the mean age was 33 years and the sex predominantly male.

In the remaining patients the mean age was 69, revealing a much older population who sustain pelvic fractures secondary to minor trauma. The younger patients, victims of high-energy trauma, showed more unstable pelvic fracture patterns, whereas the older patients with minimal trauma showed stable patterns. This research further confirms the principle that must be followed in the study of pelvic fractures; that is, we must not compare apples with oranges, or stable fracture patterns with unstable ones. The two groups noted in this epidemiologic study were different in all ways, and, as noted, the majority occurred in the older population, who sustained relatively minor trauma, and by inference required minimal treatment.

Semba and colleagues analyzed the results of 53 Malgaigne fractures over the period 1968 to 1977 (19). Nine patients died in the polytrauma period, one later of suicide, and 13 were lost to follow-up, leaving 30 patients to be followed from 2 to 12 years after injury. These 53 patients were only 6.5% of the 804 patients treated with pelvic fractures at the Hennepin County Medical Center (Minneapolis, MN) during the same period. Only two patients had isolated injuries; the remainder suffered major polytrauma. Treatment was nonoperative in all cases: 26 with minimal displacement had bed rest; five, skin traction; 17, skeletal traction; two, external fixation; and three, a pelvic sling. Of the 30 patients followed, only 11 were asymptomatic (Table 1-1). Eleven had paresthesias of the lower extremity on the ipsilateral side; nine, a gait disturbance; eight, severe back pain; four, groin pain; and two, fecal incontinence. Low back pain was always associated with a sacral or sacroiliac injury, and in no case with an iliac fracture. A correlation appeared to exist between continuing symptoms and the amount of displacement, as well as the site of the fracture. Those patients with less than 10 mm of combined displacement were all asymptomatic, whereas those with more displacement showed a high incidence of severe low back pain.

TABLE 1-1. LONG-TERM RESULTS IN 30 PATIENTS

Result	
No discomfort	11
Low back pain	8
Gait disturbance	9
Paresthesias	11
Fecal incontinence	2
Groin pain	4
Urinary incontinence	0
Sexual dysfunction	0

Source: Semba RT, Yasukawa K, and Gustilo RB. Critical analysis of results of 53 Malgaigne fractures of the pelvis. *J Trauma* 1983;23:535, with permission.

Henderson studied the long-term results of nonoperatively treated major pelvic disruption in 26 patients of a group of 366 treated at University of Iowa hospitals between January 1970 and December 1979 (20). Using Pennal's classification (21), modified by Tile (1), 10 of the 26 showed complete instability (vertical) and 16 partial (rotational) instability, four of which were caused by open-book external mechanisms and 12 to lateral compression mechanisms. The patients were re-evaluated an average of 8 years following injury (minimum 5 years). All pelvic injuries were treated nonoperatively, 16 with bed rest alone, seven with skeletal traction, five with a pelvic sling, and three with a plaster cast. Subjective complaints at the time of follow-up included low back pain (50%), localized ipsilateral dysesthesias (46%), and work disability (38%). On physical examination, objective neurologic deficit was noted in 42% and a gait disturbance in 32%. The long-term results correlated well with the amount of residual vertical displacement, the involvement of the sacroiliac joint, and the initial stability of the fracture. The author concluded that

> nonoperative treatment results in an acceptable long-term outcome if the pelvic injury is minimally displaced and stable. However, the prognosis is not so favorable with displaced unstable injuries treated nonoperatively. Further studies are necessary to determine if operative treatment improves the long-term outcome.

A number of studies examined external and internal fixation methods during the past decade. All the articles agree that stabilization is imperfect and migration of the hemipelvis is likely when an anterior external skeletal frame is used on a vertically unstable pelvis. All agree that the partial rotationally unstable pelvis with vertical stability can be stabilized adequately with an anterior external skeletal frame. Biomechanically, as is shown in Chapters 4 and 5, the partially stable lesions can be stabilized with an anterior external skeletal frame. The vertically unstable lesions cannot.

Wild and colleagues examined 45 patients with an unstable fracture of the pelvic ring (22). Only partial rotational instability was noted (18 lateral compression, 14 anteroposterior compression) in 32 of the 45. The treatment was successful and no migration occurred in these patients. Proximal migration of the hemipelvis was observed in four of 11 patients with a unilateral vertical shear-type injury.

Lansinger and coworkers examined 16 patients with unstable pelvic fractures (23). Again, an anterior frame restored stability in the external rotationally unstable anteroposterior compression fracture (Type B1). For the lateral compression fractures, reduction was anatomic in three and showed a minor rotational malalignment in three others. The clinical results were good. Anatomic reduction was not achieved in any of the five patients with a vertical shear injury. In spite of this, the authors indicate that the patients had good clinical results.

Edwards and associates reported in 1985 on 50 patients with unstable pelvic trauma treated with external skeletal frames applied anteriorly (24). The authors concluded that the vertically unstable pelvis cannot be stabilized with an anterior external skeletal frame, and 50% of their patients had continuing major symptoms, especially low back pain.

Kellam and colleague examined 53 patients with unstable pelvic disruptions treated by anterior external skeletal fixation (25). Again, adequate reduction was obtained and maintained in virtually all of the rotationally unstable fractures in the open-book and lateral compression types, but in only 27% of the vertically unstable group. The authors reiterate that the end result depends on the quality of the sacroiliac joint reduction and the stability of the pelvic ring. The anterior external skeletal fixator, by itself, could not stabilize the posterior lesion and put it in a reduced position.

The number of papers describing internal fixation of the pelvic ring has increased. These are described in Chapters 15 and 31.

Gansslen and associates (26) published a landmark paper on the epidemiology of pelvic ring injuries in which 2,551 patients gathered in a German Trauma Society multicentered trial were assessed. Of these, 61.7% were polytraumatized, and 12.2% suffered a major pelvic injury with concomitant soft tissue injury. The pelvic ring injury was classified as Stable (Type A) in 54.8%, Partially Stable (Type B) in 24.7%, and Unstable (Type C) in 20.5%. Concomitant acetabular fractures were present in 15.7%. The overall rate of pelvic operative stabilizations was 21.6%, in the Unstable C types 46.7%. The overall mortality rate was 13.4%, but it reached 31.1% in complex polytrauma with a pelvic ring injury.

Muir and colleagues (27) reported on the epidemiology of severe pelvic trauma in the Mersey region of the United Kingdom. All survivors of blunt trauma with an injury severity score (ISS) > 15 were considered. Of 831 patients, 230 (28%) died at the scene, 272 (33%) died in the hospital, and the remaining 329 (39%) survived. There were 153 pelvic fractures (18.4%), with 111 survivors to make up the study group. The findings were similar to the previous study.

SUMMARY OF THE LITERATURE

The unstable pelvic fracture is a potentially lethal injury, with 10% to 31% mortality; the morbidity may be high in survivors, in spite of modern treatment.

The literature supports the concept that the final results clearly depend on the fracture type; patients with stable fractures have few long-term problems, whereas those with unstable types often exhibit major chronic disability, usually resulting from the following factors:

1. Pain, usually lower lumbar or sacroiliac, often secondary to a sacroiliac dislocation. The literature suggests that, if the posterior sacroiliac complex or weight-bearing arch of the pelvis is disrupted and remains unstable, then the patient will continue to have pain (see Fig. 1-2).
2. Malunion causing pelvic obliquity and gait abnormalities (Fig. 1-3)
3. Nonunion causing chronic pain (Figs. 1-4 and 1-5)
4. Neurologic dysfunction, which is surprisingly common
5. Genitourinary dysfunction

However, patients with residual deformity do much worse; therefore, the surgeon should continue to strive for restoration of pelvic stability, important in the initial phase of saving the patient's life, and restoration of anatomical or

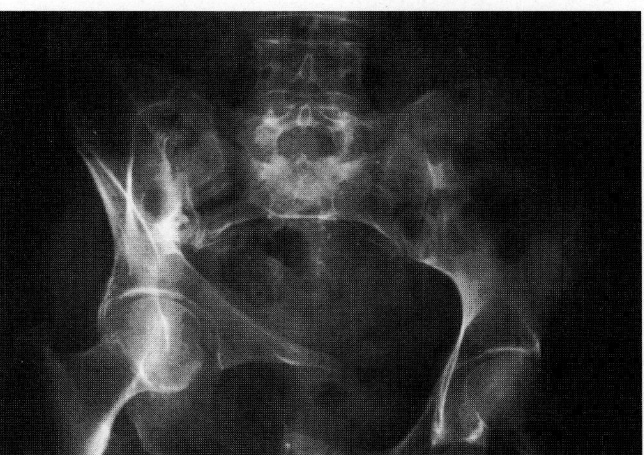

FIGURE 1-3. Radiograph of a 52-year-old woman injured in a motor vehicle accident. Note the marked internal rotation of the right hemipelvis. This malrotation occurred in this unstable injury, in spite of treatment with an external skeletal fixator. Malunion resulted in 3 cm shortening in the right leg.

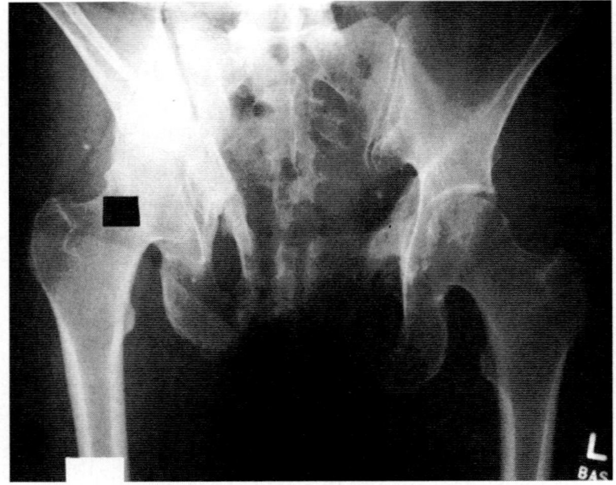

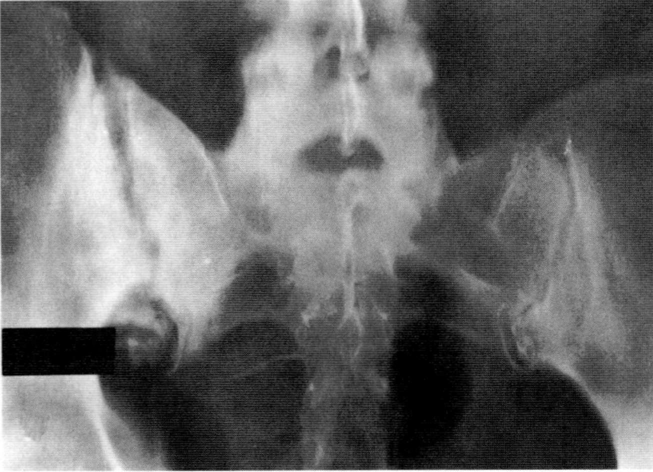

FIGURE 1-4. A: Outlet radiograph of the pelvis of a 32-year-old woman 24 months after pelvic disruption. Note the hypertrophic nonunion through the right sacroiliac joint and the nonunion of the superior and inferior pubic rami. **B:** Tomogram of the same patient, taken through the right sacroiliac complex, clearly shows the hypertrophic nonunion.

near anatomical reduction, without which the outcomes are compromised.

NATURAL HISTORY: AUTHOR'S CLINICAL STUDIES

The author, in association with Robert Lifeso, Dalton Dickinson, and Robert McBroom, attempted to characterize the natural history of pelvic ring trauma in the era prior to the current wave of internal fixation as conventional treatment for the unstable pelvic injury. Therefore, these results may serve as a clue to the natural history of the injury to which more recent results may be compared.

We carried out two clinical studies in which we considered only patients with injuries caused by major high-energy trauma; all others were eliminated. The first study, Series A, is a retrospective study of 148 patients, treated in The University of Toronto teaching hospitals and in other non–teaching hospitals in southern Ontario (28). The second, Series B, was a prospective study of 100 consecutive cases admitted to the trauma unit at Sunnybrook Medical

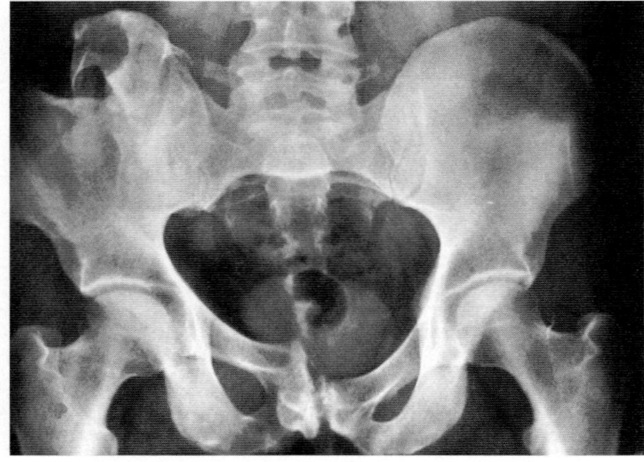

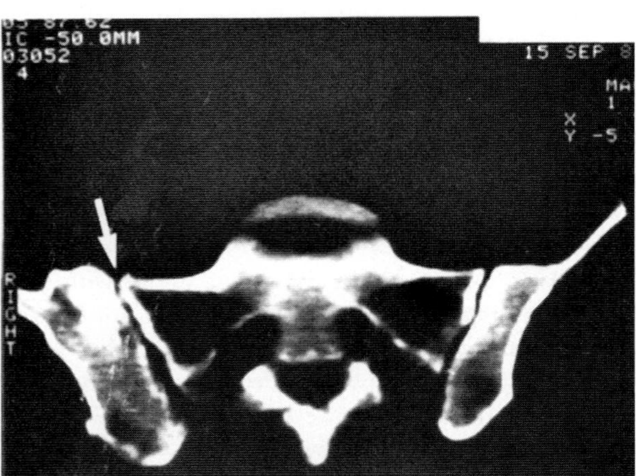

FIGURE 1-5. A: Anteroposterior radiograph of a 38-year-old man 8 years following pelvic disruption. Attempted fusion across the sacroiliac joint and symphysis pubis failed on three separate occasions, leaving him with chronic right sacroiliac pain. **B:** CT of the same patient shows the dense sclerosis around the right sacroiliac joint with hypertrophic callus formation but persistent nonunion. Instability of the symphysis pubis resulted in anterior pain.

TABLE 1-2. COMPARISON OF SERIES A AND SERIES B PATIENTS

	Series A (148 Cases)	Series B (100 Cases)
Age (range)	34.2 yr (15–81)	30.9 yr (14–85)
Sex		
Male	91	55
Female	57	45
Injury types		
Motor vehicle accidents	89 (60%)	81
Fall	17 (11.5%)	11
Crush	34 (23%)	4
Miscellaneous	8 (5.5%)	4
Workmen's Compensation Board	43 (29%)	5
Associated injuries		
Central nervous system	31 (21%)	38
Chest	19 (13%)	15
Gastrointestinal	10 (6.6%)	20
Genitourinary		
Bladder	17 (11%)	8
Urethra	6 (4%)	4
Nerve	12 (8%)	3
Musculoskeletal	63 (43%)	10
Average follow-up	5 yr	2 yr

Centre in Toronto (29). The similarities and differences of both groups are noted in Table 1-2. A study of the demographic pattern indicates that both groups are young and were victims of high-energy trauma. In Series A, there were more men, indicating a higher number of compensable industrial accidents, whereas in Series B, the sex incidence was equal, indicating a preponderance of motor vehicle accidents. In Series B, 38% of the patients had major head injuries, reflecting the admission pattern to the Sunnybrook Trauma Unit. The mortality rate was high, 17%; deaths were the result of a combination of intracranial and abdominal injury. The average follow-up periods were 60 months for Series A and 2 years for Series B.

Patients in both groups all were personally interviewed and examined, and were studied with the three standard radiographic views popularized by Pennal and Sutherland (21), the anteroposterior, inlet, and outlet views. Comparison was made to the original radiographs. Each fracture was classified according to its degree of stability and the type of force that caused it (Table 1-3).

Our results were tabulated by a point system heavily weighted to pain; lesser scores were allotted for malunion, leg length discrepancy, and nonunion. Fractures that were principally acetabular with a pelvic ring injury were eliminated from the results, which are given in Table 1-4. As suggested in the literature, the morbidity rate associated with unstable fractures of the pelvic ring is significant. We found, as did Holdsworth (6), Slatis and Huittinen (10), and others, that pain was the common factor in the unsatisfactory results (Table 1-5).

TABLE 1-3. CLASSIFICATION OF FRACTURES

- Stable
- Anteroposterior compression
- Lateral compression
- Unstable (vertical shear, Malgaigne, double vertical)
- Unilateral posterior injury
- Bilateral posterior injury
- Complex
- Acetabular involvement

Most of the pain was located in the sacroiliac area, and occasionally in the lower lumbar spine. Pain in the symphysis pubis was uncommon but certainly was not absent. The pain was most severe in the unstable sacroiliac dislocations and much less severe in the more stable types, especially the open-book fracture; however, late anterior pain was reported by a number of patients with disruption of the symphysis pubis (see Fig. 1-5). Malunion leading to a leg length discrepancy of 1 to 2 cm was common, but more than 2 cm was relatively uncommon, occurring in 5% of Series A and 2% of Series B (Table 1-6). Nonunion was present in 3% of all cases in both series and always led to an unsatisfactory result (see Fig. 1-4). Therefore, 37 of 148 (25%) patients in Series A had an unsatisfactory result, as compared with 35 of 100 (35%) patients in Series B, the prospective study. This reflects a larger number of severe high-energy injuries in the latter series, with an average ISS-17 of 37.3 and a mortality rate of 17%. If one subtracts the 17 early deaths from the total, the percentage of long-term unsatisfactory results in Series B rises to 42%.

Unsatisfactory results are most likely to occur with unstable pelvic fractures (vertical shear, Malgaigne, double vertical) (Fig. 1-6; Table 1-7). These patients have the highest risk of chronic sacroiliac pain, which is most common with a sacroiliac dislocation (60%) and less common with a sacral or iliac fracture. Again, a high-resolution CT scan reveals the malreduced sacroiliac joint as the probable cause of the pain. Also, the highest incidence of malunion leading to leg length discrepancy and nonunion was found in this group. Major associated injuries were common, often leading to

TABLE 1-4. FACTORS ASSOCIATED WITH UNSATISFACTORY RESULTS

	Series A (37/148)	Series B (35/100)
Pain	37	32
Leg length discrepancy >2 cm	7	2
Nonunion	5	3
Permanent nerve damage	9	3
Urethral symptoms	5	1
Death	—	17

TABLE 1-5. PAIN (MODERATE AND SEVERE)[a]

	Series A: 148 Cases				Series B: 100 Cases			
	N	Nil	Moderate	Severe	N	Nil	Moderate	Severe
Incidence	53 (36%)				35			
Location								
Posterior	47 (32%)				32			
Anterior	6 (4%)				3			
Severity								
Anteroposterior compression	23	14	8	1	6	3	3	
Lateral compression	86	47	35	4	69	53	16	
Unstable (shear)	9	4	2	3	25	9	13	3
Total	**118[a]**	**65**	**45**	**8**	**100**	**65**	**32**	**3**

[a]Thirty cases with major acetabular involvement were not considered in this total.

TABLE 1-6. LEG LENGTH DISCREPANCY (MALUNION)

Amount (cm)	Series A (%)	Series B (%)
0	64	68
0–1	19.5	19
1–2	11.5	11
>2	5	2

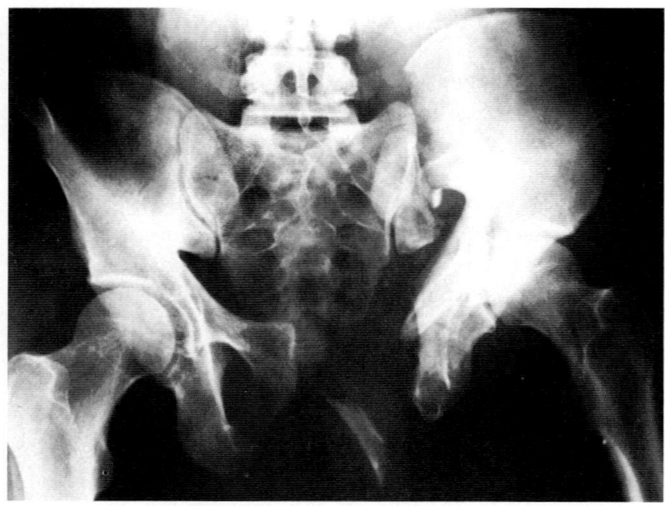

FIGURE 1-6. Anteroposterior radiograph of a 34-year-old man 18 months after he fell down a mine shaft. His open fracture resulted in bone loss at the superior and inferior pubic rami and marked gross left hemipelvic instability. In addition to chronic pain, the patient had a permanent lumbosacral plexus injury.

chronic morbidity, associated with permanent nerve or genitourinary tract damage.

Patients with lateral compression injuries usually had satisfactory results, although there were notable exceptions. First, malunion resulting from fixed rotation of the hemipelvis resulted in major leg length discrepancy in some of these patients, especially in children and adolescents. Second, patients with a particular variety of injury, in which the symphysis pubis is rotated and disrupted, often continued to complain of significant pain in the symphysis area (Fig. 1-7).

Patients with an open-book injury usually had few problems with adequate treatment. Symphysis pain, usually moderate, was a problem in a small number of cases. Patients who had proper reduction and stabilization of the pelvic ring had much better results than those whose pelvis was left unreduced.

CONCLUSION

There have been valuable additions to the literature since the first edition. All have strengthened, and indeed validated, the conclusions reached in that edition. The importance of a precise diagnosis has been stressed, because the results of the various treatment modalities depend on it. The interpretation of stable, partially stable, and unstable pelvic disruptions is of major importance, because the incidence of serious complications—early or late—is highest in the unstable group. In the early posttrauma phase, life-threatening

TABLE 1-7. RESULTS BY FRACTURE TYPE

	Series A: 148 Cases			Series B: 100 Cases		
	Total N	Satisfactory N (%)	Unsatisfactory N (%)	Total N	Satisfactory N (%)	Unsatisfactory N (%)
Anteroposterior compression	23	18 (78)	5 (22)	6	3 (50)	3 (50)
Lateral compression	114	79 (69)	35 (31)	69	53 (77)	16 (23)
Unstable (shear)	9	5 (56)	4 (44)	25	9 (36)	16 (64)

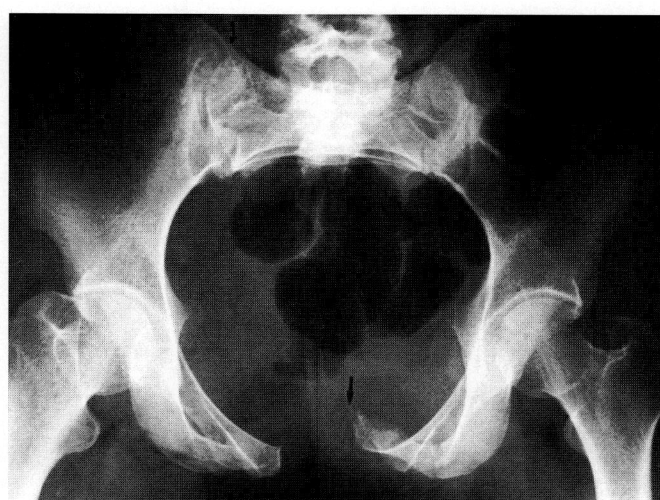

FIGURE 1-7. Inlet radiograph of the pelvis of a 31-year-old woman showed massive symphysis disruption with internal rotation of the left superior pubic ramus into the pelvis. This patient complained of chronic anterior pain and dyspareunia.

associated injuries and massive pelvic bleeding may lead to difficulties in resuscitation and a high mortality rate. A significant number of the surviving patients may be left with pain, usually sacroiliac in origin; malunion, leading to pelvic obliquity; leg length discrepancy and gait abnormality; nonunion; and the sequelae of permanent nerve or genitourinary damage. These late sequelae are much more common than is generally believed. Although the biological effect of the visceral and nerve injury may be permanent and result in a poor outcome, the poor results caused by malunion and nonunion should be largely eliminated with techniques of reduction and stabilization available to the pelvic trauma surgeon.

Significant late morbidity is more likely to occur in patients who suffer disruption of the weight-bearing portion of the pelvic ring, that is, the posterior sacroiliac complex. Because these unstable fractures are commonly associated with both early and late complications, urgent resuscitation efforts and exemplary fracture care must be performed. If we are to improve the late results we must be certain that the unstable fracture is treated concomitantly with the early associated injuries and that all of our modern techniques of external and internal fixation are used to stabilize the unstable pelvis. In the past decade, the natural history of the pelvic fracture has been further clarified. We must improve our technical abilities, decrease the prevalence of iatrogenic complications, and assess our treatment modalities by prospective clinical trials in the next decade.

REFERENCES

1. Tile M. Pelvic fractures: should they be fixed? *J Bone Joint Surg* 1988;70B:1.
2. Delal S, Burgess AR, Siegel JH, et al. *Pelvic fractures in multiple trauma. Classification by mechanism is the key to organ injury, resuscitation requirements and outcome.* Presented at the Orthopaedic Trauma Association Meeting. Dallas, TX, Oct. 27–28, 1988.
3. Melton L, Sampson J, Morrey B, et al. Epidemiologic features of pelvic fractures. *Clin Orthop* 1981;155:43.
4. Westerborn A. Beitrage zur Kenntniss der Beckenbrueche and Beckenluxationen. *Acta Chir Scand* 1928;(Suppl 8).
5. Wilenius R. Ubher Beckenbrueche. *Acta Chir Scand* 1943; (Suppl 79).
6. Holdsworth FW. Dislocation and fracture dislocation of the pelvis. *J Bone Joint Surg* 1948;30B:461.
7. Peltier LF. Complications associated with fractures of the pelvis. *J Bone Joint Surg* 1965;47A:1060.
8. Raf L. Double vertical fractures of the pelvis. *Acta Chir Scand* 1966;131:298.
9. Dunn AW, Morris HD. Fractures and dislocations of the pelvis. *J Bone Joint Surg* 1968;50A:1639.
10. Huittinen VM, Slatis P. Fractures of the pelvis, trauma mechanism, types of injury and principles of treatment. *Acta Clin Scand* 1972;138:563.
11. Slatis P, Huittinen VM. Double vertical fractures of the pelvis: a report on 163 patients. *Acta Clin Scand* 1972;138:799.
12. Slatis P, Karaharju ED. External fixation of unstable pelvic fractures: experiences in 22 patients treated with a trapezoid compression frame. *Clin Orthop* 1980;151:73.
13. Looser KG, Crombie HD. Pelvic fractures: an anatomic guide to severity of injury. *Am J Surg* 1976;132:638.
14. Reynolds BM, Balsano NA, Reynolds TX. Pelvic fractures. *J Trauma* 1973;13:1011.
15. Holm CL. Treatment of pelvic fractures and dislocations. *Clin Orthop* 1973;97:97.
16. Trunkey DD, Chapman MW, Lim RC Jr, et al. Management of pelvic fractures in blunt trauma injury. *J Trauma* 1974;14:912.
17. Monahan PRW, Taylor RG. Dislocation and fracture dislocation of the pelvis. *Injury* 1975;6:325.
18. Riska EB, von Bonsdorff H, Hakkinen S, et al. External fixation of unstable pelvic fractures. *Int Orthop* 1979;3:183.
19. Semba R, Yasukawa K, Gustilo R. Critical analysis of results of 53 Malgaigne fractures of the pelvis. *J Trauma* 1983;23:535.
20. Henderson RC. The long-term results of nonoperatively treated major pelvic disruptions. *J Orthop Trauma* 1989;3:41.
21. Pennal CF, Sutherland GO. *Fractures of the Pelvis* [motion picture]. Park Ridge, IL: American Academy of Orthopaedic Surgeons Film Library, 1961.
22. Wild JJ Jr, Hanson GW, Tullos HS. Unstable fractures of the pelvis treated by external fixation. *J Bone Joint Surg* 1982;64A: 1010.
23. Lansinger O, Karlsson J, Berg U, et al. Unstable fractures of the pelvis treated with trapezoidal compression frame. *Acta Orthop Scand* 1984;55:325.
24. Edwards CC, et al. *Results of treating 50 unstable pelvic injuries using primary external fixation.* Proceedings of the 53rd Annual Meeting of the American Academy of Orthopaedic Surgeons. Park Ridge, IL, 1986, p 434.
25. Kellam JF, McMurtry RY, Paley D, et al. The unstable pelvic fracture: operative treatment. *Orthop Clin North Am* 1987;18:25.
26. Gansslen A, Pohlemann T, Paul C, et al. Epidemiology of pelvic ring injuries. *Injury* 1996;(27 Suppl 1):S–A,13–20.
27. Muir L, Boot D, Gorman DF, et al. The epidemiology of pelvic fractures in the Mersey region. *Injury* 1996;27(3):199–204.
28. Dickinson D, Lifeso R, McBroom R, et al. Disruptions of the pelvic ring. *J Bone Joint Surg* 1982;64B(5):635.
29. McMurtry R, Walton D, Dickinson D, et al. Pelvic disruption in the polytraumatized patient. A management protocol. *Clin Orthop Rel Res* 1980;151:22–30.

2

ANATOMY OF THE PELVIC RING

MARVIN TILE

INTRODUCTION

It is not my purpose in this chapter to describe the minutiae of pelvic anatomy, which are well described in all standard anatomy texts. Rather, I concentrate on applied anatomy; that is, the important features of the anatomy of the pelvis that relate to pelvic injuries.

The pelvis is a ring structure made up of three bones, the sacrum and the two innominates. In turn, the innominate is formed by the fusion of three separate centers of ossification, the ilium, the ischium, and the pubis. They meet at the triradiate cartilage, which fuses by age 16. These three components have no inherent stability: If all soft tissues were removed from the pelvis, then it would fall apart (Fig. 2-1). Yet, *in vivo,* it is able to withstand major forces; therefore, the soft tissues must confer this stability to the pelvic girdle. Stability is the essential anatomic feature of the pelvis, whereas mobility is for the pectoral girdle.

STRUCTURAL STABILITY

The pelvic ring is formed by the connection of the sacrum to the innominate bones at the sacroiliac joints and the symphysis pubis. Because the major weight-bearing lines are transmitted across the sacroiliac joint and into the neck of the femur, it may be assumed that the major stabilizing structures are posterior (Fig. 2-2). The anterior joint, that is, the symphysis pubis, acts more like a strut, preventing collapse of the pelvis, than like a major weight-bearing, stabilizing structure. Absence of this anterior strut, as in patients with congenital extrophy of the bladder (Fig. 2-3) or trauma victims (Fig. 2-4), only minimally affects this weight-bearing function. Many mammals possess a posterior bony strut, the symphysis ischii (Fig. 2-5). In humans, this function is accompanied by the strong sacrospinous and sacrotuberous ligaments.

Posterior Pelvic Stability

Sacroiliac Joints (Fig. 2-6)

The adjacent surfaces of the ilium and sacrum are divided into two parts: a lower one, the articular surfaces, and an upper one, the tuberosities. The articular surface of the sacrum is covered with hyaline cartilage and the adjacent surface of the ilium with fibrocartilage; however, the articulation so formed is not truly a synovial joint. Embryonically, the sacroiliac joints develop not as other synovial joints do—as clefts in a continuous rod of condensed mesenchyme—but by the direct contact of the ilium and sacrum posteriorly. Some movement does occur at this joint, but this is markedly restricted by several ligaments, the strongest being the interosseous ligaments.

Interosseous Sacroiliac Ligaments
The interosseous sacroiliac ligaments, the strongest in the body, unite the tuberosities of the ilium and sacrum and confer stability on the posterior sacroiliac complex (Fig. 2-7).

Posterior Sacroiliac Ligaments (Fig. 2-2)
Two distinct bands are described: (a) the short posterior sacroiliac ligament consists of a number of fibers that pass obliquely from the tubercle or ridge of the sacrum to the posterior superior and posterior inferior spine of the ilium; and (b) the long posterior sacroiliac ligament is composed of longitudinal fibers that run from the posterior superior iliac spine to the lateral portion of the sacrum, intermingling

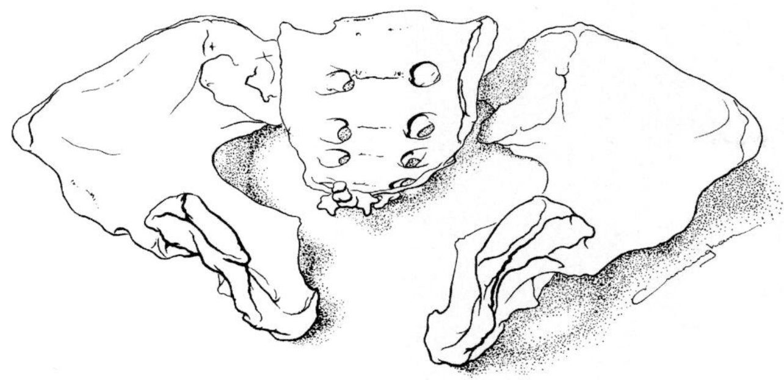

FIGURE 2-1. Removal of the ligamentous structures from the sacrum and two innominate bones would result in complete instability of the pelvic ring.

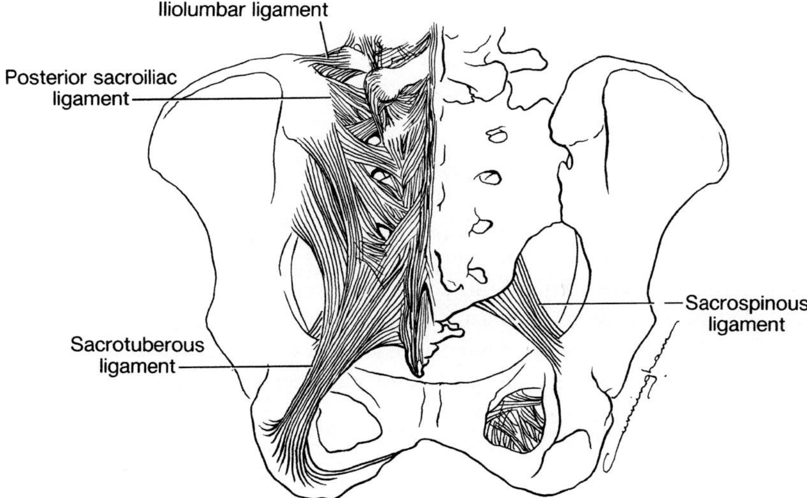

FIGURE 2-2. The major posterior stabilizing structures of the pelvic ring, that is, the posterior tension band of the pelvis, include the iliolumbar ligament, posterior sacroiliac ligaments, sacrospinous ligaments, and sacrotuberous ligaments.

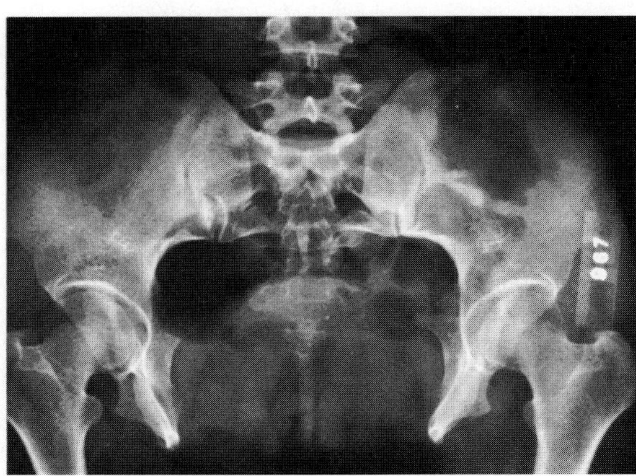

FIGURE 2-3. Radiograph of a 39-year-old woman with congenital extrophy of the bladder. Note the total lack of anterior stability because of excessive widening of the symphysis pubis. In spite of this, the sacroiliac joints have remained intact and show no evidence of instability.

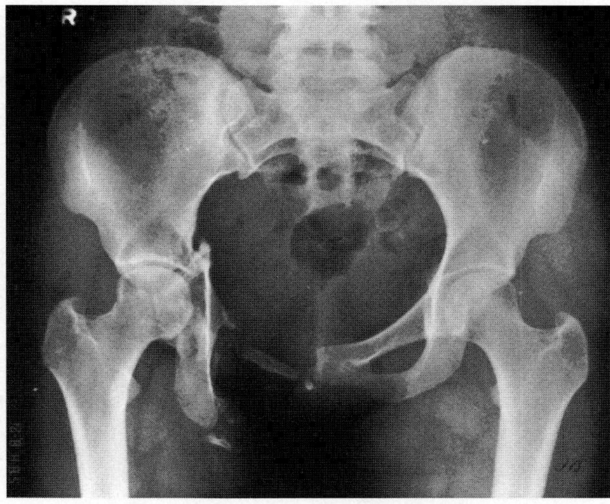

FIGURE 2-4. Anteroposterior radiograph of the pelvis of a 21-year-old woman who had previously lost a portion of the superior and inferior pubic rami in an open fracture of the pelvic ring at the age of 12. The superior ramus fracture entered the right acetabulum. No posterior instability is noted in spite of the gap in the pelvic ring. The patient has no symptoms referable to the sacroiliac joints or the gap anteriorly. She was seen for an unrelated medical problem.

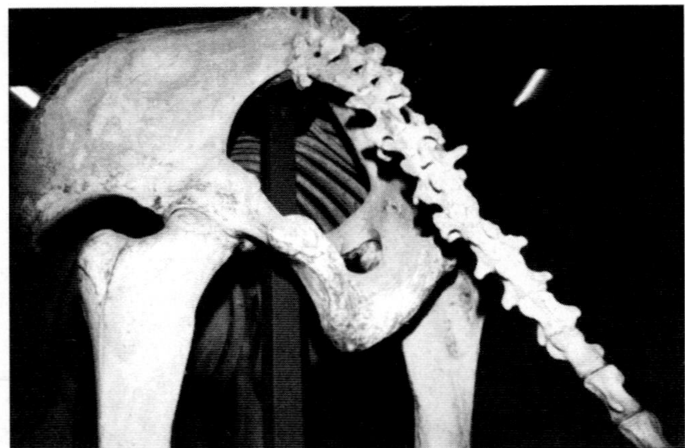

FIGURE 2-5. The bony skeleton of an elephant shows the symphysis ischium, a solid bony strut posteriorly.

with the origin of the sacrotuberous ligament and covering the short ligament.

Anterior Sacroiliac Ligaments (Fig. 2-9)

Anterior sacroiliac ligaments are strong, flat bands, composed of transverse and oblique fibers that pass from the anterior surface of the sacrum to the anterior adjacent surface of the ilium.

Connecting Ligaments

Sacrotuberous Ligament (Figs. 2-8 and 2-9)

The sacrotuberous ligament is an extremely strong, broad band extending from the lateral portion of the entire dorsum of the sacrum and the posterior surfaces of the posterior superior and inferior iliac spines to the ischial tuberosity. In some areas it covers and in others it is contiguous with the

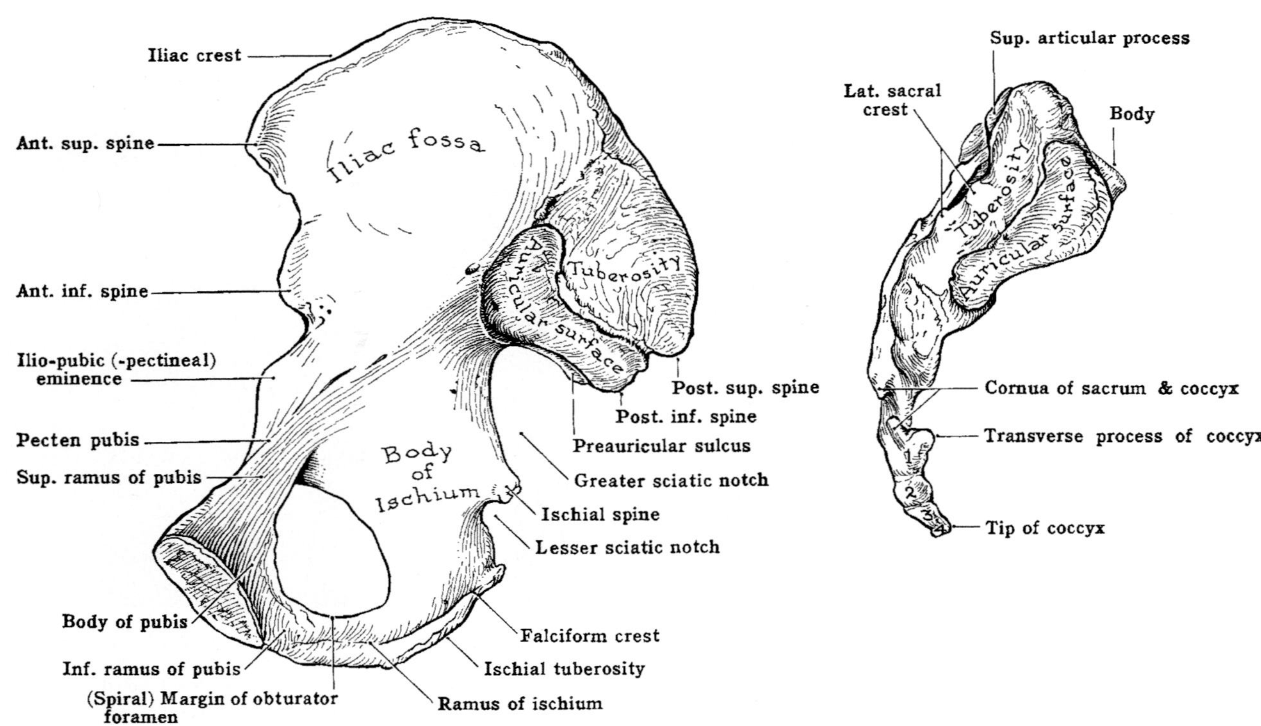

FIGURE 2-6. The adjacent surfaces of the sacroiliac joint, indicating the area of hyaline cartilage on the articular surface and fibrocartilage over the tuberosity. (From: Anderson JE. *Grant's atlas of anatomy,* 8th ed. Baltimore: Williams & Wilkins, 1983, with permission.)

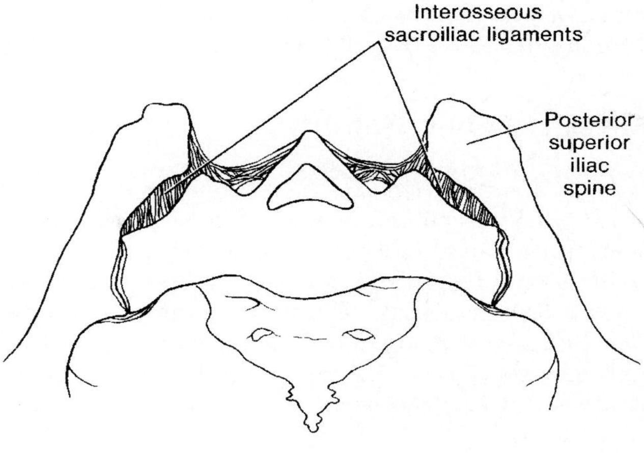

FIGURE 2-7. Cross-section through the sacroiliac joints shows the direction of the interosseous sacroiliac ligaments, considered by Grant to be the strongest ligaments in the body.

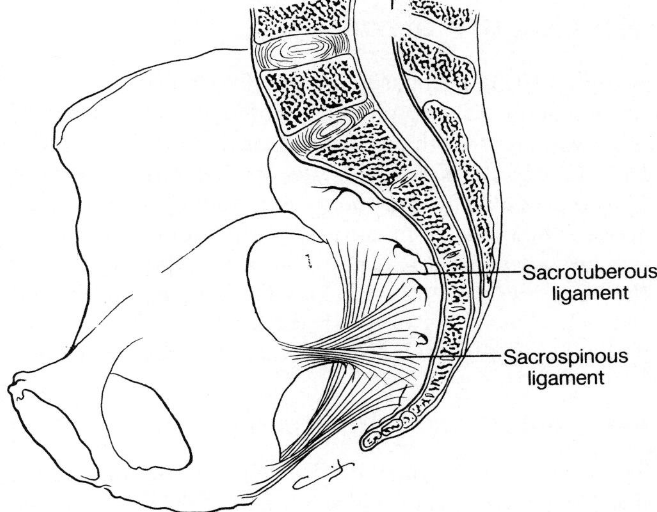

FIGURE 2-8. A sagittal view of the sacrotuberous and sacrospinous ligament indicates their attachment from the sacrum to the ischial tuberosity and ischial spine, respectively.

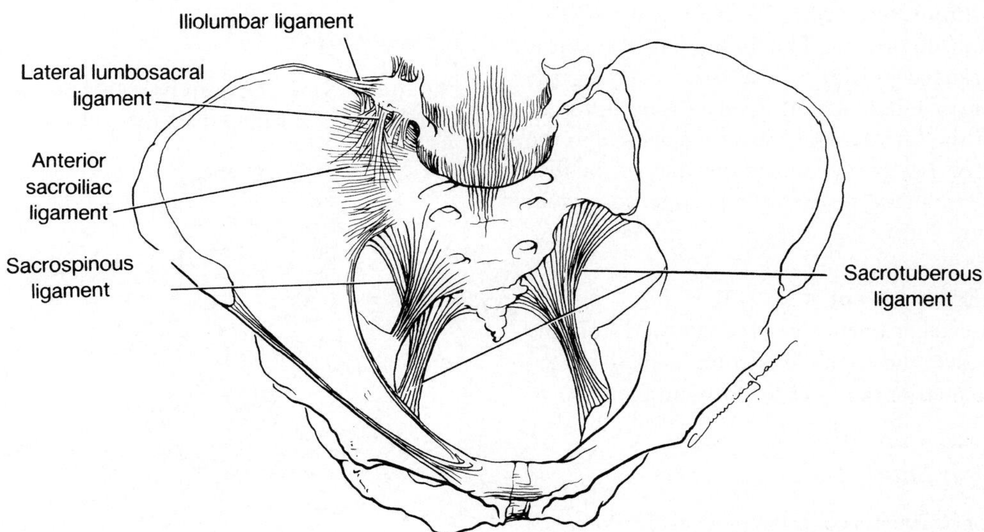

FIGURE 2-9. Anteroposterior view of the pelvis indicates that the sacrospinous ligament is a triangular strong ligament lying anterior to the sacrotuberous ligament, which is a strong broad band extending from the lateral portion of the dorsum of the sacrum to the ischial tuberosity.

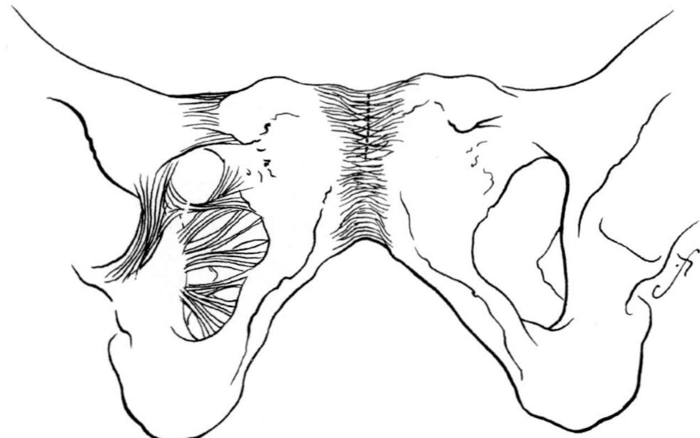

FIGURE 2-10. The symphysis pubis is the main anterior stabilizing structure, uniting the two surfaces of the pubis with a complex structure of hyaline cartilage, fibrocartilage, and fibrous tissue. A cleft often appears as part of the aging process in the fibrous tissue layer *(dotted line)*.

sacrospinous ligaments. The medial border extends as a falciform crest to the ischial tuberosity, where it is continuous with the obturator fascia. Laterally, at its superior origin, it gives attachment to the gluteus maximus. The sacrotuberous ligament forms a portion of the pelvic outlet.

Sacrospinous Ligament (Figs. 2-8 and 2-9)
The sacrospinous ligament is a strong triangular sheet arising from the lateral margin of the sacrum and the coccyx, deep to the sacrotuberous ligament, and passing to the ischial spine, dividing the ischial area into the greater sciatic notch and the lesser sciatic foramen. Its pelvic surface covers and is adherent to the coccygeus muscle.

Iliolumbar Ligaments (Fig. 2-2)
The pelvis is secured to the axial skeleton at the lumbosacral articulation. In addition to a strong intervertebral disc, two particular ligaments are present. The iliolumbar ligament is the markedly thickened portion of the fascia covering the quadratus lumborum. Bilaterally, this very strong ligament attaches the tip of the fifth lumbar transverse process to the iliac crest. Lying just below the level of the apex of the iliac crest, these transverse processes are usually large, somewhat conical, and upward tilted (Fig. 2-9).

Lateral Lumbosacral Ligament (Fig. 2-9)
The lateral lumbosacral ligament spreads downward from the L5 transverse process to the ala of the sacrum. Its sharp medial edge may abut the anterior ramus of the fifth lumbar root.

Posterior Tension Band

All of the posterior ligaments collectively form the posterior tension band of the pelvis, binding together the skeletal elements to resist deforming forces. The transversely placed ligaments, short posterior sacroiliac, anterior sacroiliac, iliolumbar, and sacrospinous resist transverse rotational forces, whereas those that are vertically placed resist longitudinal shearing forces (Figs. 2-2 and 2-7).

Anterior Pelvic Stability

Symphysis Pubis (Fig. 2-10)

In the symphysis pubis, the opposed bony surfaces of the pubis are covered by hyaline cartilage and are united by layers of fibrocartilage and fibrous tissue. In the fibrocartilage, a cleft frequently appears, often as part of the aging process. Superiorly and anteriorly, dense ligamentous fibers blend with the fibrocartilage; inferiorly, the symphysis is reinforced by a more independent structure, the inferior pubic or arcuate ligament.

INTERIOR OF BONY PELVIS

Because visceral injury is so commonly associated with disruption of the pelvic girdle, a description of the proximity of these structures to the bony skeleton is in order. *Pelvis* is Latin for basin. The basin is really divided into two sections by the pelvic brim; the true pelvis, below, and the false, above. The pelvic brim consists of the promontory of the sacrum, iliopectineal line, pubic crest, and upper portion of the symphysis pubis (Fig. 2-11). The posterior portion of the pelvic brim is extremely thick, in keeping with its weight-bearing function. No muscle crosses the pelvic brim.

False Pelvis

The false pelvis is formed by the ala of the sacrum and the iliac fossa, the fan-shaped inner surface of the ilium covered entirely by the iliacus muscle.

True Pelvis

The true pelvis is the deep basin below the pelvic brim. The lateral wall is composed of the pubis and ischium, with a

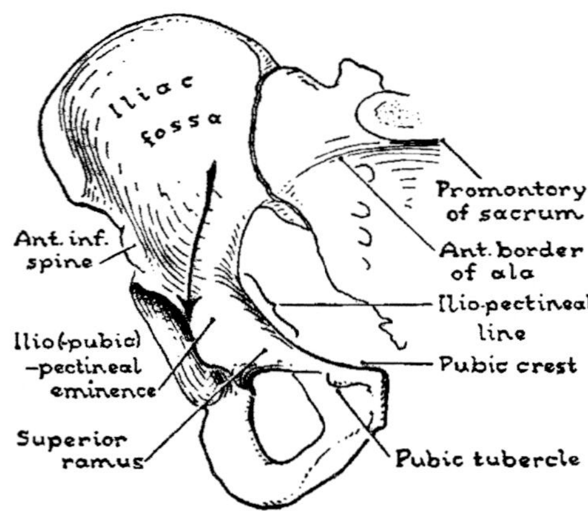

FIGURE 2-11. The false pelvis and the pelvic brim. (From: Basmajian IN. *Grant's method of anatomy,* 10th ed. Baltimore: Williams & Wilkins, 1980, with permission.)

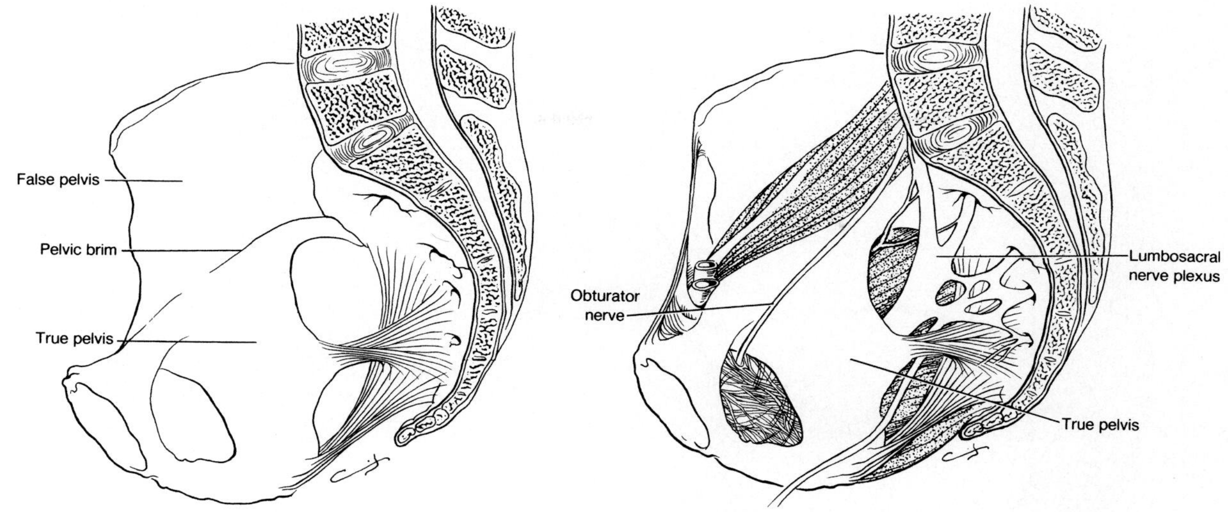

FIGURE 2-12. A: The true pelvis below the pelvic brim. **B:** The position of the obturator nerve and lumbosacral nerve plexus.

small triangular portion of the ilium, the weight-bearing portion (Fig. 2-12). The obturator foramen, separating the pubis from the ischium, is covered by a membrane, deficient only on top to allow the obturator vessels and nerve to escape from the pelvis (Fig. 2-13). At this point they are vulnerable and may be torn in pelvic trauma. The lateral wall of the pelvis below the obturator foramen is lined with obturator internus muscle and fascia, which leave the pelvis through the lesser sciatic foramen.

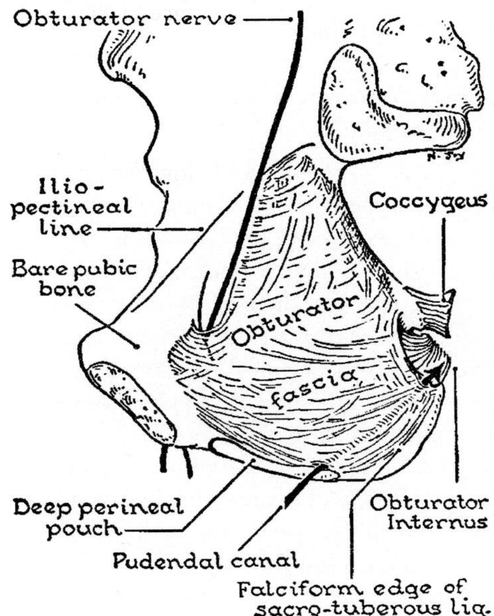

FIGURE 2-13. The lateral wall of the true pelvis, indicating the obturator internus fascia, deficient superiorly to allow the obturator nerve to escape from the pelvis. (From: Basmajian IN. *Grant's method of anatomy,* 10th ed. Baltimore: Williams & Wilkins, 1980, with permission.)

The piriformis arises from the lateral mass and anterior portion of the sacrum, leaving the pelvis through the greater sciatic notch. It is the key to the position of the sciatic nerve. In most persons, the entire nerve leaves the pelvis below this muscle; although in some the peroneal division either pierces it or, rarely, escapes above it (Fig. 2-14).

Pelvic Diaphragm

The levator ani and the coccygeus stretch across the pelvis, forming a floor to support the pelvic organs and separating them from the perineum. The diaphragm is composed of voluntary muscle and is perforated by the urethra, rectum, and vagina.

Structures at Risk

Lumbosacral and Coccygeal Nerve Plexus (Fig. 2-15)

The lumbosacral and coccygeal nerve plexuses are derived from the anterior rami of the T12-S4 spinal nerves. The L4-S1 segments are of surgical significance. Injury to all of these segments has been reported, including occasional injury to the femoral nerve. The pelvic splanchnic nerves, the nervi erigentes, arise from the anterior rami of S2, S3, and S4.

Lumbosacral Plexus (Fig. 2-15)

A branch of the L4 root crosses the L5 transverse process; L5 crosses and grooves the ala of the sacrum where it joins with L4 to form the lumbosacral trunk. The upper four anterior sacral rami leave the sacral foramina, grooving the lateral mass of the sacrum. The lumbosacral trunk and the first sacral root unite anterior to the sacroiliac joint and they in

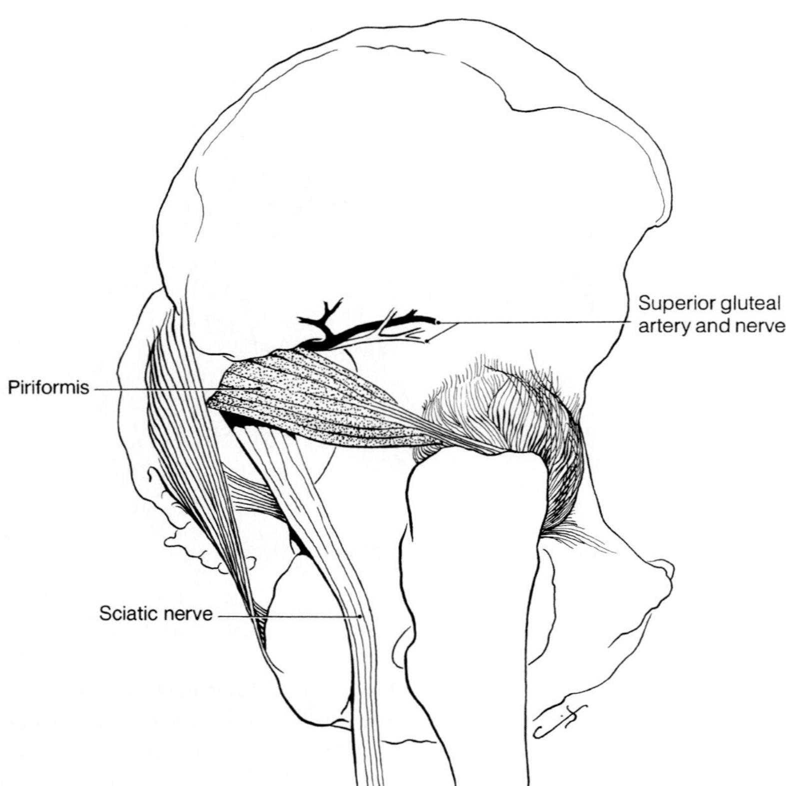

FIGURE 2-14. The piriformis divides the greater sciatic notch and is key to this region. The sciatic nerve is shown leaving the pelvis below this muscle and the superior gluteal artery, vein, and nerve above it.

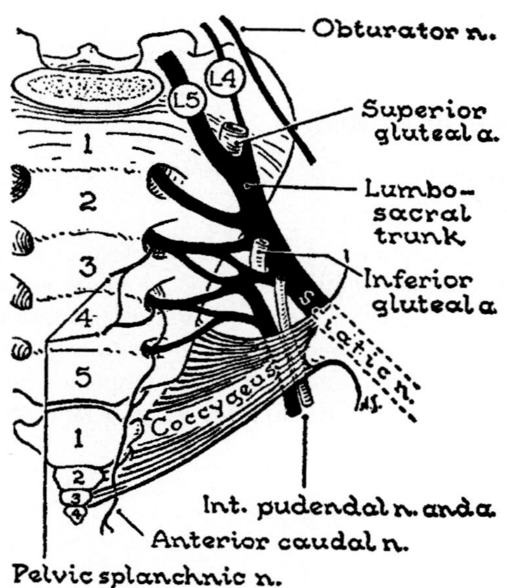

FIGURE 2-15. Sacral nerve plexus. (From: Basmajian IN. *Grant's method of anatomy,* 10th ed. Baltimore: Williams & Wilkins, 1980, with permission.)

turn unite with S2, S3, and S4 anterior to the piriformis, ending in two terminal branches, the sciatic and pudendal nerves, and many collateral branches, including the superior and inferior gluteal nerves. The branches of the sacral plexus may be grouped as follows.

Branches from the Roots of the Plexus. Rami from the roots of the plexus include muscular branches to the piriformis, levator ani, and coccygeus and the pelvic splanchnic nerve.

Branches That Pass through the Greater Sciatic Notch. The sciatic nerve forms the largest branch of the sacral plexus. It leaves the pelvis between the lower border of the piriformis and the ischial border of the greater sciatic notch. Its two divisions, the tibial and peroneal, are loosely held together. This nerve is commonly injured in pelvic trauma, especially in posterior dislocation of the hip with or without an acetabular fracture. The peroneal division is most prone to injury in this location, and the least likely to recover.

Because the major supply of the peroneal division of the sciatic nerve is the L5 root, it may be difficult to determine clinically whether the injury is to the nerve as it passes through the greater sciatic notch behind the hip joint or to the root.

The pudendal nerve (S2, S3, S4) escapes between the piriformis and coccygeus just medial to the sciatic nerve. The collateral nerves arising from the plexus include the superior gluteal, inferior gluteal, the nerve to the obturator internus (L5, S1, S2), the nerve to the quadratus femoris (L4, L5), and the posterior cutaneous nerve of the thigh (S1, S2, S3). The superior gluteal nerve (L4, L5, S1) and its artery and vein escape from the pelvis by winding around the greater sciatic notch. Injury to the nerve is uncommon, although the artery may be injured by trauma. This nerve is in jeopardy in posterior approaches to the hip joint for acetabular fractures, because application along the posterior plate may require excessive retraction, and resultant stretch of the nerve. The inferior gluteal nerve (L5, S1, S2) escapes from the pelvis beneath the piriformis and behind the sciatic nerve to supply the gluteus maximus.

Three branches that emulate the coccygeal plexus terminal branches are the perforating cutaneous branch of S2 and S3 and the perineal branch of S4. These descend anterior to the coccygeus, where they become cutaneous and supply the skin of the buttock and perineum.

Anterior Coccygeal Plexus

The anterior coccygeal plexus is formed by the anterior rami of S5 and C1, ending in the anterior caudal nerve, a sensory nerve supplying the coccygeal area.

Blood Vessels (Fig. 2-16)

Massive hemorrhage is the major complication of a pelvic disruption. Precise knowledge of the anatomy of the pelvic vasculature is essential because embolization of the bleeding vessel has emerged as one of the treatment options. The arteries of the pelvis are the median sacral, superior rectal, and internal iliac, the latter being the most surgically significant.

Median Sacral Artery

The median sacral artery is the continuation of the aorta; therefore, it hugs the vertebral column and may be injured in a sacral disruption. However, it is a small vessel and therefore not of major surgical significance.

The Superior Rectal (Hemorrhoidal) Artery

The superior rectal artery, the continuation of the superior mesenteric, is rarely involved in pelvic trauma.

The Internal Iliac Artery

The internal iliac is the vessel of major importance in pelvic trauma. It arises from the common iliac artery in the false pelvis and extends to the pelvic brim, where it splits into anterior and posterior divisions. It crosses medial to the external iliac vein, the psoas muscle, and the obturator nerve during its course. Anteriorly lies the ureter, posteriorly its vein. Severe trauma to the pelvis may disrupt the internal iliac artery or even the common iliac artery; survival is unlikely in those cases. Usually, the superior gluteal, iliolumbar, and lateral sacral arteries arise from the posterior division; all the others arise from the anterior division.

Posterior Division. Because of their location on the skeletal plane and because severe trauma to the pelvic ring usually causes posterior displacement, these vessels are most prone to damage. The superior gluteal artery is the largest branch of the internal iliac. It courses across the sacroiliac joint to

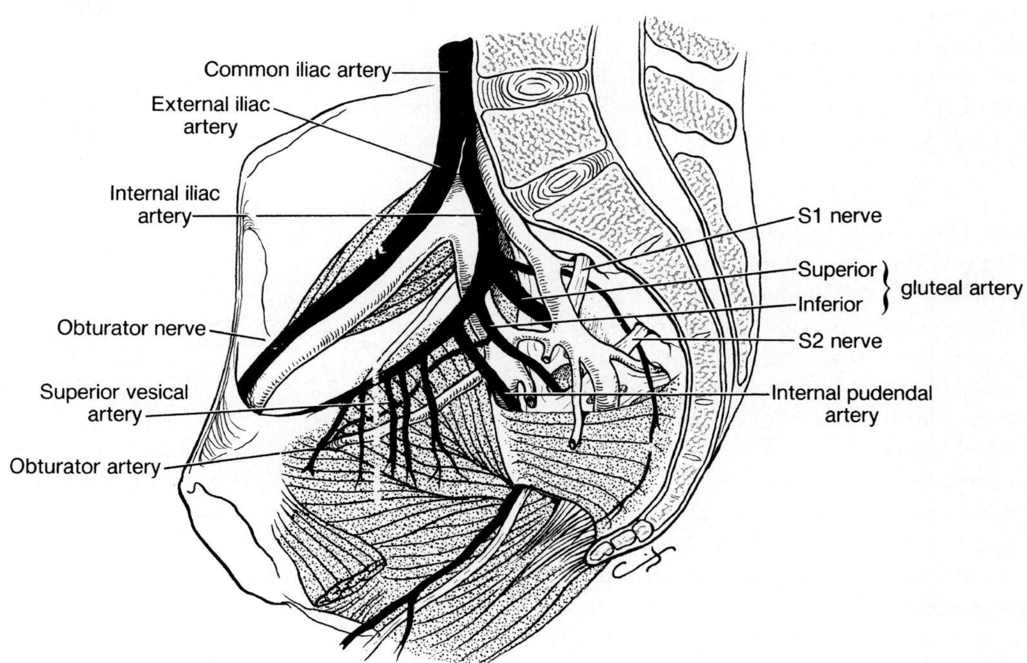

FIGURE 2-16. The internal iliac plexus of arteries and veins.

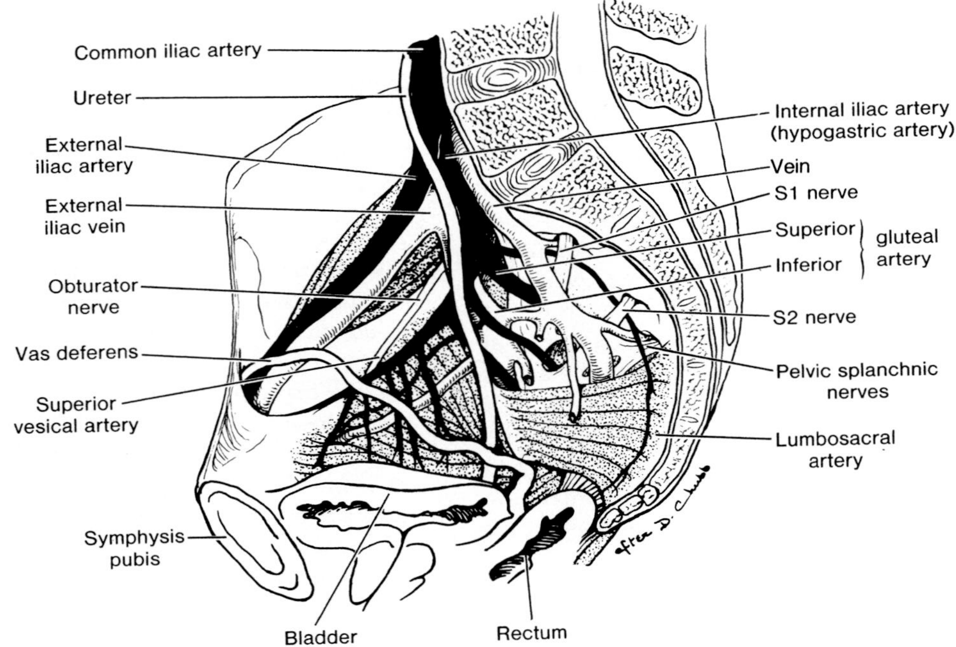

FIGURE 2-17. The internal iliac system of arteries and veins showing the position of the pelvic viscera.

the greater sciatic notch, where it lies against the ilium, making a U turn around the notch into the gluteal region, accompanied by its nerve and vein (Fig. 2-14). Damage to this large artery is a common cause of massive hemorrhage in pelvic disruption, because its course on the ilium crosses the common area of pelvic trauma. Also, traumatic aneurysm of the artery has been reported. The *iliolumbar artery* is the somatic artery of the fifth lumbar segment; therefore, it must ascend to that level. As it crosses the ala of the sacrum, it too is commonly injured. The *lateral sacral artery* descends lateral to the anterior sacral foramina and in front of the sacral plexus.

Anterior Division. The visceral branches supply the bladder, genitalia, and a portion of the rectum. They are: (a) the obliterated obturator artery, which clings to the peritoneum on the side wall of the pelvis above the level of the bladder and ends in the superior vesical arteries that supply the upper surface of the bladder; and (b) the inferior vesical and middle rectal arteries, which run in the retropubic leash of veins and supply the bladder and genitalia.

The *limb* and *perineal branches* include the internal pudendal artery and inferior gluteal artery, which descend anterior to the sacral plexus and pass between the borders of the piriformis and coccygeus into the gluteal region. The inferior gluteal artery passes between the first, second, or third sacral nerves and leaves the pelvis inferior to the piriformis to supply the gluteus maximus. The internal pudendal artery crosses the ischial spine and returns to the pelvis through the lesser sciatic foramen in the company of its own nerve. Both may be torn by trauma to this area. The obturator artery runs along the side wall of the pelvis to the obturator foramen, lying between its nerve and vein. As it leaves the pelvis through the superior defect in the obturator membrane, it may be disrupted in common injuries to the pubic rami.

The Pelvic Veins (Fig. 2-17)

The pelvic viscera lie upon a massive thin-walled venous plexus through which the arteries thread their way. Most

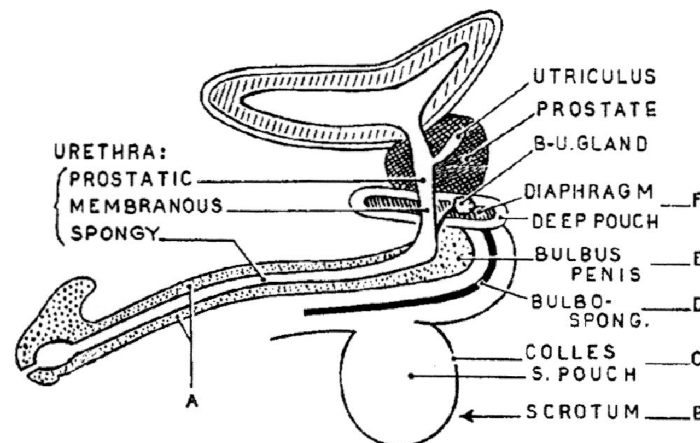

FIGURE 2-18. The male perineum. (From: Basmajian IN. *Grant's method of anatomy,* 10th ed. Baltimore: Williams & Wilkins, 1980, with permission.)

drain into the internal iliac vein, but some drain into the superior rectal, then into the inferior mesenteric, and on to the portal vein. Massive bleeding may occur from this venous plexus following pelvic trauma.

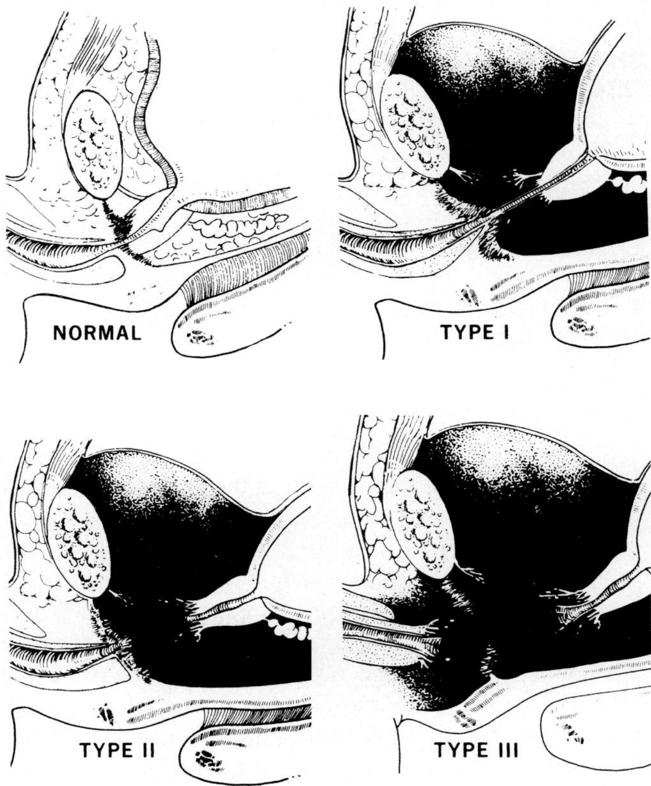

FIGURE 2-19. Classification of urethral tears. Normal: The prostate and urogenital diaphragm blend together as one unit. Type I: The clinical findings may suggest a complete rupture, but, in fact, the urethra is intact although attenuated. Type II: The classic supradiaphragmatic injury. Type III: Subdiaphragmatic rupture. A complete rupture is shown, but partial Type III rupture also occurs. In our experience, Type III injuries are common. A retrograde urethrogram in these patients shows perineal extravasation. (From: Colapinto V. Trauma to the pelvis: urethral injury. *Clin Orthop* 1980;151:46, with permission.)

Male Urethra

Because this text deals mainly with skeletal injury, a detailed description of the gastrointestinal and genitourinary systems is not in order; however, urethral injuries are so common—and so potentially devastating—that some description is in order. A controversy has arisen over the conventional anatomic description of the male urethra and newer anatomic and urologic information.

The urogenital diaphragm is depicted in most texts as in Fig. 2-18; that is, as two separate fascial layers spanning the pubic arch with skeletal muscle between. Normally, the prostate is believed to sit on the superior layer of fascia, but separate from the urogenital diaphragm, the only connection being the membranous urethra, which perforates the diaphragm at its midpoint. Obviously, if the prostate is displaced or the urogenital diaphragm suddenly shifts, the membranous urethra ruptures at this natural plane between the apex of the prostate and the superior layer of the diaphragmatic fascia. Colapinto, in a recent publication, offers a different explanation (1). In clinical studies, he found that most urethral ruptures were not of this "classic" variety, but occurred below the urogenital diaphragm (Fig. 2-19). His anatomic studies showed that the junction between the prostate and urogenital diaphragm is not a natural weak spot, but the prostate and urogenital diaphragm tend to be a single unit. The membranous urethra is strong in this region, surrounded by smooth muscle that extends into the prostatic urethra. The muscle ends abruptly at the inferior surface of the diaphragm, where the bulbous urethra begins; thus, this is the truly weak area of the urethra, and the location of the rupture of the bulbous urethra confirms a clinical truth. Based on his studies, Colapinto has classified urethral tears (Fig. 2-19) (2).

REFERENCES

1. Colapinto V. Trauma to the pelvis: urethral injury. *Clin Orthop* 1980;151:46.
2. Grant JC. *An atlas of anatomy,* 6th ed. Baltimore: Williams & Wilkins, 1972.

3

ANATOMY OF THE ACETABULUM

MARTIN D. BIRCHER
MARVIN TILE

INTRODUCTION

Hidden within the safety cage of the pelvic ring lie the acetabulae. They are the jewels within the pelvic crown. The acetabulum is the proximal half of the hip joint transferring weight and allowing movement between the legs and axial skeleton. This weight transfer takes place over a relatively small horseshoe-shaped area of articular cartilage.

The shape of the hemipelvis is complex and very three-dimensional. There are eight ossification centers. The three primary centers are the ilium, ischium, and pubis (Fig. 3-1). The five secondary centers are the crest, anterior inferior iliac spine, ischial spine, pubic symphysis, and Y cartilage of the acetabulum. The variable thickness of the bone and epiphyseal scars contribute to some degree to the standard fracture configurations. It can be seen by looking at Fig. 3-1 how a T-shaped fracture propagates in an adult.

ARTICULAR CARTILAGE

The *articular cartilage* is not replaceable. Any loss caused by injury will lead to a substandard bearing. The situation could be likened to that of the effect of primary brain damage. Cartilage cells that are lost are lost forever. An acetabular fracture will result in a variable amount of cell loss, which is often related to the violence of the injury. The goal of treatment must be to minimize secondary loss caused by cell abrasion and differential loading. One must also endeavor to provide the ideal environment for bone, cartilage, and soft-tissue healing.

The articular cartilage is thinnest anteriorly and somewhat thicker posteriorly. This may owe to the fact that we have evolved via quadrupeds. However, pressure studies have shown that all the surfaces play an important role in load sharing. Loss of even an insignificant piece of posterior wall leads to changes in joint pressures.

The joint space is approximately 4 to 5 mm wide on an AP (anteroposterior) radiograph of the hip. It has been shown that the maximum thickness of articular cartilage lies in the position of maximum load in the roof of the acetabulum.

Thus, the most important single structure in the acetabulum is the *articular cartilage,* but the shape of the acetabulum and its orientation in relation to that of the femoral head and neck are almost as important. Dysplasia and excessively retroverted and anteverted hips will lead to head/socket mismatch and an increased load on the articular cartilage. The orientation of the acetabulum may also predispose a joint to particular types of injury; for example, an increased risk of posterior dislocation in retroverted hips.

ANATOMIC STRUCTURES

One must be adept at visualizing spatial relationships in order to master the complex anatomy of the acetabulum. Inspection of the lateral aspect of the acetabulum without the femoral head clearly outlines the anatomic features (Fig. 3-2). From its lateral aspect, the acetabulum is cradled by the arms of an inverted Y (Fig. 3-3) (1).

Posterior Column

The *posterior column* is strong and triangular and is most suitable for internal fixation. Beginning at the dense bone of the greater sciatic notch—the strongest bone in the pelvis—it extends distally through the center of the acetab-

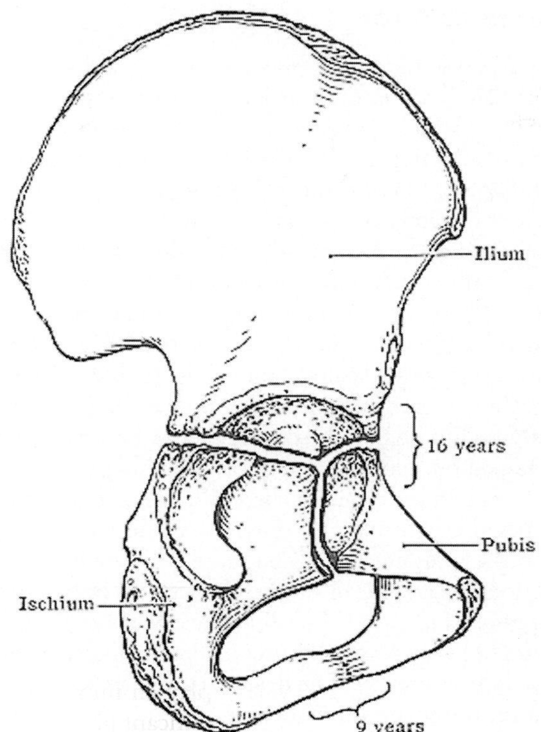

FIGURE 3-1. Primary centers of ossification of the pelvis: one each for the ischium, pubis, and ilium. They meet in the acetabulum at the triradiate cartilage and fuse between 18 and 23 years of age. (From: Anderson JE. *Grant's anatomy,* 8th ed. Baltimore: Williams & Wilkins, 1983, with permission.)

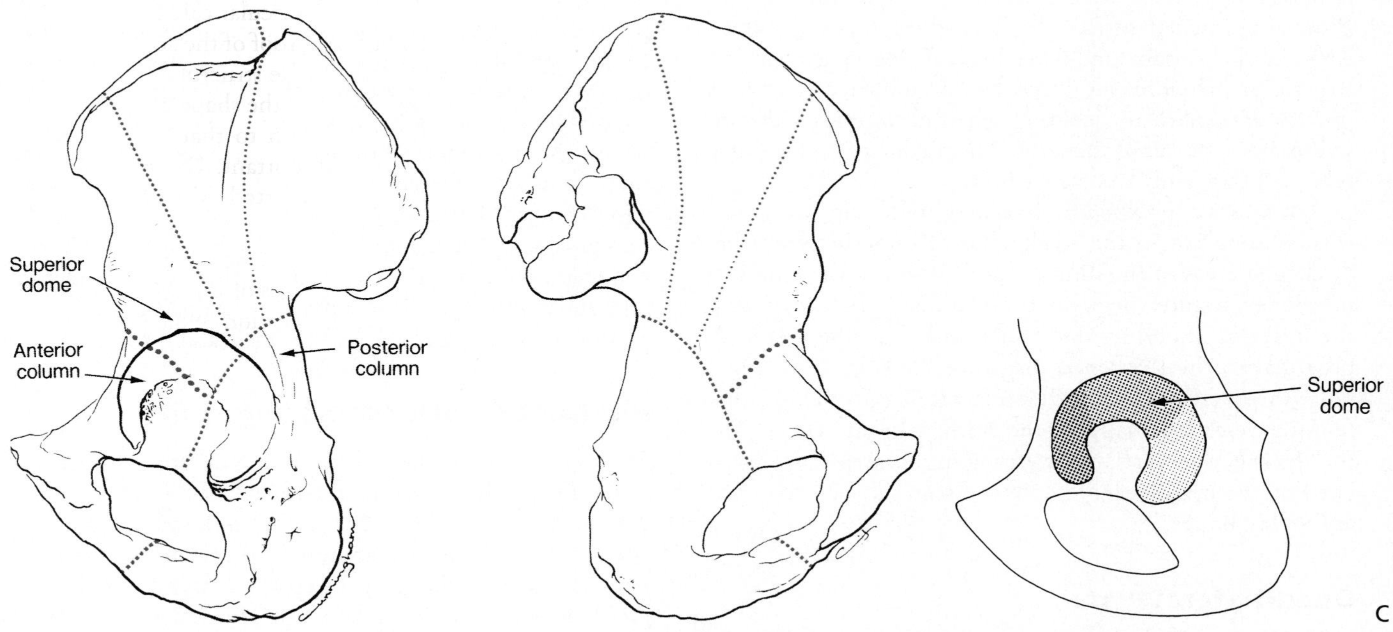

FIGURE 3-2. A: Lateral aspect of the hemipelvis and acetabulum. The posterior column is characterized by the dense bone at the greater sciatic notch and follows the *dotted line* distally through the center of the acetabulum, obturator foramen, and inferior pubic ramus. The anterior column extends from the iliac crest to the symphysis pubis and includes the entire anterior wall of the acetabulum. Fractures involving the anterior column commonly exit through weak areas in the ilium (i.e., distal to the anterior inferior iliac spine, between the anterior superior and anterior inferior iliac spines, or between the anterior superior and the iliac tubercle and proximal to the iliac tubercle). **B:** The hemipelvis from its medial aspect. **C:** The area between the posterior column and the *heavy dotted line*—a fracture through the anterior column—is often considered the superior dome fragment, which actually is represented by the middle portion.

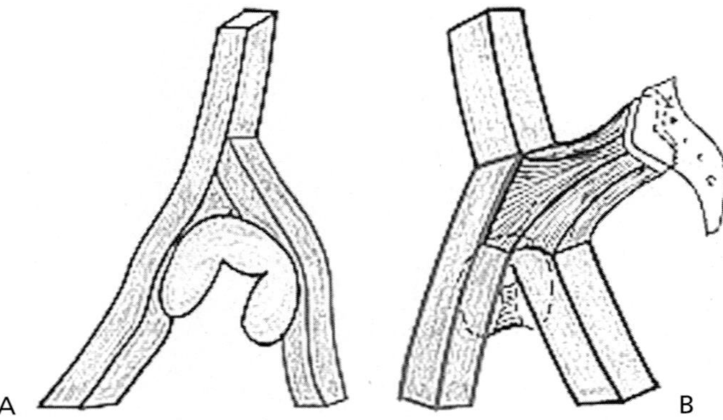

FIGURE 3-3. **A:** Diagram of the two columns supporting the two columns with inverted Y. **B:** The two columns are linked to the sacral bone by the sciatic buttress. (From: ref. 1, with permission)

ulum to include the ischial spine and ischial tuberosity. Its inner surface forms the wall of the acetabulum, and its anterior surface the posterior articular surface of the acetabulum.

Anterior Column

The *anterior column* extends from the iliac crest to the symphysis pubis and includes the anterior wall of the acetabulum. As it descends in the pelvis, the column rotates 90° just above the articular surface, to reach the symphysis pubis. The anterior surface undulates beneath the neurovascular structures; therefore, the iliopectineal eminence is an important landmark in deciding whether anterior column screws are in or out of the joint. The medial part of the anterior column is the true pelvic brim.

Commonly, *proximally,* fractures involving the anterior column exit in the weak areas of bone between the thickened areas of the ilium; that is, distal to the anterior inferior iliac spine, between the two iliac spines, between the anterior superior iliac spine and the tubercle, and proximal to the thickened iliac tubercle (Fig. 3-2). Distally, the anterior column fracture often exits behind the femoral vessels (usually in the both column types). Although the bone is relatively strong in this area, it is weakened by the pre-existing epiphyseal scar between the iliac and pubic bones.

Quadrilateral Plate

Rotation of the hemipelvis to expose the inner surface (Fig. 3-2) elucidates the three-dimensional structure of the acetabulum. The two columns cradle the acetabulum, and meet medially to form the medial surface, the *quadrilateral plate.* It is debatable whether the quadrilateral plate is an anterior or posterior column structure; it is best considered an accessory structure preventing medial displacement of the hip, the medial wall, or, if you like, a *thin third column.*

Dome or Roof

Inspection of the lateral aspect of the acetabulum reveals the important features of its articular surface, especially the superior or weight-bearing surface often referred to as the *dome* or *roof* (Fig. 3-3). This dome, which has great clinical significance, extends from the strong bone just posterior to the anterior inferior iliac spine to the posterior column.

The dome or roof of the acetabulum on AP x-rays is in reality only a very small piece of articular cartilage. However, it represents the most important part of the acetabulum as far as weight bearing is concerned. The radiographic marker in Fig. 3-4 is only 2 mm wide, yet seems to represent the whole of the weight-bearing dome. Oblique x-rays and computed tomographic scanning allow better estimation of this small but crucial piece of the acetabulum (Fig. 3-4).

The main use of newer three-dimensional scanning techniques may be that the dome-as-a-line concept inferred from the x-ray image will be supplanted by the concept of the dome as an *area* of the weight-bearing surface of the acetabulum (Fig. 3-5). These lines have been used clinically by Matta in his roof arc measurements to help decide on operative indications (2). The determinant may become the *roof area* measurement in the future.

Femoral Head

The femoral head is held between the jaws of three major pieces of acetabular cartilage (the anterior column, posterior column, and dome). Medially, these three jaws are continuous with the fovea. If the fovea is viewed externally with the femoral head removed it is noted to be nonarticular and represents the attachment of the ligamentum teres. Distally, the fovea connects at the superior limit of the obturator foramen with the quadrilateral surface of the acetabulum. If a significant force is applied to the greater trochanter, the femoral head will fracture through these jaws, producing standard fracture lines and eventually will burst through the quadrilateral place, producing the classically described "central dislocation."

Hip Joint Relationships (Fig. 3-6)

The hip capsule is attached to the circumference of the acetabulum by the relatively avascular labrum. This further deepens the acetabulum. The gluteal mass muscles hide the lateral aspect of the acetabulum and makes access to the joint extremely challenging. Deep to the muscles lie the major blood supply to the acetabulum (see Chapter 28). Anteriorly, the femoral vein and artery are extremely close to the anterior part of the acetabulum (Fig. 3-7). The iliopsoas muscle provides some protection when retractors are placed over the anterior lip of the acetabulum.

The key anterior anatomical structure is the iliopectineal fascia. This can only be visualized during anterior approaches to the acetabulum (Fig. 3-8). The iliopectineal fascia separates the femoral vessels from the femoral nerve, which itself is cradled within the iliopsoas

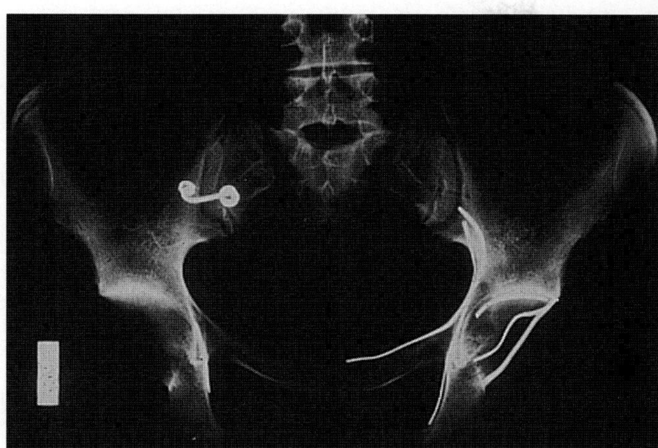

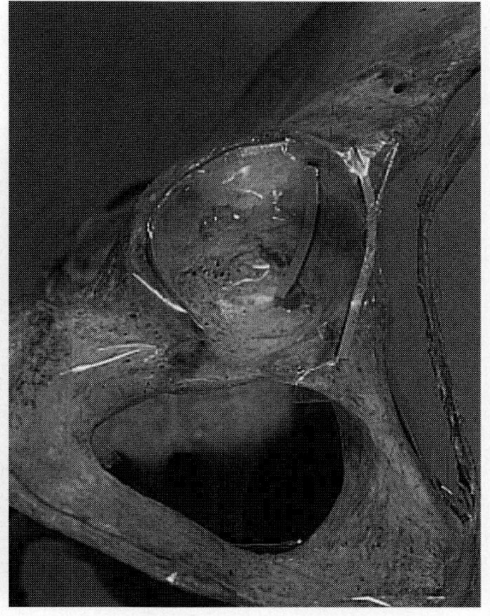

FIGURE 3-4. A: Lead markers placed on the radiographs seem to represent the whole of the weight-bearing dome. **B:** In reality, viewing the lead marker on the anatomic specimen indicates that this is only 2 mm wide. Therefore, oblique x-rays and three-dimensional scanning allow better estimation of this small but crucial piece of the acetabulum.

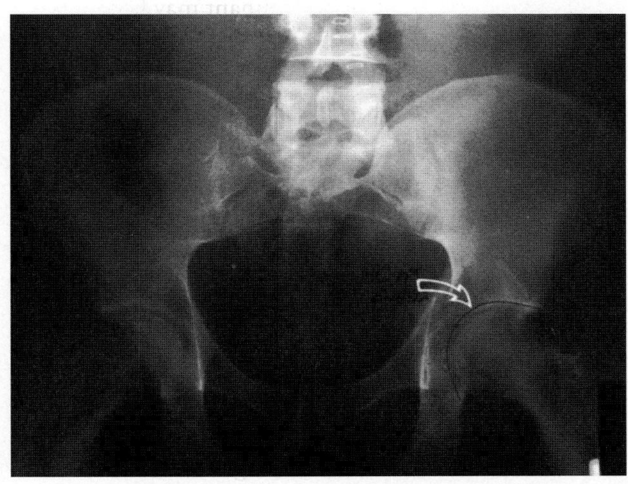

FIGURE 3-5. A: On the plain radiograph the dome or roof has a distinctive appearance *(white arrow)*; however, this appearance is deceptive because the radiographic line represents an area on the articular surface of the acetabulum that is 2 to 3 mm wide. One of the main advantages in three-dimensional computed tomography is that the true area of the weight-bearing surface is seen clearly. This is a much more realistic representation than the narrow line visible on a plain radiograph: **(B)** with the femoral head intact; **(C)** with the femoral head subtracted.

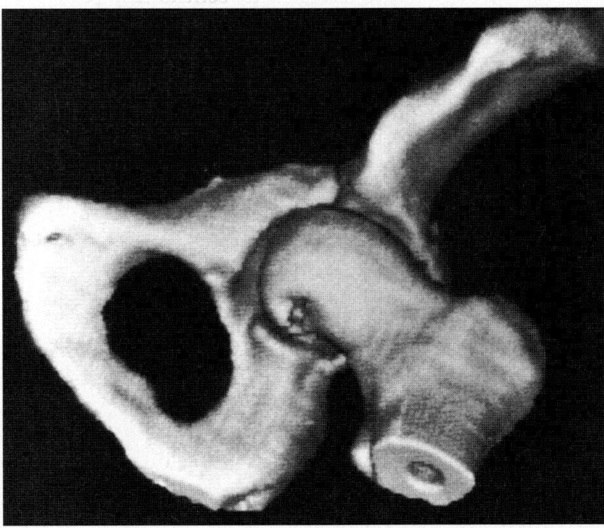

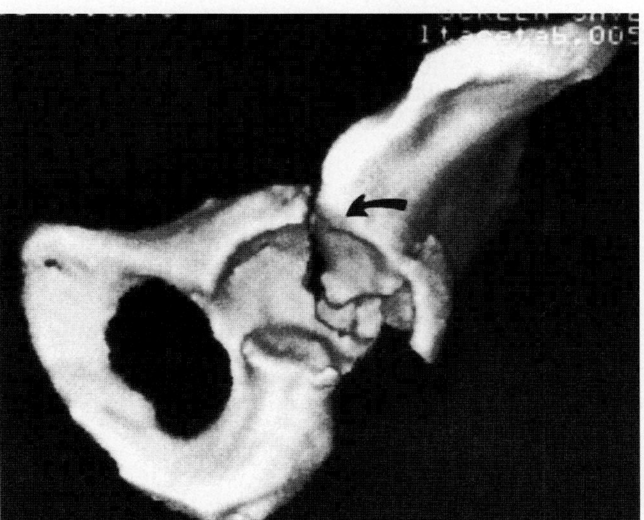

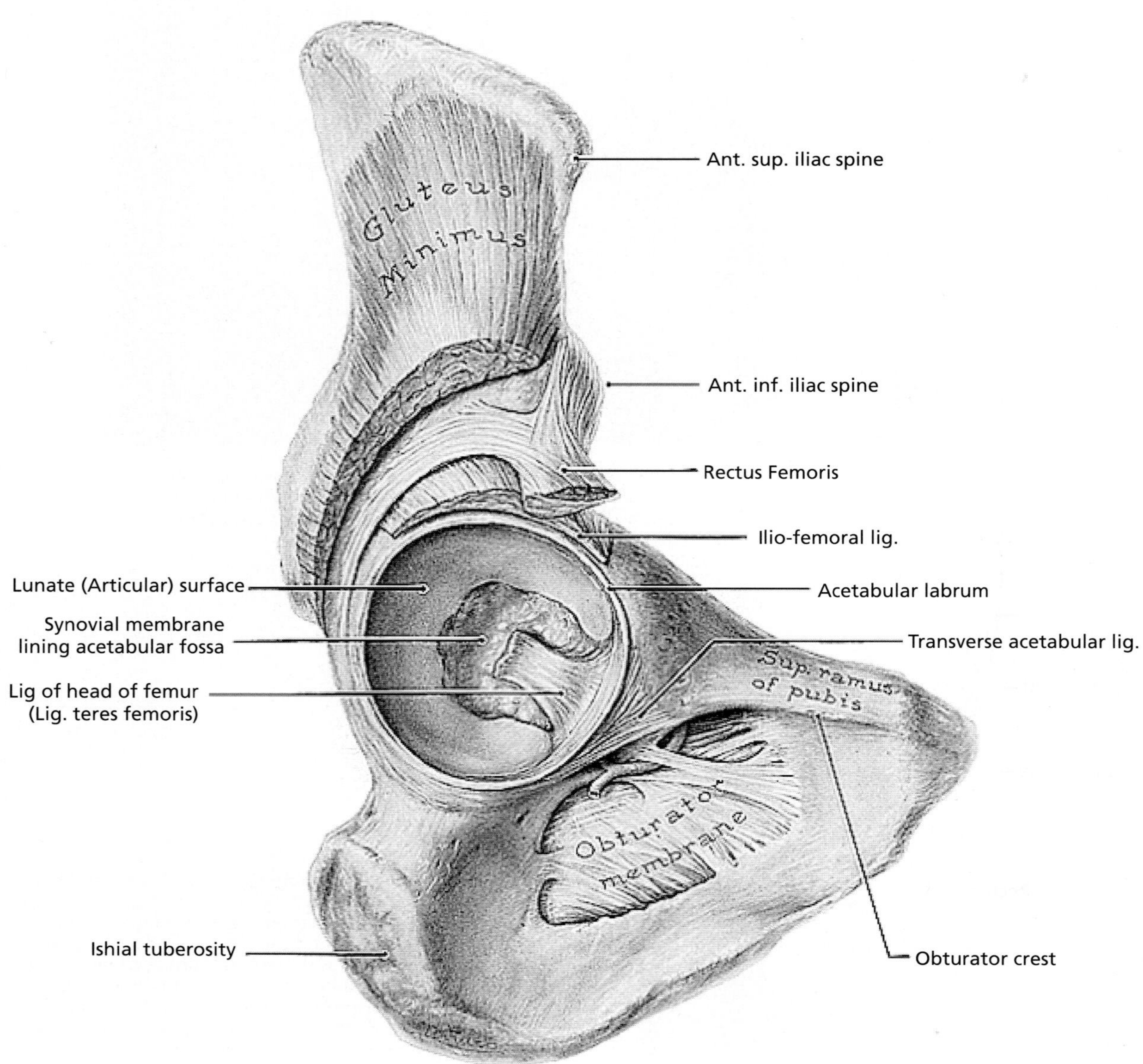

FIGURE 3-6. A view of the acetabulum with the femoral head removed. Note the circumferential nature of the labrum, which tends to effectively deepen the acetabulum. (From: Anderson IE. *Grant's atlas of anatomy,* 8th ed. Baltimore: Williams & Wilkins, 1983, with permission.)

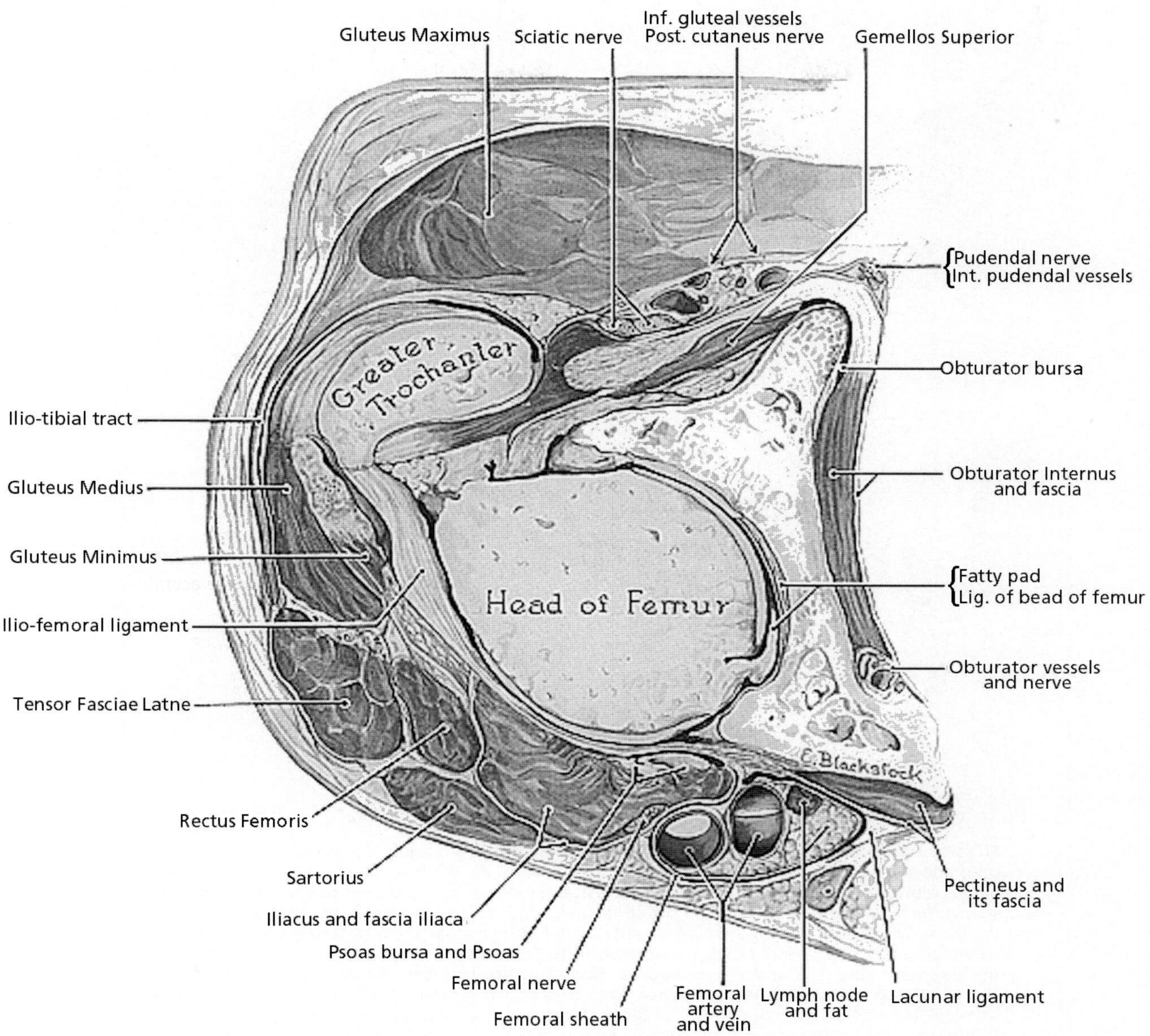

FIGURE 3-7. Transfer section through the thigh at the level of the hip joint. Note the close proximity of the femoral artery and vein to the anterior aspect of the hip joint and head of the femur. Note also the proximity of the sciatic nerve and gluteal vessels to the posterior aspect of the hip joint separated only by the gemelli and obturator externes muscle. (From: Anderson IE. *Grant's atlas of anatomy,* 8th ed. Baltimore: Williams & Wilkins, 1983, with permission.)

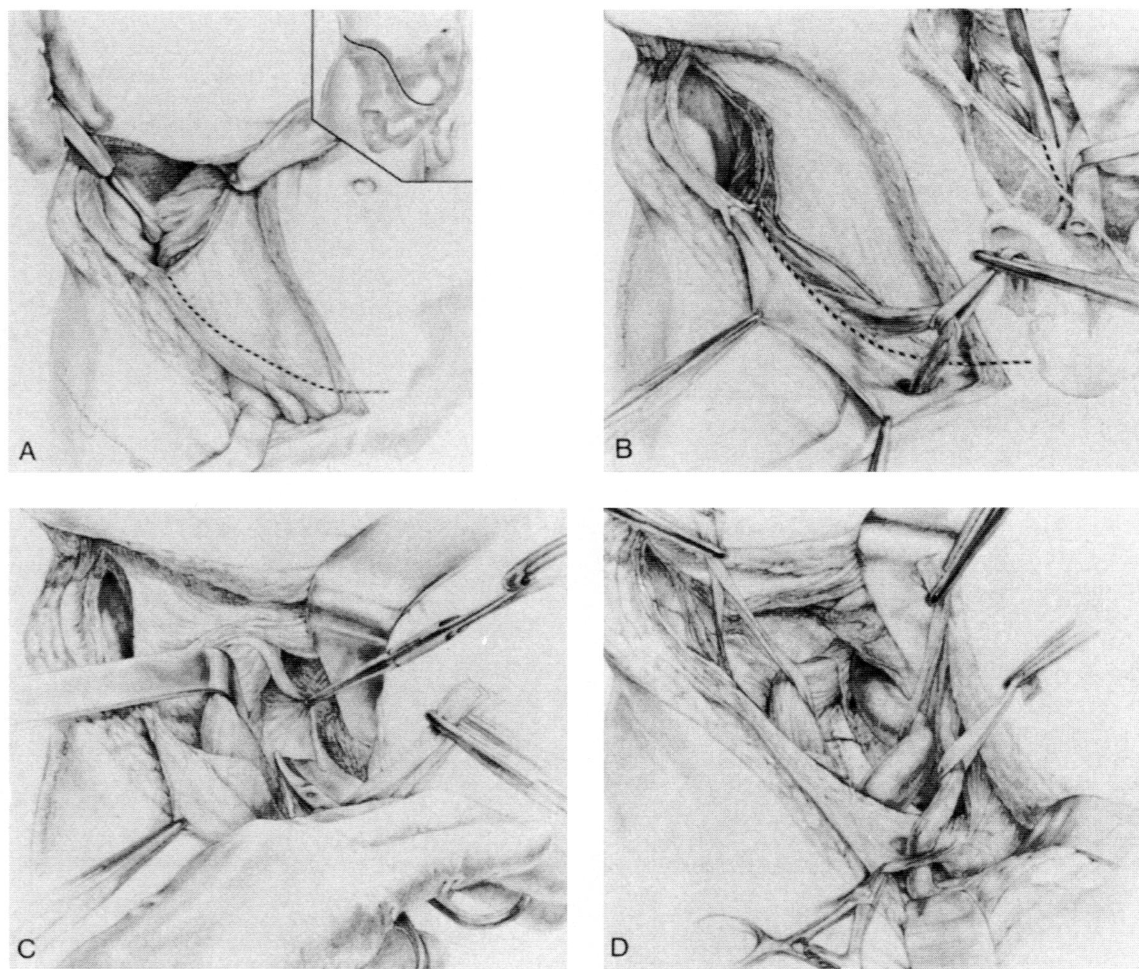

FIGURE 3-8. Note the anterior anatomic relationships in the ilioinguinal approach—a commonly used approach to the anterior aspect of the acetabulum. **A:** The inset shows the incision, which begins along the lateral aspect of the iliac crest and extends forward over the anterior superior spine. The iliacus muscle is dissected subperiosteally with an elevator from the interior aspect of the ilium. The sacroiliac joint can be exposed through this approach. The *dotted line* shows the incision through the external oblique aponeurosis. **B:** The aponeurosis has been divided, exposing the spermatic cord and underlying iliopsoas fascia. In the inset, the iliopsoas fascia is identified and divided to the iliopectineal eminence. Note the retractor around the great vessels. **C:** The position of the scissors has changed, and they now divide the iliopsoas fascia along the bony attachment in the region of the iliopectineal eminence. **D:** Tapes have been placed around the spermatic cord, femoral artery and vein, and iliopsoas muscle, to allow access to the underlying bone. The iliac crest can be identified by retracting the iliopsoas medially. The quadrilateral plate can be reached by reflecting it laterally and the vessels medially.

muscle. Distally, the fascia lies in the sagittal plane between the nerve and the artery, but it moves a little medially as it plunges down to the anterior column to blend with the periosteum. As the fascia then runs cranially it rotates gently, almost through 90 degrees, and attaches to the pelvic brim, again blending with the periosteum. It is impossible to palpate the quadrilateral surface of the acetabulum unless this structure is divided fully during anterior pelvic surgery.

It is possible to expose the whole of the superior pubic ramus from symphysis to greater sciatic notch after division of the iliopectineal fascia. Great care must be taken in raising the periosteum along the superior pubic ramus for fear of division of accessory obturator vessels (corona mortis). These connect the internal and external iliac systems via the obturator artery and vein. These accessory vessels are variable in size and position. They must be carefully ligated or clipped before division to prevent retraction into the obturator foramen, where bleeding is sometimes impossible to control (Fig. 3-9).

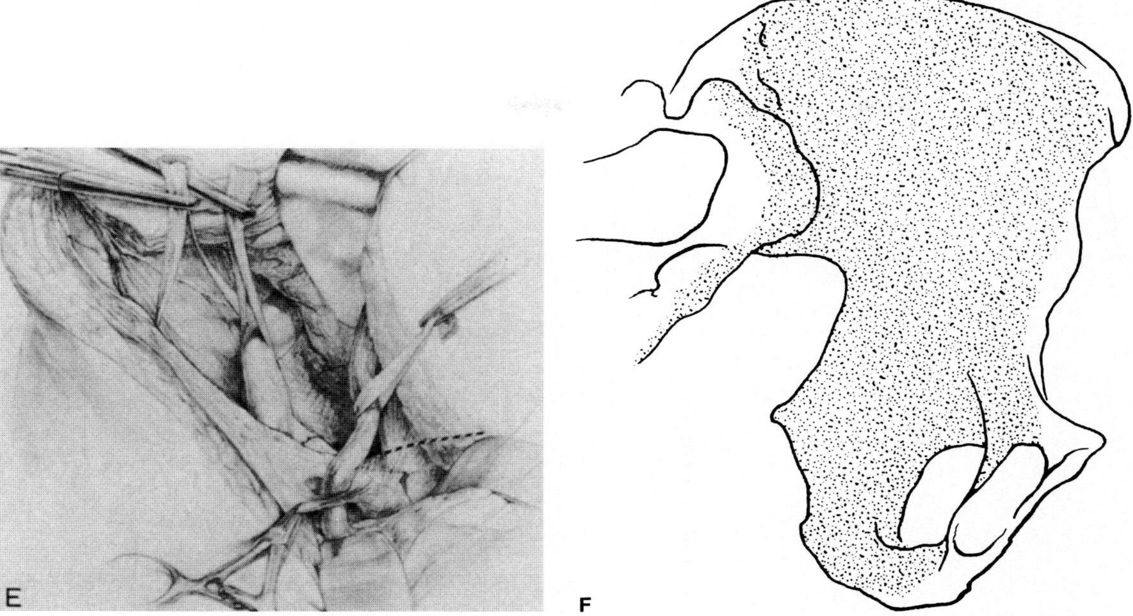

FIGURE 3-8. *(continued)* **E:** To reach the symphysis pubis, the rectus abdominis sheath is divided and the muscle is removed from its insertion into the symphysis along the *dotted line*. **F:** The *dotted area* reveals the access of the entire interior aspect of the pelvis, including the sacroiliac joint, which can be achieved through the ilioinguinal approach. (From: Steinberg M. *The hip and its disorders.* Philadelphia: WB Saunders, 1991, with permission.)

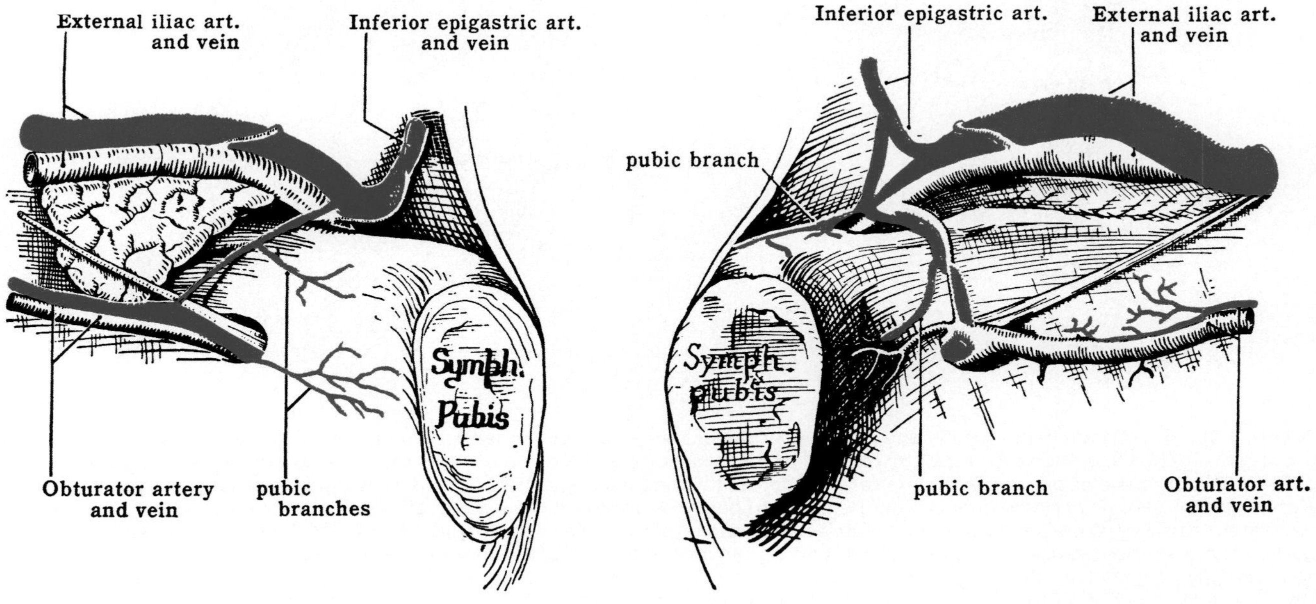

FIGURE 3-9. A: Behind the body of the pubis, the pubic branch of the obturator artery forms an anastomosis with the pubic branch of the inferior epigastric artery. **B:** The obturator artery arises from the inferior epigastric via the pubic anastomosis. In a study of 283 limbs, the obturator artery arose from the internal iliac artery in 70%, from the inferior epigastric in 25.4%, and from both equally in 4.6%. (From: Anderson IE. *Grant's atlas of anatomy,* 8th ed. Baltimore: Williams & Wilkins, 1983, with permission.)

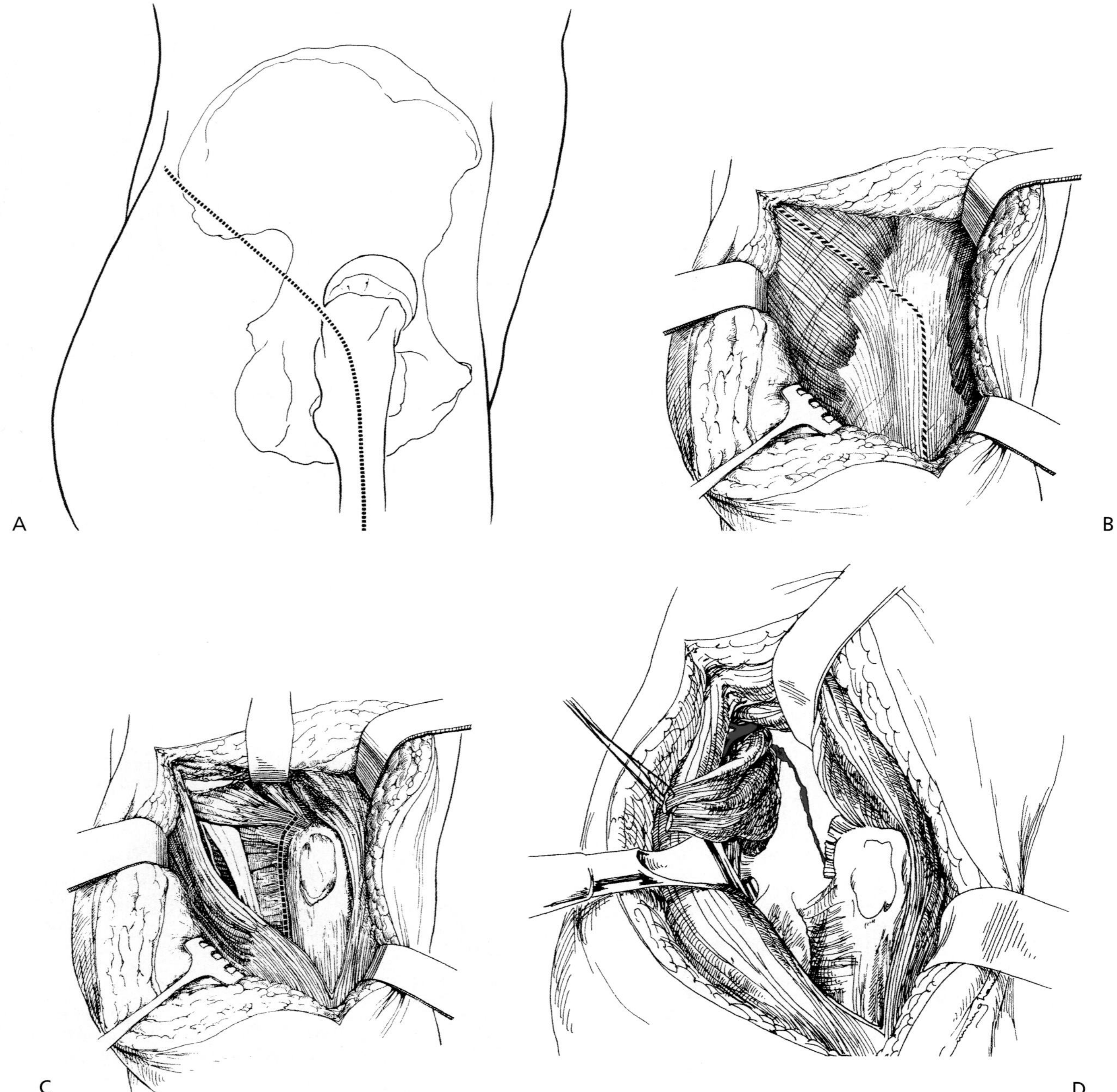

FIGURE 3-10. A: Diagram demonstrates the incisions for the posterior Kocher-Langenbeck approach. On occasion, extending the exposure anteriorly **(B)** allows increased access by removal of the trochanter and division of fibers of the tensor fasciae latae. (From: Schatzker J, Tile M. *The rationale of operative fracture care.* Heidelberg: Springer-Verlag, 1987, with permission.) Some surgeons prefer a straight lateral approach. For posterior wall fractures, the standard posterior approach **(A)** is adequate, but for complex fractures removal of the trochanter helps with exposure. **B:** The tensor fasciae latae and gluteus maximus muscle are identified following division of skin and subcutaneous tissue. These structures are divided by splitting the muscle fibers of the gluteus maximus and dividing the tensor fasciae latae longitudinally *(striped line)*. **C:** The posterior structures of the hip are identified after division of the gluteus maximus and tensor fasciae latae. These include the piriformis, short external rotators, quadratus femoris, and sciatic nerve. In this case, the sciatic nerve is exiting anterior to the piriformis and posterior to the short external rotators. On occasion, the sciatic nerve enters posterior to the piriformis or splits the muscle. The tendons of the short external rotators and the piriformis are divided along the *checked line* to achieve access to the posterior column. **D:** Elevation of the short external rotators allows identification of the obturator internus bursa and leads the surgeon to the greater and lesser notch, allowing access to the entire posterior column. Care must be taken when dissecting in the greater sciatic notch to avoid injuring the superior gluteal artery and/or nerve.

Posteriorly, it is important to understand the relationship between the short external rotators and the sciatic nerve. Considerable anatomic variation is possible; for example, a high dividing sciatic nerve. The usual configuration is with piriformis exiting the pelvis through the greater sciatic notch (Fig. 2-14). The muscle comes into view at 45 degrees and forms 1 to 2 cm of distinct tendon before obtaining attachment in the piriform fossa. Care must be taken in dividing this muscle. If it is divided too close to the bone, the ascending branch to the medial circumflex artery is in danger. When the piriformis tendon is turned outward and freed up with a finger from the greater sciatic notch, the sciatic nerve should be visible underneath. More distally, the multipennate tendon of obturator internus guides the surgeon to the posterior column of the acetabulum (Fig. 3-10). The obturator internus attaches to the femur at a right angle and is a shorter tendon, which causes the gemelli to bulge both above and below it. The sciatic nerve is partially protected when the obturator internus is retracted. As the obturator tendon is followed into the pelvis it turns around the bone, through the lesser sciatic notch beneath it, allowing movement around the notch in the obturator internus bursa. The obturator internus tendon seems to remain intact even in severely displaced posterior column injuries. The surgeon will always be led to bone and relative safety by tracing it backward.

REFERENCES

1. Letournel E. Diagnosis and treatment of non unions and malunions of acetabular fractures. *Orthop Clin North Am* 990;21:769.
2. Matta JM, Merritt PO. Displaced acetabular fractures. *Clin Orthop* 1988;May: 230–283.

4

BIOMECHANICS OF THE PELVIC RING

MARVIN TILE
TREVOR HEARN
MARK VRAHAS

INTRODUCTION

Understanding pelvic stability is the key to evaluating and managing pelvic injuries. Pelvic anatomy was described in some detail in Chapter 2. In this chapter we discuss how the anatomic elements interact to maintain pelvic stability, and how injurious forces affect these elements.

ANATOMIC STRUCTURES

Anterior Structures

The anterior pubic rami act as a strut to prevent anterior collapse of the pelvic ring during weight bearing (Fig. 4-1). However, congenital or traumatic absence of the anterior structures has little effect on pelvic stability (see Figs. 2-3 and 2-4). The intact symphysis pubis is a strong ligamentous structure that withstands external rotation, but isolated disruptions of the symphysis have little effect on stability of the pelvic ring.

Posterior Structures

Pelvic stability depends on an intact posterior sacroiliac complex. This intricate posterior complex, a masterful biomechanical structure, is able to withstand the transference of the weight-bearing forces from the spine to the lower extremities. Without this design, the sacrum would tend to displace anteriorly and the innominates posteriorly. The vital role assumed by the ligaments as posterior stabilizers may be appreciated even more by examining the bony structure of the sacroiliac joints. One might have expected the sacrum to be designed by the great biologic designer in the form of a keystone of an arch. In fact, in one plane it is quite the opposite, allowing the sacrum to fall forward, not locking it into place (Fig. 4-2). Therefore, rotation may occur through the sacroiliac joints with weight bearing, but at the expense of perfect stability. Let us now look at this intricate ligamentous arrangement in more detail.

The *anterior sacroiliac ligaments* are flat and strong, to resist external rotation and shearing forces. It is the *posterior ligamentous structures* that form the major tension band effect of the pelvic ring. The entire posterior ligamentous complex may be likened to a suspension bridge in which posterior superior iliac spines the pillars, the interosseous sacroiliac ligaments the suspension bars, and the sacrum the bridge (Fig. 4-3). The iliolumbar ligaments joining the transverse processes of L5 to the iliac crest and the intervening transverse fibers of the interosseous sacroiliac ligaments enhance the suspensory mechanism. Grant describes the posterior sacroiliac interosseous ligament as the strongest ligament in the body. When one understands its function, the reason for this becomes obvious.

The posterior sacroiliac ligamentous complex prevents posterior displacements of the pelvic ring on the sacrum, or from the alternative point of view, anterior displacements of the sacrum and axial skeleton on the pelvis. Although this

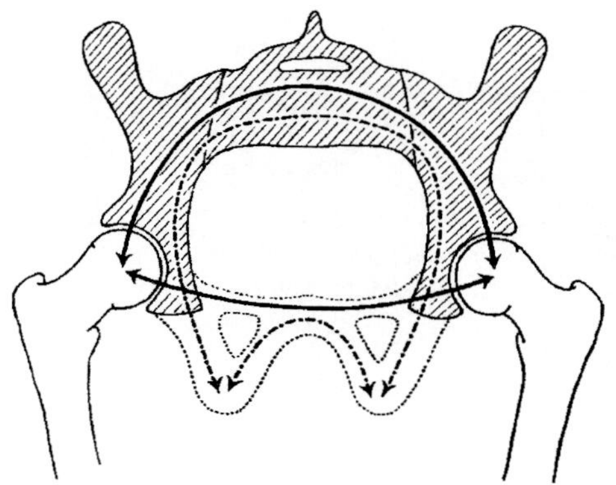

FIGURE 4-1. The major weight-bearing area is represented by the diagonal lines; the symphysis pubis acts only as an anterior strut. (After Braus.) (From Bazmajian JV. *Grant's method of anatomy,* 4th ed. Baltimore: Williams & Wilkins, 1980, with permission.)

posterior sacroiliac ligamentous complex acts as the primary stabilizer to the posterior pelvis, the caudally positioned *sacrospinous* and *sacrotuberous* ligaments as well as the *pelvic floor* augment stability (Figs. 4-4 and 4-5). Any major degree of vertical instability in the pelvic ring is associated with disruption of these ligaments and the pelvic floor.

CONCEPT OF PELVIC STABILITY

For practical purposes, the pelvic ring can be considered a single anatomic structure. The pelvis is comprised of three bony elements: two innominate bones and the sacrum. It is apparent on examining these elements that they have no inherent stability; that is, a pelvis devoid of soft tissues would immediately separate into its component parts. The bones are joined anteriorly at the symphysis and posteriorly at the sacroiliac joints (Fig. 4-6). Although the ligaments connecting these points can be considered the major stabilizing structures, it is important to remember that smaller liga-

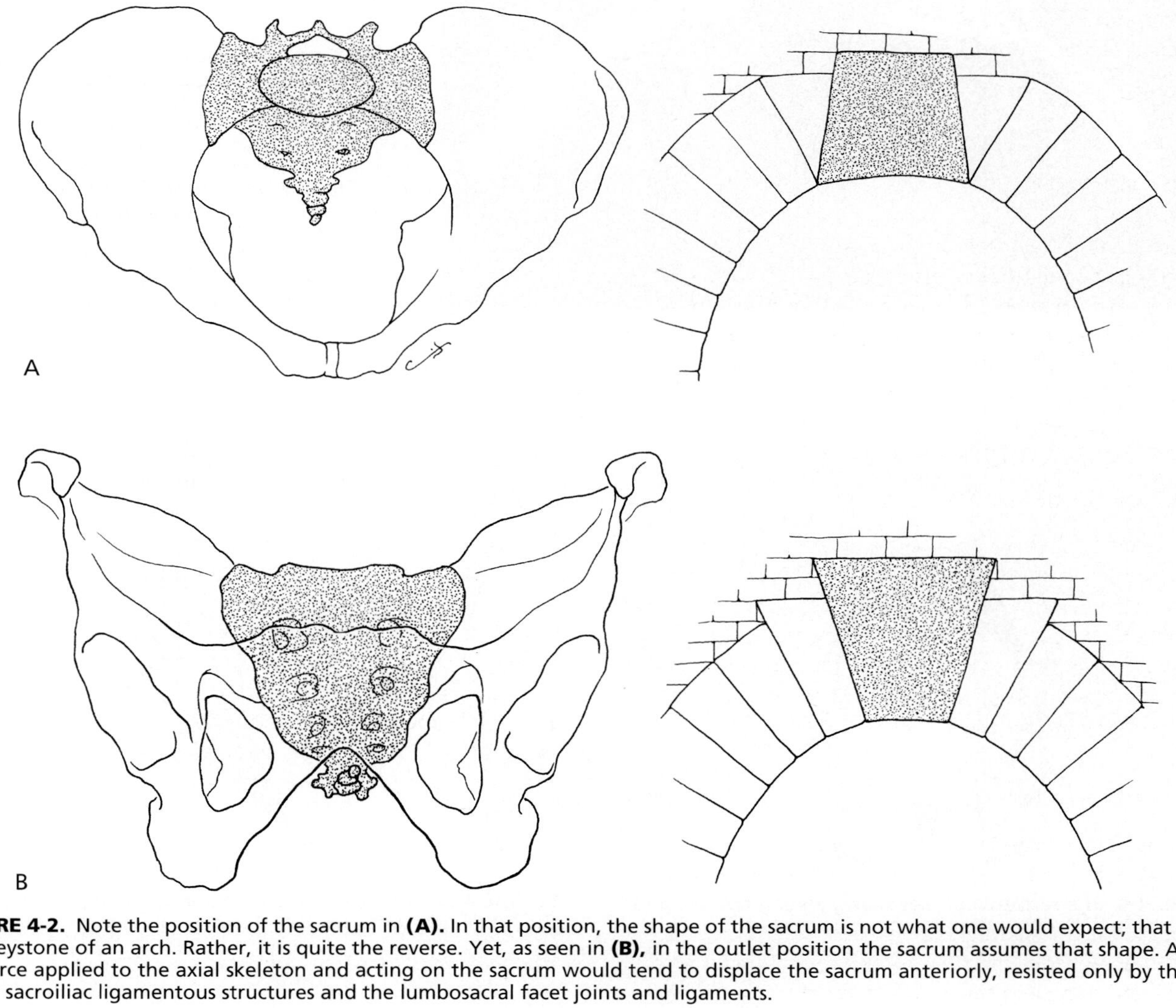

FIGURE 4-2. Note the position of the sacrum in **(A).** In that position, the shape of the sacrum is not what one would expect; that is, like the keystone of an arch. Rather, it is quite the reverse. Yet, as seen in **(B),** in the outlet position the sacrum assumes that shape. A vertical force applied to the axial skeleton and acting on the sacrum would tend to displace the sacrum anteriorly, resisted only by the posterior sacroiliac ligamentous structures and the lumbosacral facet joints and ligaments.

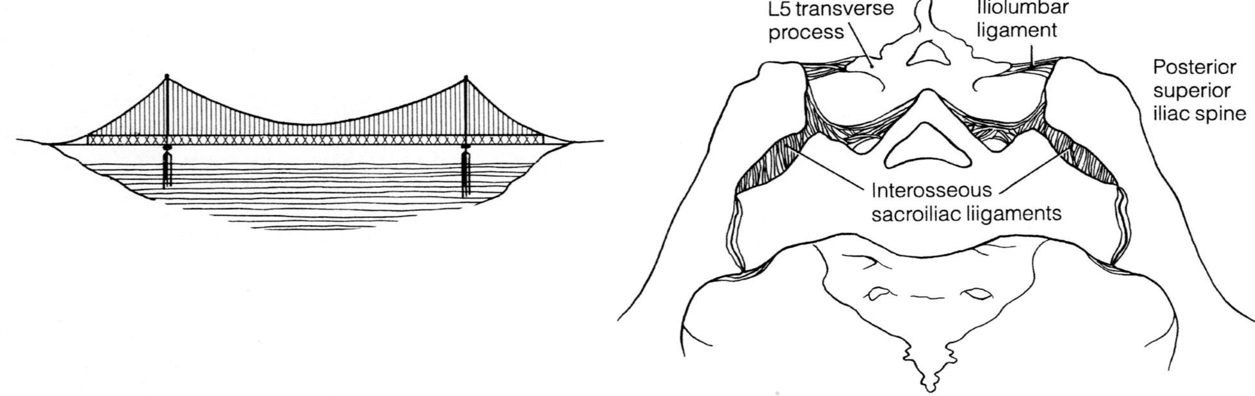

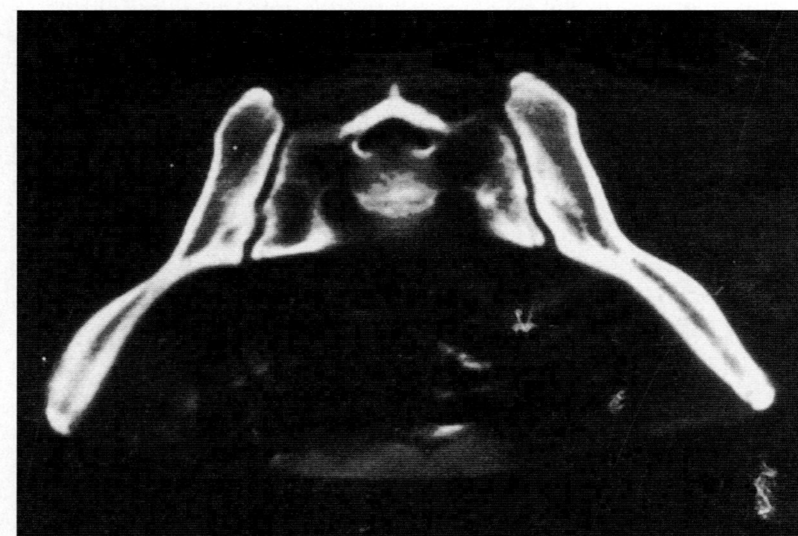

FIGURE 4-3. A: Drawing depicting the suspension bridge-like appearance of the ligaments binding the posterior sacroiliac complex. Note the vertical direction of the interosseous, posterior sacroiliac ligaments, noted by Grant to be the strongest in the body. Note also the transverse component acting as the suspension, joining the pillars, represented by the posterior superior iliac spines, to the sacrum. **B:** Computed tomographic scan demonstrating the appearance of the sacroiliac arch.

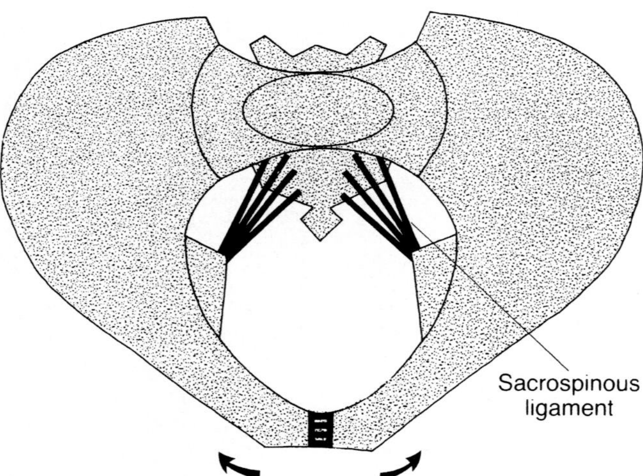

FIGURE 4-4. The sacrospinous ligaments, joining the sacrum to the ischial spines, resist external rotatory forces.

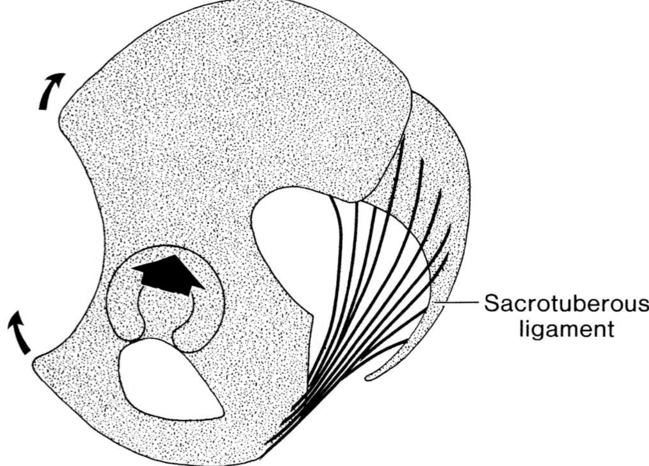

FIGURE 4-5. The sacrotuberous ligament, joining the sacrum to the ischial tuberosity, resists a shearing rotatory force *(arrows).*

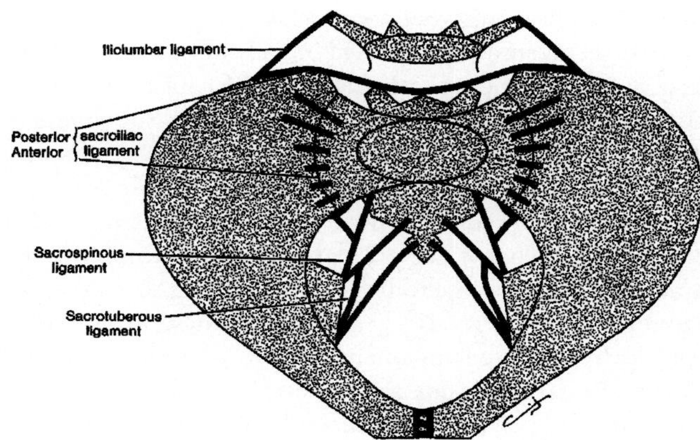

FIGURE 4-6. Diagrammatic representation of the major ligaments of the pelvis: the strong symphysis pubis anteriorly and the posterior tension band of the pelvis, including the iliolumbar, posterior sacroiliac, sacrospinous, and sacrotuberous ligaments.

ments such as the sacrotuberous and sacrospinous as well as the muscles and investing fascia of the pelvic floor also contribute to the overall stability. Disruptions in the pelvic ring, whether through the ligaments or bone, result in instability. The degree of instability is determined by the magnitude of displacements that can occur in the ring.

For convenience we often describe instability in discrete terms; that is, the pelvis is stable, partially unstable, or completely unstable. These categories form the basis for classifying injuries. In actuality, instability occurs along a continuum from completely stable to completely unstable. The elderly woman with a low-energy fall and a minimally displaced ramus fracture has a completely stable pelvis. That is, only very small displacements can occur within the pelvic ring even with full weight bearing. On the other hand, a young man who has fallen 50 feet and has disrupted the pubic symphysis and sacroiliac joints has a completely unstable pelvis. Large displacements can occur in the pelvic ring even with no weight bearing.

Analyzing pelvic stability is a critical step in managing a patient with a pelvic injury. The degree of pelvic instability correlates nicely with the energy of the insult. This is important not so much for the injury to the pelvis per se, but rather for what it means for the patient in general. A completely unstable pelvis suggests a very high-energy insult. The effects of this insult are not restricted to the bony pelvis. The pelvic blood vessels and organs would suffer the same insult as would the patient in general. Patients with unstable pelvic fractures are more likely to suffer severe pelvic blood loss as well as injury to other organ systems. Patients with unstable pelvic fractures are much more likely to die than patients with stable pelvic fractures. Moreover, an unstable pelvis should warn the clinician that the patient has suffered a very high-energy insult (1).

The degree of pelvic instability also guides the definitive treatment of the pelvic injury. The primary goal in the definitive management of pelvic injuries is to prevent deformity. The pelvis that is stable or partially stable may need only restricted weight bearing to prevent deformity. Similarly, a pelvis that has been disrupted anteriorly but not posteriorly may need only anterior surgical stabilization. The completely disrupted pelvis may need both anterior and posterior fixation.

Physiologic Instability: Pregnancy

It has long been assumed that the hormones of pregnancy allow the pelvic ligaments to relax during childbirth. However, recent evidence suggests that this effect is minor, and that there is normally very little diastasis of the symphysis during labor and delivery (Fig. 4-7). Bjorklund and colleagues measured symphyseal diastases sonographically during delivery in 24 patients. The average width of the symphysis at the onset of labor was 5.8 mm. The average distention during delivery was only 1.1 mm (2). In addition, further studies demonstrated that postpartum pelvic pain did not correlate to symphyseal distention for these normally small displacements (3).

Occasionally true pelvic disruptions occur during delivery and can be very disabling. During labor wedging of the child in the birth canal can result in rupture of the symphysial ligaments. The rupture is often accompanied by an audible crack, and postoperative x-rays demonstrate severe diastases of the symphysis greater than 4 cm. The exact incidence of this problem is not known, but it is reported to occur in from one in 600 to one in 30,000 births. In the early postpartum period patients can have extreme discomfort. Although reported series are very small, it appears that the pain and pubic diastases resolve spontaneously over several months. Pelvic binders may provide some relief (4).

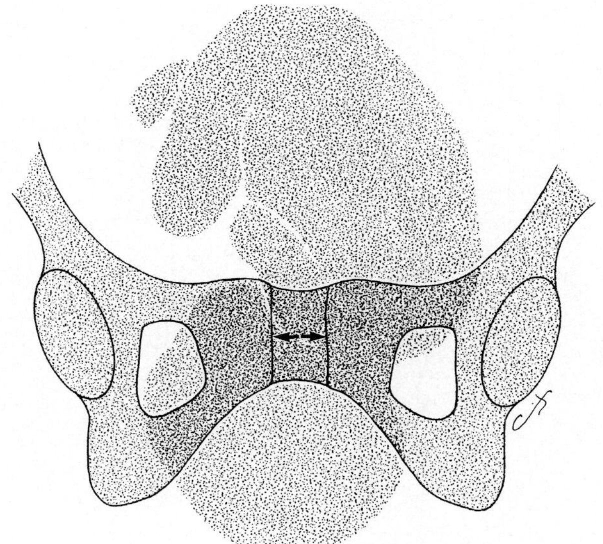

FIGURE 4-7. During normal delivery the symphysis pubis opens slightly (see text), but the posterior sacroiliac ligaments remain intact.

There have been reports of operative treatment, but there are not enough data available to determine whether surgery is more effective than nonoperative treatment.

Iatrogenic Instability: Posterior Bone Graft

In rare instances, when bone grafts are taken electively from the posterior superior iliac spine and the posterior interosseous ligaments are destroyed, marked pelvic instability may ensue (5). One might speculate that the continuing pain experienced by some patients in the donor bone graft site might result from minor degrees of pelvic ring instability.

Division of Specific Ligaments

As we have seen, a stable pelvis requires intact ligamentous structures. This point can be emphasized by cutting the ligaments and observing what happens. Although these days this exercise seems simplistic, this was not always the case. Pennal first preformed these experiments in 1961 for an American Academy of Orthopaedic Surgeons video (6). Our modern concepts of pelvic stability grew from these basic experiments.

Pennal found that cutting the pubic symphyseal ligaments alone allowed the pelvis to open only 2.5 cm. Further opening of the pelvis was prevented by the sacrospinous ligaments and anterior sacroiliac ligaments. Translations at the sacroiliac joint were also prevented by these ligaments as well as by the other ligaments of the posterior complex. When the sacrospinous and anterior sacroiliac ligaments were cut, the pelvis opened like a book until the posterior superior spines abutted the pelvis. However, because the remainder of the posterior complex remained intact, no vertical translations were possible. When the remainder of the posterior ligaments were transected, the entire hemipelvis became unstable (Fig. 4-8).

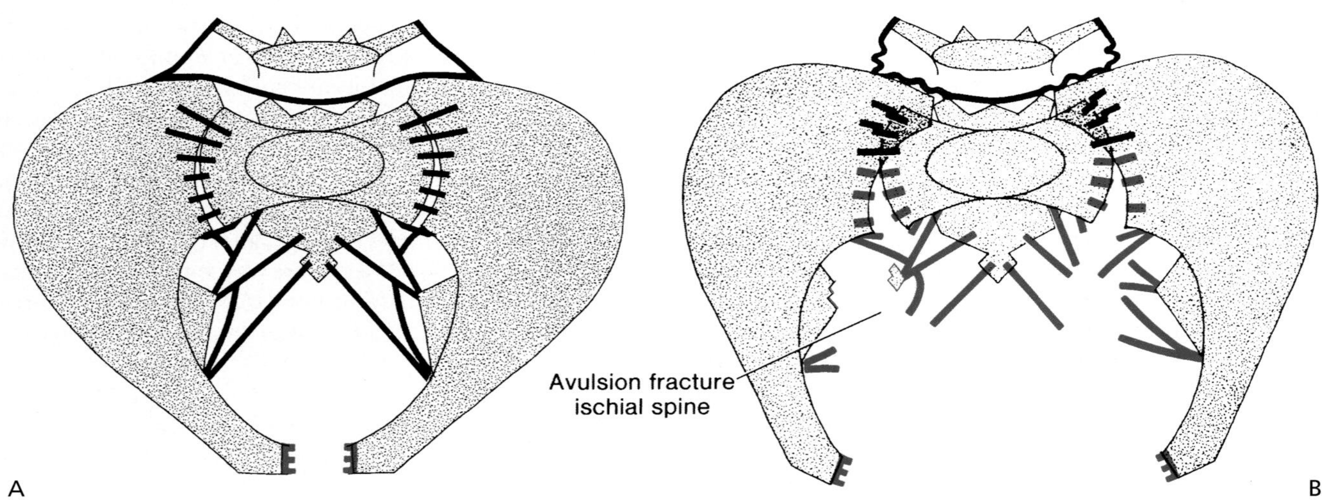

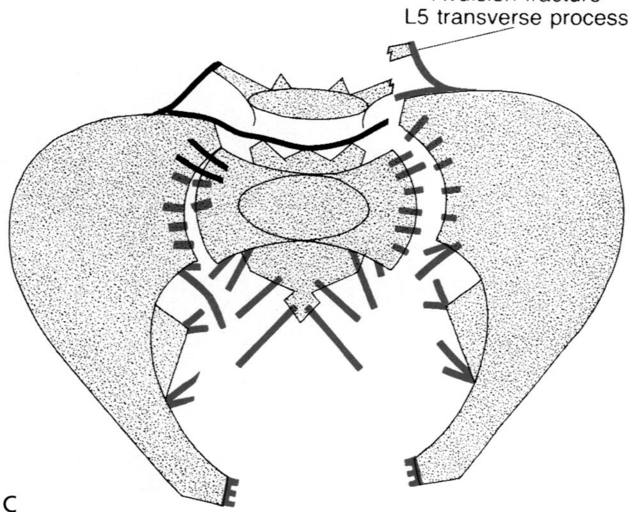

FIGURE 4-8. A: Division of the symphysis pubis allows the pelvis to open approximately 2.5 cm with no damage to any posterior ligamentous structures. **B:** Division of the anterior sacroiliac and sacrospinous ligaments, either by direct division of their fibers (noted on the left side) or by avulsion of the tip of the ischial spine (right side) allows the pelvis to rotate externally until the posterior superior iliac spines abut on the sacrum. Note, however, that the posterior ligamentous structures (i.e., the posterior sacroiliac and iliolumbar ligaments) remain intact. Therefore, no displacement in the vertical plane is possible. **C:** Division of the posterior tension band ligaments (i.e., the posterior sacroiliac) as well as the iliolumbar (left side), together with an avulsion of the transverse process of L5, causes complete instability of the hemipelvis. Note that posterior displacement is now possible. Also required for complete instability that allows vertical displacement is disruption of the sacrospinous and sacrotuberous ligaments of the pelvic floor.

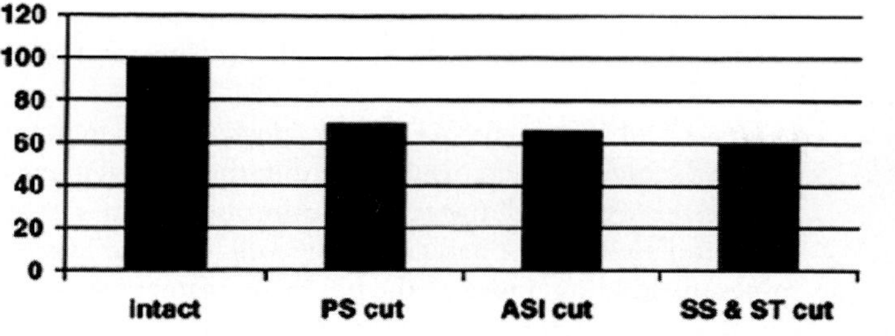

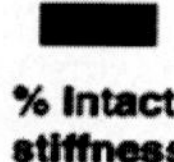

FIGURE 4-9. Stability of the pelvic ring. Effects of sectioning of ligaments.

More recent work from Tile's laboratory suggests that the actual contribution of various ligaments to pelvic stability is much more complex and is dependent on how the pelvis is loaded as well the order in which the ligaments are cut (7). In single leg stance the anterior pelvis is in compression, and the posterior pelvis is in tension. Thus, cutting the pubic symphysis causes little displacement in the pelvic ring. Conversely, if the posterior ligaments are cut, large displacements are possible at the sacroiliac joint. On the other hand, in double leg stance the anterior pelvis is in tension and the posterior pelvis is in compression. If the posterior ligaments are cut in this mode, little displacement occurs, but if the anterior ligaments are cut, the pelvis opens dramatically. These simple examples consider only the contributions of the pubic symphyseal and posterior ligaments. The complexity increases as all other ligaments and soft tissues investing the pelvis are considered. Moreover, all the ligaments interact to provide stability over a full range of physiologic activity.

In general, these experiments have shown that the posterior pelvic ligaments are most important in maintaining pelvic stability, the anterior structures (symphysis, rami) play a greater role than previously thought. In double leg stance, 60% of pelvic stability comes from the posterior structures, 40% from the anterior. Knowledge of this fact is important in methods of pelvic fixation, and also in the aftercare of patients whose pelvic fractures have been surgically stabilized. In unstable fracture types (C), fixation only, of the posterior structures, may lead to redisplacement of the hemipelvis, because 40% of pelvic instability remains resulting in compromised outcomes (8). Therefore, these patients require adequate stable fixation both front and back to allow mobilization safely (Fig. 4-9) (see Chapter 15).

Division of a Ring Structure

Because the pelvis behaves as a stable ring-like structure, it is theoretically not possible to break the pelvis in just one spot. A true ring cannot be broken in just one place. In fact, clinical literature supports this theoretical prediction. Gertzbein and Chenoweth preformed technetium bone scans on a series of patients with minimally displaced pelvic fractures (9). In each case uptake was noted in the sacroiliac region. Today, it is almost always possible to identify a posterior lesion using a computed tomographic (CT) scan. In very stable pelvic fractures there may only be a small buckle in the anterior cortical line of the sacrum. In a few cases, it is not possible to identify a posterior injury. In most of these cases a more sensitive study would identify the injury. In a few rare cases, the injury may be truly isolated to the anterior pelvis. However, it is always best to assume that there is a posterior lesion. For young people, this fact mandates that a CT scan be obtained to define the posterior injury. For older people with low-energy fractures, it is reasonable to assume that the posterior injury is stable and no further studies are necessary. However, one should not be surprised when an older patient with a "ramus fracture" complains of low back pain.

INJURIOUS FORCE PATTERNS

Typical fracture patterns develop depending on the direction of the force causing the injury. Pennal first made this observation, and defined the primary force directions and the resulting fracture patterns. He noted that in general forces tend to open the pelvis like a book, collapse it toward the midline, or cause vertical translations. He labeled the forces that cause these deformations anteroposterior compression, lateral compression, and vertical shear. These terms are still used today, and still accurately predict general fracture patterns. Given this, we often analyze the fracture pattern to get some idea of the mechanism of injury. However, it is important to remember that the actual forces that disrupted the pelvis are often complex. A person thrown from a car is likely to have forces striking the pelvis from multiple directions, and it is not unusual for a patient run over by a car to have one side of the pelvis crushed toward the midline and the other opened like a book. Moreover, although the fracture patterns give clues as to the direction of the insulting force, they do not always completely elucidate the mechanism of injury.

It is useful to review the consequences of various traumatic insults by describing what happens to the major supporting structures of the pelvis; therefore, several points should be considered. We discuss how various forces affect the major supporting ligaments in the following. However, it is not uncommon for a ligament to remain intact while the bone next to the ligament is disrupted. The effect is the same as if the ligament had been disrupted. Although certain mechanisms are more likely to result in greater degrees of instability, any mechanism can create any degree of instability. Lateral compression injuries are frequently stable; however, a very large lateral compression force can cause as much instability as a vertical shear injury.

Anteroposterior Compression/External Rotation

This term is generally used to describe forces that open the pelvis like a book. They are sometimes called *external rotatory forces,* and may be applied to the pelvis by several mechanisms.

Posterior Crush

A direct blow to the posterior superior iliac spines can externally rotate one or both ilia, causing disruption of the pelvis at the symphysis. A severe force will also disrupt one or both anterior sacroiliac ligaments (Fig. 4-10A).

Direct Pressure to the Anterior Superior Iliac Spine

An anterior posterior force located at the anterior superior iliac spine can also externally rotate the ilia causing disruption of the pubic symphysis. With further force the anterior sacroiliac ligaments and the posterior sacroiliac ligaments will rupture sequentially.

External Rotation through the Femur

A violent external rotatory force through the femur acting as a lever will disrupt the symphysis anteriorly (or fracture the rami) and with continuing force, the sacrospinous and anterior sacroiliac ligaments. The force may be unilateral or bilateral (Fig. 4-10B).

In each of these instances, if the posterior ligamentous complex remains intact, displacement in the vertical plane is not possible. Although the pelvis may be opened like a book, either unilaterally or bilaterally, only when the force overcomes the holding power of the posterior ligamentous complex does the pelvis become vertically unstable.

Lateral Compression

Lateral compressive forces generally collapse the pelvis toward the midline. The force may be applied directly to the iliac crest, or to the greater trochanter, and may also cause an associated acetabular fracture (Fig. 4-11). The major lateral thrust of this force is to the posterior sacroiliac complex. At that point, the bony trabeculae run largely parallel to the force vector; therefore, the net effect is compression of the posterior sacroiliac complex.

If bone is subjected to pure compression, with no shearing element, the surrounding posterior soft tissues remain intact (Fig. 4-12). As a result, the pelvic ring subjected to lateral compression usually remains stable. In lateral compression injury the anterior lesion may be on the same or the opposite side of the posterior lesion. Also, all four pubic rami may be fractured (straddle fracture) or the symphysis pubis disrupted. Combinations of symphysis disruption with rami fractures are also found (Fig. 4-13).

Although the anterior lesion may show internal rotation, the posterior lesion reveals impaction of cancellous bone, possibly with slight displacement but often with an intact posterior ligamentous complex. In some instances, the anterior sacrum may be crushed and the posterior ligamentous

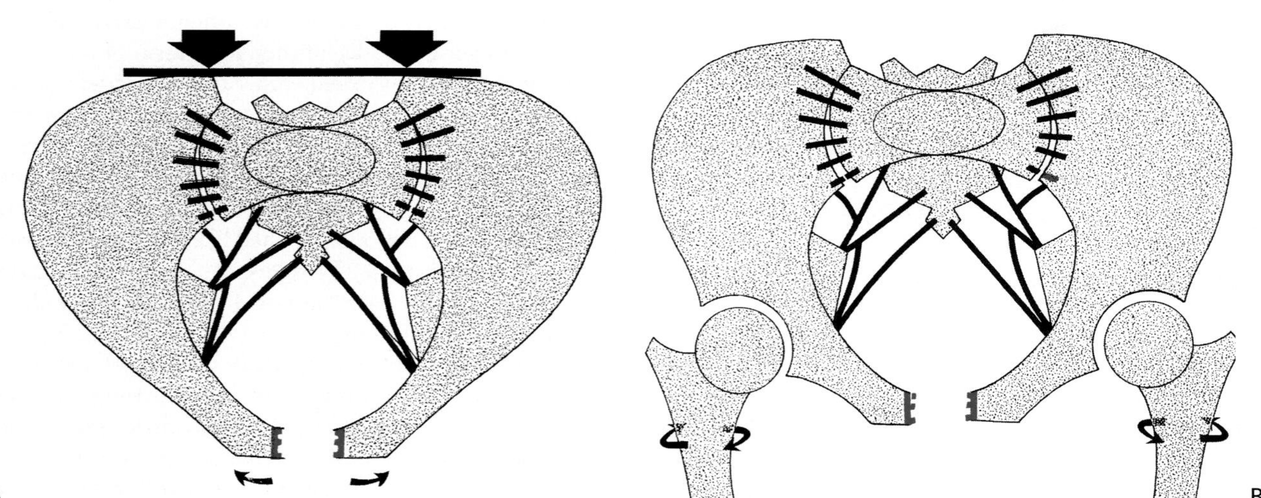

FIGURE 4-10. A: A direct blow to the posterior superior iliac spines causes the symphysis pubis to spring open. **B:** External rotation of the femora or direct compression against the anterior superior spines also causes disruption of the symphysis pubis, or equivalent fractures of the pubic rami.

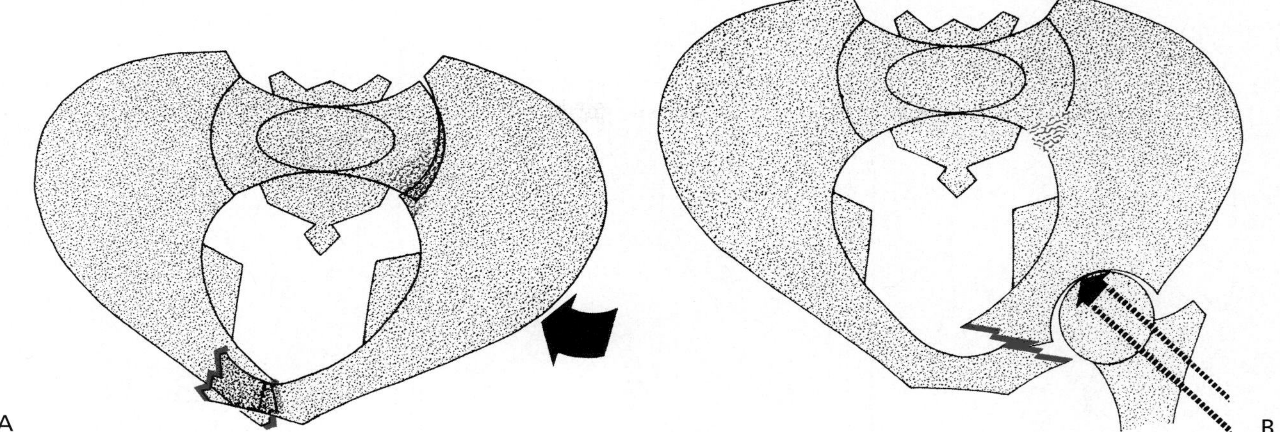

FIGURE 4-11. A: A lateral compressive force directed against the iliac crest causes the hemipelvis to rotate internally, crushing the anterior sacrum and displacing the anterior pubic rami. B: Lateral compression injury also may be caused by a force against the greater trochanter. In that situation the femoral head acts as a battering ram, dividing the pubic rami as shown, often through the anterior column of the acetabulum. The ipsilateral sacroiliac complex is also crushed in this injury.

structures, including the interosseous ligaments and sacroiliac ligaments, may be ruptured. On occasion, with this mechanism, an avulsion fracture of the transverse process of L5 is seen. A pure lateral compressive force applied to the pelvis does not usually result in vertical or translational instability. However, displacements in the sagittal plane can be substantial. More important, it is rare that the lateral force is so exactly applied as to cause pure horizontal collapse toward the midline. It is not uncommon for the pelvis to collapse in an inward and upward direction. As such, it is possible to have substantial leg length discrepancies even though the pelvis is relatively stable.

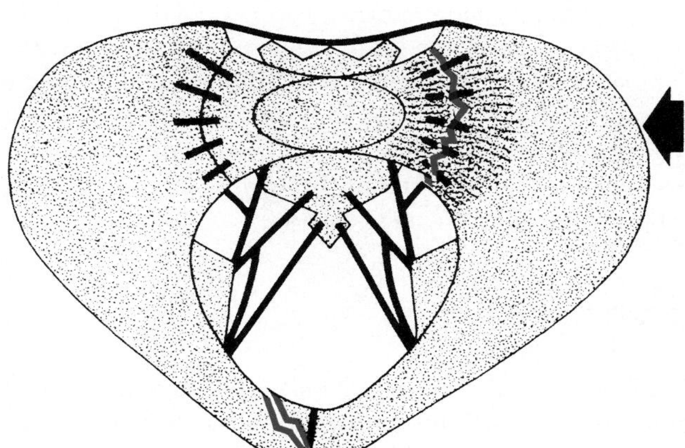

FIGURE 4-12. Lateral compressive forces are directed parallel to the bony trabeculae of the sacroiliac joint, therefore causing impaction of bone. If the force is purely lateral compression, the pelvic floor—including its major ligaments, the sacrospinous and sacrotuberous—remains intact, thus retaining pelvic ring vertical stability. The stability is maintained by the pelvic floor even if the posterior ligamentous structures rupture. In most cases of lateral compressive force the posterior structures remain intact.

As in all musculoskeletal trauma, a word of caution is in order. In younger persons who have strong cancellous bone, the strong anterior portion of the ala of the sacrum extending into the pelvic brim may resist fracturing; therefore, the continuing internal rotation force would cause a major posterior ligamentous injury (Fig. 4-14). This same phenomenon occurs in other areas, such as the tibial plateau, where it is perhaps much easier to understand. In that instance, a blow from the lateral side may, in a patient with osteoporotic bone, cause compression of the lateral tibial plateau. If the force continues, the medial collateral ligament may disrupt; however, in a young person with strong bone, a minor crack on the lateral side or even no fracture at all caused by a similar force, may result in complete disruption of the medial collateral and anterior cruciate ligaments. The same reasoning may be applied to the pelvis. Therefore, although the forces involved are lateral compression, the consequences of the force may be different depending on the relative strength of the bone and soft-tissue envelope.

Vertical Shear

A shearing force is one that crosses perpendicular to the main trabecular pattern of the posterior pelvic complex in the vertical or posterior plane (Fig. 4-15). Whereas a lateral compressive force causes impaction of the cancellous bone and retention of the ligaments, shearing forces cause marked displacement of the bone and gross disruption of the soft-tissue structures. Continuation of these forces beyond the yield strength of the soft tissues produces an unstable pelvic ring. Displacement occurs both anteriorly and posteriorly and has no finite point.

In the extreme, the entire hemipelvis may be avulsed from the body, resulting in traumatic hemipelvectomy

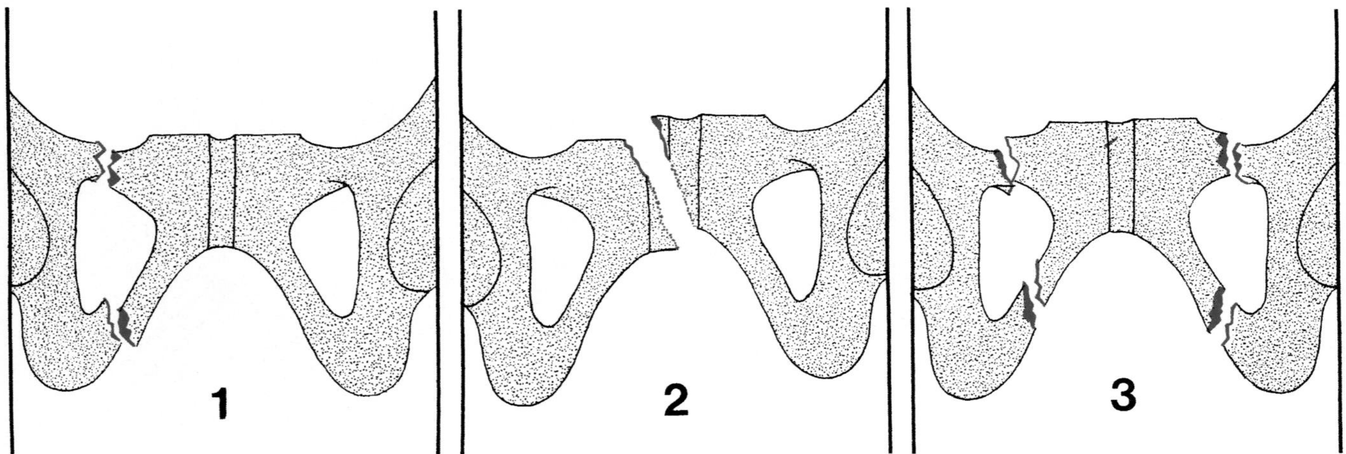

FIGURE 4-13. The anterior lesion in a lateral compression injury may be through both pubic rami (1), the symphysis pubis (2), or all four pubic rami, the so-called straddle fracture (3).

(Fig. 4-16). Sixteen patients have been reported in the literature, and we have seen two cases in our trauma unit (10–21). In virtually all of these cases the traumatic hemipelvectomy occurred as a result of a severe external rotation shearing force on the lower extremity. This is especially likely when a motorcyclist is hit on the lower extremity by an oncoming car. On impact, the pubic symphysis ruptures. Eventually the pelvic floor muscles and ligaments, including the iliopsoas, tear, as do all of the ligamentous structures posteriorly, which attach the ilium to the sacrum.

In trauma, these forces of anteroposterior compression, lateral compression, and vertical shear are rarely pure. Therefore, combinations of these forces may result in bizarre injuries.

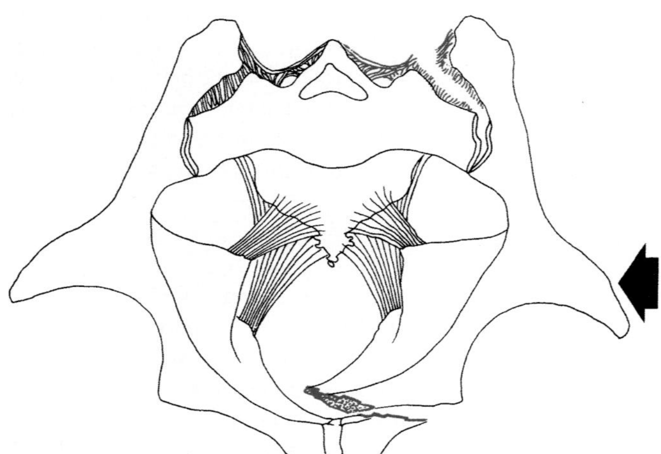

FIGURE 4-14. In some instances, a lateral compressive force may rupture the posterior ligamentous structures, especially in younger patients. In these patients the bone sacroiliac complex is extremely strong. Therefore, the internal rotation force will tend to rupture the sacroiliac ligaments posteriorly rather than fracture the strong bone. However, in such instances pelvic stability is maintained by the intact pelvic floor ligaments.

Effect of Force Patterns on Soft Tissue and Viscera

The various forces that act on the bony pelvis have a major effect on the contents of the pelvis, namely the soft tissues, arteries, nerves, and viscera. The effect on the ligaments, muscles, and fascia already has been described. It is apparent that forces of external rotation or shear will tend to tear the soft tissues of the pelvis. The viscera, blood vessels, and nerves are subjected to traction forces that tend to disrupt the vessels, cause traction injuries or avulsion of nerves, and tear the viscera (1).

Lateral compression injuries cause visceral damage by direct bony penetration. The anterior rotation of the hemipelvis in a lateral compression injury may drive the bony spike of the pubic rami into the bladder or rupture it by increasing intravascular pressure. Posteriorly, the compression injury of the sacrum through the foramina may compress any of the sacral nerve roots.

CONCLUSION

Of considerable clinical importance is the determination of the degree of instability imparted by these forces on the pelvic ring. Although this is discussed in detail in Chapter 11, some mention is in order at this time. The assessment of stability in a pelvic ring disruption depends on clinical and radiographic features. On clinical examination the stable, undisplaced, or minimally displaced pelvic ring cannot be moved abnormally, whereas the grossly unstable vertical shear fracture can. In those circumstances the unstable

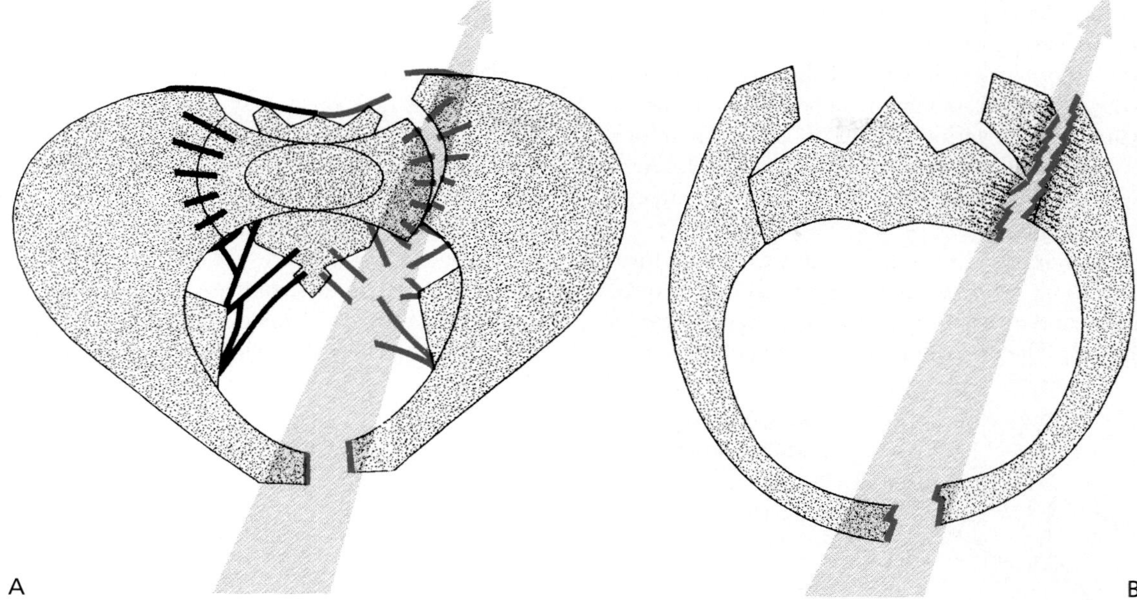

FIGURE 4-15. A shearing force *(arrows)* crosses perpendicular to the main trabecular pattern of the posterior pelvic complex in the vertical plane. These forces cause marked displacement of bone and gross disruption of the soft tissues, resulting in major pelvic instability.

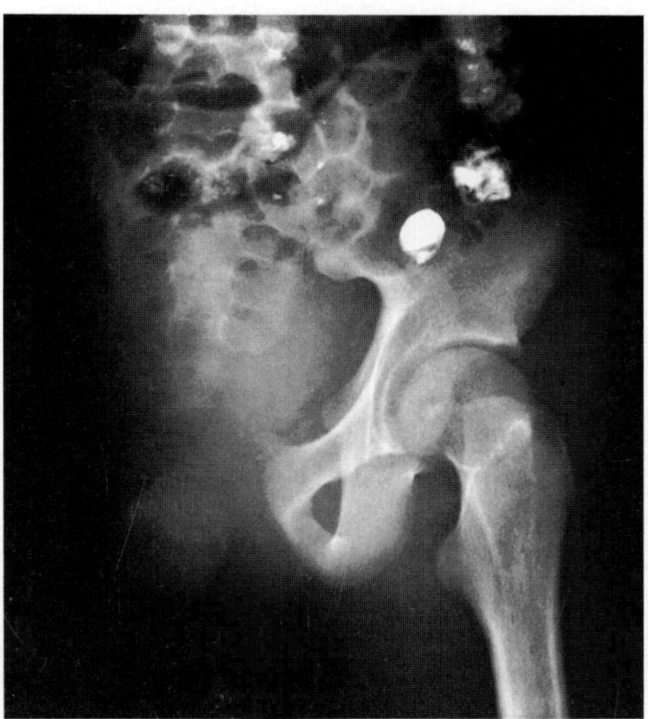

FIGURE 4-16. Pelvic radiograph of a 19-year-old man struck by a motor vehicle. His entire hemipelvis was avulsed from the body, resulting in a traumatic hindquarter amputation, the ultimate vertical shear injury.

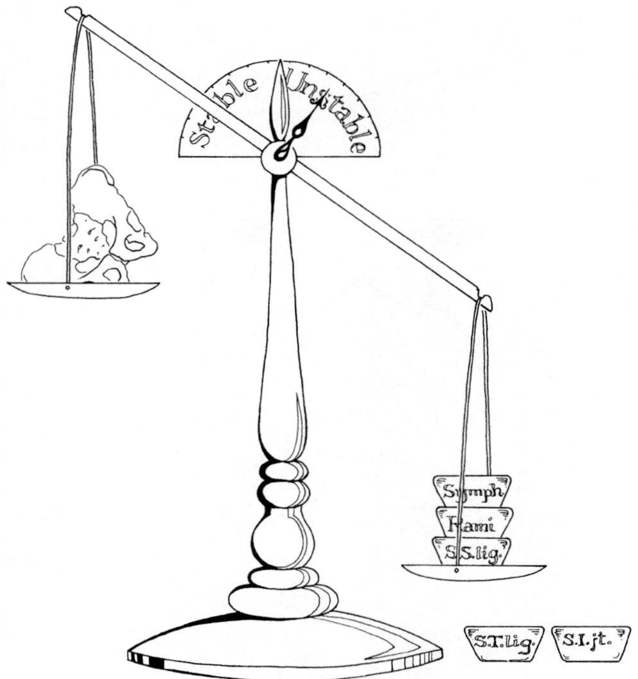

FIGURE 4-17. The "stability scale" outlining the concept of stability in pelvic injury. As each of the structures outlined on the right is injured, the scale tips more toward its unstable aspect. Each pelvic ring disruption is different and must be carefully assessed, both clinically and radiographically to determine where that particular injury lies on the stability scale.

hemipelvis can be moved into almost any position, because all of the soft tissues are disrupted.

Obviously, many cases fall between these two extremes. Therefore, the concept of stability must be considered not as black or white, but as various shades of gray. Therefore, the various types of pelvic ring disruption fall at different places on a stability scale, depending on their precise pathoanatomy (Fig. 4-17).

Although the various types of pelvic ring disruption form a continuum, three major types of pelvic stability may be noted. They form the basis of the proposed classification in Chapter 12 (22). Therefore, fractures of the pelvis may be stable, partially stable (rotationally unstable, vertically stable), or completely (vertically) unstable.

Stable fracture patterns do not disrupt the ligamentous structures of the pelvic ring. These include avulsion fractures, iliac wing fractures, undisplaced cracks through the pelvic ring, and transverse fractures of the sacrum and coccyx distal to the pelvic ring.

The partially or rotationally unstable pelvic fracture, by definition, cannot displace vertically, because either the posterior ligamentous structures are intact or the ligaments and muscles of the pelvic floor are intact.

In the common external rotation open-book variety,

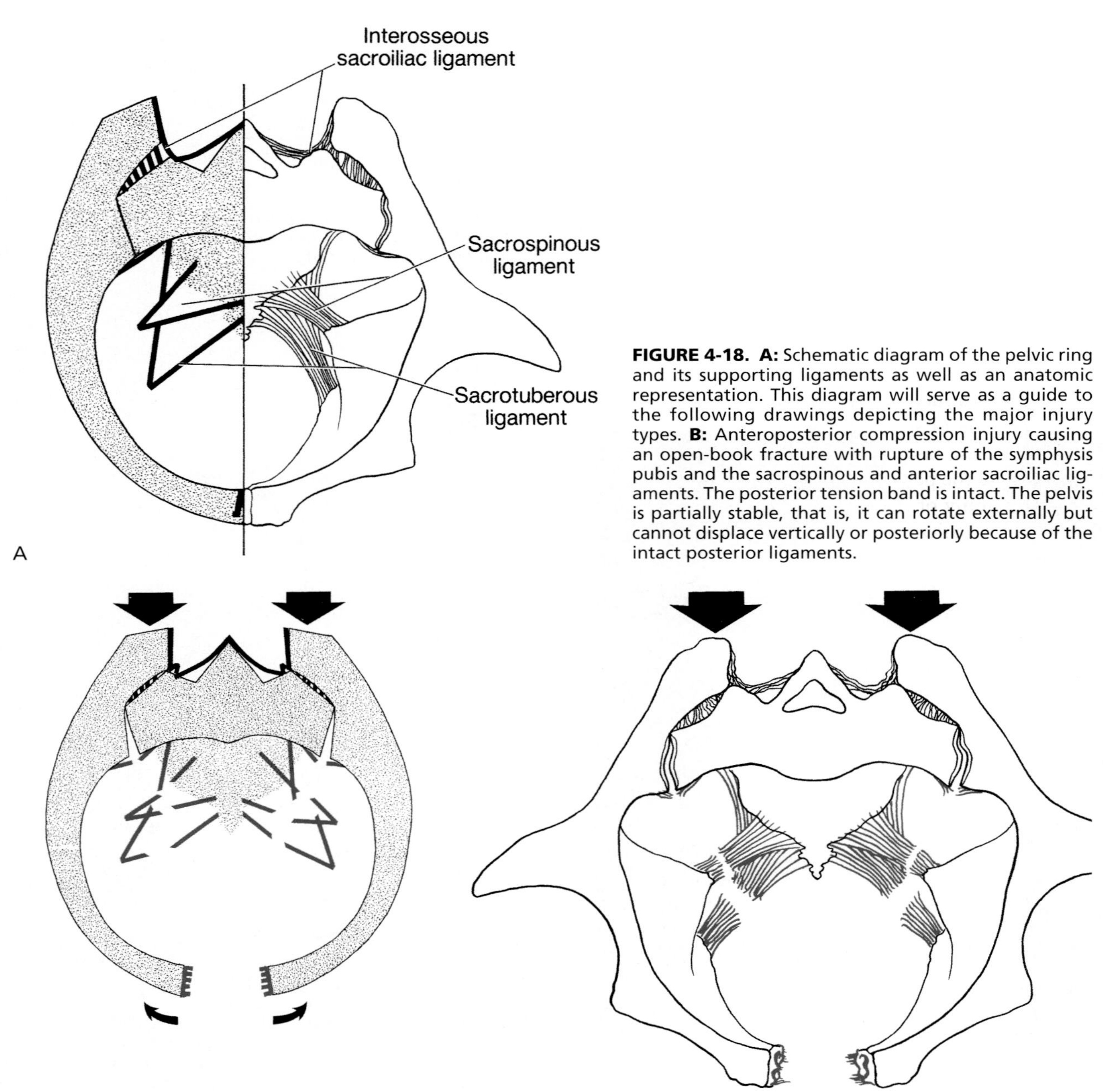

FIGURE 4-18. A: Schematic diagram of the pelvic ring and its supporting ligaments as well as an anatomic representation. This diagram will serve as a guide to the following drawings depicting the major injury types. **B:** Anteroposterior compression injury causing an open-book fracture with rupture of the symphysis pubis and the sacrospinous and anterior sacroiliac ligaments. The posterior tension band is intact. The pelvis is partially stable, that is, it can rotate externally but cannot displace vertically or posteriorly because of the intact posterior ligaments.

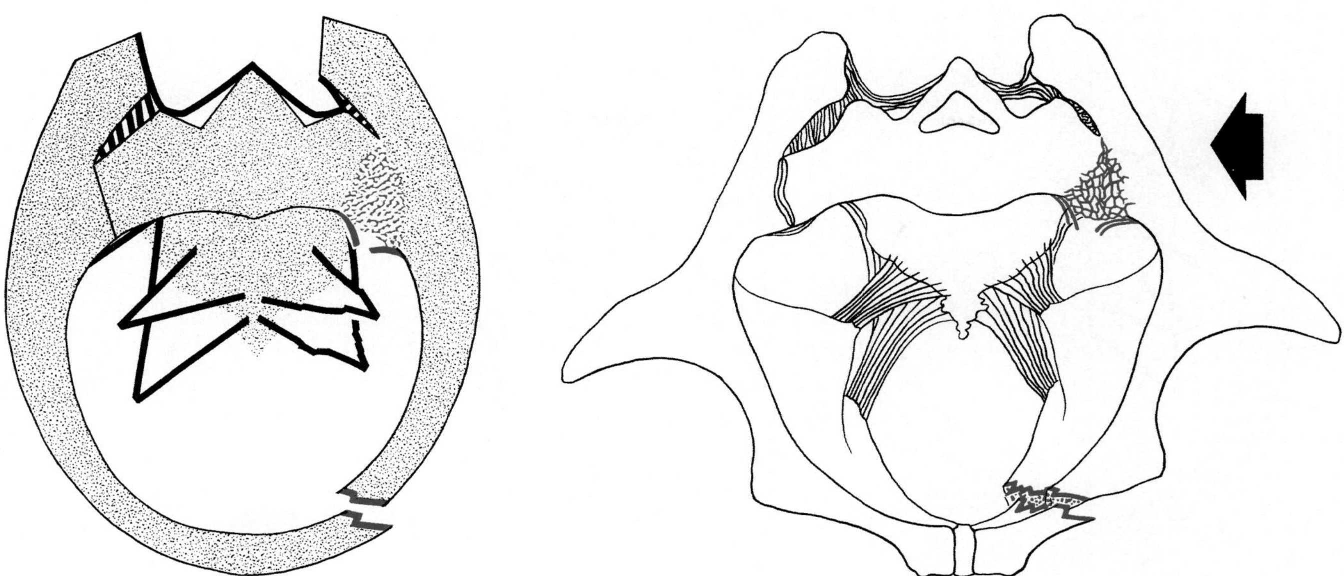

FIGURE 4-19. A lateral compression injury depicting a posterior sacral crush but no disruption of the posterior sacroiliac ligamentous complex or the pelvic ligaments; therefore, relative stability is maintained.

with disruption of the symphysis pubis, displacement beyond a finite point is not possible, owing to abutment of the posterior superior spine against the sacrum. Because the posterior ligamentous structures are intact, vertical displacement is not possible in spite of a disruption of the pelvic floor in some of these cases. Reduction by internal rotation restores stability to the pelvic ring (Fig. 4-18).

The pathoanatomy of the lateral compression may vary considerably from patient to patient. Lateral compression forces may impact the sacrum so completely that no motion at all is possible in the hemipelvis (Fig. 4-19). In other cases, the anterior hemipelvis rotates through the fractured rami, either ipsilaterally or contralaterally, causing internal rotational instability. Anterior impaction of the sacrum may occur in association with posterior disruption of the ligaments.

In the unstable shearing injury posterior displacement of more than 1 cm indicates complete disruption of the ligamentous structures (Fig. 4-20). However, if the posterior injury is relatively undisplaced, and if on clinical examination the pelvis feels stable, major instability is unlikely.

Complete vertical instability occurs when both the pelvic floor ligaments and the posterior ligamentous structures are disrupted. This may be noted clinically during physical examination and radiographically by posterior and cephalad vertical displacement of more than 1 cm.

The best method of radiographic examination of the posterior pelvic complex is CT. A comparison of the CT scans in Fig. 4-21 demonstrates this concept of stability better than the written word.

McCoy and colleagues examined the biomechanical aspects of pelvic and hip injuries in road traffic accidents (23). In this chapter, 40 cases of pelvic injury sustained in road traffic accidents, where the direction of impact on the velocity differential was known, were examined. In the total study, 2,520 vehicle occupants were included and of these, 49 sustained a fracture of the pelvis or a dislocation of the hip. However, in only 40 cases could the velocity differential (DV) be ascertained. In these cases the radiographs were available, which allowed the type of fracture to be compared to the direction of and energy involved in the impact, expressed as DV. Associated injuries and the overall severity of the injury were scored according to the abbreviated injury scale (AIS) and the ISS. In frontal motor vehicle impacts, indirect shear injuries of the pelvis were prominent, as were posterior dislocations of the hip. In side impacts, lateral compression-type injuries occurred. With increasing velocity differentials, more severe pelvic injuries occurred often in association with significant head, chest, and lower limb injuries. Side impacts were noted to produce more severe injuries at lower velocity differentials when compared with frontal crashes because there is less protection in modern motor vehicle accidents on the side. The authors conclude from this study that modifications in design are necessary to improve passenger safety and reduce the incidence of lateral compression type pelvic fractures.

This study supports many of the principles enunciated in this chapter about the importance of force patterns in both the bony and soft-tissue injury. Therefore, a quick inspection of the anteroposterior radiographs of the pelvis in the acutely polytraumatized patient may guide the attending surgeon in resuscitation (24).

The reader should turn to further studies by Alonso and

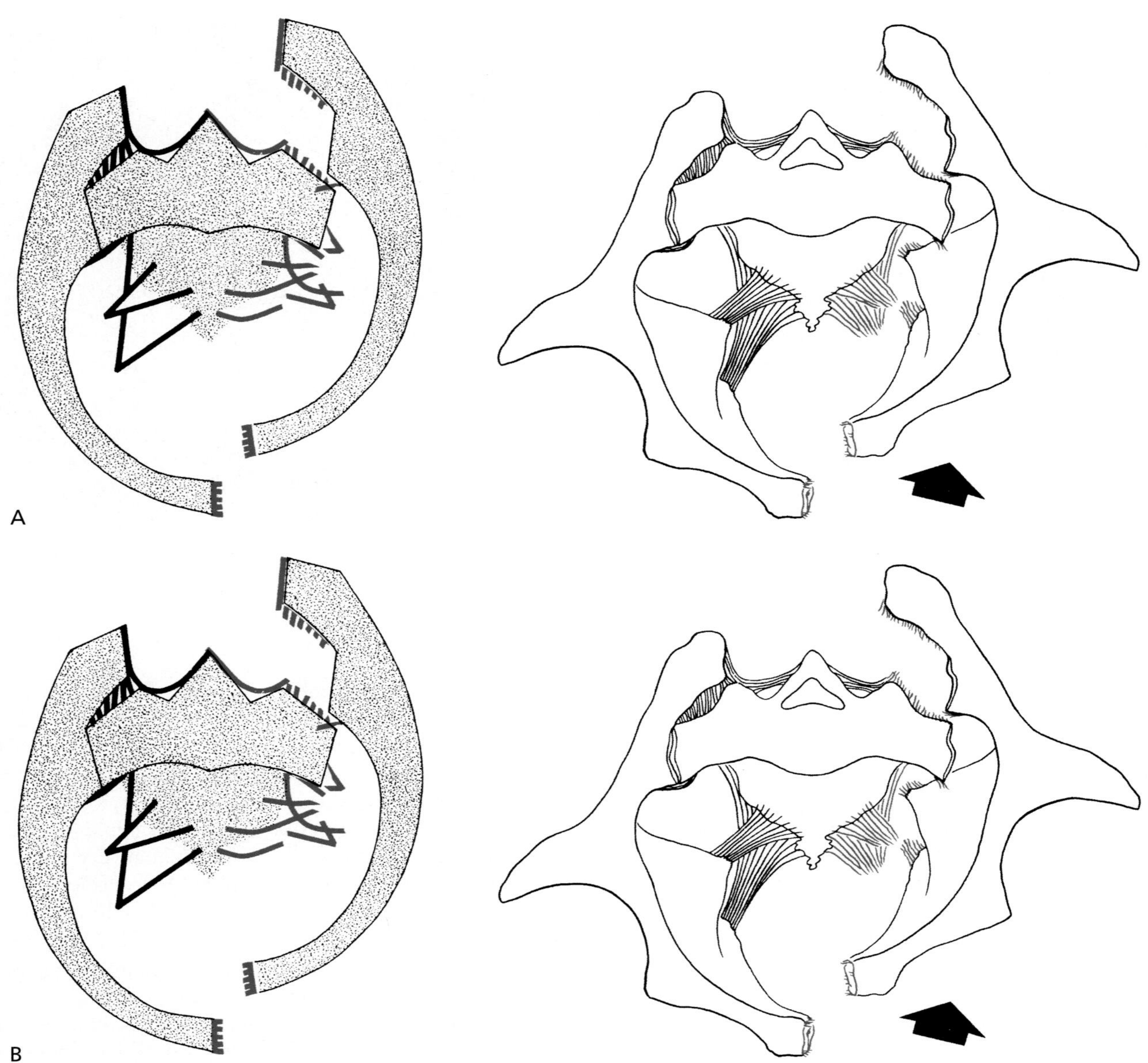

FIGURE 4-20. A: An unstable vertical shear injury causing gross disruption of both the anterior and posterior portions of the pelvis, resulting in a sacroiliac dislocation and major instability of the affected hemipelvis. **B:** A bilateral posterior lesion, the most unstable type of pelvic disruption. In this diagram, a bilateral fracture-dislocation of the sacroiliac joint is depicted.

his coworkers, as noted in Chapter 6, which also supports these concepts.

In conclusion, the stability of the pelvic ring is dependent on the integrity of its ligamentous structures, mainly the posterior ligamentous structures and the muscles, ligaments, and fascia of the pelvic floor. Trauma to the pelvic ring may occur through several force mechanisms, each with its own specific pattern of ligamentous damage. How these forces disrupt the pelvis will determine the degree of instability associated with any specific injury. As well, the force patterns may have different effects on the soft tissues and viscera of the pelvis. For example, external rotation and shearing forces have a tearing effect on the viscera, blood vessels, and nerves, whereas lateral compression injuries injure the viscera, nerves, and vessels by direct penetration of bone or by compression. Therefore, the determination of these force patterns informs the general management of the patient and the specific management of a musculoskeletal injury.

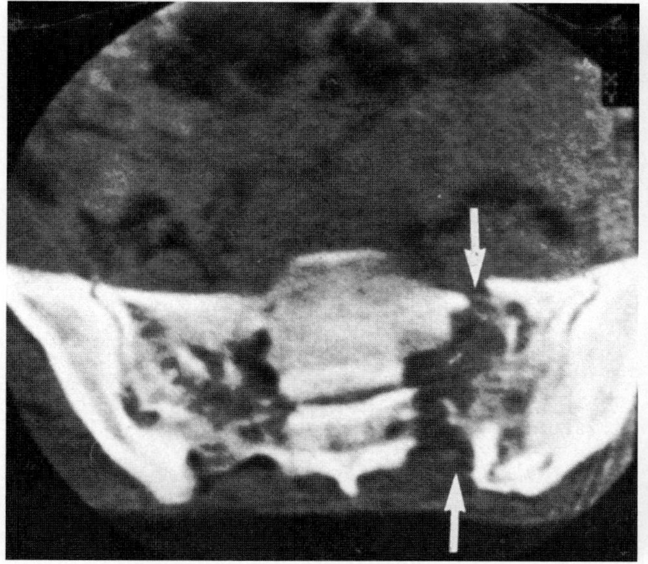

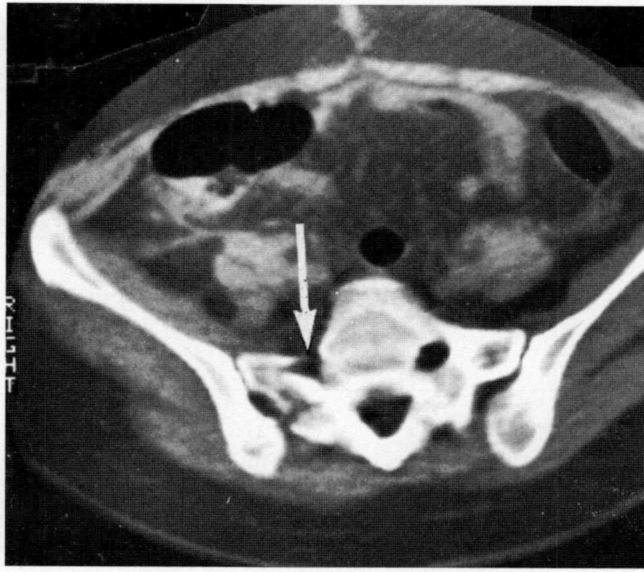

FIGURE 4-21. A: Computed tomography (CT) shows marked disruption and instability of the left sacrum as a result of a shearing force. **B:** CT shows impaction of the right sacrum from a lateral compression injury. This young woman sustained an acetabular fracture as well, confirming the mechanism of injury. Note the marked overriding of the sacral fragments on the fractured side as compared to the normal left side. Impaction was so rigid that no abnormal movement of the hemipelvis was detected on physical examination with image intensification.

REFERENCES

1. Dalal SA, Burgess AR, Siegel JH, et al. Pelvic fracture in multiple trauma: classification by mechanism is key to pattern of organ injury resuscitative requirements, and outcome. *J Trauma* 1989;(7):981–1000; discussion 1000–1002.
2. Bjorklund K, Lindgren PG, Bergstrom S, et al. Sonographic assessment of symphyseal joint distention intra partum. *Acta Obstet Gynecol Scand* 1997;76(3):227–232.
3. Bjorklund K, Nordstrom ML, Bergstrom S. Sonographic assessment of symphyseal joint distention during pregnancy and post partum with special reference to pelvic pain. *Acta Obstet Gynecol Scand* 1999;78(2):125–130.
4. Kharrazi FD, Rodgers WB, Kennedy JG, et al. Parturition-induced pelvic dislocation: a report of four cases. *J Orthop Trauma* 1997;11(4):277–281; discussion 281–282.
5. Coventry MB, Tapper M. Pelvic instability, a consequence of removing iliac bone for grafting. *J Bone Joint Surg* 1972;54A:85.
6. Pennal CF, Sutherland GO. *Fractures of the pelvis* (motion picture). Park Ridge, IL: American Academy of Orthopaedic Surgeons Film Library, 1961.
7. Vrahas M, Hearn TC, Angelo D, et al. *Ligamentous contribution to pelvic ring stiffness* (poster). Orthopaedic Research Society Meeting. Anaheim, CA, March 1991.
8. Keating JF, Werier J, Blachut P, et al. Early fixation of the vertically unstable pelvis: the role of iliosacral screw fixation of the posterior lesion. *J Orthop Trauma* 1999;13(2):107–113.
9. Gertzbein SD, Chenoweth DR. Occult injuries of the pelvic ring. *Clin Orthop* 1977;128:202.
10. Rodriguez-Morales G, Phillips T, Conn AK, et al. Traumatic hemipelvectomy: report of two survivors and review. *J Trauma* 1983;23:615.
11. Wade FV, Macksood WA. Traumatic hemipelvectomy: a report of two cases with rectal involvement. *J Trauma* 1965;5:554.
12. Johansson H, Olerud S. Traumatic hemipelvectomy in a ten-year-old boy. *J Bone Joint Surg* 1971;53A:170.
13. Langloh ND, Johnson EW, Jackson CB. Traumatic sacroiliac disruptions. *J Trauma* 1972;12:931.
14. McLean EM. Avulsion of the hindquarter. *J Bone Joint Surg* 1962;448:384.
15. McPherson JHT Jr. Traumatic hind quarter amputation. *J Med Assoc GA* 1960;49:494.
16. Meester GL, Myerley WH. Traumatic hemipelvectomy: case report and literature review. *J Trauma* 1975;15:541.
17. Oppenheim WL, Tricker J, Smith RB. Traumatic hemipelvectomy, the 10th survivor: a case report and review of the literature. *Injury* 1977;9:307.
18. Orcutt TW, Emerson CW Jr, Rhamy RK, et al. Reconstruction and rehabilitation following traumatic hemipelvectomy and brachial plexus injury. *J Trauma* 1974;14:695.
19. Palvolgyi L. Traumas hemipelvectomia. *Orv Hetil* 1969;110:970.
20. Siemens R, Flint LM Jr. Traumatic hemipelvectomy: a case report. *J Trauma* 1977;17:245.
21. Turnbull H. A case of traumatic hindquarter amputation. *Br J Surg* 1978;65:390.
22. Tile M. Fractures of the pelvic ring. Should they be fixed? *J Bone Joint Surg* 1988;708:1.
23. McCoy GF, Johnstone RA, Kenwright J. Biomechanical aspects of pelvic and hip injuries in road traffic accidents. *J Orthop Trauma* 1989;3:118.
24. Cryer HM, Miller FB, Evers BM, et al. Pelvic fracture classification: correlation with hemorrhage. *J Trauma* 1988;28:973.

5

BIOMECHANICS OF ACETABULAR FRACTURES

STEVEN A. OLSON

INTRODUCTION

Mechanical forces acting across the hip joint are complex and not easily quantified precisely. Forces across the joint itself are greatest during midstance and are derived from two primary sources: body weight and the abductor moment. During single leg stance these two forces reach equilibrium. The abductor force (ABD) is greater than body weight (BW) owing to a shorter moment arm, so that in the steady state (BW $\times$ a) = (ABD $\times$ b) (Fig. 5-1). The joint reactive force (JRF) represents the sum of mechanical forces acting across the hip joint and is also expressed as a vector on the free body diagram. Joint reactive force during stance when walking on level ground averages about 2.5 to 2.8 $\times$ BW and about 0.1 to 0.5 $\times$ BW during swing phase (1–3). This value increases to 4.8 to 5.5 $\times$ BW when jogging, and almost 8 $\times$ BW with inadvertent stumbling. However, even sedentary activities generate significant forces across the joint with straight leg raise 1.0 to 1.8 $\times$ BW and bed-to-chair transfer 0.8 to 1.2 $\times$ BW (1–3).

Although JRF is a calculated figure based on the sum of forces acting across the hip, contact pressures within the joint can be measured directly. During "normal" gait, contact pressures within the hip joint average 3 to 5 MPa during stance and about 0.5 MPa during swing phase with peak pressures of 5 to 10 MPa. When rising from a chair, peak stresses increase approximately threefold in the posterior acetabulum to 18 MPa secondary to muscle activation (1–3).

Several studies have demonstrated that the contact area within the hip joint appears to be load dependent. Dye transfer and dye exclusion techniques within the joint have demonstrated increasing contact between the femoral head and acetabulum with increasing loads (4,5). However, other investigations have demonstrated loading of the hip joint almost exclusively in the superior region, even at low loads (6–8). These reports typically use a model that explants the acetabulum from the pelvic ring and rigidly puts it on a loading jig.

The work of Bay and associates suggests that explanting the acetabulum alters the relatively uniform loading distribution seen in intact pelves loaded via an abductor mechanism to one of superior acetabulum (dome) loading with little anterior or posterior contact (9). This supports the theory of incongruence in which a small amount of elastic deformation in the intact pelvis at physiologic loads occurs. Processes that inhibit this deformation (explantation) or disrupt the structural integrity (fracture) of the acetabulum concentrate joint contact in the superior aspect of the acetabulum in the laboratory setting.

BIOMECHANICAL CONSEQUENCES OF ACETABULAR FRACTURE

The pathogenesis of posttraumatic degenerative arthritis has not been clearly elucidated, although several theories have been proposed. Clinically there is a strong correlation between articular malreduction and accelerated degenerative changes (10). Damage to the articular surface at the time of injury is difficult to quantify, but nevertheless may play a significant role in joint pathogenesis. It is unclear what factors predominate in developing arthritis, but undoubtedly biomechanical alterations in the joint are a significant component. There have been a number of studies focusing on the biomechanical consequences of acetabular fracture that can be divided into three even categories: studies focusing on intraarticular contact area and pressure, those focusing on loss of congruence or instability after fracture, and those focusing on stiffness of fracture fixation.

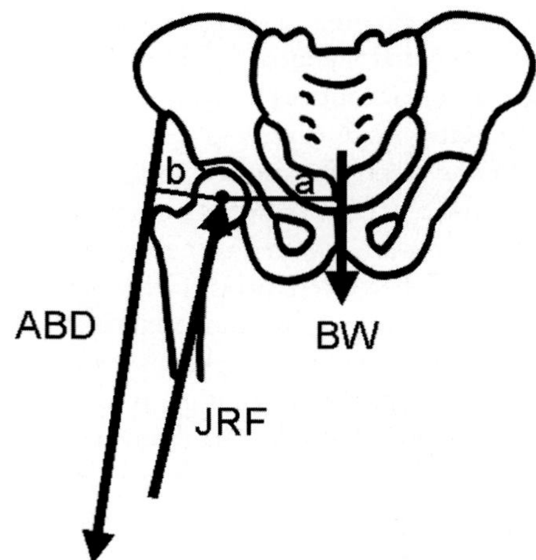

FIGURE 5-1. A line drawing of hip joint loading. The joint reaction force vector of the hip is the result of moments around the hip caused by two opposing forces. The body weight (BW) is centered in front of S2 and is distance (a) away from the center of the femoral head. The force of the abductor muscle (ABD), centered from the mid iliac wing to the greater trochanter, is distance (b) away from the femoral head. During single leg stance, the product of BW × distance (a) will equal the force of ABD × distance b. Because distance (b) is much shorter than (a), the force of the abductor mechanism is greater. (From: *Orthopaedic knowledge update, trauma 2.* Chicago: American Academy of Orthopaedic Surgeons, 2000, with permission.)

INTRAARTICULAR CONTACT CHARACTERISTICS

Those studies focusing on contact area and pressures argue increased stresses within the cartilage exceed the capacity of the tissue to adapt, initiating a cascade of degenerative changes leading to arthritis in the joint. There is clinical evidence that increased peak pressures, especially in the superior region on the acetabulum, lead to degenerative arthrosis (11).

Several studies have focused on the alteration of contact area and stresses in the joint as a result of fracture. These investigations were undertaken with a model simulating the abductor mechanism, using cadaveric pelvis with Fuji prescale film to record the intraarticular stresses. Common to all fracture patterns studied—including posterior wall, anterior wall, anterior column, and transverse—was the change from a uniform contact pattern to one of increased contact area and peak pressures in the superior acetabulum (12–16).

Fractures of the posterior wall resulted in increased peak pressure and contact area in the superior aspect of the acetabulum with concomitant decreased pressures and contact area in the anterior and posterior walls. These changes were not reversed by anatomic reduction and rigid fixation using interfragmentary lag screws and a posterior wall buttress plate (15). Varying the size of the posterior wall fragment altered contact area in a proportional amount; however, the greatest change in contact area was seen in the smallest defects (16).

Investigations of a high anterior column fracture demonstrated increased peak contact pressures with both step (10 MPa) and gap (12 MPa) malreductions (13). Fractures of a low anterior wall fracture corresponding to a 45-degree roof arc measurement had no effect on peak pressure or contact area within the superior acetabulum (14).

Juxtatectal transverse fractures with step or gap malreduction (computed tomographic [CT] subchondral arc of 9 mm) did not produce significant changes in peak contact pressures (12). However, transtectal transverse fractures (CT subchondral arc of 1 mm) produced an increased peak contact pressure (20 MPa) in fractures with step malreductions (Fig. 5-2). Increased peak pressures in the superior acetabulum with step malreductions of transtectal fractures also have been reported with an explanted acetabulum model.

All of these changes produced increased peak pressures of in excess of 10 MPa. These findings mirror the results of large clinical series of operatively treated acetabular fractures.

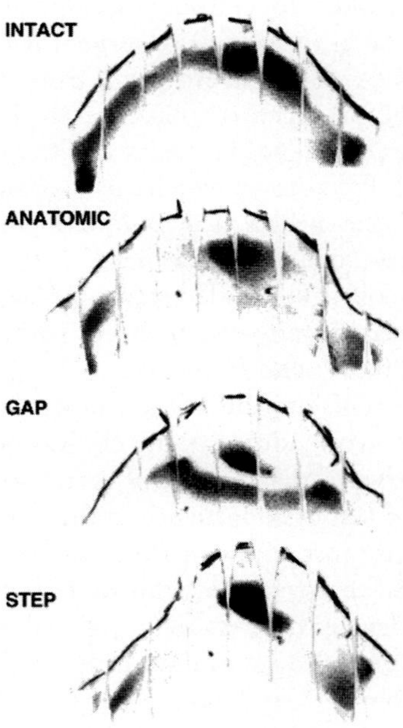

FIGURE 5-2. The articular contact pattern of the hip of a 44-year-old categoric specimen that had a simulated transtectal, transverse acetabular fracture created. Shown is the articular contact pattern in the intact condition, after anatomic reduction, and with gap and step malreduction. The thin dark line above each contact pattern represents the rim of the acetabulum. The two small dots on the contact pattern represent the reference points midway between the rim of the acetabulum and the acetabular fossa, positioned at 30 degrees on either side of the vertex of the acetabulum. With the creation of the transtectal fracture, the peripheral load distribution is lost. Step malreduction results in significantly increased articular contact pressure in the superior acetabulum in this model. (From: Hak DJ, Hamel AJ, Bay BK, et al. Consequences of transverse acetabular fracture malreduction on load transmission across the hip. *J Orthop Trauma* 1998;12:90–100, with permission.)

INSTABILITY OF THE HIP

Keith and coworkers, Calkins and coworkers, and Vailas and coworkers reported on stability of the hip following posterior wall fractures (17–19). Each measured the amount of posterior wall involved differently, but each found three groups: Group 1, small fragment–stable hip; Group 2, intermediate fragment and variable stability; and Group 3, large fragment, unstable hip. Keith and Vailas used a cadaver hip as a model, whereas Calkins reported CT data on patients with isolated posterior wall fractures.

Clinically, attempts to define the weight-bearing portion of the acetabulum have used the roof arc measurements. This measurement represents the angle formed between a vertical line drawn to the geometric center of the acetabulum, and a tangential line drawn from the geometric center to where the fracture line enters the joint on anteroposterior and Judet view radiographs. When measured on standard anteroposterior and 45-degree oblique radiographs, it can give an estimation of the amount of articular surface remaining intact. Matta and associates concluded in fractures with a roof arc of 45 degrees or greater, enough weight-bearing articular surface remained intact to consider nonoperative treatment when the femoral head remains congruent with the superior acetabulum. Subsequent investigation using CT scan reaffirmed this concept. Fractures that enter the joint 10 mm or below the vertex on CT scan correlated with a CT roof arc of 45 degrees (20). Fractures in which the femoral head remains congruous with the superior acetabulum out of traction need the criteria for nonoperative treatment.

Vrahas and colleagues loaded explanted cadaveric acetabulae with simulated transverse fractures with roof arc measurements of 30, 60, and 90 degrees (21). They measured stability based on dislocation of the femur relative to the acetabulum. This work addresses the clinical problem of the relationship between the amount of intact acetabular articular surface and loss of congruence of the femoral head and acetabulum (i.e., instability in this experimental model). They concluded that fractures with roof arc measurements of 60 and 90 degrees did not affect hip stability, but those with roof arcs of 300 degrees uniformly produced instability of the hip joint.

MECHANICS OF ACETABULAR FIXATION

There are limited data pertaining to the stability of fixation and techniques used to repair specific fracture patterns of the acetabulum. Most aim to test the relative strength or stiffness of various fixation techniques; however, there is significant variation between studies with regard to experimental loading characteristics. Goulet and coworkers investigated the rigidity and strength of four methods of fixation of comminuted posterior wall fractures using a cadaveric model (22). For posterior wall fractures with transverse comminution, interfragmental lag screws with a spanning buttress plate provided the most rigid fixation. For posterior wall fractures with concentric comminution, a buttress plate with a spring plate was optimal.

Sawaguchi and associates studied various methods of fixation of transverse fractures patterns using a cadaveric model (23). The fractures were repaired using a variety of plates/lag screw constructs. There were no differences with regard to stiffness of the implants used, and none of the constructs failed at loads up to 1,600 N (roughly two-thirds joint reactive force in stance), but significant gapping of the fractures was noted. Examination of juxtatectal transverse fractures in a synthetic pelvic model demonstrated significantly increased rigidity using a 6.5-mm anterior column screw in combination with a 3.5-mm reconstruction plate on the posterior column.

When osteotomies of the posterior column were investigated, a combination of a 3.5-mm lag screw with a spanning 3.5-mm reconstruction plate allowed less motion at the osteotomy site than combined anterior and posterior plating (24). Simonian and associates evaluated the stability of three different fixation techniques requiring anterior, posterior, or combined surgical approaches for T-type acetabular fractures (25). There was no difference between the fixation groups with regard to fracture displacement at low loads (150 N), and the author concluded that given these testing parameters, a plate with a lag screw from single approach comparable stability to dual plating from a combined approach. However, most biomechanical data suggest that joint reactive forces of (200–400 N) are typical of the swing phase of gait; thus, the loading force may have been underestimated (1–3).

The main problem with the studies available is a lack of uniformity in both testing conditions and loading parameters. There is a wide range of loading parameters, from touchdown weight bearing (100 N) to full joint reactive force (2,000 N), making comparison between studies virtually impossible. In addition, the variation in cadaveric specimens within a study makes comparison within a group difficult. More work is needed in this area.

REFERENCES

1. Bergman G, Graichen F, Rohlmann A. Hip joint loading during walking and running in two patients. *J Biomech* 1993;26: 969–990.
2. Hodge WA, Carlson KL, Fijan RS, et al. Contact pressures from an instrumented hip endoprosthesis. *J Bone Joint Surg (Am)* 1989;71:1378–1386.
3. Kotzar GM, Davy DT, Goldberg VM, et al. Telemeterized in vivo hip joint force data: a report on two patients after total hip surgery. *J Orthop Res* 1991;9:621–633.
4. Bullough P, Goodfellow J, Greenwald A, et al. Incongruent surfaces in the human hip joint. *Nature* 1968;217.
5. Greenwald A, O'Connor J. Transmission of load through the human hip joint. *J Biomech* 1971;4:507–528.

6. Brown TD, Shaw DT. In vitro contact stress distributions in the natural human hip. *J Biomech* 1983;16:373–384.
7. Day W, Swanson S, Freeman M. Contact pressures in the loaded human cadaver hip. *J Bone Joint Surg* 1975;57B:302–313.
8. Macirowski T, Tepic S, Mann RW. Cartilage stresses in the human hip joint. *J Biomech Eng* 1994;116:10–18.
9. Bay BK, Hamel AJ, Olson SA, et al. Statically equivalent load and support conditions produce different hip joint contact pressures and periacetabular strains. *J Biomech* 1997;30:193–196.
10. Letournel E, Judet R. *Fractures of the acetabulum.* New York: Springer-Verlag, 1993.
11. Hadley NA, Brown TD, Weinstein SL. The effects of contact pressure elevations and aseptic necrosis on the long-term outcome of congenital hip dislocation. *J Orthop Res* 1990;8:504–513.
12. Hak DJ, Hamel AJ, Bay BK, et al. Consequences of transverse acetabular fracture malreduction on load transmission across the hip joint. *J Orthop Trauma* 1998;12(2):90–100.
13. Konrath G, Hamel A, Sharkey N, et al. Biomechanical consequences of anterior column fracture of the acetabulum. *J Orthop Trauma* 1998;12:547–552.
14. Konrath GA, Hamel AJ, Sharkey NA, et al. Biomechanical evaluation of a low anterior wall fracture: correlation with the CT subchondral arc. *J Orthop Trauma* 1998;12:152–158.
15. Olson SA, Bay BK, Chapman MW, et al. Biomechanical consequences of fracture and repair of the posterior wall of the acetabulum. *J Bone Joint Surg (Am)* 1995;77:1184–1192.
16. Olson SA, Bay BK, Pollak AN, et al. The effect of variable size posterior wall acetabular fractures on contact characteristics of the hip joint. *J Orthop Trauma* 1996;10:395–402.
17. Calkins MS, Zych G, Latta L, et al. Computed tomography evaluation of stability in posterior fracture dislocation of the hip. *Clin Orthop Rel Res* 1988;227:152–163.
18. Keith JE Jr, Brashear HR Jr, Guilford WB. Stability of posterior fracture-dislocations of the hip. Quantitative assessment using computed tomography. *J Bone Joint Surg (Am)* 1988;70:711–714.
19. Vailas JC, Hurwitz S, Wiesel SW. Posterior acetabular fracture-dislocations: fragment size, joint capsule, and stability. *J Trauma* 1989;29:1494–1496.
20. Olson S, Matta J. The computerized subchondral arc: a new method of assessing acetabular articular congruity after fracture: a preliminary report. *J Orthop Trauma* 1993;7:402–413.
21. Vrahas MS, Widding KK, Thomas KA. The effects of simulated transverse anterior column and posterior column fractures of the acetabulum on the stability of the hip joint. *J Bone Joint Surg* 1999;81A:966–974.
22. Goulet JA, Rouleau JP, Mason DJ, et al. Comminuted fractures of the posterior wall of the acetabulum. A biomechanical evaluation of fixation methods. *J Bone Joint Surg (Am)* 1994;76(10): 1457–1463.
23. Sawaguchi T, Brown TD, Rubash HE, et al. Stability of acetabular fractures after internal fixation. A cadaveric study. *Acta Orthop Scand* 1984;55:601–605.
24. Schopfer A, DiAngelo D, Hearn T, et al. Biomechanical comparison of methods of fixation of isolated osteotomies of the posterior acetabular column. *Int Orthop* 1994;18:96–101.
25. Simonian PT, Routt ML Jr, Harrington RM, et al The acetabular T-type fracture. A biomechanical evaluation of internal fixation. *Clin Orthop Rel Res* 1995;18:234–240.

6

PATHOANATOMY OF THE PELVIC RING

JORGE E. ALONSO

INTRODUCTION

Pathologic verification of the lesions seen radiographically has been insufficient until recent years, for two reasons: (a) few cases of pelvic disruption have been subjected to posterior open reduction and internal fixation; and (b) direct autopsy material has rarely been studied. This picture has changed in the past decade. Open reduction is being done more frequently now, and more autopsy material has been examined and reported.

A retrospective review was conducted of all decedents examined at the Jefferson County (Alabama) Coroner/Medical Examiner's Office between 1994 and 1996 with the primary or underlying cause of death owing to motor vehicle accident (1). The medical examiner's statute charges the office with the responsibility of investigating all sudden and unexpected deaths that have occurred in Jefferson County and that have been caused by events that transpired in Jefferson County. Information was abstracted from the medical examiner's files, including age, cause of death, blood alcohol level, other substances detected, and circumstances surrounding death. A computer database search for deaths caused by motor vehicle accident resulted in 392 cases. As we wished to study pelvic trauma in the absence of a significant interval of survival, 32 cases in which the decedent received evaluation and treatment at a hospital were excluded. Another five were excluded because police records could not be found. In Jefferson County all decedents from motor vehicular accidents get a set of trauma radiographs, lateral of the neck, anteroposterior of the chest, and an anteroposterior of the pelvis. Radiographs (anteroposterior) of the remaining cases were reviewed to identify the presence of pelvic trauma and the type of pelvic fracture. In addition to the radiograph other variables were included: cause of death, position of decedent in the motor vehicle accident (MVA), direction of impact, use of seatbelt, and substance abuse. These were correlated with the presence and type of pelvic fracture according to Tile's classification.

Of the remaining 355 cases, 82 of the decedents suffered pelvic fractures (23%). The radiographs were suitable for scoring in 73 of the 82 cases of pelvic fracture (89%). Findings are summarized in Table 6-1.

Further stratification into type of fracture, position of decedent in the MVA, and the cause of death are shown in Table 6-2. The majority of the decedents were drivers (50%), with passengers being second (24%).

According to direction of impact, decedents who sustained pelvic fractures (n = 82) were found to be involved in a head-on impact in 44 cases, a side impact in 21 cases, and in rollover accidents in two cases. The direction of impact was unknown in five cases. The automobile was totaled in 32 cases. We see the direction of the impact in Table 6-3, frontal collision being the most common type.

We can see that the majority of decedents in MVAs were not seatbelted. Table 6-4 shows that a seatbelt was used in 21% (n = 17) of the cases of decedents with pelvic fractures. No seatbelt was used in 39% (n = 32), use was undetermined in 16% (n = 13), and use of a seatbelt was not applicable (e.g., cases of pedestrians or motorcyclists) in 24% (n = 20).

The decedent was found to be intoxicated with ethanol, cocaine, or a combination of both in 26% of the cases of decedents with pelvic fractures (n = 21).

After reviewing the radiographs, only an anteroposterior view could be reviewed and classified. Again the fractures were classified with only one anteroposterior radiograph. The results are shown in Table 6-5.

TABLE 6-1. DEMOGRAPHICS

Study years	1994–1996	
Number of cases reviewed	392	
Cases excluded	37	
Delayed death	32	
No police record	5	
Number of cases available for study	355	
Pelvic fracture present	82	23%
Cases with radiographs suitable for scoring	73	89%
Pelvic fracture was cause of death	63	77%
Mean age of decedents with pelvic fractures	44 ± 25 years	

TABLE 6-2. RELATIVE POSITIONS OF DECEDENTS WITH PELVIC FRACTURES

Position of Decedent	N	(%)
Driver	41	(50)
Passenger	20	(24)
Pedestrian	18	(22)
Motorcycle driver	2	(2)
Undetermined	1	(1)
Total	**82**	

TABLE 6-3. TYPE OF FRACTURE BASED ON FORCE DIRECTION[a]

Direction of Impact	N
Front	44
Side	21
Rollover	2
Unknown	5
Total	**32**

[a]Note that the sum of these is greater than the number of cases because of multiple impacts in some cases.

TABLE 6-4. SEATBELT USE IN THOSE WITH PELVIC FRACTURES

N	(%)
Seatbelt used	17 (21)
Not used	32 (39)
Undetermined	13 (16)
Not applicable (Pedestrians and motorcyclist)	20 (24)

Sixty-two fractures were classified as Type Cs. As expected, the more severe high-energy types are the ones that produced death. Type C1s were more common than C2s and C3s after reviewing the Type C and the year of occurrence.

In 1981 Bucholz reported that of 150 consecutive persons killed in MVAs examined at the time of autopsy, 147 (31%) had a pelvic injury (2). Radiography of the pelvis and postmortem examination were performed in 32 of the victims; of those, 22 had a unilateral double vertical fracture, four had a bilateral fracture, and the remainder had an acetabular or complex pattern. His findings mirror, and indeed confirm, our biomechanical concepts. Disruption of the pelvic ring always occurred in two locations, anteriorly and posteriorly.

In his Group I (14 cadavers), no posterior lesion could be demonstrated radiologically in the presence of an anterior lesion, yet all had an undisplaced vertical fracture of the sacrum or a tear of the anterior sacroiliac ligament on postmortem examination. This confirms the study of Gertzbein and Chenoweth, whose findings using technetium polyphosphate scanning were identical (3). These authors found increased uptake of technetium polyphosphate in the sacroiliac area of all patients in whom an apparently undisplaced anterior fracture of the pubic rami was diagnosed ra-

TABLE 6-5. DISTRIBUTION OF PELVIC RING DISRUPTION BY TYPE (TILE CLASSIFICATION)

Type	Number of Cases
A1	2
A2	3
A3	0
B1	7
B2	10
B3	1
C1	38
C2	11
C3	13

A
B
C

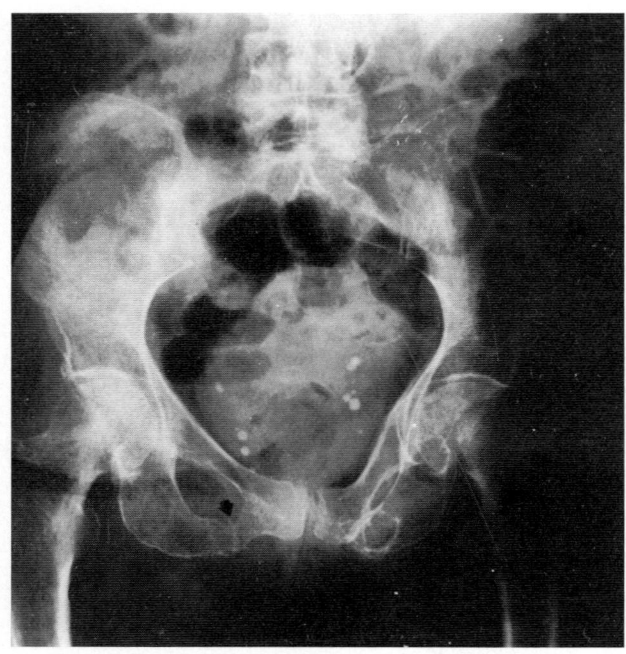

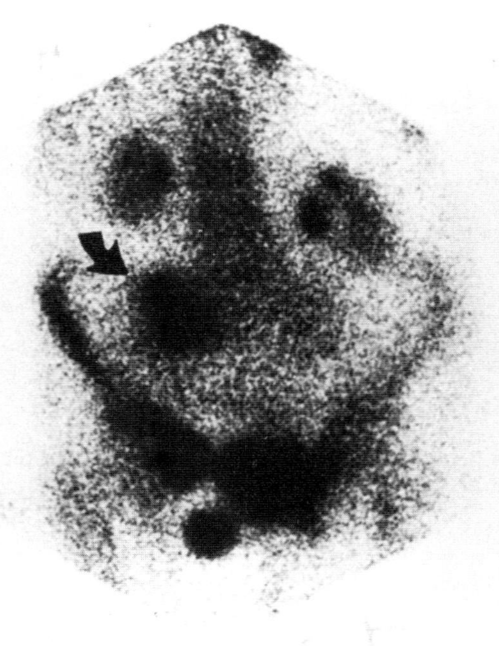

FIGURE 6-1. A: Radiograph of a patient with an apparently undisplaced fracture of the inferior and superior pubic rami on the right side *(black arrow).* No lesion is seen posteriorly. The deformity on the left hemipelvis represents malunion of an old left acetabular fracture. **B:** Technetium polyphosphate bone scan of the same patient clearly shows the increased uptake of the superior and inferior pubic rami fracture anteriorly but also massively increased uptake of the right sacroiliac joint, indicating a posterior lesion. (Courtesy of Dr. Stanley Gertzbein.)

diographically (Fig. 6-1), thereby confirming the dictum that if a ring structure is broken in one area, a lesion must be present at another site in the ring.

In Bucholz's Group II (five cadavers), in addition to an anterior lesion of the pelvic ring there was radiographic evidence of a posterior injury (usually avulsion of the anterior sacroiliac ligaments) but sparing of the strong posterior ligaments. Using autoradiographs, Chenoweth's group showed that the technetium polyphosphate was deposited in these microligamentous avulsions (Fig. 6-2) (3,4). In this particular group, the pelvic ring remained relatively stable because of the intact posterior ligamentous structures.

Both of these groups represent variants of the so-called open-book injury caused by external rotatory forces. The relatively stable nature of these injuries is confirmed by these studies. As well, the principle that the ring must be broken anteriorly and posteriorly in all cases is further enhanced by the observation that all of the straddle injuries, characterized by fractures of all four pubic rami, were accompanied by a posterior lesion.

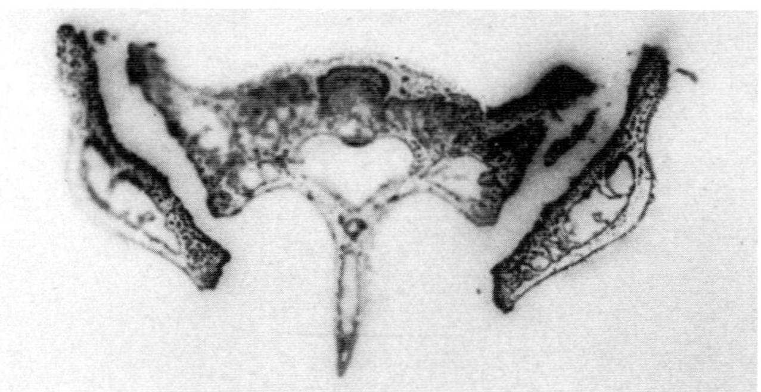

FIGURE 6-2. Autoradiograph of the sacroiliac joint of a rabbit shows technetium polyphosphate deposited in microligament avulsions in the right side.

In the Group III injuries (11 cadavers), complete disruption of both the anterior and posterior sacroiliac ligaments occurred, allowing marked cephalad and posterior displacement, as well as external rotation of the affected hemipelvis. The involved hemipelvis was completely unstable, owing to the loss of all of its soft-tissue support. Bucholz did not mention the sacrotuberous or sacrospinous ligaments in his studies, but in our studies these ligaments must be torn to allow triplane displacement.

This type of injury, the vertical shear, has been subjected to posterior open reduction and internal fixation. Our findings were identical to those of Bucholz. In those cases, the only intact posterior structure is the skin, which was also torn in some instances of open fracture (Fig. 6-3).

At surgery, once the skin is incised, the surgeon is confronted with a completely torn posterior ligament complex, already described as the strongest in the body. Through the widely displaced fracture or dislocation, the surgeon may easily palpate the posterior peritoneum and the pelvic contents, including the rectum. If exposed relatively soon after injury, reduction may be accomplished by removing any interposed

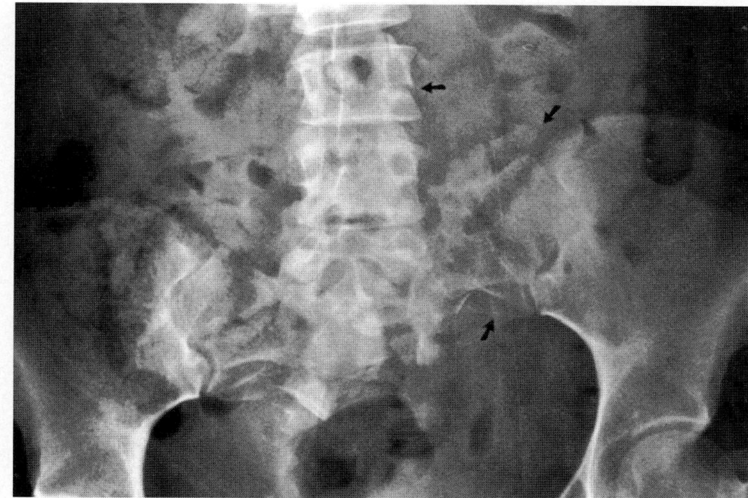

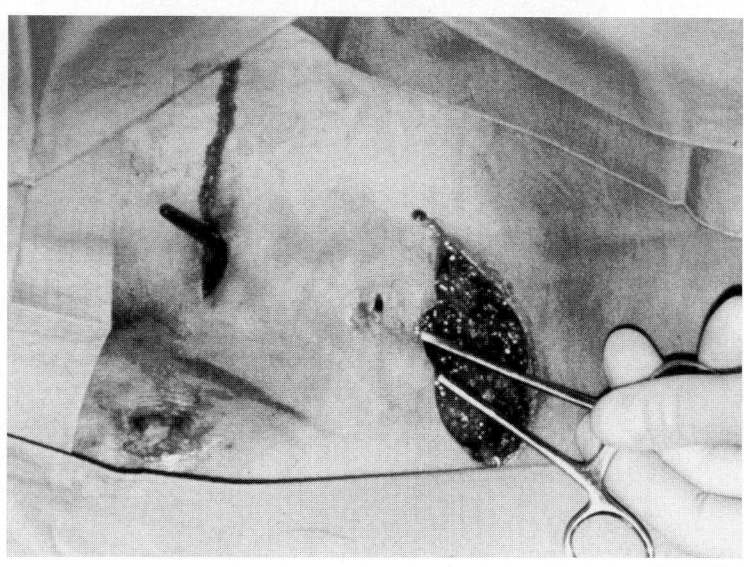

FIGURE 6-3. A: Radiograph of a disrupted pelvis of a 19-year-old woman injured after jumping from a bridge. Note the marked posterior displacement through the sacrum and fracture of the L3 vertebral body. **B:** Clinical photograph of the same patient showing two large communicating lacerations posteriorly. An examining finger inserted through the wound could palpate the pelvic viscera, because all the ligaments were completely torn.

soft tissue. Bucholz has found reduction of unstable fractures difficult because of the common ligamentous interposition.

SITE OF LESIONS

The precise site of the lesion is less important than its effect on the stability of the ring, because some of these patients have several injuries, anterior and posterior.

Anterior Lesions

The anterior lesion may run through the symphysis pubis or the superior and inferior pubic rami, unilaterally or bilaterally. Also, a diastasis of the symphysis may be combined with a fracture of the inferior and superior pubic rami. The symphysis diastasis, although often through ligamentous tissue alone, may occur as a bony avulsion. In our studies at the Department of Engineering at the University of Alabama in Birmingham, we have found that these injuries might not be as severe as expected because the symphysis can recoil back to almost any anatomic position (Fig. 6-4). Preinjured symphysis pubis were placed in a joint stiffness jig and tested (Fig. 6-5) (5).

This fixture made it possible to apply tension and compression in plane axial loads, as well as bending moments to the joints in the transverse and sagittal planes using the MTS machine. Load, displacement, and bending angle data were sampled and recorded by a personal computer–based data acquisition system (Fig. 6-6).

The mean stiffness values for impacted joints and nonimpacted joints were consistently lower for impacted specimens. The higher loading rate (100 mm/s) produced a larger stiffness response, as well as a greater ultimate failure strength compared to a low loading rate (0.01 mm/s), as shown in Fig. 6-7.

The biomechanical data showed us that even though the anterior pathology might look benign in the radiographs, a

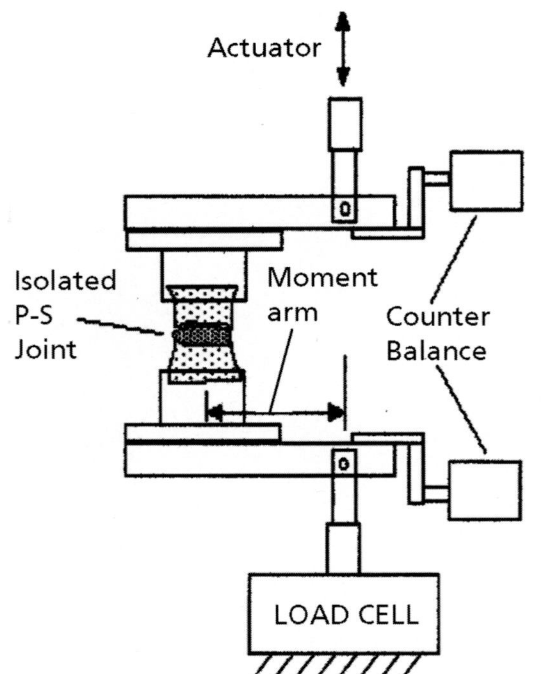

FIGURE 6-4. Joint stiffness jig placed in the MTS machine.

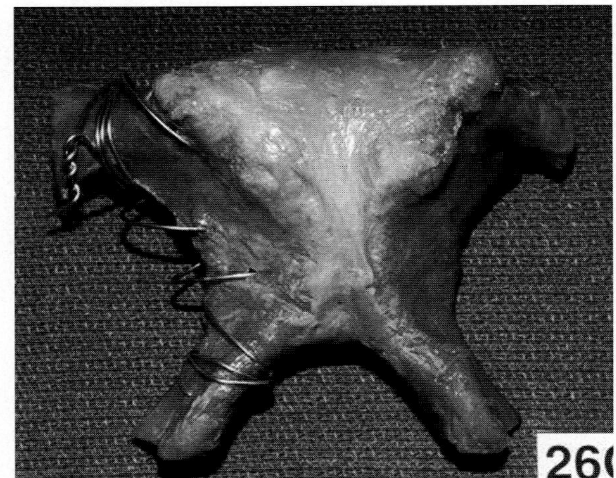

FIGURE 6-5. Cadaveric specimen tested.

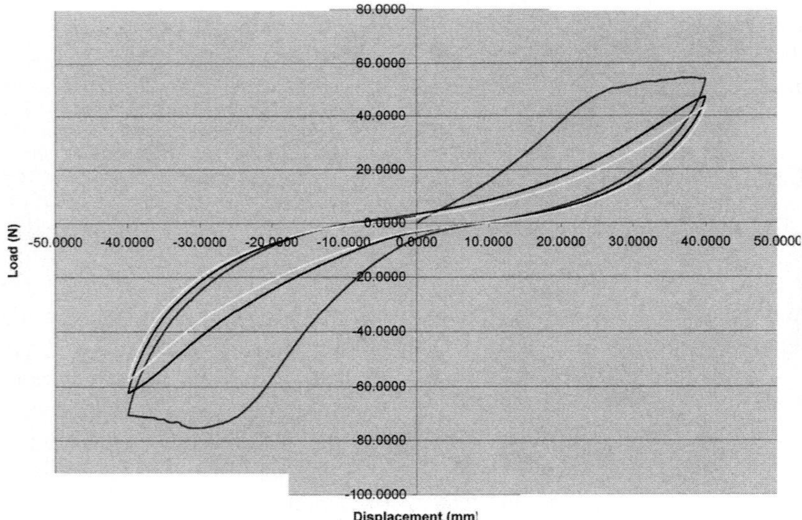

FIGURE 6-6. Load and displacement data during testing and the recoil back to near normal position.

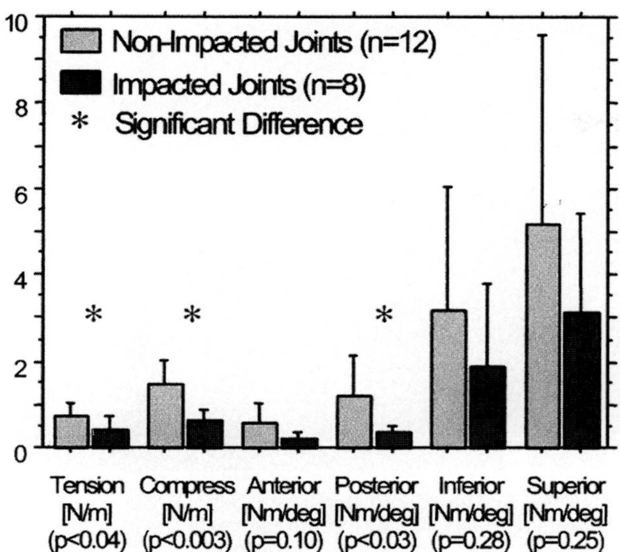

FIGURE 6-7. Impacted and nonimpacted symphysis, their failure strength compared to the loading rate.

lot of soft-tissue damage and displacement occurred during the impact, recoiling back to the near anatomic position before the accident.

Posterior Lesions

Posteriorly, the lesion may be a sacroiliac dislocation, a sacral fracture (usually through the sacral foramina), an iliac fracture, or a sacroiliac fracture-dislocation. In fracture-dislocations, a common pattern is a dislocation of the articular surface of the joint with a fracture extending posteriorly through the ilium in the region of the posterior superior iliac spine (Fig. 6-8). A fracture through the sacrum is less common anteriorly, dislocating the joint posteriorly.

TABLE 6-6. SITE OF PATHOLOGIC LESION

Lesion	N
Anterior	
Bilateral rami	12
Unilateral pubic rami	8
Diastasis symphysis pubis	6
Combined	4
Posterior	
Sacroiliac dislocation	19
Sacral fracture	6
Iliac fracture	1
Combined	4

Source: Bucholz RW. The pathological anatomy of Malgaigne fracture-dislocations of the pelvis. *J Bone Joint Surg* 1981;63A:400, with permission.

Vertical fractures of the sacrum may occur lateral to the sacral foramina, through the sacral foramina, or medial to the sacral foramina (6). Occasionally, the longitudinal vertical fracture occurs in the midline. Other patterns include a bilateral injury or an H-type injury with bilateral vertical extensions and a transverse extension as well. Sacral fractures and sacroiliac joint dislocations, with or without a fracture, are approximately equal in most literature reports and together make up more than 90% of posterior lesions, the remainder being fractures of the ilium. The sites of injury are summarized in Table 6-6. The precise pathologic lesion in

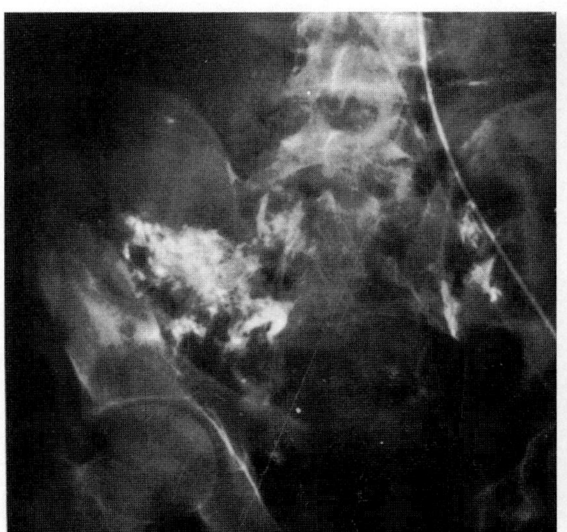
A

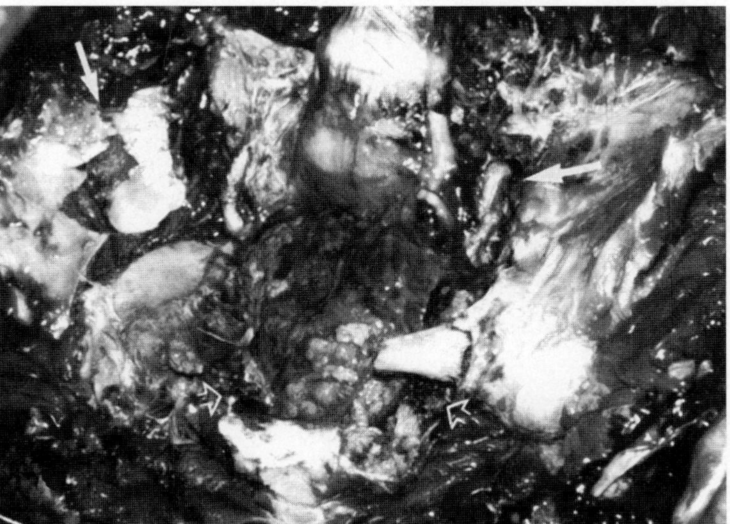
B

FIGURE 6-8. A: An anteroposterior radiograph and arteriogram of a 19-year-old man involved in a motorbike injury. Note the marked disruption, both anteriorly and posteriorly, and the marked extravasation of dye, indicating major arterial lacerations. **B:** Postmortem dissection of the pelvis of the same patient, who died of associated injuries. Note the completely unstable anterior fracture involving all four pubic rami, resulting in a floating straddle fragment. On the right side the entire iliac wing is crushed through bone but the sacroiliac joint is intact. On the left side there is a complete disruption and posterior dislocation of the sacroiliac joint.

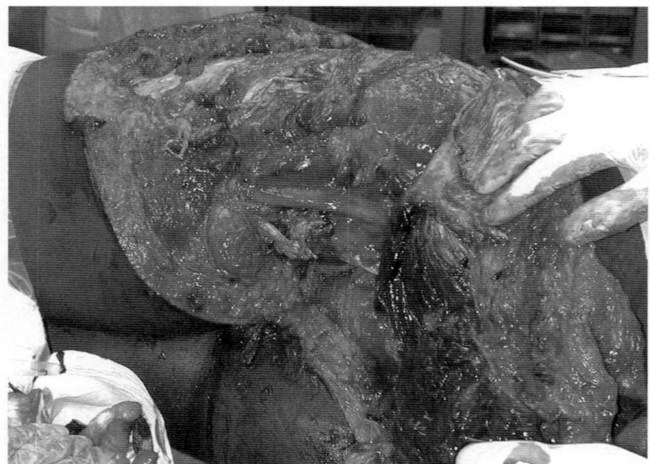

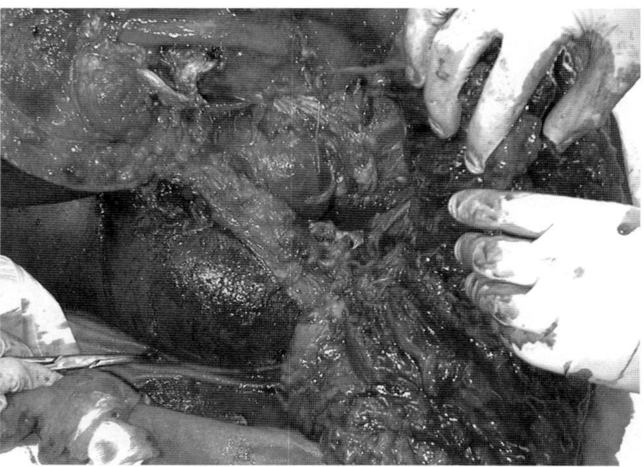

FIGURE 6-9. A 28-year-old man involved in a high velocity motor vehicle accident sustained an open pelvic fracture. The posterior pathology, a transforaminal sacral fracture on the left with completely torn ligaments, and exposure of the pelvic organs. You can see the rectum and left sciatic nerve.

cases of dislocation varies, as it does in the anterior lesion (Fig. 6-9). Ligamentous disruption as well as minor or major bony avulsions may be present. In children or adolescents, massive instability may be associated with complete avulsion of the iliac apophysis at the posterior superior spine.

REFERENCES

1. Adams JE. Analysis of the incidence of pelvic trauma in 392 consecutive fatal automobile accidents in Jefferson County, Alabama 1994–1996. *Am J Forens Pathol,* submitted.
2. Bucholz RW. The pathologic anatomy of Malgaigne fracture-dislocations of the pelvis. *J Bone Joint Surg* 1981;63A:400.
3. Gertzbein SD, Chenoweth DR. Occult injuries of the pelvic ring. *Clin Orthop* 1977;128:202.
4. Chenoweth DR, Cruickshank B, Gertzbein SD, et al. A clinical and experimental investigation of occult injuries of the pelvic ring. *Injury* 1981;12:59.
5. Dakin GJ, Arbelaez RA, Molz FJ 4th, et al. Elastic and viscoelastic properties of the human pubic symphysis joint: effect of lateral impact joint holding. *J Biomech Eng* 2001;123(3):218–226.
6. Denis F, Davis S, Comfort T. Sacral fractures: an important problem. *Clin Orthop Rel Res* 1988;227:67.

7

PATHOANATOMY OF THE ACETABULUM

JORGE E. ALONSO

INTRODUCTION

We cannot talk about pathoanatomy of the acetabulum without giving full credit to Emile Letournel, whose initial cadaveric studies of the acetabulum gave us an understanding of the anatomy, a radiographic evaluation, and the guidelines for managing these difficult fractures.

Compared to the pelvic ring, there are no cadaveric studies after acetabular fractures. What we have learned comes from cadaveric testing after impacts in the biomechanical labs. Our surgical experience has become more extensive in the last 20 years since additional surgeons have been trained to manage these fractures.

MECHANISM OF INJURY

Fractures of the acetabulum are caused by forces that drive the femoral head into the pelvis. For this reason, damage to the articular surface of the femoral head must always be suspected with any acetabular fracture. Because the force is often distributed through the flexed knee, injuries to the patella and the posterior cruciate ligament are common—and often overlooked.

The type of acetabular fracture depends on the position of the femoral head at the moment of impact; this accounts for the myriad possible fracture types (Fig. 7-1). The injurious force may be applied to the flexed knee—as in the dashboard injury—to the greater trochanter, foot, or lumbosacral area (Fig. 7-2).

The following general statements may be made:

1. Dashboard injuries cause a preponderance of posterior wall fractures of all types, including those associated with posterior column or transverse fractures. Posterior dislocation of the hip is also prevalent with this injury.

2. The resolution of forces applied directly to the great trochanter determines the type of acetabular fracture (Fig. 7-2). In general, external rotation of the head disrupts the anterior part of the acetabulum and internal rotation of the head disrupts the posterior part. Also, the abducted head will fracture the inferomedial area; and the adducted head will fracture the superolateral area. Classic acetabular fractures have been difficult to produce in the laboratory (Pennal GF, Garside H. unpublished data); however, there is good clinical correlation between the type of fracture and the force that created it.

SITE OF LESIONS

We have reported our results of acetabular patterns associated with motor vehicle crash information and verified the type of impact to the type of fracture (Fig. 7-3). They correlate similarly to the biomechanical studies done by Letournel (1). As we have seen, many variables can cause the different types of fracture: sitting position, impact, and load of the impact.

The sitting position is important because the position of the hip joint in sitting can affect the type of fracture. Internal rotation/external rotation, abduction/adduction, or flexion/extension and their degree at the time of injury can produce different types of fractures. Another variable is the size of the individual—the effect of an impact is different in a petite woman than a large truck driver.

The impact also depends on frontal, lateral, or off-axis loading. In our study we evaluated 83 patients with fractures—41 women and 42 men—who had a combined average age of 32.8 years. Femoral shaft axis loading fractures (frontal impact) correlated significantly with male sex and trucks. Greater trochanter loading fractures occurred statis-

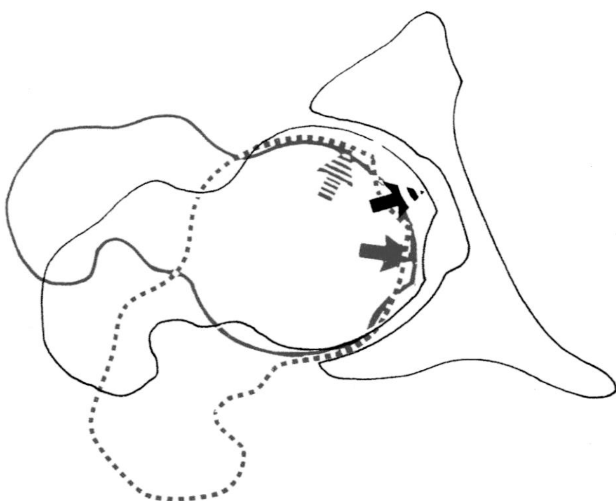

FIGURE 7-1. The type of acetabular fracture sustained depends on the position of the femoral head at the moment of impact. If externally rotated *(striped arrow),* the anterior column will be involved; if internally rotated *(solid arrow),* the posterior column will be involved.

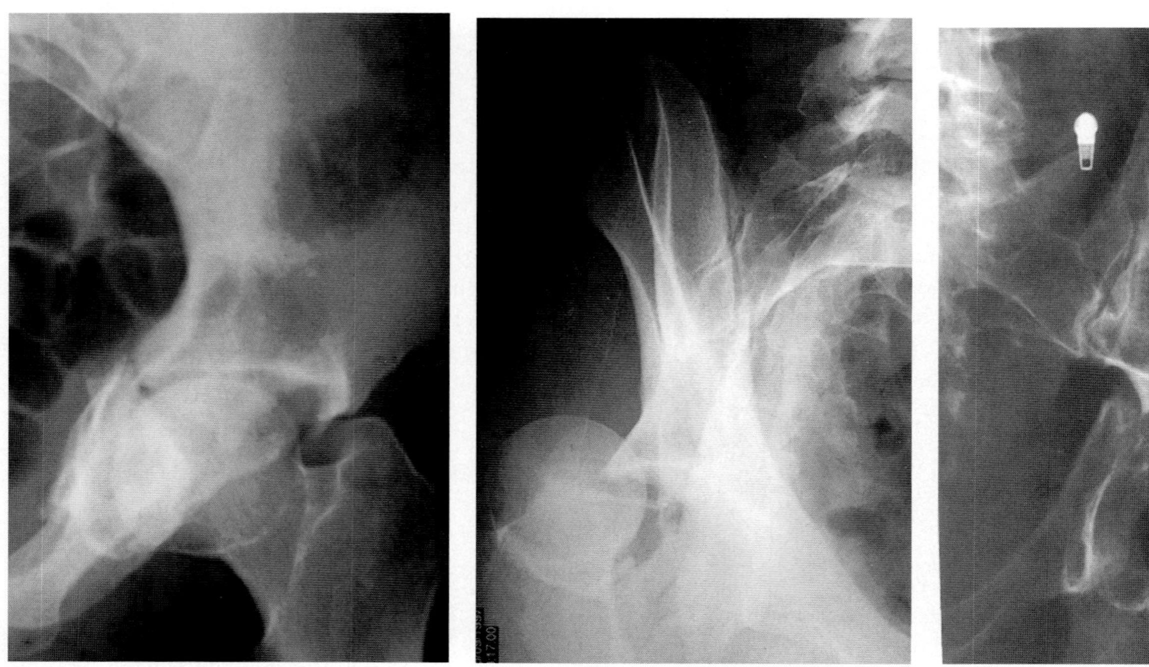

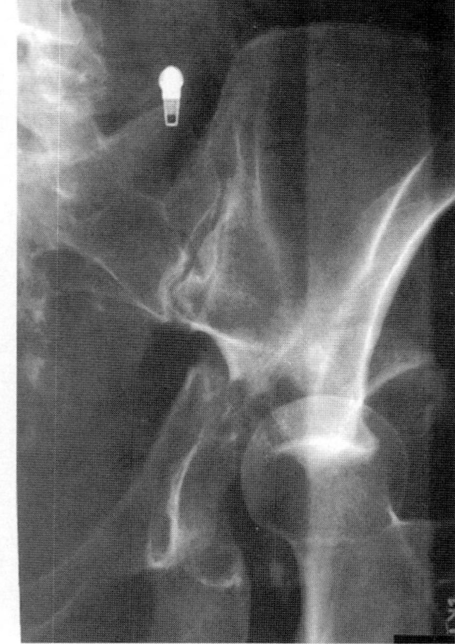

A, B C

FIGURE 7-2. Three radiographs depicting the different types of acetabular fractures according to their mechanism of injury. **A:** Posterior wall fracture secondary to a frontal impact. **B:** A transverse fracture secondary to a lateral impact. **C:** A transverse posterior wall secondary to an off-axis injury.

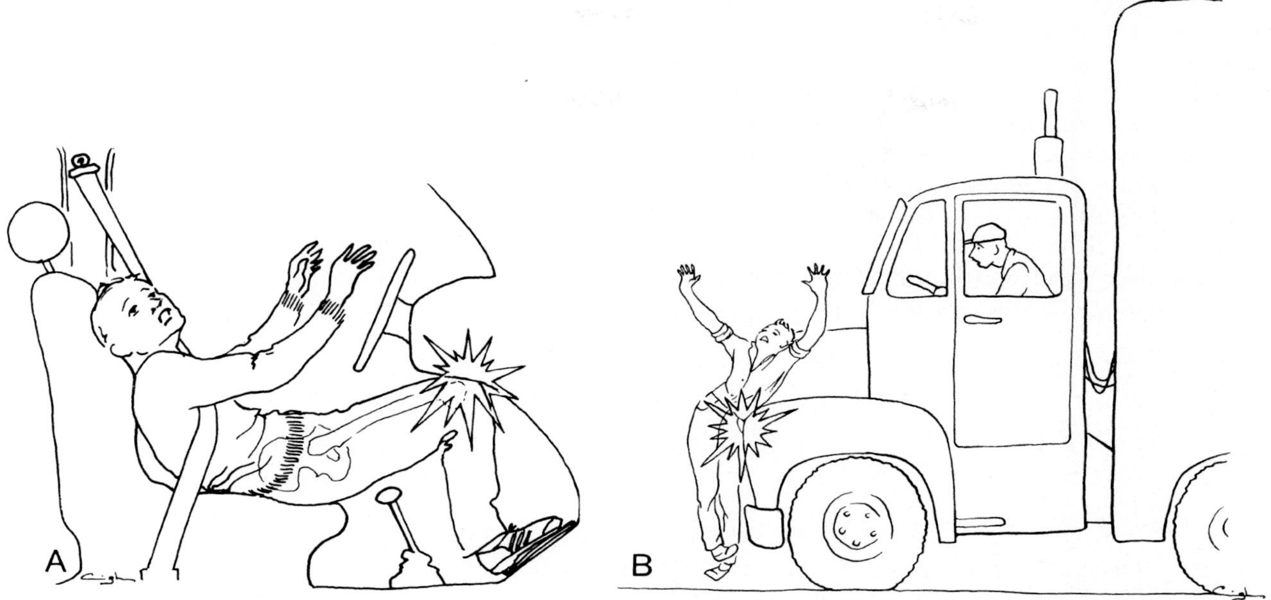

FIGURE 7-3. The injurious force may be applied to the flexed knee **(A),** thereby causing a common pattern of patellar fracture, posterior subluxation of the knee, posterior cruciate instability, and posterior wall fractures of the acetabulum. Alternatively, the force may be applied directly to the greater trochanter **(B),** producing transverse and anterior types of acetabular disruption.

tically more frequently in side impacts (the typical transverse fracture). Women received a higher rate of off-axis loading fractures, in smaller vehicles (with an increase of the transverse posterior wall) (2).

We are currently evaluating the type of injury with type of restraint. Preliminary results show that the worst fracture patterns are with front airbags alone without wearing seatbelts. Our theory is that although the airbag averts death by preventing head or thoracic injuries, the passenger, who is not held in place by the seatbelt, slides under the airbag and sustains severe injuries to the pelvis and lower extremities. The load is also important. A high load in a short period of time gives the worst injuries.

Finite modeling of the acetabulum (Figs. 7-4 and 7-5) with lateral impacts in our laboratory has shown that it takes just 55 ms to produce an acetabular fracture.

We have to keep in mind that it is not only the acetabulum that suffers with these types of trauma. A close evalua-

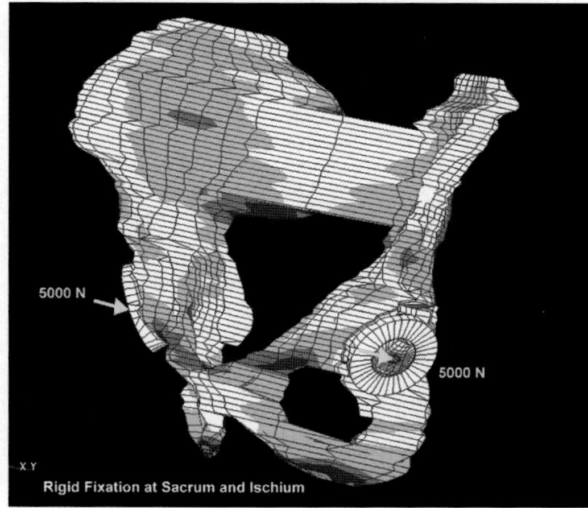

FIGURE 7-4. Finite element modeling showing the effect of a lateral impact through the greater trochanter, the loads in symphysis, and both sacroiliac joints.

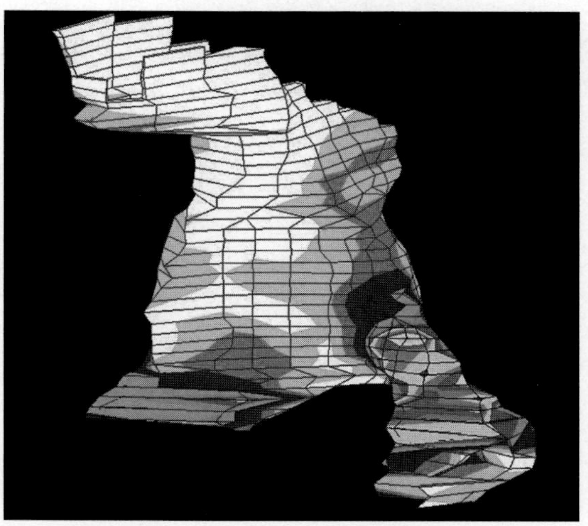

FIGURE 7-5. Finite element of the acetabulum after a lateral impact showing the high concentration areas of force in the weakest portion of the acetabulum.

tion of the symphysis and sacroiliac joint should always be thought of when there is pain after acetabular repair. Good reconstructions of the acetabular fracture have been performed when there is pain in the hip 3 to 4 years after surgery if excellent radiographs and range of motion exist. These patients underwent total hip arthroplasty without pain relief, and were evaluated later and diagnosed with sacroiliac arthritis. After injection and arthrodesis the pain subsided.

More studies are required in the pathoanatomy of the acetabulum. Because its fractures are more complex in nature than pelvic fractures, additional biomechanical and cadaveric studies should be performed in order to understand the mechanism more thoroughly.

REFERENCES

1. Judet R, Judet J, Letournel E. Fractures of the acetabulum: classification and surgical approaches for open reduction. *J Bone Joint Surg* 1964;46A:1615.
2. Dakin GJ, Eberhardt AW, Alonso JE, et al. Acetabular fracture patterns: associations with motor vehicle crash information. *J Trauma* 1999;47(6):1063–1071.

8

GENERAL ASSESSMENT AND MANAGEMENT OF THE POLYTRAUMA PATIENT

WOLFGANG K. ERTEL

INTRODUCTION

Polytrauma defines a syndrome of multiple injuries that exceed an injury severity score (ISS) of 17 points with consecutive systemic reactions that may lead to dysfunction or failure of remote—primarily uninjured—organs and vital systems (1). Thus, polytrauma is a systemic disease rather than a combination of local injuries. Most deaths occur at the scene, during the first 24 hours after admission, and in the second and third week ("trimodal mortality") (Fig. 8-1). Although the mortality at the scene can only be influenced by the motor industry with improved security technology, mortality owing to hemorrhage during the first 24 hours after admission and late mortality owing to septic multiple organ failure (MOF) can be influenced significantly through an appropriate emergency management and treatment algorithm.

Fractures of the "central bones" (pelvis, spine, femur) frequently occur in patients with high-energy trauma. Pelvic fractures are predominantly present (10% to 20%) in blunt multiple trauma and represent a significant source of morbidity and mortality (2–5). The pelvis as a central part of the skeleton possesses exceptional inherent strength because of its strong ligaments and bony structures. Major forces are required to fracture the normal pelvis. In this light, pelvic ring disruption, more than any other fracture of a bony structure of the body, can lead to severe complications, including massive bleeding and organ injuries. Exsanguinating hemorrhage represents the most dreaded acute complication of pelvic fractures. In addition, because of its function as a bony basin for different organs, the cauda equina and essential nerves for the lower extremity, serious injuries of those structures significantly increase the total trauma impact of the multiply injured patient with a pelvic injury. The unstable untreated pelvis enforces immobility and does not allow appropriate positioning of those patients with chest and brain injuries for their necessary intensive care.

The importance of the pelvic fracture varies with the severity of the fracture, both in terms of how severely the patient is otherwise injured and how much compromise is caused by the fracture itself. In general, pelvic disruption with sacrogluteal arch displacement presents a more serious problem, both for patient management and pelvic fracture care. The mortality rate approximates 50% if the fracture is open (compound) or associated with major vessel injury (6,7).

Interestingly, in the multiply injured patient with associated pelvic fracture, the outcome is more related to associated organ injuries and complications rather than the pelvic fracture. Poole and coworkers (8,9) found more deaths in those patients owing to head injury or nonpelvic hemor-

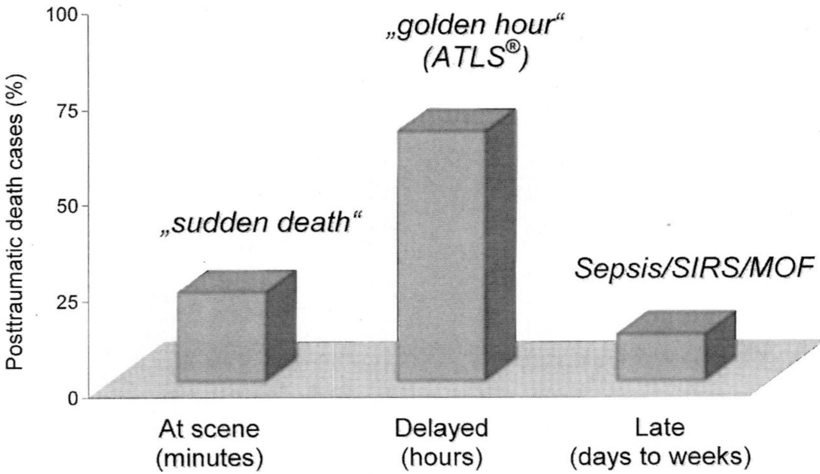

FIGURE 8-1. Trimodal distribution of death after severe injury.

rhage. The pelvic fracture was responsible for only one seventh of the deaths. Similar results are reported by various other groups with a pelvic injury related mortality between 7% and 18% in multiply injured patients (10–15). Studies from our own group revealed that parameters predicting mortality were the age, the ISS, and the existence of severe hemorrhage rather than the type of pelvic ring injury or the APACHE II score at admission (16). Although this is surprising on the first view, it is quite clear that the severity of pelvic ring disruption reflects the total trauma impact as well as contributes to severity of hemorrhage.

Most treatment concepts previously reported have focused on isolated pelvic ring disruption. They are widely accepted and include a rapid evaluation, identification, and control of the source of major blood loss, as well as reduction and primary fixation of the pelvis. Because additional injuries require a more variable scheme of diagnostic and therapeutic approaches, the order of emergent treatments, the procedures of bleeding control, and the time point of pelvic fixation in multiply injured patients are different compared to the isolated pelvic ring injury. Therefore, the general diagnostic and treatment algorithm of the polytrauma patient are reviewed and the interactions of pelvic fracture management with associated injuries are discussed.

GENERAL PRINCIPLES

The primary objective in the initial care of the multiply injured patient is survival with normal cognitive functions. The understanding of the pathophysiologic alterations occurring after severe injuries is mandatory for successful outcome (Fig. 8-2). The host reacts to severe injury with a systemic trauma reaction (host defense response), which represents a physiologic response to tissue injury, hypotension, hypoxemia, pain, and stress (antigenic load). However, if the emergency treatment does not rapidly eliminate or at least significantly decreases the so-called antigenic load, the host defense response converts to the host defense failure disease. This pathophysiologic response of the host results in lifelong defects or even death.

Therefore, rapid and adequate resuscitation and treatment of life-threatening injuries has the highest priority rather than precise reconstruction of fractures (1,16). The stepwise approach and the close interaction between diagnostic and emergency procedures to save the patient's life depend predominantly on the structure and the experience of the emergency team. This can be successfully achieved using a trauma leader who is experienced in both trauma and orthopedic surgery or, as recently stated, a multidisciplinary approach with joint emergency department presence of the attending trauma surgeon, orthopedic surgeon, and anyone else deemed necessary by the trauma team captain (17). The evolution of a multidisciplinary pathway coordinating the resources of a Level 1 trauma center and directed by joint decision making between trauma surgeons and other sub-

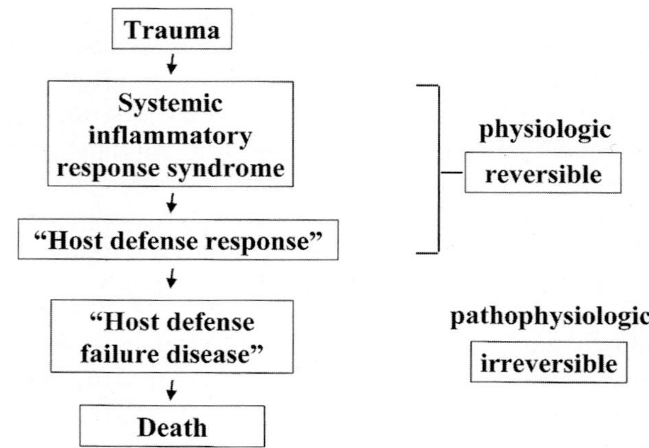

FIGURE 8-2. Immunological reaction of the host after severe injury.

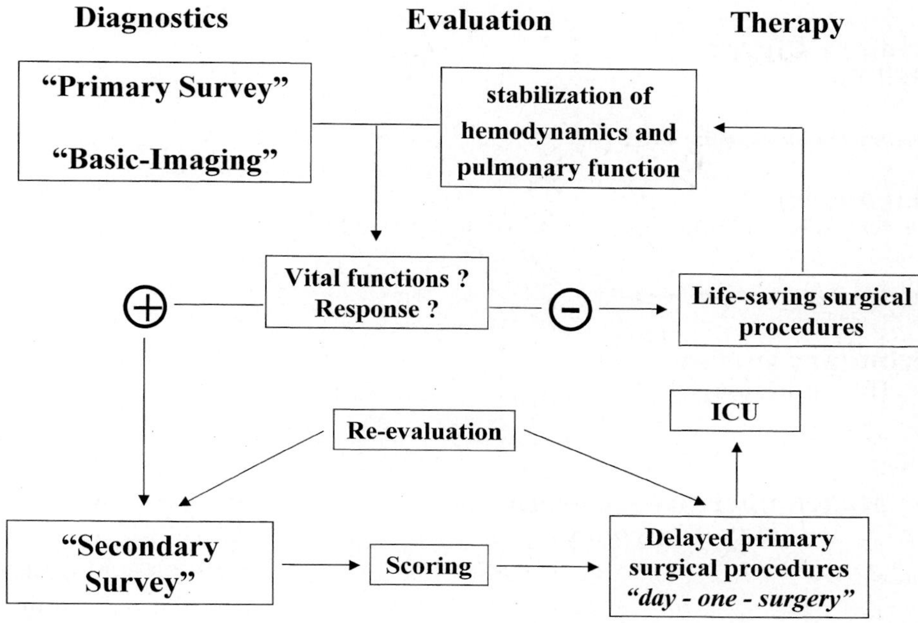

FIGURE 8-3. Stepwise approach of diagnostic and surgical procedures during the "golden hour."

speciality traumatologists has resulted in significantly improved patient survival (17).

The first hour ("golden hour") after admission to the emergency room (ER) is most critical in terms of survival and reduction of morbidity. The need for a planned treatment protocol for multiply injured patients is important, although a flexible approach in the presence of specific injuries cannot be overstated. Multiply injured patients should have immediate evaluation of their vital organ functions, resuscitation, focused and rapid diagnostic procedures, and appropriate surgical treatment, including damage control followed by stabilization of their vital organ functions in the intensive care unit (ICU) (1).

The analysis of causes of mortality in multiply injured patients reveals a pattern dependent on the time of death and clearly indicates the objectives of emergency treatment. Although exsanguination and severe head injury dominate during the first 24 hours after admission, isolated or multiple organ failure are responsible for late mortality (Fig. 8-1). Based on these data, the fundamental objectives of primary treatment are rapid recognition and control of severe hemorrhage as well as the acute evacuation of intracranial hematoma. In this light, a stepwise algorithm, including diagnostic and therapeutic procedures to maximize the vital organ functions, has been developed (Fig. 8-3) (1,16). The major objective is the rapid diagnosis of life-threatening injuries in the shortest time possible. In the case of acute circulatory and/or pulmonary failure, the diagnostic procedures have to be stopped immediately and the patient transported to the operating room for damage control, which includes decompression of body cavities as well as control of hemorrhage and contamination.

PRINCIPLES OF RESUSCITATION

Resuscitation of the multiply injured patient starts at the accident scene. Early intubation and aggressive fluid replacement are mandatory (Fig. 8-4). After admission to the ER, simultaneous resuscitation that combines restoration and maintenance of vital functions with damage control procedures rather than sequential care is the hallmark of a proper trauma system. Many algorithms have been published re-

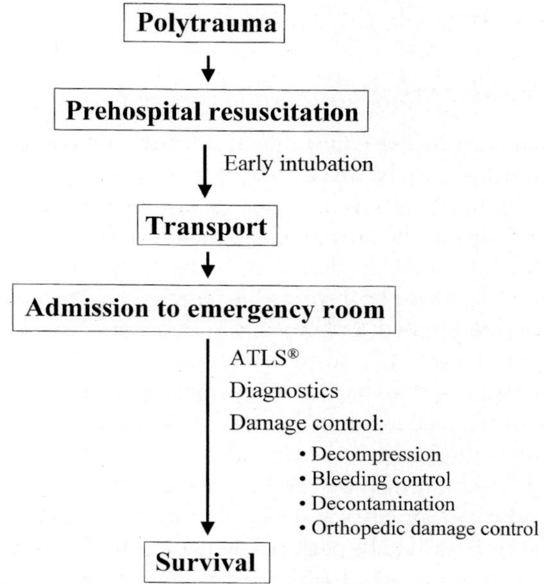

FIGURE 8-4. Algorithm for the treatment from the scene to the intensive care unit.

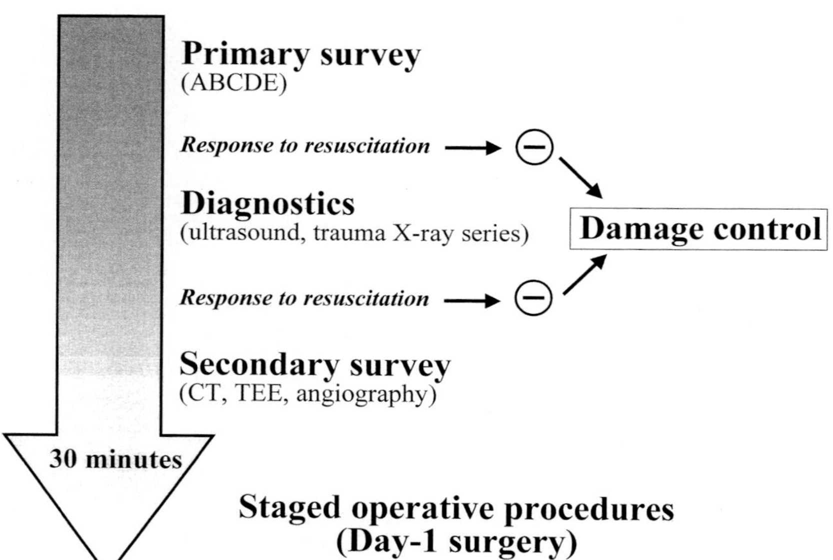

FIGURE 8-5. Continuous reevaluation of vital organ functions during the diagnostic workup and immediate damage control in the case of a negative response to resuscitation.

cently, but the best is that of the American College of Surgeons in the Advanced Trauma Life Support (ATLS) program (18).

Primary Survey

Ideally, the trauma team consists of a trauma leader experienced in all injury patterns, or a trauma surgeon, orthopedic surgeon, anesthesiologist, two nurses, and any other subspecialist required by the trauma team leader. The primary survey should take 3 to 5 minutes. In multiply injured patients with signs of torrential hemorrhage or absence of vital signs, resuscitation has to be carried out simultaneously with the primary survey (Fig. 8-5).

Airway and Breathing

A patent airway is the most urgent priority, and the respiratory system must be assessed from the lips to the alveoli. First, the upper airway must be determined to be patent from the lips to the larynx. The patient's upper airway can be most expeditiously cleared by a jaw thrust or chin lift. The mouth should be inspected for foreign bodies or vomitus, suction applied and foreign bodies removed. At this point it is important to stress that excessive movement of the cervical spine should be avoided, because as many as 15% of unresponsive patients may have an unstable cervical spine. The lower respiratory system should be assessed by first exposing the chest, then by checking the adequacy of ventilation. Adequate air entry and exchange must be ensured.

The chest should be palpated meticulously to identify lesions such as fractured ribs, fractured sternum, flail segments, or costochondral separations. Fractured ribs in a patient who is ventilated or requires ventilation are an indication for a chest tube. If chest tubes are already in place, one must be sure that they are functioning and that there are no technical problems, such as inadequate seal or tube fenestration outside the chest.

Cardiovascular System

In most multiply injured patients the cardiovascular system is hurt by hypovolemic shock resulting from bleeding. Assessment, including vital signs, should be carried out clinically, and simultaneously starting the resuscitation. The quality of the carotid, femoral, and peripheral pulses, together with tissue perfusion assessment by such methods as the capillary return tests, are performed. Obvious sites of bleeding are controlled by direct pressure. The use of tourniquets is contraindicated.

The key problem in young patients with multiple injuries is their ability to tolerate >30% loss of their blood volume without obvious signs of hemorrhage such as significant hypotension and tachycardia. Moreover, if the interval between the time point of injury and the admission to the ER is short, the decrease of hemoglobulin and hematocrit does not correlate with the true blood loss (18). This can lead to underestimation of the real hemodynamic status of the patient with fatal consequences. The rapid detection of so-called "hidden shock" can be achieved easily by using blood gas analysis and looking at either the base deficit or blood lactate levels. Previous studies of critically ill and severely injured patients have suggested that the ability to maintain lactate at normal levels correlates with the true state of hemorrhage and consequently with the probability of survival (19–22). Pathophysiologically, lactate production is increased in the case of decreased pyruvate oxidation during tissue hypoxia. The amount of lactate produced is believed to correlate with the total oxygen debt, which is dependent on the magnitude of hypoperfusion and severity of hemorrhagic shock (21). Therefore, blood lactate levels seem to better correlate with hypovolemia-induced tissue perfusion changes and local oxygen debt than hemoglobin and hematocrit, as recently demonstrated (23).

Central Nervous System

Rapid neurologic assessment should be carried out at this stage, including assessment of pupillary reaction and determination of the Glasgow Coma Scale (GCS) (24). More detailed neurologic assessment is contraindicated at this stage. The GCS obtained in the ER always should be compared with those values registered at the scene and during transport of the patient. If there is suspicion of intracranial lesions, rapid computed tomography (CT) is mandatory, especially in the presence of different pupillary reactions between both eyes.

Exposure

The primary survey should include a complete exposure of the patient by cutting off clothes in a standard pattern on the patient's arrival.

Resuscitation

The resuscitation period should take 10 to 15 minutes, or significantly less depending on the urgency of the situation (Fig. 8-5). Although the treatment options are described in a sequential fashion, as far as possible these maneuvers should be carried out simultaneously.

Airway

Impaired pulmonary gas exchange through severe chest injury and circulatory shock results in decreased oxygen delivery to injured organs, aggravates the hypoxic tissue damage, induces the release of cytokines with a subsequent activation of macrophages and neutrophils, precipitates pulmonary and systemic microvascular alterations, and leads to the development of multiple organ failure. Acute respiratory distress syndrome (ARDS) is frequently the precursor of MODS, suggesting that altered pulmonary function has a key role in subsequent organ failure. In the presence of severe head injury, persistent, untreated hypoxemia and/or hypotension are responsible for secondary brain damage with high mortality (Table 8-1) (25,26).

Most upper airway problems can be managed in the primary survey phase. Endotracheal intubation is warranted in most multiply injured patients. There are three essential indications: (a) impairment of pulmonary gas exchange and/or respiratory mechanics; (b) presence of hypovolemic shock; and (c) presence of central nervous system disorders associated with severely altered airway reflexes. In addition, early intubation reduces stress and allows adequate analgesia. In the presence of a potentially unstable cervical spine, nasotracheal intubation is the safest way to achieve tracheal intubation, because there is less need to position the head. Obviously, a degree of expertise is essential before attempting this method, and this can best be gained by the use of an intubation mannequin. In about 1% of patients, surgical control of the airway is necessary. The recommended method is cricothyrotomy, because it is the simplest and surest way to secure an airway surgically. Tracheostomy should be deferred to more elective circumstances.

As far as the lower airway is concerned, 90% of blunt chest trauma can be managed with chest tubes. They are indicated whenever there is reasonable suspicion of the presence of air or blood in the pleural space. Using a scalpel, a Kelly clamp, and the finger, a single large-bore (32 to 36 French) chest tube should be inserted into the fourth or fifth interspace in the midaxillary line. Trocars for insertion of chest tubes are contraindicated, because they are unnecessary and potentially dangerous. The chest tube should be

TABLE 8-1. INFLUENCE OF SYSTEMIC HYPOTENSION ON THE OUTCOME AFTER SEVERE TRAUMATIC BRAIN INJURY

	N	Death or Vegetative State (GOS 1–2) (%)	Favorable Outcome (GOS 4–5) (%)
No hypotension	307	17	64
Early hypotension (from injury through resuscitation)[a]	248	55	40
Late hypotension (in the intensive care unit)[a]	117	66	20
Early and late hypotension[a]	39	77	15

[a]Systemic blood pressure <90 mm Hg.
Source: Chesnut et al. *Acta Neurochir* 1993;59:121–125.

connected to drainage and the drainage monitored. Excessive air or blood may indicate the necessity for thoracotomy. A preliminary drainage of 1,000 mL, a total drainage exceeding 1,500 mL, or more than 250 to 300 mL per hour of blood for 4 hours are all indications for thoracotomy to control bleeding. Continuous bubbling or failure of the lung to expand may indicate a bronchopleural fistula that requires surgical repair.

Cardiovascular System

The first step in managing hypovolemia, the most common cause of shock in the trauma patient, is the insertion of at least two large-bore needles for intravenous infusions (i.e., 16-gauge or larger). They should be placed distally, one above and one below the diaphragm, and not in a limb with a proximal fracture. Failure to achieve percutaneous infusion after two attempts should lead to a venous cutdown at both ankles. Initially, a combination of crystalloid and colloid solutions with a ratio of 3:1 in favor of crystalloids should be run at the maximum capacity of the intravenous line (27). Hypovolemic shock should not be treated by vasopressors or sodium bicarbonate.

In the presence of severe or even torrential hemorrhage, universal donor blood should be used immediately. Type-specific blood may be used if available; beyond that, cross-matched blood may be given. Two to three units of fresh-frozen plasma and 7 to 8 units of platelets should be given for every 5 L of replacement the patient receives. The coagulation status of the patient must be monitored, including the partial thromboplastin time, prothrombin time, platelet count, and tests for fibrin split products. Intravenous fluids should be warmed through appropriate devices to avoid hypothermia. Continuing acidosis documented through a persistent elevation of lactate levels represents inadequate fluid replacement and persisting cellular hypoxia and should be treated as such.

Simultaneously, blood should be drawn for appropriate tests, including cross-matching for a minimum of 6 units of blood, hemoglobin, hematocrit, white cell count, blood glucose, urea nitrogen, and serum electrolytes. Preferably, tests should also include serum creatinine and arterial blood gases, the latter being an invaluable aid for assessing the degree and longevity of shock initially, and monitoring the patient subsequently.

Cardiogenic shock in injured patients is either caused by cardiac tamponade or compression of the pericardium from tension pneumothorax, or to cardiac contusion with extended myocardial infarction. If the origin of pump failure is a tension pneumothorax or cardiac tamponade, the insertion of a chest tube or a pericardiocentesis should be carried out immediately. Drugs with positive inotropic action may be effective in the case of myocardial contusion with significant reduction in blood pressure.

Spinal shock occurs in injured patients with a fracture of the spine and compression or dissection of the spinal cord. In the management of injured patients with spinal shock, where significant blood loss into the areas of injury surrounding the cord is often found, a balanced therapy of fluid administration and vasopressors is recommended.

Diagnostics and Secondary Survey

At this point a systemic review of all vital systems should be carried out (Figs. 8-3 and 8-5). The diagnostic algorithm is always carried out simultaneously with ATLS rather than sequentially. However, each diagnostic procedure and especially procedures that need transport of the multiply injured patient have to be carefully evaluated with regard to the vital functions of the multiply injured patient.

The diagnostic algorithm in Table 8-2 for a multiply injured patient is divided into primary and secondary diagnostic procedures. Although primary diagnostic procedures can be rapidly performed in the ER within minutes, for secondary diagnostic procedures the patient has normally to be transported to specific suites. Additionally, those procedures are time-consuming and do not allow quick access to surgery in a life-threatening failure of vital organ functions.

The importance of blood gas analysis for evaluation of pulmonary dysfunction and rapid detection of "hidden"

TABLE 8-2. PRIMARY AND SECONDARY DIAGNOSTIC PROCEDURES

Primary Procedures	Secondary Procedures
Mandatory	Computed tomography (with contrast)
Body examination	Angiography
Blood gas analysis (lactate, base deficit)	
Ultrasound	
Chest and pelvis radiograph	
Computed tomography of the head, if high suspicion for compressive lesion	
Dependent on specific injuries	
Electrocardiogram	
Transesophageal echocardiography	
Retrograde urethrogram	

hemorrhagic shock has been described under Principles of Resuscitation.

For detection of free fluid, ultrasound of the abdomen and chest, and chest x-ray are performed to detect hemoperitoneum, hemothorax, and hemopericardium. Diagnostic peritoneal lavage (DPL) is still used in some centers for this indication, although ultrasound has become the standard test in expert hands. In the presence of obesity or subcutaneous emphysema, DPL may be helpful to detect blood in the peritoneal cavity. Using four cuts to evaluate the complete abdomen and chest an experienced physician needs 2 to 3 minutes to recognize free fluid and judge its amount. In the case of free fluid (>500 mL) but stable hemodynamics, a CT of the chest, abdomen, and pelvis is recommended. In the presence of significant hemoperitoneum (>1,000 mL of intraabdominal free fluid) on ultrasound examination and hemodynamic instability, it is not recommended to further continue the diagnostic algorithm with a CT of the abdomen. The patient should be transferred immediately to the operating room for abdominal exploration and bleeding control.

An anteroposterior chest radiograph is obtained to exclude intrathoracic injury, especially pneumothorax or tension pneumothorax. Clinical examination and anteroposterior pelvic radiograph are used to determine whether the patient has unstable pelvic injury. It is important to emphasize that the pelvic radiograph obtained in the ER often does not allow precise evaluation of posterior ring injury except in the presence of gross dislocation. If confirmed, the pelvic volume is closed by securing sheets tightly around the pelvis, and taping the knees and ankles together in light flexion and inner rotation of the knee joints. Clues such as anterior rib fractures or sternal injuries should direct suspicion toward myocardium contusion. If so, an electrocardiogram should be performed. An area of contused myocardium can compromise cardiac function. Myocardial contusion is a relatively common yet often unrecognized complication in trauma.

The single most reassuring sight for the trauma leader is copious amounts of clear urine. Under such circumstances, one feels that "urine is gold." It is important to emphasize that a lower urinary tract injury must be ruled out before passing a urinary catheter. If there is any blood in the urethral meatus following milking of the urethra in males, a retrograde urethrogram is warranted. A urethrogram is also indicated if there is a high floating prostate on rectal examination, perineal hematoma, or unstable pelvic fracture type "open book" or "vertical shear." If time does not permit these maneuvers, catheterization should be deferred and central venous pressure (CVP) used to monitor cardiac output. With pelvic fractures, there is a 13% incidence of bladder or urethral injury. In women, bladder injury is more frequent, whereas in men, urethral injury, usually of the membranous urethra, is more common. As far as the upper urinary tract is concerned, the presence of hematuria is an indication for CT and an anteroposterior abdomen radiogram to exclude a renal injury or a tear of the ureter.

CT and angiography represent the gold standard for diagnosis of organ injuries and arterial bleeding, respectively. Despite major advances in technology and the introduction of spiral CT, in most hospitals the patient has to be transferred to the CT suite. The same is true for angiography, although angiography also can be used interventionally for bleeding control. CT is used, if there is suspicion of head, chest, abdominal, and/or pelvic injury. With the possibility of spiral CT technology, a rapid examination of all body cavities in less than 40 seconds can be achieved. Moreover, an evaluation of grossly displaced spine and extremity fractures is possible.

Recent studies have shown the diagnostic value of contrast-enhanced CT in localizing arterial bleeding. Contrast found in the gluteal region usually means superior gluteal arterial bleeding (Fig. 8-6), whereas contrast in the obturator area indicates obturator artery bleeding. Therefore, the simple addition of contrast to the CT protocol greatly alerts the clinician to the presence of pelvic arterial bleeding that, in turn, may lead to earlier intervention, such as embolization. The use of arterial angiography for either diagnostic and/or therapeutic purpose is controversial. Because <10% of all bleeding sources is generated because of an injury of small-bore arteries rather than caused by bleeding from venous plexus or cancellous bone, its primary use is questionable and is discussed later under treatment options. It can be helpful to use angiography, if ultrasound and/or CT do not reveal free fluid or do not allow localization of the bleeding source, but the patient requires ongoing blood transfusion. It should be emphasized that a patient with signs of severe hemorrhagic shock should not be transported for any diagnostic procedure.

PRINCIPLES OF DAMAGE CONTROL

"Damage control" is a term coined by Rotondo and coworkers in 1993 and has been most often used for devastating abdominal injury (Table 8-3) (28). By using this philosophy, only major injuries resulting in significant blood loss are addressed at the time of initial laparotomy. Intestinal injuries are stapled, and packing is often used as an adjunct to hemostasis. The patient is then transferred as quickly as possible to the ICU for rewarming, monitoring, and ongoing resuscitation. Generally 24 to 48 hours later, when the patient is adequately resuscitated, euthermic, and has a normal coagulation profile, he or she is taken back to the operating room and unpacked. Gastrointestinal reconstruction can be performed at that time. This principle of care can be used for injuries outside of the abdomen as well. Applying this technique to the multiply injured patient with a pelvic injury and severe hemorrhage, acute stabilization of the pelvic ring by external means, thus minimizing the operative time

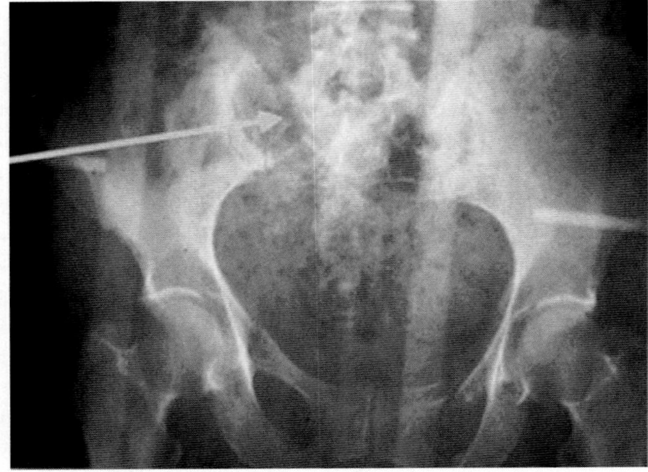

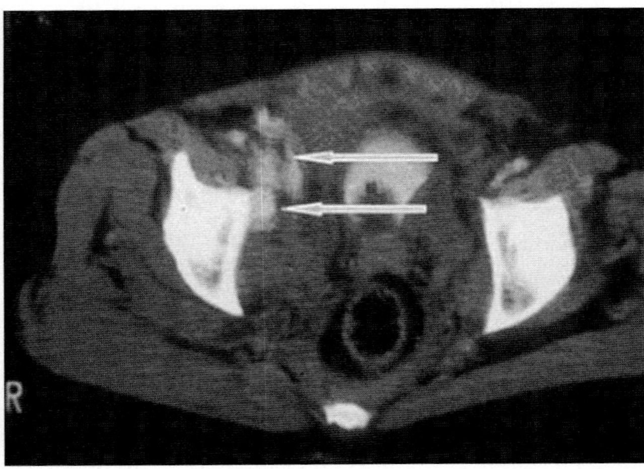

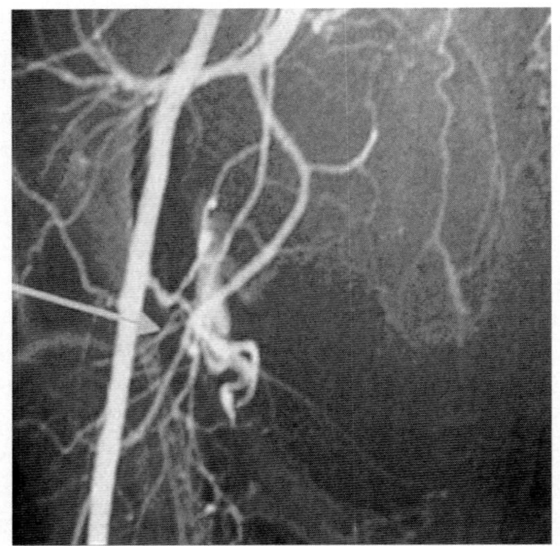

FIGURE 8-6. A 70-year-old female struck by a car sustained an unstable C-type pelvic fracture. She was in shock, with no obvious source. **A:** Skeletal traction was applied to her right leg. **B:** A contrast-enhanced CT showed extravasation that correlated with angiographic findings indicating bleeding from the obturator artery. **C:** 9 hours post -injury shows successful angiographic embolization of obturator artery. (Courtesy of Dr. David Stephen)

and preventing heat and blood loss, would be done. Following this, the patient should then be taken to the ICU. Once resuscitated, they are returned to the operating room for more elective definitive fracture fixation.

TABLE 8-3. PELVIC DAMAGE CONTROL

Closed reduction of the pelvis at admission
External fixation
- Wrapping pelvis with sheets with inner rotation and slight flexion of knees
- External fixator
- Pelvic C-clamp
- Pneumatic Antishock Garment

Control of hemorrhage
- Pelvic packing
- Angiography

Control of contamination
- Repair of genitourinary and rectal injuries
- Debridement of necrotic tissue in the case of open injury

The admission of multiply injured patients under resuscitation still remains a challenge for every ER team. Resuscitative thoracotomy has become an established treatment for those patients with acute cardiopulmonary arrest after severe injury. It should be performed only in trauma patients with absent vital signs either at the very moment of admission or when in proximity to the hospital under rapid transportation. The knowledge of mechanism of trauma and signs of major injuries may help to decide. The best survival rates are seen in penetrating trauma, whereas the outcome in patients with blunt trauma is still disappointing.

Decompression of Body Cavities

Tension Pneumothorax

The presence of a tension pneumothorax should already have been recognized during the primary survey and must be immediately decompressed.

Cardiac Tamponade

When cardiac tamponade is suspected, puncture of the pericardium may confirm diagnosis and temporarily solve the problem. The puncture is performed through the paraxyphoid route. In the case of crash laparotomy, the release of a cardiac tamponade is performed under vision through the subxiphoid membranous diaphragm route.

Intracranial Mass Lesion

The importance of severe head injury is documented by the fact that secondary brain edema is the major factor for mortality in patients <40 years. The primary goal of treatment, therefore, is to avoid secondary brain damage or at least decrease its severity. Restoration and maintenance of adequate cerebral perfusion and oxygenation of the brain is pivotal. Moreover, repeated periods of hypotension and/or hypoxemia significantly increase the risk of secondary brain edema (25,26). Small epidural or subdural hematoma can be closely observed by repeated CT. Epidural as well as subdural hematomas that are causing brain tissue compression need immediate evacuation. Under specific circumstances, such as increasing mydriasis, the emergency burr hole on the side of the enlarged pupil without further CT can be life saving. Continuous monitoring of the intracranial pressure (ICP) is performed regularly in every patient with: (a) GCS below 8 points after initial resuscitation; (b) a GCS of 8 points or higher with positive CT findings, if the patient is intubated or neurologic assessment is impossible; or (c) a neurologic deficit in patients in which neurologic reevaluation is impossible because of long-term sedation. An intraventricular catheter is used as the primary monitoring device, except in patients with continuous bleeding and a breakdown of the coagulation system. In those patients, a subdural epiarachnoidal catheter is implanted.

Bleeding Control

Massive Hemathorax

Emergency thoracotomy is indicated when the blood loss through the chest tube exceeds 1,500 mL at the time of thoracostomy, 500 mL within 1 hour, or >200 mL/h for 4 hours. Injuries of great vessels are controlled by cross-clamping and repaired with suture. Often, associated lacerations of lung tissue are repaired by suture or partial lung resection using a stapler device.

Massive Hemoperitoneum

Abdominal injuries are a common problem in polytrauma patients. They frequently occur with pelvic fractures (2,3,11). Bleeding from intraabdominal organs in combination with bleeding from the pelvis is particularly lethal. Patients with hypotension and significant free fluid in the abdominal cavity require emergency laparotomy through a midline incision. This is the only incision that guarantees free access to the complete abdominal cavity and retroperitoneum. Additionally, it allows an extension into the chest and down to the symphysis. After opening, all four quadrants are examined followed by packing to stop venous bleeding. Cross-clamping of the subdiaphragmatic aorta has to be carried out immediately in patients with ongoing hemorrhage despite packing or those under resuscitation. The concept of "damage control" includes in the presence of specific organ injuries splenectomy, packing of liver tears, and resection of ruptured small bowel areas using stapler technique, but without primary anastomosis. Patients in extremis have a better chance of survival when definitive repair of intraabdominal injuries is delayed until effective resuscitation and stabilization of vital organ functions in the ICU has occurred.

The abdomen should be left open, especially if packs are used, to avoid abdominal compartment syndrome (29). It is advisable to measure urinary bladder pressure in those patients to rapidly recognize upcoming abdominal compartment syndrome.

Massive Retroperitoneal Bleeding

The initial management of retroperitoneal bleeding is dependent on the hemodynamic stability of the patient and potential location of the injury. It involves a rapid decision to perform an exploratory laparotomy in the case of continuous hemorrhagic shock. CT is recommended in patients with stable hemodynamics and suspicion of retroperitoneal injuries. The retroperitoneum is classified into zones for intraoperative evaluation in blunt trauma, whereas the retroperitoneal hematoma always needs surgical exploration in penetrating injury. Retroperitoneal hematomas in the central zone should be explored in blunt trauma. Flank or perirenal hematomas are explored if CT reveals a renal injury requiring repair or if the hematoma is expanding.

Control of Contamination

The control of contamination includes the treatment of all hollow viscus organ injuries. Leakage of the stomach, duodenum, small bowel, or colon needs suturing to control the contamination of the peritoneal cavity. Suturing does not have to be definite at this point, especially if the injured patient is in shock, but should be done rapidly so that other serious injuries can be diagnosed and repaired.

Orthopedic Damage Control

Fractures are often relegated to the end of the priority list, but it must be stressed that they can often figure importantly in the mortality and morbidity of patients. Orthopedic damage control in the severely injured patient with critical organ injuries involves external stabilization of pelvic disruption, long bone fractures, and unstable large joints on day of admission, repair of peripheral arterial injury, radical debridement of soft-tissue injury, cleaning of fragments in the presence of open fractures, and release of compartment syndrome. This concept minimizes operative time and prevents heat and blood loss. The advantages of early provisional stabilization of long bone fractures are the facilitation of nursing care, early mobilization with improved pulmonary function, shorter ventilation time, and reduced morbidity and mortality (30,31).

The use of external fixation of the pelvis, tibia, and humerus is commonplace (32). In contrast, external fixation of femur fractures is controversial, even in critically injured patients. In North America, femur fractures often are treated with primary nailing regardless of the patient's condition (33–36). European trauma centers try to involve dysfunctions of vital organs in their treatment concept (37–38). There is abundant experimental and clinical evidence demonstrating that intramedullary nailing increases intramedullary pressure. In turn, this leads to a significant passage of emboli into the lung, which can be impressively demonstrated by transesophageal echocardiography (38). The embolization of fat particles to the already injured lung may worsen pulmonary dysfunction even to the extent of acute pulmonary failure (37,38).

Scalea and coworkers (36) suggest a sophisticated treatment concept of stabilization of femur fractures in multiply injured patients that is in line with the concept of staged surgery (1). Primary nailing is only recommended for multiply injured patients without significant chest injury and stable hemodynamics. In the case of orthopedic damage control in traumatized patients in critical condition, the femur similar to the pelvis and other long bones is stabilized using an external fixator. Plating may be a good alternative in some patients, if soft-tissue injury requires debridement, fasciotomy, or active control of local hemorrhage.

RELATION OF PELVIC FRACTURES TO INJURIES IN OTHER SYSTEMS

Pelvic fractures present a thorny and stubborn therapeutic challenge. Most are caused by blunt trauma, and massive forces are required to produce an unstable pelvic injury in young people. Thus, other or associated injuries are frequent (2–4), both in adjacent anatomic areas and more remote sites. This set of circumstances—that is, violent forces and high frequency of injury to other systems—contributes to the related problems of obscuring of diagnosis and hemorrhage. When confronted by the formidable task of managing these patients, it is essential to have some foreknowledge of the problems that will arise, in particular a knowledge of the most lethal combinations of injuries (14,40,41).

For patients with pelvic fractures who died (3,42), associated head injury was identified as a major cause of death. The combination of pelvic fracture and mass lesion requiring neurosurgical intervention has an associated mortality of 50% (2). Similarly, pelvic fracture associated with intraperitoneal injuries with significant blood loss demanding laparotomy has a mortality rate of 52% (2). When the combination of all three exists (i.e., pelvic fracture, mass lesion intracranially, and intraperitoneal pathology), the chance at survival is very small, less than 10%. By contrast, pelvic fractures associated with thoracic, urologic, or other musculoskeletal injuries have a mortality rate of 20%(2).

The exact explanation for these statistics is uncertain, but one might speculate that, with head injuries, the die is cast at the time of injury (43). In many cases, simultaneous diagnosis and treatment of both lesions is essential early in the course of management. Similarly, the sorting out of a patient with combined intraperitoneal and extraperitoneal sources of bleeding demands a firm protocol and decisive surgery for success. As discussed subsequently, this is not a dilemma that readily lends itself to a solution. Priority must be given to that source of bleeding associated with the greatest blood loss, but there are no clear guidelines by which to establish which one that might be; therefore, the debate continues (44).

SPECIFIC TREATMENT OF PELVIC DISRUPTION IN A MULTIPLY INJURED PATIENT

It is very helpful in multiply injured patients associated with pelvic ring disruption to adapt the diagnostic and therapeutic algorithm according to the hemodynamic status at admission and its development during resuscitation (Fig. 8-7) (16,23). The most complex patients are those "in extremis" with either absent vital signs or with signs of torrential hemorrhage. These patients need mechanical resuscitation or catecholamines despite complete blood volume replacement within 120 minutes (>12 units of blood/2 h) (2). A regular diagnostic workup is not possible. Most of those patients need immediate resuscitative thoracotomy and/or laparotomy, aortic clamping, and abdominal/pelvic packing. The second group includes patients with persistent signs of hemorrhagic shock (systolic blood pressure <90 mm Hg, pulse >100 beats/min, CVP <5 cm H_2O, urine output <30 mL/h) despite adequate fluid replacement and blood transfusions over a period of 2 hours. Diagnostics include ultrasound or diagnostic peritoneal lavage (DPL) and x-rays of chest and pelvis. CT is not indicated in most of those patients except in the presence of head injury. Most patients need emergency laparotomy and surgical control of bleeding. Multiply injured patients with stable hemodynamics undergo the complete diagnostic algorithm.

The therapeutic interventions (pelvic damage control) that are appropriate in the management of a multiply injured patient associated with pelvic injury in the presence or absence of bleeding are: (a) closed reduction; (b) external fixation; (c) control of hemorrhage by laparotomy and pelvic packing, or angiography; (d) and control of contamination (Table 8-3).

Closed Reduction

In the case of an obvious opening pelvic ring disruption a gross reduction of the displaced hemipelvis should be carried out immediately in the ER. Both legs are slightly flexed at the hips and knees and internally rotated. The pelvic ring is closed by pushing the iliac crest from both sides and wrapping a broad bandage or sheet around the pelvis and clamping it together over the midline of the patient (hip spica) (Fig. 8-8). The effectiveness of this simple procedure is shown in Fig. 8-9. Specific pelvic binders are commercially available for this technique. Also useful is a vacuum operat-

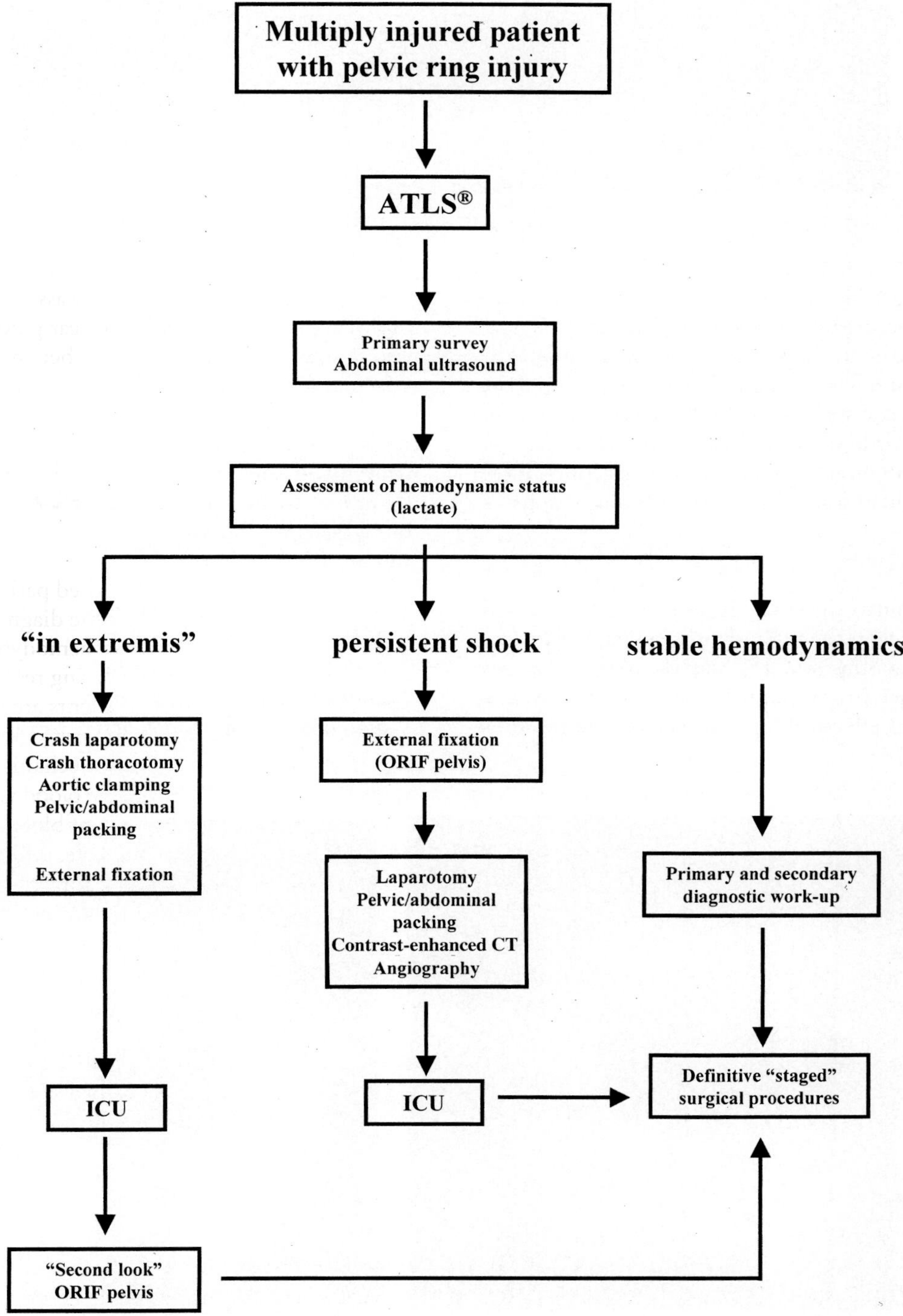

FIGURE 8-7. Orthopedic damage control of pelvic injury.

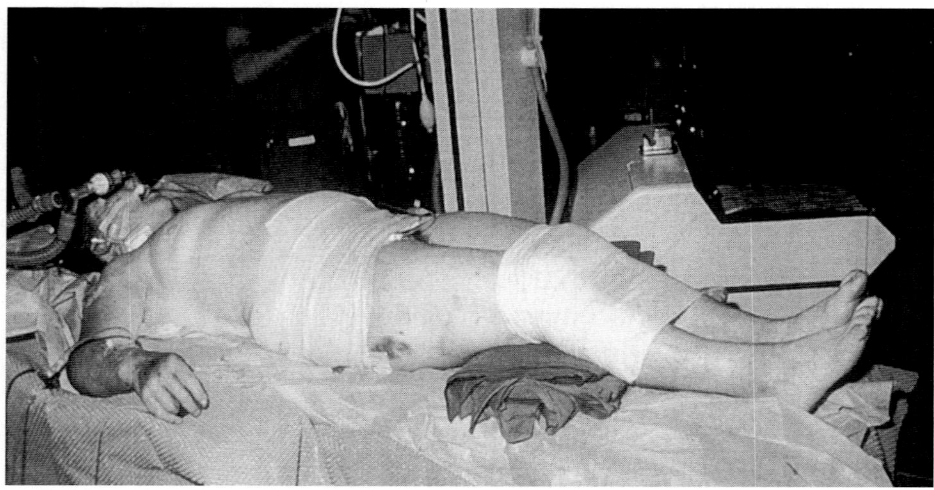

FIGURE 8-8. Positioning of the patient with pelvic ring disruption in the emergency room.

ing room positioner or total body vacuum splint. The patient lies on it and then the splint is pushed up about the flanks and ilium, and when a reduction is accomplished the splint is exhausted and will then hold the reduction. This allows the anterior abdominal wall to remain uncovered. If time permits, the application of longitudinal traction on the involved side will help control any posterior translation.

External Fixation

Primary and definitive internal fixation of the disrupted pelvis is not possible in the multiply injured patient in critical condition. In contrast, external fixation of the pelvis has been demonstrated to temporarily stabilize an unstable pelvic fracture and effectively restore pelvic volume, thus improving survival (45,46). Moreover, if pelvic packing is used, a stable posterior ring is mandatory to give sufficient resistance for effective packing of the true pelvis. The application of external fixation has become a resuscitative tool that should be applied as soon as possible even before laparotomy (47,48). Three potential mechanisms may explain the role of pelvic stabilization for the control of retroperitoneal bleeding, although this effect does not work in every patient (49).

1. Stabilization of the pelvic ring can prevent dislodgement of hemostatic clots, especially when transferring the patient for diagnostic procedures (50,51).
2. Fracture reduction reopposes bleeding osseous surfaces, thus promoting clot formation and decreasing blood loss (47).

A

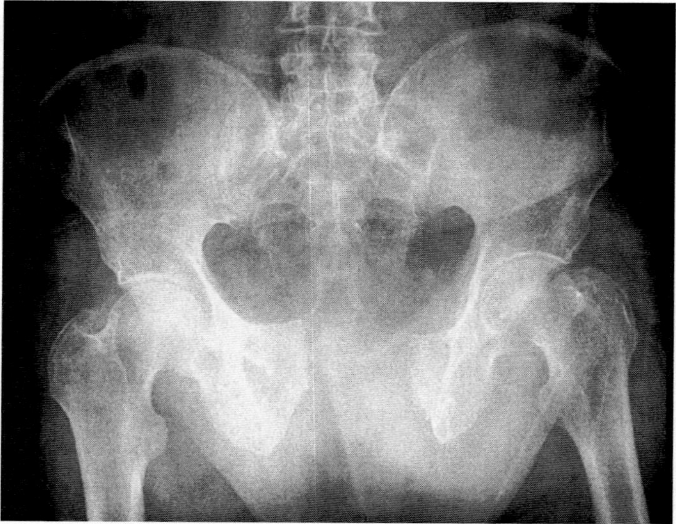

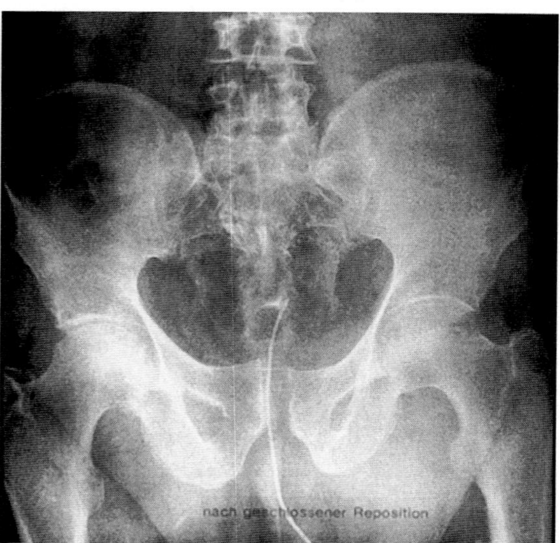

B

FIGURE 8-9. Patient with "open-book" type injury before and after closed reduction and wrapping the hip and knee joints. **A:** Before closed reduction. **B:** After closed reduction.

3. Reducing the diastasis will significantly decrease the volume of a widened pelvis (52–54).

Although some authors believe in a spontaneous retroperitoneal tamponade of hemorrhage from nonarterial sources (47,53–55), there is sufficient potential space for significant continued bleeding along the lacunae distally and cranially toward the chest (23, 32). In multiply injured patients with pelvic disruption it can be fatal to rely on retroperitoneal self-tamponade. Moreover, dramatic hemorrhage despite external fixation can continue in patients with open fractures and fractures in which there is no significant reduction in the pelvic volume (32).

Different techniques are available to externally fix the unstable pelvic ring. The external fixator only gives sufficient stability in patients with an open-book type injury. Although many different anterior frames have been described in the past, none of those effectively stabilizes the posterior ring in type C pelvic ring instability (56). Therefore, in the presence of a completely unstable type C injury (APC III, Bucholz 3) the pelvic C-clamp is recommended (57). If, however, the expertise for the pelvic C-clamp or the instrument itself is not available, then external fixation in combination with traction may be used.

External Fixator

The external fixator represents an important tool of resuscitation with hemorrhage control in multiply injured patients with associated pelvic ring instability (58). Moreover, it is a temporary treatment for the anterior pelvic ring instability, allows mobilization of the patient on the ICU, and reduces pain and stress. In certain situations—such as open pelvic ring injury or associated injury of genitourinary organs—the external fixator may be used as primary definitive treatment, but only for stabilization of the anterior pelvic ring.

Frame constructions have been simplified over the past years, especially in the emergency situation. It should be emphasized again that frames of any construction or multiple pins do not allow control of vertical instability. Two routes of pin placement can be applied: (a) the upper pin placement in the crest behind the anterior superior iliac spine; and (b) the lower pin placement at the anterior inferior iliac spine. The first route described should be used in patients in extremis, because the placement of pins into the iliac crest is simple and an image intensifier is not necessary. However, at least two pins on each side of the pelvis have to be placed to achieve a sufficient hold. The lower pin placement provides a better hold and one pin on each side of the pelvis is enough to obtain sufficient strength. However, there are potential dangers, such as intraarticular positioning of the pin and injuries of vessels and nerves. Therefore, this technique is best reserved for less urgent or elective situations (58).

Pelvic C-Clamp

The pelvic C-clamp (57,59) is a device that is applied posteriorly (Fig. 8-10). Pressure is applied through pins placed in the area of the pelvis lateral to the sacroiliac joints. The C-clamp as a posterior device is mechanically superior to any anterior frame, especially in the case of C-type injuries (56). It can be applied within 15 minutes with sufficient stability of the pelvic ring, including for pelvic packing. Although the application is not very difficult, its use should be practiced first in the anatomy laboratory. In contrast to previous studies (60), no loss of reduction or loosening of the pins was observed in our own series (23). Additionally, none of the complications, such as vascular and nerve injuries or displacement of the unstable hemipelvis into the true pelvis, were noted (23). The pelvic C-clamp may not be used in the presence of iliac wing fracture.

Pneumatic Antishock Garment

The application of the pneumatic antishock garment (PASG) is not limited to the pre-hospital phase of treatment, where it has had the widest use, but it also has a role in the in-hospital management of patients (Fig. 8-11) (61). The physiologic effects of the device are best reviewed by Pelligra and Sandberg (62). In their article they review 75 years of clinical reports and experience on the use of "circumferential pneumatic compression." One can summarize the principal clinical effects of the PASG as these: (a) short-lasting hemostasis (tamponade); (b) autotransfusion; and (c) increased peripheral vascular resistance.

The hemostatic effect is thought to be related to the external pressure, reducing the vessel wall pressure in a bleeding vessel as well as its radius. The combined effects of lowered vessel wall tension and diminished flow owing to the reduced radius, allow the patient's own, often "marginal, clotting mechanisms to take over" (62). By the same mechanism of reducing vessel radius, there is an increase in peripheral vascular resistance. In terms of the autotransfusion effect, the volume obviously depends on the size of the patient and has been variously estimated to be equivalent to 250 to 1,000 mL of "autotransfusion" (62). The combination of these three effects—hemostasis, autotransfusion, and increased peripheral vascular resistance—results in: (a) a decrease of ongoing blood loss; (b) a measurable increase in venous return and CVP; and (c) a significant improvement in mean arterial pressure. The garment also acts as a splint to reduce the displaced hemipelvis as well as any associated long bone lower extremity fractures. The advantages as well as numerous disadvantages of the device are summarized in Table 8-4.

To our mind, the PASG should only be used in the prehospital phase in countries with long transport times. In the ER, external fixation with fixator or C-clamp has much more advantages and allows more surgical treatment options in the multiply injured patient (23). All advantages of the PASG can be achieved with external fixator or C-clamp without the massive disadvantages (Table 8-4). The effect of the PASG is only short lasting. Its prolonged use can cause compartment syndrome of the lower extremity and it is very hard to apply in the case of fractures (63). Finally, it can dramatically

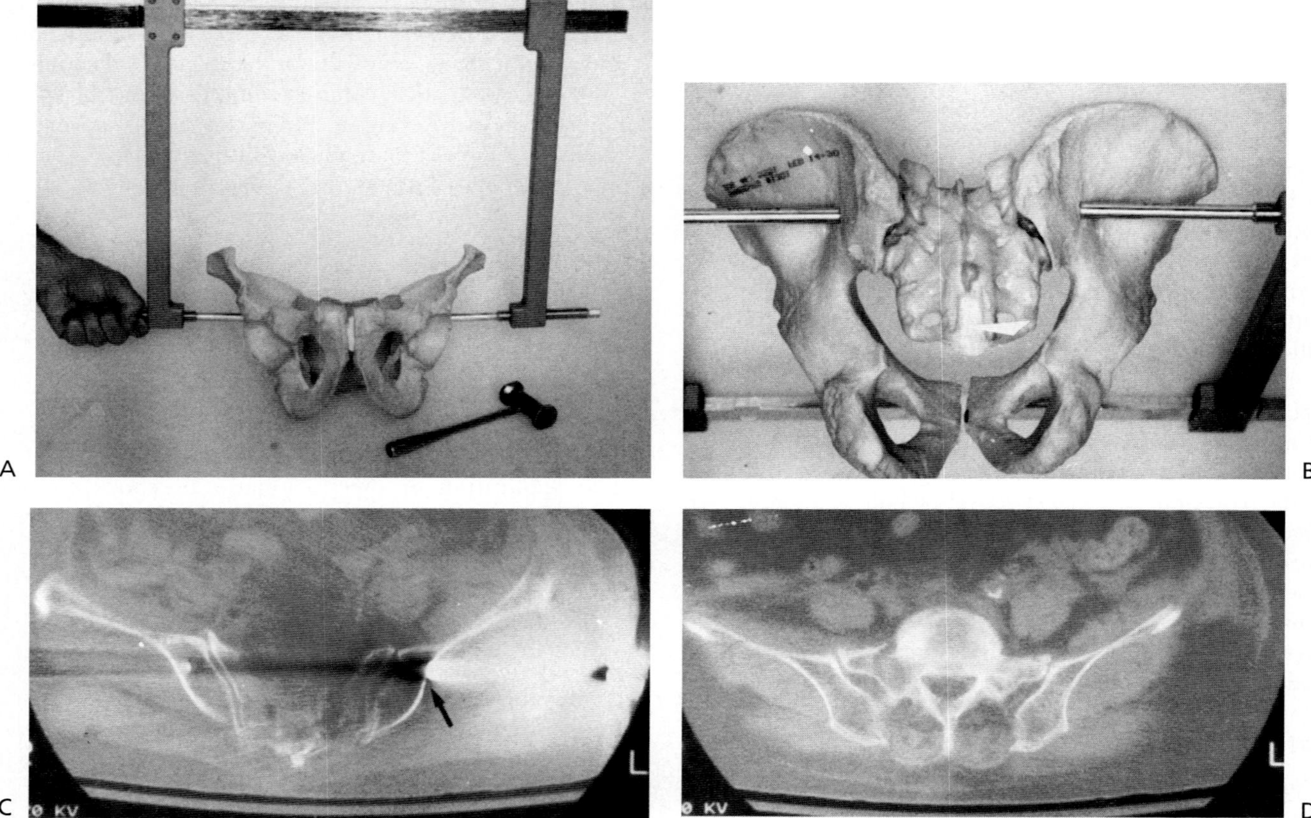

FIGURE 8-10. **A:** The AO pelvic clamp. **B:** The clamp is applied in the axis of the sacroiliac joints by hammering the spikes into the outer table of the ilium. **C:** Compression can then be obtained across the posterior lesion, stabilizing the pelvic ring, as noted in the computed tomography. This woman sustained a markedly displaced sacral fracture and had uncontrollable bleeding from the retroperineal space. **D:** Application of the clamp *(black arrow, C)* allowed restoration of the posterior sacral fracture and stabilization of the patient, who survived.

worsen chest and/or brain injuries through increased intrapulmonary pressure and reduced lung compliance.

Control of Pelvic Hemorrhage

The origin of bleeding after pelvic injury can be an injury of pelvic arteries, the venous plexus, and/or the cancellous bone in the case of sacral fracture and iliac wing fractures. The most common pelvic artery injured after blunt trauma is the superior gluteal artery, followed by the internal pudendal, obturator, and lateral sacral arteries. Contrast-enhanced CT, a noninvasive procedure, has allowed the earlier diagnosis of arterial bleeding. However, arterial injuries causing significant pelvic bleeding only occur in about 10% of cases. In contrast, pelvic venous hemorrhage occurs often and may be severe. The mechanism can involve retrograde flow of blood through the valveless portal venous system into the inferior mesentery vein and then to the "pelvic vascular sink." Major disruption of the presacral and/or pre-

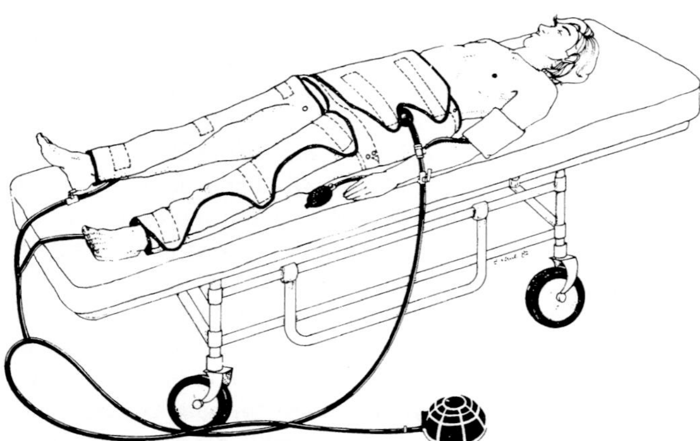

FIGURE 8-11. Diagram of a patient wearing a pneumatic antishock garment.

TABLE 8-4. PNEUMATIC ANTISHOCK GARMENT

Advantages	Disadvantages
Simple	Short-lasting volume effect
Rapid	Compartment syndrome of lower extremity
Reversible	Decreased access to abdomen and lower extremity
Accessible and available	Decreased visibility of abdomen and lower extremities
Safe	Fracture of lower extremity
	Decreases lung compliance

vesical plexus often needs surgical intervention, including pelvic packing. Bleeding from cancellous bone occurs in the presence of sacral and iliac fractures. Reduction of those fractures and compression with an external device such as a C-clamp allow immediate bleeding control.

It is believed that reduction and stabilization of the pelvic ring results in spontaneous hemostasis of retroperitoneal bleeding by decreasing pelvic volume and consequent tamponade-like effect. The intraoperative findings of our own study (23) revealed that the self-tamponade of the retroperitoneal bleeding can fail despite external fixation of the pelvic ring independently of the device used. Pelvic ring disruption dependent on the forces leads to severe damage of the constraining ligaments of the pelvic ring and also of the pelvic floor and the iliopectineal fascia. The loss of these ligamentous structures hampers the body's natural effort to achieve effective retroperitoneal self-tamponade. Moreover, the retroperitoneal space around the pelvis is not separated cranially by constraining compartments. Thus, the retroperitoneal hematoma can drain through the ruptured pelvic floor not only into the two lacunae, but also into the abdomen or chest. Although not occurring in all patients, circulatory decompensation owing to continuous bleeding can lead to a fatal outcome. Therefore, in patients with persistently increased lactate levels despite external fixation, laparotomy and pelvic packing seem to be the most effective techniques of bleeding control.

Pelvic Packing

The rationale for pelvic packing follows:

1. Bleeding from the venous plexus can be effectively controlled only by local packing.
2. Arterial bleeding also can be successfully treated by pelvic packs.
3. Bleeding from large-bore vessels can only be controlled surgically.
4. Complex pelvic injuries are often combined with intraperitoneal lesions that can be treated through the same approach.

A midline incision from the xiphoid down to the symphysis is carried out for pelvic packing in multiply injured patients with associated pelvic ring disruption and hemorrhage. The retroperitoneum is opened after evaluation of the abdominal cavity and mobilization of the colon on both sides. In the majority of patients, all parapelvic fascias and ligamentous structures are ruptured. A direct manual access down to the sacrum and the sacroiliac joints is possible without sharp dissection. Normally, a huge hematoma is present on the side of injury. This is removed. Primary orientation includes a check for an arterial bleeding or a tear of large bore vessels, which is rare. If such an injury is present, in most patients resulting from critical condition, ligation of the vessel, even of a large bore vein, is advisable. Only a tear of the common or external iliac artery should be repaired. In the presence of massive bleeding a transient cross-clamping of the infrarenal part of the aorta should be performed. A specific source of bleeding cannot be identified in the majority of patients because the origin of the bleeding is either diffuse or generated from an injury of the presacral and prevesical plexus. The presacral and prevesical regions are packed with 5 to 10 swabs on both sides of the pelvis. Although some authors recommend an extraperitoneal approach, to our mind this technique does not allow sufficient packing of the fracture side, because bleeding will continue to the contralateral side. This area cannot be reached via the extraperitoneal approach. The effectiveness of the tamponade is checked. The base deficit and lactate should decrease. The abdomen is left open after packing to avoid abdominal compartment syndrome (29). The patient is transported to the ICU for stabilization of his or her vital organ functions.

Contrast-Enhanced Computed Tomography

Early diagnosis of arterial bleeding is desirable for optimizing therapeutic intervention in the pelvic trauma patient. Contrast-enhanced CT of the pelvis, which is often performed for hemodynamically stable trauma patients, is a noninvasive procedure that is highly accurate in determining the presence or absence of ongoing pelvic hemorrhage (Fig. 8-6) (64,65). This information can be invaluable in the timing of diagnostic tests, such as angiography, and therapeutic interventions, such as timely selective embolization of mid-sized pelvic arteries, such as the gluteals, or obturator.

Angiography: Indications

Angiography as a diagnostic and therapeutic tool has been recommended as an alternative for the control of pelvic hemorrhage. It is primarily used in North America and in those countries in which a multidisciplinary approach for the management of multiply injured patients exists. In addition, the patient population seen in the ER of Level I trauma centers in North America may differ from that found in European centers. Because of the high density of rescue and transport devices and short transport times, the number of patients in extremis who need open surgery rather than lesser invasive techniques may be higher in Europe than in North America. Moreover, the indication for angiography should also take into account the location of posterior ring instability and the extent of the trauma impact.

The North American approach at the beginning is similar to that in European trauma centers. The patient who has a severe pelvic injury with hemorrhage is treated primarily with an emergency external fixation. The fixator may be applied in these emergent situations in the ER or the operating suite in 15 to 30 minutes while the angiography suite is prepared. In North American trauma centers, angiographic intervention is undertaken if the patient's hemodynamic profile does not improve with application of the fixator and there is no evidence of intraabdominal bleeding, whereas in our institution the patient would undergo emergency laparotomy. With a positive ultrasound or grossly bloody abdominal lavage specimen and a high-risk pelvic injury, either fixator or laparotomy may be performed first. However, if packing is going to be needed, then an external frame must be applied prior to the retroperitoneal packing.

The disadvantages of angiography are obvious. In the study of Agolini and coworkers (66), only 1.9% of patients with pelvic ring injury required embolization. Although the authors could successfully stop bleeding in all of their embolized patients, the mortality rate was high. Moreover, if angiography is not available in the ER, then the hemodynamically unstable patient has to be transported to the angiography suite. This represents a high risk for the patient if vital organ functions suddenly fail because of increasing bleeding. Therapeutic angiography is time consuming and needs the 24-hour service of an expert radiologist. Finally, embolization can cause gluteal muscle necrosis, which has a high mortality because of septic complications (67).

Diagnostic Arteriography

The procedure usually is done with the patient under local anesthesia, although general anesthesia is readily used as an alternative if the patient is unable to cooperate. General anesthesia is maintained if the patient is being transferred directly from the operating room.

A multihole catheter is inserted percutaneously through a femoral artery and advanced into the lower abdominal aorta. If the patient is hypertensive or in shock, there may be severe generalized constriction of the arteries; therefore, the femoral pulses may be difficult to palpate. This does not preclude performance of the procedure. The location of the femoral arteries varies minimally from patient to patient, and "blind" catheterization is almost always successful.

The first diagnostic angiogram is the pelvic aortogram (Fig. 8-12A–D). This gives some knowledge of the major arterial anatomy and may demonstrate the bleeding site. Selective internal iliac arteriography then is performed. This frequently allows more precise localization of bleeding sites and may also demonstrate clinically significant bleeding that was not apparent at all on the initial study. The bleeding site is identified by focal extravasation of contrast material in the arterial phase, usually persisting well into the capillary and venous phases. Associated findings may be focal arterial spasm, displacement, draping, and compression of vessels owing to hematoma. If findings of arteriography are normal, it is assumed that major bleeding was arterial and has stopped spontaneously, or is venous, or both. Venography is useless for detection of venous bleeding and should not be performed.

Therapeutic Angiography

Embolization may be performed using a variety of materials, according to the preference of the clinician, including autologous clot, Gelfoam, or metal coils (Fig. 8-12E).

Immediately following catheterization of the aorta, 25 mL of blood is withdrawn and placed in a sterile beaker. Formation of the typical gelatin-like clot occurs in about 15 minutes. If the patient has received multiple blood transfusions, then a clot may not form at all. In some of these cases, a few drops of thrombin added to the blood quickly produce a good clot, but if this does not occur within another 15 minutes, small pieces of Gelfoam are used as the occluding agent. Gelfoam tends to produce permanent occlusion of arteries, and inadvertent embolization of important nonbleeding arteries could have serious consequences, in contrast to an autologous clot, which would lyse within 12 hours in a nontraumatized blood vessel. Therefore, autologous clot is our agent of choice, and Gelfoam is reserved for patients whose blood cannot form a good clot.

Transcatheter occlusion of bleeding arteries ideally involves subselective catheterization. The prevention of tissue infarction obviously is of some concern, and the risk is inversely proportional to the degree of selectivity of the arterial occlusion. When the tip of the angiographic catheter is in satisfactory position, pieces of autologous clot 1 cm in diameter (or pieces of Gelfoam 3 mm in diameter) are formed with a scissors, mixed with radiographic contrast material in a plastic syringe, and eased with gentle pressure through the catheter into the artery. The contrast material allows us to carefully monitor the path of the occluding agent as well as the efficacy of occlusion, alerting us to reflux backout of the branch, which might produce inadvertent embolization of nonbleeding branches. Although this may not always be prevented, the technique usually is free of harmful sequelae, because there are multiple sources of collateral flow in the pelvis. Embolization is continued with fluoroscopic monitoring until it is felt that no further extravasation is present and the feeding vessel or vessels are occluded, as confirmed by arteriography. It is important to note that the clinical significance of arterial bleeding may not necessarily correlate well with the amount of extravasation demonstrated on the arteriogram. In view of this, all sites of extravasation must be embolized before concluding that definitive treatment has been completed. The concern with autologous clot and Gelfoam is the recanalization of the vessel in 5 to 10 days and then a significant rebleeding episode. The use of a permanent nonresorbable metallic coil avoids this problem and is recommended for selective embolization.

For the rare laceration of an internal iliac artery, em-

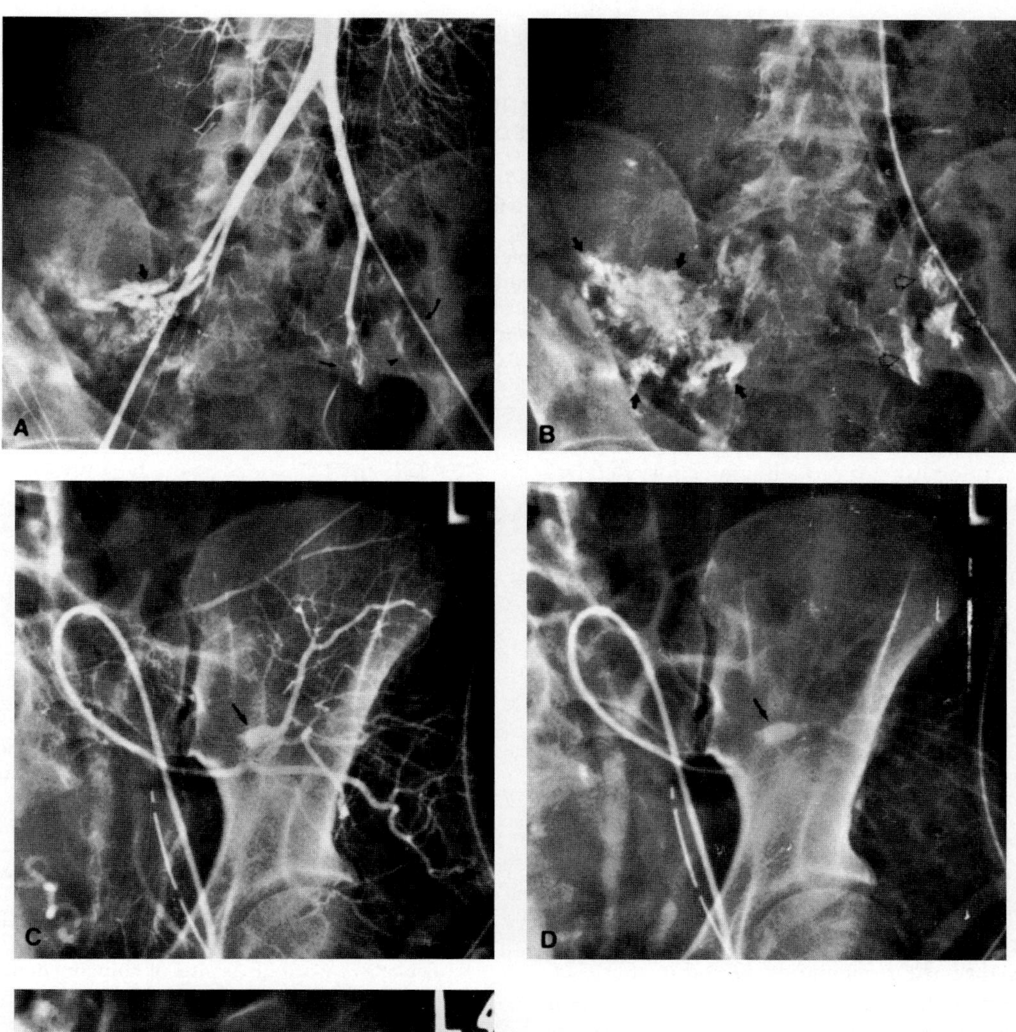

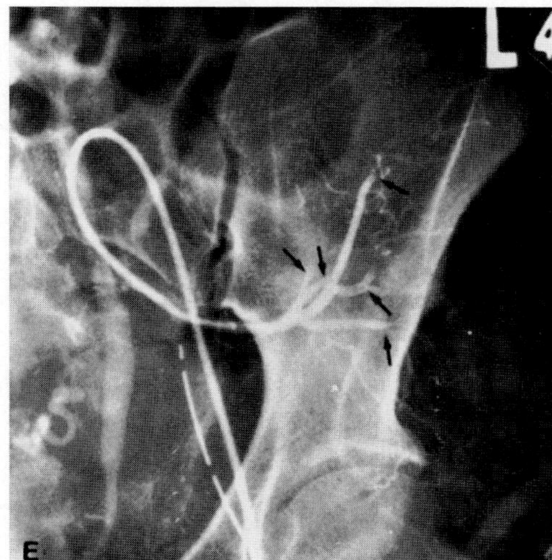

FIGURE 8-12. A: Pelvic aortography done via left femoral catheterization *(curved arrows).* Note massive extravasation from right internal iliac artery *(thick arrow)* and spasm of branch of left internal artery *(thin arrow).* A catheter is present in left iliac vein *(arrowheads).* **B:** Venous phase of the same aortogram shows massive extravasation from both internal iliac arteries. **C:** Ovoid collection of extravasated contrast shown in midarterial phase of selective superior gluteal arteriogram. **D:** Extravasation persists well into venous phase of superior gluteal arteriogram. **E:** The branches of the superior gluteal artery have been occluded, and no further extravasation is seen.

TABLE 8-5. TIMING OF SECONDARY SURGICAL PROCEDURES

Physiological Status	Surgical Intervention	Timing
Response to resuscitation	⊖ → Life saving surgery	D 1
	(?) → "Damage control"	
	⊕ → Delayed primary surgery	
Hyperinflammation	"Second look" only!	D 2–4
Window of opportunity	Scheduled definitive surgery	D 5–14
Immunosuppression	No surgery!	Wk 3
Recovery		

TABLE 8-6. CRITERIA FOR JUDGING THE MOST ESSENTIAL ORGAN FUNCTIONS OF THE MULTIPLY INJURED PATIENT BEFORE PERFORMING SECONDARY PROCEDURES

Chest radiograph	No evidence for increasing infiltration of both lungs
Pao_2/Fio_2	>250
Arterial blood pressure	Stable within normal limits
Fluid balance	Negative or at least balanced
Intracranial pressure	<15 cm H_2O
Temperature	Normothermic
Platelet counts	>100,000 and increasing
Leukocytes	>2,000 or <15,000 (no signs of sepsis)

bolization with autologous clot or Gelfoam is not effective, because the agent merely passes out of the lumen through the laceration. In this case, one might use tissue adhesives such as 2-isobutylcyanoacrylate. Laceration of the common or external iliac arteries must be dealt with surgically. Recently the use of intraarterial stents has been successful in the management of larger-caliber arterial injuries. Rupture of major veins also is not amenable to embolization because of the direction of blood flow and embolic material away from the bleeding site toward the lungs.

DEFINITIVE FRACTURE CARE IN THE MULTIPLY INJURED PATIENT

The primary care with diagnostic and damage control procedures is followed by the regeneration period in the ICU. Hemodynamic and pulmonary stability is an assumption for the planned secondary procedures. Moreover, during the first 4 days after trauma the host reacts with a whole body inflammation to trauma, shock, ischemia-reperfusion injury, mass transfusions, and stress (Table 8-5). During this period, long-lasting orthopedic procedures with high blood loss should be avoided, because the wrong time point can contribute to the onset of organ failure ("second-hit phenomenon")(68). However, evacuation of hematoma, extensive debridement of soft-tissue necrosis, and elimination of septic foci is mandatory at this stage to prevent deterioration of organ functions. Careful assessment of the patients condition using generally accepted criteria for evaluation support decision making (Table 8-6).

Operative treatment then normally starts at the end of the first week, including definite open reduction and internal fixation of all fractures, joint reconstruction, and additional reconstructive procedures. If possible, all secondary procedures should be finished at the end of the second week, because thereafter the risk of infection significantly increases owing to immunosuppression.

In the case of a perfect trauma management system, the patient is in the weaning period or even extubated during week 3 after trauma. The patient should be free from sedation and only require low levels of analgesic medication. An intensive rehabilitation program can begin. This is started after discharge from the ICU and should be continued to allow for complete rehabilitation and social reintegration.

REFERENCES

1. Platz A, et al. Assessment: principles and management of major trauma beyond ATLS. *Curr Orthop* 2001;15:167.
2. McMurtry RY, Walton D, Dickinson D, et al. Pelvic disruption in the polytraumatized patient: a management protocol. *Clin Orthop* 1980;151:22.
3. Gilliland MD, Ward RE, Barton RM, et al. Factors affecting mortality in pelvic fractures. *J Trauma* 1982;22:691.
4. Rothenberger DA, Fischer RP, Strate RG, et al. The mortality associated with pelvic fractures. *Surgery* 1978;84:356.
5. Demetriades D, et al. Pelvic fractures: epidemiology and predictors of associated abdominal injuries and outcomes. *J Am Coll Surg* 2002;195:1.
6. Richardson JD, Harty J, Amin M, et al. Open pelvic fractures. *J Trauma* 1982;22:533.
7. Beal SL, Blaisdell FW. Traumatic hemipelvectomy: a catastrophic injury. *J Trauma* 1989;29:1346.
8. Poole GV, Ward EF, Muakkassa FF, et al. Pelvic fracture from major blunt trauma. *Ann Surg* 1991;213:532.
9. Poole GV, Ward EF. Causes of mortality in patients with pelvic fractures. *Orthopedics* 1994;17:691.
10. Mucha P Jr. Recognizing and avoiding complications with pelvic fractures. *Infect Surg* 1985;4:53.
11. Trunkey DD, Chapman MW, Lim RC, et al. Management of pelvic fractures in blunt trauma injury. *J Trauma* 1974;14:912.
12. Looser KG, Crombie, H.D. Pelvic fractures: an anatomic guide to severity of injury. Review of 100 cases. *Am J Surg* 1976; 132:638.
13. Chong K, et al. Pelvic fractures and mortality. *Iowa Orthop J* 1997;17:110.
14. Dalal SA, Burgess AR, Siegel JH. Pelvic fracture in multiple trauma: classification by mechanism is key to pattern of organ injury, resuscitative requirements, and outcome. *J Trauma* 1989; 29:981.
15. Fox MA, Mangiante EC, Fabian TC, et al. Pelvic fractures: an analysis of factors affecting pre-hospital triage and patient outcome. *South Med J* 1990;83:785.
16. Ertel W, et al. Therapeutic strategies and outcome of polytraumatized patients with pelvic injuries—a six year experience. *Eur J Trauma* 2000;6:278.
17. Biffl WL, Smith WR, Moore EE, et al. Evolution of a multidisciplinary clinical pathway for the management of unstable patients with pelvic fractures. *Ann Surg* 2001;233:843.
18. Collicott PE, Hughes I. Training in advanced trauma life support. *JAMA* 243:1156, 1980.
19. Abramson D, Scalae TM, Hitchcock R, et al. Lactate clearance and survival following injury. *J Trauma* 1993;35:584.
20. Davis JW. The relationship of base deficit to lactate in porcine hemorrhagic shock and resuscitation. *J Trauma* 1994;36:168.
21. Mizock BA, Falk JL. Lactic acidosis in critical illness. *Crit Care Med* 1992;20:80.
22. Rashkin MC, Bosken C, Baughman RP, et al. Oxygen delivery in critically ill patients: relationship to blood lactate and survival. *Chest* 1985;87:580.

23. Ertel W, Keel M, Eid K, et al. Control of severe hemorrhage using C-clamp and pelvic packing in multiply injured patients with pelvic ring disruption. *J Orthop Trauma* 2001;15:468.
24. Teasdale G, Jennett B. Assessment of coma and impaired consciousness: a practical scale. *Lancet* 1974;2:81.
25. Chesnut RM, Marshall LF, Klauber MR, et al. The role of secondary brain injury in determining outcome from severe head injury. *J Trauma* 1993;34:216.
26. Chesnut RM, Marshall SB, Pick J, et al. Early and late systemic hypotension as frequent and fundamental source of cerebral ischemia following severe brain injury in the traumatic coma data bank. *Acta Neurochir* 1993;59:121.
27. Ertel W, et al. Causes of shock in the severely traumatized patient: emergency treatment. In: Goris RJA, Trentz O, eds. *The integrated approach to trauma care.* New York: Springer-Verlag, 1995.
28. Rotondo M, et al. Damage control: an approach for improved survival in exsanguinating penetrating abdominal injury. *J Trauma* 1993;35:375.
29. Ertel W, Oberholzer A, Platz A, et al. Incidence and clinical pattern of the abdominal compartment syndrome following "damage-control" laparotomy in 311 patients with severe abdominal and/or pelvic trauma. *Crit Care Med* 2000;28:1747.
30. Bone LB, Johnson KJ, Weigelt, JA, et al. Early versus delayed stabilization of femoral fractures. *J Bone Joint Surg* 1989;71-A:336.
31. Behrmann SW, et al. Improved outcome with femur fractures: early versus delayed fixation. *J Trauma* 1990;30:792.
32. Riemer BL, Butterfield SL, Diamond DL, et al. Acute mortality associated with injuries to the pelvic ring: the role of early patient mobilization and external fixation. *J Trauma* 1993;35:671.
33. Reynolds MA, Richardson JD, Spain DA, et al. Is the timing of fracture fixation important for the patient with multiple trauma? *Ann Surg* 1995;222:470.
34. Boulanger BR, Stephen D, Brenneman FD, et al. Thoracic trauma and early intramedullary nailing of femur fractures: are we doing harm? *J Trauma* 1997;43:24.
35. Bosse MJ, MacKenzie EJ, Reiner, BL, et al. Adult respiratory distress syndrome, pneumonia, and mortality following thoracic injury and a femoral fracture treated either with intramedullary nailing with reaming or with a plate. *J Bone Joint Surg* 1997;79-A:799.
36. Scalea TM, Boswell SA, Scott JD, et al. External fixation as a bridge to intramedullary nailing for patients with multiple injuries and with femur fractures: damage control orthopedics. *J Trauma* 2000;48:613.
37. Pape HC, Auf'm'Kolk M, Paffrath T, et al. Primary intramedullary femur fixation in multiple trauma patients with associated lung contusion: a cause of posttraumatic ARDS? *J Trauma* 1993;34:540.
38. Pape HC, Regal G, Dwenger A, et al. Influences of different methods of intramedullary femoral nailing on lung function in patients with multiple trauma. *J Trauma* 1993;35:709.
39. Wenda K, Runkel M, Degreif J, et al. Pathogenesis and clinical relevance of bone marrow embolism in medullary nailing—demonstrated by intraoperative echocardiography. *Injury* 1993; 24-S3:73.
40. Burgess AR. Fractures of the pelvic ring. In: Rockwood CA, Green DP, eds. *Fractures in adults,* 3rd ed. Philadelphia: JB Lippincott, 1990.
41. Young JWR, Burgess AR. *Radiologic management of pelvic ring fractures: systemic radiographic diagnosis.* Baltimore: Urban & Schwarzenberg, 1987.
42. Wright CS, McMurtry RY, Pickard J. A postmortem review of trauma mortalities: a comparative study. *J Trauma* 1984;24:67.
43. Wright CS, McMurtry RY, Hoyle M, et al. Preventable deaths in multiple trauma: a review of trauma unit mortalities—the Sunnybrook experience. *Can J Surg* 1983;26:20.
44. Peltier IE. Open pelvic fractures: discussion. *J Trauma* 1982; 22:537.
45. Gylling SF, Ward RE, Holcroft JW, et al. Immediate external fixation of unstable pelvic fractures. *Am J Surg* 1985;150:721.
46. Latenser BA, Gentilello LM, Tarver AA, et al. Improved outcome with early fixation of skeletally unstable pelvic fractures. *J Trauma* 1991;31:28.
47. Kellam JF. The role of external fixation in pelvic disruptions. *Clin Orthop* 1989;241:66.
48. Ghanayem AJ, Wilber JH, Lieberman JM, et al. The effect of laparotomy and external fixator stabilization on pelvic volume in an unstable pelvic injury. *J Trauma* 1995;38:396.
49. Ghanayem AJ, Stoverr MD, Goldstein JA, et al. Emergent treatment of pelvic fractures. *CORR* 1995;318:75.
50. Brotman S, Soderstrom CA, Oster-Granite M, et al. Management of severe bleeding in fractures of the pelvis. *Surg Gynecol Obstet* 1981;153:823.
51. Failinger MS, McGanity PL. Unstable pelvic fractures. *J Bone Joint Surg* 1992;74-A:781.
52. Mears DC, Fu FH. Modern concepts of external skeletal fixation of the pelvis. *Clin Orthop* 1980;151:65.
53. Tile M. Pelvic ring fractures: should they be fixed? *J Bone Joint Surg* 1988;70-B:1.
54. Trafton PG. Pelvic ring fractures. *Surg Clin North Am* 1990; 70:655.
55. Flint LM Jr, et al. Definitive control of mortality from severe pelvic fracture. *Ann Surg* 1990;211:703.
56. Pohlemann T, Krettek C, Hoffman R, et al. Biomechanical comparison of various emergency stabilization measures of the pelvic ring. *Unfallchirurg* 1994;97:503.
57. Ganz R, et al. The anti-shock pelvic clamp. *Clin Orthop* 1991;167:71.
58. Bircher MD. Indications and techniques of external fixation of the injured pelvis. *Injury* 1996(Suppl 27);2:S-B3.
59. Heini PF, Witt J, Ganz R, et al. The pelvic C-clamp for the emergency treatment of unstable pelvic ring injuries: a report on clinical experience of 30 cases. *Injury* 1996;27:S-A38.
60. Bartlett C, Asprinio D, Louis S, et al. Intrapelvic dislocation of the left hemipelvis as a complication of the pelvic C-clamp: a case report and review. *J Orthop Trauma* 1997;11:540.
61. Crile GW. *Blood pressure in surgery: experimental and clinical research.* Philadelphia: JB Lippincott, 1903.
62. Pelligra R, Sandberg ED. Control of intractable abdominal bleeding by external counter pressure. *JAMA* 1979;241:708.
63. Aprahamian C, Gessert G, Banclyk DF, et al. MAST-associated compartment syndrome (MACS): a review. *J Trauma* 1989;29:549.
64. Stephens DJ, Kreder HJ, Day AC, et al. Early detection of arterial bleeding in acute pelvic trauma. *J Trauma* 1999;47(4): 638–642.
65. Shanmuganathan K, Mirvis SE, Sover ER. Value of contrast-enhanced CT in detecting active hemorrhage in patients with blunt abdominal or pelvic trauma. *AJR* 1993;161:65–69.
66. Agolini SF, Shahk, Jaffe J, et al. Arterial embolization is a rapid and effective technique for controlling pelvic fracture hemorrhage. *J Trauma* 1997;43:395.
67. Takahira N, Shindo M, Tamaka K, et al. Gluteal muscle necrosis following transcatheter angiographic embolisation for retroperitoneal hemorrhage associated with pelvic fracture. *Injury* 2001;32:27.
68. Tscherne H, Regel G, Pape HC, et al. Internal fixation of multiple fractures in patients with polytrauma. *CORR* 1998;347:62.

9

PELVIC TRAUMA AND VENOUS THROMBOEMBOLISM

WILLIAM H. GEERTS
RICHARD M. JAY

INTRODUCTION

Among hospitalized patients, those who have sustained major trauma experience the greatest risk for venous thromboembolism (VTE) (1–3). Objectively documented deep vein thrombosis (DVT) is detected in 40% to 80% of major trauma patients who do not receive thromboprophylaxis (1,4). Death from pulmonary embolism (PE), reported in 0.4% to 2.0% of patients following major trauma (1,5,6), often occurs without warning as patients are recovering from their injuries (7). Among 13,000 admissions to six regional trauma centers, 17% of the preventable deaths were caused by pulmonary emboli related to failure to use thromboprophylaxis (8). Thromboembolic complications of trauma delay hospital discharge, lead to readmissions, and increase the cost of care (9,10). In the face of high thromboembolic risks and published prophylaxis guidelines, this issue also has important medical—legal significance (11).

This chapter reviews the risks of DVT and PE as well as the diagnosis, treatment, and prevention of venous thromboembolism in pelvic trauma patients. Algorithms for the diagnosis and prophylaxis of thromboembolic complications after pelvic fractures are presented.

EPIDEMIOLOGY OF VENOUS THROMBOEMBOLISM IN PELVIC TRAUMA

There is considerable evidence that patients with pelvic and other lower extremity fractures have a particularly high risk of thromboembolic complications (1,12,13). The prevalence of DVT in pelvic fracture patients not receiving any prophylaxis has been assessed in several small prospective studies (Table 9-1) (1,4,14–16). Maliska and colleagues performed bilateral contrast venography in 11 patients with pelvic fractures an average of 1 week after injury and before surgery; DVT was found in 36% (14). Kudsk and coworkers diagnosed DVT in five of the eight pelvic fracture patients who had venography between 7 and 12 days after admission (4). In another study, 16% of 50 major pelvic fracture patients who underwent serial duplex ultrasonography were found to have DVT (15). DVT was reported in

TABLE 9-1. PROSPECTIVE STUDIES OF DEEP VEIN THROMBOSIS (DVT) PREVALENCE USING OBJECTIVE SCREENING TESTS IN PELVIC FRACTURE PATIENTS NOT RECEIVING THROMBOPROPHYLAXIS

Author, Year (Ref)	Screening Test	N	DVT (%)	Proximal DVT (%)
Maliska, 1985 (14)	Venography d 7	11	4 (36)	NR
Kudsk, 1989 (4)	Venography d 7–12	8	5 (63)	NR
White, 1990 (15)	DUS weekly until discharge	50	8 (16)	6 (12)
Geerts, 1994 (1)	Venography d 7–21	100	61 (61)	29 (29)
Fisher, 1995 (16)	DUS d 5–7, Doppler studies every 5 d	38	NR	4 (11)

DUS, duplex ultrasonography; NR, not reported.

11% of pelvic fracture patients who were assessed using a single duplex scan and serial venous Doppler examinations (16). In the largest of these studies, our group obtained bilateral contrast venograms in 349 trauma patients with an injury severity score of 9 or greater, none of whom received mechanical or pharmacologic thromboprophylaxis (1). Among the 100 patients with pelvic fractures, DVT was found in 61% and proximal DVT was diagnosed in 29%.

Routine preoperative venous ultrasound screening of 197 patients with acetabular fractures who were prophylaxed with compression stockings and pneumatic compression devices detected DVT in 6% (17). A recent study assessed complications associated with the operative repair of acetabular fractures in 131 patients (18). Despite the perioperative use of combined anticoagulant and mechanical prophylaxis, DVT was the most common complication, occurring in 27% of patients.

Several investigators have recently used magnetic resonance venography (MRV) to assess the presence of venous thrombosis in patients with pelvic fractures (19–22). Montgomery and his associates obtained MRV in 101 acetabular fracture patients; 34% were considered to have proximal DVT based on the MRV (19,20). Forty-nine percent of the thrombi were located in the pelvic veins—internal iliac (29%), external iliac (12%), and common iliac (4%). If these MR abnormalities truly represented thrombi, most would not have been detected by the more commonly used venous imaging test, Doppler ultrasound (DUS). Another study, which compared two mechanical prophylaxis options in pelvic fracture patients, found that almost half of the abnormalities that were called proximal DVT by MRV or DUS were in the pelvic veins (22).

To date, the diagnostic accuracy of MRV as a screening test has not been established. Of great concern is a study in which pelvic trauma patients had both MRV and contrast computed tomography (CT) scans of the pelvis; venography was obtained in the patients with positive tests (21). There was no correlation between the venous abnormalities found in the two positive CT scans and the four positive MRV studies. Furthermore, venography confirmed only one of the positive CT scans and none of the abnormal MRVs.

The majority of venous thrombi occur ipsilateral to the lower extremity injury (20,23,24), but there are many exceptions to this generalization in orthopedic trauma patients (20,25,26).

Prior to the routine use of thromboprophylaxis, PE was reported to be the most common cause of death after pelvic fractures (25,27). In 1961, Sevitt and Gallagher published a classical autopsy study of injured patients (25). Among the 40 patients with pelvic fractures who died, pulmonary emboli were detected in 27%. The risk of symptomatic pulmonary embolism in patients who have had a pelvic fracture has been reported as 2% to 12% (28–36), and fatal PE has been reported in 0% to 10% (17,27–35,37–39). A retrospective review of 60 consecutive patients with minor pelvic fractures (defined as isolated, stable injuries not requiring surgery and allowing mobilization within 48 hours of injury) reported PE in 12% and fatal PE in 6 (10%) (29). In another retrospective review, clinically suspected PE was confirmed by pulmonary angiography in 8% of the 108 pelvic fracture patients, most of whom had received prophylaxis (30). The PE rate in the pelvic trauma patients was almost five times greater than in trauma patients without pelvic fractures. Among 486 patients with fractures of the pelvis or acetabulum who were prophylaxed with subcutaneous heparin plus compression devices, the rates of DVT, PE, and fatal PE were 6%, 2%, and 0.6%, respectively (35).

The risk of symptomatic PE associated with pelvic fracture was 4.5 to 6.9 times greater than that observed in patients without a pelvic fracture among more than 9,000 trauma patients given DVT prophylaxis (40). In a statewide study of 318,554 trauma patients, PE was diagnosed three times more often following pelvic fractures than in the entire trauma cohort (41). The case fatality rate among trauma patients who have had PE is 20% to 50% (32,38,40,41).

Symptomatic VTE and fatal PE are most common in the second to sixth weeks after trauma although, rarely, trauma patients may have fatal PE within a few days of injury and patients may present several months after the initial insult (24,30,40,42–47). Of particular concern to the pelvic surgeon is massive PE occurring intraoperatively during delayed pelvic repair (48,49).

Risk Factors for Venous Thromboembolism in Trauma and Pelvic Fracture Patients

The risk factors predisposing general trauma patients to VTE have been addressed in a number of studies (Table 9-2) (1,4,15,23,24,30,44,50–52). Age is an independent risk factor for thrombosis in trauma patients (1,4,6,23,24,30,43,44,50,52–56). However, young age per se is not an adequate protection against important thromboembolic complications and prophylaxis should not be withheld simply because the patient is below some arbitrary age. Spinal cord injury is associated with a very high thromboembolic risk (1,2,33,44,52), whereas the presence of lower extremity fractures also confers a high risk (1,4,24,33,40,46,53,56–60). The need for one or more surgical interventions (1,23,51), use of a femoral venous line (61,62) or lower extremity venous injury (44,63), and the extent and duration of immobilization (1,23,64) are additional risk factors. The risk of VTE is not related to the severity of the injury in most studies (1,4,6,23,56), although it is in others (41,52,54). This suggests that the patient's specific injuries are more important than injury severity in predicting VTE risk.

In pelvic fracture patients, few studies have specifically addressed risk factors for VTE, although age (12,15,22) and the presence of concomitant lower extremity fractures (1,12,15,32,41,51), appear to be important. Surprisingly, there is no evidence that the risk of VTE correlates with the severity of the pelvic fracture (12). It does not appear that the presence of other injuries (head, thoracic, or abdominal) (12,51), delays in fracture fixation, or the method of treatment (12,15) are predisposing factors in this trauma subgroup.

Among the 100 unprophylaxed pelvic fracture patients we investigated with contrast venography, the DVT and proximal DVT rates did not differ between those that had major injuries (defined as requiring either external or open fixation or with an Abbreviated Injury Scale for the pelvis of three or more) and those that had minor injuries. DVT was found in 40% of patients with isolated pelvic fractures or with additional nonorthopedic injuries, but the rate increased to 84% with concomitant lower extremity fractures. The DVT rates in patients managed with external fixation, with internal fixation, and nonoperatively were 46%, 56%, and 66%, respectively.

TABLE 9-2. RISK FACTORS FOR VENOUS THROMBOEMBOLISM IN GENERAL TRAUMA

Increasing age
Spinal cord injuries
Lower extremity/pelvic fractures
Surgical procedure performed
Femoral venous line
Lower extremity venous injury
Blood transfusion
Prolonged immobilization

TABLE 9-3. FACTORS CONTRIBUTING TO VENOUS THROMBOSIS RISKS IN PELVIC FRACTURE PATIENTS

Venous stasis
Compression of lower extremity and pelvic veins by hematoma, local soft-tissue swelling and increased tissue pressure
Bed rest, traction
Lower extremity immobilization—external fixation devices, plaster casts
Paralysis
Activation of coagulation
Response to the injury
Surgery
Transfusion
Sepsis
Systemic inflammatory response syndrome
Venous endothelial injury
The injury itself
Surgical positioning and manipulation
Femoral venous access catheters
Venous repair

Identifying risk factors for individual patients is not particularly useful because all patients with pelvic fractures have a moderate or high risk of VTE and there is no evidence that altering prophylaxis for pelvic fracture patients with different estimated risks reduces adverse outcomes (38). As discussed below, the use of thromboprophylaxis in these patients is associated with a reduced frequency of VTE (15,65).

Pathophysiology

Patients who have sustained a pelvic fracture are at high risk for venous thrombosis because of the simultaneous occurrence of each of the three criteria (venous stasis, endothelial injury, and coagulation activation) described by Rudolph Virchow in 1856 (Table 9-3) (66). Pelvic fracture and other types of major trauma are profound stimuli for the activation of the coagulation system (67–77). Immobilization is particularly common after pelvic and lower extremity injuries and may be prolonged, leading to venous stasis (78). Finally, endothelial injury of the pelvic or leg veins also occurs commonly following lower extremity trauma (79,80). The role of inherited coagulation disorders in trauma patients is unknown.

It is generally believed that the initiation of thrombosis occurs at or shortly after injury. Most venous thrombi in high-risk patients begin in the deep veins of the calf, do not extend proximally, and remain asymptomatic (Fig. 9-1) (1,25,81–83). It has been estimated that 10% to 20% of calf thrombi do extend into the proximal veins (81,84). Proxi-

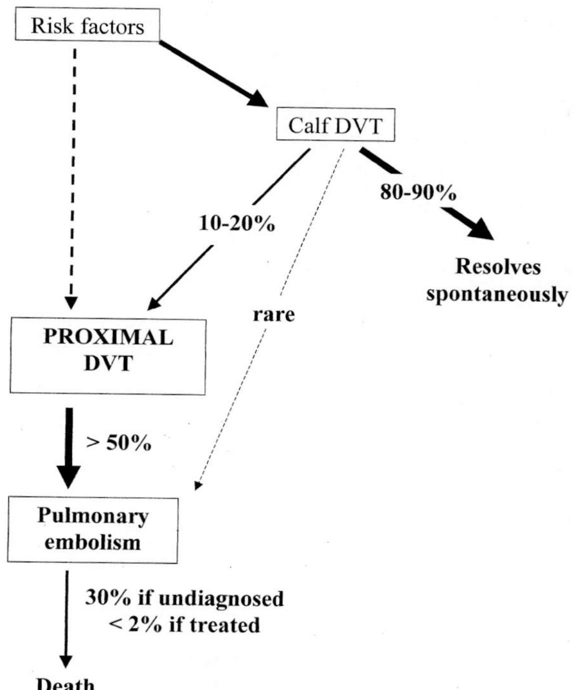

FIGURE 9-1. Pathophysiology of venous thromboembolism.

mal thrombi are considerably more serious since at least 50% of these thrombi lead to pulmonary embolism (81,85,86). It has also been estimated that approximately 10% of patients with PE die of this complication (87–89). In trauma patients, the majority of both proximal DVT and pulmonary emboli are also clinically silent (1,30,82). Almost all pulmonary emboli (and certainly all hemodynamically important PE) arise in the proximal deep veins, generally in the popliteal and femoral veins (90). The corollary is also generally true—that is, without proximal DVT, pulmonary embolism is very uncommon. In major trauma, the thrombi are more likely to originate in the proximal veins owing to adjacent injuries (91). At the same time, the consequences of calf thrombi in these patients may be more serious than those that occur following elective surgical procedures because trauma patients often remain immobilized for prolonged periods of time (92,93).

The frequency and clinical significance of isolated iliac vein thrombosis in patients with pelvic fractures are unknown. The studies using MRV suggest that pelvic fracture patients are predisposed to developing isolated iliac vein thrombosis (19,20). These thrombi may be particularly relevant in patients who undergo delayed fixation because intraoperative manipulation may result in major embolization from these large thrombi. However, the frequency of such thrombi is in some dispute and clinically important pelvic vein thrombosis may well be uncommon in these patients if appropriate prophylaxis has been given. In trauma, venous thrombosis and pulmonary emboli may also arise in the jugular and subclavian systems because of the frequent presence of central venous catheters (43,94).

After a proximal DVT, 25% to 50% of patients have chronic or episodic leg swelling, sometimes accompanied by pain, hyperpigmentation, and ulceration (95–99). The societal costs associated with this outcome are substantial (97,100,101).

DIAGNOSIS OF CLINICALLY SUSPECTED VENOUS THROMBOEMBOLISM

A consideration of possible DVT or PE arises very commonly in major trauma patients. The difficulty in diagnosing VTE in nontrauma patients is magnified in the trauma setting because of the well-known risks of these complications as well as the high frequency of lower extremity injuries and chest complications that produce clinical manifestations that closely mimic DVT or PE. The clinical diagnosis of DVT or PE, therefore, is even less reliable in trauma patients. A definitive objective diagnostic test is always required to confirm or exclude suspected VTE. Excellent, recent reviews of the diagnosis of DVT and PE can be found elsewhere (102–105). A brief review is presented here from the perspective of patients with pelvic trauma.

For clinically suspected DVT, compression duplex ultrasonography remains the test of choice (Fig. 9-2) (102–104,

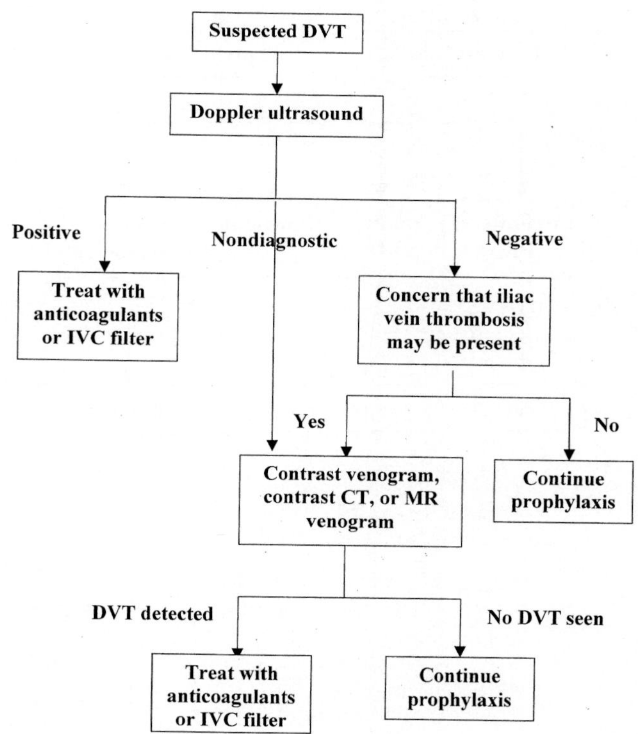

FIGURE 9-2. Approach to investigation of suspected deep vein thrombosis in pelvic trauma patients.

106). Among patients with a clinical suspicion of DVT, the sensitivity and specificity of DUS both exceed 95% (106). If a technically adequate DUS of the proximal veins cannot be performed because of the patient's injuries or if there is a clinical suspicion of pelvic vein thrombosis with a DUS that does not adequately visualize these veins, an appropriate alternative is contrast venography using a common femoral vein approach. Contrast enhanced CT and magnetic resonance imaging (MRI) also may be useful if DUS cannot be performed reliably, although there are limited data validating either of these newer diagnostic modalities for this indication (21,107–109).

The investigations are more complex and less reliable for clinically suspected PE (102–105). This is in large part because of the frequent occurrence, in trauma patients, of soft-tissue injuries to the chest wall, rib fractures, pulmonary contusion, pleural effusion, atelectasis, systemic inflammatory response syndrome, and pneumonia. Arterial blood gases have no diagnostic value in patients with suspected PE (110,111). In trauma patients, a chest radiograph should be obtained to help exclude other causes of the symptoms. However, the presence of another abnormality on the chest radiograph does not exclude the diagnosis of PE. Ventilation-perfusion lung scanning has little value in major trauma patients because the majority of the scans will be nondiagnostic and because the lung scan has no potential to provide the alternate diagnosis in the majority of patients who do not have PE (112). A ventilation-perfusion scan

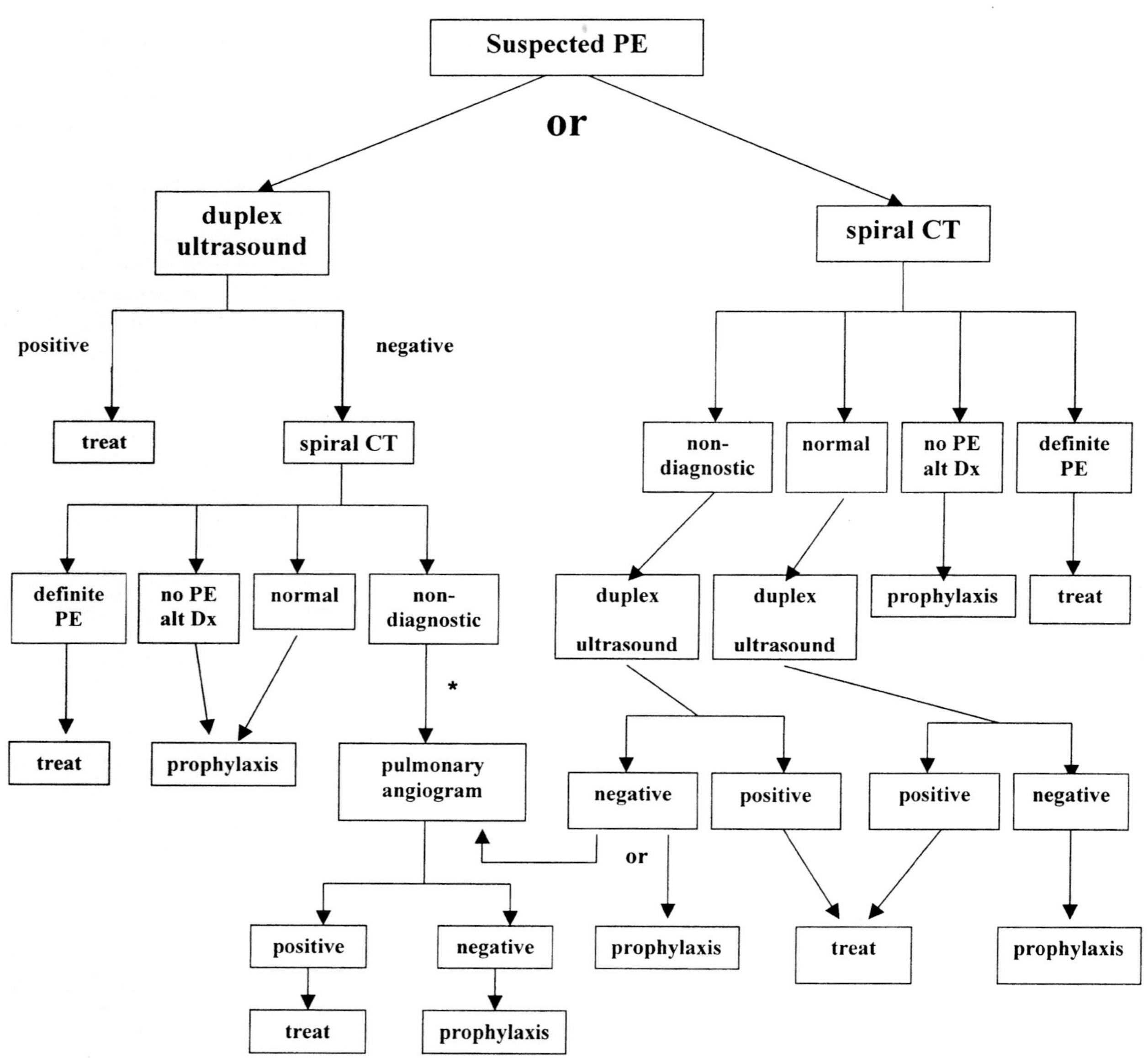

FIGURE 9-3. Approach to investigation of suspected pulmonary embolism in pelvic trauma patients (*, see text for alternate approach).

could be considered in patients with no thoracic injuries and a normal chest radiograph. Even in this setting, a high proportion of scans will be nondiagnostic. In trauma patients, therefore, the diagnosis of PE generally should be based on a spiral CT scan and/or DUS of the leg veins (Fig. 9-3). Pulmonary angiography is rarely required using this approach.

The first diagnostic decision is whether to start with spiral CT or Doppler ultrasonography. We start with a DUS if a patient with suspected PE also has leg (or arm) signs compatible with DVT, there is a relative contraindication to a contrast CT (contrast allergy or renal insufficiency), or an anticoagulation decision must be made urgently. If positive, treatment is indicated, whereas if negative, there is less urgency to investigate because it is very unlikely that major PE will ensue in the short term. Because a negative DUS in this context does not exclude a diagnosis of PE, a spiral CT scan would generally be ordered next.

If the initial test is a spiral CT scan, and the scan is diagnostic of PE in one or more segmental or lobar pulmonary arteries, then treatment is appropriate (113–115). If the CT does not demonstrate PE but does reveal an alternate cause for the patient's clinical suspicion of PE, then no further investigations are needed and continued thromboprophylaxis is indicated. If the CT is normal, a DUS of the legs (and the arms, if a subclavian or jugular central venous line has been in place) is suggested because CT misses small emboli. Further investigation is required, usually with DUS, for a spiral CT scan that is technically nondiagnostic or if subsegmental emboli are suggested. If patients with a nondiagnostic scan and normal DUS are hemostatically stable, we often simply continue "aggressive" prophylaxis rather than investigate further (see the following).

TREATMENT OF VENOUS THROMBOEMBOLISM IN PELVIC TRAUMA PATIENTS

The use of aggressive thromboprophylaxis in trauma patients is associated with a few symptomatic thromboembolic events. These "breakthrough" episodes usually occur at least several days (and usually longer) after the injury when the risk of bleeding with therapeutic anticoagulation is generally low. The treatment of proximal DVT and major pulmonary emboli, therefore, is generally similar to that in nontrauma patients, with an immediately acting anticoagulant such as intravenous (i.v.) heparin or therapeutic doses of subcutaneous low molecular weight heparin followed by longer-term, full-dose anticoagulation with warfarin (116–118). This therapy is highly effective in decreasing morbidity and mortality (119–122). The traditional acute treatment of VTE is i.v. heparin using a 5,000 U bolus and a starting infusion rate of 18 to 20 U/kg per hour. The activated partial thromboplastin time (aPTT) should be targeted to 2.0 to 3.0 times the control value (118,123). Inadequate doses of heparin, especially in the first 24 hours, are associated with a high risk of thrombus recurrence (124,125). Therefore, the use of a heparin dosing nomogram is strongly recommended because it results in more rapid and efficient anticoagulation than physician-ordered heparinization (126,127). Daily platelet count monitoring should be performed for all patients receiving full-dose heparin to screen for heparin-induced thrombocytopenia (HIT), a life-threatening complication (128). Investigation for HIT and cessation of all sources of heparin should occur if the platelet count falls more than 30% without an alternate, more plausible explanation.

The current preferred treatment for most patients with acute DVT or PE is full-dose, subcutaneous low molecular weight heparin (LMWH) (117,129). The dose of LMWH is based on body weight but no laboratory monitoring or subsequent dosage adjustment is required (118). LMWH is at least as effective as i.v. heparin, results in more rapid resolution of DVT, produces less bleeding, and is associated with substantial cost savings (130–132). Several LMWHs have been adequately studied for this indication, including: dalteparin 100 U/kg s.c. b.i.d. or 200 U/kg s.c. once daily, enoxaparin 1 mg/kg s.c. b.i.d., and tinzaparin 175 U/kg s.c. once daily. Patients who are clinically unstable or require interruptions in anticoagulation for invasive procedures probably should be managed with i.v. heparin because the anticoagulant effect is readily reversible with cessation of the infusion.

There is no evidence that patients with recent DVT require bed rest or a reduction in their mobilization, and physiotherapy generally can continue (133). Although unproved, it is prudent for patients with a very recent, iliofemoral DVT—especially a thrombus with a nonadherent proximal tail—to have aggressive leg manipulation curtailed for several days after anticoagulation has been initiated.

If no further invasive procedures requiring reversal of anticoagulation are planned, most trauma patients with VTE can be started on oral anticoagulants at the same time as the LMWH or i.v. heparin and with an overlap of at least 4 days (until the INR remains in the therapeutic range for 2 days) (118,134,135). The target intensity of anticoagulation with warfarin is an INR of 2.0 to 3.0. Use of a warfarin nomogram is highly recommended because it produces more rapid and simpler anticoagulation than physician-adjusted therapy. The duration of treatment in this setting remains controversial but probably should be 3 months if the patient is fully mobile by then and the thrombus has largely resolved; if either of these conditions is not met, anticoagulation should continue for approximately 6 months (118). Patients with a proven proximal DVT and an absolute contraindication to anticoagulation should generally have an inferior vena caval filter inserted to prevent massive and fatal PE until therapeutic anticoagulation can be started (136–138). Our practice is to use a permanent filter except in women of childbearing potential, in whom we use a removable filter (139). This avoids the additional morbidity and costs of the filter removal procedure in the majority of patients. Therapeutic anticoagulation should be started as soon as the bleeding risk allows (usually only a few days) because the filter does not prevent the extension of the DVT for which it was inserted. However, the presence of the filter alone does not prolong the duration of oral anticoagulation.

Upper extremity venous thrombosis is treated in a similar manner to those originating in the lower extremities (140,141).

PREVENTION OF VENOUS THROMBOEMBOLISM IN PELVIC TRAUMA

The most effective strategy to reduce fatal and symptomatic thromboembolic complications is the routine use of "aggressive" thromboprophylaxis. Venous thromboembolism occurs commonly after pelvic trauma; most DVT are clinically silent until they are extensive or have resulted in pulmonary embolism or sudden death, and there is no way to predict which specific patients will develop clinically important VTE (142). In 2001, the Agency for Healthcare Research and Quality (AHRQ) published a report entitled, *Making Health Care Safer: A Critical Analysis of Patient Safety Practices* (143). This systematic review ranked 79 patient safety interventions based on the impact and strength of evidence supporting more widespread implementation of these practices. The highest ranked safety practice was the "appropriate use of prophylaxis to prevent venous thromboembolism in patients at risk." This is based on strong evidence that thromboprophylaxis reduces adverse patient outcomes as well as overall costs (142,144).

A number of prophylaxis options warrant consideration in pelvic surgery patients (Table 9-4). Unfortunately, there are only two published randomized trials of thromboprophylaxis specifically conducted in patients with pelvic fractures (16,22).

Depending on the nature of the injuries, active or passive leg movements and mobilization may be of general benefit to these patients but these strategies provide little or no protection against venous thrombosis.

TABLE 9-4. THROMBOPROPHYLAXIS OPTIONS IN PELVIC FRACTURE PATIENTS

Mechanical methods of prophylaxis
Active or passive leg movements, physiotherapy
Graduated support stockings (GCS)
Intermittent pneumatic compression devices (IPC)
Venous foot pump (VFP)
Vena caval filter
Pharmacologic methods of prophylaxis
Low-dose unfractioned heparin (LDUH)
Low molecular weight heparin (LMWH)
Oral anticoagulants
Combined pharmacologic and mechanical prophylaxis
LDUH + IPC and/or GCS
LMWH + IPC and/or GCS

Mechanical Methods of Prophylaxis

Mechanical prophylaxis is widely used in trauma patients primarily because it does not cause bleeding. All of these methods act by reducing venous stasis and increasing flow velocity in the proximal deep veins. There is evidence that graduated compression stockings and/or *intermittent pneumatic compression devices* reduce the incidence of DVT in patients at low or moderate thromboembolic risk (e.g., following general or neurologic surgery) (142). Unfortunately, mechanical methods of prophylaxis have not been evaluated nearly as rigorously as anticoagulant methods, especially in higher-risk patients.

Mechanical prophylaxis methods have a number of important limitations. Intermittent pneumatic compression devices are relatively ineffective when used alone for prophylaxis in major trauma patients (16,23,24,50,51, 54,62,145–149). When these devices have been shown to be efficacious, they tend to prevent small calf thrombi without reducing the frequency of more clinically relevant proximal thrombi (150).

Fisher and colleagues randomized 73 patients with pelvic fractures to either thigh-length pneumatic compression devices or no prophylaxis (16). Duplex ultrasonography was obtained on days 3 to 5 and simple venous Doppler studies were obtained every 5 days until the patients were ambulatory. Proximal DVT or PE was diagnosed in 10.5% of the controls and 6.0% of the IPC patients ($p = 0.67$). A recent trial randomized patients with surgical repair of pelvic fractures to a thigh-length sequential compression device and a foot + calf compression device (22). Both a DUS and MRV were attempted prior to discharge in 107 patients. Proximal DVT was diagnosed in 18.5% of the patients given the thigh-length compression devices, and in 9% of those prescribed the foot + calf device ($p = 0.16$). Unfortunately, there were frequent disagreements between the two screening tests that were not resolved by obtaining additional imaging.

Pneumatic compression devices cannot be used in 35% of limbs because of lower extremity injuries (50), and some patients do not tolerate the devices. These devices do not provide protection if not used properly and consistently. Outside of a clinical trial, compliance with these devices both by nursing staff and patients is poor (151,152). In a prospective study among trauma patients in whom IPC was ordered, compliance with their actual use occurred on only 73% of days for patients in the critical care unit and only 46% of days in the intermediate care unit (152). Although mechanical prophylaxis cannot be recommended as routine, single-modality prophylaxis in pelvic trauma patients, they are potentially useful in the following situations:

1. Early after injury and possibly in the perioperative period in patients for whom evidence of primary hemostasis has not yet been obtained while waiting to commence anticoagulant prophylaxis

2. For patients who also have intracranial bleeding or ongoing, active bleeding at other sites until the high bleeding risk resolves
3. Combined with anticoagulant prophylaxis in an attempt to provide more effective protection in patients at very high risk (153,154)

There is no direct evidence that electrically powered pneumatic compression devices are more effective than much cheaper graduated compression stockings (155), although these modalities have never been compared in trauma patients. Finally, if mechanical prophylaxis is to be used, it must be applied to both legs, not to the uninjured leg only or to the upper extremities. There is evidence that pneumatic compression devices do not enhance systemic fibrinolytic function as was previously believed (156).

The *plantar foot pump* is potentially advantageous in orthopedic trauma patients because it only requires access to the feet. However, the foot pump is also unlikely to be as efficacious in major trauma as in some other patient groups (62,157–161). In a prospective study of 135 major trauma patients prophylaxed with the venous foot pump, the DVT rate by venography was 57%, and 11% of the patients had proximal DVT (161). Furthermore, many patients do not tolerate the devices and compliance in one trauma study was only 59% (62,162).

Pharmacologic Methods of Prophylaxis

These prophylaxis methods act at various steps in the coagulation process to inhibit the formation and extension of thrombi.

Low dose unfractionated heparin (LDUH), the most common method of prophylaxis for the past 30 years, has been shown to be highly effective and safe in preventing DVT, PE, and all-cause mortality in low-to-moderate risk general surgical patients (142,144). However, LDUH is much less effective in high-risk patients including those having hip and knee surgery (145,163,164), and spinal cord injury (165), and is not recommended for any of these groups (142). Studies in trauma have generally found that, compared with no prophylaxis, LDUH provides little or no protection against DVT (23,24,43,50,53,54,65,148,149,166). A recent metaanalysis found that PE was three times more likely to occur in a trauma patient randomized to LDUH than to LMWH (149).

Low molecular weight heparins (LMWH) have a number of pharmacologic properties that make them more attractive than LDUH for thromboprophylaxis (Table 9-5). Compared with unfractionated heparin, LMWH have greater bioavailability, longer half-life, reduced protein binding, and dose-independent clearance (129). Therefore, LMWH produce a more predictable anticoagulant response and can be administered once or twice daily without lab monitoring. LMWH have evolved as the prophylaxis modality of choice for most major trauma patients and have been recommended in the clinical practice guidelines produced by the Eastern Association for the Surgery of Trauma and the American College of Chest Physicians (142,148).

TABLE 9-5. PROPERTIES OF LOW MOLECULAR WEIGHT HEPARINS AND THE RESULTANT CLINICAL BENEFITS COMPARED WITH HEPARIN

Biologic Property	Clinical Benefit
Greater bioavailability Less nonspecific binding to plasma proteins and blood cells	More predictable dose–response effect; lab monitoring not required
Longer half-life	Less frequent dosing
Less binding to platelets	Lower rate of heparin-induced thrombocytopenia

We have conducted a double-blind, randomized trial comparing low dose heparin (5,000 U s.c. b.i.d.) and LMWH (enoxaparin 30 mg s.c. b.i.d.), both started within 36 hours of injury, in 344 major trauma patients without frank intracranial bleeding (65). Bilateral contrast venography between day 10 and 14 was the primary outcome measure. DVT was found in 44% of the patients given LDH and in 31% of those who received LMWH ($p = 0.01$). More importantly, the corresponding rates for proximal DVT were 15% and 6% ($p = 0.01$). There were no significant differences in bleeding, transfusions, or changes in hematocrit. In this trial, there were 47 patients with pelvic fractures. The relative risk reduction with LMWH over LDH in these patients was 47% for DVT and 77% for proximal DVT (13). There were no prophylaxis-related bleeding events.

A multicenter Belgian trial compared fixed doses of the LMWH, nadroparin, to weight-adjusted doses of the same drug for up to 6 weeks after injury (167). Nine percent of the patients had a pelvic fracture. At 10 days after injury, the DVT rates were 0% and 3% in the fixed-dose and adjusted-dose groups, respectively. Major bleeding was seen in 3.5% of patients in both groups.

There is evidence that early initiation of LMWH prophylaxis is important in pelvic trauma patients. Low molecular weight heparin started within 24 hours after injury was associated with a sevenfold lower rate of proximal DVT compared with delayed prophylaxis (3% versus 22%, $p < 0.01$) (168). Major bleeding was not encountered in either group. As a result of these trials and evidence from other high-risk groups, we can conclude that LMWH is more efficacious than LDH in high-risk patients, which includes major trauma patients, those with spinal cord injuries, and patients undergoing major hip or knee surgery (142). A cost analysis concluded that, compared with no prophylaxis, the institutional cost per thromboembolic event prevented was

$279 with routine use of LMWH (169). Another cost-effectiveness study in patients with lower extremity trauma concluded that the use of LMWH versus LDUH resulted in a societal cost of only $751 for each DVT or PE prevented and a cost per life-year saved of only $1,017 (170). A third analysis concluded that the use of LMWH was actually cheaper than LDH in major trauma patients (171,172).

Since pelvic fracture patients have a high prevalence of concomitant intraabdominal and pelvic organ injuries, and because retroperitoneal hematoma is the rule after major pelvic fractures, a prolonged concern about anticoagulant prophylaxis-related bleeding has been a major deterrent to the institution of effective thromboprophylaxis in these patients. Clearly, management of active bleeding takes precedence over preventing thrombosis in major trauma. However, in the vast majority of pelvic trauma patients, the risk of further bleeding decreases rapidly after stabilization of the pelvic and other fractures, whereas the risk of clinically important venous thrombosis is usually delayed for at least several days after injury. *This provides a window of opportunity to initiate antithrombotic prophylaxis once bleeding has been controlled and there is evidence that primary hemostasis has taken place (based on clinical examination, volume of blood in surgical drains, and hemoglobin values, supplemented, if needed, by imaging).* The delayed use of anticoagulant prophylaxis can still effectively prevent thrombus propagation, embolization, and fatal pulmonary embolism, even if venous thrombosis is already present. In our experience, the incidence of delayed, significant bleeding with anticoagulant prophylaxis is extremely low once primary hemostasis has been demonstrated.

Oral anticoagulants have rarely been assessed in the acute phase after major trauma because of their unpredictable anticoagulant effect, delayed onset of action, long duration of action, difficulty with reversal for surgical or other invasive procedures, multiple drug interactions, and the potential for bleeding. However, warfarin may be very useful in preventing thromboembolic complications beyond the acute phase. The delayed commencement of full-dose oral anticoagulation may be used effectively as prophylaxis in major trauma patients who meet the following criteria: The patient has a continued thrombosis risk; there is evidence that hemostasis has been achieved; no further invasive or surgical procedures are planned in the near future; and it is expected that hospitalization (including rehabilitation) is likely to continue for at least 2 more weeks. For pelvic fracture patients who meet these criteria, we commence warfarin approximately 5 to 7 days after injury, we aim for a target INR of 2.0 to 3.0, and we continue oral anticoagulation until the patient is discharged from acute care or rehabilitation. Among 197 patients with acetabular fractures who received perioperative mechanical prophylaxis followed by 3 weeks of oral anticoagulation, the incidence of symptomatic DVT or PE was 4% with no fatal emboli (17). Thromboembolic rates in comparable patients with other methods of prophylaxis are unknown.

Combined Pharmacologic and Mechanical Prophylaxis

The combination of mechanical prophylaxis and prophylactic anticoagulants may well be more efficacious than either alone because this approach protects against two of the three components of Virchow's triad. There is also some evidence of greater benefit with combined prophylaxis than with either alone (51,142,153). A prospective study randomized 112 patients at Tampa General Hospital with pelvic and/or femoral fractures to either IPC + GCS or to the combination of IPC + GCS and heparin 5,000 U every 8 hours followed by oral anticoagulation (51). Duplex ultrasonography was performed every 5 to 7 days until discharge. Proximal DVT was detected in 16% of the IPC + GCS group and 2% in the mechanical + anticoagulant prophylaxis group, $p = 0.02$. However, another study found that the combination of IPC + LDH was as ineffective as IPC alone (47). A recent report of the longitudinal practice of a German trauma center suggested that the combination of IPC and LMWH was more effective at preventing VTE than either alone (173). These studies suggest that combining mechanical and pharmacologic prophylaxis may improve effectiveness but the selection of pharmacologic agent may be the critical factor.

Inferior Vena Caval Filters as Primary Prophylaxis

The prophylactic insertion of inferior vena caval filters (IVCF) has been advocated in selected trauma patients because of the known high risk of VTE in these patients, because traditional prophylaxis with IPC or LDUH have been largely ineffective, and because of concerns about bleeding with anticoagulant prophylaxis (20,24,33,38,40,44,47, 174–180). Furthermore, these devices are generally easy to insert with little procedure-related morbidity (181).

There are no randomized trials of the use of IVCF in trauma patients, and the available studies all have major methodologic limitations (12). IVCF are likely to provide temporary protection against symptomatic PE in high-risk trauma patients receiving either no or inadequate thromboprophylaxis (although even this has not been proven). However, there is no evidence that filters are necessary in patients managed in trauma units with a policy of providing the best prophylaxis that can be offered currently and they are very unlikely to be cost effective (182,183). Spain and coworkers performed an analysis of 2,868 trauma patients with either high or low risk for VTE and determined that routine use of IVCF in high-risk patients may have prevented one nonfatal PE but would not have prevented any deaths (184). They concluded that prophylactic IVCF insertion was not justified.

Additional problems with prophylactic vena caval filter use include:

1. Inability to predict which patients are at sufficient risk to warrant this intervention (183)

2. Failure to prevent DVT; in fact, there is an increased risk of subsequent DVT in patients who have had an IVCF inserted (136,179,185–187)
3. The fact that patients still have PE and, rarely, may have fatal PE (136,174,179,180,183,188,189)
4. Delay of the provision of effective primary prophylaxis (patients with IVC filters still require thromboprophylaxis)
5. High cost (177)
6. Short-term complications, including hematomas, air embolism, faulty placement, early migration, and infection (138,178,185,190)
7. Long-term complications including late migration, IVC occlusion, and chronic leg swelling (38,138,174,180, 185,187,190,191)

A recent multicenter, randomized trial evaluated the added benefit of IVC filter insertion to anticoagulation in patients with proximal DVT (136). Although there were fewer pulmonary emboli in the filter group, mortality was not reduced and the patients treated with a filter plus anticoagulation experienced a significant excess of recurrent DVT. Patton and coworkers noted chronic DVT in 47% and postthrombotic syndrome in 37% of trauma patients who had prophylactic filter insertion (185). There is an increasing trend away from using vena caval filters to prevent PE in trauma (10,20,147,183,184,192). At our center, IVC filters have never been used as primary prophylaxis in trauma patients. However, as discussed, we do arrange to have an IVCF inserted in the uncommon situation of a patient who requires major pelvic surgery and has evidence of a proximal DVT on the preoperative screening venous ultrasound examination (193). In this case, we generally have a temporary filter inserted before surgery, commence anticoagulants postoperatively as soon as it is safe to do so, and then have the filter removed 5 to 7 days later when the patient has been fully anticoagulated (188). If possible, the jugular route is preferred because this avoids common femoral vein thrombosis associated with the filter insertion.

Duration of Thromboprophylaxis

The risk of VTE following pelvic fracture extends into the rehabilitation and postdischarge phases. Unfortunately, the duration of prophylaxis in trauma patients has never been studied. Postdischarge anticoagulant prophylaxis may appear to be justified by the high thromboembolic risk and frequent reduced mobility; however, we are not aware of any data to support this approach. In our experience, trauma patients who have been aggressively prophylaxed in the hospital phase of their recovery have a very low rate of symptomatic thromboembolic events after discharge, even if they are not fully mobile at that time.

Prophylaxis Use in Pelvic Trauma Patients

The use of thromboprophylaxis in patients with pelvic fractures has been assessed in two surveys (194,195). In 1992, approximately 5,000 American orthopedic surgeons were surveyed about their DVT prophylaxis practices following trauma (194). Prophylaxis was given to only 62% of patients with pelvic/acetabular fractures compared with 92% of patients who had undergone hip arthroplasty, 89% of those having knee arthroplasty, and 73% of patients who had repair of a hip fracture. The most commonly reported prophylaxis modalities in pelvic fracture patients were oral anticoagulants (38%) and combined pharmacologic/mechanical prophylaxis (25%). In 1998, a survey of members of the Orthopaedic Trauma Association who performed pelvic surgery was conducted (195). Preoperative screening was performed by 48% of the surgeons; 82% used DUS, 27% physical examination, and 8% used MRV. Preoperative thromboprophylaxis was administered by 88% of respondents. The modalities used were: compression devices (by 78% of surgeons), LMWH (45%), LDUH (29%), vena caval filters (22%), and combined methods (50%). Postoperative prophylaxis was used by 99% of the surgeons. Again, compression devices were the most commonly used (by 72%), followed by LMWH (55%), oral anticoagulants (49%), LDUH (17%), vena caval filters (10%), and aspirin (7%). Eighty percent of the surgeons used more than one modality postoperatively. Prophylaxis was continued for 3 weeks or more by half of the surgeons.

SCREENING FOR ASYMPTOMATIC DEEP VEIN THROMBOSIS

Screening trauma patients for silent DVT is often considered for the following combination of reasons: knowledge that DVT is prevalent in these patients; prophylaxis may not be possible in some patients; despite the use of prophylaxis, DVT is still common; and detection of silent DVT might reduce the frequency of symptomatic and fatal PE by selecting patients for therapeutic anticoagulation or IVC filter insertion. Regular examination of the legs is not an effective means to reduce clinically important thromboembolic complications in trauma patients (1,4,6,35,91,196,197). Duplex ultrasound is highly accurate for the detection of DVT in symptomatic patients (106) and has a number of properties that make it attractive as a screening test for DVT in trauma patients (15,23,24,43,44,48,62). It is noninvasive, can be performed serially, and, if necessary, can be performed at the bedside. Furthermore, DUS may identify large and, therefore, clinically important proximal thrombi.

We are not aware of any direct comparison between DUS and the gold standard reference test, contrast venography, in trauma patients. There is limited evidence of the accuracy of screening DUS in patients with pelvic trauma. White and coworkers found a positive predictive value of 100% (11/11) and a negative predictive value of 95% (20/21) for DUS compared with venography in a small study of pelvic fracture patients ($n = 60$) (15). However, among patients undergoing major orthopedic surgery, screening DUS has been shown to have a sensitivity of only 62% for proximal DVT and 48% for calf DVT and was not shown to be useful in preventing thromboembolic outcomes (106,198).

Further limitations of DUS screening for silent DVT in trauma patients include the inability to perform complete studies in a high proportion of patients with lower extremity injuries (23,24,43,44,199), the need for serial examinations, the need for therapeutic anticoagulation if DVT is found, the time involved, and the substantial costs (196,199). Ten percent of ultrasound examinations reported by Satiani and coworkers were nondiagnostic (200), whereas Greenfield and coworkers reported inadequate visualization of 11% to 41% of the proximal deep veins of the leg (55). In a third study, when 136 high-risk trauma patients were screened with serial DUS, 32% of the required proximal venous segments could not be adequately visualized (199).

Among trauma patients in general, serial screening for DVT fails to detect the majority of patients before they have symptomatic or fatal PE (1,23,35,39,40). A prospective DVT prophylaxis trial, which used routine serial DUS screening, found 12 thromboembolic events but only three were detected by the screening ultrasounds (23). In another study, despite serial screening with venous Doppler and duplex ultrasonography, there were three fatal pulmonary emboli among 395 trauma patients reported by Dennis and coworkers (44). Finally, a study of 486 pelvic fracture patients screened with DUS and/or MRV also concluded that routine screening failed to protect against PE or fatal PE (35).

Routine screening of trauma patients has not been shown to be cost effective (10,200). Brasel and colleagues performed a cost-effectiveness analysis in high-risk trauma patients (10). With the use of LMWH prophylaxis, the addition of either serial DUS screening or insertion of a vena caval filter, would cost more than $100,000 per PE prevented; therefore, LMWH was the most cost-effective intervention. Two recent studies concluded that, with the use of prophylaxis as early as was felt to be safe, routine screening was not required (197,201).

The use of a single or serial Doppler ultrasound examination of the leg veins in selected patients may be indicated in the following situations:

1. Preoperatively, in patients having delayed pelvic surgery
2. Patients with a combination of bleeding risks that have precluded the early use of anticoagulant prophylaxis, and lower extremity injuries that preclude the use of bilateral mechanical methods
3. Multiple risk factors for thrombosis in a patient who has received suboptimal prophylaxis

MRV has also been proposed as a screening test for DVT in patients with pelvic injuries because it is noninvasive and may allow imaging of the pelvic veins (19,22). MRV appears to be accurate for the diagnosis of symptomatic proximal DVT but its accuracy as a screening test in asymptomatic patients remains unproved, inter-observer disagreement between radiologists is high, and the cost is prohibitive for many centers (21,35,202,203). For these reasons, more research is required before the role of MRV in these patients can be determined.

PRACTICAL ASPECTS OF THROMBOSIS PREVENTION IN PELVIC FRACTURE PATIENTS

1. Routine thromboprophylaxis should be considered standard of care in all major trauma patients, including those with pelvic fractures (13,142,148,204)
2. Each trauma unit should have a written thromboprophylaxis policy based on the available evidence and local factors, including case mix and resource availability. The strategies that follow have been employed in the Trauma Unit of Sunnybrook & Women's College Health Sciences Centre for the past 10 years with only a single fatal pulmonary embolism.
3. Clearly, in the resuscitation phase and the early acute care phase after pelvic trauma, assessment and management of bleeding and the use of interventions to achieve hemostasis are the primary concerns of the trauma care team.
4. Shortly after admission, all pelvic trauma patients also should be assessed for thromboembolic risk and consideration should be given to thromboprophylaxis. Patients at high risk for VTE include those with pelvic fractures, spinal cord injuries, lower extremity fractures, major venous injuries or the use of a femoral venous line. Prophylaxis is indicated in the moderate- and high-risk trauma groups, which includes all patients with pelvic fractures.
5. For pelvic fracture patients who do not have active bleeding, we recommend prophylaxis with a low molecular weight heparin as soon as it is considered safe to do so. For about 80% of major trauma patients, this occurs within 36 hours following the injury.
6. For pelvic trauma patients, if there is evidence of active bleeding or if the patient is at very high risk for bleeding, mechanical prophylaxis should be commenced if it can be applied to both lower extremities. We do not believe that pneumatic compression devices applied to the noninjured leg or arms provide sufficient protection to be considered in this situation.
7. Apart from evidence of ongoing bleeding, the conditions we consider to represent a high bleeding risk include frank intracranial or perispinal hemorrhage and major liver or spleen lacerations that are not surgically treated. We do not consider the presence of a head in-

jury without frank intracranial bleeding, a retroperitoneal hematoma alone, or nonoperative solid organ lacerations to be contraindications to anticoagulant prophylaxis if there is evidence that primary hemostasis has occurred based on physical examination, hemoglobin levels, transfusion requirements, and surgical drain volumes.

8. High bleeding risk patients who are unable to have bilateral lower extremity mechanical prophylaxis are assessed daily to determine if LMWH can be commenced. In the high-risk group, if 5 to 7 days pass without prophylaxis, we obtain a single screening duplex ultrasound and then commence LMWH if the DUS is negative. For patients who have received prophylaxis, we do not routinely obtain a screening ultrasonography either serially or predischarge.
9. If combined mechanical and pharmacologic prophylaxis is used, we recommend that the mechanical device or graduated compression stockings commence as soon as possible after admission.
10. We generally do not withhold LMWH for surgical procedures, including laparotomy, internal fixation of limb fractures, incision and drainage, or skin grafting. However, we do not administer LMWH on the day of surgery for patients undergoing pelvic (or spinal) surgery.
11. When highly potent antiinflammatory agents, such as indomethacin, are used to prevent heterotopic bone formation in pelvic fracture patients, we add a gastrointestinal protective agent, either misoprostol or a proton pump inhibitor, to reduce the potential for upper gastrointestinal bleeding.
12. Some patients with major chest or pelvic injuries have an epidural catheter inserted for pain control. We use LMWH concomitantly with epidural analgesia with the following precautions:
    a. We look for and correct any other systemic bleeding risks, including severe thrombocytopenia and clotting factor depletion.
    b. The epidural catheter is inserted at a time when there is no LMWH effect on board. For twice daily LMWH dosing, this will be at least 10 hours after a dose; for once daily LMWH this will be at least 20 hours after a dose.
    c. After the epidural catheter has been inserted, if the procedure has been uncomplicated, the next dose of LMWH is delayed for at least 2 hours after the insertion.
    d. LMWH, given every 12 hours, is administered while the epidural is in place.
    e. We do not allow concomitant antiplatelet agents and we never use oral anticoagulants with an epidural in place.
    f. Removal of the epidural catheter is done 10 to 12 hours after a twice daily dose of LMWH and the next dose is then given no sooner than 2 hours after the removal.
13. For pelvic trauma patients who will remain in acute care for more than 2 weeks or be transferred to a rehabilitation center, we convert the LMWH to full-dose oral anticoagulation if no further invasive procedures are anticipated and the gastrointestinal tract is functioning.
14. For pelvic fracture patients who are discharged home from the hospital, we do not continue prophylaxis at home because we are not aware of any evidence to support such a practice, because of the costs, logistic difficulties, and potential risks involved, and because symptomatic venous thromboembolism is very uncommon in our experience when these patients have received aggressive prophylaxis as outlined in the preceding and in Fig. 9-4.

SUMMARY

Venous thromboembolism is a common complication after pelvic fractures, sometimes leading to lethal consequences. Without prophylaxis, the incidence of DVT in these patients is approximately 60%. Although the majority of these thrombi are clinically silent, large, proximal thrombi occur commonly and may result in major or fatal pulmonary emboli, usually without any warning.

The diagnosis of symptomatic DVT and PE is particularly difficult after pelvic fracture and other major trauma. A clinical suspicion of DVT generally can be investigated by duplex ultrasonography. If an adequate ultrasound examination is technically not possible, alternate approaches include CT venography, contrast venography, or MRV.

A clinical suspicion of PE can generally be investigated by CT pulmonary angiography and/or duplex ultrasonography.

Pelvic fracture patients with proven DVT or PE should be treated with full-dose i.v. heparin or full-dose, body-weight adjusted LMWH followed by at least 3 months of oral anticoagulation.

Aggressive thromboprophylaxis is essential after pelvic fracture. Although the number and quality of thromboprophylaxis studies in this patient group are limited, it appears that the use of low dose heparin or mechanical devices alone do not provide sufficient protection for such a high-risk group and are not recommended. Either LMWH or the combination of pharmacologic and mechanical prophylaxis modalities is recommended.

Although the prophylaxis should be initiated as early as possible after admission, there should be evidence that primary hemostasis has occurred before anticoagulant prophylaxis is commenced.

The duration of prophylaxis in pelvic fracture patients is unknown, although we recommend that prophylaxis continue for at least the duration of stay in acute care and reha-

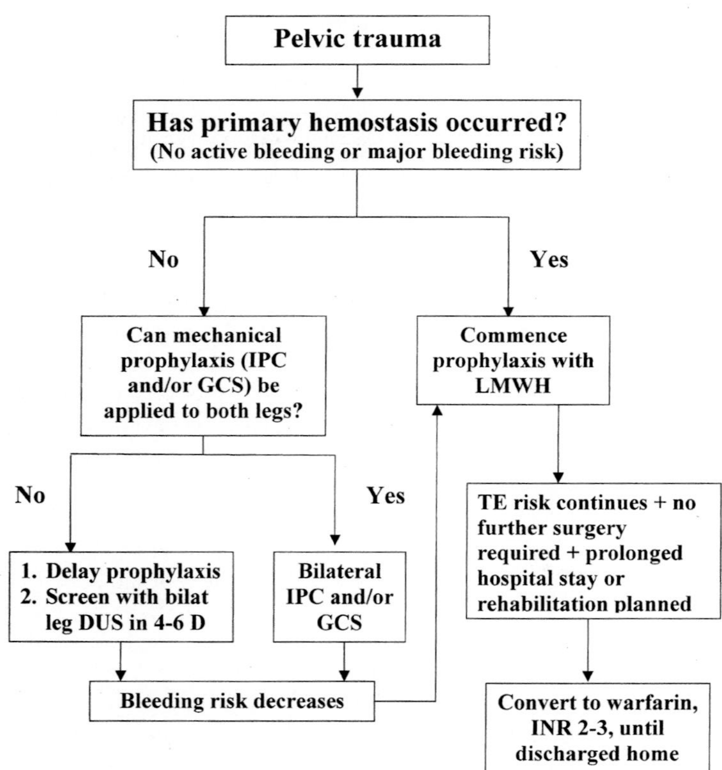

FIGURE 9-4. Approach to thromboprophylaxis in pelvic fracture patients.

bilitation. We are not aware of any evidence that pelvic trauma patients should have prophylaxis continued after discharge, even if they are not fully mobile at that time.

Routine screening with Doppler ultrasound or MRI is not recommended because there is no evidence that either is clinically effective or cost effective. However, proximal venous imaging may be appropriate in selected patients who have had inadequate prophylaxis or require delayed major pelvic surgery. All patients transferred to a specialty center for surgery should have preoperative DUS screening.

It is unlikely that vena caval filters are necessary in pelvic fracture patients who have received appropriate prophylaxis. Vena caval filter insertion is only recommended in patients with proven proximal DVT and either an absolute contraindication for anticoagulation or who require major surgery in the near future.

Among pelvic fracture patients, effective prophylaxis provides clinicians with the opportunity to reduce the morbidity and mortality associated with unprevented VTE while reducing costs.

REFERENCES

1. Geerts WH, Code KI, Jay RM, et al. A prospective study of venous thromboembolism after major trauma. *N Engl J Med* 1994;331:1601–1606.
2. Attia J, Ray JG, Cook DJ, et al. Deep vein thrombosis and its prevention in critically ill adults. *Arch Intern Med* 2001;161: 1268–1279.
3. Rogers FB. Venous thromboembolism in trauma patients: a review. *Surgery* 2001;130:1–12.
4. Kudsk KA, Fabian TC, Baum S, et al. Silent deep vein thrombosis in immobilized multiple trauma patients. *Am J Surg* 1989;158:515–519.
5. Smith RM, Airey M, Franks AJ. Death after major trauma: can we affect it? The changing cause of death in each phase after injury. [abstract] *Injury* 1994;25(Suppl):SB23–SB24.
6. Piotrowski JJ, Alexander JJ, Brandt CP, et al. Is deep vein thrombosis surveillance warranted in high-risk trauma patients? *Am J Surg* 1996;172:210–213.
7. Acosta JA, Yang JC, Winchell RJ, et al. Lethal injuries and time to death in a level 1 trauma center. *J Am Coll Surg* 1998;186: 528–533.
8. Davis JW, Hoyt DB, McCardle MS, et al. The significance of critical care errors in causing preventable death in trauma patients in a trauma system. *J Trauma* 1991;31:813–819.
9. Battistella FD, Torabian SZ, Siadatan KM. Hospital readmission after trauma: an analysis of outpatient complications. *J Trauma* 1997;42:1012–1017.
10. Brasel KJ, Borgstrom DC, Weigelt JA. Cost-effective prevention of pulmonary embolus in high-risk trauma patients. *J Trauma* 1997;42:456–462.
11. McIntyre K. Medicolegal implications of the consensus conference. *Chest* 2001;119(Suppl):337S–343S.
12. Montgomery KD, Geerts WH, Potter HG, et al. Thromboembolic complications in patients with pelvic trauma. *Clin Orthop* 1996;329:68–87.
13. Montgomery KD, Geerts WH, Potter HG, et al. Practical management of venous thromboembolism following pelvic fractures. *Orthop Clin North Am* 1997;28:397–404.

14. Maliska P, Tiercelin G, Vallee C, et al. Routine preoperative venography for patients undergoing delayed surgery for limb trauma. *Ann Fr Anesth Réanim* 1985;4:23–26.
15. White RH, Goulet JA, Bray TJ, et al. Deep-vein thrombosis after fracture of the pelvis: assessment with serial duplex-ultrasound screening. *J Bone Joint Surg* 1990;72-A:495–500.
16. Fisher CG, Blachut PA, Salvian AJ, et al. Effectiveness of pneumatic leg compression devices for the prevention of thromboembolic disease in orthopaedic trauma patients: a prospective, randomized study of compression alone versus no prophylaxis. *J Orthop Trauma* 1995;9:1–7.
17. Fishmann AJ, Greeno RA, Brooks LR, et al. Prevention of deep vein thrombosis and pulmonary embolism in acetabular and pelvic fracture surgery. *Clin Orthop* 1994;305:133–137.
18. Russell GV, Nork SE, Routt MLC. Perioperative complications associated with operative treatment of acetabular fractures. *J Trauma* 2001;51:1098–1103.
19. Montgomery KD, Potter HG, Helfet DL. Magnetic resonance venography to evaluate the deep venous system of the pelvis in patients who have an acetabular fracture. *J Bone Joint Surg* 1995;77-A:1639–1649.
20. Montgomery KD, Potter HG, Heflet DL. The detection and management of proximal deep venous thrombosis in patients with acute acetabular fractures: a follow-up report. *J Orthop Trauma* 1997;11:330–336.
21. Stover MD, Morgan SJ, Blosse MJ, et al. Prospective comparison of contrast enhanced computed tomography vs magnetic resonance venography in the detection of occult deep vein thrombosis in patients with pelvic and acetabular fractures. *Orthop Trauma* 2002;16:613–621.
22. Stannard JP, Riley RS, McClenney MD, et al. Mechanical prophylaxis against deep-vein thrombosis after pelvic and acetabular fractures. *J Bone Joint Surg* 2001;83-A:1047–1051.
23. Knudson MM, Collins JA, Goodman SB, et al. Thromboembolism following multiple trauma. *J Trauma* 1992;32:2–11.
24. Knudson MM, Lewis FR, Clinton A, et al. Prevention of venous thromboembolism in trauma patients. *J Trauma* 1994;37: 480–487.
25. Sevitt S, Gallagher N. Venous thrombosis and pulmonary embolism: a clinico-pathological study in injured and burned patients. *Br J Surg* 1961;48:475–489.
26. Hill SL, Berry RE, Ruiz AJ. Deep venous thrombosis in the trauma patient. *Am Surg* 1994;60:405–408.
27. Letournel E, Judet R. *Fractures of the acetabulum.* Berlin: Springer-Verlag, 1993:540.
28. Trunkey DD, Chapman MW, Lim RC, et al. Management of pelvic fractures in blunt trauma injury. *J Trauma* 1974;14: 912–923.
29. Spencer JD, Lalanadham T. The mortality of patients with minor fractures of the pelvis. *Injury* 1985;16:321–323.
30. O'Malley KF, Ross SE. Pulmonary embolism in major trauma patients. *J Trauma* 1990;30:748–750.
31. Poole GV, Ward EF, Griswold JA, et al. Complications of pelvic fractures from blunt trauma. *Am Surg* 1992;58:225–231.
32. Buerger PM, Peoples JB, Lemmon GW, et al. Risk of pulmonary emboli in patients with pelvic fractures. *Am Surg* 1993;59:505–508.
33. Rogers FB, Shackford SR, Wilson J, et al. Prophylactic vena cava filter insertion in severely injured trauma patients: indications and preliminary results. *J Trauma* 1993; 35:637–641.
34. Matta JM. Operative treatment of acetabular fractures through the ilioinguinal approach. A 10-year perspective. *Clin Orthop* 1994;305:10–19.
35. Borer DS, Rao AV, Starr AJ, et al. *Deep vein thrombosis in patients with pelvic or acetabular fractures: a review of 486 patients.* Abstract presented at the 16th Annual Meeting of the Orthopaedic Trauma Association, 2000, San Antonio, TX.
36. Deo SD, Tavares SP, Pandey RK, et al. Operative management of acetabular fractures in Oxford. *Injury* 2001;32:581–586.
37. McMurtry R, Walton D, Dickinson D, et al. Pelvic disruption in the polytraumatized patient: a management protocol. *Clin Orthop* 1980;151:22–30.
38. Webb LX, Rush PT, Fuller SB, et al. Greenfield filter prophylaxis of pulmonary embolism in patients undergoing surgery for acetabular fracture. *J Orthop Trauma* 1992;6:139–145.
39. Helfet DL, Schmeling GJ. Complications. In: Tile M, ed. *Fractures of the pelvis and acetabulum,* 2nd ed. Baltimore: Williams & Wilkins, 1995:252–253.
40. Winchell RJ, Hoyt DB, Walsh JC, et al. Risk factors associated with pulmonary embolism despite routine prophylaxis: implications for improved protection. *J Trauma* 1994;37:600–606.
41. Tuttle-Newhall JE, Rutledge R, Hultman CS, et al. Statewide, population-based, time-series analysis of the frequency and outcome of pulmonary embolus in 318,554 trauma patients. *J Trauma* 1997;42:90–99.
42. Racanalli J, Powell JN, Bucholz R, et al. *Thromboembolism in pelvic fractures: B-Mode doppler ultrasound and MRI as imaging techniques.* Abstract presented at the Annual Meeting of the Orthopaedic Trauma Association, Toronto, Canada, 1990.
43. Burns GA, Cohn SM, Frumento RJ, et al. Prospective ultrasound evaluation of venous thrombosis in high-risk trauma patients. *J Trauma* 1993;35:405–408.
44. Dennis JW, Menawat S, Von Thron J, et al. Efficacy of deep venous thrombosis prophylaxis in trauma patients and identification of high-risk groups. *J Trauma* 1993;35:132–139.
45. Owings JT, Kraut E, Battistella F, et al. Timing of the occurrence of pulmonary embolism in trauma patients. *Arch Surg* 1997;132:862–867.
46. Kelly K, Abdel-Al N, Moritz M, et al. Deep venous thrombosis occurs early in lower extremity fracture. [abstract] *J Trauma* 1998;45:1111.
47. Velmahos GC, Nigro J, Tatevossian R, et al. Inability of an aggressive policy of thromboprophylaxis to prevent deep venous thrombosis (DVT) in critically injured patients: are current methods of DVT prophylaxis insufficient? *J Am Coll Surg* 1998;187:529–533.
48. Gruen GS, McClain EJ, Gruen RJ. The diagnosis of deep vein thrombosis in the multiply injured patient with pelvic ring or acetabular fractures. *Orthopedics* 1995;18:253–257.
49. Kozak TKW, Diebold R, Beaver RJ. Massive pulmonary thromboembolism after manipulation of an unstable pelvic fracture: a case report and review of the literature. *J Trauma* 1995;38: 366–367.
50. Shackford SR, Davis JW, Hollingsworth-Fridlund P, et al. Venous thromboembolism in patients with major trauma. *Am J Surg* 1990;159:365–369.
51. Stickney JL, Helfet DL, Otero PR. Deep vein thrombosis in orthopedic trauma patients. [abstract] *J Orthop Trauma* 1991;5: 227.
52. Velmahos GC, Kern J, Chan LS, et al. Prevention of venous thromboembolism after injury: an evidence-based report. Part II: Analysis of risk factors and evaluation of the role of vena caval filters. *J Trauma* 2000;49:140–144.
53. Ruiz AJ, Hill SL, Berry RE. Heparin, deep venous thrombosis, and trauma patients. *Am J Surg* 1991;162:159–162.
54. Napolitano LM, Garlapati VS, Heard SO, et al. Asymptomatic deep venous thrombosis in the trauma patient: is an aggressive screening protocol justified? *J Trauma* 1995;39:651–659.
55. Greenfield LJ, Proctor MC, Rodriguez JL, et al. Posttrauma thromboembolism prophylaxis. *J Trauma* 1997;42:100–103.
56. Headrick JR, Barker DE, Pate LM, et al. The role of ultrasonography and inferior vena cava filter placement in high-risk trauma patients. *Am Surg* 1997;63:1–8.

57. Kujath P, Spannagel U, Habscheid W. Incidence and prophylaxis of deep venous thrombosis in outpatients with injury of the lower limb. *Haemostasis* 1993;23(Suppl 1):20–26.
58. Hoyt DB, Simons RK, Winchell RJ, et al. A risk analysis of pulmonary complications following major trauma. *J Trauma* 1993;35:524–531.
59. Abelseth G, Buckley RE, Pineo GE, et al. Incidence of deep-vein thrombosis in patients with fractures of the lower extremity distal to the hip. *J Orthop Trauma* 1996;10:230–235.
60. Carter YM, Caps MT, Meissner MH. Deep venous thrombosis and ABO blood groups are unrelated in trauma patients. *J Trauma* 2002;52:112–116.
61. Meredith JW, Young JS, O'Neil EA, et al. Femoral catheters and deep venous thrombosis: a prospective evaluation with venous duplex sonography. *J Trauma* 1993;35:187–191.
62. Knudson MM, Morabito D, Paiement GD, et al. Use of low molecular weight heparin in preventing thromboembolism in trauma patients. *J Trauma* 1996;41:446–459.
63. Cargile JS, Hunt JL, Purdue GF. Acute trauma of the femoral artery and vein. *J Trauma* 1992;32:364–371.
64. Eisele R. Drug prophylaxis of deep vein thrombosis in outpatients after trauma or surgery: a new management. [abstract] *Thromb Haemost* 1999;82(Suppl):201.
65. Geerts WH, Jay RM, Code KI, et al. A comparison of low-dose heparin with low-molecular-weight heparin as prophylaxis against venous thromboembolism after major trauma. *N Engl J Med* 1996;335:701–707.
66. Virchow R. Phlogose und Thrombose im Gefaβsystem. In: Virchow R, ed. *Gessamelte Abhandlungen zur Wissenschaftlichen Medicin.* Frankfurt: Meidinger Sohn, 1856.
67. Gando S, Tedo I, Kubota M. Posttrauma coagulation and fibrinolysis. *Crit Care Med* 1992;20:594–600.
68. Schmidt U, Enderson BL, Chen JP, et al. D-dimer levels correlate with pathologic thrombosis in trauma patients. *J Trauma* 1992;33:312–319.
69. Sorensen JV, Rahr HB, Jensen HP, et al. Markers of coagulation and fibrinolysis after fractures of the lower extremities. *Thromb Res* 1992;65:479–486.
70. Miller RS, Weatherford DA, Stein D, et al. Antithrombin III and trauma patients: factors that determine low levels. *J Trauma* 1994;37:442–445.
71. Dries DJ. Activation of the clotting system and complement after trauma. *New Horiz* 1996;4:276–288.
72. Engelman DT, Gabram SGA, Allen L, et al. Hypercoagulability following multiple trauma. *World J Surg* 1996;20:5–10.
73. Owings JT, Bagley M, Gosselin R, et al. Effect of critical injury on plasma antithrombin activity: low antithrombin levels are associated with thromboembolic complications. *J Trauma* 1996;41:396–406.
74. Selby R, Geerts WH, Ofosu FA, et al. Biology of the hypercoagulable state following major trauma. [abstract] *Blood* 1999; 94(suppl 1):240a.
75. Boldt J, Papsdorf M, Rothe A, et al. Changes of the hemostatic network in critically ill patients: is there a difference between sepsis, trauma, and neurosurgery patients? *Crit Care Med* 2000;28:445–450.
76. Pape HC, Schmidt RE, Rice J, et al. Biochemical changes after trauma and skeletal surgery of the lower extremity: quantification of the operative burden. *Crit Care Med* 2000;28: 3441–3448.
77. Meissner MH, Chandler WL, Elliott J. Venous thromboembolism in trauma: a local manifestation of systemic hypercoagulability. [abstract] *J Trauma* 2002;52:196.
78. Nemerson Y, Turitto VT. The effect of flow on hemostasis and thrombosis. *Thromb Haemost* 1991;66:272–276.
79. Ikegami K, Suzuki Y, Yukioka T, et al. Endothelial cell injury, as quantified by the soluble thrombomodulin level, predicts sepsis/multiple organ dysfunction syndrome after blunt trauma. *J Trauma* 1998;44:789–795.
80. Siemiatkowski A, Koczko J, Rogowski F, et al. Effect of severe trauma on endothelial cell activity. [abstract] *Intens Care Med* 1998;24(Suppl 1):S17.
81. Kakkar VV, Flanc C, Howe CT, et al. Natural history of postoperative deep-vein thrombosis. *Lancet* 1969;2:230–233.
82. Moser KM, LeMoine JR. Is embolic risk conditioned by location of deep venous thrombosis? *Ann Intern Med* 1981; 94:439–444.
83. Philbrick JT, Becker DM. Calf deep venous thrombosis: a wolf in sheep's clothing? *Arch Intern Med* 1988;148:2131–2138.
84. Kazmers A, Groehn H, Meeker C. Acute calf vein thrombosis: outcomes and implications. *Am Surg* 1999;65:1124–1127.
85. Lagerstedt CI, Olsson C-G, Fagher BO, et al. Need for long-term anticoagulant treatment in symptomatic calf-vein thrombosis. *Lancet* 1985;2:515–518.
86. Meignan M, Rosso J, Gauthier H, et al. Systematic lung scans reveal a high frequency of silent pulmonary embolism in patients with proximal deep venous thrombosis. *Arch Intern Med* 2000;160:159–164.
87. Anderson FA, Wheeler HB, Goldberg RJ, et al. A population-based perspective of the hospital incidence and case-fatality rates of deep vein thrombosis and pulmonary embolism. The Worcester DVT Study. *Arch Intern Med* 1991;151:933–938.
88. Carson JL, Kelley MA, Duff A, et al. The clinical course of pulmonary embolism. *N Engl J Med* 1992;326:1240–1245.
89. Goldhaber SZ, Visani L, DeRosa M, for ICOPER. Acute pulmonary embolism: clinical outcomes in the International Cooperative Pulmonary Embolism Registry (ICOPER). *Lancet* 1999;353:1386–1389.
90. Havig O. Source of pulmonary emboli. *Acta Chir Scand* 1977; 478(Suppl):42–47.
91. Van den Berg E, Bathgate B, Panagakos E, et al. Duplex screening as a method of quality assurance of perioperative thromboembolism prophylaxis. *Int Angiol* 1999;18:210–219.
92. Lohr JM, James KV, Deshmukh RM, et al. Calf vein thrombi are not a benign finding. *Am J Surg* 1995;170:86–90.
93. Sharpe RP, Gupta R, Gracias VH, et al. Incidence and natural history of below-knee deep venous thrombosis in high-risk trauma patients. *J Trauma* 2002;53:1048–1052.
94. Hingorani A, Ascher E, Lorenson E, et al. Upper extremity deep venous thrombosis and its impact on morbidity and mortality rates in a hospital-based population. *J Vasc Surg* 1997;26:853–860.
95. Prandoni P, Lensing AWA, Cogo A, et al. The long term clinical course of deep venous thrombosis. *Ann Intern Med* 1996; 125:1–7.
96. Bermudez KM, Knudson MM, Nelken NA, et al. Long-term results of lower-extremity venous injuries. *Arch Surg* 1997; 132:963–968.
97. Shami SK, Sarin S, Scurr JH. Chronic venous insufficiency disease. *Int J Angiol* 1997;6:30–48.
98. Mohr DN, Silverstein MD, Heit JA, et al. The venous stasis syndrome after deep venous thrombosis or pulmonary embolism: a population-based study. *Mayo Clin Proc* 2000;75:1249–1256.
99. Ziegler S, Schillinger M, Maca TH, et al. Post-thrombotic syndrome after primary event of deep venous thrombosis 10–20 years ago. *Thromb Res* 2001;101:23–33.
100. Bergqvist D, Jendteg S, Johansen L, et al. Cost of long-term complications of deep venous thrombosis of the lower extremities: an analysis of a defined patient population in Sweden. *Ann Intern Med* 1997;126:454–457.
101. Kahn SR, Solymoss S, Lamping DL, et al. Long-term outcomes after deep vein thrombosis: postphlebitic syndrome and quality of life. *J Gen Intern Med* 2000;15:425–429.

102. American Thoracic Society. The diagnostic approach to acute venous thromboembolism. Clinical Practice Guideline. *Am J Respir Crit Care Med* 1999;160:1043–1066.
103. Chunilal SD, Ginsberg JS. Strategies for the diagnosis of deep vein thrombosis and pulmonary embolism. *Thromb Res* 2000; 97:V33–V48.
104. Perrier A, Bounameaux H. Cost-effective diagnosis of deep vein thrombosis and pulmonary embolism. *Thromb Haemost* 2001; 86:475–487.
105. Rodger M, Wells PS. Diagnosis of pulmonary embolism. *Thromb Res* 2001;103:V225–V238.
106. Kearon C, Julian JA, Newman TE, et al. Noninvasive diagnosis of deep venous thrombosis. *Ann Intern Med* 1998;128: 663–677.
107. Lomas DJ, Britton PD. CT demonstration of acute and chronic iliofemoral thrombosis. *J Comput Assist Tomogr* 1991;15: 861–862.
108. Laissy J-P, Cinqualbre A, Loshkajian A, et al. Assessment of deep venous thrombosis in the lower limbs and pelvis: MR venography versus duplex Doppler sonography. *AJR* 1996; 167:971–975.
109. Fraser DGW, Moody AR, Morgan PS, et al. Diagnosis of lower-limb deep venous thrombosis: a prospective blinded study of magnetic resonance direct thrombus imaging. *Ann Intern Med* 2002;136:89–98.
110. Stein PD, Goldhaber SZ, Henry JW, et al. Arterial blood gas analysis in the assessment of suspected acute pulmonary embolism. *Chest* 1996;109:78–81.
111. Rodger MA, Carrier M, Jones GN, et al. Diagnostic value of arterial blood gas measurement in suspected pulmonary embolism. *Am J Respir Crit Care Med* 2000;162:2105–2108.
112. The PIOPED Investigators. Value of the ventilation/perfusion scan in acute pulmonary embolism: results of the Prospective Investigation of Pulmonary Embolism Diagnosis (PIOPED). *JAMA* 1990;263:2753–2759.
113. Harvey RT, Gefter WB, Hrung JM, et al. Accuracy of CT angiography versus pulmonary angiography in the diagnosis of acute pulmonary embolism. *Acad Radiol* 2000;7:786–797.
114. Mullins MD, Becker DM, Hagspiel KD, et al. The role of spiral volumetric computed tomography in the diagnosis of pulmonary embolism. *Arch Intern Med* 2000;160:293–298.
115. Rathbun SW, Raskob GE, Whitsett TL. Sensitivity and specificity of helical computed tomography in the diagnosis of pulmonary embolism: a systematic review. *Ann Intern Med* 2000; 132:227–232.
116. Hirsh J, Anand SS, Halperin JL, et al. Guide to anticoagulant therapy: heparin. A statement for healthcare professionals from the American Heart Association. *Circulation* 2001;103: 2994–3018.
117. Hirsh J, Warkentin TE, Shaughnessy SG, et al. Heparin and low-molecular-weight heparin. Mechanisms of action, pharmacokinetics, dosing, monitoring, efficacy, and safety. *Chest* 2001;119(Suppl):64S–94S.
118. Hyers TM, Agnelli G, Hull RD, et al. Antithrombotic therapy for venous thromboembolic disease. *Chest* 2001;119(Suppl): 176S–193S.
119. Barritt DW, Jordan SC. Anticoagulant drugs in the treatment of pulmonary embolism: a controlled trial. *Lancet* 1960;1: 1309–1312.
120. Brandjes DPM, Heijboer H, Buller HR, et al. Acenocoumarol and heparin compared with acenocoumarol alone in the initial treatment of proximal-vein thrombosis. *N Engl J Med* 1992; 327:1485–1489.
121. Hull RD, Raskob GE, Rosenbloom D, et al. Heparin for 5 days as compared with 10 days in the initial treatment of proximal venous thrombosis. *N Engl J Med* 1990;322:1260–1264.
122. Douketis JD, Kearon C, Bates S, et al. Risk of fatal pulmonary embolism in patients with treated venous thromboembolism. *JAMA* 1998;279:458–462.
123. Regan ME, Vanderheyden BA, Buck BD, et al. Development of a weight-based heparin dosing nomogram in trauma patients (TP). [abstract] *Crit Care Med* 1999;27(Suppl):A179.
124. Hull RD, Raskob GE, Hirsh J, et al. Continuous intravenous heparin compared with intermittent subcutaneous heparin in the initial treatment of proximal-vein thrombosis. *N Engl J Med* 1986;315:1109–1114.
125. Hull RD, Raskob GE, Brant RF, et al. Relation between the time to achieve the lower limit of the APTT therapeutic range and recurrent venous thromboembolism during heparin treatment for deep vein thrombosis. *Arch Intern Med* 1997; 157:2562–2568.
126. Raschke RA, Reilly BM, Guidry JR, et al. The weight-based heparin dosing nomogram compared with a 'standard care' nomogram. *Ann Intern Med* 1993;119:875–881.
127. Bernardi E, Piccioli A, Oliboni G, et al. Nomograms for the administration of unfractionated heparin in the initial treatment of acute thromboembolism—an overview. *Thromb Haemost* 2000; 84:22–26.
128. Warkentin TE. Heparin-induced thrombocytopenia: a clinicopathologic syndrome. *Thromb Haemost* 1999;82:439–447.
129. Weitz JI. Low-molecular-weight heparins. *N Engl J Med* 1997;337:688–698.
130. Gould MK, Dembitzer AD, Doyle RL, et al. Low-molecular weight heparins compared with unfractionated heparin for treatment of acute deep venous thrombosis. A meta-analysis of randomized, controlled trials. *Ann Intern Med* 1999;130: 800–809.
131. Gould MK, Dembitzer AD, Sanders GD, et al. Low-molecular weight heparins compared with unfractionated heparin for treatment of acute deep venous thrombosis. A cost-effectiveness analysis. *Ann Intern Med* 1999;130:789–799.
132. Dolovich LR, Ginsberg JS, Douketis JD, et al. A metaanalysis comparing low-molecular-weight heparins with unfractionated heparin in the treatment of venous thromboembolism. Examining some unanswered questions regarding location of treatment, product type, and dosing frequency. *Arch Intern Med* 2000; 160:181–188.
133. Aschwanden M, Labs K-H, Engel H, et al. Acute deep vein thrombosis: early mobilization does not increase the frequency of pulmonary embolism. *Thromb Haemost* 2001;85:42–46.
134. Gage BF, Fihn SD, White RH. Management and dosing of warfarin therapy. *Am J Med* 2000;109:481–488.
135. Ansell J, Hirsh J, Dalen J, et al. Managing oral anticoagulant therapy. *Chest* 2001; 119(Suppl):22S–38S.
136. Decousus H, Leizorovicz A, Parent F, et al. A clinical trial of vena caval filters in the prevention of pulmonary embolism in patients with proximal deep-vein thrombosis. *N Engl J Med* 1998;338:409–415.
137. Greenfield LJ, Proctor MC. Twenty-year clinical experience with the Greenfield filter. *Cardiovasc Surg* 1995;3:199–205.
138. Streiff MB. Vena caval filters: a comprehensive review. *Blood* 2000;95:3669–3677.
139. Millward SF. Temporary and retrievable inferior vena cava filters: current status. *J Vasc Interv Radiol* 1998;9:381–387.
140. Haire WD. Arm vein thrombosis. *Clin Chest Med* 1995;16: 341–351.
141. Hicken GJ, Ameli FM. Management of subclavian-axillary vein thrombosis: a review. *Can J Surg* 1998;41:13–25.
142. Geerts WH, Heit JA, Clagett GP, et al. Prevention of venous thromboembolism. *Chest* 2001;119(Suppl):132S–175S.
143. Shojania KG, Duncan BW, McDonald KM, et al, eds. *Making health care safer: a critical analysis of patient safety practices.*

Evidence Report/Technology Assessment No. 43 (Prepared by the University of California at San Francisco-Stanford Evidence-Based Practice Center under contract no. 290-97-0013). AHRQ Publication No. 01-E058, Rockville, MD: Agency for Healthcare Research and Quality, July 2001 *www.ahrq.gov/clinic/ptsafety/*

144. Collins R, Scrimgeour S, Yusuf S, et al. Reduction in fatal pulmonary embolism and venous thrombosis by perioperative administration of subcutaneous heparin. Overview of results of randomized trials in general, orthopedic, and urologic surgery. *N Engl J Med* 1988;18:1162–1173.
145. Montrey JS, Kistner RL, Kong AYT, et al. Thromboembolism following hip fracture. *J Trauma* 1985;25:534–537.
146. Gersin K, Grindlinger GA, Lee V, et al. The efficacy of sequential compression devices in multiple trauma patients with severe head injury. *J Trauma* 1994;37:205–208.
147. Cafferata HT, Morrison S, Duer C, et al. Venous thromboembolism in trauma patients: standardized risk factors. *J Vasc Surg* 1998;28:250–259.
148. Pasquale M, Fabian TC, and the EAST Ad Hoc Committee on Practice Management Guideline Development. Practice management guidelines for trauma from the Eastern Association for the Surgery of Trauma. *J Trauma* 1998;44:941–957.
149. Velmahos GC, Kern J, Chan LS, et al. Prevention of venous thromboembolism after injury: an evidence-based report. Part I: Analysis of risk factors and evaluation of the role of vena caval filters. *J Trauma* 2000;49:132–139.
150. Francis CW, Pellegrini VD, Marder VJ, et al. Comparison of warfarin and external pneumatic compression in prevention of venous thrombosis after total hip replacement. *JAMA* 1992; 267:2911–2915.
151. Comerota AJ, Katz ML, White JV. Why does prophylaxis with external pneumatic compression for deep vein thrombosis fail? *Am J Surg* 1992;164:265–268.
152. Huk M, Lynsky D, O'Callaghan T, et al. Compliance of sequential compression device for deep vein thrombosis prophylaxis in the adult trauma patient: surgical intensive care unit vs. intermediate care. [abstract] *Crit Care Med* 1998;26(Suppl): A47.
153. Wille-Jorgensen P. Prophylaxis of postoperative thromboembolism with a combination of heparin and graduated compression stockings. *Int Angiol* 1996;15(Suppl 1):15–20.
154. Amarigiri SV, Lees TA. Elastic compression stockings for prevention of deep vein thrombosis (Cochrane Review). In: The Cochrane Library, Issue 1, 2001. Oxford: Update Software.
155. Turpie AGG, Hirsh J, Gent M, et al. Prevention of deep vein thrombosis in potential neurosurgical patients. A randomized trial comparing graduated compression stockings alone or graduated compression stockings plus intermittent pneumatic compression with control. *Arch Intern Med* 1989;149:679–681.
156. Cahan MA, Hanna DJ, Wiley LA, et al. External pneumatic compression and fibrinolysis in abdominal surgery. *J Vasc Surg* 2000;32:537–543.
157. Purtill L, Gens DR, Joseph LA, et al. Randomized prospective comparison of foot pumps versus calf pumps for deep venous thrombosis prophylaxis in trauma patients. [abstract] *J Trauma* 1997;43:197.
158. Anglen JO, Bagby C, George R. A randomized comparison of sequential-gradient calf compression with intermittent plantar compression for prevention of venous thrombosis in orthopedic trauma patients: preliminary results. *Am J Orthop* 1998;27:53–58.
159. Blanchard J, Meuwly J-Y, Leyvraz P-F, et al. Prevention of deep-vein thrombosis after total knee replacement: randomised comparison between a low-molecular-weight heparin (nadroparin) and mechanical prophylaxis with a foot-pump system. *J Bone Joint Surg* 1999;81-B:654–659.
160. Elliott CG, Dudney TM, Egger M, et al. Calf-thigh sequential pneumatic compression compared with plantar venous pneumatic compression to prevent deep-vein thrombosis after non-lower extremity trauma. *J Trauma* 1999;47:25–32.
161. Geerts W, Jay R, Code K, et al. Venous foot pump as thromboprophylaxis in major trauma. [abstract] *Thromb Haemost* 1999;82(Suppl):650.
162. Anglen JO, Goss K, Edwards J, et al. Foot pump prophylaxis for deep venous thrombosis: the rate of effective usage in trauma patients. *Am J Orthop* 1998;27:580–582.
163. Planes A, Vochelle N, Mazas F, et al. Prevention of postoperative venous thrombosis: a randomized trial comparing unfractionated heparin with low molecular weight heparin in patients undergoing total hip replacement. *Thromb Haemost* 1988; 60:407–410.
164. Nurmohamed MT, Rosendaal FR, Buller HR, et al. Low-molecular-weight heparin versus standard heparin in general and orthopaedic surgery: a meta-analysis. *Lancet* 1992;340: 152–156.
165. Green D, Lee MY, Lin AC, et al. Prevention of thromboembolism after spinal cord injury using low-molecular-weight heparin. *Ann Intern Med* 1990;113:571–574.
166. Upchurch GR, Demling RH, Davies J, et al. Efficacy of subcutaneous heparin in prevention of venous thromboembolic events in trauma patients. *Am Surg* 1995;61:749–755.
167. Haentjens P and the Belgian Fraxiparine Study Group. Thromboembolic prophylaxis in orthopaedic trauma patients: a comparison between a fixed dose and an individually adjusted dose of a low molecular weight heparin (nadroparin calcium). *Injury* 1996;27:385–390.
168. Dodenhoff RM, Steele N, Ward AJ. Thromboprophylaxis in pelvic and acetabular fracture surgery: the role of early treatment. [abstract] *J Bone Joint Surg* 1999;81-B(Suppl III): 290–291.
169. Wade WE, Chisholm MA. Deep venous thrombosis prophylaxis in trauma: cost analysis. *Blood Coag Fibrinol* 2000;11: 101–106.
170. Devlin JW, Petitta A, Shepard AD, et al. Cost-effectiveness of enoxaparin versus low-dose heparin for prophylaxis against venous thrombosis after major trauma. *Pharmacotherapy* 1998;18:1335–1342.
171. Shorr AF, Ramage AS. Enoxaparin for thromboprophylaxis after major trauma: potential cost implications. *Crit Care Med* 2001;29:1659–1665.
172. Selby R, Geerts WH. Venous thromboembolism prophylaxis after trauma: dollars and sense. *Crit Care Med* 2001;29: 1839–1840.
173. Van den Berg E, Wennmacher M, Meissner A. Duplex screening for deep venous thrombosis and optimization of perioperative thromboembolism prophylaxis: results from Postoperative Thromboembolism Intervention Study (POTIS II). [abstract] *Thromb Haemost* 2001;86(Suppl):abstract CD3593.
174. Rohrer MJ, Scheidler MG, Wheeler HB, et al. Extended indications for placement of an inferior vena cava filter. *J Vasc Surg* 1989;10:44–50.
175. Leach TA, Pastena JA, Swan KG, et al. Surgical prophylaxis for pulmonary embolism. *Am Surg* 1994;60:292–295.
176. Rosenthal D, McKinsey JF, Levy AM, et al. Use of the Greenfield filter in patients with major trauma. *Cardiovasc Surg* 1994; 2:52–55.
177. Greenfield LJ. Venous thromboembolism in trauma patients. *J Am Coll Surg* 1995;180:725–726.
178. Khansarinia S, Dennis JW, Veldenz HC, et al. Prophylactic Greenfield filter placement in selected high-risk trauma patients. *J Vasc Surg* 1995;22:231–236.
179. Rogers FB, Shackford SR, Ricci MA, et al. Routine prophylac-

tic vena cava filter insertion in severely injured trauma patients decreases the incidence of pulmonary embolism. *J Am Coll Surg* 1995;180:641–647.

180. Rodriguez JL, Lopez JM, Proctor MC, et al. Early placement of prophylactic vena caval filters in injured patients at high risk for pulmonary embolism. *J Trauma* 1996;40:797–802.
181. Greenfield LJ, Proctor MC, Michaels AJ, et al. Prophylactic vena caval filters in trauma: the rest of the story. *J Vasc Surg* 2000;32:490–497.
182. O'Malley KF, Marberger S, Ross SE. Prevention of pulmonary embolism after pelvic fracture: rational use of inferior vena caval filters. [abstract] *J Trauma* 1996;40:182.
183. McMurtry AL, Owings JT, Anderson JT, et al. Increased use of prophylactic vena cava filters in trauma patients failed to decrease overall incidence of pulmonary embolism. *J Am Coll Surg* 1999;189:314–320.
184. Spain DA, Richardson JD, Polk HC, et al. Venous thromboembolism in the high- risk trauma patient: do risks justify aggressive screening and prophylaxis? *J Trauma* 1997;42: 463–469.
185. Patton JH, Fabian TC, Croce MA, et al. Prophylactic Greenfield filters: acute complications and long-term follow-up. *J Trauma* 1996;41:231–237.
186. Blebea J, Wilson R, Waybill P, et al. Deep venous thrombosis after percutaneous insertion of vena caval filters. *J Vasc Surg* 1999;30:821–829.
187. Wojcik R, Cipolle MD, Fearon I, et al. Long-term follow-up of trauma patients with a vena caval filter. *J Trauma* 2000;49: 839–843.
188. Lorch H, Welger D, Wagner V, et al. Current practice of temporary vena cava filter insertion: a multicenter registry. *J Vasc Intervent Radiol* 2000;11:83–88.
189. David W, Cross WS, Colaiuta E, et al. Pulmonary embolus after vena cava filter placement. *Am Surg* 1999;65:341–346.
190. Becker DM, Philbrick JT, Selby JB. Inferior vena cava filters: indications, safety, effectiveness. *Arch Intern Med* 1992;152: 1985–1994.
191. Alexander JJ, Yuhas JP, Piotrowski JJ. Is the increasing use of prophylactic percutaneous IVC filters justified? *Am J Surg* 1994;168:102–106.
192. Quirke TE, Rotota PC, Swan KG. Inferior vena caval filter use in U.S. trauma centers: a practitioner survey. *J Trauma* 1997; 43:333–337.
193. Collins DN, Barnes CL, McCowan TC, et al. Vena caval filter use in orthopaedic trauma patients with recognized preoperative venous thromboembolic disease. *J Orthop Trauma* 1992;6: 135–138.
194. Janku GV, Paiement GD, Green HD. Prevention of venous thromboembolism in orthopaedics in the United States. *Clin Orthop* 1996;325:313–321.
195. Morgan SJ, Jeray KJ, Phieffer LS, et al. Attitudes of orthopaedic trauma surgeons regarding current controversies in the management of pelvic and acetabular fractures. *J Orthop Trauma* 2001;15:526–532.
196. Meyer CS, Blebea J, Davis K, et al. Surveillance venous scans for deep venous thrombosis in multiple trauma patients. *Ann Vasc Surg* 1995;9:109–114.
197. Schwarcz TH, Quick RC, Minion DJ, et al. Enoxaparin treatment in high-risk trauma patients limits the utility of surveillance venous duplex scanning. *J Vasc Surg* 2001;34:447–452.
198. Robinson KS, Anderson DR, Gross M, et al. Ultrasonographic screening before hospital discharge for deep venous thrombosis after arthroplasty: the Post-Arthroplasty Screening Study. A randomized, controlled trial. *Ann Intern Med* 1997;127:439–445.
199. Hammers LW, Cohn SM, Brown JM, et al. Doppler color flow imaging surveillance of deep vein thrombosis in high-risk trauma patients. *J Ultrasound Med* 1996;15:19–24.
200. Satiani B, Falcone R, Shook L, et al. Screening for major deep vein thrombosis in seriously injured patients: a prospective study. *Ann Vasc Surg* 1997;11:626–629.
201. Cipolle MD, Wojcik R, Seislove E, et al. The role of surveillance duplex scanning in preventing pulmonary embolism in trauma patients. *J Trauma* 2002;52:453–462.
202. Polak JF, Fox LA. MR assessment of the extremity veins. *Semin Ultrasound CT MRI* 1999;20:36–46.
203. Morgan SJ, Stover MS, Stackhouse DJ, et al. Magnetic resonance venography: interobserver variability in the identification of pelvic vein thrombosis. [abstract] *J Orthop Trauma* 2000;14:147.
204. Meissner MH. Deep venous thrombosis in the trauma patient. *Semin Vasc Surg* 1998;11:274–282.

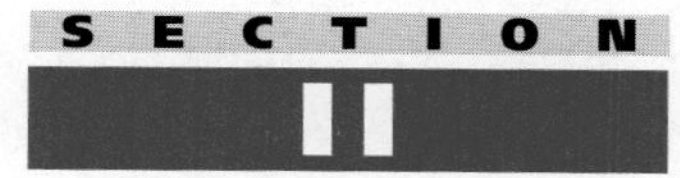

DISRUPTION OF THE PELVIC RING

10

DEFINING THE INJURY: ASSESSMENT OF PELVIC FRACTURES

MARVIN TILE
JOEL RUBENSTEIN

INTRODUCTION

The importance of determining the degree of instability in any pelvic injury was stressed in Chapter 2. The proposed classification and management protocol depend entirely on this important fact. In this chapter we deal with the assessment of stability in a given pelvic injury so that logical management will follow.

CLINICAL ASSESSMENT

History

As in all areas of clinical medicine, an accurate history is essential, because one may suspect what type of pelvic injury is present from the history alone. A history always can be obtained, either directly if the patient is conscious, or from the ambulance attendant or relatives if the patient is unconscious. This important first step directs the initial attending physician to suspect an emergent or less emergent problem. If the force causing the injury is low energy in nature (e.g., a simple fall at home), then the outlook for the patient is markedly different than if the force is high energy (e.g., that associated with motor vehicle trauma, falls from heights, or industrial accidents). Therefore, a complete history should include the following observations.

Patient Profile

Age

The age of the patient has an important effect on the structure of bone. Persons older than 40 years lose cancellous bone, thus diminishing the strength of the pelvis. Consequently, an injury to the pelvis of an older patient may have been caused by a much less violent force than a similar injury in a younger patient. As in all musculoskeletal injuries, especially those involving cancellous bone, this fact has a direct bearing on the degree of associated soft-tissue trauma. In young patients, minor fractures in those sites may be associated with major soft-tissue disruption and ensuing joint instability, whereas the same fracture may have no soft-tissue disruption and be relatively stable in older patients. Therefore, in young patients even minor degrees of displacement may be associated with major soft-tissue injury causing instability to the pelvic ring and increasing numbers of associated injuries to the pelvic and abdominal viscera, nerve, and blood vessels.

Sex

Male. Because of the course of the male urethra, injuries to that structure always should be suspected with trauma to the male pelvis. These injuries may be particularly disastrous to a young man because of the high incidence of impotence.

Female. Urethral injuries are uncommon in women; however, an equally disastrous complication may be overlooked and therefore should always be suspected; that is, a vaginal tear that converts a closed pelvic fracture to an open fracture, with the high attendant morbidity and mortality rate.

Medical History

Knowledge of illness, medications, and drug or alcohol abuse is important, if available.

Associated Injuries

The history of injury to other body systems is important in determining the amount of trauma inflicted on the bony pelvis, as indicated in Chapter 8.

Injury Profile

Magnitude of Force

The magnitude of the force causing the injury is an important historical determination. It is obvious that injuries caused by violent shearing forces are associated with the highest degree of pelvic ring instability as well as the largest number of associated injuries. These high-energy forces of immense magnitude usually are associated with motor vehicle or industrial accidents, such as heavy construction or mining, depending on the geographic area.

Direction of Force

Because our classification of pelvic disruption is based partly on the direction of force causing the injury, the determination of that force assumes some importance, and surprisingly this information often is available.

Anteroposterior forces produce open-book type patterns, often leaving the posterior ligamentous structures intact.

Lateral compressive forces can cause several injury patterns. On occasion, the posterior sacroiliac complex is disrupted and rigidly impacted, similar to most os calcis or tibial plateau fractures, thus causing confusion to the unwary observer who may expect gross instability from the history of a violent injury. As in most impacted cancellous fractures, reduction may cause instability, owing to the resultant large gap. Lateral compressive forces also may cause pelvic injuries of major importance, which on initial radiographic examination, appear innocuous because of the elastic recoil of the tissues following injury. Again, this may lull the unwary into a false sense of security so that potentially unstable injuries may be overlooked.

Violent shearing forces, acting perpendicular to the main axis of the cancellous surfaces, produce grossly unstable patterns. The cancellous bone is not compressed but is torn apart by this force, often leaving marked displacement and a gap at the fracture site. Soft tissues, including nerves, vessels, and viscera, are often injured; therefore, important associated injuries are the rule rather than the exception. A history of this type of force should suggest to the astute surgeon that the patient is at risk if immediate resuscitation is not initiated, and that the musculoskeletal injury itself may be difficult to manage.

Physical Examination

The physical examination ranks at least equal in importance to the radiologic assessment in determining the degree of pelvic instability. One may easily be misled by the radiographic appearance, but it would be unusual to be misled after a careful physical examination. The essence of the physical examination, as described by Apley (1) is: look, feel, move, and listen.

Look

The patient must be completely undressed at this stage; otherwise important physical findings will be missed.

Wounds

All wounds should be carefully assessed. Of utmost importance is the diagnosis of an open pelvic fracture; therefore, open wounds in the vicinity of the pelvic disruption must be regarded as communicating with the fracture until it is proven otherwise. Failure to recognize an open pelvic disruption often leads to a disastrous outcome.

Contusions

The careful observer notes the position of the contusions and abrasions, which may indicate the direction of the injurious force.

Bleeding Genitalia

In men, blood escaping from the urethral meatus suggests a urethral rupture; in women, blood from the urethra or vagina suggests an occult open fracture of the pelvis (Fig. 10-1).

Displacement of Pelvis or Lower Extremities

If there is no other fracture in the leg, its degree of rotation and shortening suggest to the surgeon what type of pelvic fracture is present. If the extremity is obviously shortened, internally rotated, and displaced at the posterior iliac spine, the pelvic injury is most likely a lateral compression type injury with posterior impaction (Fig. 10-2). Displacement of the posterior superior iliac spine may be striking, giving the appearance of a large bony mass (Fig. 10-3). The fracture in this young woman was so firmly impacted on the day of injury that it could not be reduced, even when she was given general anesthesia. Conversely, if the extremity is externally rotated and shortened, and no lower limb fracture is noted, the pelvic injury is most likely a severe unstable vertical shear type. Careful inspection of the level and rotation of the anterior superior and posterior superior iliac spines also aids in the determination of the fracture pattern.

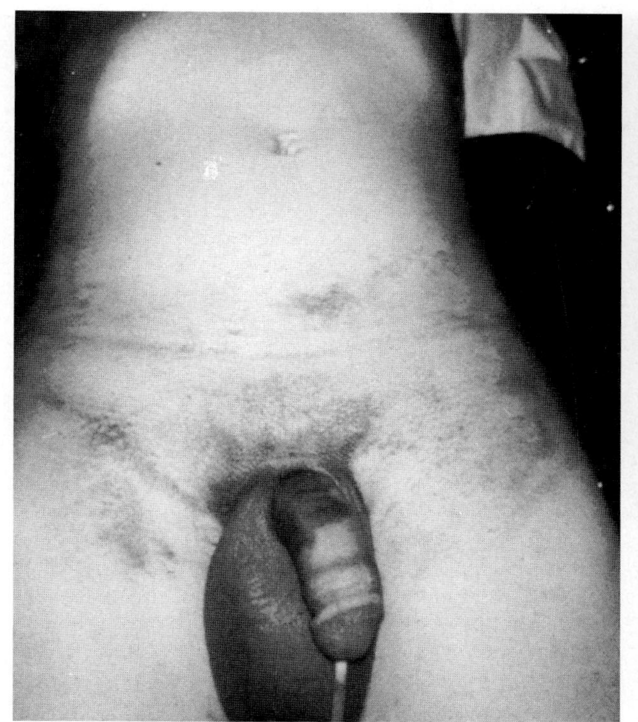
A

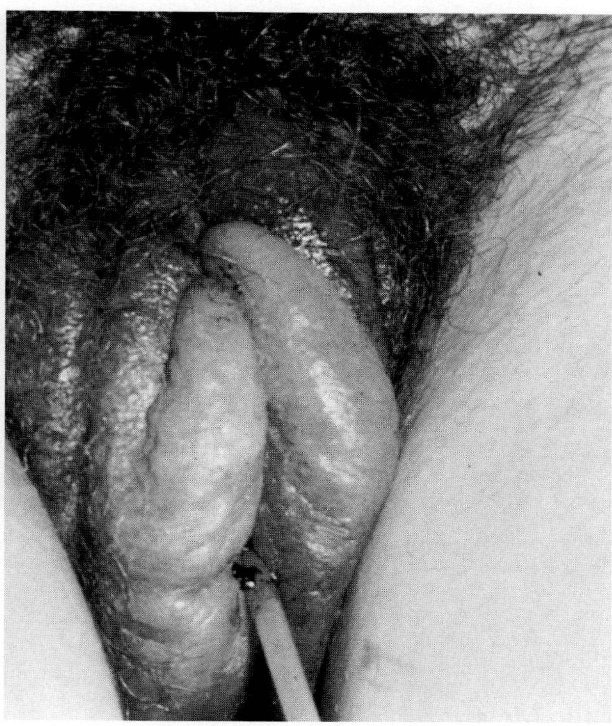
B

FIGURE 10-1. A: Massive ecchymosis and hemorrhage into the scrotum and penis as a result of a severe pelvic disruption with bladder rupture. **B:** Massive swelling of the labia majora as a result of a disruption of the symphysis pubis in an unstable type of pelvic disruption. This 16-year-old girl also sustained a laceration of her vagina, indicating an occult open fracture of the pelvis.

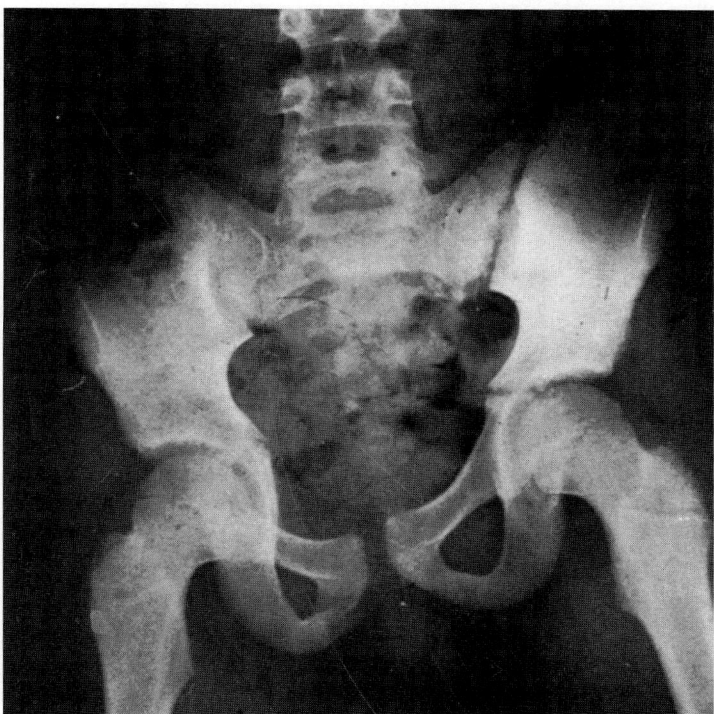
A

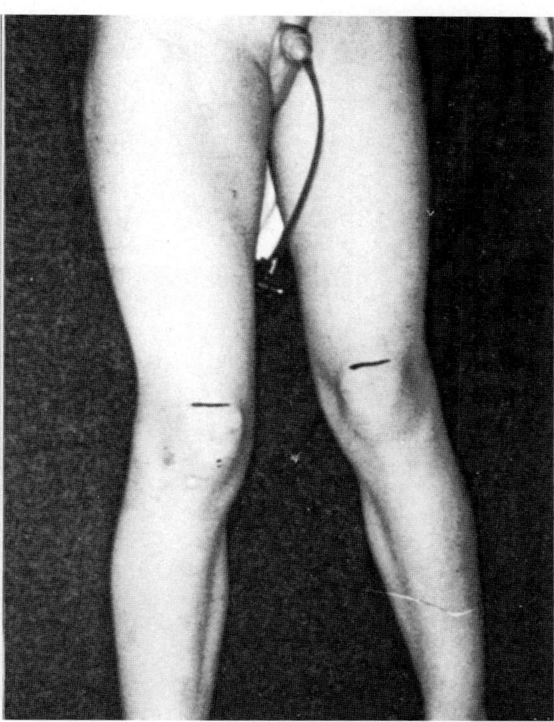
B

FIGURE 10-2. A: Anteroposterior radiograph of a young man with a severe pelvic disruption. **B:** Clinical examination indicates an internally rotated shortened left lower extremity.

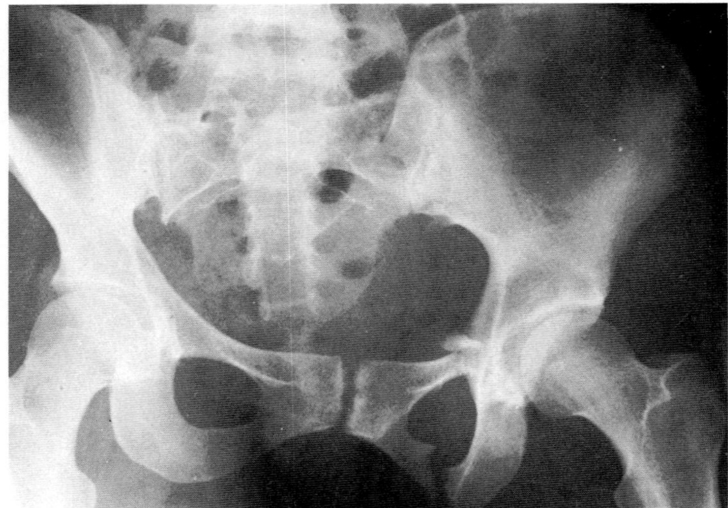
A

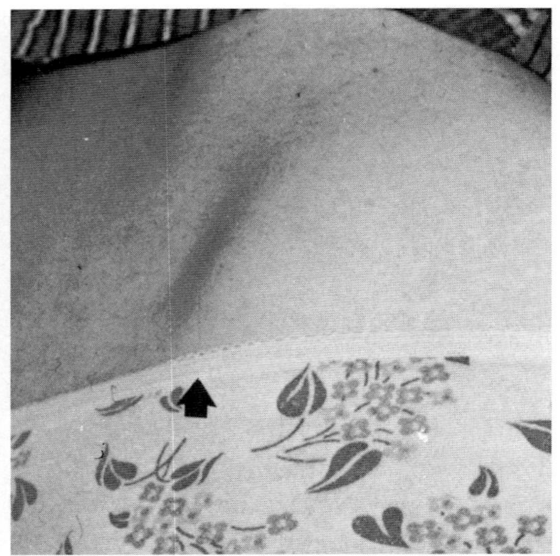
B

FIGURE 10-3. A: Anteroposterior radiograph of a lateral compression type of pelvic disruption with marked impaction of the right sacroiliac complex. Note the marked internal rotation of the right hemipelvis. **B:** Clinical photograph of the same patient showing the large bony mass posteriorly. This bony mass is caused by the internal rotation of the right hemipelvis with displacement of the posterior superior iliac spine.

Feel and Move

Following careful observation, the examiner should go on to palpate the injured area.

Palpation

Careful palpation of the pelvis may reveal crepitus or abnormal motion in the hemipelvis, either one indicative of instability. The hemipelvis should be rotated carefully by pushing medially on the iliac crests to determine abnormal movement (Fig. 10-4). Also, the same maneuver may be accomplished by internally and externally rotating the femora. Direct palpation of the symphysis may reveal a large gap, indicating disruption of the symphysis (Fig. 10-5). Occasionally, in spite of obvious deformity, no crepitus or abnormal motion is found. Careful radiographic correlation usually indicates posterior impaction owing to lateral compression.

Palpation reveals the presence or absence of further injury to the lower extremities, because injuries to the hip, femur, and knee are not infrequently associated with pelvic disruption. An internally rotated limb, although it often indicates only a lateral compression injury to the pelvis, also may indicate a concomitant posterior dislocation of the hip or acetabular disruption.

Fractures of the femur usually are obvious, but injuries to the knee, unfortunately, are commonly missed. Posterior knee instability is especially common in pelvic injuries where the injurious force has been applied through the femora.

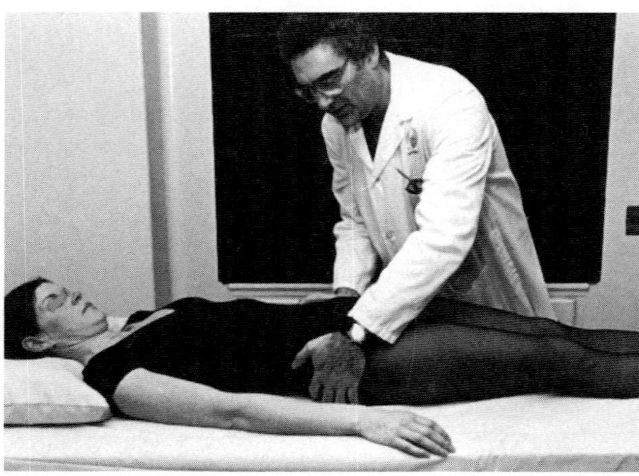

FIGURE 10-4. Direct palpation of the iliac crest reveals crepitus or abnormal motion, which, if present, is the best indicator of instability of the pelvis.

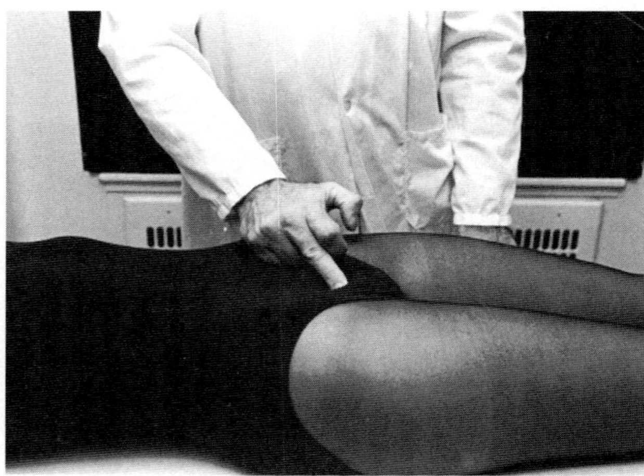

FIGURE 10-5. Direct palpation of the symphysis pubis may reveal a gap and ecchymosis, indicating a symphysis disruption.

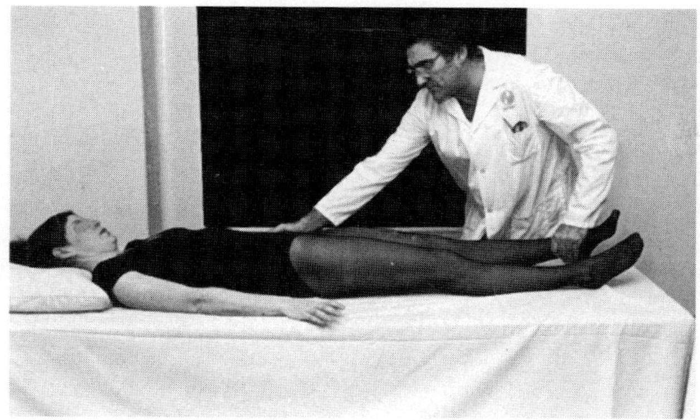

FIGURE 10-6. With one arm controlling the injured hemipelvis and the second arm applying traction, one can again determine the amount of instability present.

Traction

Traction to the extremity is an important maneuver; first to rule out an injury to the extremity, and second, if none exists, to determine the degree of pelvic instability (Fig. 10-6). If no extremity injury exists and shortening is present, traction on the extremity may have one of two effects. (a) The hemipelvis will reduce as traction is applied, indicating the gross instability of that hemipelvis. The instability can be appreciated readily by palpating the iliac crests during the maneuver or by direct visualization on the image intensifier. (b) Traction has no effect on the hemipelvis, indicating impaction of the posterior complex. These maneuvers are as important as radiographs for determining pelvic instability, and they must be performed to aid in the proper management of the injury.

Rectal and Vaginal Examination

Both rectal and vaginal examination are essential for complete patient assessment. Very often the fracture can be palpated by either of these routes, to further assess the stability of the pelvic ring. Of equal importance, of course, is the presence or absence of vaginal or rectal lacerations.

Neurologic Examination

Injury to the lumbosacral plexus, especially the L5 root, is common; therefore, a careful neurologic examination is mandatory. Lesions of the S1 root and the pudendal nerve are less common. Nerve injuries of all types are much more common in shear-type fractures; therefore, they suggest gross pelvic instability.

Summary

In summary, a careful history and physical examination lead the examiner to a correct diagnosis of pelvic instability. If gross instability of the hemipelvis is present, simple traction applied through that extremity easily reduces the deformity. Palpation of the anterior and posterior iliac spines and application of both internal and external rotational forces through the iliac spines also may reveal gross abnormal motion, through one hemipelvis or both. In the most unstable examples, the affected hemipelvis may be moved to almost any position, because motion is limited only by the skin and subcutaneous tissue.

It is almost always possible to make this determination in a conscious patient. If, however, palpation is difficult in a conscious patient because of pain, the patient may be put under general anesthesia. Because most of these patients undergo general anesthesia for an associated injury, the attending surgeon should use that opportunity to assess the degree of stability of the pelvic ring, checking it with image intensification, if possible. As stressed in the following, definitive management of the fracture should be carried out at that time, immediately following management of the associated injuries.

In some cases with gross deformity and shortening, the pelvis is completely stable; that is, no amount of rotatory force applied to the pelvis reduces the hemipelvis and no amount of traction through the lower extremity reduces the short extremity. Manipulation under image intensification confirms the stable nature of the injury.

In those cases, either the important posterior tension band of the pelvis, that is, the posterior sacroiliac ligaments, is intact, or the posterior bony complex, although displaced, has been so impacted by the lateral compression force that it is rendered stable and immovable. This concept is akin to the concept of compression of cancellous bone in any other part of the body, such as fractures of the os calcis, tibial plateau, and neck of the humerus. Experienced orthopedic surgeons recognize that, in many situations where cancellous bone is impacted and surgery is necessary to restore normal anatomy, for example, in the tibial plateau fracture, the impacted bone is often so stable that it has to be pried out with an elevator or even hammered out with a bone punch. This is in marked contrast to shearing injuries through cancellous bone, which cause instability and, often, delayed union.

It should be readily apparent following a careful physical examination that one is dealing with either a displaced or undisplaced pelvic disruption and whether that disruption is inherently stable or unstable. This clinical determination is extremely important even before radiologic assessment, because the anticipated associated injuries to other body systems are much greater in patients with an unstable pelvic injury, as carefully outlined by McMurtry and coworkers (2). However, the precise recognition of the patterns of displacement demands special radiographic techniques.

RADIOLOGIC ASSESSMENT

Plain Radiography

A single anteroposterior radiograph, commonly used in most trauma centers, is often sufficient in the acute situation

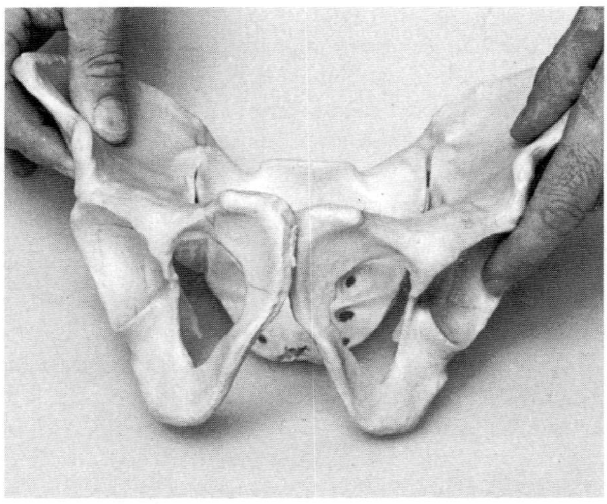

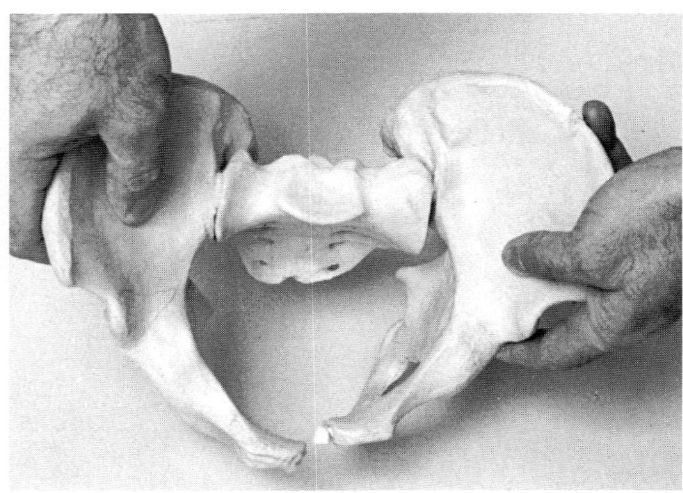

FIGURE 10-7. A: When placed in the anteroposterior plane, the skeleton appears intact, when in fact, the left hemipelvis is displaced posteriorly. **B:** Therefore, the anteroposterior radiograph of the pelvis may be misleading and the inlet view is the best view for determining posterior displacements.

to determine the presence or absence of pelvic ring instability. In most instances, when dealing with life-threatening injuries in a polytrauma patient, resuscitation should be instituted immediately on the basis of this single anteroposterior radiograph. If displacement has occurred in the sacroiliac area, major hemorrhage must be suspected and resuscitation expedited. However, the single anteroposterior radiograph may be misleading. Reliance on this view alone may mislead the surgeon into believing that little or no posterior displacement exists, when in truth, major displacement may be present. The best view for disclosing posterior displacement is the inlet view (Fig. 10-7). Therefore, for accurate definitive treatment of the pelvic ring injury, more detailed radiologic information is required.

Anatomically, the plane of the true pelvic brim lies oblique to the axis of the trunk, subtending an angle of 45° to 60°. Therefore, the usual anteroposterior radiograph is oblique to the pelvic brim (Fig. 10-8). To obtain more information on anterior, posterior, or rotatory displacements of the pelvic ring, other radiographic projections are required. Because the lateral radiograph is of little value, three anteroposterior projections, as described by Pennal and Sutherland (3), are more informative.

Anteroposterior Projection

With the patient supine on the x-ray table, the beam is directed perpendicular to the midpelvis and radiographic plate (Fig. 10-9). A careful inspection of the anteroposterior radiograph may give a wealth of information. The surgeon should examine the film for the type of anterior lesion, that is, a symphysis disruption or rami fractures, or both, and for the type of posterior lesion, anatomically and morphologically. The posterior lesion may disrupt the ilium, sacroiliac joint (often with a portion of ilium attached), or sacrum (often through the weakest area, the sacral foramina). Also, the posterior lesion may be grossly displaced with a large gap between the fragments, indicating instability, or conversely, may be severely impacted, indicating immediate stability of the fragments. However, this latter type of injury may exhibit displacement of the prior sacroiliac area in spite of the inherent stability.

Other telltale signs of instability may be noted on the standard radiograph. Of major importance is the presence of a displaced avulsion fracture of the tip of the transverse process of the fifth lumbar vertebra, almost always indicative of pelvic instability. The presence of a displaced avulsion fracture of either end of the sacrospinous ligament (e.g., the ischial spine, or a fragment of the adjacent sacrum) is indicative of instability of that hemipelvis. Bilateral posterior

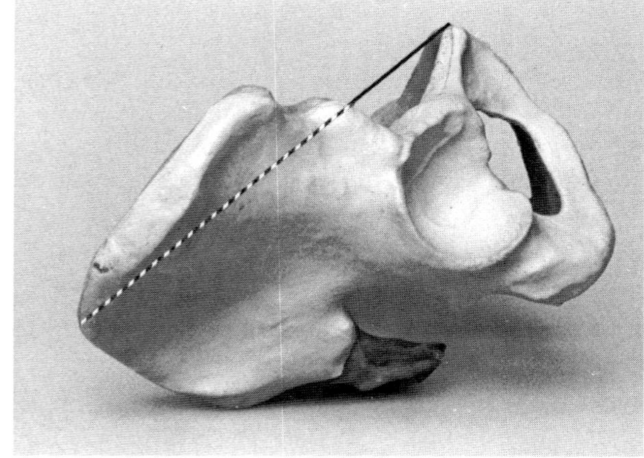

FIGURE 10-8. The plane of the true pelvic brim lies oblique to the axis of the trunk, subtending an angle of 45° to 60°.

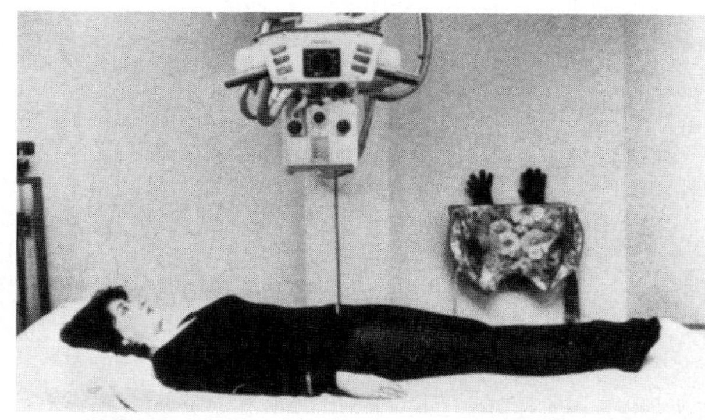

A

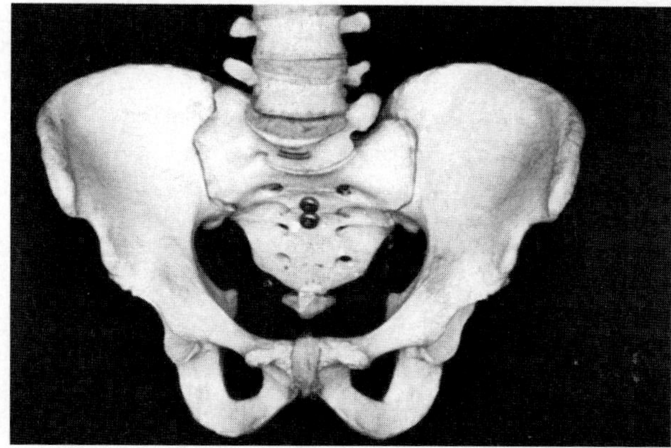

B

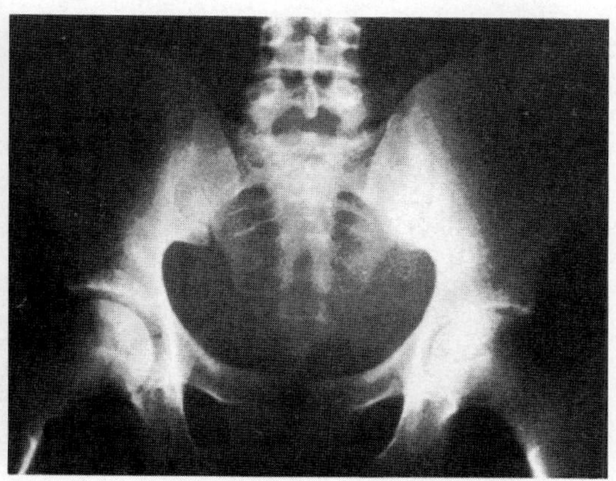

C

FIGURE 10-9. A: For the anteroposterior projection, the beam is directed perpendicular to the midpelvis and the radiographic plate. **B:** Anatomic appearance of the pelvis in the anteroposterior plane. **C:** Radiographic appearance of the pelvis in the anteroposterior plane.

pelvic disruptions, always difficult and dangerous to deal with, may be suspected on the standard radiograph.

Inlet Projection

With the patient supine, this view is obtained by directing the x-ray beam from the head to the midpelvis at an angle of 60° to the x-ray table (Fig. 10-10). This projection, which is perpendicular to the pelvic brim, shows the true pelvic inlet. This view shows anterior and posterior displacements of the pelvis better than any other, and is, in my opinion, the most useful pelvic projection. The usual posterior displacements through the sacroiliac complex are best seen on this projection. Also seen are inward rotation associated with lateral compression injuries and outward rotation often seen in shearing injuries or in acetabular fractures.

Outlet Projection

With the patient supine on the x-ray table, the beam is directed from the foot to the symphysis at an angle of 45° to the radiographic plate (Fig. 10-11). The tangential view is helpful in disclosing superior displacements of the posterior half of the pelvis and either superior or inferior displacement of the anterior portion of the pelvis. Thus, rotational deformity of the bucket-handle type can often be seen on the outlet view. On this view, true elevation of the hip joint is reflected in a leg length discrepancy; therefore, this view helps in determining the necessity for reduction.

Posterior displacement, as seen on the inlet view, does not necessarily indicate significant limb shortening, in contrast to the shortening associated with elevation of the acetabulum in the outlet view.

The inlet and outlet views are approximately at right angles to each other, satisfying in part the prerequisite for adequate radiologic assessment. Most displacements of the pelvis can be determined by careful observation of the three radiologic views.

Theoretically, these displacements may be anterior or posterior, lateral or medial, superior or inferior. Rotation may also occur about any axis parallel to or perpendicular to the pelvic brim; however, the perpendicular axis is usually through the sacroiliac joint. By carefully scrutinizing all avulsion fractures, gross instability may be suspected and correlated to the clinical findings.

Oblique Projection

The injury to the posterior complex is often most important in considering fracture management. Oblique views taken through the sacroiliac joint may be most helpful in determining the displacement of the fracture or dislocation through the joint, and whether indeed the fracture is of the impacted or the shear variety (Fig. 10-12).

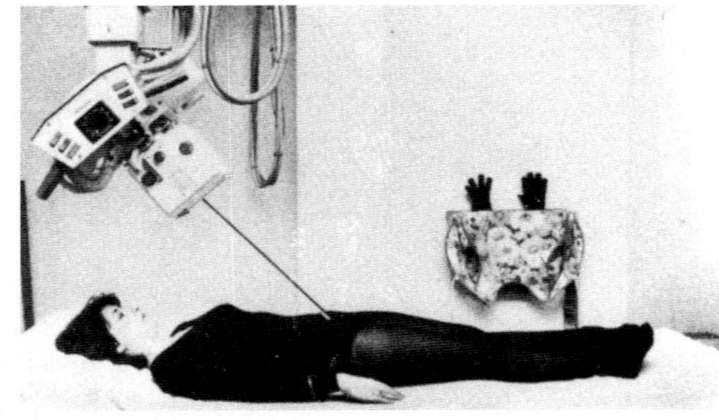

A

FIGURE 10-10. A: For the inlet projection the beam is directed from the head to the midpelvis at an angle of 60° to the plate. B: Anatomic appearance in the inlet projection. C: Radiologic appearance in the inlet projection.

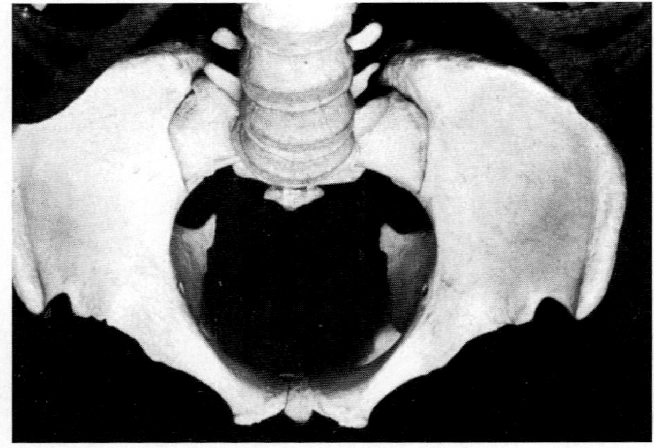

B

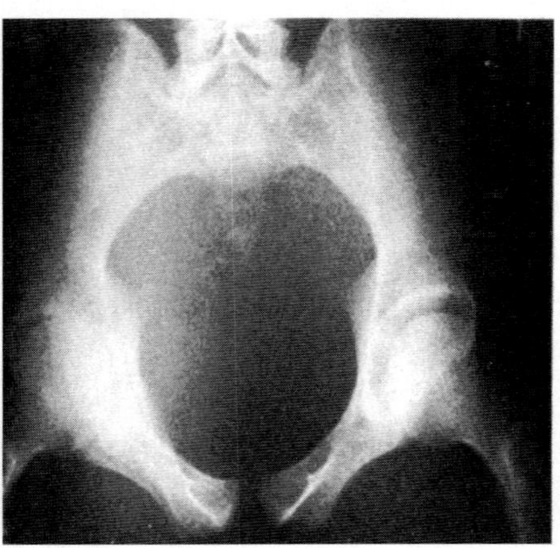

C

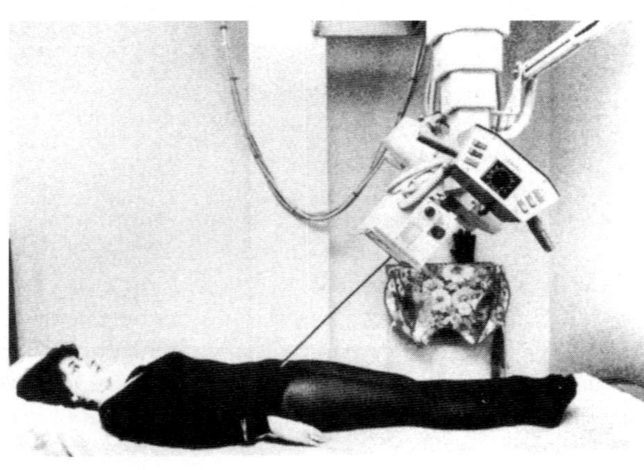

A

FIGURE 10-11. A: For the outlet projection, the beam is directed from the foot to the symphysis at an angle of 45° to the plate. B: Anatomic appearance in the outlet projection. C: Radiologic appearance in the outlet projection.

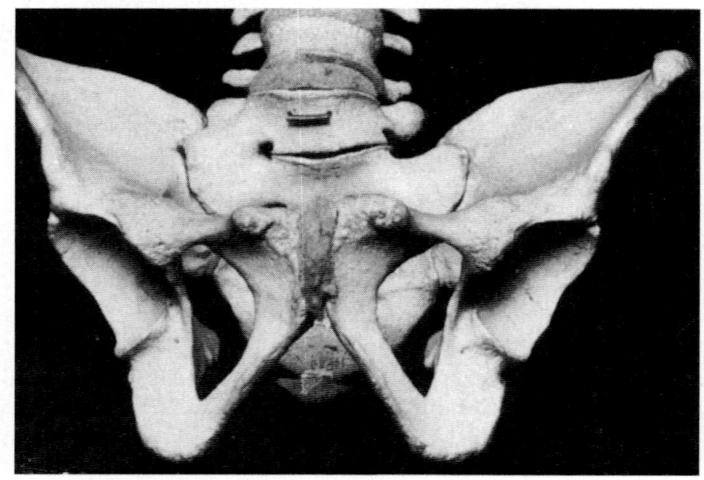

B

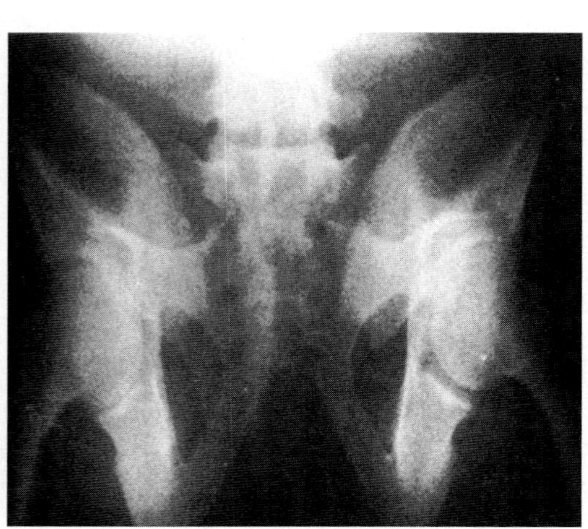

C

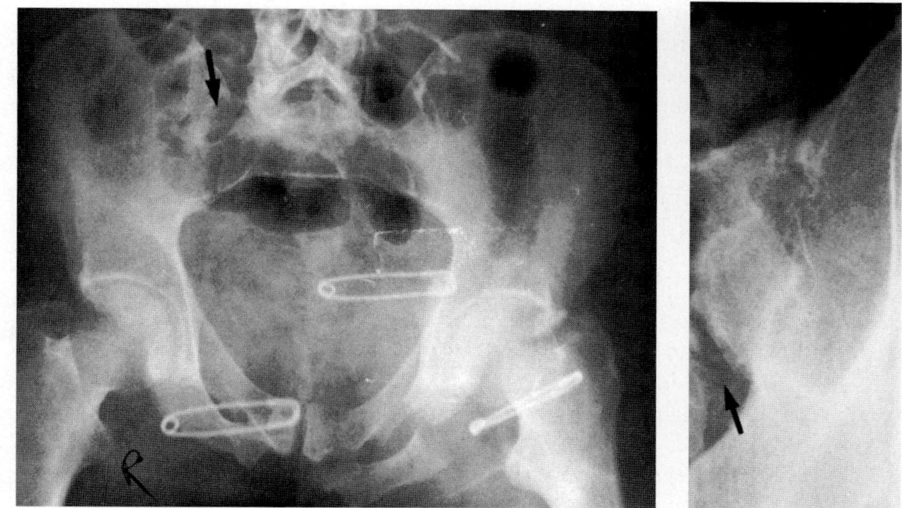

FIGURE 10-12. A: Anteroposterior radiograph of a 33-year-old man involved in a mine injury. The *black arrow* points to the right sacroiliac joint, where very little disruption can be seen. Note the inferior pubic ramus displacement. This patient sustained a complete disruption of his urethra. **B:** Oblique view of the sacroiliac area shows the disruption through the sacrum. This view outlines the pathology much better than the standard anteroposterior view. This patient also sustained an injury to the L5 and S1 nerve roots.

Tomography

Tomograms may also be helpful in the assessment of the posterior fracture complex and may show gross disruption through the sacral foramina. The advent of computed tomography (CT), where available, has rendered standard tomography obsolete in most cases (Fig. 10-13).

Nuclear Scanning

Technetium polyphosphate bone scanning has only limited value in the early diagnosis and treatment of pelvic fractures; however, as shown by Gertzbein and Chenoweth (4), occult lesions of the pelvic ring can be determined by technetium scanning. Experimental work by Gertzbein and Chenoweth

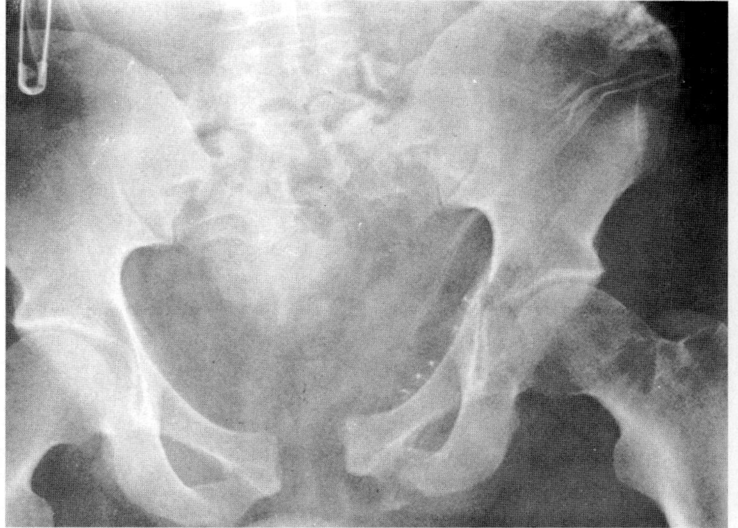

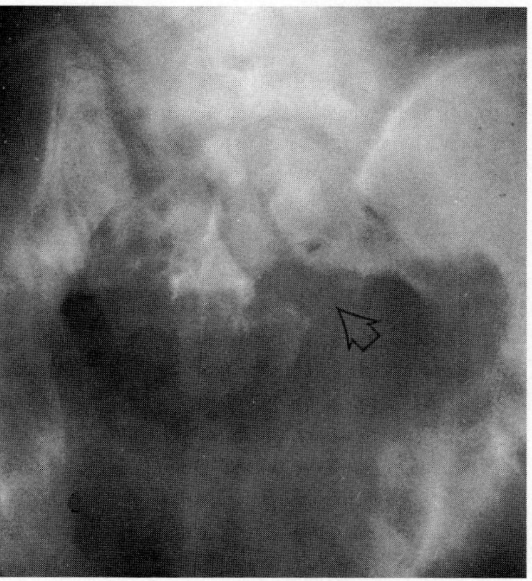

FIGURE 10-13. A: Anteroposterior radiograph shows marked pelvic disruption of the unstable type. **B:** A tomogram through the sacrum shows the massive posterior disruption much better than the anteroposterior projection. This girl sustained an open fracture posteriorly, eventually leading to sepsis and nonunion.

has proven that the technetium accumulates in the subchondral bone of the sacroiliac joint in areas demonstrated histologically to be osteoblastic. The nature of the sacroiliac lesion in these occult cases appears to be microavulsion fractures of the subchondral bone. The injury, therefore, occurs when small portions of bone are avulsed with Sharpey's fibers at the insertion of the sacroiliac ligaments.

Computed Tomography

Dramatic advances in CT imaging have been made since the previous edition of this book. Quadsection CT technology, which became available in 1998, allows images to be obtained eight times faster than with the original multisection techniques that were introduced in 1992. This newer CT technology also provides images with better spatial and temporal resolution, decreased image noise, and increased concentration of intravascular contrast, while permitting longer areas of anatomic coverage than with conventional single-section helical (spiral) CT scanners. In patients with acute trauma, these advantages are particularly important because diagnostic examinations are obtained more quickly and because factors such as accurate positioning of the pelvis are less critical.

CT adds an important dimension to the determination of the displacement of the pelvic ring injury, by demonstrating the osseous and soft-tissue elements of the pelvis in cross section, and to the assessment of pelvic stability (Fig. 10-14). Perhaps most important is its value in the assessment of pelvic ring stability. No other imaging technique shows so vividly the detail of the sacroiliac area, where injuries are difficult to visualize with standard radiologic technique (Fig. 10-15). The cross-sectional CT images clearly indicate whether the posterior injury is impacted and stable or disrupted and unstable (Fig. 10-16). Because of the cross-sectional nature of the CT image, rotational deformities are best seen by this method. This knowledge is indispensable in formulating a treatment plan for these patients.

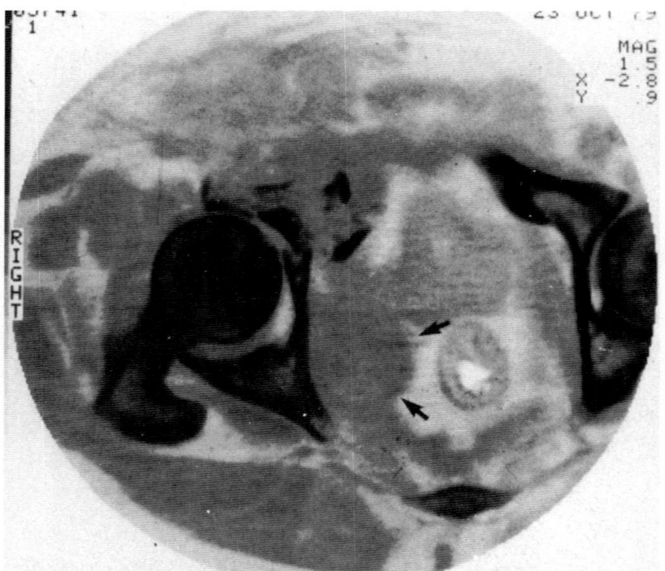

FIGURE 10-14. Computed tomography indicates a marked disruption of the anterior column of the acetabulum. Note the massive pelvic hematoma displacing the visceral contents of the pelvis to the left side.

Multiplanar Reconstruction and Three-Dimensional Computed Tomography

The series of axial images obtained with conventional CT provides additional details about the fracture pattern; however, integration of these images into a three-dimensional (3D) concept is difficult, even for the experienced observer. Therefore, computer software programs for multiplanar reconstruction (MPR) and three-dimensional computed tomography (3DCT) provide an alternative method for displaying the same information but allow a more immediate appreciation of the fracture pattern and some of its associated complications. These latter two techniques are particularly useful in deciding which fractures require surgery and in planning the operative treatment of those injuries.

The ability to obtain thin section CT images allows the creation of high-quality MPR images with excellent spatial resolution. For extraarticular pelvic fractures the protocol at our institution uses 2.5-mm helical axial sections from the iliac crests to the ischial tuberosities. In selected cases, ultrathin sections (i.e., 5.0 mm) can be obtained to achieve truly isotropic voxels, such than the reformatted images have the same resolution as the original axial sections. This allows the MPR images to be displayed in any plane with essentially no loss of diagnostic information, although coronal and sagittal MPR images generally are considered the most valuable for routine imaging. Curved reformations also can be produced, which is of particular value in assessing structures such as the sacrum.

A variety of computer algorithms have been described to produce 3DCT images from CT data sets; however, three methods are most commonly used (shaded surface display, maximum intensity projection, and volume rendering) (5–9). The surface-rendering technique was developed earliest and provides the most 3D appearance to the 3DCT image by using a subset of the available data representing the boundaries of a given object, but is limited by its failure to show subcortical detail. The major shortcoming of maximum intensity projection images is that they misrepresent spatial relationships because the projected data ignore spatial location, thus necessitating extensive editing if clinically useful images are to be produced. The volume rendering techniques use all the CT data and generally are considered superior to the other two methods, providing better detection of subsurface abnormalities and internal contours

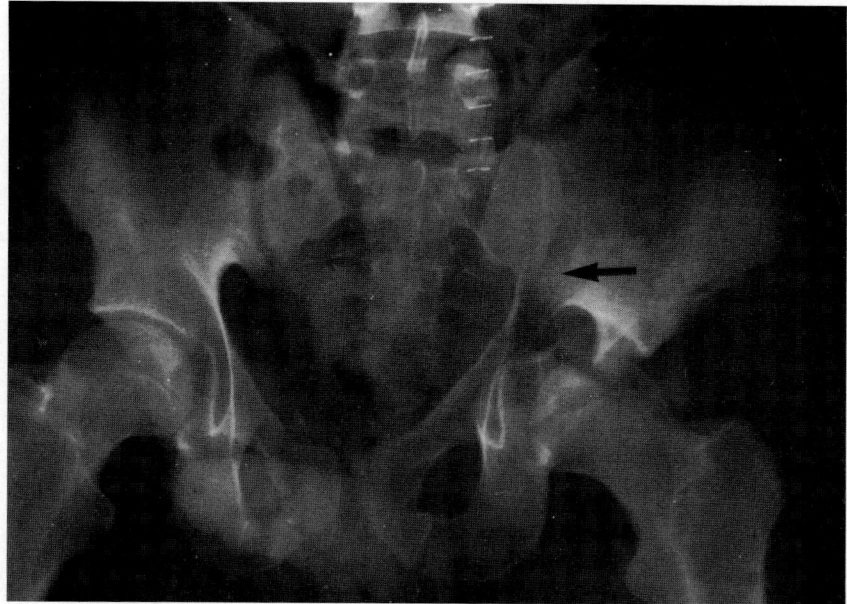

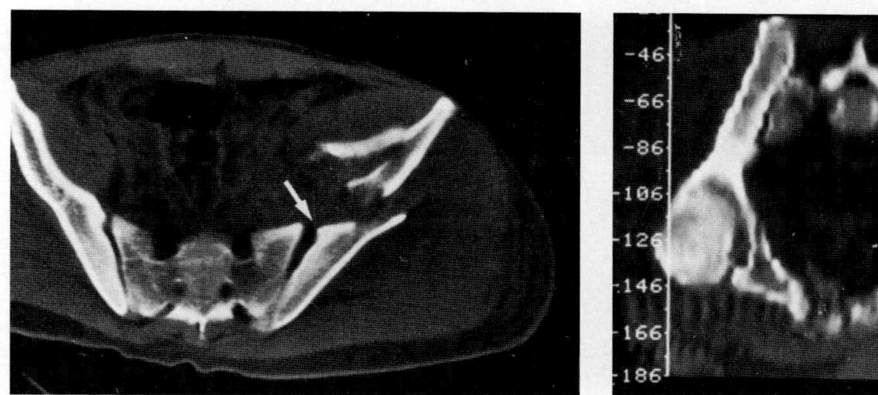

FIGURE 10-15. **A:** Anteroposterior radiograph demonstrates a marked pelvic disruption through the left sacroiliac joint *(arrow),* the left acetabulum, and the right pubic ramus. **B:** Computed tomography through the sacroiliac joint clearly shows the external rotatory displacement of the left ilium and the fracture into the acetabulum. **C:** Computed tomographic reconstruction again shows the left ilium to be externally rotated by the femoral head, which is displaced into the pelvis. This type of reconstruction is invaluable in determining the exact displacement of the pelvic ring.

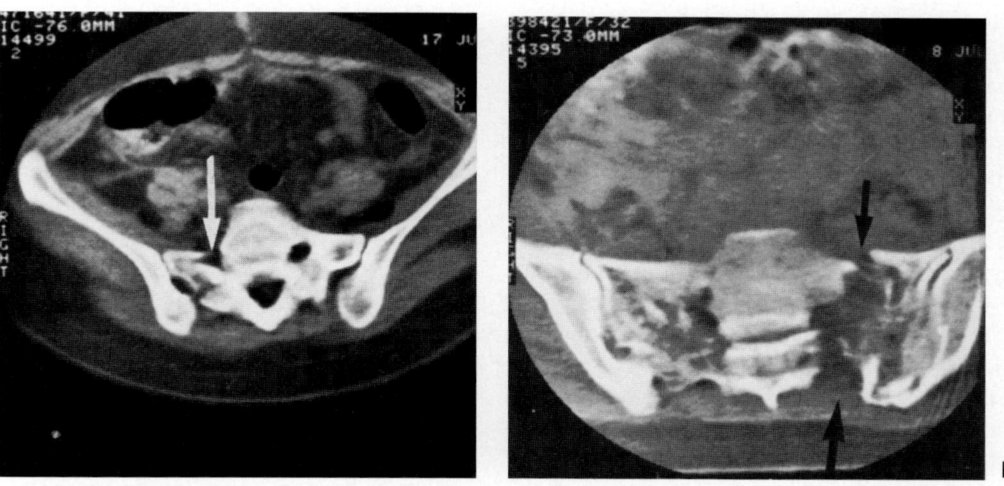

FIGURE 10-16. **A:** Computed tomography through the sacroiliac joint indicates an impacted lateral compression type fracture of the sacrum *(white arrow).* **B:** A computed tomographic scan through the sacroiliac joint indicates a complete disruption of the sacrum on the left side *(black arrow).*

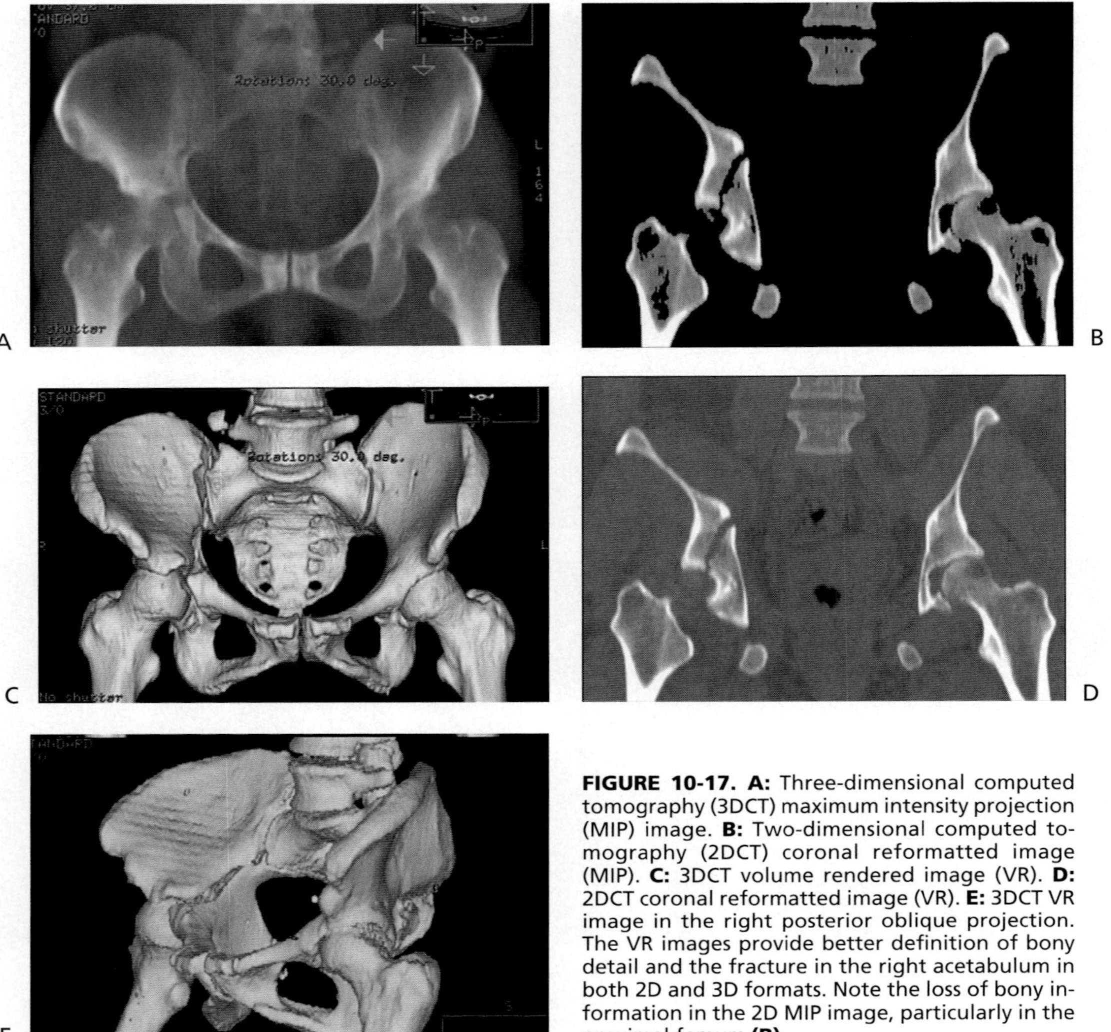

FIGURE 10-17. **A:** Three-dimensional computed tomography (3DCT) maximum intensity projection (MIP) image. **B:** Two-dimensional computed tomography (2DCT) coronal reformatted image (MIP). **C:** 3DCT volume rendered image (VR). **D:** 2DCT coronal reformatted image (VR). **E:** 3DCT VR image in the right posterior oblique projection. The VR images provide better definition of bony detail and the fracture in the right acetabulum in both 2D and 3D formats. Note the loss of bony information in the 2D MIP image, particularly in the proximal femurs **(B).**

(Fig. 10-17). One study of simulated femoral neck fractures compared volume rendered and surface rendered images: Volumetric rendering provided accurate depiction of fracture gaps, whereas surface rendering either caused spurious fusion of fracture gaps or false holes in adjacent bone, depending on software window and level settings (10).

Although the 3DCT image provides no new information over that of the axial images, 3DCT does enhance the surgeon's understanding of each fracture by simulating the gross anatomy of the injury. Rotational deformities and displacements of the pelvis, in particular, are best appreciated with 3DCT (Fig. 10-18). These 3D images can be rotated in any plane to produce real-time sequences that permit examination of each fracture from any perspective, further assisting the preoperative planning (Fig. 10-19). Many software programs also allow editing for selective dissection of the anatomy to visualize areas that are obscured or overlapped by other structures (11–14).

Although 3DCT is a useful and exciting diagnostic tool, the disadvantages of this technique should be kept in mind. To maximize the detail of these images, thin slices (2.5 mm or less) are recommended, which increases the number of axial cuts, the cost, the time of the examination, and the radiation dose to the patient. The smoothing algorithm, available with many software packages, is another factor that can result in loss of information and misleading appearances. Although it provides an esthetically more pleasing image, this may be at the sacrifice of eliminating subtle abnormalities.

Computed Tomography Angiography (Contrast-Enhanced Computed Tomography)

When evidence of active bleeding in the pelvis is present, CT angiography, consisting of multisection CT combined with intravenous contrast injection, provides high-resolution

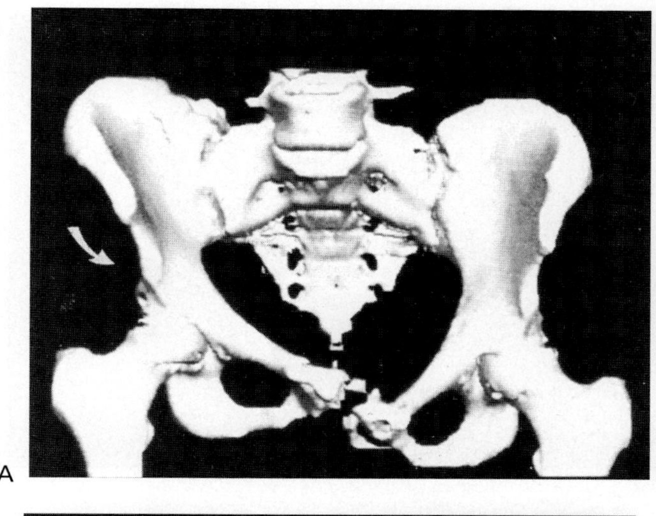

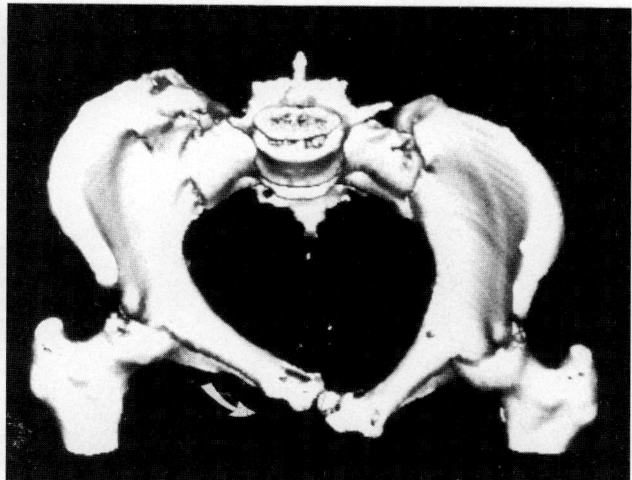

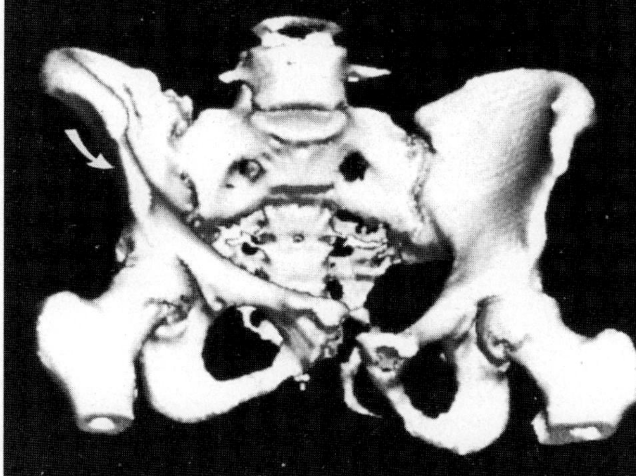

FIGURE 10-18. Anteroposterior **(A)**, inlet **(B)**, and outlet **(C)** projections clearly define internal rotation of the right hemipelvis *(white arrows)*, with posterior and superior displacement occurring through the pubic symphysis and right sacroiliac area.

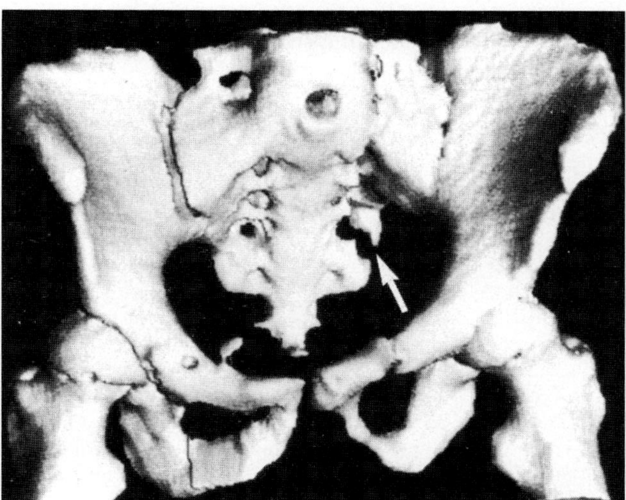

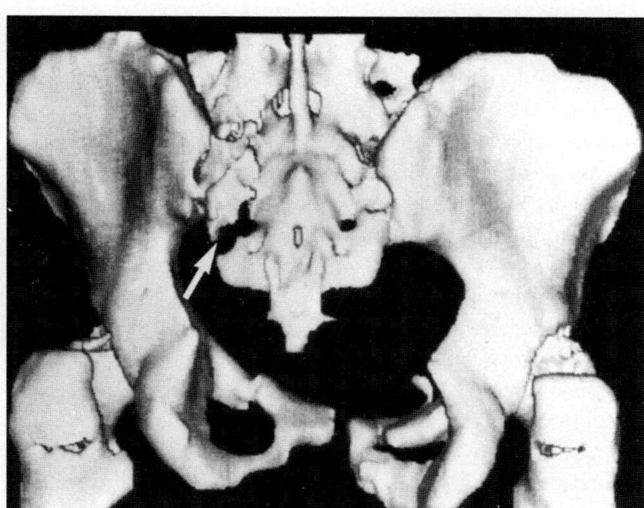

FIGURE 10-19. Anteroposterior **(A)** and posterior-anterior **(B)** projections of the pelvis demonstrate bilateral pubic rami fractures plus an impacted fracture of the left sacral ala. Displacement and rotation of the left hemipelvis through the pubic symphysis and left sacrum *(white arrows)* also can be appreciated.

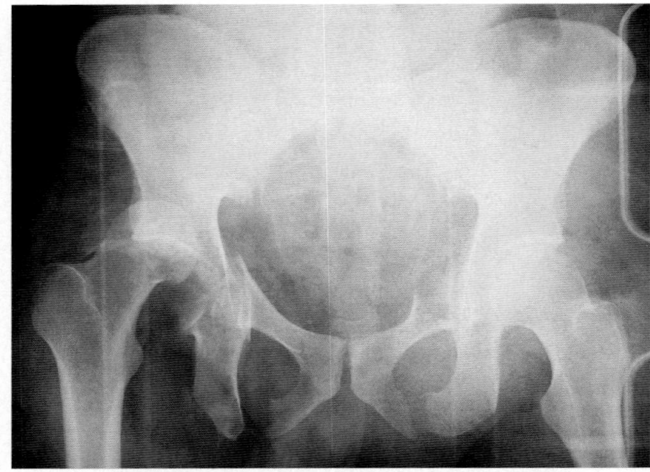

A

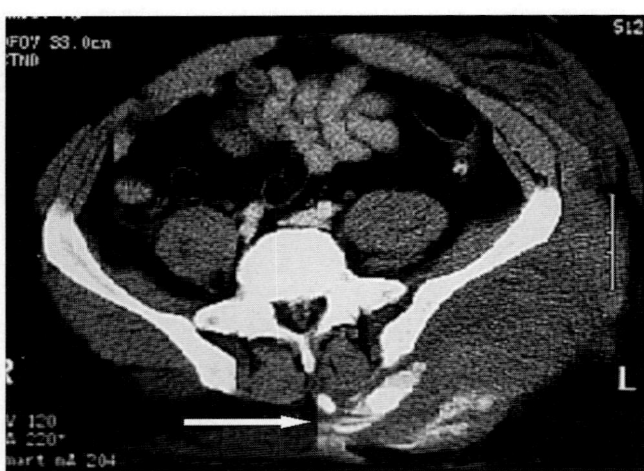

B

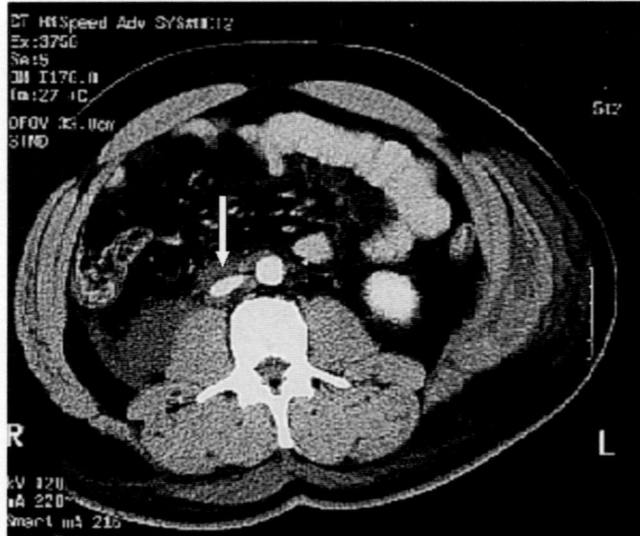

C

FIGURE 10-20. A: Anteroposterior radiograph of a C-type pelvic fracture with the patient in shock. **B:** Contrast-enhanced computed tomography showing a blush in the gluteal region *(arrow)* indicating massive arterial bleeding from the superior gluteal artery. **C:** Note the oval-shaped inferior vena cava *(arrow)* indicating severe blood volume depletion.

images that can be obtained over long anatomic areas (e.g., the entire abdomen and pelvis can be examined in a single scan) (Fig. 10-20). The protocol at our institution consists of injecting nonionic contrast material (iodine, 300 mg/cc) at a rate of 4 cc/sec to a total volume injected of 130 to 150 cc. Image contrast enhancement is maximized using a Smart-Prep technique in which an area of interest is identified (e.g., the iliac crest) and the scan is initiated when a contrast peak is reached at that site of interest. In cases of polytrauma, abdominal and pelvic CT is a frequently ordered test. The addition of contrast is a valuable adjunct, and will facilitate the diagnosis of arterial bleeding, allowing for earlier, more effective intervention (15).

In summary, a careful history and meticulous physical examination leads the attending surgeon to suspect a major pelvic ring disruption and determine the degree of instability. Precise radiologic techniques, including anteroposterior, inlet, and outlet views as well as oblique views of the sacroiliac joints and CT, when possible, confirm the type of lesion, the presence or absence of instability, and the precise nature of the displacement.

REFERENCES

1. Apley AG. *System of orthopedics and fractures,* 5th ed. London: Butterworths, 1978.
2. McMurtry RY, Walton D, Dickinson D, et al. Pelvic disruption in the polytraumatized patient: a management protocol. *Clin Orthop* 1980;151:22.
3. Pennal CF, Sutherland GO. *Fractures of the pelvis* (motion picture). Park Ridge, IL: American Academy of Orthopedic Surgeons Film Library, 1981.
4. Gertzbein SD, Chenoweth DR. Occult injuries of the pelvic ring. *Clin Orthop* 1977;128:202.
5. Totty WG, Vannier MW. Complex musculoskeletal anatomy: analysis using three dimensional surface reconstruction. *Radiology* 1984;150:173.
6. Herman GT, Vose WF, Gomori JM, et al. Stereoscopic computed three-dimensional surface displays. *Radiographics* 1985;5:825.
7. Sutherland CJ. Practical application of computer-generated

three-dimensional reconstructions in orthopedic surgery. *Orthop Clin North Am* 1986;17:651.
8. Altman NR, Altman DH, Wolfe SA, et al. Three-dimensional CT reformation in children. *AJR* 1986;146:1261.
9. Fishman EK, Drebin B, Magid D, et al. Volumetric rendering techniques: applications for three-dimensional imaging of the hip. *Radiology* 1987;163:737.
10. Drebin RA, Magid D, Robertson DD, et al. Fidelity of three-dimensional CT imaging for detecting fracture gaps. *J Comput Assist Tomogr* 1989;13:487.
11. Brewster LJ, Trivedi SS, Tuy HK, et al. Interactive surgical planning. *IEEE Comp Graphics Appl* 1984;4:31.
12. Kuhlman JE, Fishman EK, Ney DR, et al. Nonunion of acetabular fractures: evaluation with interactive multiplanar CT. *J Orthop Trauma* 1989;3:33.
13. Rydberg J, Buckwalter KA, Caldemeyer KS, et al. Multisection CT: scanning techniques and clinical application. *Radiographics* 2000;20:1787.
14. Calhoun PS, Kuszyk BS, Heath DG, et al. Three-dimensional volume rendering of spiral CT data: theory and method. *Radiographics* 1999;19:745.
15. Stephen DJG, Kreder HJ, Day AC, et al. Early detection of arterial bleeding in acute pelvic trauma. *J Trauma* 1999:47(4): 638PA.

11

BIOMECHANICS AND METHODS OF PELVIC FIXATION

JOHN GORCZYCA
TREVOR HEARN
MARVIN TILE

INTRODUCTION

The previous chapters have established the significance of the unstable pelvis fracture in terms of mechanism of injury, associated injuries, as well as the long-term impact of pelvic ring instability. There is more detail on the indications and techniques of surgical intervention in the chapters on external fixation and internal fixation.

Stable pelvis fractures (Type A) are those that do not displace significantly with physiologic loading. These injuries often require protective weight bearing and limitation of activities until significant healing of the fracture has occurred. With proper protection from forces such as weight bearing, however, they do not require operative stabilization in order to heal properly.

Rotationally unstable injuries (Type B) are those in which significant rotational instability of the pelvic ring is present, but there is sufficient residual ligamentous stability to prevent vertical displacement of the posterior pelvis. These injuries, especially the open-book (B1) types, benefit from stabilization of the anterior pelvic ring. If satisfactory reduction and stabilization of the anterior pelvic ring is achieved, both the anterior and posterior pelvic injuries remain reduced until the injury has healed.

The vertically unstable (Type C) pelvic injuries have disruption of the anterior and posterior pelvic ring and require more complex fixation in order to maintain anterior and posterior reduction of the pelvis. Most often, stabilization of the anterior pelvis should be achieved by internal or external means, and stabilization of the posterior pelvis should be obtained by internal fixation. There are several techniques by which the surgeon can achieve pelvic stability, and it is of extreme importance to understand the biomechanics of the injury and the fixation techniques in order to choose the treatment that best matches that particular patient.

EVALUATION OF BIOMECHANICAL STUDIES OF PELVIC FIXATION

Numerous biomechanical studies have been performed to evaluate methods of stabilizing the unstable pelvis. It is essential that the surgeon understand the seemingly small, but significant, differences in design between various studies. These differences may limit the valid extrapolation of *in vitro* mechanical data to the treatment of patients *in vivo.* Furthermore, comparison of results from studies with different designs may not be valid.

Studies may differ by the type of bone or bone composite that is used, the injury pattern that is created for testing, the means by which load is applied to the pelvis, and the means by which displacement is measured. Each of these should influence the reader's interpretation of the data.

Type of Bone Used

Most pelvic studies use cadaveric human bone for testing. Commonly, the cadaveric bone is obtained from elderly persons who donate their body for medical science. Thus, the bone tends to be osteoporotic and weaker than that typical of trauma patients. Furthermore, there is a large degree of variability in the strength of bone obtained from osteoporotic cadavers. Consequently, there tends to be a high variability in the fixation strength or stability achieved with cadaveric bone, making it more difficult to demonstrate that an observed difference in fixation strength or stability is a statistically significant one.

Pelvic bone specimens obtained from organ donors, on the other hand, come from younger patients who have healthier bone. This correlates better with the bone one sees when treating trauma patients. The reverse caveat is true with these studies: High fixation strength obtained in strong cadaveric bone must not be extrapolated to the clinical situation of treating an elderly, osteoporotic person with an unstable pelvis fracture.

When used for mechanical testing, composite bone or sawbones have the advantage that they are less expensive and have less individual variability in measured strength and stiffness. Thus, it becomes easier to demonstrate that an observed difference in fixation strength or stability is statistically significant. The way that artificial bone models fail, however, can be quite dissimilar to the way that human bone fails. Artificial bone can be an acceptable means by which to measure stiffness (i.e., ratio of applied load to displacement in response to that load) of a fixation construct, but is a less reliable means by which to compare fixation strength (i.e., load at which failure occurs).

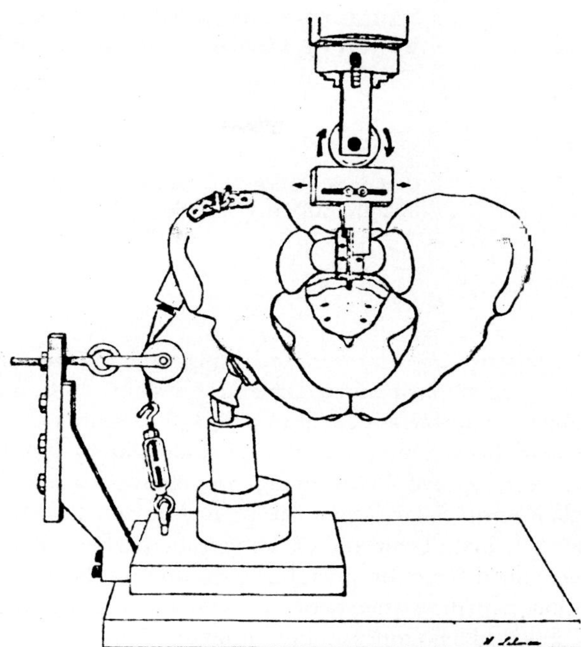

FIGURE 11-2. Unilateral stance testing model with pelvis in anatomic position and load applied through L5 vertebra. Pulley system simulates abductor contraction that maintains level pelvis in unilateral stance.

Means of Applied Force and Means of Measurement

The means by which force is applied to the pelvis and the means by which measurements are obtained are other important variables. The surgically stabilized pelvis may be subjected to gravitational forces, muscle forces, and joint reaction forces. To represent upright stance, the properly loaded pelvis should be oriented in the position that best represents standing (i.e., with the anterior superior iliac spines and the pubic tubercle in a coronal plane) (1). Furthermore, the testing should be performed without lateral constraint to pelvic motion (Fig. 11-1). Otherwise, friction between the bone or joint surfaces will artifactually increase stability of the fixation device measured. Loading of the injured pelvis model should be applied in a means analogous to the *in vivo* situation. Thus, load should be applied through the top of the S1 vertebra, preferably through an L5 vertebra, which remains attached to the sacrum by its ligaments. Also, the injured pelvis model will behave differently in response to loading in single-leg stance versus bilateral stance (Fig. 11-2). When loaded vertically, the sacroiliac joints are subjected primarily to shear. However, in unilateral stance there is compression inferiorly and distraction superiorly, whereas in bilateral stance, there is greater compression across the sacroiliac joint, with distraction inferiorly (Table 11-1). There are relatively small shearing forces across the pubic symphysis, with compression when loaded in single-leg stance and distraction in bilateral stance in general.

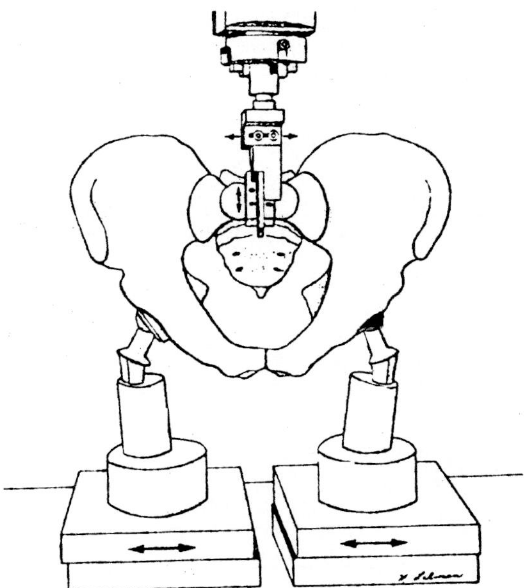

FIGURE 11-1. Bilateral stance testing model with pelvis in anatomic position, load applied through L5 vertebra, and unconstrained lateral motion.

Stability of pelvic fixation is quantified by measuring fracture displacement in response to a specific load. *Stiffness* is the ratio of applied force to displacement of the repaired

TABLE 11-1. RELATIVE FORCES ACTING ACROSS THE PELVIC JOINTS DURING VERTICAL LOADING, IN UNILATERAL AND BILATERAL STANCE

	Sacroiliac Joint			
	Overall	Superior	Inferior	Pubic Symphysis
Unilateral stance	Shear	Distraction	Compression	Compression, ↓ shear
Bilateral stance	Shear	↑↑ Compression	Distraction	Distraction, ↓ shear

pelvis construct. Most often, the displacement is measured from the actuator of a materials testing system. Thus, measurement of stiffness is easier to obtain, but is not as accurate in evaluating motion at the injury site. Strength of fixation is measured by applying progressive load to the implant until "failure" is visualized. Failure may be defined differently in different studies. Some studies define failure as the maximal force, or strength, withstood by the fracture fixation construct, whereas others use fracture displacement of a specified amount as an indication of failure.

The single most important determinant of the biomechanics of the pelvis is its ring structure (2,3). Just as complete disruption of the ring results in the greatest reduction in biomechanical measures of stiffness, surgical reconstruction of the complete ring has the greatest restorative effect. The biomechanics of fixation at multiple sites then is highly interrelated. In particular, anterior stability greatly affects loads and displacements in the posterior aspects of the ring. Therefore, it is important to consider the biomechanics of each site of fixation in the context of the pelvic ring as a whole.

Thus, several variables are present in each biomechanical study of pelvic fixation. It is essential that the surgeon interpreting the results of a study understands its particular details in order that the information obtained be used to the benefit of each patient's unique injury.

METHODS OF PELVIC FIXATION

Early Resuscitation

Resuscitation of the polytrauma patient with an unstable pelvis often necessitates use of techniques to stabilize the pelvis injury quickly with the goal of controlling hemorrhage. Sheets or straps tightened around the pelvis, military antishock trousers (MAST), spica casts, traction, emergency external fixation, and pelvic clamps have been reported to be helpful during the resuscitation of the hemodynamically unstable patient with an unstable pelvic injury (Fig. 11-3) (4–12). Pelvic slings and spica casts also have been used to stabilize the injury until it has healed (11,13), but today, have been abandoned largely for definite treatment, because of the high complication rate. Therefore, most of these methods should be used only temporarily; long-term use of each of these methods has been associated with complications such as pressure ulcers and pelvic malunion or nonunion, and carries the morbidity associated with prolonged immobilization.

Biomechanical evaluations of the many temporary-stabilizing devices applied to the hemodynamically unstable patient have not been performed. However, Simonian and coworkers compared the stability provided by a two-pin external fixator to that of a pelvic clamp in a vertically unstable cadaveric pelvis model (14). They concluded that neither method provided significant stability compared to the intact pelvis. The two constructs provided a similar degree of stability, although the external fixator provided more stability at the pubic symphysis and the pelvic clamp provided more stability at the sacroiliac joint (Fig. 11-4).

The benefits of definitive stabilization of the pelvis are that the patient can be mobilized with less pain and less risk of displacing the pelvic injury. Thus, unstable injuries that, in the early course of patient resuscitation, are provisionally stabilized with one or more of the aforementioned techniques, should be evaluated for definitive stabilization using internal and/or external fixation. The goal of definitive stabilization is to obtain and maintain satisfactory reduction of

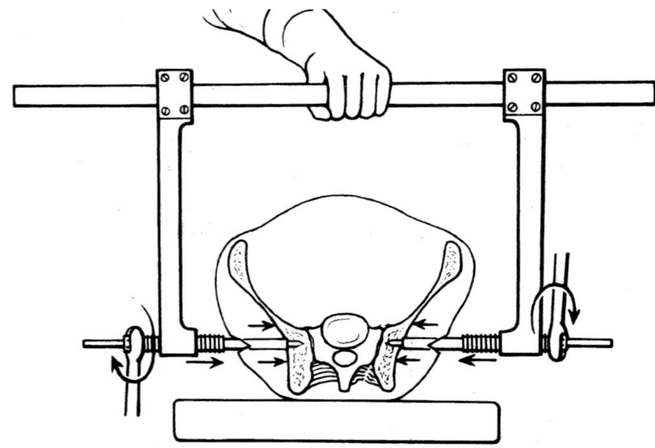

FIGURE 11-3. The Ganz pelvic clamp, which compresses the sacroiliac joint when tightened after proper positioning. (From: Ganz R, Krushell RJ, Jakob RP, et al. The antishock pelvic clamp. *Clin Orthop* 1991;267:74, with permission.)

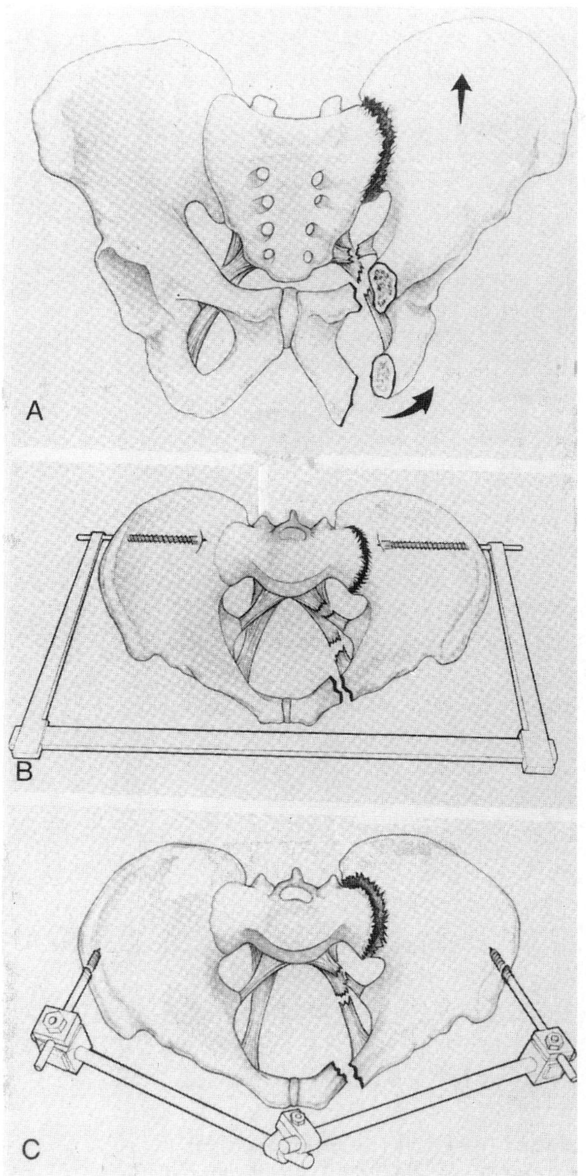

FIGURE 11-4. A: Vertically unstable pelvis model tested with emergency fixation methods. **B:** Placement of Ganz clamp. **C:** Simple anterior external fixator frame. Both fixation methods provide a comparable, but significant, degree of stability to the injured pelvis. (From: Simonian PT, Routt MLC Jr, Harrington RM, et al. Anterior versus posterior provisional fixation in the unstable pelvis. *Clin Orthop* 1995;310:247, Philadelphia: JB Lippincott, with permission.)

the pelvis injury, safely, to improve the overall care of the patient.

Definitive Fixation

Anterior External Fixation

Anterior external fixation has several uses in the treatment of pelvis fractures. Indications for its use include: (a) emergency stabilization of an unstable fracture in a patient with hemodynamic instability; (b) definitive stabilization of the rotationally unstable injury (B types); and (c) definitive stabilization of the vertically unstable injury with concomitant internal fixation posteriorly (see also Chapter 14) (4,8, 15–21).

Anterior external fixation is one of the treatment options for definitive treatment of the rotationally unstable open-book injury (B1, B3-1). All biomechanical studies to date have indicated that external fixation provides adequate stability for patient mobilization, but is not strong enough to allow unrestricted weight bearing through a rotationally unstable sacroiliac joint in the early postoperative period.

Both Dahners and colleagues and McBroom and coworkers have demonstrated that the design of a pelvic external fixation frame affects stability (22,23). Multiple configurations of external fixators appear in the literature (Fig. 11-5). The differences in stability provided by external fixators of different manufacturers do not appear to be significant enough to have clinical impact, provided a basic understanding of external fixator biomechanics is used in planning frame construction (22–25). McBroom's biomechanical study has demonstrated that in the partially stable anteroposterior compression (open-book) cadaveric model, external fixators provided sufficient but limited stability of the pelvis. However, this stability is far less than that gained by fixing the symphysis with two plates (Fig. 11-6A).

McBroom's testing of the cadaveric vertical shear injury has shown that external fixators provide minimal stability to posterior displacement (Fig. 11-6B). Even the addition of two symphyseal plates to an external fixator resulted in only limited posterior stability. This underscores the significance of the ring construct of the pelvis, and adds biomechanical data to support the clinical observation of superior stability of internal over external fixation (15,26).

In general, the stability of an external fixator can be improved by using large (5- to 6-mm diameter) external fixator pins, by decreasing the distance between the external fixator bars and the bone, using two or more pins in each ilium, and increasing the number of bars anteriorly (13,22,27). In some cases, the patient's bone morphology and habitus limit the possibilities of pin placement and bar positioning, thereby limiting the stability that can be achieved with external fixation (28). Kim and coworkers have demonstrated that external fixator pins placed into the dense bone in the supraacetabular region between the anterior-superior and the anterior-inferior iliac spines obtain better purchase than those placed through the iliac crest (29). This improved purchase results in greater stability to resist displacement of the posterior pelvis (Fig. 11-7).

Biomechanical studies measuring the strength of different fixation methods do not exist for lateral compression injuries (B2). The rotationally unstable lateral compression injury may be associated with extraperitoneal bladder disruption caused by significant internal rotation of the pubis.

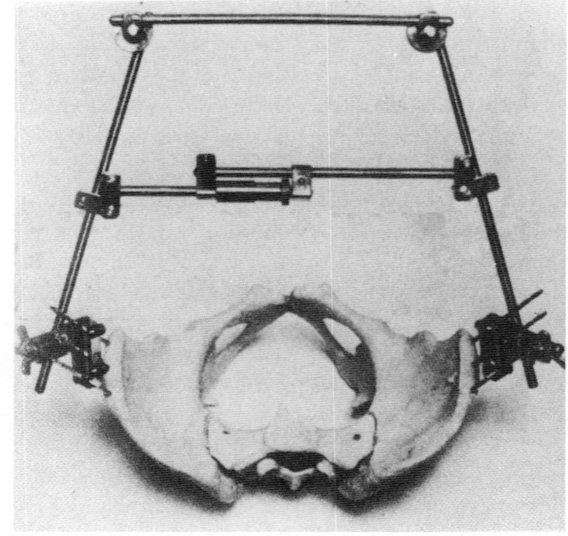

A

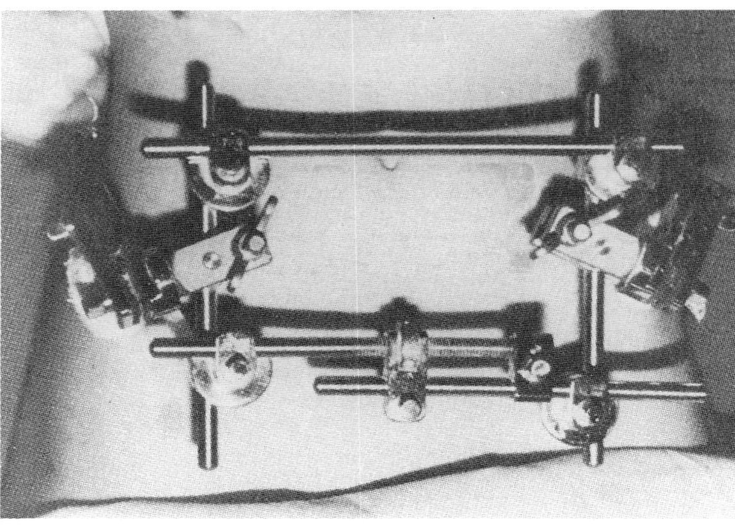

B

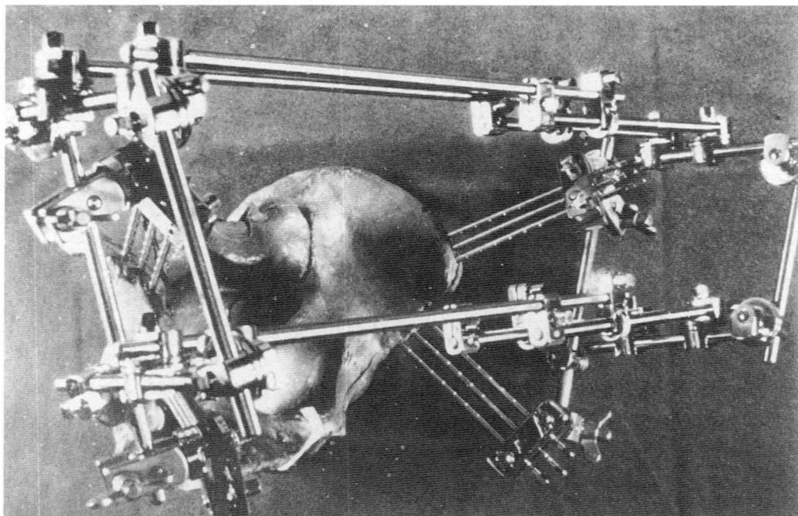

C

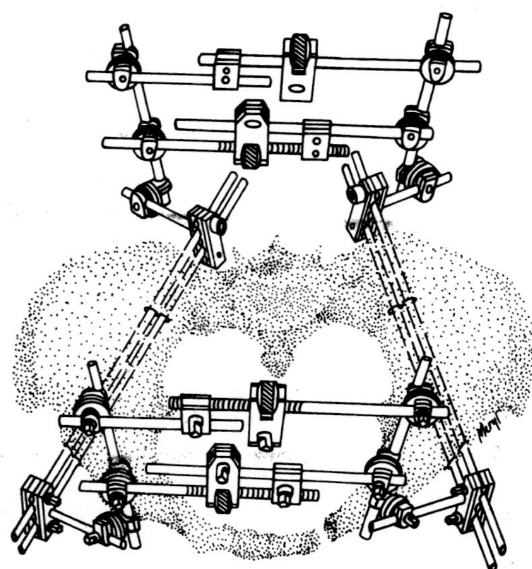

D

FIGURE 11-5. Different external fixator frame constructs. **A:** Trapezoidal (Slätis) frame. (From: Mears DC. *External skeletal fixation.* Baltimore: Williams & Wilkins, 1983:379, with permission.) **B:** Rectangular frame. (From: Tile M, Pennal G. Pelvic disruption: principles of management. *Clin Orthop* 980;151:158. Baltimore: Williams & Wilkins, with permission.) **C:** Double cluster ("triangular") frame. (From: Mears DC. *External skeletal fixation.* Baltimore: Williams & Wilkins, 1983:380, with permission.) **D:**"Thru and thru" fixator. (From: Mears DC. *External skeletal fixation.* Baltimore: Williams & Wilkins, 1983:381, with permission.)

In a true partially stable (B2) injury, sufficient ligamentous stability remains to limit vertical migration or posterior translation of the hemipelvis. Most *isolated* lateral compression (B2) injuries can be treated by nonoperative symptomatic care with satisfactory results. In polytraumatized patients with this injury, external fixation may greatly aid in the overall management of the patient. Satisfactory reduction of the pelvis usually can be obtained by external rotation maneuvers, when this is not possible, internal fixation may be necessary.

Open Reduction and Internal Fixation (ORIF) of Pubic Symphysis

Many studies have demonstrated that internal fixation of the pubic symphysis provides stronger and/or more stable fixation than external fixation, in both the open-book fracture model and the vertically unstable model (2,23,26).

Numerous methods have been described for stabilizing the pubic symphysis with internal fixation. The open-book injury can be satisfactorily treated by any of these means pro-

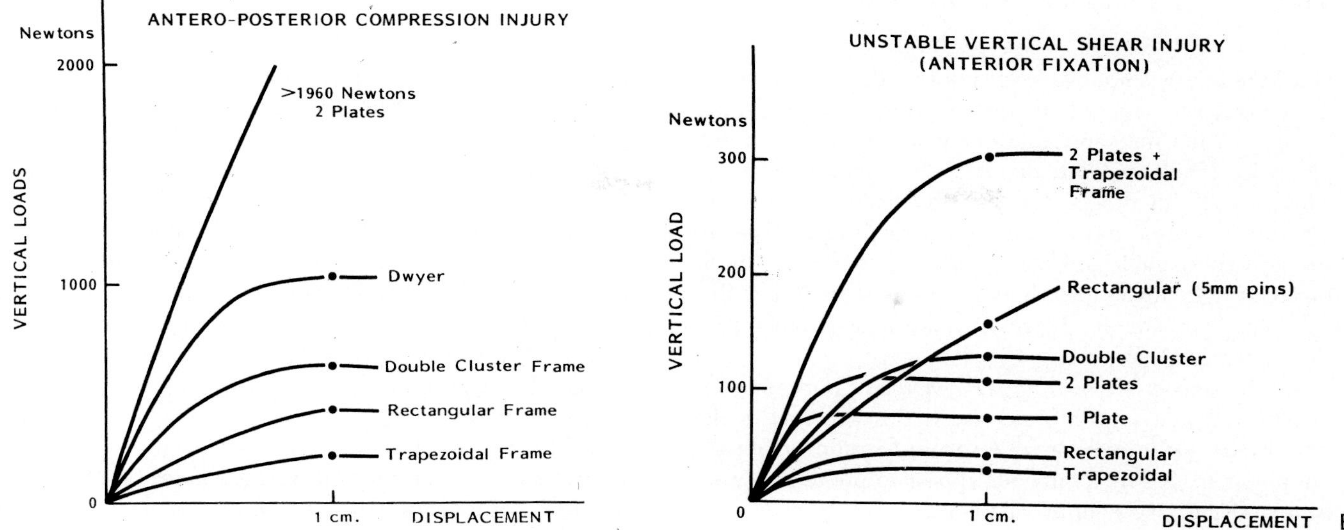

FIGURE 11-6. Stability of pelvis injuries provided by external fixation. **A:** Graph demonstrates stability provided by different fixation constructs in cadaveric unstable open-book injury model. Note that internal fixation with two symphyseal plates provides significantly more stability than any other form of fixation. **B:** Graph demonstrates stability provided by different anterior fixation constructs in cadaveric vertical shear injury model. Note that minimal stability is provided by external fixation, and only limited stability is gained by the addition of symphyseal fixation to external fixation in this injury model. (From: Tile M. *Fractures of the pelvis and acetabulum,* 2nd ed. Baltimore: Williams & Wilkins, 1995, with permission.)

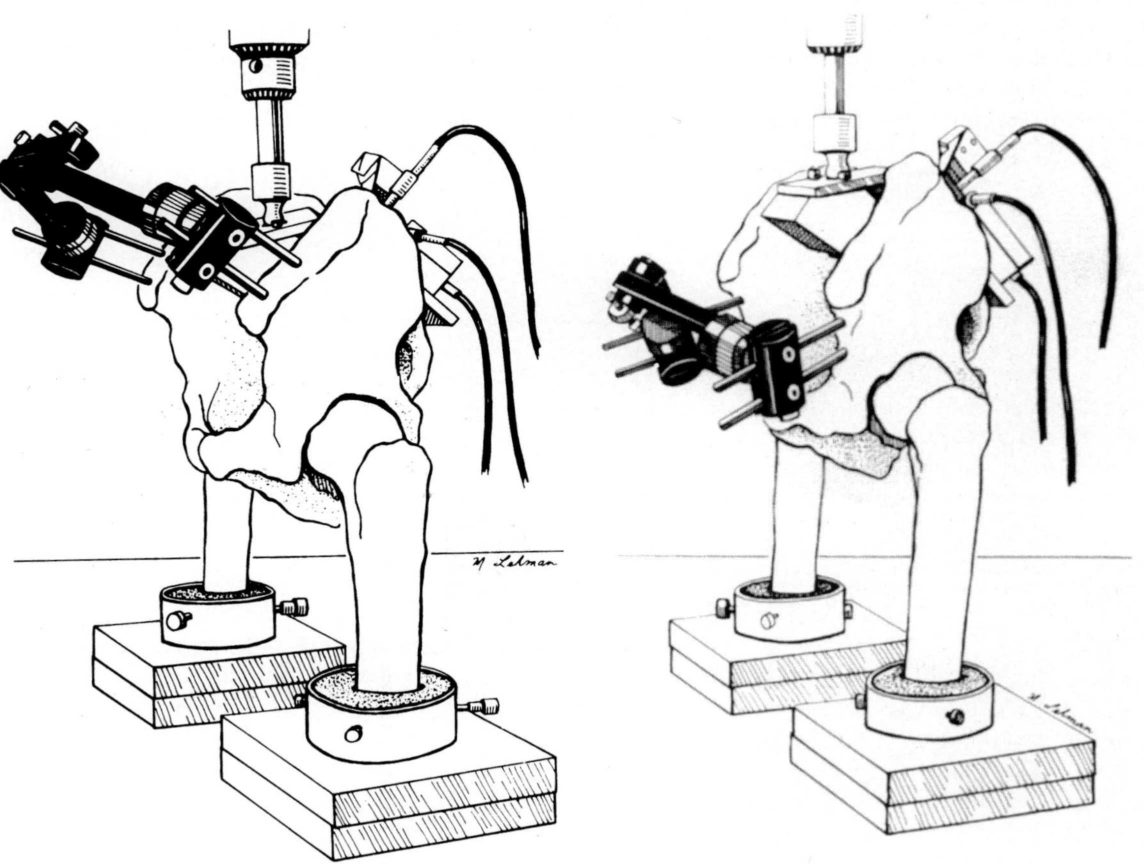

FIGURE 11-7. Testing model comparing stability of fixator frames with: **A:** pins located in iliac crest; and **B:** pins located between anterior superior iliac spine and anterior inferior iliac spine. (From: Kim W-Y, Hearn TC, Seleem O, et al. Effect of pin location on stability of pelvic external fixation. *Clin Orthop Rel Res* 1999;361:239,240. Baltimore: Lippincott Williams & Wilkins, with permission.)

vided the injury is not overloaded during the healing phase. Two plates, one superior and one anterior, provided greater stability than a single plate, as one would expect (21). Box plates have been devised to make this technique easier. These specifically designed plates, which allow biplanar insertion of screws, have been shown to provide fixation strength comparable to that provided by two plates positioned at right angles to each other (30), but are more difficult to apply; therefore, there is little advantage to their routine use (Fig. 11-8).

Other methods for treating the symphyseal disruption include cerclage wiring (around screws on each side of the symphysis) and nonabsorbable suture fixation across the symphysis (31). These methods appear to provide fixation comparable to two symphyseal plates.

Pubic Rami Fractures. Biomechanical comparisons of external and internal fixation for anterior ring injuries concentrate on pubic symphyseal disruptions. In this injury model, one or two plates are biomechanically superior to an external fixator (21,23). In a clinical situation, however, the anterior injury may consist of unilateral or bilateral pubic ramus fractures. These ramus fractures often have some intrinsic stability owing to the surrounding muscle and ligamentous attachments, which may remain completely or partially intact. Furthermore, the surgeon's ability to obtain strong fixation through a limited dissection becomes increasingly compromised the farther the fracture is located from the midline on one or both sides. Preliminary studies, however, have shown that even for unstable, bilateral proximal ramus fractures, ORIF with a single, long plate provides fixation that is stronger and stiffer than external fixation (32). However, the advantages of internal fixation for pubic ramus fractures become less significant the further the fracture occurs from the pubic symphysis. Thus, in some fractures anterior external fixation of vertically unstable injuries with pubic ramus fractures is a better option than anterior ORIF. Routt has used a retrograde ramus screw to stabilize these injuries (33).

ORIF Posterior Pelvis

Unstable Iliac Fractures. An excellent indication for ORIF of the posterior pelvis is the *unstable vertical shear injury with a fracture passing from the greater sciatic notch,* through the pelvic brim, and out the iliac wing. This *"unstable iliac fracture"* must be stabilized to provide enough stability for healing in the anatomic position. Routt's laboratory has shown that the use of two properly positioned lag screws (one at the iliac crest, the other at the pelvic brim), provides fixation stability comparable to that of a lag screw and a reconstruction plate in this fracture model (20). Use of a single lag screw at the iliac crest provided less stability, but the difference was not shown to be statistically significant because of the variability of bone quality between the specimens. This study did not measure fixation strength.

A

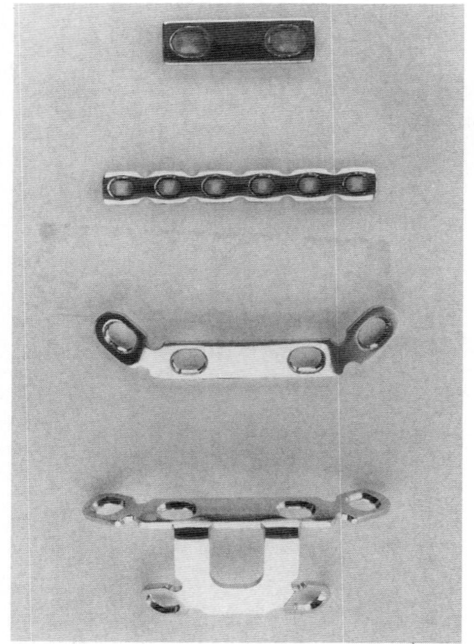

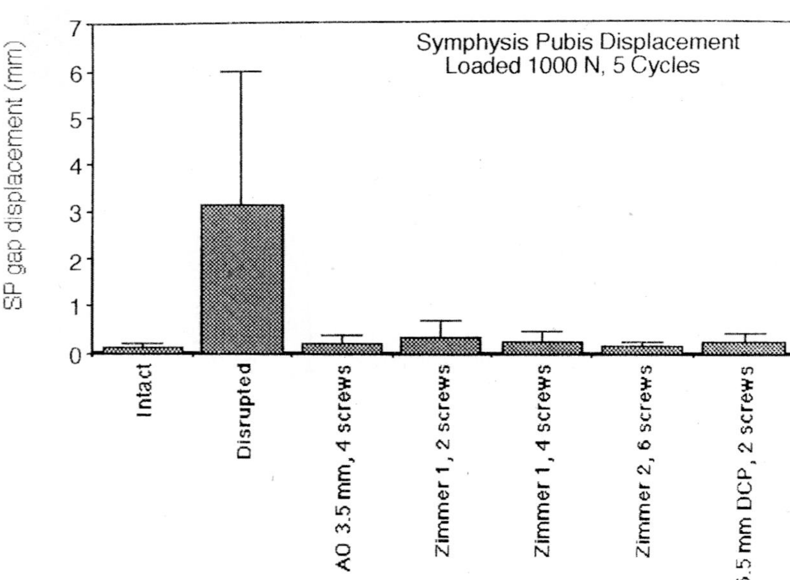

B

FIGURE 11-8. A: Types of plates available for symphyseal fixation. **B:** Comparative displacement in response to 1000 Newton loads. (From: Simonian PT, Schwappach JR, Routt MLC Jr, et al. Evaluation of new plate designs for symphysis pubis internal fixation. *J Trauma* 1996;41:499–500, with permission.)

Thus, for the unstable iliac wing fracture, internal fixation with lag screw fixation and/or plates appears to provide sufficient stability. It is intuitive that fixation of the injury at both the crest and pelvic brim would provide optimal stability.

Crescent Fracture. Fracture dislocations of the sacroiliac joint with dislocation of the inferior sacroiliac joint and fracture through the posterior iliac crest have been termed *crescent* fracture-dislocations. Because of the easy access to the posterior ilium from anterior or posterior approaches, these injuries can be treated successfully by a variety of methods. As with all vertically unstable injuries, satisfactory stability mandates use of anterior and posterior fixation. Anterior fixation can be achieved with internal or external fixation. Although biomechanical studies using this fracture model have not been performed, extrapolation of data from other vertically unstable pelvis models indicates that stability is improved with use of internal fixation anteriorly, coupled with internal fixation posteriorly.

Stabilization of the crescent fracture in the posterior ilium can be achieved with plates and screws inserted through posterior or anterior incisions. In some cases, the iliac injury extends through or near the location through which an iliosacral screw would be placed. In these situations, the fixation achieved with iliosacral screws would be biomechanically insufficient owing to the compromised bone strength.

Anterior fixation of the sacroiliac joint with plates and screws can be used alone or in conjunction with plating of the crescent fracture for stability. Biomechanical studies comparing these fixation methods for this injury pattern have not been performed. It seems prudent, however, to supplement internal fixation of the posterior ilium with anterior plating of the sacroiliac joint or iliosacral screw fixation if the stability achieved at the time of iliac plating appears, in the judgment of the surgeon, to be insufficient.

Sacroiliac Dislocations. Purely ligamentous disruptions through the sacroiliac region require anterior and posterior pelvic stabilization. The goal in treatment should be anatomic reduction and stable fixation.

Posterior fixation of the disrupted sacroiliac joint can be achieved with iliosacral screws, anterior plating, transiliac bars, or transiliac plating (Fig. 11-9) (17,34–38). Each of these methods, when coupled with accurate anatomic reduction and stable anterior fixation of the anterior injury, has been shown in the laboratory to restore sufficient stability to the sacroiliac joint (23,34,35). The technical considerations of these procedures and the judgment and experience of the treating surgeon guide treatment.

Hearn and coworkers, in the Sunnybrook Biomechanics Laboratory, sequentially tested 12 combinations of internal and external fixation of cadaveric pelvises with sacroiliac dislocation and pubic symphyseal disruption (2). Posterior fixation methods included two iliosacral lag screws; transiliac bars; and double plating of the anterior aspect of the sacroiliac joint. Anterior fixation methods included superior symphyseal plate fixation; anteroinferior plate fixation; double symphyseal plate fixation; and anterior external fixation. Pelvic ring stiffness and triaxial displacement of the sacroiliac joint were measured during loading in bilateral stance.

The combination of two plates across the symphysis with any form of posterior fixation yielded the greatest overall ring stiffness, a fact that stressed the importance of stable anterior fixation in this model (Fig. 11-10). The combination of external fixation with transiliac bars was least stable. In this model, iliosacral screws provided the best protection

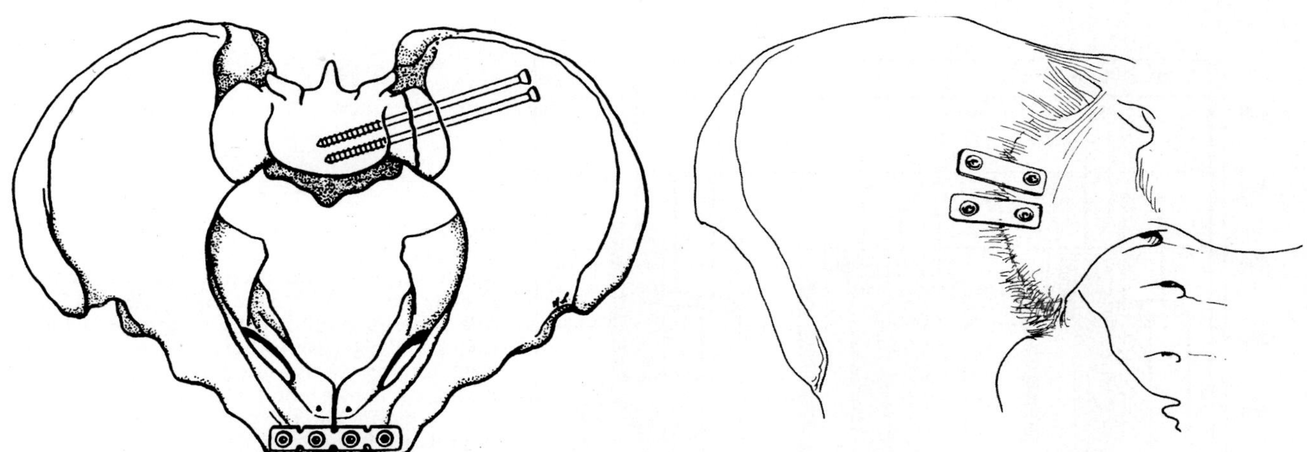

FIGURE 11-9. Methods for stabilizing posterior pelvic disruptions. **A:** Iliosacral screws. (From: Gorczyca JT, Varga E, Woodside T, et al. The strength of iliosacral screws and transiliac bars in the fixation of vertically unstable pelvic fractures with sacral fractures. *Injury* 1996;27:561–564, New York: Elsevier Science, with permission.) **B:** Fixation of a sacroiliac dislocation by two, 2-hole 4.5-mm DC plates.

(Figure continues)

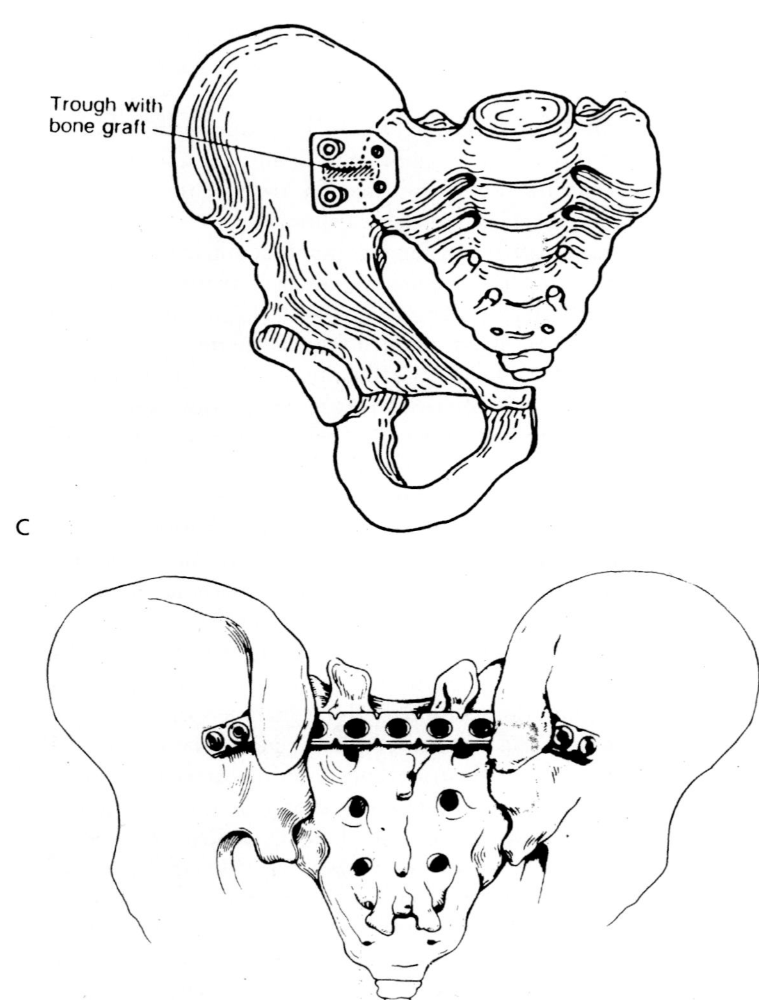

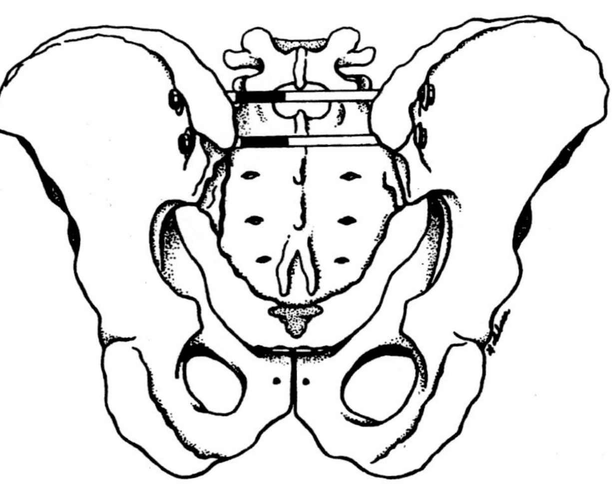

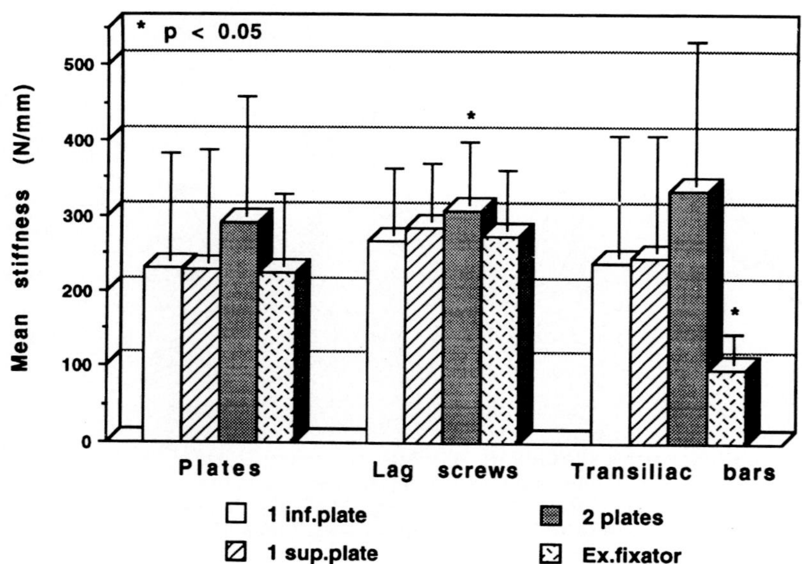

FIGURE 11-9. ***(continued)*** **C:** Anterior sacroiliac plate. (From: Leighton R, Waddell J, Bray TJ, et al. Biomechanical testing of new and old fixation devices for vertical shear fractures of the pelvis. *J Orthop Trauma* 1991;5:315, New York: Raven Press, with permission.) **D:** Transiliac bars. (From: Gorczyca JT, Varga E, Woodside T, et al. The strength of iliosacral screws and transiliac bars in the fixation of vertically unstable pelvic fractures with sacral fractures. *Injury* 1996;27:561–564, New York: Elsevier Science, with permission.) **E:** Transiliac plating. (From: Albert MJ, Miller ME, MacNaughton M, et al. Posterior pelvic fixation using a transiliac 4.5-mm reconstruction plate: a clinical and biomechanical study. *J Orthop Trauma* 1993;3:228, New York: Raven Press, with permission.)

FIGURE 11-10. Graph indicates the main stiffness of the pelvis (in newton meters) achieved with various forms of anterior fixation, noted by the bars; namely, one inferior plate on the symphysis pubis, one superior plate on the symphysis pubis, two plates, and external fixation. In each case, the anterior fixation was associated with anterior sacroiliac plates, lag screws, and transiliac *(sacral bars)*. Note that no matter what form of posterior fixation was used, two plates across the symphysis *(dark bars)*, yielded the highest values of overall ring stiffness, stressing the importance of stable anterior fixation in this model. (From: Hearn TC, et al. *The effects of ligament sectioning and internal fixation of bending stiffness of the pelvic ring.* Proceedings of the 13th International Conference on Biomechanics. Perth, Australia, Dec. 9–13, 1991, with permission.)

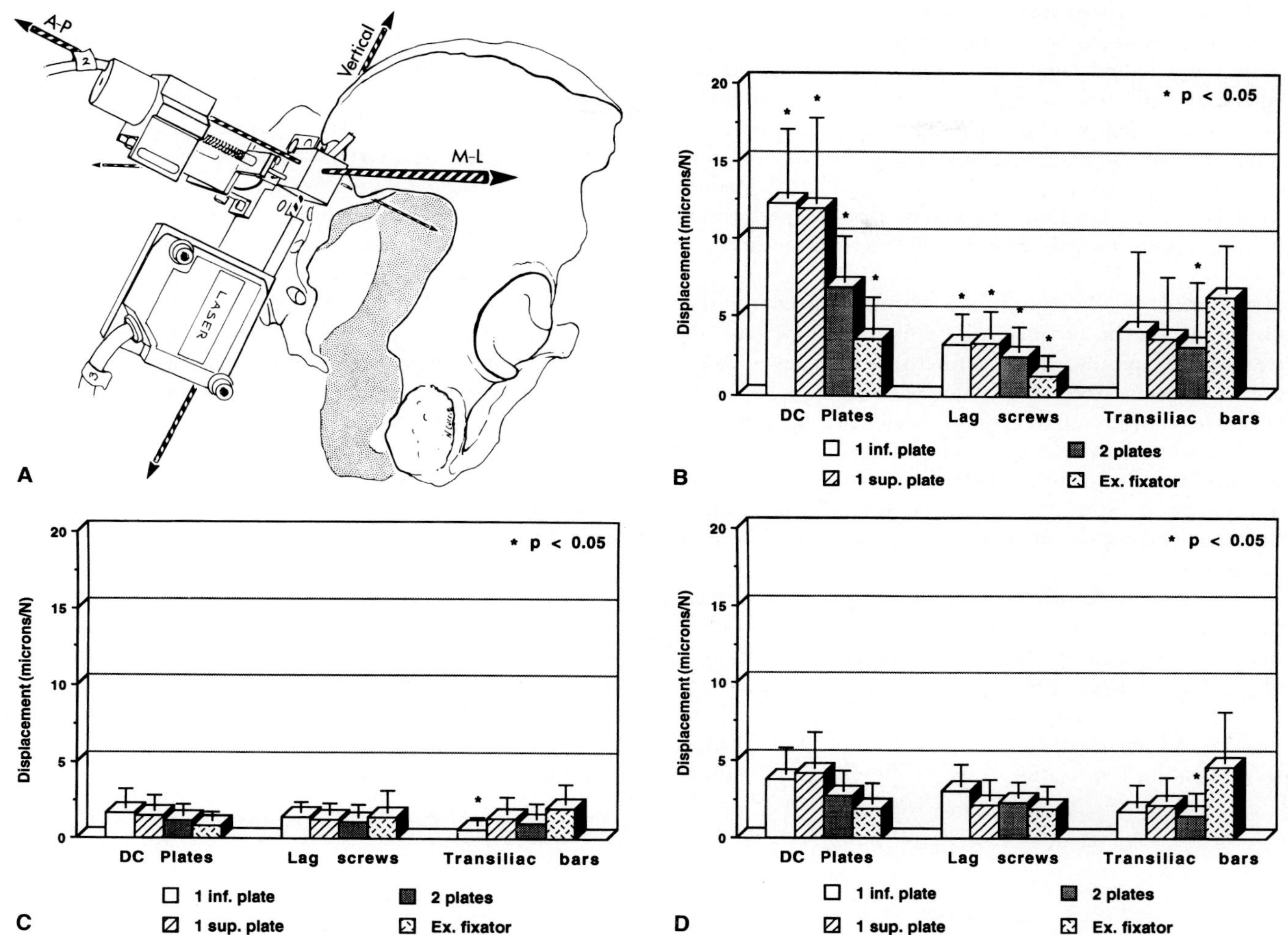

FIGURE 11-11. A: Schematic representation of displacement transducers and target, aligned with three orthogonal sacroiliac axes. **B:** Mean displacement, in micrometers per newton applied axial load (±SD), in the medial-lateral axis, corresponding to sacroiliac joint separation. Values are grouped by posterior fixation, showing anterior fixation within each group (n = 8). **C:** Mean anteroposterior displacement (±SD), in micrometers per newton applied axial load, corresponding to shear displacements of the sacroiliac joint in the direction of the longitudinal axis of the sacrum. Values are grouped by posterior fixation, showing anterior fixation within each group (n = 8). (From: Hearn TC, et al. *The effects of ligament sectioning and internal fixation of bending stiffness of the pelvic ring.* Proceedings of the 13th International Conference on Biomechanics. Perth, Australia, Dec. 9–13, 1991, with permission.)

against lateral displacement of the ilium (Fig. 11-11). These laboratory data are consistent with clinical observations (15).

Kraemer and coworkers studied the pullout strength of 7-mm diameter iliosacral lag screws in cadaveric pelvises (39). They noted that long-threaded (32-mm) screws had significantly greater pullout strength than short-threaded (16-mm) screws, and that pullout strength of screws placed into the first sacral body was significantly greater than those placed into the sacral ala. A particularly significant finding was that long-threaded screws in the first sacral body had a purchase strength almost ten times greater than short-threaded screws in the sacral ala. Although pure pullout forces are not applied to the stabilized pelvis *in vivo,* resistance to sacroiliac shearing loads depends largely on the amount of compression that the screws can generate across the fracture. This study provides important information on the quality of fixation that can be achieved with short- and long-threaded screws in different regions of the sacrum.

It should be noted that symphyseal plating coupled with external fixation has been shown to provide more strength than either method alone, but does not appear to provide adequate strength to the sacroiliac joint to allow patient mobilization on crutches. Thus, this technique would be a reasonable means by which to temporarily improve stability of the unstable pelvis injury, but patients treated by this method should be referred to a surgeon who is capable of performing definitive posterior stabilization of the sacroiliac injury.

Sacral Fracture. Posterior injuries through the sacrum that do not involve the sacroiliac joint can present new issues for treatment. Typically, these fractures pass obliquely through the transforaminal region. Fracture patterns produced in the laboratory, however, have typically been made right through the foramina. Furthermore, in the clinical situation, these fractures are often comminuted. Because of the risk of nerve injury from compressing the comminuted fracture, interfragmentary compression may not be a good option in some patients (40).

Several methods of fixation can be used effectively for these injuries. Anterior internal or external fixation optimizes stability of the pelvic ring construct. Posterior fixation of the sacral fracture can be achieved with transiliac bars, sacral plating, iliosacral screws, or direct exposure of the fracture and open reduction internal fixation. Several studies comparing the fixation achieved by different methods have been performed. Pohlemann and coworkers have shown that direct posterior exposure of the sacrum and internal fixation of the transforaminal fracture with small fragment screws and plates (Fig. 11-12) provides fixation comparable to both transiliac bars and an internal spine (Olerud) fixator in a cadaveric model tested in unilateral stance (41). Gorczyca and associates have shown that transiliac bars provide stronger fixation than iliosacral screws in osteoporotic pelvises fixed anteriorly with two symphyseal plates and tested in bilateral stance (42). The difference in fixation strength, however, was not statistically significant. Simonian and coworkers have shown comparable fixation stability using iliosacral screws, transiliac plates, or a combination of these in a cadaveric transforaminal sacral fracture model in which the anterior pelvis was not disrupted (Fig. 11-13) (37,43).

Bilateral Posterior Injuries. Type C3 injuries, with bilateral vertically unstable pelvis injuries, require special consideration. It is well established in the clinical setting that posterior fixation that is achieved simply by fixing the two ilia to each other (i.e., transiliac bars or transiliac plating) is insufficient. If this treatment option is used, the sacrum has little restraint to displacement because of the lack of ligamentous attachments on each side. Thus, fixation of the sacrum to one or both ilia with iliosacral screws or anterior plating of the sacroiliac joint is essential.

A
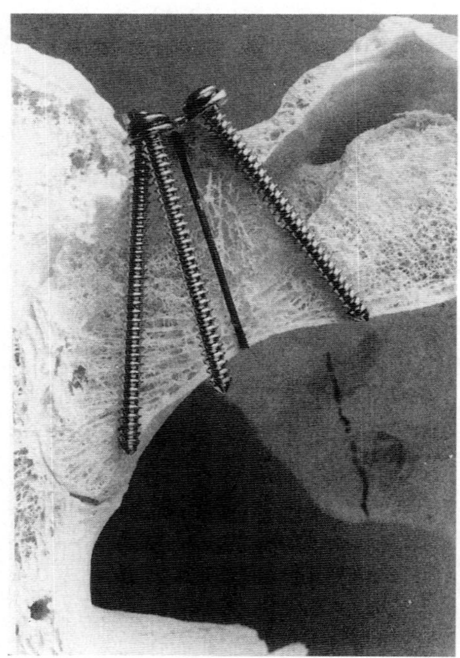

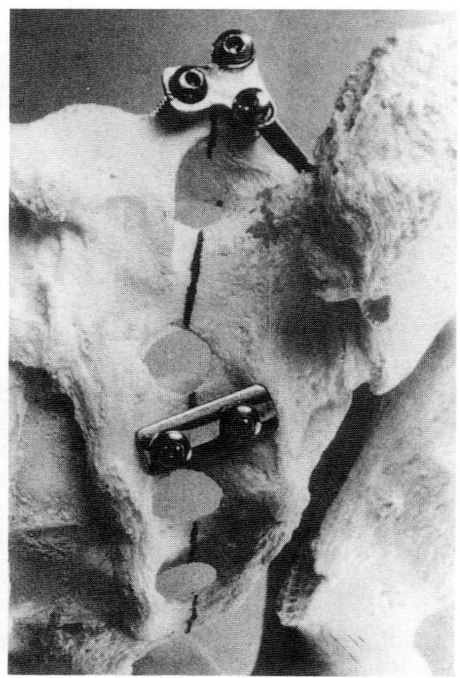
B

FIGURE 11-12. Cadaveric model of internal fixation of unstable transforaminal sacral fracture using small fragment screws through posterior approach. **A:** Superior view of sacrum, dissected to show screw orientation at first sacral pedicle. **B:** Posterior view of sacrum. (From: Pohlemann T, Angst M, Schneider E, et al. Fixation of transforaminal sacrum fractures: a biomechanical study. *J Orthop Trauma* 1993;7:112, New York: Raven Press, with permission.)

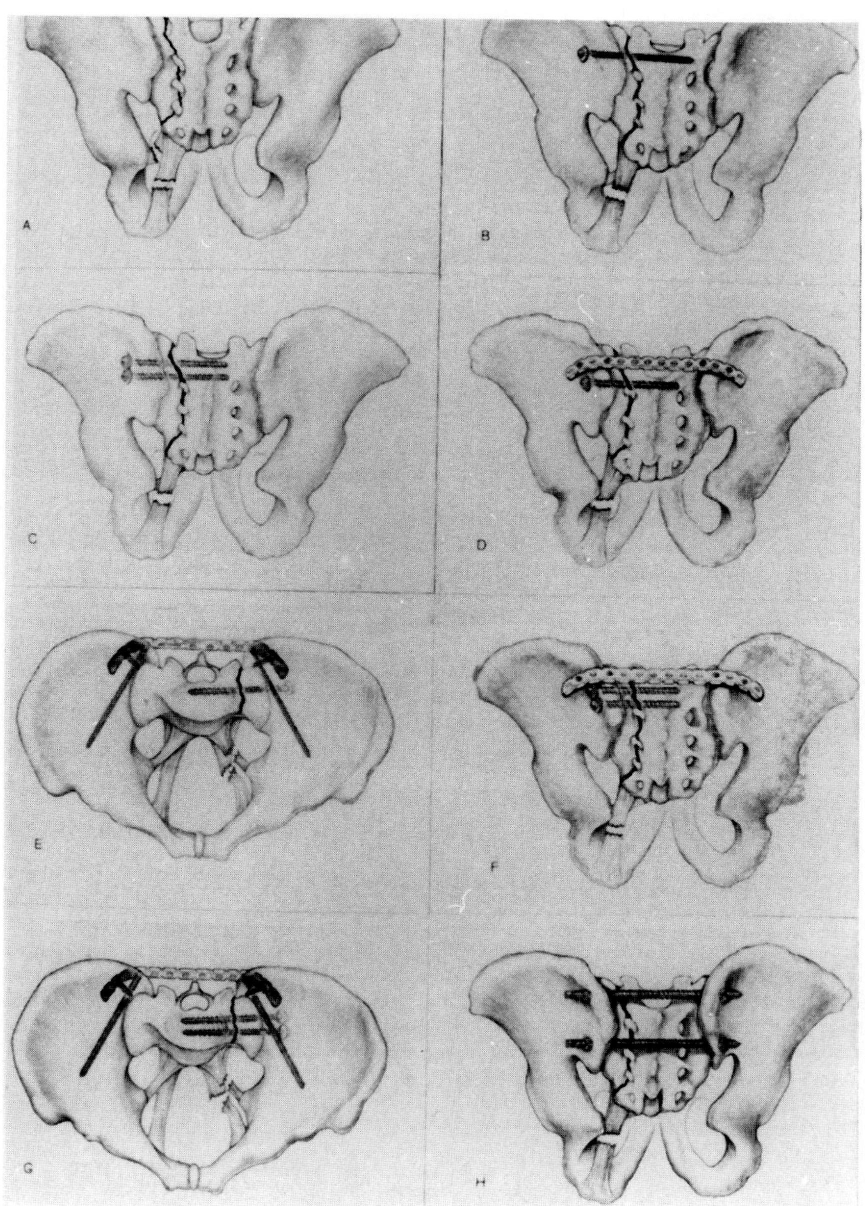

FIGURE 11-13. A: Transforaminal sacral fracture model used by Simonian and coworkers to compare stability of posterior fixation methods. **B:** Single 7-mm cannulated cancellous fully threaded iliosacral screw. **C:** Two 7-mm screws. **D,E:** Single 7-mm screw and 3.5-mm reconstruction plate between posterior iliac wings in tension band configuration. **F,G:** Two 7-mm screws with 3.5-mm plate. **H:** Two parallel 6-mm diameter transiliac bars. (From: Simonian PT, Routt MLC Jr, Harrington RM, et al. Internal fixation for the transforaminal sacral fracture. *Clin Orthop Rel Res* 1996;323:205, New York: Lippincott-Raven, with permission.)

CONCLUSION

1. An understanding of the details of laboratory studies is necessary before the biomechanical findings of these studies are extrapolated to the treatment of patients with unstable pelvis injuries.
2. The biomechanics of each site of fixation should be considered in the context of the pelvic ring as a whole.
3. Fixation of the anterior pelvis is stronger with internal fixation than with external fixation. Both methods, when coupled with appropriate posterior internal fixation, provide adequate stability to mobilize a patient with an unstable pelvis injury.
4. Vertically or translationally unstable injuries (Type C) cannot be adequately stabilized by external fixation alone.
5. Maximal stability from internal rotation is gained by reconstituting the anterior and posterior portions of the ring through internal fixation.
6. For the unilateral sacroiliac dislocation or fracture dislocation, iliosacral compression screw fixation, transiliac rod, transiliac plating, and anterior sacroiliac plating all restore adequate stability to the posterior pelvis for patient mobilization, if the anterior pelvis is stabilized. Studies to date have shown the iliosacral screw coupled with two symphyseal plates to be the most biomechanically stable.

7. For transforaminal sacral fractures, adequate stability can be achieved with iliosacral screws, transiliac bars, transiliac plates, or direct posterior sacral exposure and internal fixation, again, only if the anterior pelvis has been stabilized.
8. With bilateral posterior pelvic injuries, at least one side of the posterior injury must be fixed to the axial spine to provide adequate stability for maintenance of sacral reduction with patient mobilization. Combining an iliosacral screw with transiliac bars or plates provides a biomechanical advantage in resisting sacroiliac displacement bilaterally.
9. Stability of anterior external fixators can be improved by placing Shanz pins between the anterior superior and anterior inferior iliac spines through the supraacetabular bone.
10. Iliosacral screws obtain maximal strength if long-threaded screws are placed into the sacral body.
11. In the completely unstable pelvic disruption, really considered an internal hemipelvectomy, fixation both anteriorly and posteriorly may be insufficient to allow unrestricted weight bearing. Redisplacement may occur because this fixation only withstands 1.5 × body weight. Postoperative regimes must take this into account.

REFERENCES

1. Anderson JE. *Grant's atlas of anatomy,* 7th ed. Baltimore: Williams & Wilkins, 1978.
2. Hearn TC, Schopfer A, D'Angelo D, et al. *The effects of ligament sectioning and internal fixation on bending stiffness of the pelvic ring.* Proceedings of the 13th International Conference on Biomechanics. Perth, Australia, Dec. 9–13, 1991.
3. Vrahas M, Hearn TC, D'Angelo D, et al. Ligamentous contribution to pelvic ring stiffness. *Orthopedics* 1995;18:271–274.
4. Alexander RH, Proctor HJ. *Advanced trauma life support student manual.* Chicago: American College of Surgeons, 1993.
5. Cotler HB, LaMont JG, Hansen ST. Immediate spica cast for pelvic fractures. *J Orthop Trauma* 1988;2:222.
6. Ganz R, Krushell RJ, Jakob RP, et al The antishock pelvic clamp. *Clin Orthop* 1991;267:71–78.
7. Karaharju RO, Slätis P. External fixation of double vertical fractures with a trapezoidal compression frame. *Injury* 1978;10:142.
8. McMurtry RY, Walton D, Dickinson D, et al. Pelvic disruption in the polytraumatized patient: a management protocol. *Clin Orthop* 1980;151:22.
9. Slätis P, Karaharju EO. External fixation of unstable pelvic fractures: experiences in 22 patients treated with a trapezoid compression frame. *Clin Orthop* 1980;151:73.
10. Slätis P, Huittinen VM. Double vertical fractures of the pelvis, a report on 163 patients. *Acta Chir Scand* 1972;138:799.
11. Tile M. *Fractures of the pelvis and acetabulum.* Baltimore: Williams & Wilkins, 1984.
12. Vrahas MS, Wilson SC, Cummings PD, et al. Comparison of fixation methods for preventing pelvic ring expansion. *Orthopedics* 1998;21:285–290.
13. Mears DC, Rubash HE. *Pelvic and acetabular fractures.* Thorofare, NJ: Slack, 1986.
14. Simonian PT, Routt MLC Jr, Harrington RM, et al. Anterior versus posterior provisional fixation in the unstable pelvis. *Clin Orthop* 1995;310:242–251.
15. Keating JF, Werier J, Blachut P, et al. Early fixation of the vertically unstable pelvis: the role of iliosacral screw fixation of the posterior lesion. *J Orthop Trauma* 1999;13:107–113.
16. Kellam JF, McMurtry RY, Paley D, et al. The unstable pelvic fracture: operative treatment. *Orthop Clin North Am* 1987;18:25.
17. Matta JM, Saucedo T. Internal fixation of pelvic ring fractures. *Clin Orthop* 1989;242:83.
18. Mears DC, Rubash HE, Nelson DD. External fixation of the pelvic ring: the use of the Pittsburgh triangular frame. *Contemp Orthop* 1982;5:21.
19. Pennal GF, Tile M, Waddell JP, et al. Pelvic disruption: assessment and classification. *Clin Orthop* 1980;151:12.
20. Routt MLC Jr, Simonian PD, Swiontkowski MF. Stabilization of pelvic ring disruptions. *Orthop Clin North Am* 1997;28:369–388.
21. Schied DK, Kellam JF, Tile M. Open reduction and internal fixation of pelvic fractures. *J Orthop Trauma* 1991;5:226.
22. Dahners LE, Jacobs RR, Jayaraman G, et al. A study of external fixation systems for unstable pelvic fractures. *J Trauma* 1984;24:876.
23. McBroom R, Tile M. Disruption of the pelvic ring. *Orthop Trans* 1982;6:493.
24. Bell AL, Smith RA, Brown TD, et al. Comparative study of the Orthofix and Pittsburgh frames for external fixation of unstable ring fractures. *J Orthop Trauma* 1988;2:130.
25. Mears DC, Fu FH. Modern concepts of external skeletal fixation of the pelvis. *Clin Orthop* 1980;151:65.
26. Stocks GW, Gabel GT, Noble PC, et al. Anterior and posterior internal fixation of vertical shear fractures of the pelvis. *J Orthop Res* 1991;9:237.
27. Mears DC. *External skeletal fixation.* Baltimore: Williams & Wilkins, 1983.
28. Hupel TM, McKee MD, Waddell JP, et al. Primary external fixation of rotationally unstable pelvic fractures in obese patients. *J Trauma* 1998;45:111–115.
29. Kim W-Y, Hearn TC, Seleem O, et al. Effect of pin location on stability of pelvic external fixation. *Clin Orthop Rel Res* 1999; 361:237–244.
30. Simonian PT, Schwappach JR, Routt MLC Jr, et al. Evaluation of new plate designs for symphysis pubis internal fixation. *J Trauma* 1996;41:498–502.
31. Varga E, Hearn T, Powell J, et al. Effects of method of internal fixation of symphyseal disruptions on stability of the pelvic ring. *Injury* 1995;26:75–80.
32. Gorczyca JT, Watt PM, Goltz M, et al. *A mechanical comparison of anterior internal fixation vs. external fixation for unstable pelvic injuries with iliosacral screws* (poster). Orthopaedic Trauma Association. San Antonio, TX, October 2000.
33. Simonian PT, Routt MLC Jr, Harrington RM, et al. Internal fixation of the unstable anterior pelvic ring: a biomechanical comparison of standard plating techniques and the retrograde medullary superior pubic ramus screw. *J Orthop Trauma* 1994; 8:476–482.
34. Albert MJ, Miller ME, MacNaughton M, et al. Posterior pelvic fixation using a transiliac 4.5-mm reconstruction plate: a clinical and biomechanical Study. *J Orthop Trauma* 1993;3:226–232.
35. Leighton R, Waddell J, Bray TJ, et al. Biomechanical testing of new and old fixation devices for vertical shear fractures of the pelvis. *J Orthop Trauma* 1991;5:313–317.
36. Mears DC, Capito CP, Deleeuw H. Posterior pelvic disruptions managed by the use of the double cobra plate. *AAOS, Instructional Course Lectures* 1988;37:143.
37. Simonian PT, Routt MLC Jr, Harrington RM, et al. Internal fixation for the transforaminal sacral fracture. *Clin Orthop Rel Res* 1996;323:202–209.

38. Simpson LA, Waddell JP, Leighton RK, et al. Anterior approach and stabilization of the disrupted sacroiliac joint. *J Trauma* 1987; 12:1332.
39. Kraemer W, Hearn T, Tile M, et al. The effect of thread length and location on extraction strengths of iliosacral lag screws. *Injury* 1994;25:5-9.
40. Denis F, Davis S, Comfort T. Sacral fractures: an important problem. *Clin Orthop* 1988;227:61.
41. Pohlemann T, Angst M, Schneider E, et al. Fixation of transforaminal sacrum fractures: a biomechanical study. *J Orthop Trauma* 1993;7:107–117.
42. Gorczyca JT, Varga E, Woodside T, et al. The strength of iliosacral screws and transiliac bars in the fixation of vertically unstable pelvic fractures with sacral fractures. *Injury* 1996;27: 561–564.
43. Simonian PT, Routt MLC Jr. Biomechanics of pelvic fixation. *Orthop Clin North Am* 1997;28:351–367.

12

DESCRIBING THE INJURY: CLASSIFICATION OF PELVIC RING INJURIES

MARVIN TILE

INTRODUCTION

Relevance of Classification

In Chapter 10 we discussed defining the injury leading to an injury personality type.

Defining the injury requires a careful assessment of both patient factors and the injury factors in the pelvis. Only by looking at all of these factors can a logical decision be made with respect to treatment of any given patient. Defining the injury, looking at the personality of the injury type, is different than classifying the injury. To define the injury we must examine all aspects, including the following:

- Degree of displacement
- Stability of the pelvic ring
- Force direction
- State of the soft tissues, including whether the fracture is open or closed
- The anatomic injury in the pelvis
- The associated injuries

A classification is essentially a description of the bony injury so that no one classification can include all of those factors. Classifications are important, especially for academic study so that we can compare like-type injuries as closely as possible, not chalk with cheese, or apples with oranges. The problem is that there are very many types of apples. Classifications could become minutiae if we attempt to incorporate each and every factor. Therefore, they are compromises at the very best.

An excellent exercise for any surgeon treating a patient with a pelvic fracture is to actually write all of these factors down on a board or sheet of paper. Looking at all of these factors makes the treatment decisions relatively straightforward.

In each individual case when attempting to assess it, we may find that we need to put a square peg in a round hole on occasion.

The present classifications when used this way, that is, combining the classification with all of the other defining factors, can help with decision making. A clear-cut definition of the injury patterns is now possible with a precise physical examination, careful history, and the use of the more exacting imaging techniques now available. The *personality* of each fracture now can be more clearly defined.

The documentation of any fracture is useful only if it aids in the management of the patient; otherwise it is simply an academic exercise. In the past, precise definition of the injury patterns to the pelvis has been difficult, but now this has become possible with more exacting radiologic techniques, including computed tomography (CT). Both anterior and posterior lesions and their effects on the degree of stability of the pelvic ring—in effect, the *personality of the fracture*—can be carefully assessed.

Historical Considerations

Most of the early classifications were based on anatomic injuries.

It was the pioneering work of George Pennal in the late 1950s that led to the present-day classifications. After studying 359 pelvic ring disruptions (1), Pennal and Sutherland suggested that the major force vectors of anteroposterior compression, lateral compression, and vertical shear produce typical and reproducible injury patterns. Laboratory studies confirmed their suspicions, and a classification based on these forces was suggested and visualized in a movie produced for The American Academy of Orthopaedic Surgeons in 1961, which is still available from the Academy's film library.

The original Pennal classification, modified by Tile (2), is based purely on force direction and included the anteroposterior compression type, the lateral compression types, and the vertical shear.

The Young-Burgess classification (3) is based almost entirely on the original Pennal classification with the addition of one extra grouping—complex.

In the original classification the problem of instability of the pelvic ring was not clearly addressed in the film; therefore, the suggested classification required revision. As well, our further study of 248 cases of pelvic disruption detailed in Chapter 1, indicated other patterns of injury, which have now been added to the revised classification (2).

It also must be clearly understood that, although the various forces applied to the pelvis produce fairly typical injury patterns, all may be associated with complex forces that cause instability in a portion of the pelvic ring. For example, the typical anteroposterior compression injury causes a disruption of the symphysis pubis and thereby opens the pelvis like a book. Usually, the posterior sacroiliac ligaments remain intact; therefore, the posterior pelvic tension band is maintained and the pelvis is relatively stable. In some cases, however, the magnitude of the force overcomes the tensile strength of the posterior sacroiliac ligaments, rendering the pelvic ring unstable. Also, remember that the degree of instability is more likely to depend on the degree of soft-tissue trauma, a concept important in all musculoskeletal injuries.

Our proposed classification first published in 1988 also includes the original Pennal types. It is based on the concepts of force direction and stability. The A types are undisplaced stable pelvic injuries. B types—including the B1 open book, anteroposterior compression, external rotation, and B2 lateral compression (internal rotation)—show partial stability; and the C types are completely unstable, irrespective of force direction. It is often difficult to define the original force direction in the completely unstable C type.

Therefore, although this classification has proven useful in patient management, it must be strongly emphasized that each patient and each fracture is different and must be carefully and individually studied to determine the exact personality of the fracture. Only then can we hope to institute logical management.

Before discussing the classification, including examples of the various types, I must again emphasize that an injury to any part of the pelvic ring is associated with an injury somewhere else in that same ring. It was believed that undisplaced pelvic ring fractures, especially to the rami, were not necessarily accompanied by another injury to the posterior complex. A publication by Chenoweth and coworkers has shown that, in virtually all of these undisplaced fractures, one could expect a positive technetium polyphosphate bone scan, indicative of an occult injury to the posterior complex (4). Also, in his publications, Bucholz confirmed the presence of a posterior lesion in all of his postmortem material (5). Therefore, it is fallacious to speak of an *isolated* anterior or posterior injury, when, in almost all cases, both are present.

The closest example of an exception to this rule would be those rare cases where the entire pelvic ring is avulsed from the sacrum; that is, a bilateral shearing sacroiliac dislocation unaccompanied by an anterior ring injury. These patients always have a bilateral posterior injury but no injury to the anterior portion of the pelvic ring. Other exceptions include simple avulsion fractures of portions of the pelvis (e.g., the anterior superior spine in adolescents, or isolated iliac wing fractures). These are, by definition, not pelvic ring disruptions; therefore, they are not relevant to this discussion.

Finally, we have adapted our classification to the universal classification nomenclature suggested by Müller and coworkers and to the AO group (6). In this classification, fractures are grouped according to increasing severity (Types A, B, or C) and many subgroups are possible. In my article in the January 1988 *Journal of Bone and Joint Surgery,* I first suggested this new nomenclature as it relates to the previous classification; in other words, the principles have remained, but the coding has changed. Further refinements to this coding recently have been suggested by Helfet. Tile, Kellam, Ganz, and Isler have been adopted by Müller as the AO classification (7).

DEFINING THE INJURY TYPES

Before discussing this classification, the anatomic types of lesions found anteriorly and posteriorly in pelvic disruption and the importance of the degree of displacement in determining the stability of the pelvic ring are outlined.

Anterior Lesions

Symphysis

The anterior lesion may be a *disruption* of the symphysis pubis. In most cases, this disruption is an avulsion from bone;

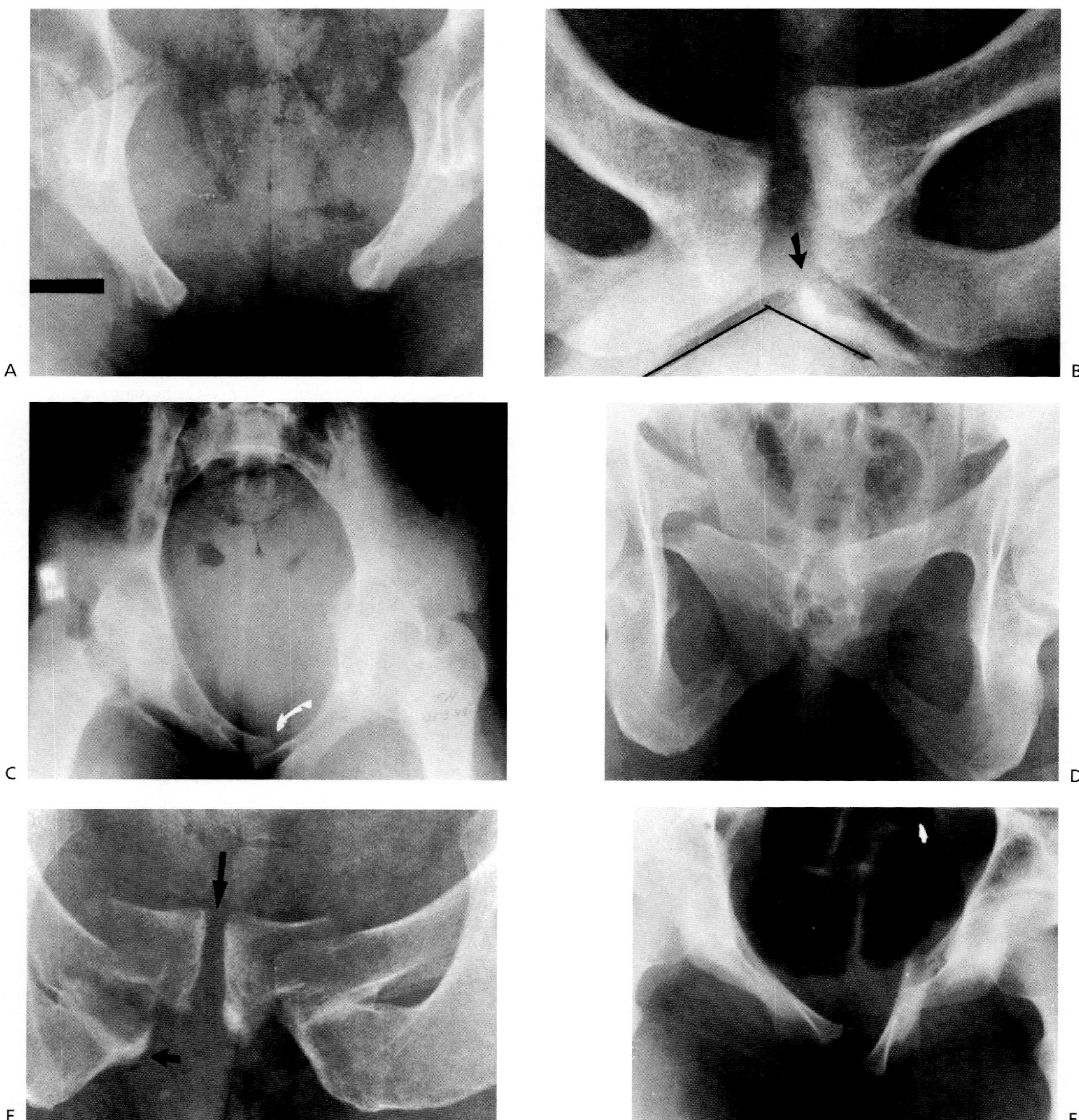

FIGURE 12-1. The anterior pelvic lesion may be: **A:** A disruption of the symphysis pubis through soft tissue. **B:** An avulsion of the entire symphysis from one or other pubis *(arrow).* **C:** A locked, overlapped symphysis *(white arrow)* in a lateral compression- type injury. **D:** A fracture of the superior and inferior pubic rami on the same side. **E:** A disruption of the symphysis associated with an anterior avulsion of the insertion of the rectus abdominis muscle *(large arrow).* **F:** Combinations of all of the preceding, as noted in this example of a symphysis disruption, associated with fractures of the superior and inferior pubic rami on the left side *(tilt fracture).*

that is, the symphysis itself becomes avulsed from one or other hemipelvis. Also, the symphysis may tear in midsubstance, as may any other ligamentous structure. The symphysis may be overlapped and locked if the mechanism of injury is lateral compression (Fig. 12-1A–C).

Pubic Rami

The anterior lesion may be a fracture of both pubic rami, and occasionally a fracture of the superior pubic ramus with an extension into the symphysis. Various combinations of symphysis and pubic rami lesions are noted and are described later in this chapter. This fracture pattern through the superior ramus may extend into the anterior column of the acetabulum (Fig. 12-1D).

Avulsion of Insertion of Rectus Abdominis

Occasionally, a small anterior fragment of bone, representing the insertion of the rectus abdominis muscle, may be avulsed from the symphysis. Disruption of the symphysis proper usually accompanies this fracture (Fig. 12-1E).

Combined Lesions

Several of the fracture patterns to be described have combinations of the aforementioned lesions, including fractures to all four pubic rami and fractures to two pubic rami associated with a symphysis disruption (the tilt fracture) (Fig. 12-1F).

Posterior Lesions

The importance of the posterior lesion cannot be overstated. Several questions immediately come to mind concerning posterior lesions: Where is the lesion? Is it unilateral or bilateral? Is it displaced or undisplaced? Is it stable or unstable?

Location

The posterior lesion may involve the ilium, sacroiliac joint, or sacrum.

Ilium

An iliac fracture usually extends from the greater sciatic notch to the iliac crest, but on occasion it extends into the posterior column of the acetabulum (Fig. 12-2A,B).

Sacroiliac Joint

A sacroiliac lesion may be a pure dislocation, but more commonly it includes a portion of ilium or the sacrum in the fracture-dislocation pattern (Fig. 12-3A–D).

Sacrum

Fractures of the sacrum may be vertical or transverse below the sacrogluteal line. Vertical fractures are common in pelvic ring disruption; transverse fractures are really spinal injuries (Fig. 12-4A). The vertical fracture may occur through the sacral foramina (Fig. 12-4B), lateral (Fig. 12-4C) or medial (Fig. 12-4D) to them. Occasionally, sacral fractures are complex, with transverse and vertical components, the so-called H fracture associated with falls from a height (Fig. 12-4E).

The vertical fractures may be caused by lateral compression, causing impaction of the cancellous bone of the sacrum; or by shear, causing a gap in the cancellous bone (Fig. 12-4F,G). These two types are vastly different, including their associated injuries, degree of stability, and final outcome.

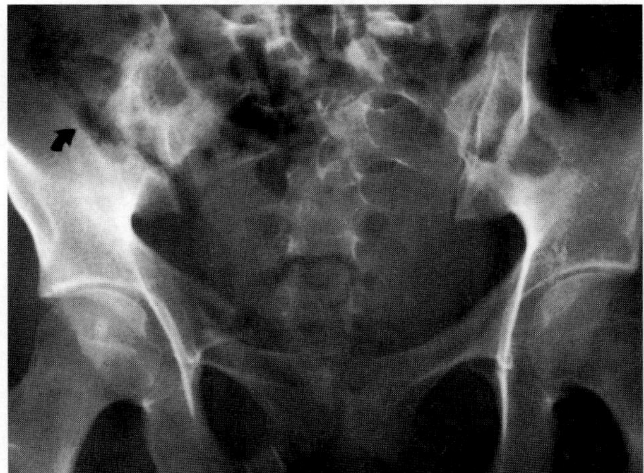

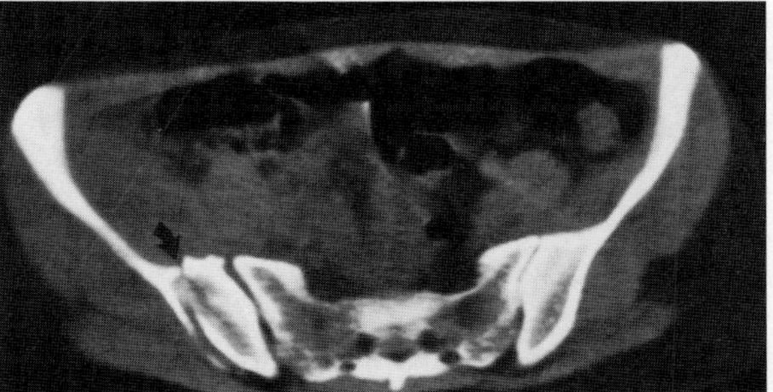

FIGURE 12-2. A: The posterior lesion may be a fracture of the ilium, as shown on the anteroposterior radiograph of the pelvis. **B:** It also may be shown by computed tomography.

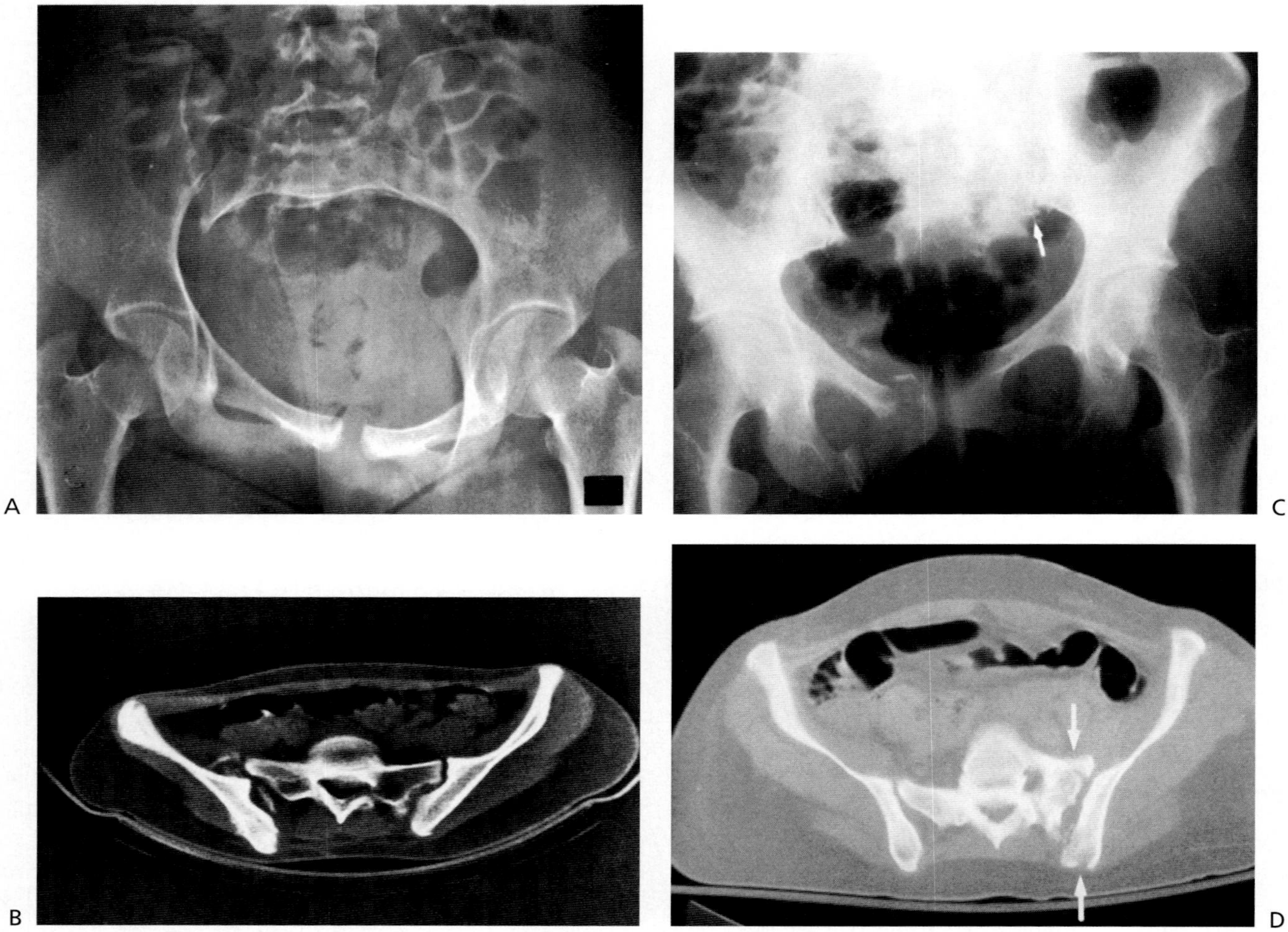

FIGURE 12-3. **A:** A dislocation of the sacroiliac joint suspected in the radiograph and confirmed on computed tomography (CT). **B:** Only small flakes of bone are noted on the CT. **C:** The anteroposterior radiograph shows a lateral compression injury of the contralateral type. **D:** Without CT the surgeon could not tell that this sacroiliac dislocation includes a fracture of the sacrum and a fracture of the ilium *(white arrows).*

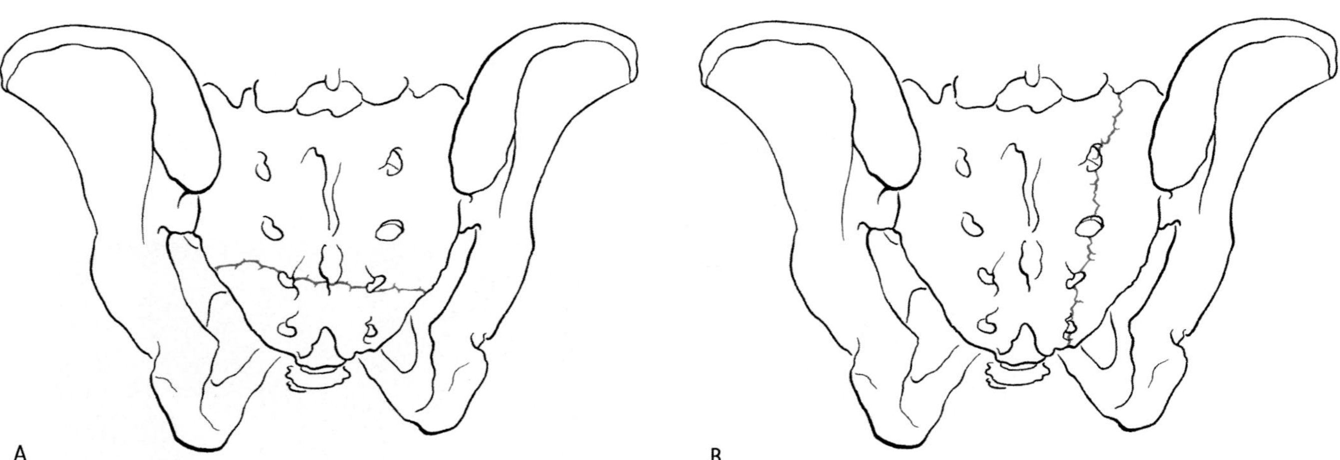

FIGURE 12-4. **A:** Fractures of the sacrum may be vertical or horizontal. The horizontal or transverse fractures are really spinal injuries, whereas the vertical fractures are part of pelvic ring disruption. The vertical fractures may be: **B:** through the foramina; **C:** lateral; or **D:** medial to it. **E:** Finally, fractures of the sacrum may be markedly comminuted in an H fashion, often caused by falls from a height. The posterior lesion may be stable or unstable.

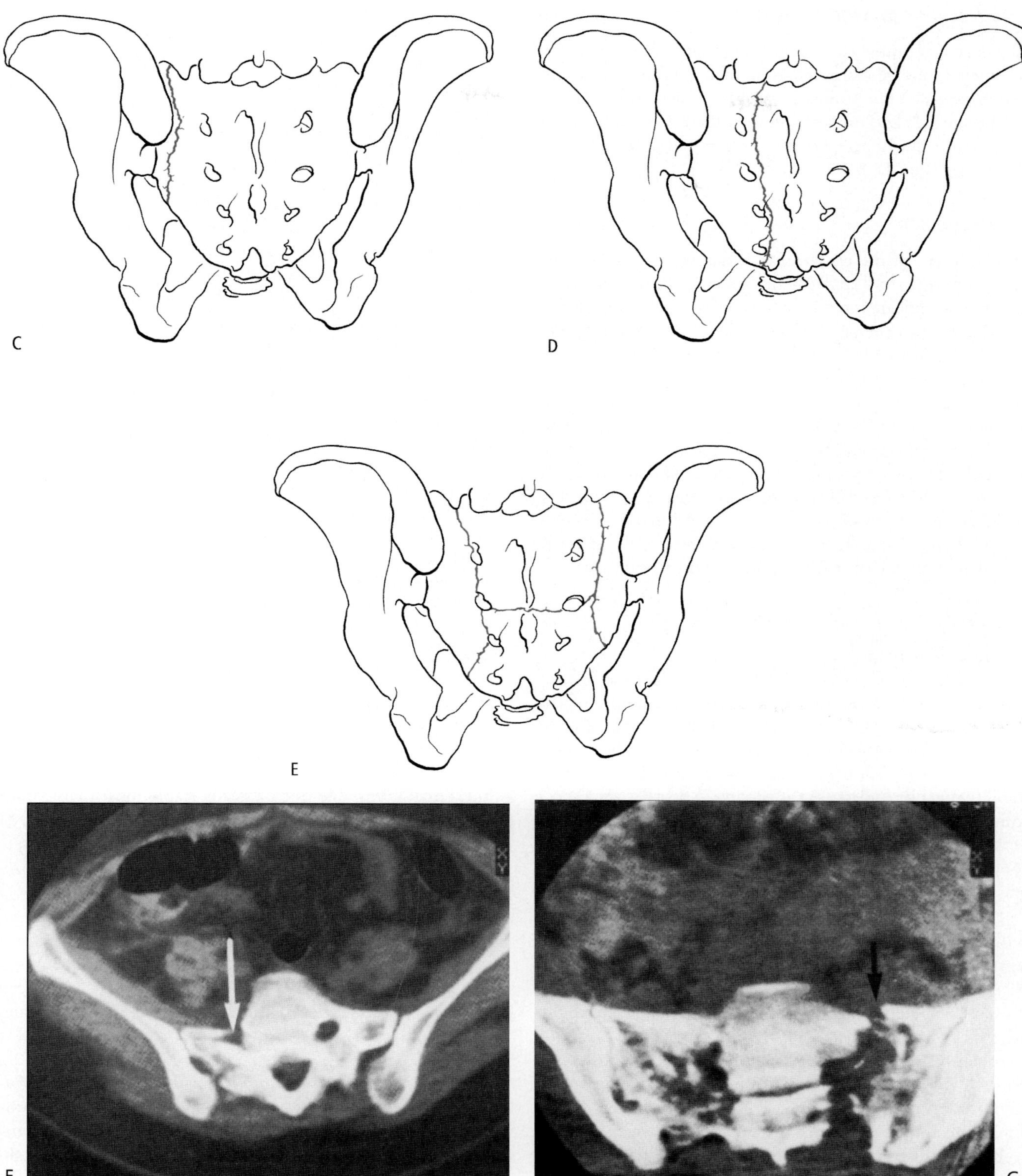

FIGURE 12-4. (*continued*) **F:** Here, the impacted right sacrum is clearly seen *(white arrow)*. There is at least 1 cm of overlap between the two fragments. This posterior lesion is stable and cannot be moved. **G:** The left sacral lesion is grossly unstable. All soft tissues are disrupted as well as the displacement at the fracture.

Unilateral or Bilateral Injury

The posterior injury may be bilateral; that is, both sacroiliac complexes may be disrupted. The bilateral posterior lesion may be unstable on both sides, stable on both sides, or stable on one side and unstable on the other. A bilateral lesion has a significant impact on the management of the unstable pelvic ring (Fig. 12-5).

Displacement

Displacement of the posterior complex is the most important prognostic indicator for the general assessment of the patient. As indicated in Chapter 8, the presence of posterior displacement in the pelvic ring increases the mortality and morbidity rates significantly. The inlet view is ideal for assessing posterior displacement, but is rarely obtained in a crisis situation. In those circumstances, the standard anteroposterior view suffices. The sacrogluteal line (Fig. 12-6) should be carefully outlined; if it is discontinuous, gross posterior displacement should be suspected. CT and an inlet view of the pelvis confirm these suspicions. As well on the anteroposterior view of the pelvis, a disruption of the second sacral foraminal arcuate line with the iliopectineal line at the sacroiliac joint is indicative of posterior disruption (3).

Stability

General Assessment

As it relates to musculoskeletal trauma, stability is a difficult concept to grasp. A simple definition is, "the ability of the anatomic structure to withstand physiologic forces *without deformation*." It is obvious that the concept cannot be applied absolutely: Every lesion is not either unstable or stable; rather, stability must be understood as varying in degree over a spectrum. Also, one must decide whether to describe the stability of the pelvis at the time of injury or following reduction. This concept applies to all musculoskeletal injuries and must be grasped before logical fracture management can be initiated.

For example, an impacted Colles fracture is stable until it is disimpacted, at which time its stability depends on the integrity of the soft-tissue envelope. The same is true of the impacted posterior injury of the pelvis caused by lateral compression. It is stable in the impacted state, but if reduced, the degree of stability depends on the integrity of the posterior sacroiliac ligaments and the ligaments and fascia of the pelvic floor. These structures are relatively intact in a true lateral compression injury; therefore, it is almost inconceivable to destabilize an impacted posterior sacroiliac injury.

Because disruption and displacement of the posterior sacroiliac complex are associated with increased risk of hemorrhage and associated soft-part injuries, an understanding of this concept is crucial to the management of the patient and the fracture.

As described in Chapters 4 and 6, the key to the stability of the pelvic ring is the integrity of the posterior weight-bearing arch and the integrity of the pelvic floor. Because there is no inherent stability in the unattached bony structures, the stability is imparted by the soft tissues, mostly the ligaments. The posterior ligamentous structures joining the sacrum to both ilia have a unique configuration; if viewed on cross section, the area resembles a suspension bridge (Fig. 12-7), with the two posterior superior spines resembling the pillars; the sacrum, the span; and the interosseous sacroiliac ligaments, the suspension. Therefore, the posterior weight-bearing arch is maintained by the sacroiliac complex with the addition of the iliolumbar ligaments, which join the transverse processes of L5 to the ilium. Together, these structures may be considered as the *posterior tension band of the pelvis.* Also, the muscles, fascia, and ligaments of the pelvic floor play a major role in determining pelvic stability. The sacrospinous ligament limits external rotation. The sacrotuberous ligament limits rotation in the sagittal plane; both insert anterior to the line of the sacroiliac joint.

External rotatory and shearing forces tend to disrupt the pelvic floor, whereas lateral compression forces do not (Fig. 12-4F,G). Following trauma, several scenarios are possible, depending on which soft tissues and bones are injured. Vertical and posterior pelvic stability is ensured if the integrity of the posterior tension band is maintained or the pelvic floor is intact. The degree of ligamentous disruption varies from case to case, and so must the degree of instability of the pelvic ring.

Types of Stability

All pelvic injuries may be placed on the *stability scale* (Fig. 12-8), depending on the degree of posterior bony and/or ligamentous damage. These injuries can be classified as stable, rotationally unstable but vertically stable, or unstable both rotationally and vertically. Determination of the degree of stability of any particular injury depends on an accurate clinical and radiographic assessment (see Chapter 10).

Stable Lesions

The lesions considered to be stable are those with intact soft tissues around the bony pelvis or those that do not involve the pelvic ring itself (e.g., iliac wing injuries). Undisplaced fractures of the pelvic ring do not displace if all soft tissues are intact (Fig. 12-9A).

Partially Stable (Rotationally Unstable, Vertically and Posteriorly Stable) Lesions. Partially stable lesions, by definition, cannot be significantly displaced vertically or posteriorly because of the intact posterior ligaments, and/or an intact pelvic floor. Two types of rotational instability are recognized, external rotatory (open book) and internal rotatory (lateral compression). In each, stability is maintained by either mechanism, that is, intact posterior ligaments and/or an intact pelvic floor.

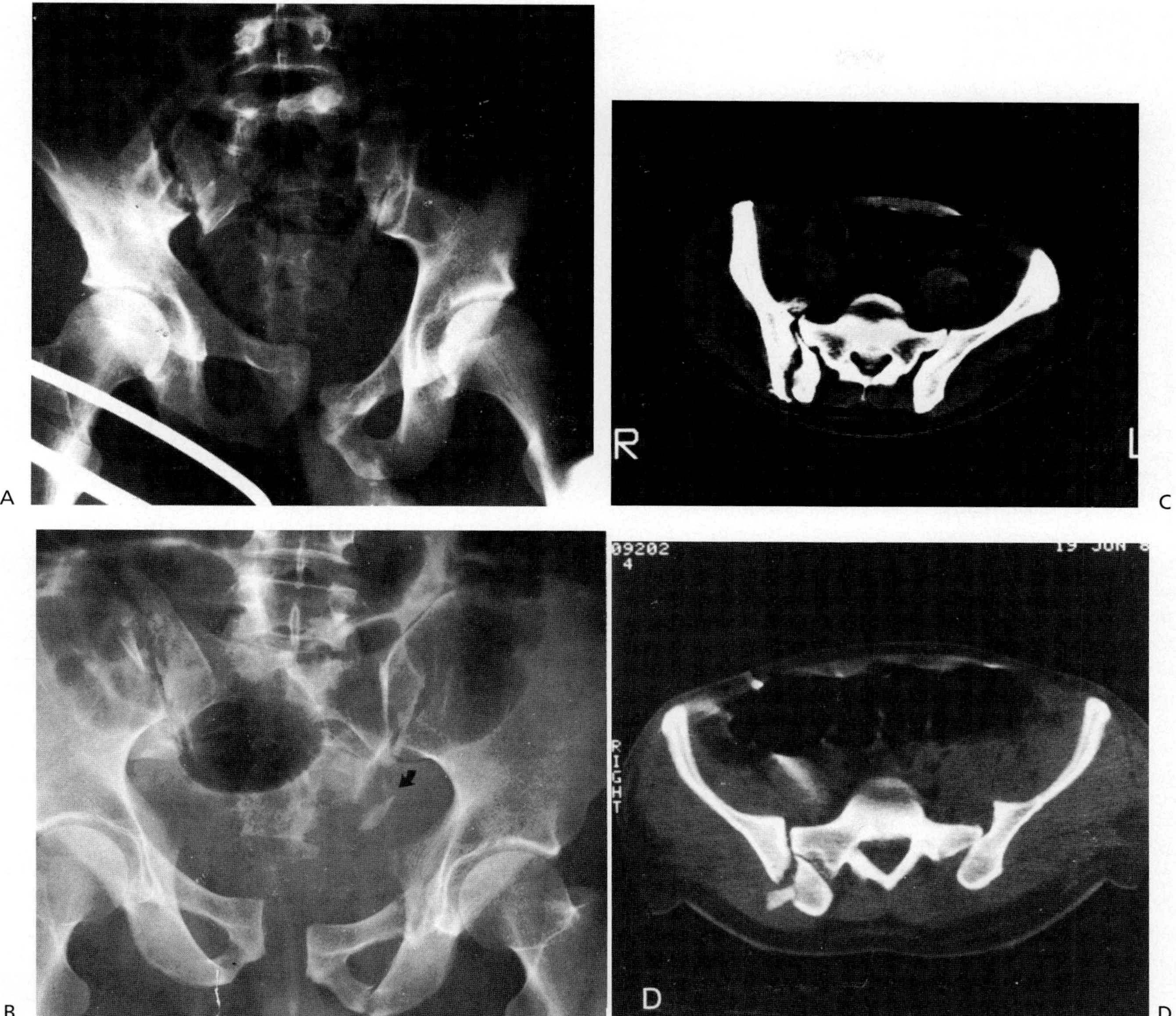

FIGURE 12-5. **A:** The posterior lesion may be unilateral or bilateral. **B:** A unilateral fracture dislocation of the sacroiliac joint is noted and confirmed on computed tomography (CT). **C:** A bilateral sacroiliac lesion, a most unstable type of pelvic disruption. The *black arrow* points to an avulsion of the left lateral aspect of the sacrum, representing the sacral attachment of the sacrospinous ligament. The posterior displacement of the right sacroiliac joint is clearly noted, as is the disruption of the symphysis pubis. **D:** CT scan through the sacroiliac joint of the same patient shows the degree of displacement of the left sacroiliac joint, suspected by the avulsion of the sacrum but certainly not seen clearly in the radiograph. The fracture-dislocation on the right side is a typical pattern.

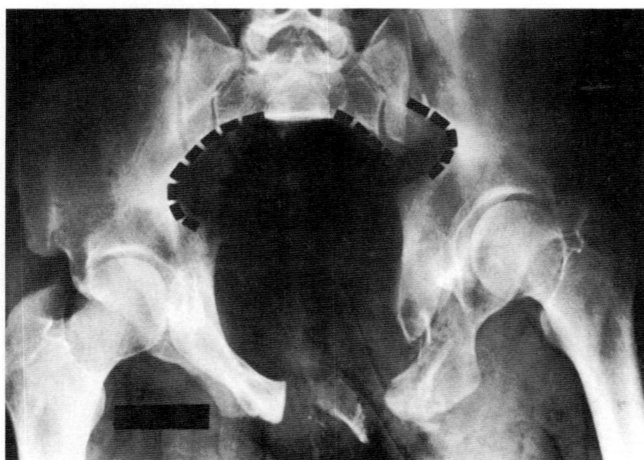

FIGURE 12-6. The dotted line on the right side represents the sacrogluteal line on this inlet view of the pelvis. Any break in the continuity of this line, as noted on the left side, represents displacement of the posterior complex, an ominous prognostic indicator.

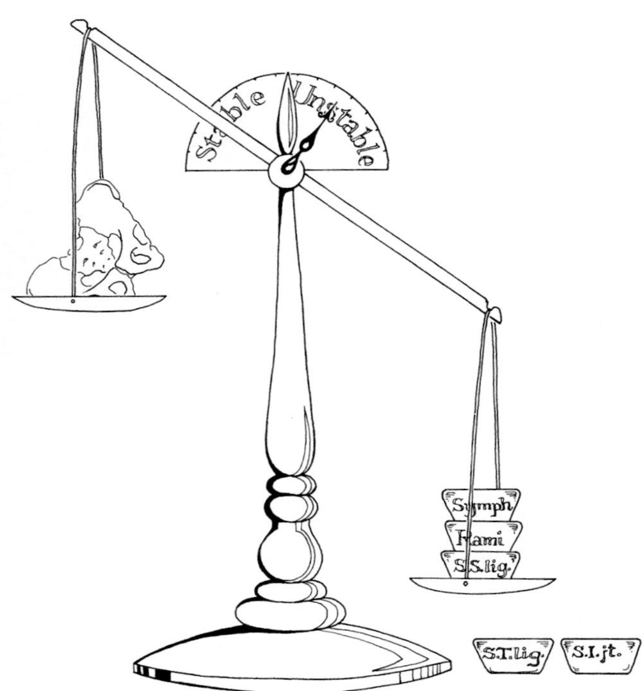

FIGURE 12-8. The stability scale may be tipped in favor of instability by division of ligamentous structures, including the symphysis pubis and sacrospinous, sacrotuberous, and sacroiliac ligaments.

Intact Posterior Ligaments. Intact posterior sacroiliac ligaments ensure the stability of the pelvic ring in spite of anterior pelvic ring disruption. In the so-called open-book injury, caused by *external rotational forces,* the symphysis pubis may be disrupted and displaced, but the posterior structures remain intact. Therefore, "closing the book" restores full stability to the pelvic ring (Fig. 12-9B).

Intact Pelvic Floor. As well, *lateral compressive forces* tend to decompress rather than tear the pelvic floor; therefore, vertical and posterior stability are maintained by this mechanism even in cases in which the posterior tension band ligaments are disrupted. This is akin to the flexion compression type of vertebral fracture in which the vertebral body is compressed, the interspinous ligament is torn, but the anterior soft tissues are intact. Stability is maintained by a

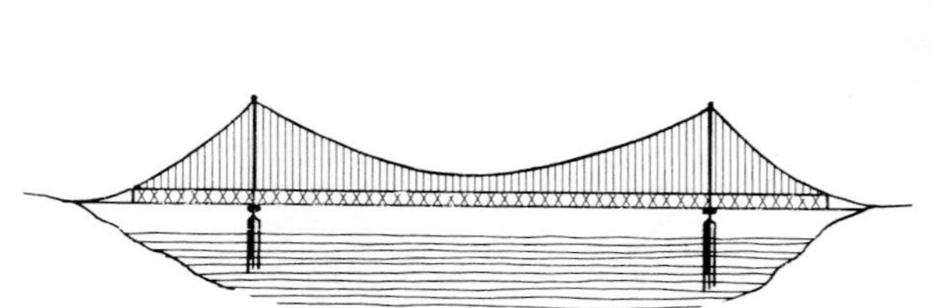

A

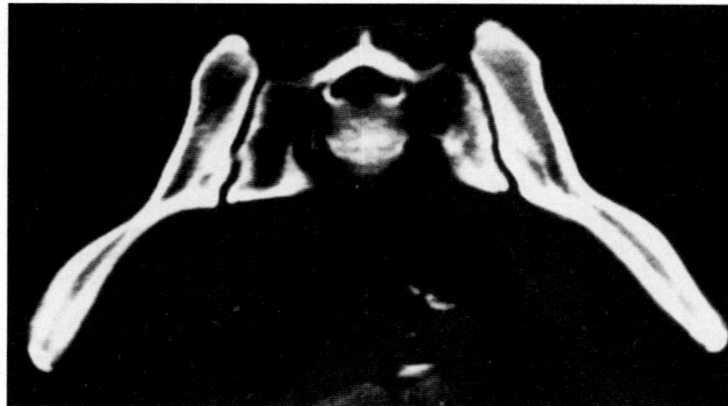

B

FIGURE 12-7. Skeletal and posterior skeletal ligamentous structures joining the sacrum to both ilia have a unique configuration, resembling a suspension bridge. **A:** The two posterior superior spines resemble the pillars, the sacrum the span, and the interosseous sacroiliac ligaments the suspension. **B:** The posterior weight-bearing arch is maintained by the sacroiliac complex, with the addition of the iliolumbar, sacrospinous, and sacrotuberous ligaments, the so-called posterior tension band of the pelvis.

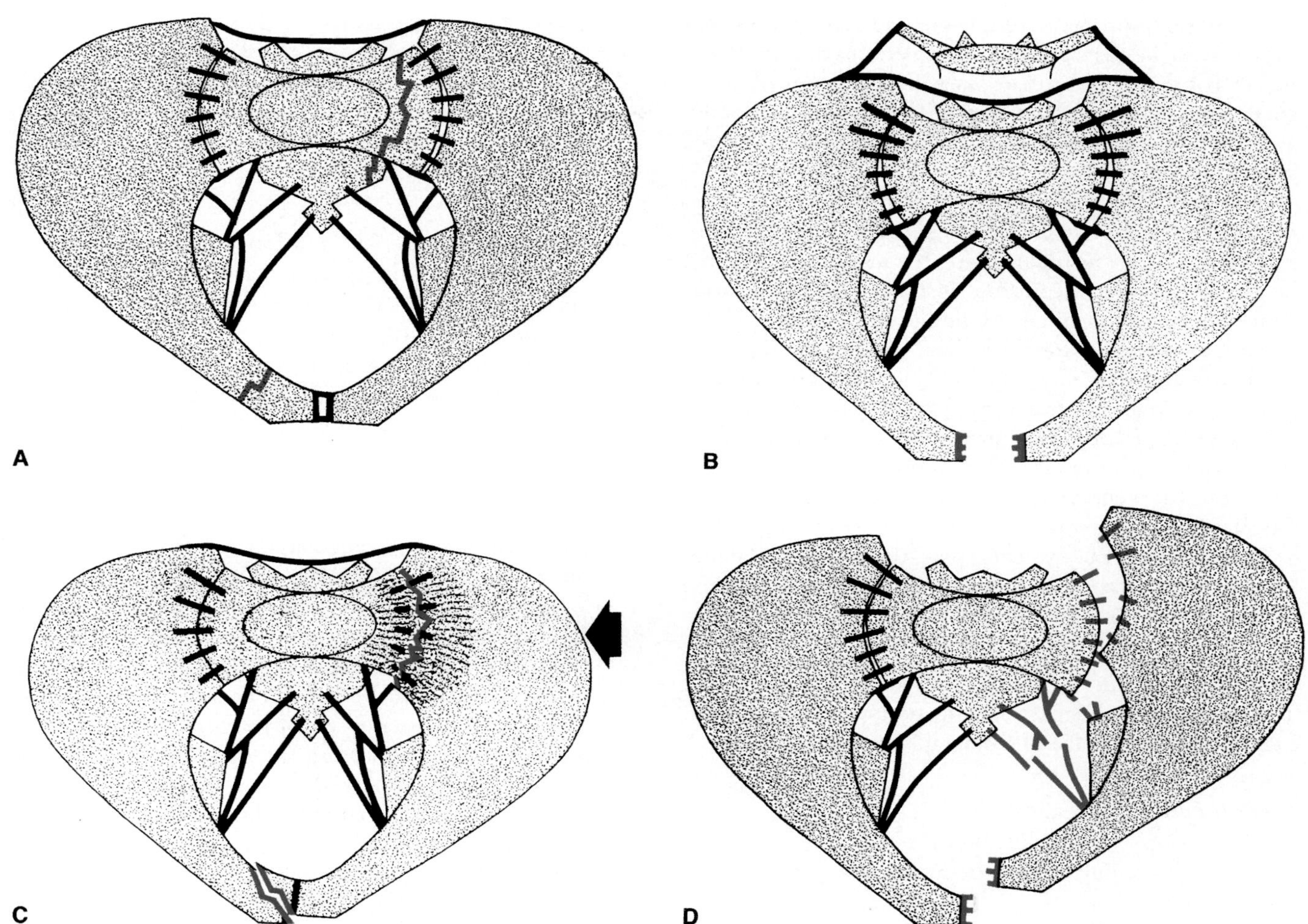

FIGURE 12-9. A: Stable Type A. Stable lesions are those with intact soft tissues around the bony pelvis. Undisplaced fractures of the pelvic ring will not be displaced if all soft tissues are intact, as in the drawing. **B:** Type B is partially stable with the intact posterior ligaments. Intact posterior sacroiliac ligaments ensure the stability of the pelvic ring in spite of disruption of the anterior pelvis. This is best noted in the so-called open-book injury caused by external rotation forces. **C:** The pelvic floor is intact. Lateral compressive forces disrupt and displace the pelvic rami anteriorly and impact or compress the posterior sacroiliac complex. In this injury the posterior ligaments may hold or disrupt. In either case, pelvic stability is maintained by the intact pelvic floor. No major displacement can occur in the vertical or posterior plane. **D:** In unstable Type C fractures of the pelvic ring, both the pelvic floor and posterior sacroiliac complex are disrupted.

combination of the intact soft tissues of the pelvic floor and the compression injury to the sacrum. In this injury, the posterior ligaments may hold, especially in older patients, so that simple bed rest in the supine position restores stability to the pelvic ring with elastic recoil of the tissues (Fig. 12-9C).

Therefore, vertical stability is maintained with external rotation forces because the "posterior tension band" remains intact, allowing the "book" to open to the finite point, whereas with internal rotation (lateral compression) the pelvic floor is relatively intact, even if the posterior tension band is disrupted.

Unstable (Rotationally, Vertically and Posteriorly) Lesions. At the opposite, or unstable, end of the stability scale is the lesion of the posterior pelvic complex, characterized by disruption or avulsion of the posterior sacroiliac ligaments as well as the pelvic floor, resulting in gross displacement. Shearing forces usually cause this lesion, which may be unilateral or bilateral. Clinical examination reveals apparent gross abnormal motion of the affected hemipelvis and radiographic examination, especially the inlet view or CT, reveals posterior or vertical displacement of the pelvic ring (Fig. 12-9D).

The cancellous bone of the sacrum or ilium or the sacroiliac joint may be markedly separated by the shearing forces

(Fig. 12-4G). Both the sacrotuberous and sacrospinous ligaments must be disrupted for complete instability of the hemipelvis to occur; therefore, an avulsion fracture of the ischial spine or adjacent portion of the sacrum, indicating avulsion of the sacrospinous ligament, is a pathognomonic sign of instability (Fig. 12-10A,B).

The degree of instability may be almost complete (i.e., the affected hemipelvis may be held together only by skin and subcutaneous tissue; in effect, the lesion is an internal hemipelvectomy) or incomplete, if some of the ligamentous attachments may remain in continuity.

Patients with gross instability have almost three times the morbidity and mortality rates and require more intensive general care than patients with a stable pelvic ring injury. They lose up to three times the amount of blood; therefore, the diagnosis of instability has important clinical implications for the general management of the patient (see Chapter 8).

By combining the two concepts—the degree of stability of the posterior sacroiliac complex and the direction of the injurious force—a meaningful classification is developed.

Signs of Instability

The stability scale (Fig. 12-8) is tipped toward the unstable side by certain clinical and radiographic features.

Clinical Factors. These include:

1. Severe displacement, including rotation of the pelvis and/or shortening of the extremity noted on physical examination
2. Marked posterior disruption characterized by bruising and swelling
3. Gross instability of the hemipelvis on manual palpation
4. Severe associated injuries to viscera, blood vessels, or nerves
5. An associated open wound

Radiographic Factors. These include:

1. Displacement of the posterior sacroiliac complex >1.0 cm, either by a fracture, dislocation, or combination of the two (Fig. 12-10)
2. The presence of a gap rather than impaction posteriorly (Fig. 12-4G). If the injury is through cancellous bone, the presence of a gap implies gross soft-tissue disruption and, therefore, instability; whereas impaction of cancellous bone along the lines of the major trabeculae implies preservation of the soft-tissue envelope. The compressed bone may have inherent stability, so that no abnormal movement can be detected on clinical examination. A dislocation of the sacroiliac joint must be unstable, because the extremely strong interosseous sacroiliac ligaments must be ruptured, whereas a subluxation may have retained ligamentous structures. The forces that cause disruption of the posterior weight-bearing complex cross the major trabeculae, shearing the cancellous bone of the sacrum or ilium with the adjacent soft tissues or disrupting the ligaments only, causing a dislocation. These forces usually are a combination of external rotation and shear. Forces directed laterally against the iliac crest or the greater trochanter cause compression of the posterior complex.

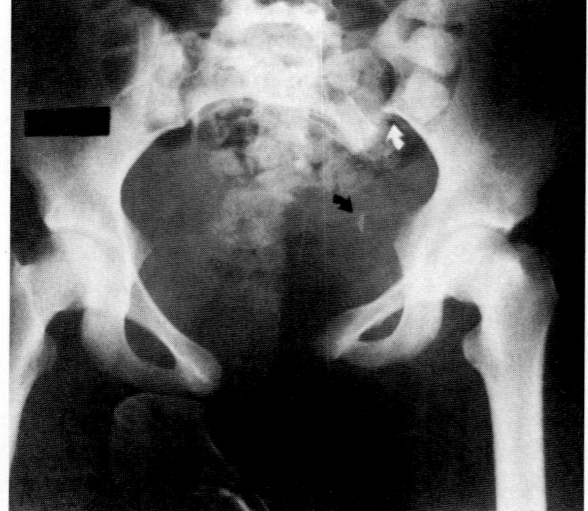
A

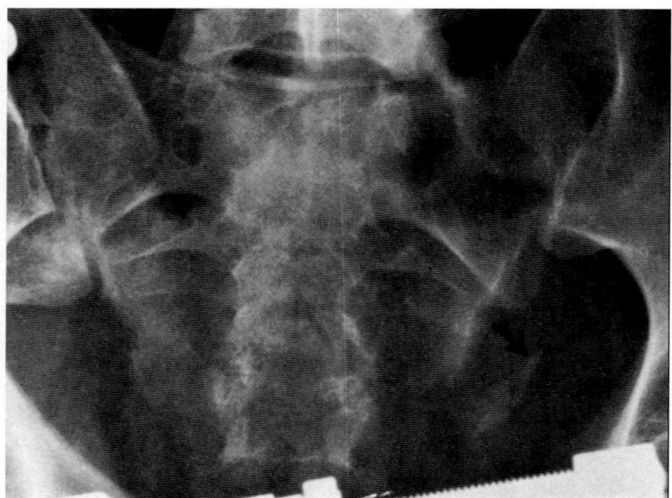
B

FIGURE 12-10. A: Radiographic signs of instability include posterior displacement of the left sacroiliac joint *(white arrow)* and avulsion of the tip of the ischial spine, representing an avulsion of the sacrospinous ligament *(black arrow).* **B:** The left hemipelvis in this young woman is completely unstable. Posterior displacement of the sacroiliac joint is shown, and in this case an avulsion of the sacral end of the sacrospinous ligament.

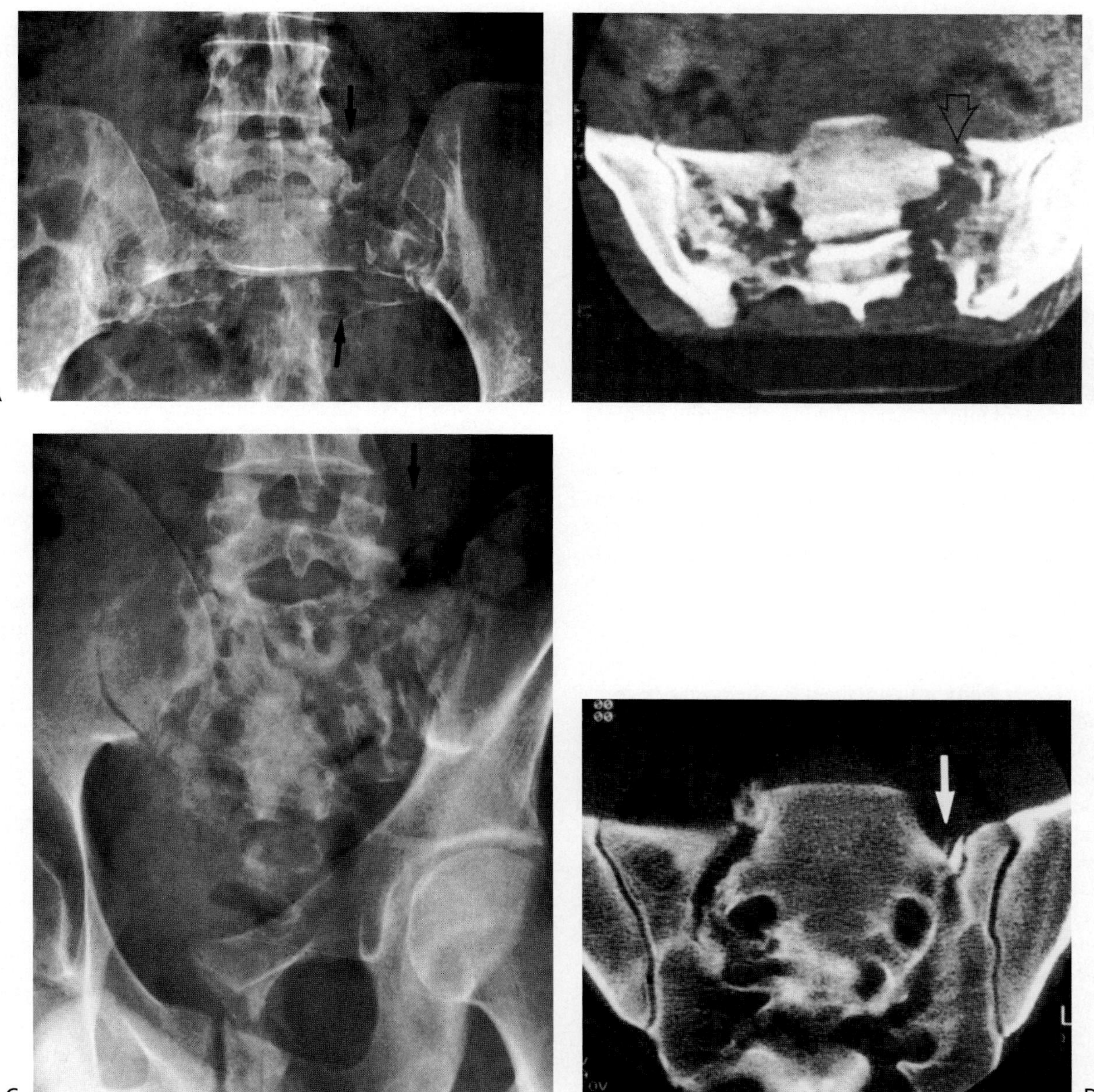

FIGURE 12-11. A: The avulsed L5 transverse process *(superior black arrow)* in the radiograph is associated with a markedly unstable sacral fracture. **B:** This is best seen on computed tomography (CT) *(arrow).* **C:** Whereas the avulsion of the transverse process of L5 in the radiograph is associated with a more stable lateral compression injury seen by the internally rotated left hemipelvis and overlapped symphysis in the radiograph **(C)** and the sacral crush on CT (**D,** *white arrow).*

3. The presence of avulsion fractures of the sacral or ischial end of the sacrospinous ligament (Fig. 12-10)
4. Avulsion fractures of the transverse process of L5 may be a sign of either an unstable posterior complex, if associated with a posterior gap (Fig. 12-11), or a lateral compression injury, if associated with impaction of the sacrum.
5. Vertical fractures through the pubic and ischial rami

Effect of Pelvic Injury on the Viscera, Vessels, and Nerves

Pelvic injuries if displaced that tend to tear the pelvis apart—anteroposterior compression or external rotation—often are associated with major visceral injury, severe bleeding, and traction injuries to nerves. Lateral compression injuries often are associated with puncture of the viscera; for example, a bladder causing bleeding because the pelvic floor tends to remain intact and nerve injury is often entrapment. These factors have been carefully studied in a landmark paper by Dalal and coworkers (8). The effect on viscera in the pelvic injury is discussed in more detail in the following section on classification.

CLASSIFICATION

Introduction

The present classification (Table 12-1) maintains the underlying principle of correlation between pelvic stability and the mechanism of injury; that is, the force direction required to produce the injury. It was first proposed in the classifications of Pennal, modified by Tile in 1988, and incorporated in the second edition of this book. The second principle was to modify the classification to conform with the nomenclature proposed by Müller and colleagues adopted by the AO-ASIF groups.

The classification is based on the integrity of the posterior sacroiliac complex, most important for the retention of pelvic stability. Recent biomechanical work has shown that 60% of pelvic stability is maintained by the posterior complex, and 40% by the anterior complex, anterior to the hip joints (9). Therefore, main subgroups are divided into Type A, preserves stability of the posterior pelvic ring; Type B, partial posterior stability; and Type C, complete loss of posterior stability.

Stability, however, is not a black-and-white concept but is seen as shades of gray. The stability scale is noted in Chapter 10 and is tipped in favor of instability by division of ligamentous structures. All pelvic fractures may fall along this stability scale (Fig. 12-8B).

The anatomic lesions, that is, fractures of the sacrum, the sacroiliac joint, fractures or fracture dislocations, and fractures of the ilium, as well as unilateral and bilateral rami fractures, are included in this classification.

The anatomic lesions in the anterior pelvic ring, also important for academic purposes, and therefore in this alphanumeric classification to be used for academic purposes, are included for completeness. It is obvious that disruptions of the symphysis may have different treatment methodologies and problems than displaced fractures of the rami. Therefore, although we may use a relatively simple classification in our clinical practice, extensive descriptive classification following the anatomic lesions should be captured for documentation and outcome purposes.

Many types of fractures defy precise classification because of complex force resolutions, usually the result of major motor vehicle trauma. In these cases, which are usually major Type C unstable injuries, the pelvic ring may be disrupted in a very bizarre pattern. With careful thought, however, all cases should fit into the proposed classification.

For a clinical practice the following classification is proposed as seen in Table 12-1. The classification in Table 12-1 serves the practitioner, because it is based on the concepts of pelvic stability, increasing severity, and increasing mortality and morbidity as one reaches the Type C fractures.

In recent literature there is a tendency to group all of the Type B fractures, the partially stable fractures, together. The B1 open-book types, even though the integrity of the posterior ring is relatively intact, produce very different visceral type injuries than the lateral compression types. Therefore, it is extremely important when reporting these injuries to differentiate between the B1 open-book types, whether they be unilateral B1 or bilateral B3, and the B2 lateral compression injuries, which are discussed subsequently in this chapter.

The comprehensive classification that follows classifies for academic purposes, so that as closely as possible when we are discussing the literature we will be comparing apples to apples and not apples to oranges.

TABLE 12-1. CLASSIFICATION

Type A: stable pelvic ring injury
Type B: partially stable pelvic ring injury
- B1: Open book injury (AP compression, external rotation)
- B2: Lateral compression (internal rotation)
- B3: Bilateral injuries

Type C: completely unstable (allows all degrees of translational displacement)

COMPREHENSIVE CLASSIFICATION

The comprehensive classification is based on the preceding with the inclusion of modifiers for the anterior lesion and more detail for the posterior lesion. The Young-Burgess classification is a popular system also, based on the original Pennal classification. A correlation of the comprehensive classification with the Young-Burgess is discussed.

Type A: Stable

Type A fractures are fractures with no major instability of the posterior ring (Fig. 12-9A).

Stable Type A fractures of the pelvis fall into two broad categories. First, those fractures that do not involve the ring, namely, avulsion fractures, fractures of the iliac wing, and transverse fractures of the sacrum and coccyx. Second, those fractures involving the ring but with so little bone displacement that the soft tissues are virtually intact. This stable Type A fracture can be further classified as follows.

A1: Avulsion Fractures

Avulsion fractures usually occur in adolescents at the end of their growth period, but they are not limited to adolescents; they also occur in adults. The avulsions occur through the apophysis, most commonly the anterior superior spine (Fig. 12-12).

Avulsion fractures of the anterior superior spine (A1-1) almost always occur in the adolescent age group as a result of resistance against the acutely flexed hip. As a result, the sartorius muscle pulls a portion of the iliac apophysis from the ilium. Most of these injuries can be managed with bed rest with the hip in the flexed position. Rarely, surgery may be indicated to replace the fragment in avulsions with major displacement. Avulsions of the anterior inferior iliac spine (A1-2) usually occur in sprinters, adolescents, or adults. They are caused by sudden contraction of the rectus femoris against resistance. Avulsions of the pubic spine (A1-3) and iliac crest (A2) are less common.

Avulsions of the ischial tuberosity (A1-3) may be either acute or chronic, and are caused by sudden contraction of the hamstrings against resistance. We most frequently encounter this in water skiers. In adolescents, the healing may be incomplete and may produce a syndrome of chronic pain, especially on sitting, very much akin to the so-called Osgood-Schlatter's disease of the tibial tubercle. Occasionally adults suffer a massive avulsion of the entire tuberosity, including a portion of the inferior pubic ramus (Fig. 12-13; Table 12-2).

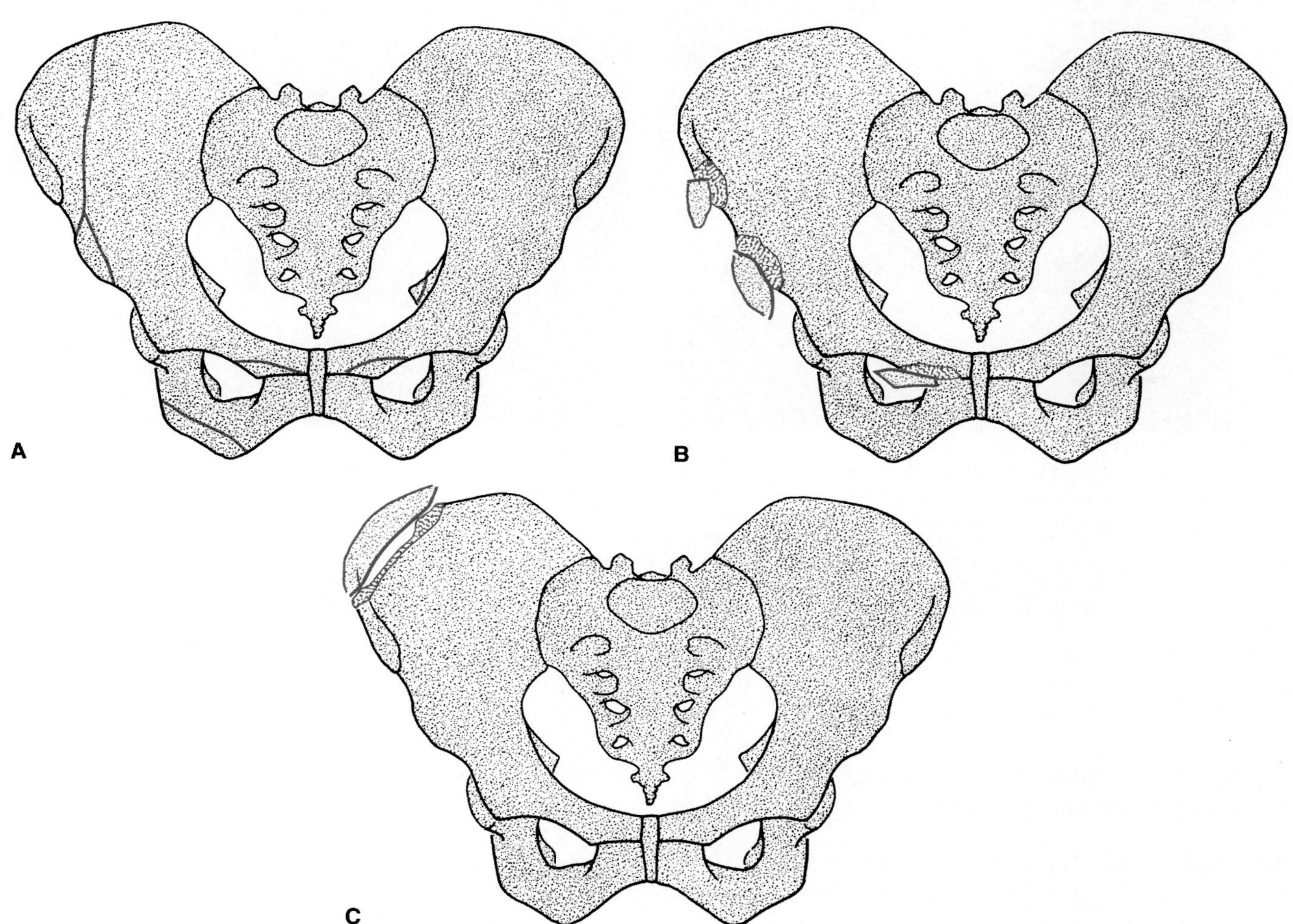

FIGURE 12-12. Avulsion fractures of the pelvic ring. **A:** Avulsion fractures usually occur in adolescents at the end of their growth period and, as noted in the diagram, may involve the anterior superior, anterior inferior, or ischial spine. Avulsions also may occur at the pubic tubercle and iliac crest. **B:** Avulsions of the anterior superior spine caused by the sudden contraction of the sartorius, the anterior inferior spine caused by rectus femoris contraction, and pubic tubercle by pectineus are demonstrated. **C:** Occasionally, avulsion of a major portion of the iliac crest occurs.

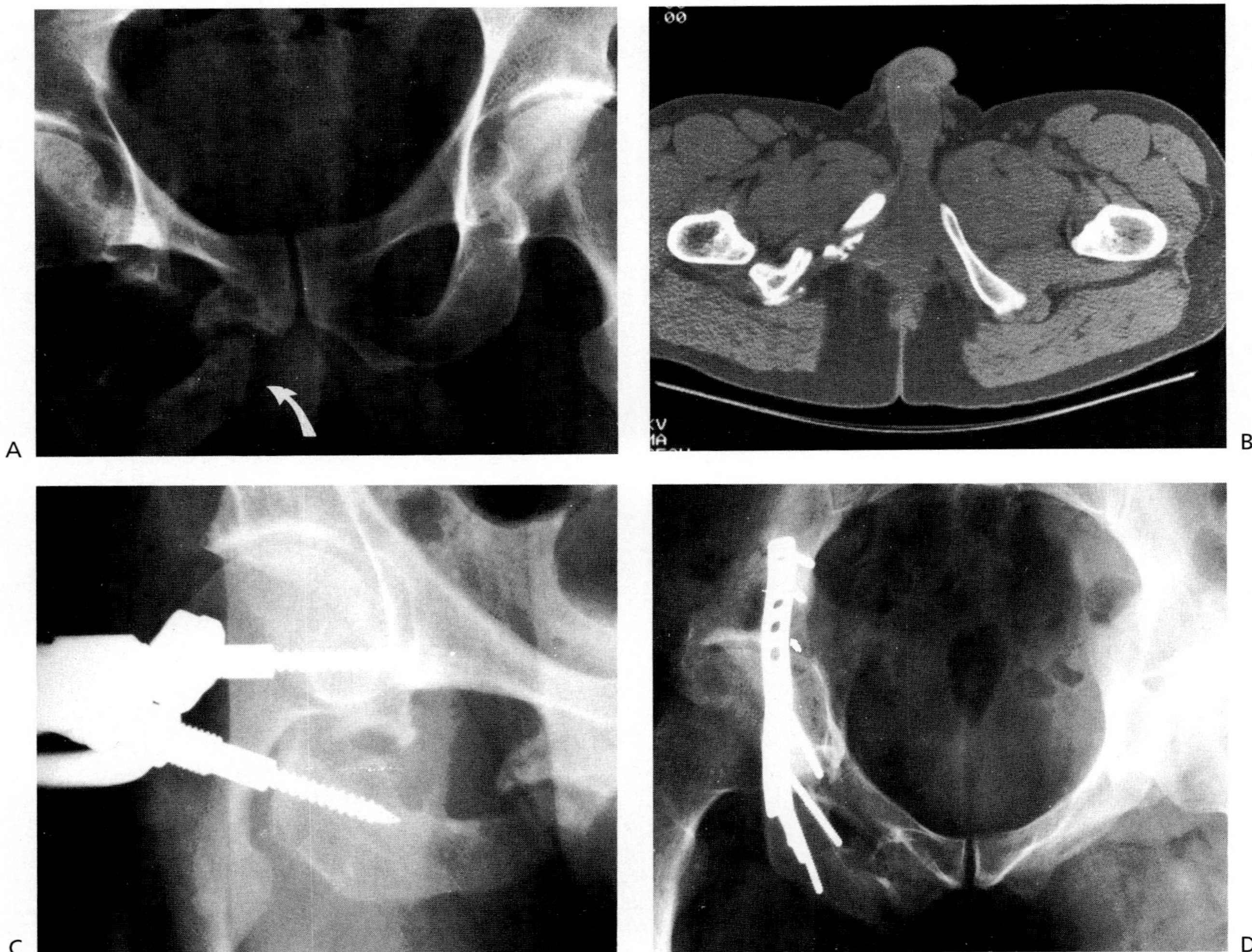

FIGURE 12-13. A: This patient sustained a massive avulsion of the entire ischial tuberosity, including a portion of the inferior pubic ramus while water skiing *(arrow)*. Note the nonunion of the inferior ramus and the large gap, causing nonunion at the ischial tuberosity. **B:** The nonunion is confirmed on the computed tomography. The patient was having both pain on sitting and sciatic nerve irritation symptoms. **C:** At surgery, the sciatic nerve was dissected freely from the nonunion and a new pelvic compression device was inserted. **D:** A cancellous bone graft was used, and the nonunion ultimately healed. The patient's sciatic nerve symptoms also abated.

A2: Stable Iliac Wing Fractures or Minimally Displaced Fractures of the Pelvic Ring

A2-1: Isolated Iliac Wing Fractures (Fig. 12-14A)

These injuries are caused by a direct blow to the ilium. They do not involve the pelvic ring, which remains stable; therefore, most can be managed nonoperatively (Fig. 12-14B,C). However, in some cases the iliac wing is so deformed that open reduction and internal fixation are desirable. These fractures also may have significant soft-tissue injury to the overlying abdominal and pelvic girdle muscle, as well as bleeding consequences because of the disruption of the large cancellous surface of the iliac wing.

A2-2: Stable, Undisplaced, or Minimally Displaced Fractures of the Pelvic Ring

This fracture pattern (Fig. 12-15) is relatively common, usually occurring in elderly women with osteoporosis as the result of a fall. The mechanism is lateral compression, cracking the pubic rami and crushing the sacrum at the sacroiliac joint. Because of the marked osteopenia of the pelvis, the fracture occurs as a result of very low energy, so the soft tis-

TABLE 12-2. CLASSIFICATION OF PELVIC RING DISRUPTION

Comprehensive Classification	Young and Burgess Classification
Type A: Stable pelvic ring injury	No equivalent
A1: Avulsion of the innominate bone	No equivalent
A2: Stable iliac wing fracture or stable minimally displaced ring fractures	No equivalent
A3: Transverse fractures of the sacrum and coccyx	No equivalent
Type B: Partially stable	
B1: Open-book injury	APC 1, APC 11
B2: The lateral compression injury	LC1, LC11, crescent fracture
B3: Bilateral B injuries	Windswept, complex
Type C: Complete unstable	
C1: Unilateral	APC 111, vertical shear
C2: Bilateral, one side B, one side C	Complex
C3: Bilateral C lesions	Complex

Source: Tile, *JBJS,* Jan 1988.

sues are intact. The posterior injury usually cannot be seen on plain radiographs but can be diagnosed on technetium bone scan or CT (4) (see Fig. 4-1).

A2-3: Isolated Anterior Ring Injuries (Four-Pillar)

This injury is also called the *straddle,* or *butterfly fracture* because it involves all four pubic rami anteriorly, with no posterior injury. In these rare instances, the rami fractures are caused by a direct blow without a concomitant posterior lesion. This is rarely the case in our series and in our experience. Most of these injuries are variations of lateral compression (Type B2) or Type C shearing with an associated posterior lesion (Fig. 12-16A–C). The examiner should not be misled by a rather innocent-looking four-ramus fracture. It almost always represents a high-energy injury of shearing or lateral compression. In our review, it was usually associated with high rates of morbidity and mortality. Physicians should not be misled by the plain radiographs, which may not show the posterior lesion; they must always examine by CT, which does reveal the lesion.

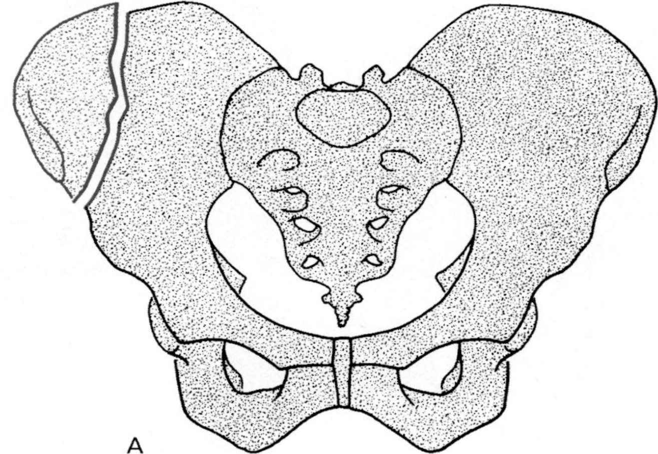

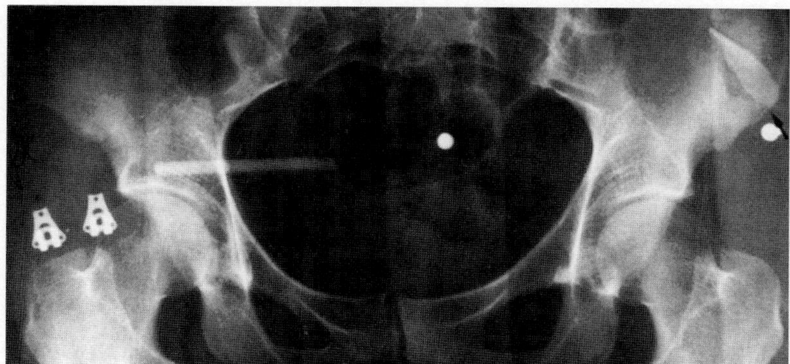

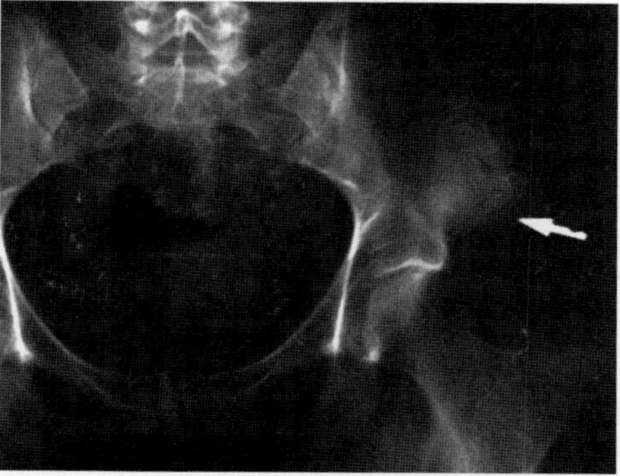

FIGURE 12-14. A: This drawing depicts an isolated fracture of the iliac wing, without involvement of the ring; therefore, this is an A2 isolated iliac wing fracture. **B:** The anteroposterior radiograph demonstrates such a fracture without involvement of the ring *(white arrow).* **C:** Nonoperative symptomatic treatment resulted in healing with a large calcified mass on the ilium.

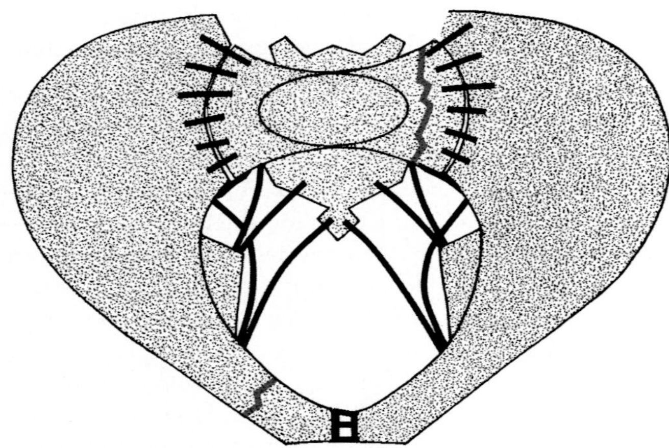

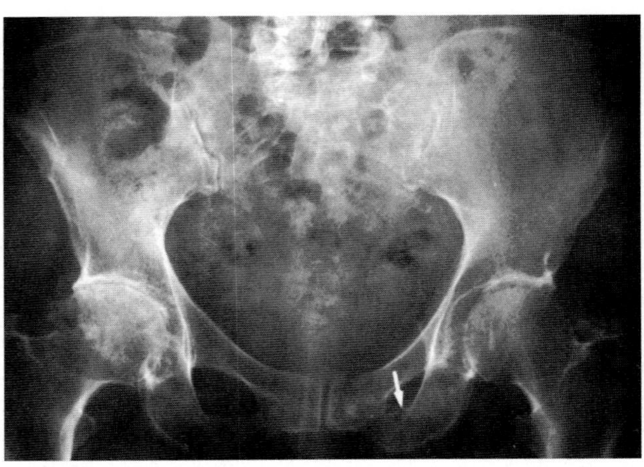

FIGURE 12-15. Type A2-2. **A:** A drawing of a stable undisplaced fracture of the ring with intact soft tissues. **B:** The anteroposterior radiograph of the pelvis shows a minimally displaced fracture of the pelvic ring anteriorly in the rami and posteriorly through the sacrum. An incidental finding is an osteoarthritic right hip.

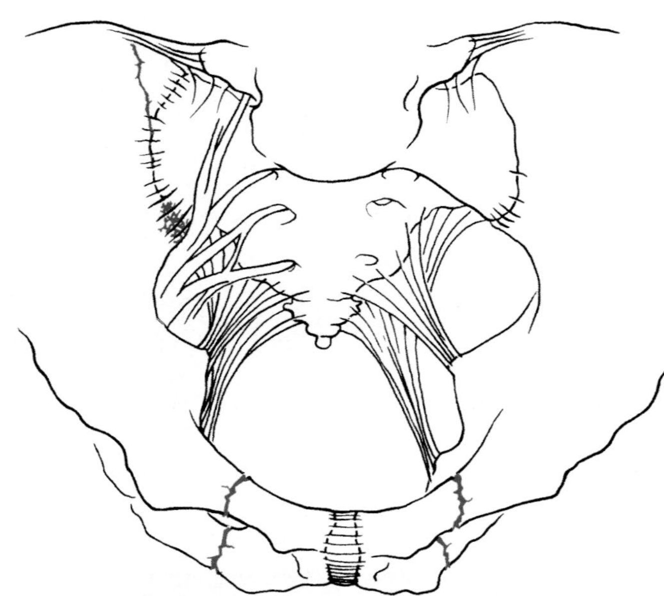

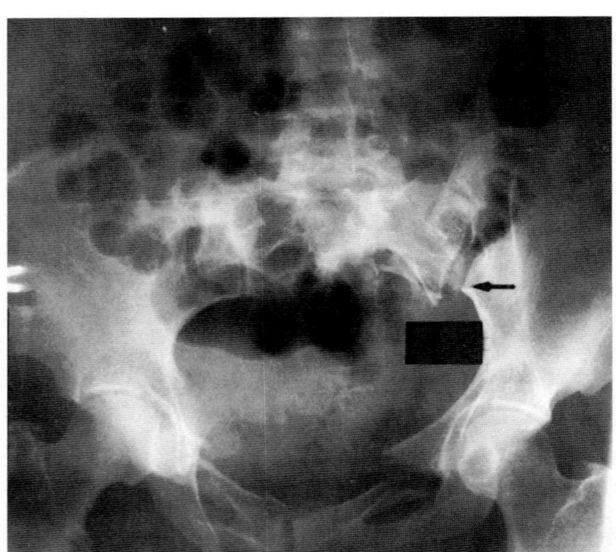

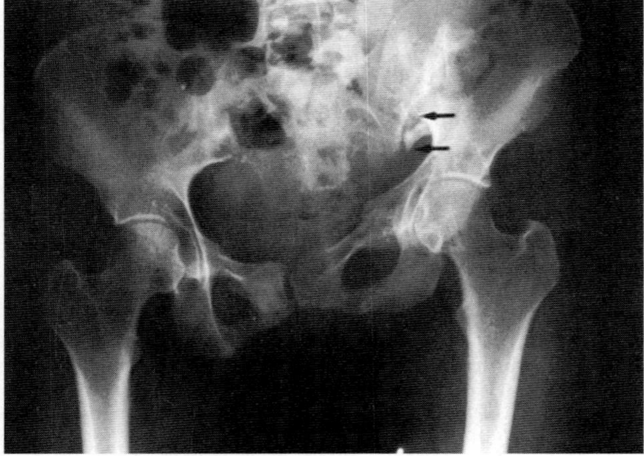

FIGURE 12-16. A: Note the fracture of all four pubic rami. Although this so-called straddle, or butterfly, fracture may be caused by anteroposterior compression and may be an isolated and stable injury, in almost all cases, as in this case, a posterior lesion is present. **B:** Note the marked disruption of the left sacroiliac joint on the radiograph. **C:** Two years later the fractures are healed, but with considerable posterior displacement of the left sacroiliac joint, resulting in a 2-cm leg length discrepancy.

The displacement of the floating anterior fragment is usually superior and may persist with contraction of the rectus abdominis muscle. The patient in Fig. 12-1E with this type of injury was given a general anesthetic for application of an external skeletal fixator. At the time, we were watching the event on the image intensifier. When the patient coughed as the endotracheal tube was being inserted, the anterior fragment floated up to the level of the umbilicus, owing to the violent contraction of the rectus abdominis muscle. Displacement occasionally may persist because of the unopposed pull of this muscle, if the patient is not managed in some degree of hip flexion or if the symphysis is not stabilized.

A3: Transverse Fractures of the Coccyx and Sacrum

A3-1: Fractures of the Coccyx or Sacrococcygeal Dislocation

A3-1 Lesions are common and may be a source of prolonged pain in some patients, but neurologic disability is not present (Fig. 12-17A).

A3-2 and A3-3: Transverse Fractures of the Sacrum

Transverse fractures of the sacrum distal to the sacrogluteal line (usually below S2) are not truly fractures of the pelvic ring. They may occur from simple falls, especially in older persons, but may also be associated with high-energy violence, such as falls from a height. In those instances they should be considered more as spinal injuries than pelvic ring disruptions. The undisplaced transverse sacral fracture (A3-2), usually resulting from a fall, has a relatively good prognosis with nonoperative treatment; however, the displaced transverse sacral fracture (A3-3), often caused by high-energy violence, may be associated with a major neurologic deficit involving the sacral portion of the cauda equina. In those instances, open reduction of the fracture, usually combined with a sacral laminectomy, to decompress the nerve roots maybe considered (Fig. 12-17B,C).

Type B: Partially Stable

These fractures are rotationally unstable but vertically and posteriorly stable (Fig. 12-9B,C). They may have anterior displacement through the symphysis and/or pubic rami but

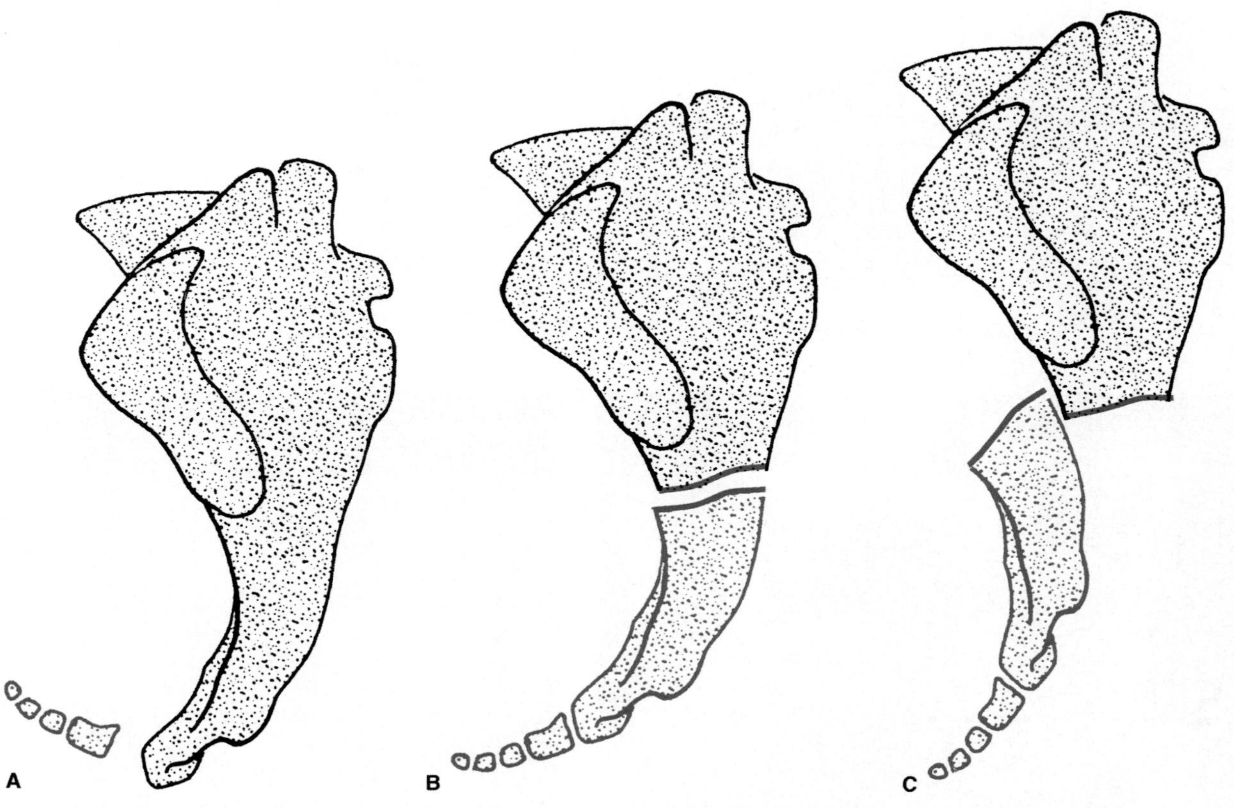

FIGURE 12-17. A: Fractures of the coccyx are common and may be a source of prolonged pain in some patients. Sacrococcygeal dislocation may occur. **B:** Transverse fractures of the sacrum distal to the sacrogluteal line do not usually involve the pelvic ring and preferably are classified as spinal injuries. In Type A3-2 the transverse fracture is undisplaced and rarely causes neurologic abnormalities. **C:** In Type A3-3 the marked displacement or translation of the distal fragment often causes injury to the sacral nerve roots.

no vertical or posterior displacement other than that allowed by rotation of the hemipelvis, usually less than 1 cm. Greater than 1 cm of posterior displacement at the sacroiliac complex represents a completely unstable Type C lesion. The rotationally unstable, but translationally stable Type B lesions may be caused by external rotatory (anteroposterior compression) or internal rotatory forces (lateral compression). They may be unilateral or bilateral. The Type B lesions are characterized by either an intact posterior tension band; that is, by retention of the posterior sacroiliac ligaments, and/or pelvic floor by solid impaction of bone through the sacrum or fracture of the ilium, with an intact pelvic floor.

In the universal nomenclature, the *bilateral* Type B lesions are all put into the B3 classification, whereas the B1 and B2 types are all unilateral. For teaching purposes it is much simpler to keep the open-book injuries together and the lateral compression injuries together, but I indicate the universal nomenclature for these lesions.

B1: The Open-Book Injury (External Rotational Instability)

The Typical Lesion

Anteroposterior compressive forces applied to the anterior superior iliac spines of the fixed pelvis or forces applied through the externally rotated femora (to the pelvis) may open the pelvis like a book. Conversely, a posterior blow against the posterior superior iliac spines may produce a similar injury. A disruption of the symphysis pubis, associated with anterior unilateral or bilateral sacroiliac joint disruption, characterizes this injury (Fig. 12-18). The strong posterior sacroiliac ligaments remain intact, maintaining the posterior tension band of the pelvic ring in this injury pattern.

The open-book injury may be further characterized as follows, depending on the displacement of the symphysis: Experimentally, a symphysis pubis separation of <2.5 cm has no associated disruption of the pelvic floor or the

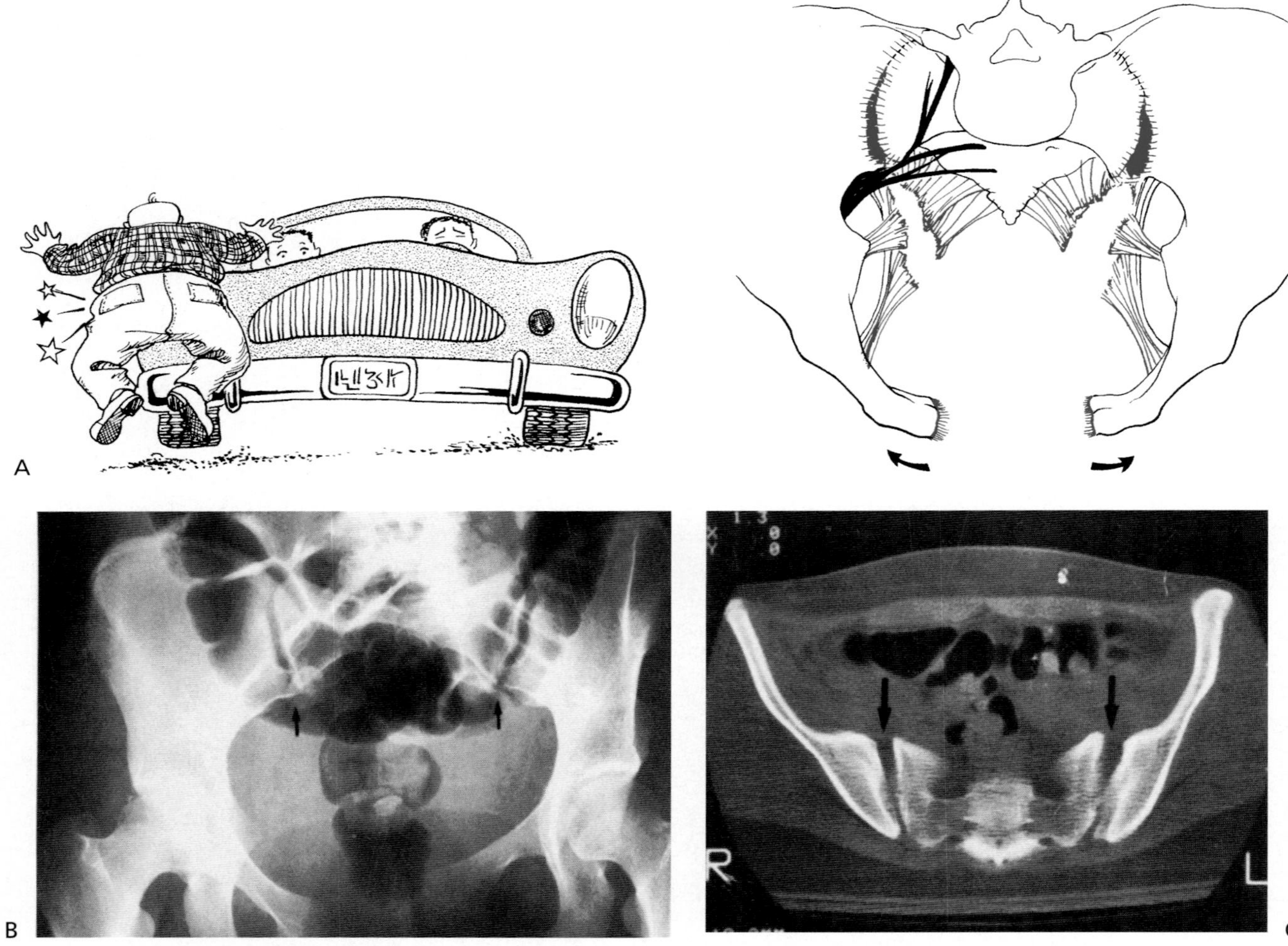

FIGURE 12-18. Type B1 open-book injury. **A:** The typical open-book injury is usually caused by anteroposterior compression or external rotation of the femora, resulting in a disruption of the symphysis pubis and anterior sacroiliac ligaments as well as the pelvic floor. With the posterior sacroiliac ligaments intact, this injury exhibits external rotational instability but no posterior or vertical instability. **B:** The anteroposterior radiograph shows the anterior widening of the sacroiliac joints and the displaced symphysis pubis. **C:** This is confirmed on the computed tomography.

sacrospinous ligament, whereas a separation of the symphysis of >2.5 cm always is associated with disruption of the sacrospinous ligament and pelvic floor. Also, disruption of the pelvic floor is associated with a much higher incidence of visceral injury (10).

Symphysis Disruption Less Than 2.5 cm

Although rare, this injury may be more troublesome clinically than one might expect (Fig. 12-19A). The patient in Fig. 12-19B was a 31-year-old hockey player who crashed into the boards, striking his posterior sacroiliac area. He noted immediate pain at the symphysis pubis, which radiographically was separated 1.5 cm. Three months after the injury, calcification is noted at the symphysis (Fig. 12-19C). Eventually, he became pain free and returned to competitive hockey (Fig. 12-19D). This is the Young-Burgess Anterior/Posterior Compression Injury I.

Symphysis Disruption Greater Than 2.5 cm

Continuation of the external rotation or anteroposterior force causes a disruption of the symphysis pubis >2.5 cm. This is associated with disruption of the pelvic floor, fascia,

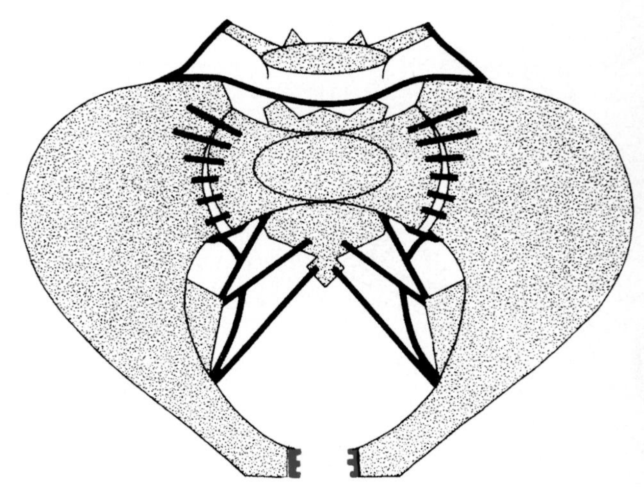

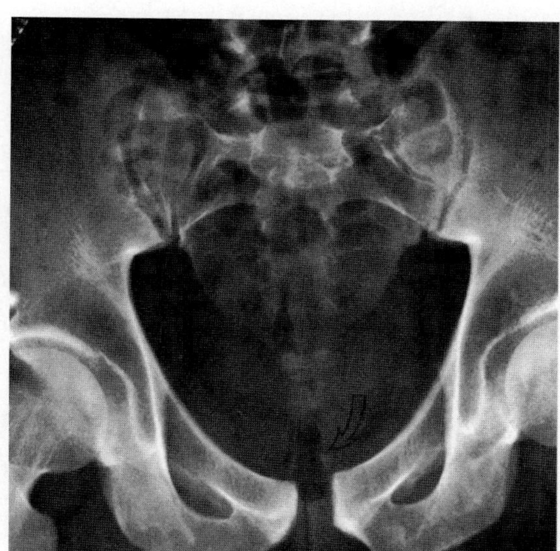

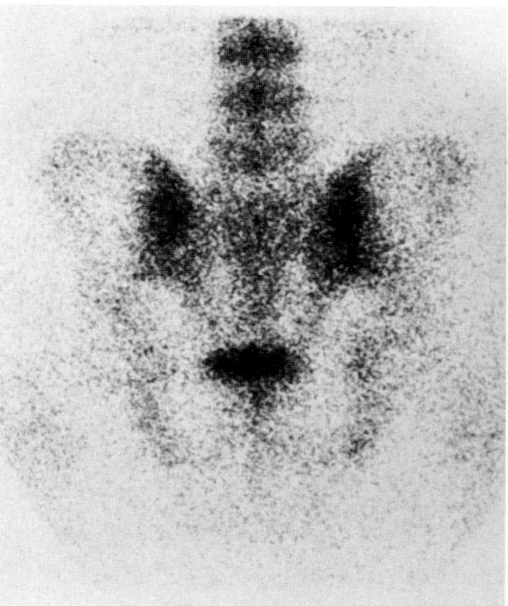

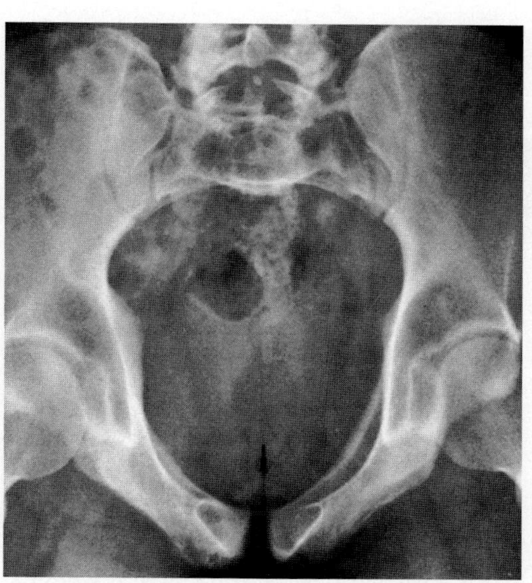

FIGURE 12-19. Symphysis disruption <2.5 cm. This injury is uncommon but it can clinically be more troublesome than one might expect. **A:** The drawing shows the intact soft tissues other than the disrupted symphysis. **B:** An anteroposterior radiograph of a hockey player who sustained a direct blow to the posterior sacroiliac area bilaterally and noted immediate pain anteriorly at the symphysis pubis. The arrow shows a minimal disruption of the symphysis pubis with no major opening of the sacroiliac joints posteriorly. **C:** The technetium bone scan indicates markedly increased uptake at the symphysis. **D:** The radiograph 12 weeks after injury shows calcification *(black arrow)* and a stable pelvis.

sacrospinous ligaments, and anterior sacroiliac ligaments (Fig. 12-18). This injury may be unilateral B1 or bilateral B3-1. This is the Young-Burgess Anterior/Posterior Compression Injury II.

Unilateral B1 injury (Fig. 12-20) is usually caused by violent external rotation of one femur; for example, when a motorcyclist or a snowmobiler puts a leg out for balance and gets caught on a stationary object such as a tree or rock. The external rotation force usually disrupts the symphysis, and as the external rotational force continues, the pelvic floor, fascia, and sacrospinous and anterior sacroiliac ligaments are disrupted. If the force stops at that point, the hemipelvis exhibits external rotational instability only and cannot be vertically or posteriorly displaced because of the intact posterior sacroiliac ligaments.

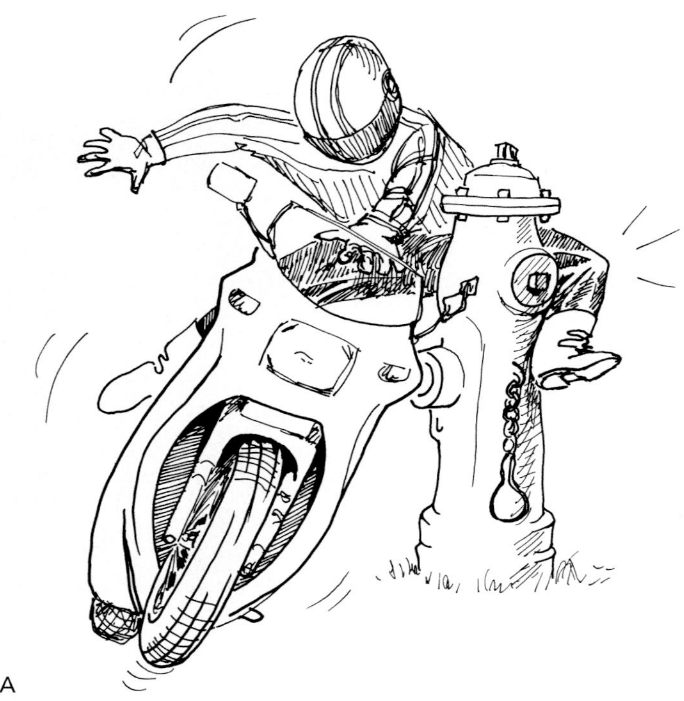
A

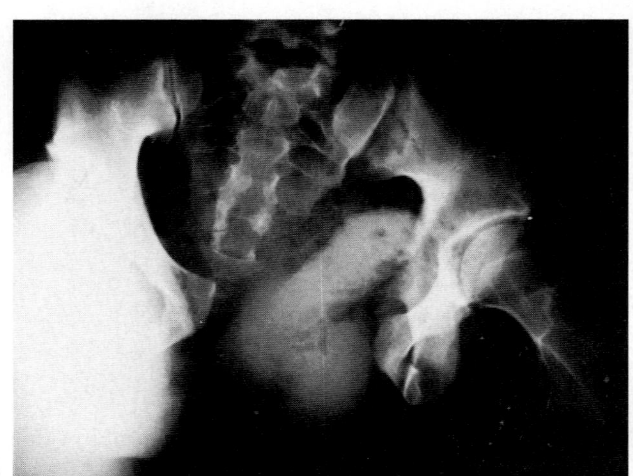
B

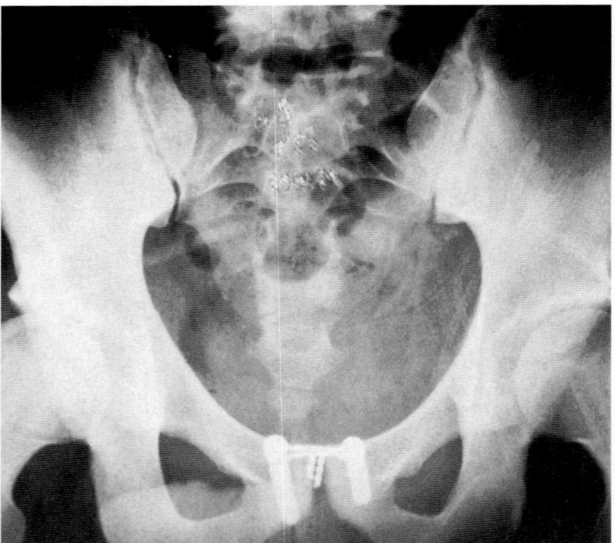
C

FIGURE 12-20. Unilateral injury Type B1. **A:** This injury is usually caused by a violent external rotation of one femur, for example the cyclist. **B,C:** The anteroposterior radiograph shows marked external rotation and disruptions of the left hemipelvis in a skier who caught the tip of his ski in a protective net. Treatment consisted of stabilization of the symphysis, which restored stability to the pelvis. (Courtesy Dr. J. Schatzker.)

B3-1: Bilateral Injury

Type B3-1 is the classic open-book injury (Fig. 12-18A). Because of the pelvic floor disruption, visceral injuries are common (Fig. 12-18B), in spite of the relative stability of the pelvic ring. To be classified as a B3-1 injury, no posterior or vertical displacement may be seen on the plain radiographs or CT. The posterior ligaments remain intact in this type (B3-1); therefore, relative vertical and posterior stability of the pelvic ring is maintained through the pelvis but is unstable in external rotation. Therefore, as noted in our treatment protocol, simply "closing the book"—closing the pelvic ring—reduces the fracture, which is restored to stability if maintained in that position (Fig. 12-18C).

Atypical Lesions

Variations of the open-book injury are common. As in the usual type, the symphysis pubis is disrupted anteriorly but the posterior lesion is a fracture of the ilium, either unilaterally or bilaterally, rather than an anterior disruption of the sacroiliac joints (Fig. 12-21A–C). Also, the anterior lesion may be rami fractures rather than a symphysis disruption (Fig. 12-21D,E). All fractures of the open-book variety maintain the integrity of the posterior pelvic complex. These variations are easily classified in the universal classification by using the modifiers.

The open-book injury is relatively uncommon. Symphysis disruptions >2.5 cm are more commonly associated with severe unstable Type C injuries, which may require much more aggressive treatment.

Therefore, *a word of caution,* which also applies to other injury patterns, is in order. The forces of external rotation and shear may overcome the tensile strength of the posterior sacroiliac ligaments, thereby rupturing them and rendering the hemipelvis unstable (Fig. 12-22). These injuries should properly be classified as Type C *unstable shear injuries,* but the radiographs may be misleading. These are also the Young-Burgess Anterior/Posterior Compression Injury III. The physician must not be misled by the radiographs but be guided by the clinical assessment and more precise radiographic techniques, such as CT.

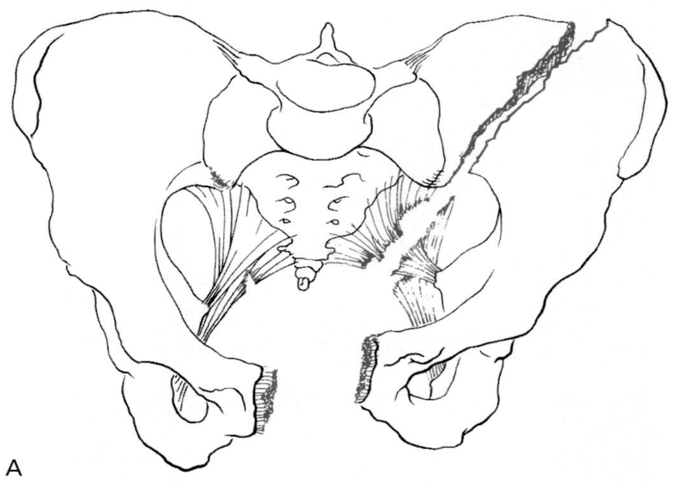

FIGURE 12-21. A: A common variation of the open-book injury. The right sacroiliac joint is open, whereas the injury on the left side is a fracture through the ilium. **B:** This injury is mirrored in the anteroposterior pelvic radiograph, clearly showing the open right sacroiliac joint and the fractured left ilium. **C:** Nineteen months after injury, the radiograph shows the fusion across the right sacroiliac joint and the healed fracture on the left.

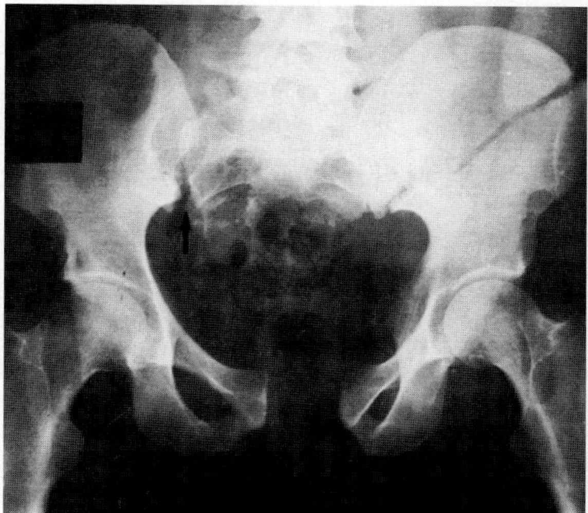

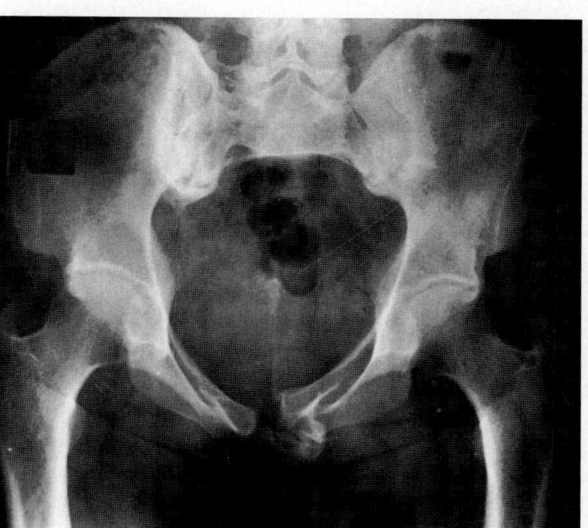

(Figure continues)

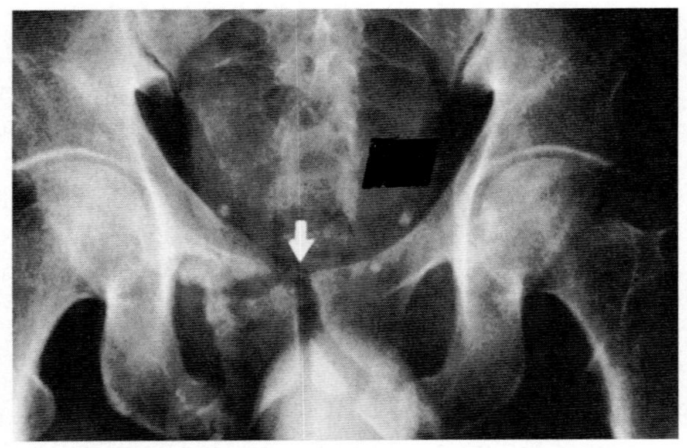

D

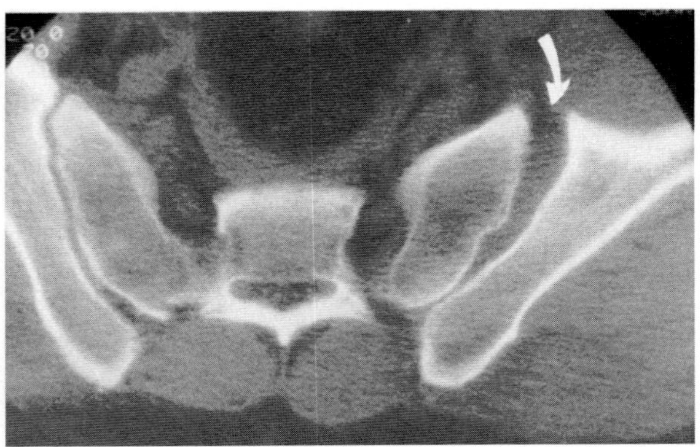

E

FIGURE 12-21. *(continued)* **D,E:** Another variation is noted in the anteroposterior radiograph and on computed tomography (CT). In this particular injury multiple fractures in the symphysis pubis are associated with the symphyseal disruption, but the CT clearly shows that this is an open-book (B1) type of injury *(white arrow).*

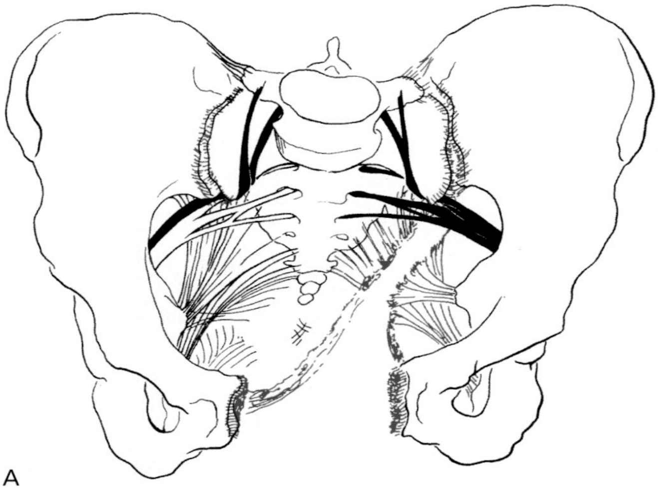

A

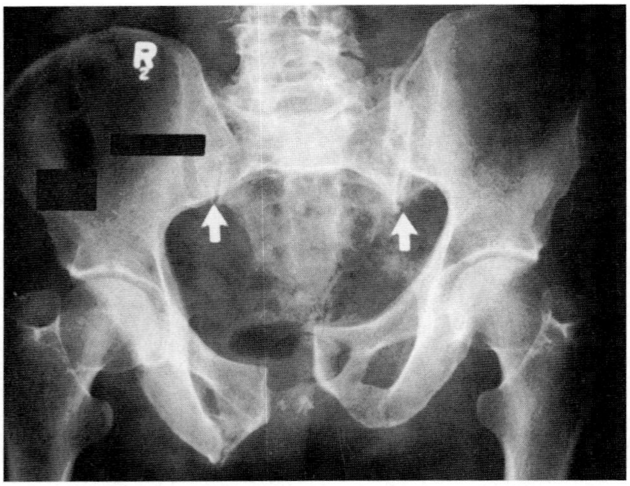

B

C

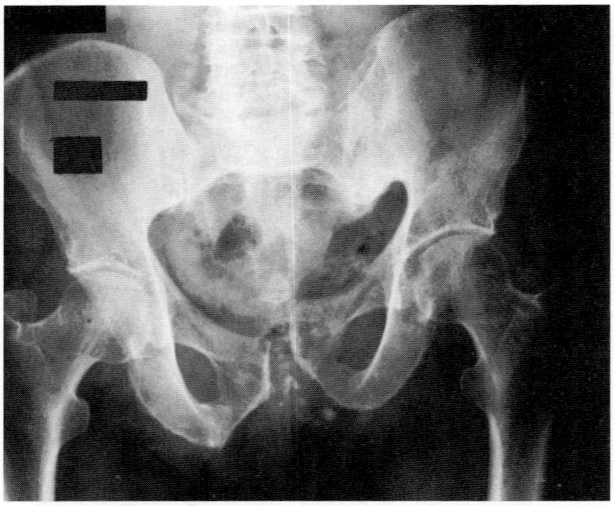

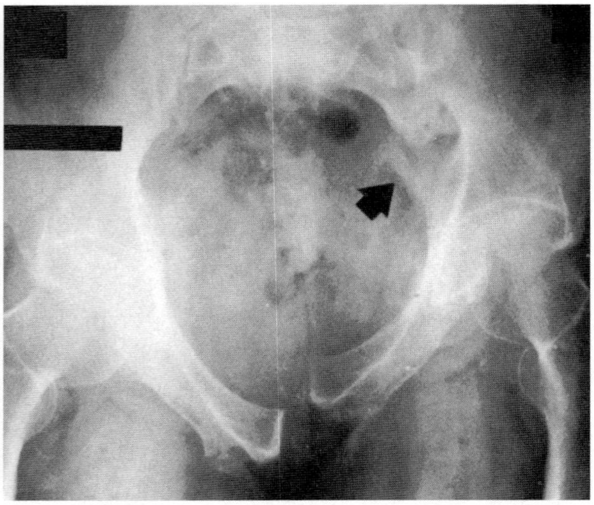

D

FIGURE 12-22. Continuation of the external rotation force that produced the open-book injury may cause disruption of the posterior sacroiliac ligaments. **A:** This renders the hemipelvis unstable. **B:** The anteroposterior pelvic radiograph shows the open right sacroiliac joint, but the left sacroiliac joint is not only open but also posteriorly displaced. **C:** Ten months later the left sacroiliac joint shows evidence of bony fusion. **D:** This is seen more clearly in the inlet view. On that view, calcification of the sacrospinous ligament on the left side is clearly noted *(black arrow).*

Symphysis Rupture in Obstetric Patients (see also Chapter 18)

Symphysis displacement is seen in obstetric patients. In some countries, division of the symphysis is performed for difficult labor, apparently with few long-term ill effects. Also, symphysis displacement of 2.5 cm may be seen in the postpartum period. In most cases, these women have no symptoms, and if they do, they usually disappear within 4 to 8 weeks postpartum.

Occasionally, an acute disruption of the symphysis occurs during a difficult delivery. In the example in Fig. 12-23, a loud crack was heard by the obstetrician and anesthetist. An immediate postpartum pelvic radiograph revealed a massive symphyseal disruption. With nonoperative symptomatic treatment, the pelvis returned to a normal state within 8 weeks. Because this lesion occurs when the patient is under the influence of relaxing hormones, surgical intervention is not indicated in the acute phase. Symptomatic nonoperative care usually results in a satisfactory outcome.

Rarely, symphyseal pain may continue for several months, and may become a chronic permanent disability that requires surgical intervention. Those resistant cases may be associated with an osteitis pubis or "false" joint formation at the symphysis. Treatment of these latter cases may be arthrodesis or (my preference) excision of the inflammatory tissue in the symphysis plus a small amount (1 cm) of bone. Similarly, in posttrauma cases, symptoms of anterior symphyseal pain may persist many months, requiring treatment similar to that already described.

B2: The Lateral Compression Injury

These injuries are characterized by unilateral partial disruption of the posterior arch maintaining vertical and posterior stability (internal rotational).

Lateral compressive forces cause the greatest number of fractures of the pelvis. Some of these injuries have been produced in the laboratory and others have clear clinical documentation. For example, one patient, a 35-year-old man, was standing sideways and was crushed by a truck. The radiograph clearly shows a standard lateral compression injury (Fig. 12-24). A lateral compressive force directed at the pelvic ring may cause two types of injury, one in which the anterior and posterior lesions are on the same side of the pelvis (ipsilateral) and one in which the displacement is on the opposite side (contralateral, bucket-handle) (Fig. 12-25; Table 12-3). Stability is maintained, because the lateral

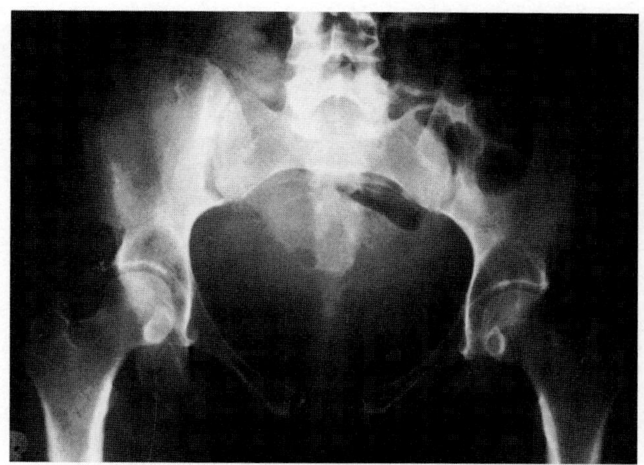
A

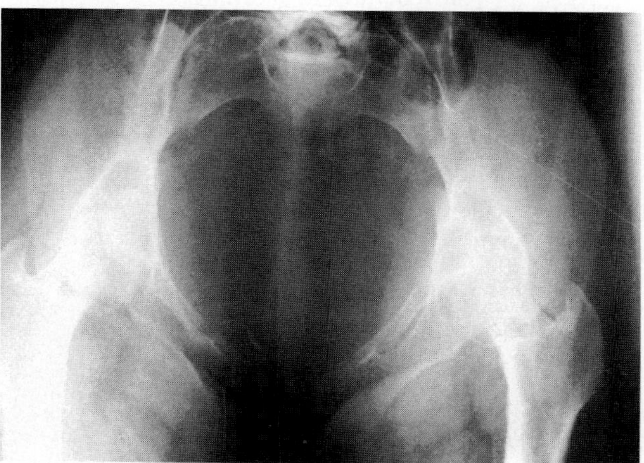
B

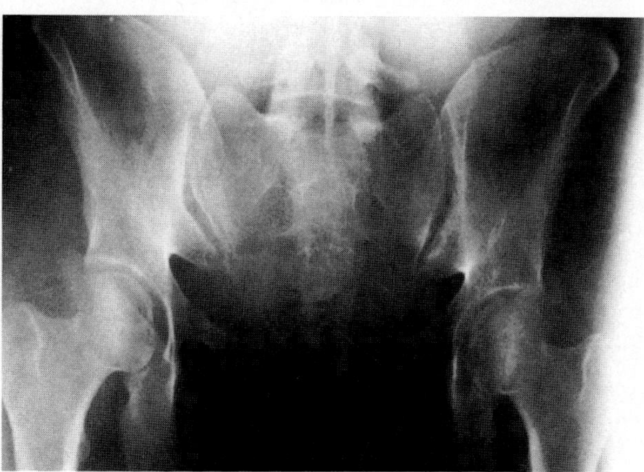
C

FIGURE 12-23. Acute disruption of the symphysis pubis during obstetric labor. **A:** Anteroposterior, **B:** inlet, and **C:** outlet radiographs of the pelvis show disruption of the symphysis pubis and anterior opening of the sacroiliac joints during a difficult labor. The patient, anesthetist, and obstetrician all heard a loud crack during the delivery.

(Figure continues)

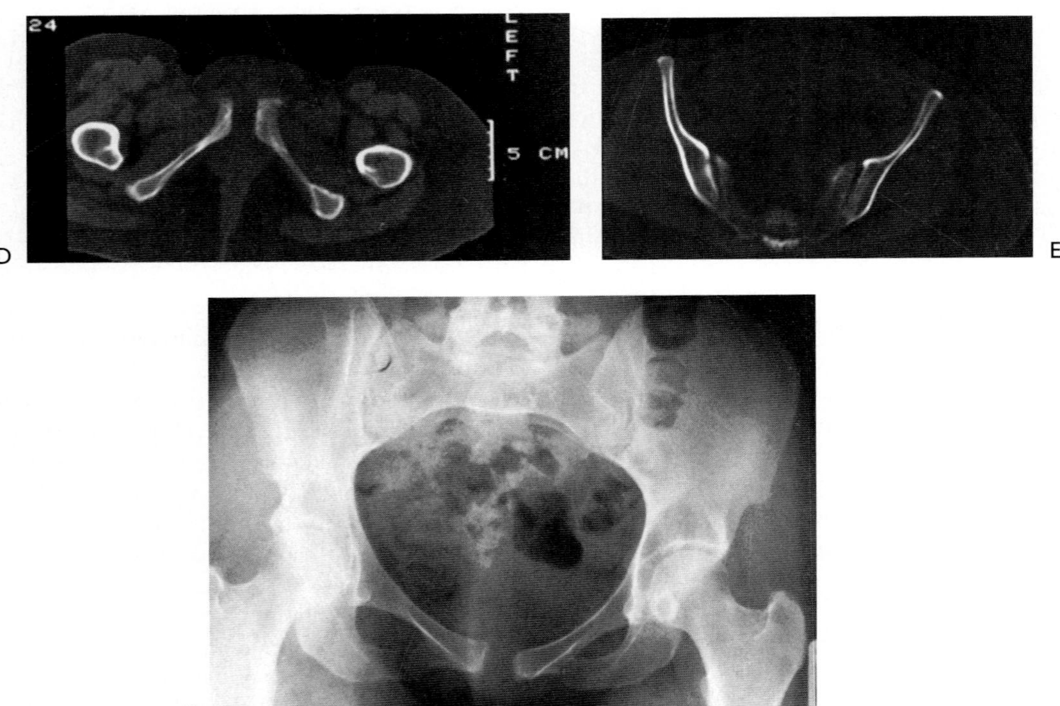

FIGURE 12-23. *(continued)* **D,E:** The lesion was confirmed on computed tomography. **F:** Nonoperative symptomatic care resulted in the symphysis stabilizing, albeit in a slightly widened position. (Courtesy Dr. S. Cartan.)

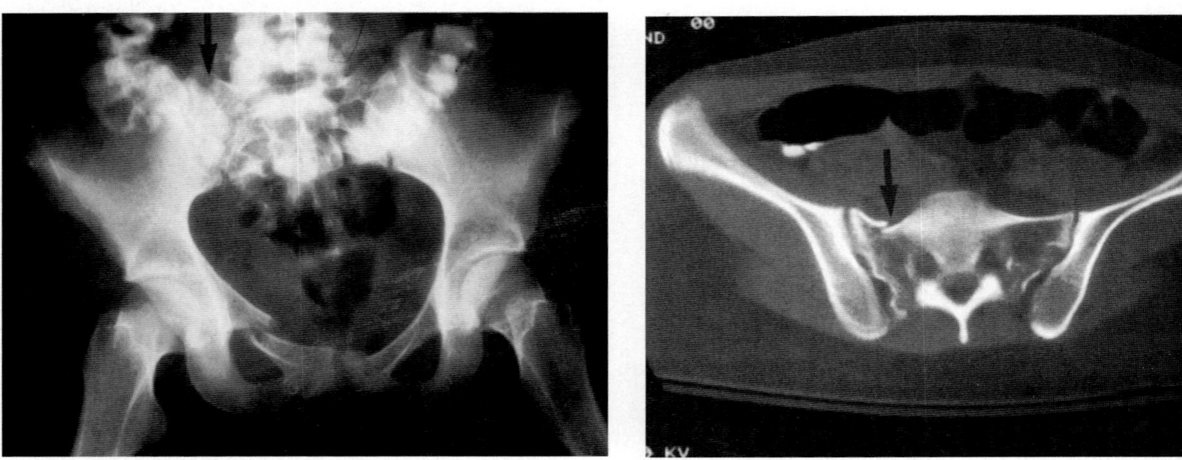

FIGURE 12-24. Typical lateral compression injury. **A:** The anteroposterior radiograph shows the fracture of the superior and inferior pubic rami with internal rotation of the right hemipelvis noted by the overlap of the superior ramus fracture. Note also the compression fracture on the left side of the symphysis pubis. This radiograph also shows a crush injury to the sacrum *(black arrow)*. **B:** The compressive nature of the sacral fracture is best seen on the computed tomography *(black arrow)*. Note how the anterior surface of the sacrum is crushed by 0.5 cm compared to the normal left side.

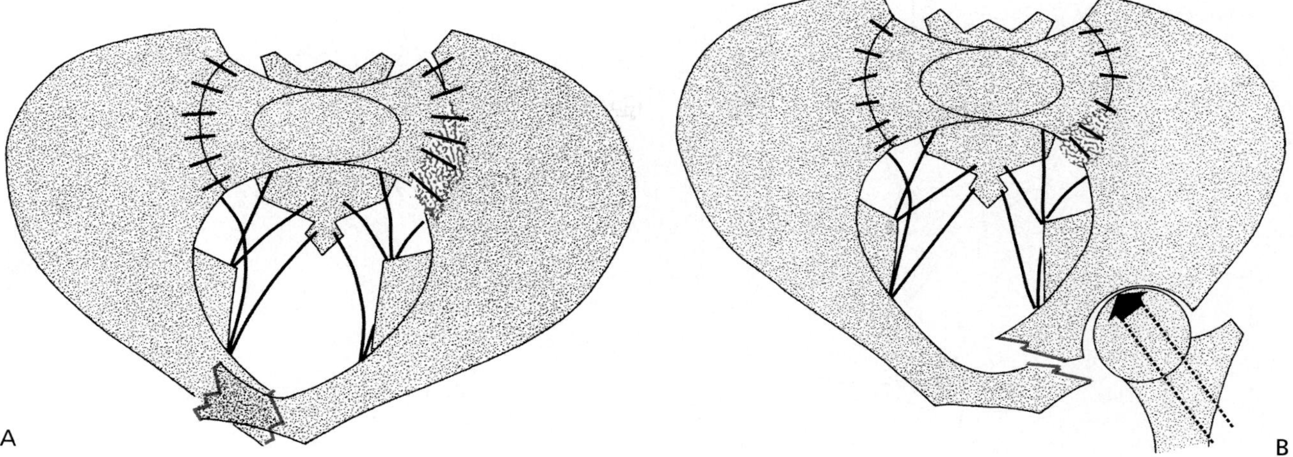

FIGURE 12-25. A lateral compressive force directed against the iliac crest causes the hemipelvis to rotate internally, producing a posterior compressive lesion to the sacrum and a lesion to the **(A)** contralateral **(B)** or ipsilateral anterior structures.

compressive force, by its very nature, causes impaction of the posterior pelvic complex, usually leaving the posterior ligaments intact. More important, the compressive force does not tear the muscles and ligaments of the pelvic floor; therefore, vertical or posterior stability is ensured. For that reason, especially in younger patients with strong sacral cancellous bone, even if the lateral compressive force disrupts the posterior sacroiliac ligaments, the intact pelvic floor prevents vertical and posterior displacement of the hemipelvis.

Any of the lateral compression fracture types may have a combination of posterior crush injury and ligament damage. This is very similar to the situation in the tibial plateau fracture, because older patients with poor cancellous bone may have a crush of the lateral tibial plateau from a valgus force, whereas younger ones with strong cancellous bone may have a minimal crush and major medial ligament disruption. The same is true when lateral compressive forces are applied to the pelvis. The posterior complex may be impacted in the displaced position with intact posterior sacroiliac ligaments or may sustain a minor posterior crush with major ligament damage (Fig. 12-26). Again, the emphasis must be on careful individual assessment of the specific injury. Biomechanically (9), several types of anterior and posterior lesions may be produced, and most have a clinical counterpart.

TABLE 12-3. TYPE B2: LATERAL COMPRESSION INJURIES

B2-1	Ipsilateral Anterior and posterior injury
B2-2	Contralateral Anterior and posterior injury

Types of Lesions

Anterior. The anterior lesions produced by a lateral compression force include double rami fractures on the same side as the posterior injury, double rami fractures on the side opposite the posterior injury, four rami fractures, a locked symphysis, and a fracture of the superior ramus rotated through the symphysis (tilt fracture).

Posterior. The posterior lesions all have an element of compression to the sacroiliac complex and include anterior crush of the sacrum at the sacroiliac joint with an intact posterior tension band; an impacted, compressed, posterior complex, either through the sacrum or ilium, with intact posterior ligaments; and an impacted compressed posterior complex with disrupted posterior ligaments.

Pelvic Floor. The integrity of the pelvic floor muscles, fascia, and ligaments is maintained, although some parts of it may be penetrated by the rotating rami (Fig. 12-26).

A study of these fracture patterns reveals the typical types of lateral compression injuries.

B2-1: Ipsilateral Anterior and Posterior Injury

As the lateral compressive force is applied to the iliac crest, the affected hemipelvis is subjected to an inward rotational stress, causing an anterior lesion to the pelvic ring. Commonly, this lesion may be a fracture of the superior and inferior pubic rami, or less commonly a locked symphysis or tilt fracture. At the moment of impact, the pelvic rami may rotate and strike the opposite hemipelvis. As the force continues medially, the anterior sacrum is crushed, but the posterior sacroiliac ligaments may remain intact (Fig. 12-27A). Also, the integrity of the pelvic floor is maintained, preventing vertical and posterior migration of the

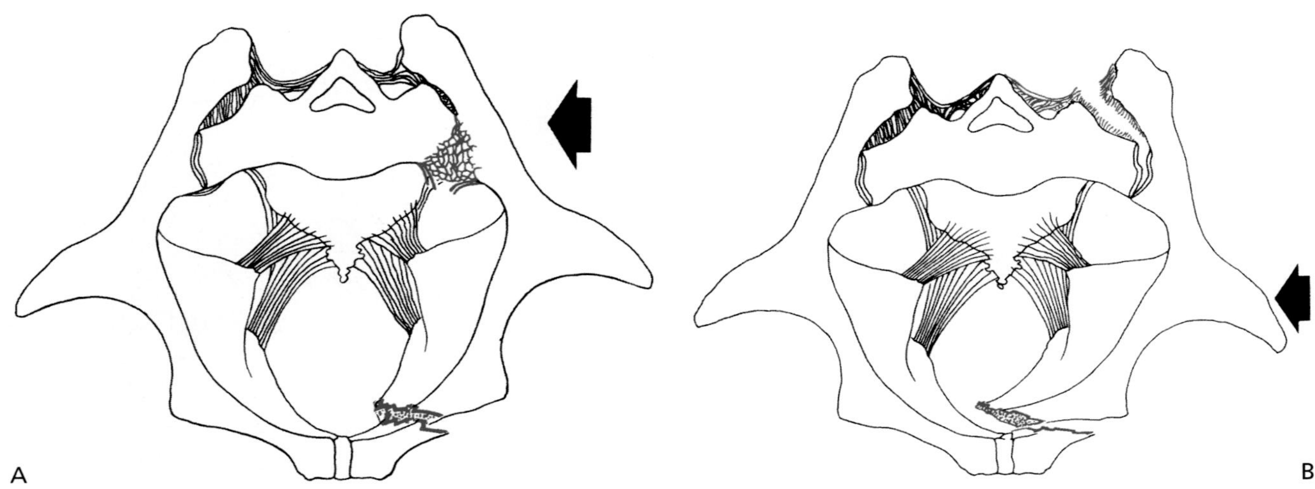

FIGURE 12-26. With all B2 lateral compression injuries the integrity of the pelvic floor is maintained except for penetration by the rotating rami. **A:** The pelvic floor is intact, as are the posterior ligamentous structures. **B:** In the diagram, the posterior ligamentous structures are ruptured, but vertical and posterior pelvic stability is maintained by the intact pelvic floor.

hemipelvis. This is a Young-Burgess Lateral Compression Injury I.

If the patient is nursed in the supine position, displacement is not common and usually not clinically relevant (Fig. 12-27B–E). The posterior lesion may be difficult to visualize, but it is always present. Only by erroneously reproducing this force during management, as with a pelvic sling, or nursing the patient on the side, may the original displacement be known (see Fig 13-13).

Therefore, although the intact posterior sacroiliac ligaments and pelvic floor confer an element of stability to the pelvic ring, the amount of original displacement of the ring may be greatly underestimated by the apparently innocent appearance of the fracture. Many apparently undisplaced fractures have caused rupture of the bladder. A most interesting example is the patient in Fig. 12-28, who sustained a seemingly undisplaced lateral compression injury to the pelvis, and yet had a ruptured bladder when seen in the emergency department (ED). A review of her cystogram revealed that the bladder had been caught in the fracture as it spontaneously reduced, indicating the amount of lateral displacement that was present, even in this apparently undisplaced fracture.

Locked Symphysis. Any of the lateral compression injuries may disrupt the symphysis anteriorly instead of fracturing the pubic rami. Although rare, this injury does occur. In Fig. 12-29, the patient, a fireman, fell 20 feet from a ladder onto his side. The overlapped symphysis remained locked, and closed manipulation under general anesthesia was required for reduction.

Tilt Fracture. The anterior lesion may be a fracture of the superior pubic ramus, often involving the anterior column of the acetabulum. As the lateral compressive force continues, the superior ramus rotates through the symphysis pubis, which ultimately ruptures through the symphysis, causing a tilt fracture (Fig. 12-30). The ramus assumes a vertical position in the most extreme cases. Distally at the symphysis, impingement may occur in the perineum or the inferior pubic ramus, causing the significant disability of dyspareunia in women. This fragment often requires open reduction because of its displacement.

B2-2: Contralateral (Bucket-Handle) Type

A different pattern is produced when the lateral compressive force is combined with a rotatory component, usually through the hip joint. The anterior lesion—either a symphysis disruption or a fracture of both or all four of the superior and inferior pubic rami—is associated with an injury to the posterior complex on the opposite side. The posterior complex usually is firmly impacted, and the posterior ligaments may be disrupted or intact (Fig. 12-31). As in all lateral compression types, vertical and posterior stability is maintained by a relatively intact pelvic floor. The resultant displacement of the hemipelvis is superior and medial rotation, like the handle of a bucket (Fig. 12-31). Clinically, the leg is often in the internally rotated, shortened position.

This fracture may cause clinically significant malrotation of the pelvic ring and considerable shortening of the affected limb. Therefore, these injuries, so common in young people, pose many management problems. This particular in-

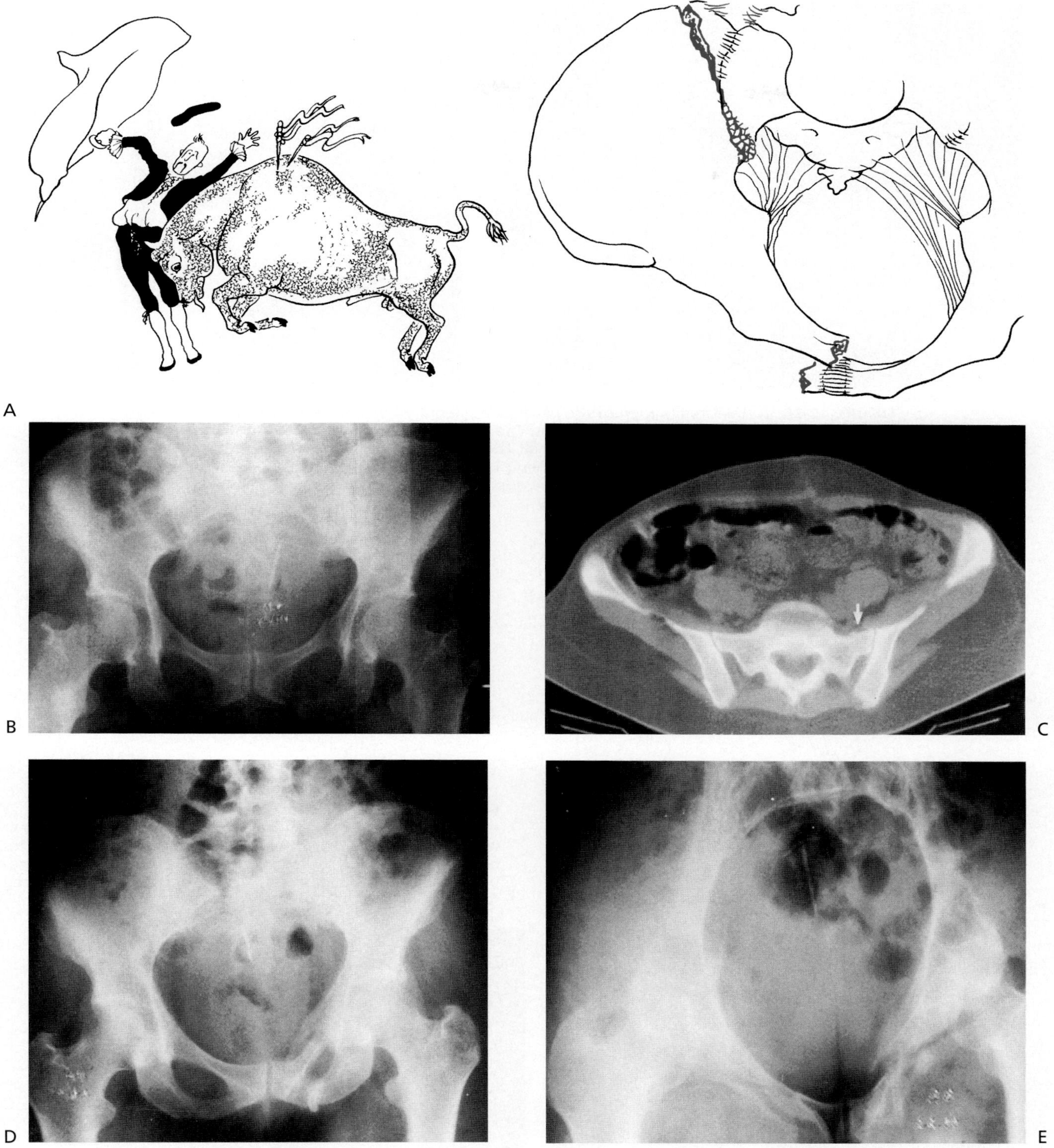

FIGURE 12-27. A: The diagram shows atypical ipsilateral type of lateral compression injury, showing a posterior injury and an anterior disruption of the pubic rami with rotation of the hemipelvis. Note the intact pelvic floor, which imparts relative stability to this pelvic ring injury. **B:** The anteroposterior radiograph shows lateral compression of the left hemipelvis with fractures of the superior and inferior pubic rami. **C:** The posterior lesion can be seen only on the computed tomography, the *white arrow* indicating the compressive nature of the sacral fracture. Nonoperative care resulted in excellent healing of the fracture, seen on **(D)** the anteroposterior radiograph and **(E)** the inlet view. A slight amount of internal rotation is of little consequence to the normal function of the patient.

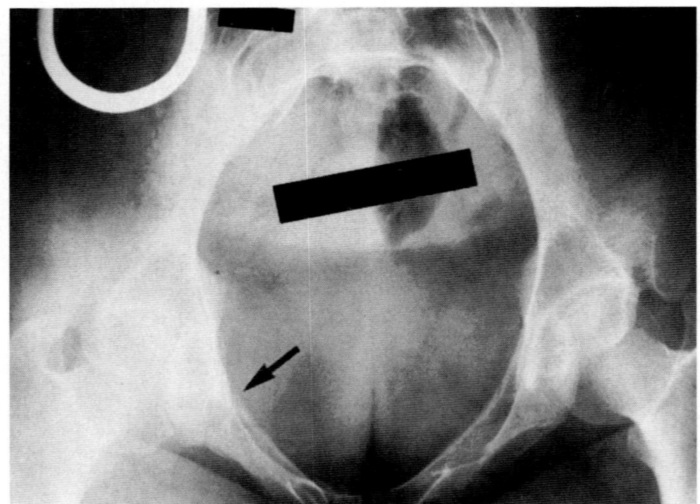

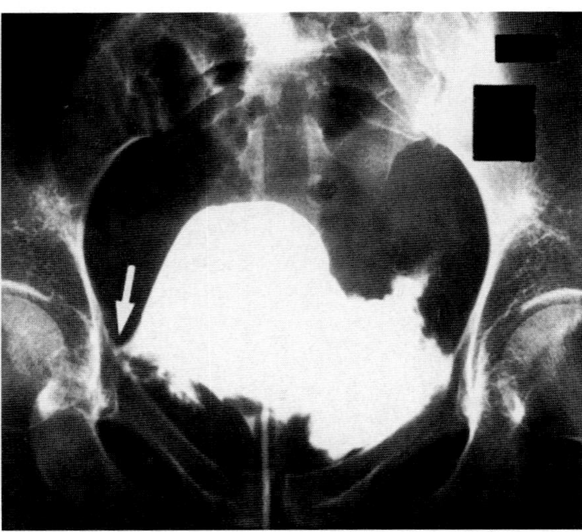

FIGURE 12-28. A: Inlet radiograph of the pelvis of a patient who sustained a seemingly undisplaced lateral compression injury to the pelvis. The fracture is barely perceptible *(black arrow)*. Clinically, this patient had a ruptured bladder. **B:** The cystogram shows that the bladder wall has been pulled into the fracture line as it spontaneously reduced following the injury. This indicates the amount of lateral displacement even in this apparently undisplaced fracture.

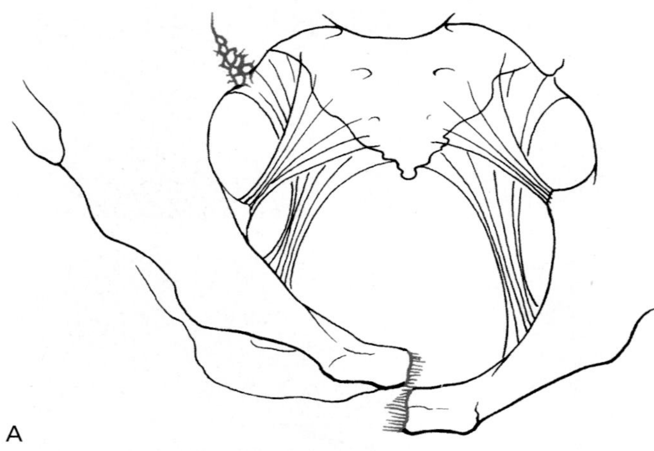

FIGURE 12-29. A: Drawing of a lateral compression injury that resulted in a locked symphysis pubis anteriorly. **B:** The patient was a fireman who fell 20 feet from a ladder directly onto his right side. The rigidly locked symphysis is seen on the **(B)** anteroposterior and **(C)** outlet views. General anesthesia was required for reduction of the dislocation.

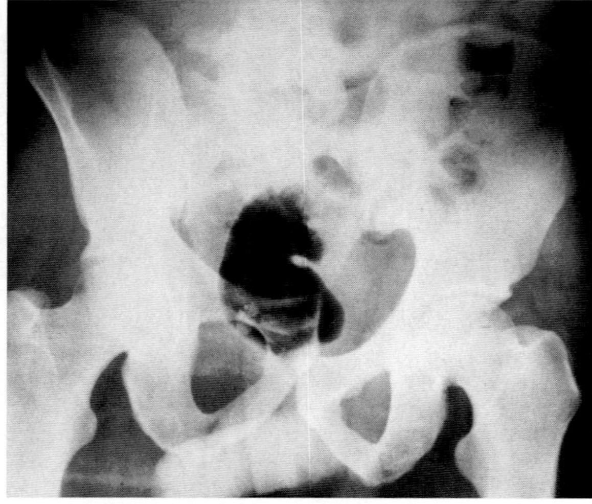

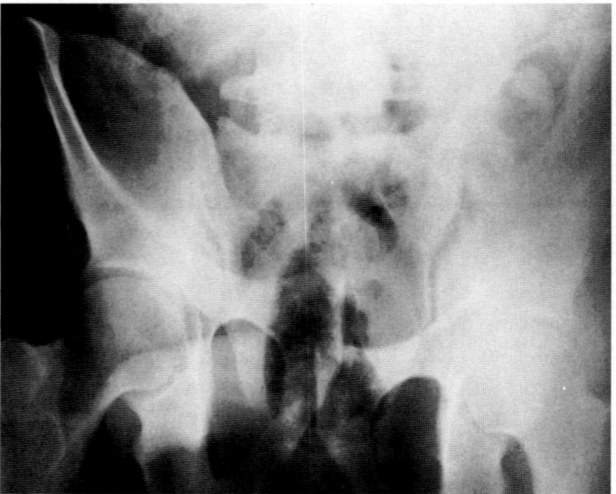

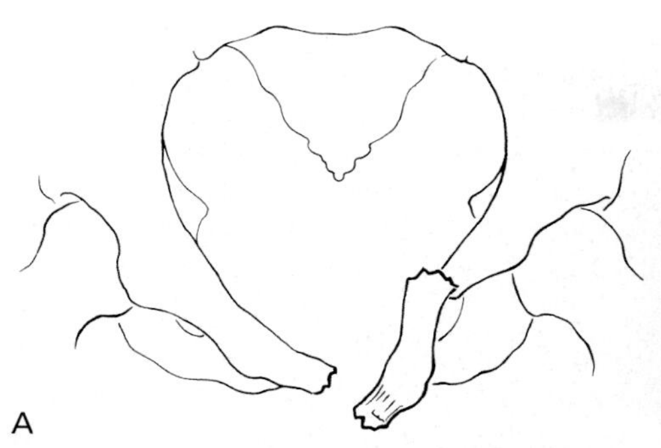

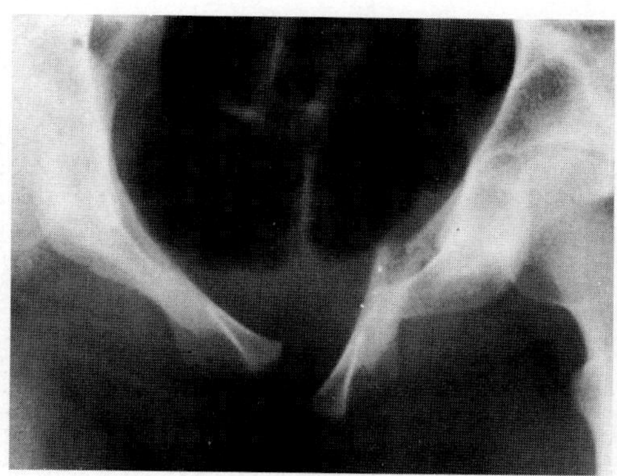

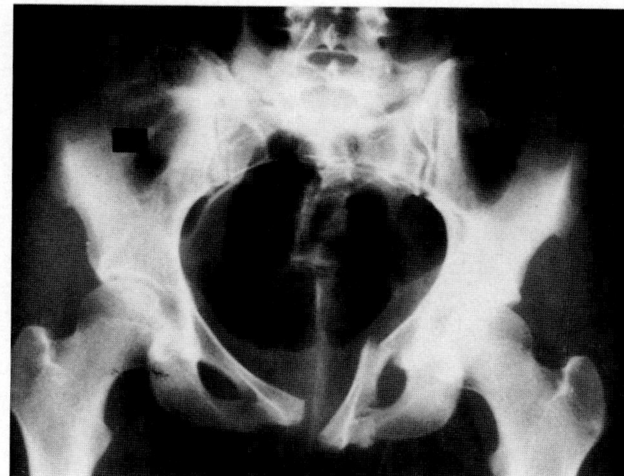

FIGURE 12-30. A: Diagram of a variant of the Type B2 injury, often seen in young women. The lateral compression force fractures the superior ramus, often through the anterior column of the acetabulum. Continuing lateral compression rotates the distal fragment through the symphysis pubis, thereby disrupting it. **B,C:** In most cases the distal fragment assumes a vertical position and may impinge on the perineum, as demonstrated in the radiographs, showing the typical displacement.

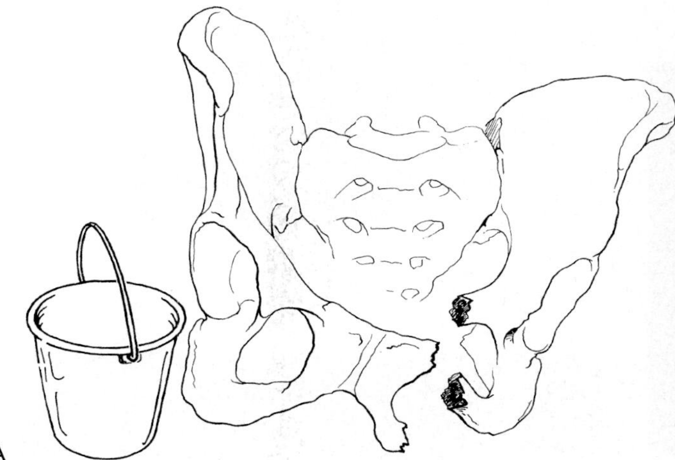

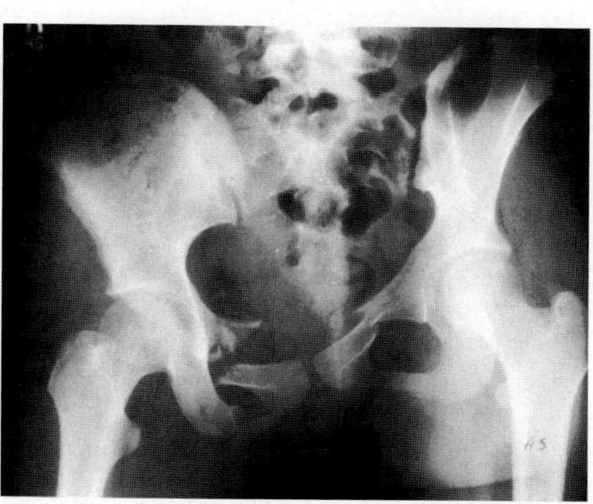

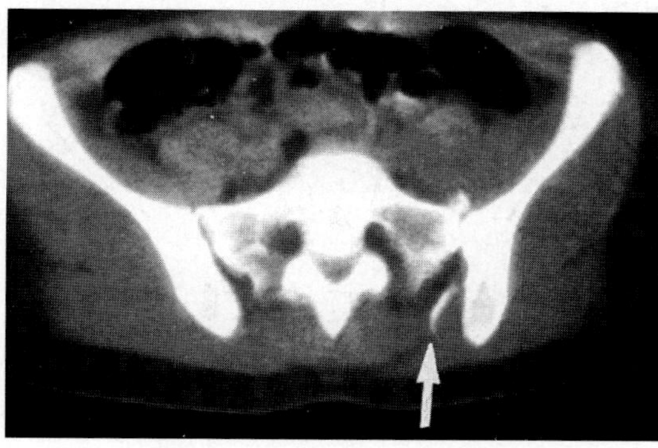

FIGURE 12-31. Type B2-2 contralateral bucket-handle type of lateral compression injury. **A:** The drawing shows the posterior injury to be on the side opposite the anterior rami fractures. Displacement is not only internal but also superior in rotation, like the handle of a bucket. **B:** A typical example is noted in the anteroposterior radiograph of a 16-year-old girl struck from the side in a motor vehicle. Note that the left hemipelvis is internally rotated, the superior rotation is noted by the superior position of the femoral head, also indicating leg length discrepancy. **C:** The lesion is more clearly seen on computed tomography, showing internal rotation of the left hemipelvis, anterior crush at the sacroiliac joint, and an avulsion of the posterior apophysis *(white arrow).*

jury was associated with the largest number of bowel, bladder, and major vessel injuries in the lateral compression group. Because it appears to be caused by more powerful forces, many of the patients exhibit severe impaction of the posterior complex. Displacement of the sacrogluteal line was the rule rather than the exception, but it was always <1 cm.

Clinically, the displacement is suspected by an internally rotated, shortened extremity. The affected posterior superior iliac spine often is elevated and displaced, so that a tender bony mass in that site is easily palpable. Impaction of the posterior cancellous complex is usual with continuing lateral compressive force. Stability of the pelvic ring is maintained in the unreduced position if impaction has occurred. In some cases, the continuing rotational force may cause disruption of the posterior ligaments. Even if the posterior ligaments are disrupted, the intact pelvic floor maintains vertical and posterior stability of the hemipelvis.

The maneuver of reducing an impacted fracture in this area is fraught with many hazards, including the possibility of further vessel and nerve damage. Unless gross leg length discrepancy and malrotation are present in a young person, it is more prudent to use the principle of "judicious neglect" and to allow the fracture to heal in the im-

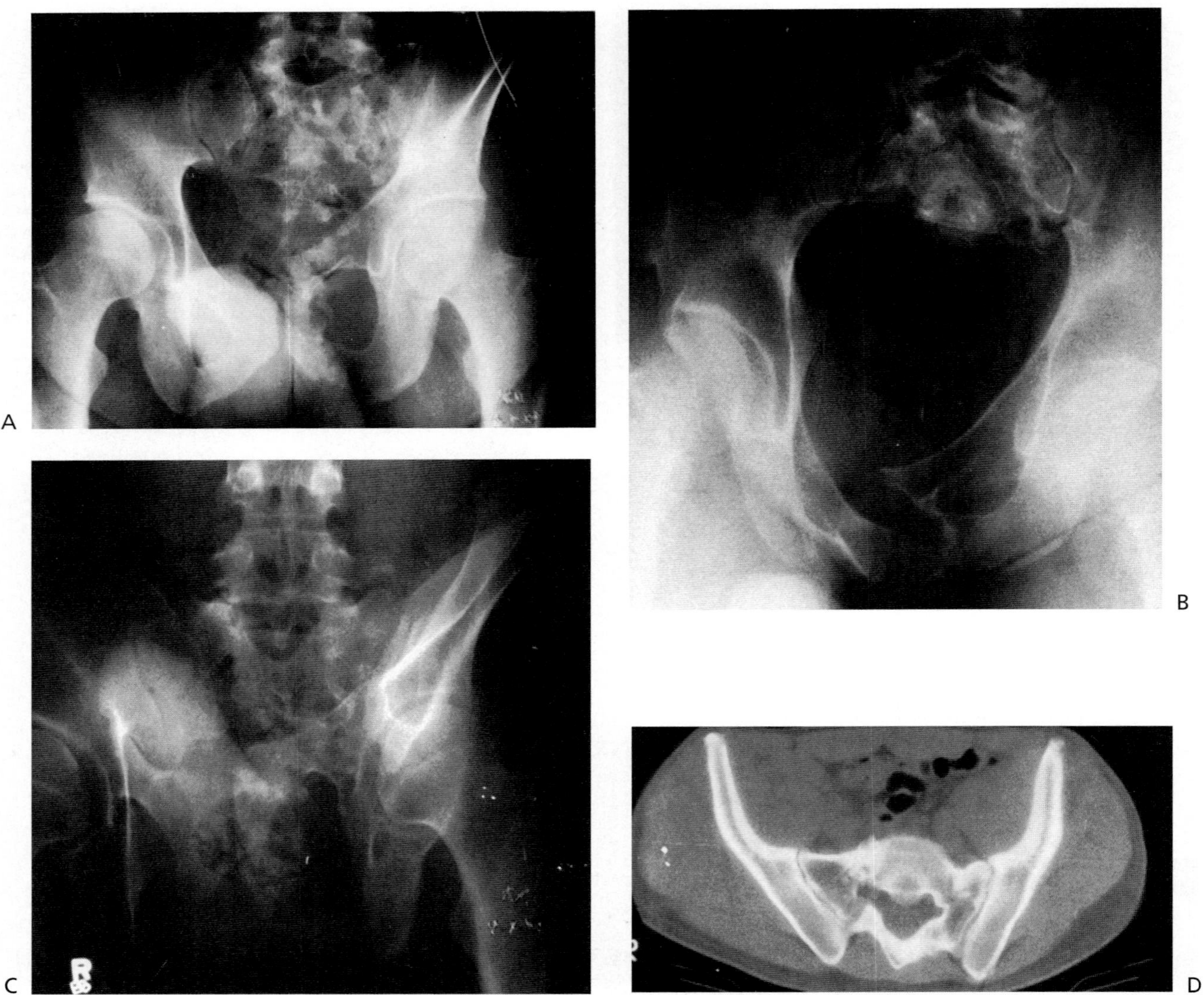

FIGURE 12-32. (A) Anteroposterior, **(B)** inlet, and **(C)** outlet radiographs of a 27-year-old man seen 6 months following lateral compression injury. **D:** Note the amount of internal rotation of the left hemipelvis on the three radiographs and especially on computed tomography. At that time, the sacral compression fracture was solidly united in the internally rotated position. Clinically, the patient had a prominence of the left posterior iliac spine, and minimal shortening of the left leg. He eventually regained full motion in his hip joint, which exceeded the internal rotation deformity. This allowed him to walk with minimal disability, and no secondary surgical intervention was necessary.

pacted position. The surgeon may be guided by the degree of hip joint rotation. If the rotation allows 20° to 30° of external rotation, nonoperative methods may suffice, but fixed internal rotation deformity should be corrected (Fig. 12-32). However, this fracture pattern also can lead to a progressive internal rotation deformity if not recognized and followed closely.

Young and Burgess describe a similar fracture pattern secondary to lateral force directed more anteriorly on the iliac crest. The injury, the Lateral Compression Injury II, is recognized by medial rotation and associated crushing of the anterior sacrum with either disruption of the posterior sacroiliac ligaments (LC-IIA) or a fracture through the iliac wing, the crescent fracture (LC-IIB).

B3: Bilateral B Type Injuries

Bilateral lesions may occur with both sides being vertically stable. The most common type of B3 injury is the open-book injury with posterior stability, the bilateral open-book injury with opening of the sacroiliac joints, disruption of the anterior sacroiliac ligaments and the pelvic floor and usually a disruption of the symphysis pubis. These lesions have been dealt with in the section on B1 open-book type injuries.

With lateral compressive forces bilateral B2 lesions are usual. Rarely, a B1 unilateral open-book injury on one side is associated with B2 lateral compression on the other side. This is described by Young-Burgess as the Lateral Compression Injury III or the windswept pelvis.

Type C: Unstable

The Type C unstable injury is a complete disruption of the posterior sacroiliac complex, involving vertical shear forces. This fracture, which can be unilateral or bilateral, is almost always caused by severe trauma such as falls from heights, crushing injuries, or motor vehicle accidents. The displacement indicates that the forces involved are usually in the vertical or posterior plane and therefore, of necessity, shearing in nature. By their very nature, these shearing forces cause massive disruption of the pelvic ring as well as the surrounding soft tissues (Fig. 12-33). The anterior lesion may disrupt the symphysis pubis, and/or two pubic rami or all four.

The pathognomonic feature of the Type C unstable injury is gross disruption of the posterior sacroiliac complex. Gross displacement and instability occur through the sacrum, sacroiliac joint, or ilium. Each of these lesions is distinctive, and they form the basis of the subgroups, iliac fractures Type C1-1, sacroiliac dislocation or fracture dislocation C1-2, and sacral fractures C1-3. Often, all of the tissues except the skin and subcutaneous tissues are torn, indicating extreme instability. In some cases, even the posterior skin is torn, thus completing the spectrum. This injury should be thought of almost as an internal hemipelvectomy. This is the Young-Burgess Anterior/Posterior Compression Injury III or vertical shear.

For the affected hemipelvis to be completely unstable, the sacrotuberous and sacrospinous ligaments, that is, the pelvic floor, must be torn (Fig. 12-33A). As well, the ante-

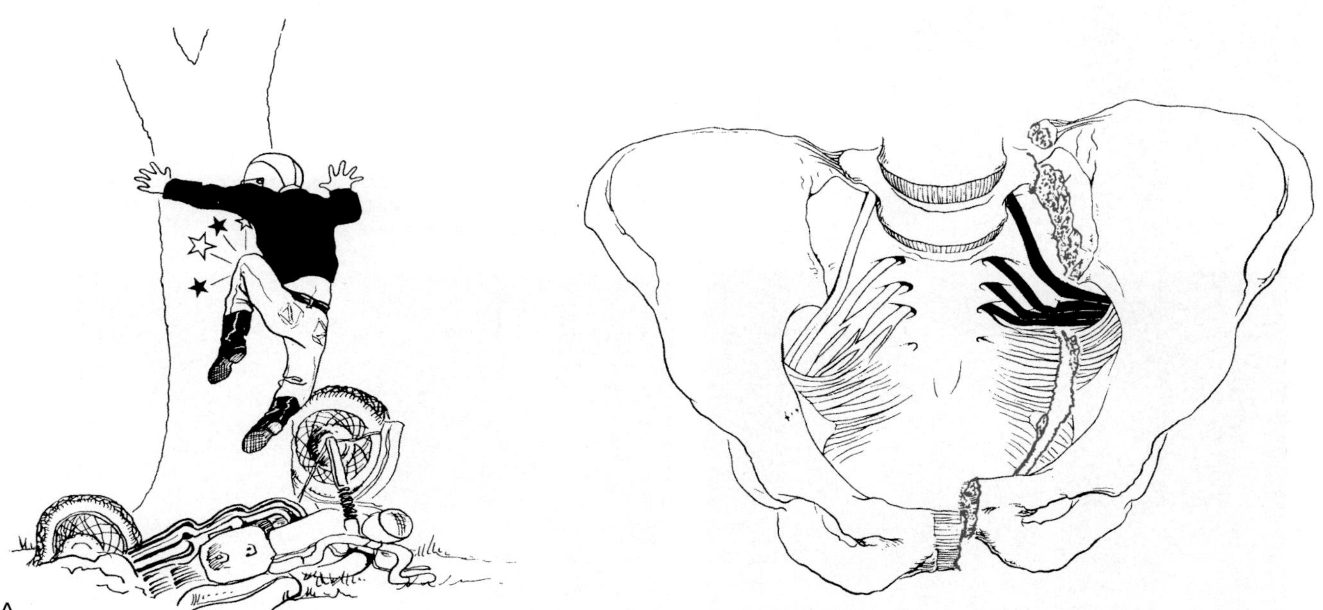

FIGURE 12-33. A: The drawing demonstrates a unilateral unstable (vertical shear, Malgaigne) fracture. The shearing forces cause massive disruption of the pelvic ring, including its soft-tissue contents and surroundings.

(Figure continues)

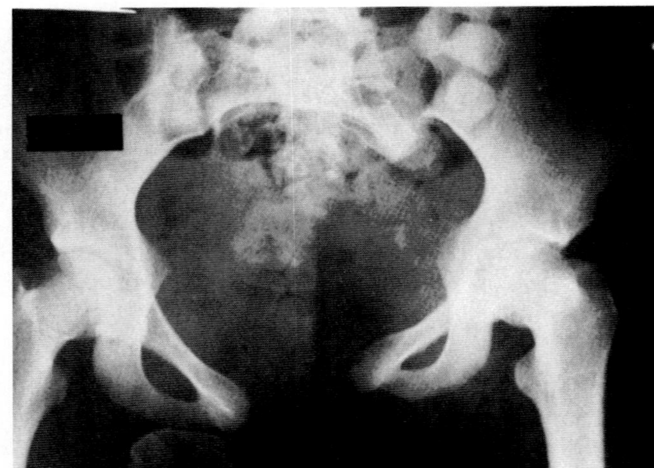

B

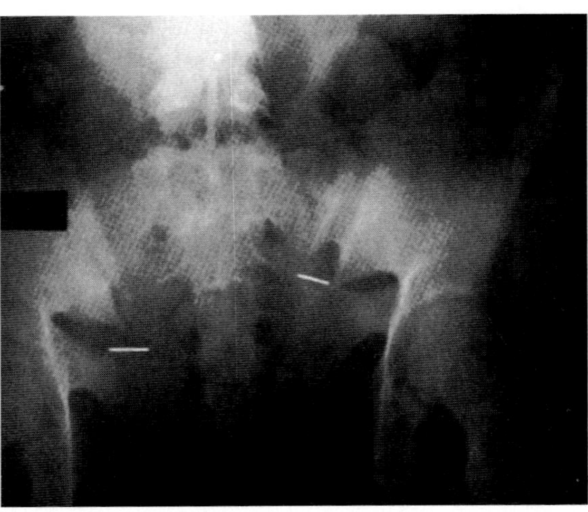

C

FIGURE 12-33. *(continued)* **B:** The inlet view of the pelvis shows the severe posterior displacement and total disruption of the soft tissues on the left side, indicated by the avulsion of the ischial spine. **C:** The outlet view indicates upward displacement anteriorly at the symphysis pubis, outlined by the *white lines.*

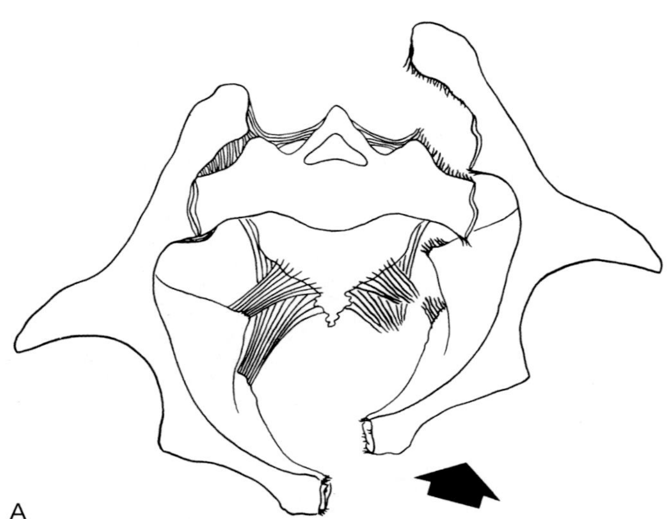

A

FIGURE 12-34. Type C-1. **A:** The diagram indicates a unilateral unstable left hemipelvis with disruption of posterior ligaments and pelvic floor. The posterior lesion is a sacroiliac dislocation. **B,C:** The anteroposterior radiograph and computed tomography show unilateral grossly unstable right hemipelvis, the posterior lesion being a sacral fracture.

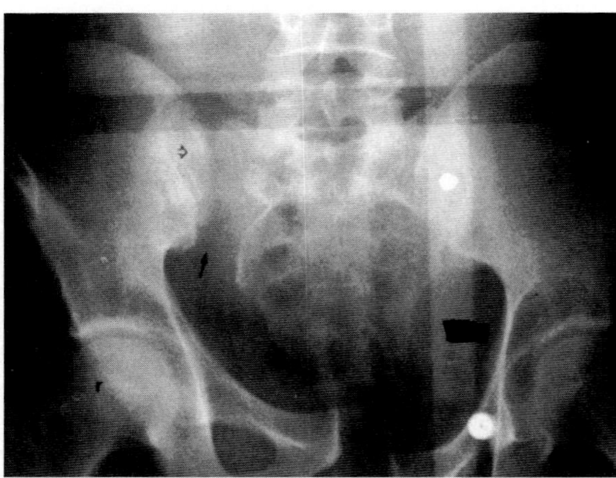

B

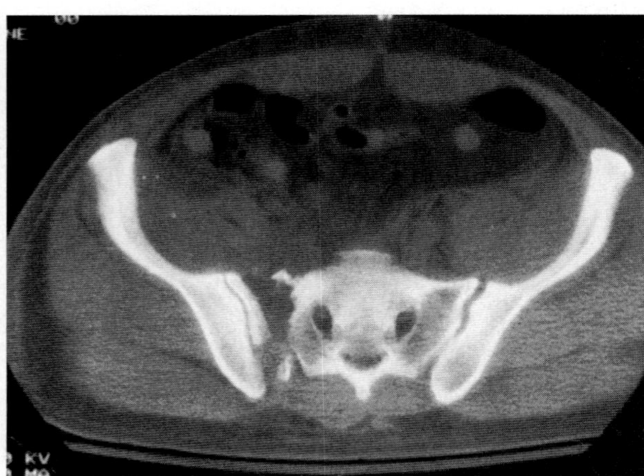

C

rior and posterior portions of the pelvic ring must be disrupted. Because the forces required to disrupt the strong pelvic ligaments are considerable, these same forces may also be expected to disrupt other vital pelvic and abdominal soft tissues. This injury, therefore, has the greatest number of associated injuries to the gastrointestinal, genitourinary, vascular, and nervous systems (9).

Because of the sinister specter raised by this fracture, "Beware the massive posterior pelvic disruption" should be the motto of all trauma surgeons, and immediate resuscitative measures instituted.

The posterior lesion may be unilateral Type C 1 (Fig. 12-34) or bilateral (Types C2 and C3; Fig. 12-35), the latter being *the most unstable* variety of pelvic disruption. Both the degree of instability and bilateral lesion have important implications for their management.

If one posterior complex is disrupted and the other intact, the disrupted hemipelvis may be stabilized against the intact hemipelvis by various forms of treatment modalities; however, if both hemipelvis are unstable, management becomes very difficult indeed. It must also be recognized that fixation of an unstable vertical shear fracture by an anterior external skeletal frame will not rigidly stabilize the posterior lesion. This unstable lesion must be diagnosed both clinically and radiologically. The clinical signs are gross instability on direct manual palpation and easy reduction of the hemipelvis with traction on the affected leg. In bilateral cases, each hemipelvis may be individually manipulated and may move independently of the other.

Plain radiographs and CT show disruption and displacement >1 cm, both anteriorly and posteriorly. Avulsions of the transverse process of L5 associated with a posterior gap in the sacroiliac complex or the ischial spine are definitive evidence of gross instability (Fig. 12-33A).

C1: Unilateral

See Fig. 12-36.

C1-1: Fractures of the Ilium

Fractures of the ilium are the least common and least troublesome of the posterior injuries (Fig. 12-2). Fractures usu-

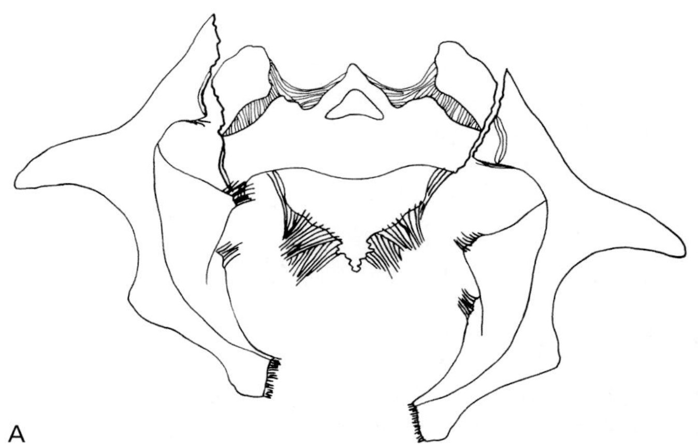

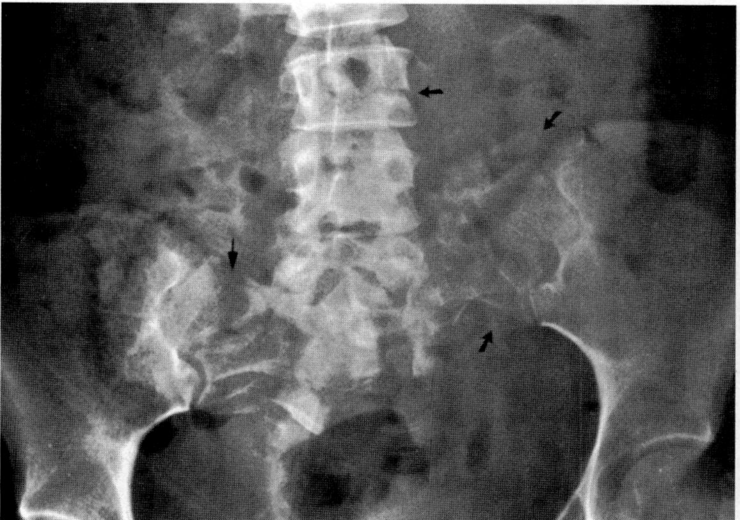

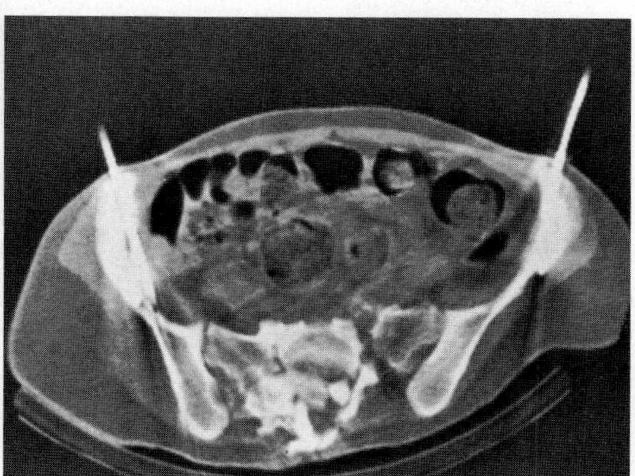

FIGURE 12-35. A: The diagram indicates a bilateral posterior lesion, a most unstable type of pelvic disruption and the most difficult to treat. **B:** The patient jumped from a bridge and sustained a severe disruption of the sacrum on the left side with gross posterior displacement and a lumbosacral plexus avulsion. The fracture of the opposite sacrum also is noted, as well as a fracture of the body of the L3 vertebra. **C:** Computed tomography of the same patient shows the marked displacement of the left sacral fracture.

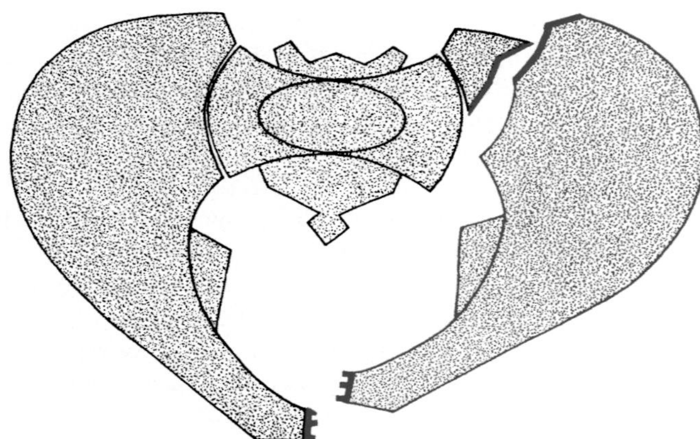

FIGURE 12-36. Type C1: unilateral unstable injury of the hemipelvis. This drawing shows symphysis disruption and sacroiliac fracture dislocation.

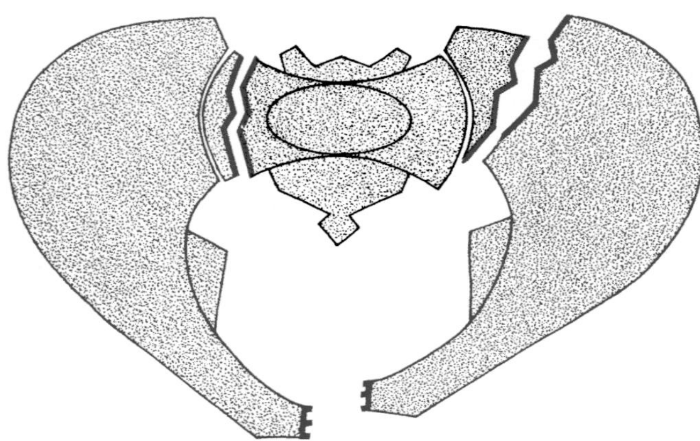

FIGURE 12-37. Type C2: bilateral injury to the pelvic ring in which one side is partially stable Type B injury, in this drawing a sacral fracture, and the opposite an unstable C injury, in this case an iliac fracture.

ally begin at the inferior aspect of the sacroiliac joint and run to the iliac crest posteriorly. In this pure lesion, the sacroiliac joint is intact. Injuries to the nerves and vessels associated with a pure iliac fracture also are rare.

Therefore, the prognosis for this injury is generally good compared to unstable fractures of the sacrum because in sacral fractures nerve injury is common, whereas it is rare in iliac fractures.

C1-2: Sacroiliac Dislocation or Fracture Dislocation

Pure dislocations (C1-2a2) of the sacroiliac joint are associated with extreme violence (Fig. 12-3C,D). Because the sacroiliac ligaments are among the strongest in the human body, disruption usually is caused by severe shearing forces associated with external rotation. As the posterior superior iliac spine abuts on the back of the sacrum, the continuing external rotation force tears the ilium free from the sacrum.

Fracture dislocations through the sacroiliac joint are more common than pure dislocations, and also are usually caused by shearing forces. The most common fracture dislocation is a dislocation of the anterior aspect of the sacroiliac joint associated with a posterior iliac fracture (C1-2a1). In some instances the fracture is in the coronal plane. A fracture through the sacrum associated with a sacroiliac dislocation (C1-2a3) is less common. The ala of the sacrum is extremely strong, making this combination unlikely.

C1-3: Fractures of the Sacrum

The most common posterior Type C injury is the sacral fracture, again caused by shearing forces. Fractures of the sacrum (Fig. 12-4) may be of several types. The sacral fracture occurs most commonly through the sacral foramina (C1-3a2), the weakest point in the sacrum; however, fractures may occur lateral to the sacral foramina (C1-3a1), or medial to them (C1-3a3). The incidence of nerve injury increases as the fracture nears the midline. The incidence of nerve injury approaches 50% in unstable sacral fractures. These injuries are traction injuries with a very guarded prognosis.

Complex fractures of the sacrum are seen especially in patients who fall from a great height. In that particular high-energy injury a so-called H-type fracture may be seen; that is, two vertical fractures joined with a transverse fracture line. These are difficult to classify but usually fall into the bilateral category (Type C3) (Fig. 12-35).

Pure transverse fractures of the sacrum below the sacral gluteal line are not injuries of the pelvic ring, and are, therefore, Type A2 or A3 injuries.

C2: Bilateral, One Side Type B, The Other Side Type C

In this pattern one posterior lesion is partially unstable only; that is, it is either a B-1 open-book unilateral injury or a B-2 lateral compression injury. The opposite side is an un-

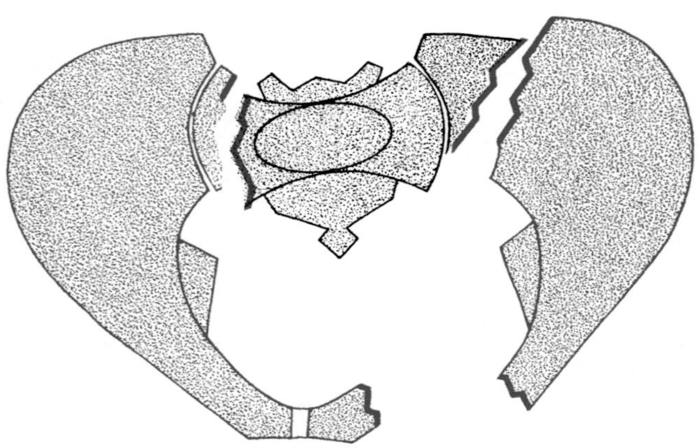

FIGURE 12-38. Type C3: a bilateral injury in which both hemipelves are unstable.

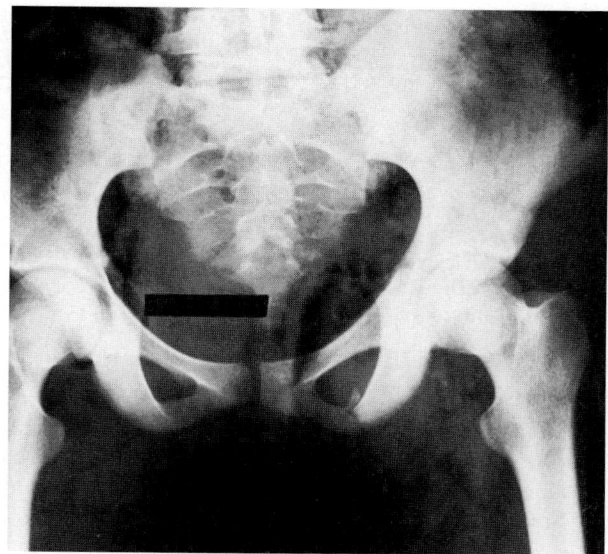

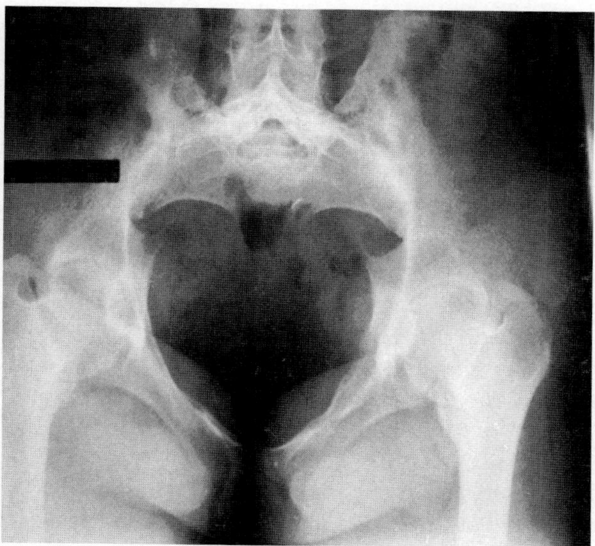

FIGURE 12-39. A: Radiograph of a 19-year-old woman demonstrates a bilateral sacroiliac dislocation with an insignificant anterior ramus injury. This unusual injury occurred while she was crushed by a horse (in the hyperflexed position). **B:** Four years later both sacroiliac joints have fused, as seen on the inlet view.

stable Type C lesion, through the ilium, the sacroiliac joint, or the sacrum (Fig. 12-37).

C3: Bilateral, Both Sides Type C

This pattern, always caused by high energy, produces the most unstable type of pelvic disruption and has the worst prognosis (Figs. 12-35 and 12-38). Each hemipelvis is a Type C unstable pattern; therefore, the entire pelvic floor is disrupted bilaterally. Visceral, nerve, and arterial injuries are common.

C3 Variant: Bilateral Sacroiliac Dislocations with an Intact Anterior Arch

This injury (Fig. 12-39), really a Type C3 variant, has been seen four times in our series, and I have consulted on two other cases. The lesion is caused by a force delivered to the sacrum when the patient is hyperflexed, forcing the complete sacral body into the pelvis. Radiologically, the anterior complex remained intact, but both sacroiliac joints were dislocated posteriorly. Clinically, the posterior deformity is evident, with posterior bruising, crepitus, and deformity. The hyperflexed attitude drives the sacroiliac posteriorly, whereas the flexed thigh seems to protect the anterior complex.

PELVIC RING DISRUPTION ASSOCIATED WITH ACETABULAR FRACTURE

Most displaced acetabular fractures, as will be noted in Chapter 24, have either an associated pelvic ring fracture or a disruption of the sacroiliac joint (Fig. 12-40). Many of the acetabular fractures also have associated pelvic ring disruptions on the contralateral side, indicating a lateral compression mechanism. CT has clarified these lesions considerably.

Each should be discussed as a separate entity because the prognosis depends more on the acetabular component than on the pelvic ring disruption. In the review of acetabular fractures by Pennal and colleagues (Pennal GF, Garside H, unpublished data) (11), a major acetabular fracture associated with a severe disruption of the pelvic ring had a poorer

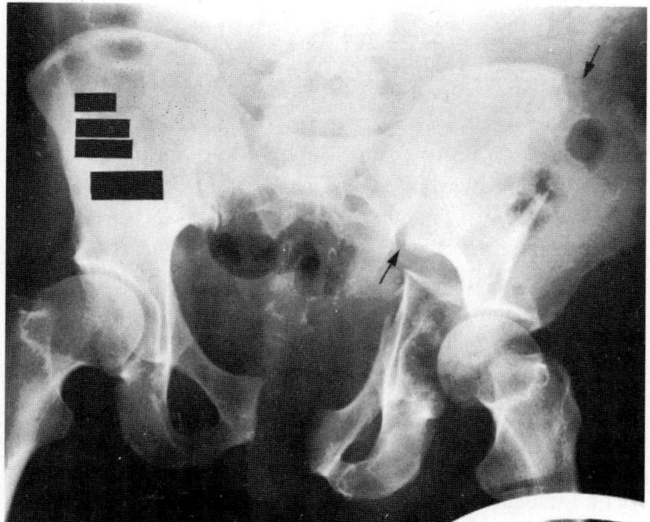

FIGURE 12-40. Anteroposterior pelvic radiograph indicates a severe left acetabular disruption associated with a pelvic ring disruption, characterized by avulsion of the symphysis pubis and an injury to the left sacroiliac joint and left ilium.

prognosis than many other types. These injuries should be classified as both acetabular and pelvic ring fractures.

CLINICAL RELEVANCE OF CLASSIFICATION TO SOFT-TISSUE INJURY

The classification just described is based on a concept of pelvic stability related to the direction of force causing the injury. It is based on the Müller-AO system of fracture classification, in which severity increases from Type A to Type C (5). It is clear that this classification, now widely accepted, is relevant to the management of the bone injury. Is it also relevant to the soft-tissue injury, and does it have some prognostic value?

This aspect has been addressed by several authors in the past decade, all of whom concluded that there was relevance and prognostic value in this classification. McCoy and colleagues, using a modification of this classification, examined pelvic fractures and correlated them to the type and extent of injury with both accident information obtained from examination of vehicles at the scene of accidents and injury information obtained from examination or resulting casualties (12). The CRASH (Calspan Reconstruction of Accident Speeds on the Highway) computer program composed by Henry and Lynch was used to determine the force of the crash. From the detailed dimensions of the vehicle deformation measured and deformation data known for standard vehicles, the program allowed calculation of the change of velocity (ΔV) at the moment of collision. The authors felt that the calculation was more relevant to injury causation than preaccident velocity. Of the 2,520 subjects studied, 49 (1.9%) had fractures and dislocations of the pelvis and hip. Of these, the ΔV could be calculated for 40. The authors found a definite relationship between the direction of impact and the pattern of pelvic injury. Posterior dislocation of the hip most frequently resulted from frontal impact, with or without associated fracture of the acetabulum. Serious additional injuries to the head, chest, and abdomen tended to be associated with high-energy frontal impact. When the ΔV was <15 mph pelvic injury was rare, but the incidence was >40% when the ΔV was >35 mph. Thus, these head-on collisions, which produce posterior dislocation of the hip and or shearing fractures of the pelvis (Type C), are associated with extremely high energy.

The pattern of injuries observed from side impacts was markedly different. The pelvic injury was usually a lateral compression type (Type B2) and was often associated with ipsilateral femoral or tibial fractures. Passenger compartment intrusion is much more common in the side crash; therefore, significant injury may occur with low-speed impact (Table 12-4). The authors conclude that there is a relation between force direction, magnitude of the force, and type of pelvic fracture. They also recommend that the possibility of injury in lateral compression could be reduced by strengthening the doors and side columns of motor vehicles.

TABLE 12-4. DISTRIBUTION OF INJURIES IN SIDE IMPACTS

	ΔV (mph)		
	<15	15–30	>30
Same side impacts			
Total pelvic fractures	3	7	2
Minor pelvic injury (ilium/pubic rami)	3	3	1
Major pelvic injury (bucket handle pelvis/"stove-in" pelvis)	—	4	1
Significant injury (AIS = 4) to			
Head	—	3	1
Chest	—	4	2
Contralateral side impacts			
Total pelvic fractures	1	1	3
Minor	1	1	1
Major	—	—	2
Fracture femur/tibia	—	1	—
Significant injury to . . .			
Head	—	—	2
Chest	—	—	1

Source: McCoy GF, Johnstone RA, and Kenright J. Biomechanical aspects of pelvic injuries in road traffic accidents. *J Orthop Trauma* 1989;3:118, with permission.

Wright and coworkers, studying a series of 98 pelvic fractures, found a direct correlation with the Injury Type and the Injury Severity Score, and subsequently the mortality rate of the patients (13). Completely unstable (Type C) injuries had an average Injury Severity Score of 36, as compared with 29 for the Types A and B, three times the mortality, and three times the amount of blood required (5.8 units as compared with 15.5 units).

Cryer and associates concluded that, with the amount of hemorrhage, abdominal injury, and pelvic arterial injury this pelvic fracture classification was highly predictive (14). They attempted further correlation to a single anteroposterior pelvic film in the ED and found a direct correlation.

Dalal and colleagues studying 343 polytrauma patients with major pelvic ring disruption, concluded that the mechanical force type and severity of the pelvic fracture (that is, unstable) are the keys to the expected organ injury pattern, resuscitation needs, and mortality (8). Their classification was a modification of the original Pennal and Sutherland and Tile modifications (1), and included anteroposterior compression, lateral compression, vertical shear, combined mechanical injuries, and acetabular fractures. Also, each of these types was graded according to severity (Table 12-5). Their final conclusion was that classification by mechanism is a key to the pattern of organ injury, resuscitation requirements, and outcome.

It would appear, therefore, that the literature supports a relationship between this classification based on force direction and stability and the outcome of the bone and soft-tissue injury and their sequelae. As indicated in the previous

TABLE 12-5. MECHANISMS OF INJURY PRODUCING PELVIC FRACTURE AND THEIR SEVERITY FRACTURE

	N	%	% Total
Lateral compression			
3	5	1.5	
2	22	6.4	41.4
1	115	33.5	
Anteroposterior compression			
3	27	7.9	
2	30	8.7	25.7
1	31	9.0	
Vertical shear	16	4.7	
Combined mechanism injury	34	9.9	
Acetabular fracture	63	18.4	
TOTAL	**343**	**100.0**	

Source: Dalal SA, et al. Pelvis fractures in multiple trauma: classification by mechanism is key to pattern of organ injury, resuscitative requirements, and outcome. *J Trauma* 1989;29:981, with permission.

section, pelvic injuries caused by external rotation or shearing forces caused disruption of soft tissues. In the open-book Type B1 injury, the external rotation force stops short of rendering the entire hemipelvis vertically unstable, whereas in the unstable Type C injury massive forces are reflected in a higher incidence of soft-tissue injury, namely hemorrhage and visceral damage (Fig. 12-33A).

In lateral compression injuries (Type B2) the main mass of the pelvic floor is not violated. Injuries to the viscera are caused by penetration by bone; for example, the internally rotating pubic rami may puncture the bladder. Nerve injury posteriorly may be produced by compression rather than traction.

Thus, a classification based on stability and force direction is relevant not only for the management of the bone injury but also for overall management of the patient. By definition, all Type A fractures have an intact stable pelvic ring; therefore, in general, treatment of the bony injury does not affect the general status of the patient. However, Type B and C fractures have either partial or complete instability. Specific management of the bone injury has a major effect on the patient's outcome.

CONCLUSION

This classification is presented to the practicing surgeon as a guide to management. When confronted with a severe pelvic disruption, the astute surgeon carefully defines the "personality" of the lesion.

The clinical signs of instability include obvious deformity of the pelvis of the lower extremity with leg length discrepancy. Direct palpation of the pelvis reveals abnormal motion, and traction to the uninjured extremity corrects the displacement in the markedly unstable pelvic ring disruption.

Radiographic evidence of instability includes posterior displacement of the sacrogluteal line >1 cm, marked disruption or gapping of the posterior complex on a plain radiograph or, especially, on CT, or avulsion of the ischial or sacral end of the sacrospinous ligament. Avulsion of the transverse process of L5 may also indicate instability of the hemipelvis, although in some cases the transverse process may be avulsed in the B2-type lateral compression injury. The presence of instability should alert physicians to the possibility of major associated injuries and the necessity for immediate action.

After general resuscitation, careful assessment of the "personality" of the injury suggests what type of injury is present (that is, whether it is stable, partially stable, or unstable) and the force that produced it. In turn, this should suggest the proper management for the musculoskeletal injury.

REFERENCES

1. Pennal GF, Sutherland GO. *Fractures of the pelvis* (motion picture). Park Ridge, IL: American Academy of Orthopaedic Surgeons Film Library, 1961.
2. Kellam JF, McMurtry RY, Paley D, et al. The unstable pelvic fracture: operative treatment. *Orthop Clin North Am* 1987;18:25.
3. Young JWR, Burgess AR. *Radiologic management of pelvic ring fractures.* Baltimore: Urban and Schwarzenberg, 1987:45.
4. Chenoweth DR, et al. A clinical and experimental investigation of occult injuries of the pelvic ring. *Injury* 1981;12:59.
5. Bucholz RW. The pathological anatomy of Malgaigne fracture-dislocation of the pelvis. *J Bone Joint Surg* 1981;63A:400.
6. Müller ME, Allgower M, Schneider R, et al. *Manual of internal fixation,* 3rd ed. Berlin: Springer-Verlag, 1990.
7. Helfet D, Tile M, Kellam J, et al. *Comprehensive classification of fractures: pelvic fractures.* Berne: Maurice E. Müller Foundation; Helfet D, Tile M, Kellam J, et al. Fractures and fracture compendium. *J Orthop Trauma* 1996;10(Suppl 1):66–69.
8. Dalal SA, Burgess AR, Siegel JH, et al. Pelvic fracture in multiple trauma: classification by mechanism is key to pattern of organ injury, resuscitative requirements, and outcome. *J Trauma* 1989; 29:981–1000.
9. Schopfer A, DiAngelo D, Hearn T, et al. Biomechanical comparison of methods of fixation of isolated osteotomies of the posterior acetabular column. *Int Orthop* 1994;18:96–101.
10. Tile M. Disruptions of the pelvic ring. In: *AO manual of internal fixation,* 3rd ed. Berlin: Springer-Verlag, 1990.
11. Pennal GF, et al. Results of treatment of acetabular fractures. *Clin Orthop* 1980;151:115.
12. McCoy GF, Johnstone RA, Kenwright J. Biomechanical aspects of pelvic injuries in road traffic accidents. *J Orthop Trauma* 1989;3:118.
13. Wright CS, et al. Preventable deaths in multiple trauma: a review of trauma unit mortalities—the Sunnybrook experience. *Can J Surg* 1983;26:20.
14. Cryer HM, Miller FB, Evers M. Pelvic fracture classification: correlation with hemorrhage. *J Trauma* 1988;28:973.

13

MANAGEMENT OF PELVIC RING INJURIES

MARVIN TILE

INTRODUCTION

Careful clinical and radiologic assessment should make the precise characteristics of a skeletal injury apparent to the surgeon. Other factors to consider are the expertise of the health care team and the desires and expectations of the patient. When clear alternatives to treatment exist, these should be outlined precisely to the patient, who should share in the management decision.

The principles of management of any skeletal injury depend on precise diagnosis. Each injury has a peculiar pattern, that is, its "personality" (Fig. 13-1); therefore, several methods of management may be used for what seem to be similar injuries.

Factors to be considered in determining the personality of the injury include not only the skeletal injury type but also the patient's profile. Of special significance is the age of the patient and his or her hemodynamic status. The principles of management of the skeletal injury are noted in the accompanying algorithm (Table 13-1), which should serve as a guide, and if followed should make management decisions more logical.

DECISION MAKING: HEMODYNAMIC AND FRACTURE STATUS

In the acute trauma management phase the patient's injury personality includes the hemodynamic status and pelvic fracture description, in particular the fracture's stability. Decisions in treatment at this stage may permanently compromise the surgeon's ability to achieve the best possible patient outcome with minimal complications. It is important to have a long-term surgical tactic in mind even in the early phases of care to avoid this compromise. The personality of the injury may be defined by the *patient's hemodynamic stability* associated with the *stability of the injury.* Four possible scenarios exist:

1. Stable hemodynamics and stable pelvic injury
2. Unstable hemodynamics and stable pelvic injury
3. Stable hemodynamics and unstable pelvic injury
4. Unstable hemodynamics and unstable pelvic injury

Each scenario has a specific plan to assure that the final outcome will be the best possible for the injury. In the patient who is *stable hemodynamically with a stable pelvic ring*

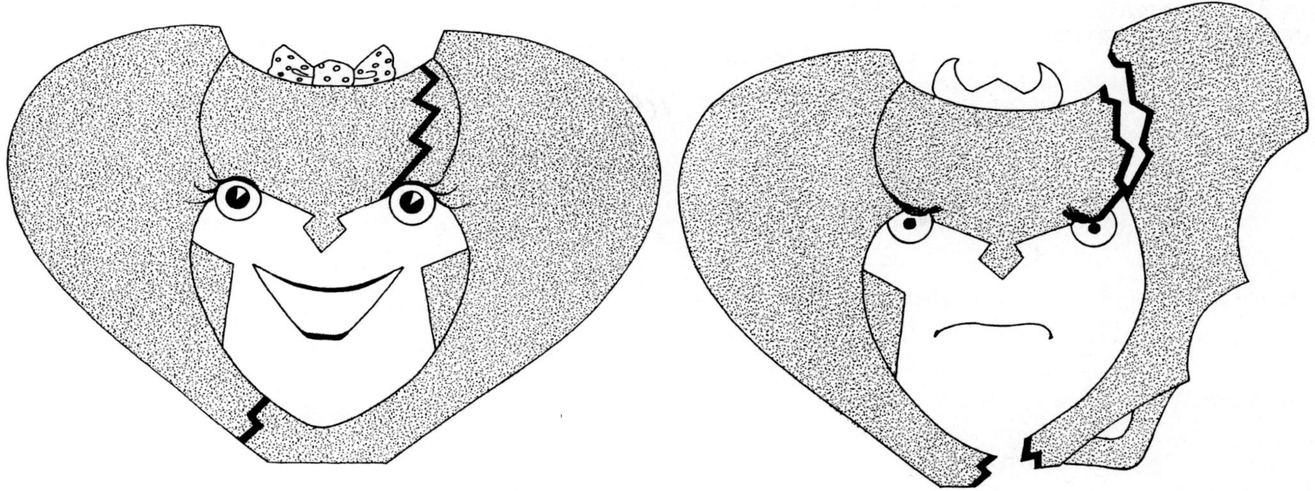

FIGURE 13-1. The management of any pelvic ring disruption depends on a clear evaluation of the personality of the disruption, including the type of fracture, the severity of the associated injuries, the general status of the patient, and the expertise of the health care team. The management and ultimate prognosis of the "good" personality types depicted on the left is vastly different from the "bad" personality on the right.

injury, the most important early decision is by the appropriate investigations, to assure that the injury is stable and has acceptable displacement. The plan is to mobilize the patient based on the symptoms. In the patient who is *hemodynamically unstable with a stable pelvic ring injury,* the priorities first rest with the saving of life. Because the pelvic ring injury is stable it requires no further concern until such time as the patient becomes hemodynamically stable. Once stable, further clinical examination and investigation will confirm that the injury is stable with acceptable displacement and can be treated nonoperatively with mobilization of the patient, depending on symptoms. Occasionally a stable injury is displaced to a degree that leaves the patient with an unacceptable deformity. In this case, an early closed reduction (within 5 to 7 days) and stabilization are indicated.

The patient who is *hemodynamically stable with an unstable pelvic ring injury* requires close observation for 24 to 48 hours to assure that no occult or late pelvic vascular bleeding occurs. The radiographic investigations must be completed as soon as possible and a decision made as to the next stage in care. A traction pin in the involved leg will reduce any translational displacement as well as maintain the reduction until surgery is available. It is imperative that any external fixator applied as a nondefinitive method be removed as soon as possible to minimize the chance of pin tract sepsis. Consultation with an orthopedic surgeon specializing in pelvic trauma must be done early so as to facilitate the care plan and not delay treatment. The *hemodynamically unstable patient with an unstable pelvic ring* is the most problematic injury for both the surgeon and patient. The first priority is the resuscitation and critical care management of the hemodynamically unstable patient. The treatment of unstable pelvic ring injury may be a part of the resuscitation procedure. This may involve the application of a noninvasive pelvic stabilization device along with a traction pin in the distal femur or proximal tibia and, when time permits, a conventional external fixator frame and embolization of the pelvic arterial vasculature if needed to stop the bleeding. The pelvis should be maintained in a reduced position so as to help the surgeon with the later reduction and definitive fixation. Once the patient is hemodynamically stable, the surgeon must be prepared to operatively reduce and stabilize the pelvic ring injury. The faster this can be done the less chance of pin tract sepsis affecting the patient with an external frame in place. If a delay is encountered it might be prudent to remove the pins and frame, maintaining the reduction through traction until surgery can be scheduled.

TYPE A: STABLE FRACTURES

Type A fractures are characterized by a completely stable pelvic ring. Type Al fractures are avulsion fractures that do not disturb the pelvic ring. Type A2 fractures involve either the iliac wing or the pubic rami without disturbing the pelvic ring's stability. Alternatively, they are ring fractures so minimally displaced that the soft-tissue envelope around the pelvic ring is undisturbed. Finally, Type A3 fractures involve the sacrum and coccyx distal to the sacrogluteal arch; thus, they have no effect on pelvic ring stability.

TABLE 13-1. MANAGEMENT PROTOCOL FOR PELVIC RING DISRUPTION

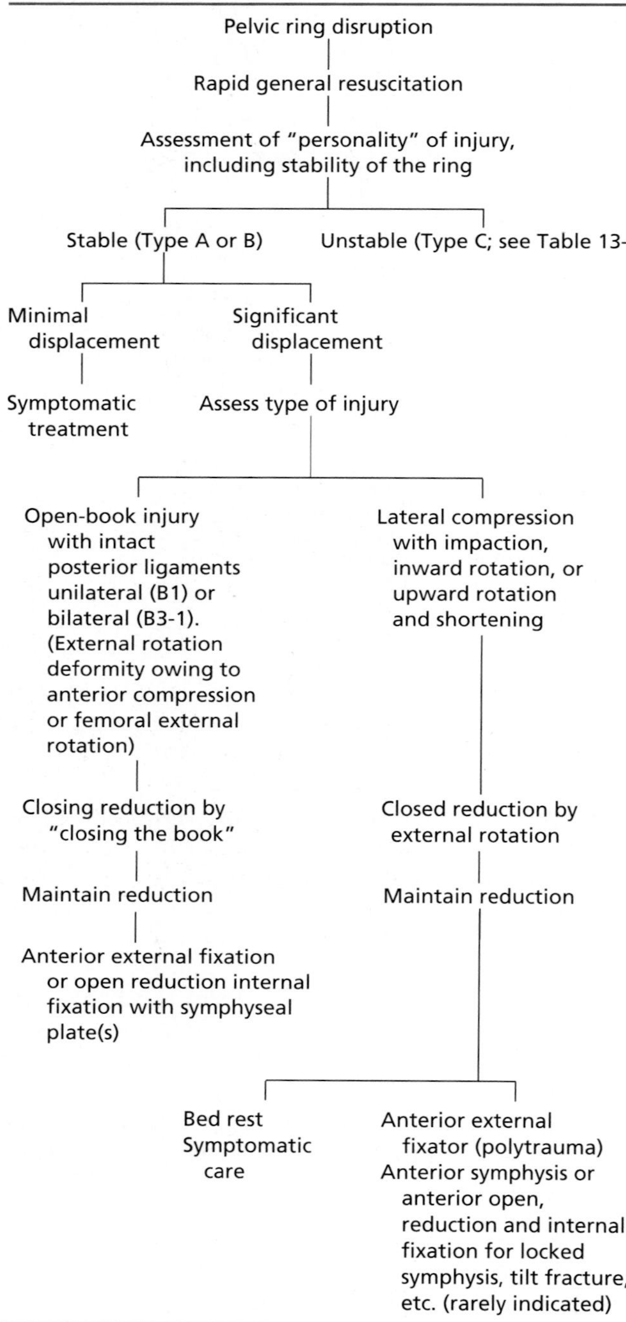

A1: Avulsion Fractures

Pelvic avulsion fractures typically occur in adolescents and represent avulsions of portions of the iliac apophysis. An avulsion may occur through the anterior superior spine (A1-1), the anterior inferior spine (A1-2), or the pubic spine (A1-3). Avulsions also may occur at the iliac crest (A1-2) or ischial tuberosity (A1-3). In adolescents, most can be managed nonoperatively with satisfactory results; however, each case must be determined on its own merit. If the avulsion is massive and the displacement great, open reduction and internal fixation restores function.

Less commonly, these avulsions may occur in the adult age group. Fractures of the anterior inferior spine represent an avulsion of the rectus femoris attachment. This injury is seen in sprinters and may affect their performances. Massive avulsions of the ischial tuberosity occur from contraction of the hamstrings against resistance. This may occur in water skiing, when the skier arises from the water. Again, each case needs to be examined on its own merit. If major displacement is noted, open reduction and internal fixation may be indicated. Otherwise, significant limitation of function, and even nonunion, may occur (see Fig. 12-13).

A2: Isolated Iliac Wing or Minimally Displaced Ring Fractures

A2-1: Isolated Iliac Wing Fractures

Isolated fractures of the iliac wing are relatively common. By definition, they do not involve the pelvic ring and are always caused by a direct blow to the iliac wing. Because the bony pelvis is surrounded by massive muscles—the iliacus medially and the gluteal muscles laterally—some displacements may be accepted; therefore, nonoperative treatment usually is indicated. On occasion these fractures produce major deformities along the iliac crest. If the displacement is major, then open reduction and internal fixation of the fragment may be recommended to maintain the function of the hip muscles and for cosmetic purposes (Fig. 13-2). In those circumstances the patient must be fully informed of the risks and benefits and must share in the decision. An open fracture must be debrided and stabilized internally to provide the contused skin and soft tissue with a stable framework to facilitate healing.

A2-2: Stable Undisplaced or Minimally Displaced Fractures of the Pelvic Ring

These fractures (Fig. 13-3) commonly occur in elderly persons with osteopenia. In this particular circumstance, the soft tissues around the pelvis are completely intact, the fracture is not displaced, and the patient can be treated symptomatically. If the fracture is isolated and not associated with other major system injuries, bed rest suffices until the patient is comfortable. Analgesia may be required for pain, which should be minimal in this situation. All of the aggressive measures necessary to prevent thromboembolic disease and the other complications of bed rest should be vigorously pursued, including frequent turning in bed and deep breathing exercises.

In young patients, seemingly stable minimally displaced fractures may be caused by high-energy insults. A careful physical examination must be performed to rule out *occult*

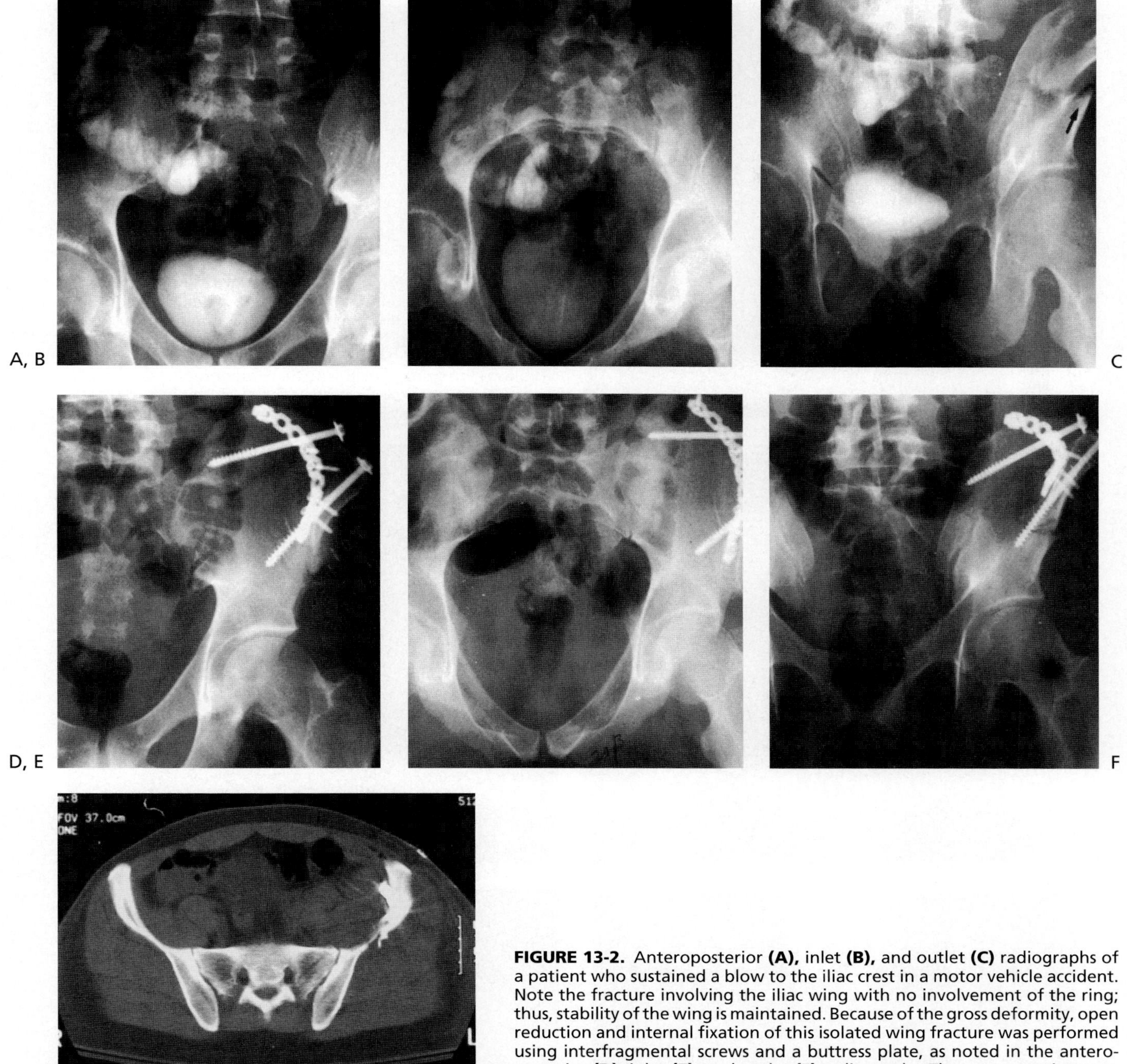

FIGURE 13-2. Anteroposterior **(A),** inlet **(B),** and outlet **(C)** radiographs of a patient who sustained a blow to the iliac crest in a motor vehicle accident. Note the fracture involving the iliac wing with no involvement of the ring; thus, stability of the wing is maintained. Because of the gross deformity, open reduction and internal fixation of this isolated wing fracture was performed using interfragmental screws and a buttress plate, as noted in the anteroposterior **(D),** inlet **(E),** and outlet **(F)** radiographs. The postoperative computed tomography shows the restoration of the anatomy of the ilium **(G).**

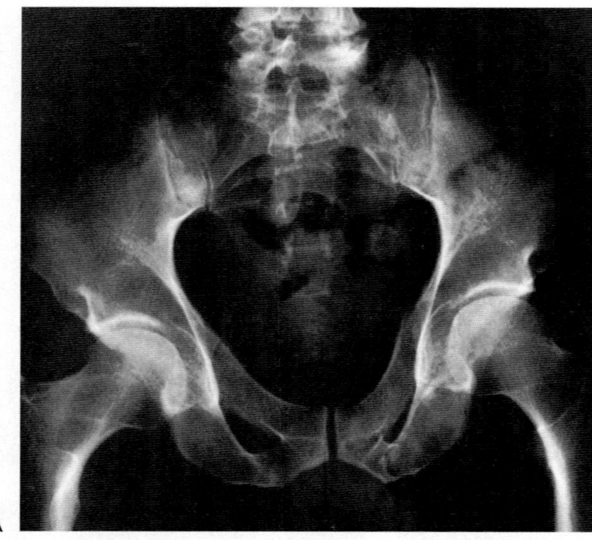

A

FIGURE 13-3. Anteroposterior **(A),** inlet **(B),** and outlet **(C)** views of a stable, minimally displaced pelvic disruption. In spite of the lack of displacement, all four pubic rami are fractured in this young male patient, so a major visceral injury must be suspected. **D:** Gross displacement of the bladder is visible on the cystogram. **E:** The final radiograph, taken 1 year after the injury, shows sound union with minimal displacement. The patient was asymptomatic at that time.

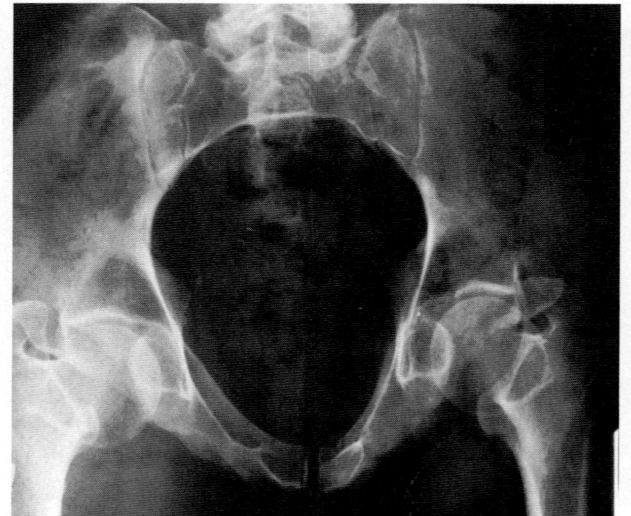

B

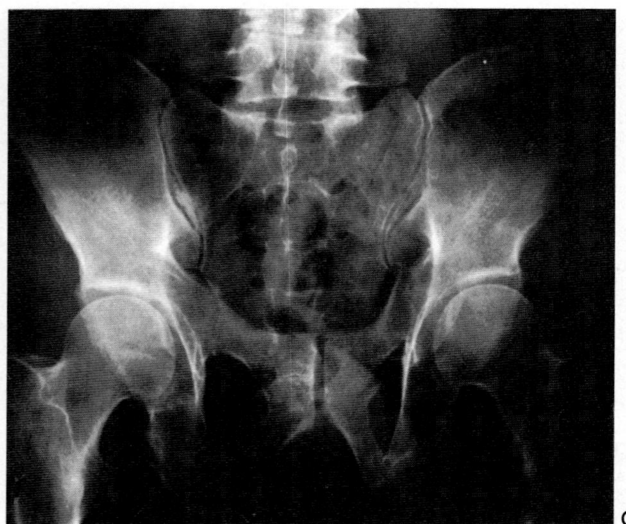

C

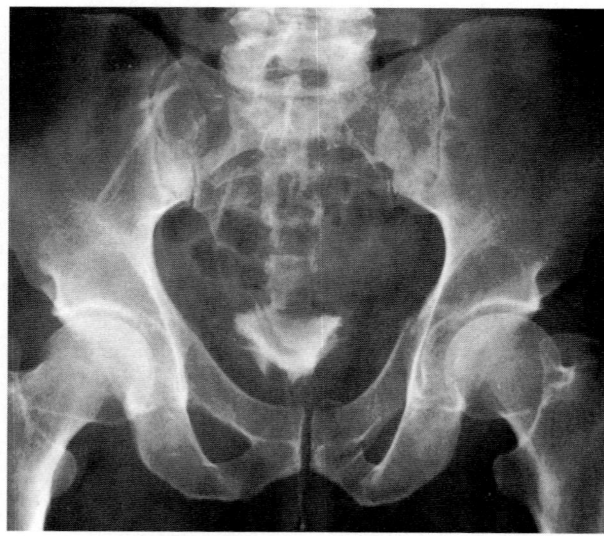

D

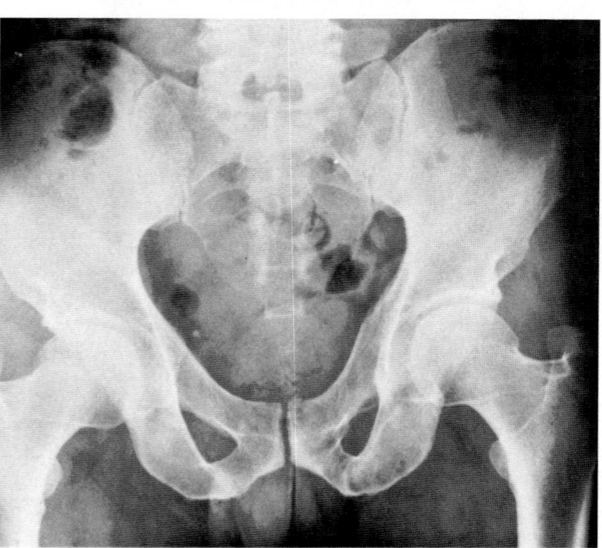

E

instability. If the pelvis is stable on careful physical examination (performed under image intensification if necessary), then nonoperative symptomatic treatment is indicated. Polytrauma patients often have major chest problems that require that they remain upright. Because these patients have minimally displaced and stable fractures, there is no contraindication to nursing them in that position; further displacement is unlikely.

A2-3: Isolated Anterior Ring Injuries

A so-called straddle or four-pillar injury anteriorly with no posterior involvement is rare and usually is caused by a direct blow anteriorly. If the pubic rami are in reasonable apposition, a good result may be expected from nonoperative treatment. The position does not need to be anatomic. Wide displacements through the pubic rami often result in nonunion, which can be disabling. In that circumstance, open reduction and internal fixation are indicated. A pubic ramus fracture also may be associated with a laceration to the femoral artery, vein, or nerve. It is advisable to internally fix the ramus at the same time if these structures are being repaired.

A3: Transverse Fractures of the Sacrum and Coccyx

These injuries do not affect pelvic ring stability because they are located distal to the pelvic ring.

A3-1: Coccygeal Fracture or Sacrococcygeal Dislocation

Type A3-1 fractures, which are common and are caused by falls, usually heal; although disability may be prolonged and may be related to nonunion in some cases.

A3-2: Undisplaced Transverse Sacral Fractures

Transverse fractures occur below the sacral gluteal arch; therefore, they do not affect the stability of the pelvic ring. Nonoperative treatment is recommended for minimal displacement.

A3-3: Displaced Transverse Sacral Fractures

Displaced transverse sacral fractures are really spinal injuries. They may be associated with severe neurologic deficit of the sacral nerve roots. Treatment depends on the presence or absence of such a deficit. If the patient has a neurologic deficit, the fracture should be reduced openly, a procedure usually combined with sacral laminectomy to protect the nerve roots during manipulation. If the patient is neurologically intact, nonoperative treatment usually suffices.

TYPE B: PARTIALLY STABLE (ROTATIONALLY UNSTABLE, VERTICALLY AND POSTERIORLY STABLE) LESIONS

Type B injuries are characterized by rotational instability but, by definition, are vertically and posteriorly stable; that is, they cannot significantly be displaced vertically or posteriorly by physiologic forces. All Type B injuries maintain vertical and posterior stability by a combination of an intact posterior tension band, compression of the posterior bony elements (usually the sacrum), and/or an intact pelvic floor. The plain radiographs may indicate up to 1 cm of displacement as a result of rotational forces, but clinical examination and further radiographic studies, including computed tomography (CT), confirm the diagnosis. The rotational instability may be of two types, external (B1) or internal (lateral compression B2). The injuries are considered separately here because the mechanisms, pathoanatomy, and treatment are very different.

Type B1: Unilateral Open-Book Injury; and Bilateral B3-1: External Rotationally Unstable, Vertically and Posteriorly Stable Injury

General Considerations

The common form of an open-book injury, caused by an anteroposterior compression injury of the pelvis or an external rotation force through the hip joint, disrupts the symphysis pubis, opening the pelvis like a book. A continuum of injury may be noted, as in all pelvic disruptions. The original force avulses the symphysis pubis, either through its fibers or with a thin shell of bone. As the force continues, the pelvic floor fascia tears, and the anterior sacroiliac ligaments rupture, either unilaterally or bilaterally, but the posterior ligaments remain intact, maintaining vertical stability. Other variants of the anteroposterior compression injury include fracture of the ilium instead of disruption of the anterior sacroiliac ligaments. Also anteriorly, the pubic rami may fracture instead of the symphysis avulsion.

The mere presence on the radiograph of a wide disruption of the symphysis pubis does not always mean that the pelvic ring is stable. The external rotation and shearing forces may overcome the tensile strength of the posterior sacroiliac ligaments, creating an unstable hemipelvis. This must be carefully sought on clinical examination by looking for extreme local tenderness of the posterior sacroiliac complex, and on radiographic examination for posterior displacement of the one hemipelvis. By definition, such a lesion is not a Type B, but an unstable Type C injury.

Variations of the Open-Book Injury

Many variations of the open-book (B1) lesion are possible and need to be precisely diagnosed. Such injuries may be unilateral or bilateral, and displacement of the symphysis may be minimal (<2.5 cm) or major (>2.5 cm) measured on radiograph or calibrated CT. In the universal nomenclature, all are accounted for by using modifiers for the degree of displacement and by using the designation B1 for the unilateral types and B3-1 for the bilateral types.

The posterior sacroiliac lesion is virtually always an anterior opening of the sacroiliac joint with intact posterior ligamentous structures, but some variations of posterior lesions may occur, such as iliac or sacral fractures or fractures associated with anterior opening of the sacroiliac joint.

Management of the Open-Book Injury

Management depends on the precise subgroup. The most important consideration is the width of the symphysis disruption. For the purpose of this discussion, open-book injuries are divided into two groups: (a) those with symphyseal disruption of <2.5 cm, whether the posterior lesion is unilateral or bilateral; and (b) those in which the symphysis is disrupted >2.5 cm, again, whether the posterior lesion is unilateral or bilateral.

Symphyseal Disruption Less Than 2.5 cm

When the symphysis pubis is disrupted <2.5 cm the muscles, fascia, and ligaments of the pelvic floor usually are intact, as is the anterior sacroiliac ligament. The posterior lesion may be bilateral or unilateral and is typically an anterior opening of the sacroiliac joint. Obviously, as in all trauma, the pathologic anatomy ranges widely. If the force stops with symphysis disruption only, then the soft tissues of the pelvic floor remain intact, but if the force continues there may be partial disruption of the pelvic floor. It has been found experimentally that the pelvis can open 2.5 cm while the pelvic floor and sacroiliac ligaments remain intact. Massive bleeding and major visceral injuries are uncommon because the forces in this injury are relatively mild.

Patients with minimal displacement through the symphysis pubis caused by trauma may be managed nonoperatively and symptomatically in anticipation of a good final result. Often, the symphyseal gap closes. There is a biomechanical explanation for this. We have found in our laboratory testing that, with an intact posterior pelvic arch, the symphysis is subjected to compressive forces in double stance gait. Therefore, once pain has been controlled, these patients should be allowed to walk with supports as needed.

Some of these patients may have prolonged and significant pain and tenderness in the region of the symphysis. This is well illustrated in Fig. 13-4. The patient, a 31-year-old professional hockey player, was knocked into the boards while playing hockey. He noted immediate pain in the region of the symphysis pubis. A slight diastasis at the symphysis was noted, but there were no posterior symptoms or evidence of posterior disruption. The patient's symptoms were prolonged; he felt pain and tenderness for 6 months. The repair reaction at the symphysis was characterized by heterotopic ossification and a hot technetium polyphosphate bone scan. Eventually, the patient was able to return to professional hockey without surgical intervention. Surgical intervention is rarely necessary for this particular injury, whether unilateral or bilateral, because the outcome usually is satisfactory with less invasive methods.

Symphyseal Disruption in Obstetrical Patients

There are situations in clinical medicine that mimic this injury, namely, physiologic stretching of the symphysis during normal childbirth or iatrogenic division of the symphysis in obstetrics to facilitate a difficult delivery (see Chapter 18). Neither situation requires surgery to stabilize the pelvic ring, because pelvic contraction occurs when the hormonal effects of childbirth have disappeared, although patients may complain of pain for many months in the postpartum period. Even an acute rupture of the symphysis, which rarely occurs in childbirth, usually returns to normal with symptomatic treatment.

Symphyseal Disruption Greater Than 2.5 cm

If the symphysis pubis is widely displaced, either associated with unilateral or bilateral posterior lesions, then one must assume disruption of the pelvic floor fascia, including the sacrospinous ligaments and the anterior sacroiliac ligaments. As the pelvic book opens, the posterior superior spine of the ilium abuts the sacrum. If the force stops at that point, the posterior sacroiliac ligaments remain intact. Therefore, this injury is rotationally unstable to the point of contact between the posterior superior iliac spine and the sacrum but vertically stable. Reduction is desirable for this injury. Massive bleeding and visceral injuries are common because the external rotation or anteroposterior compression force disrupts the soft tissues of the pelvic floor. Early reduction is important to restore the tamponade effect of the bony pelvis, otherwise the patient may exsanguinate. The volume of a sphere is $\frac{3}{4}\pi r^3$; therefore, restoration of the normal anatomy of the bony pelvis by reducing the volume into which blood may pour is essential (Fig. 13-5A,B).

Reduction

Reduction may be achieved simply by placing the patient in the lateral position, thus closing the book (Fig. 13-5C,D). Because the posterior tension band of the pelvis (i.e., the posterior sacroiliac ligaments) is intact, the anterior portion of the pelvic ring reduces anatomically and cannot over-reduce (Fig. 13-5E–G). In addition, the femora may be used as levers to achieve full internal rotation of both hip joints.

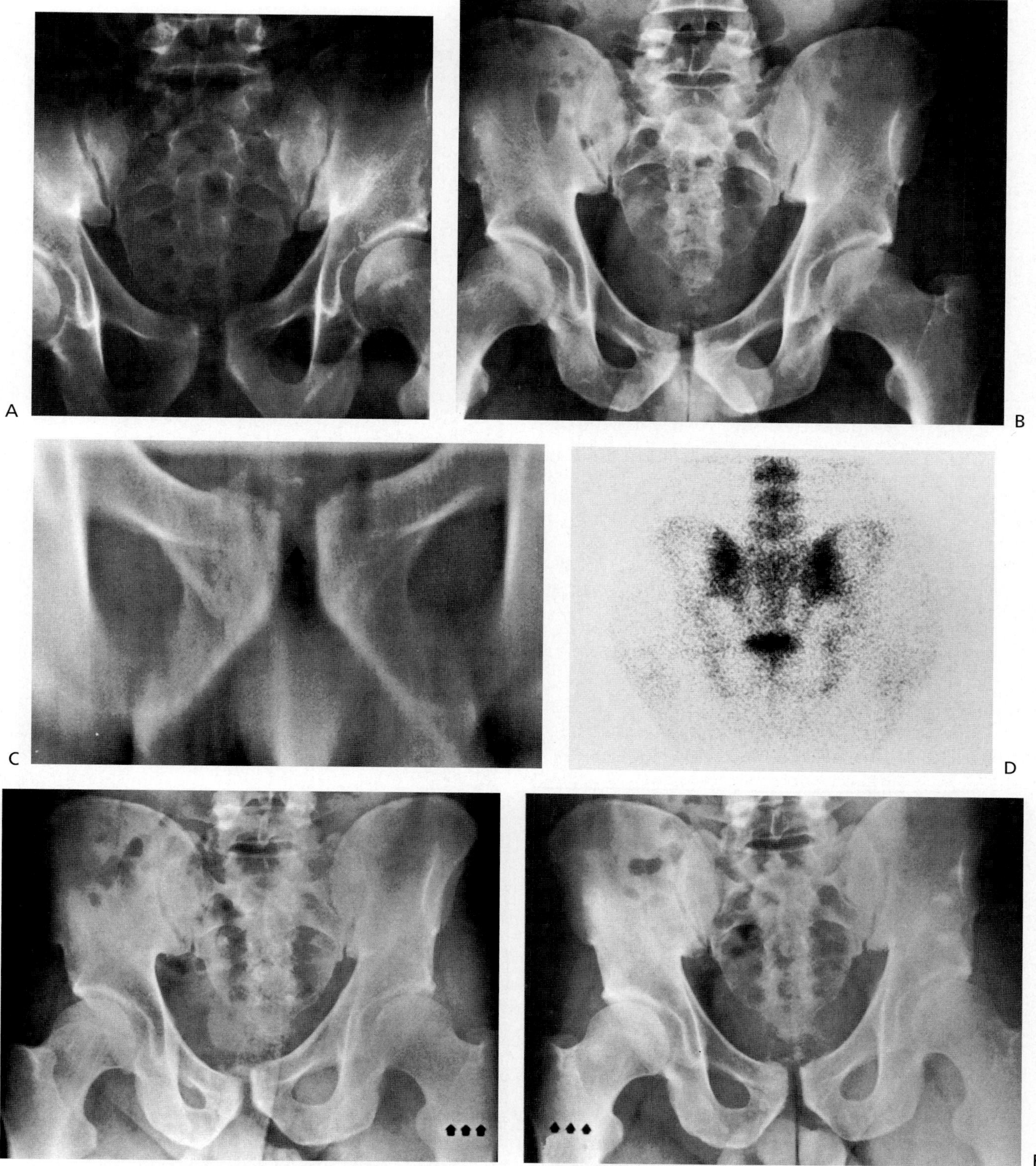

FIGURE 13-4. This patient was struck into the boards while playing hockey and noted immediate pain in the region of the symphysis pubis. The first anteroposterior radiograph of the pelvis **(A)** shows a diastasis of the symphysis with no evidence of posterior disruption. At 3 months, the patient had severe symptoms and could not return to prolonged skating. A radiograph **(B)** and a tomogram **(C)** of the symphysis pubis show a major repair reaction at the symphysis with heterotopic ossification. The technetium polyphosphate bone scan **(D)** shows an extraordinarily "hot" area along the symphysis pubis. Eventually, the symptoms settled and the patient returned to playing professional hockey without surgical intervention. The final radiographs **(E)** and **(F)** were taken with the patient standing, successively on his left and then his right foot. No major instability is noted, although slight movement has occurred when standing on the left leg. The posterior sacroiliac complex is intact.

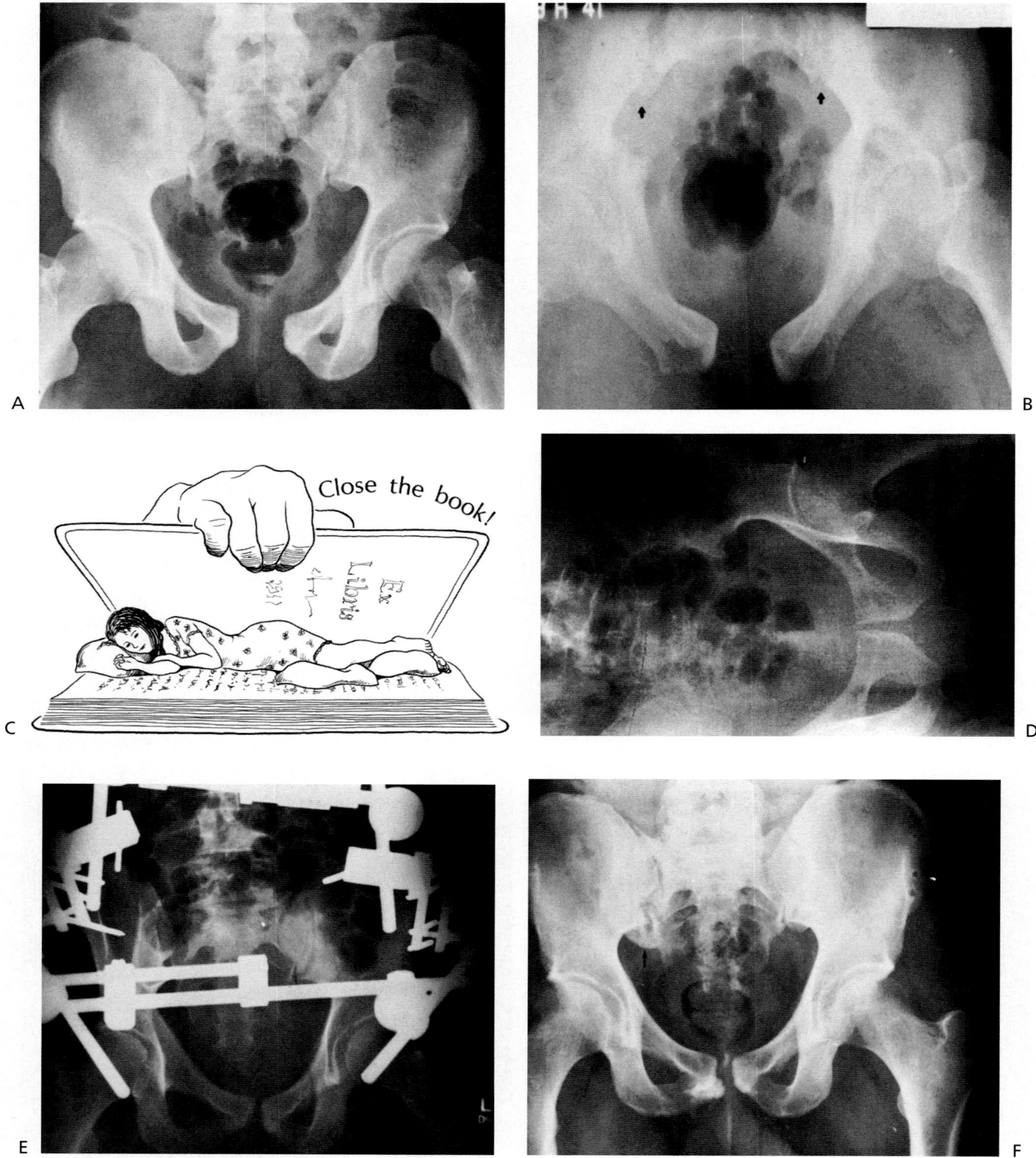

FIGURE 13-5. The anteroposterior **(A)** and inlet **(B)** radiographs show a typical open-book type of pelvic disruption. The displacement of the sacroiliac joints is indicated by two *black arrows.* Reduction of this open-book injury is easy: Just close the book **(C).** This is accomplished simply by placing the patient in the lateral position **(D).** Note on this radiograph, in lateral recumbency, that the position of the symphysis pubis has become "anatomic." Reduction can be maintained with an external skeletal fixator **(E).** The final result shows healing anteriorly and calcification across the right sacroiliac joint posteriorly **(F,G).** The clinical result was excellent. *(continued on next page)*

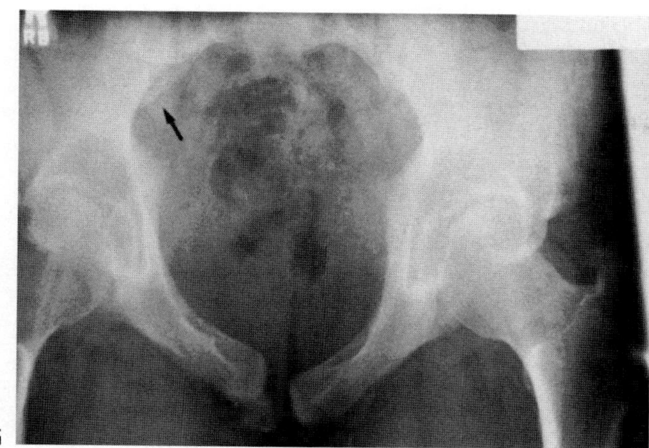

G

FIGURE 13-5. *(continued)*

If an external fixator is to be used for definitive treatment, an internal rotation force applied directly to the anterior skeletal pins also effectively reduces the pelvic ring (Fig. 13-6A). *Great care* must be taken with this maneuver, because excess stress of the pins, especially if poorly placed, may dislodge them. It is preferable to compress the hemipelvis manually and then tighten the assembled anterior frame (Fig. 13-6B).

Maintenance of Reduction

Once the book is closed, several methods are available for maintaining this reduction. The precise method chosen, either operative or nonoperative, depends on the details of the case.

Nonoperative Treatment

Pelvic Sling. The anteroposterior compression injury is the only pelvic ring disruption that logically can be managed by a pelvic sling. The pelvic sling closes the symphysis pubis, and if the sling is retained until the anterior ligaments have healed, a good result may be anticipated.

However, nursing a patient in a pelvic sling for the 6 to 12 weeks required for stabilization is difficult and is rarely tolerated by either the patient or the nursing staff. Thus, this method is rarely used. If a sling is chosen the patient must be turned frequently, so that decubitus skin ulcers are prevented.

Hip Spica. A full hip spica with the lower extremities in the internally rotated position can hold the symphysis pubis in the reduced position. In less than ideal circumstances, as in remote areas or a war zone, this would be the treatment of choice. It is easy to apply and yields good results, but it requires a long period of immobilization in a most awkward position, and today, few patients are willing to tolerate this type of treatment (1).

Operative management usually is indicated because nonoperative management is fraught with difficulties. The method chosen—internal fixation or external skeletal fixation—depends on other factors. If the patient requires a laparotomy or urologic procedure, the symphysis should be plated at that time unless there is fecal contamination. The presence of urine, especially in a male, does not preclude internal fixation, but physicians should be wary of a suprapubic tube, which poses a high risk for infection. If no urinary or abdominal operation is planned, external skeletal fixation is safe and effective or open reduction and internal fixation may be an option, but the patient must be informed of the risks of each option.

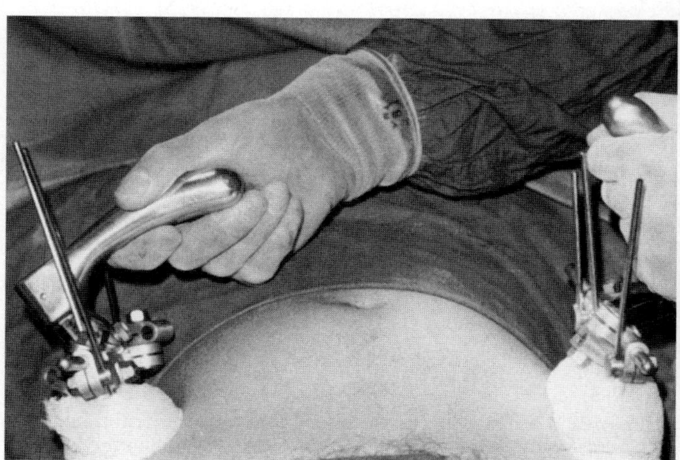

A

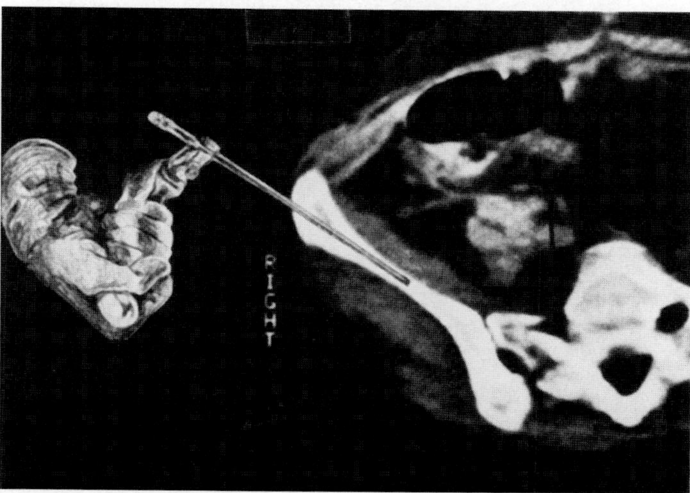

B

FIGURE 13-6. A: The photograph demonstrates the type of leverage one can obtain by placing handles on the crossbars of the external fixation device to allow for both internal and external rotation of the unstable hemipelvis. **B:** The diagram on a computed tomography scan indicates the type of direct leverage one can bring to bear on the affected hemipelvis.

Operative Treatment

The surgeon has two surgical options for stabilization of the symphysis disruption: external or internal fixation. Each has its indications, risks, and benefits.

External Skeletal Fixation. External skeletal fixation is a safe and effective method of stabilizing the symphysis pubis. This particular injury has been recreated in our laboratory by cutting the symphysis pubis (see Chapter 14). Subsequent biomechanical studies have shown that an external skeletal fixator offers adequate stabilization for this type of injury, allowing early ambulation without risk of redisplacing the fracture (see Chapter 14). Because posterior stability is retained, anterior stability can be ensured with any type of anterior external fixator, thus effectively stabilizing the pelvic ring (Fig. 13-7). After application of the external skeletal pins, reduction is obtained by placing the patient in the lateral position, and the crossbars on the frame are tightened to maintain the reduction. Full weight bearing may be instituted as soon as it is tolerated by the patient. The pins are retained until healing has occurred across the symphysis pubis, usually 8 to 12 weeks. The use of the external frame for this injury is simple, safe, and logical for this injury if no urinary tract or abdominal surgery is planned. The major contraindication is the variant of this injury in which a fracture goes through the ilium to the crest. If the fracture line extends too far anteriorly, the external pins may cross it, converting a closed fracture to an open one. In that situation, one should choose open reduction and internal fixation of the symphysis and ilium.

Usually, 6 to 8 weeks must pass before sufficient healing has occurred and the pins can be removed. To test the stability of the pelvis at that time, the crossbars should be loosened and inlet, outlet, and anteroposterior radiographs

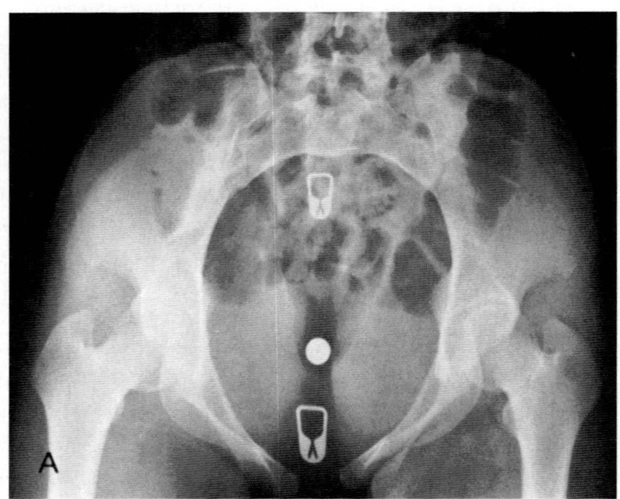

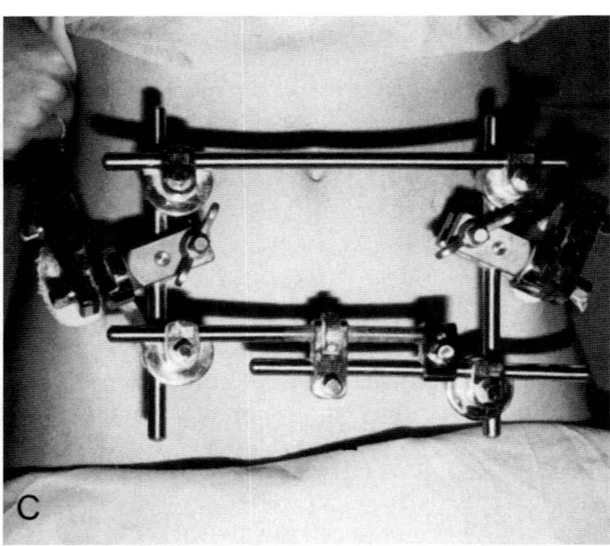

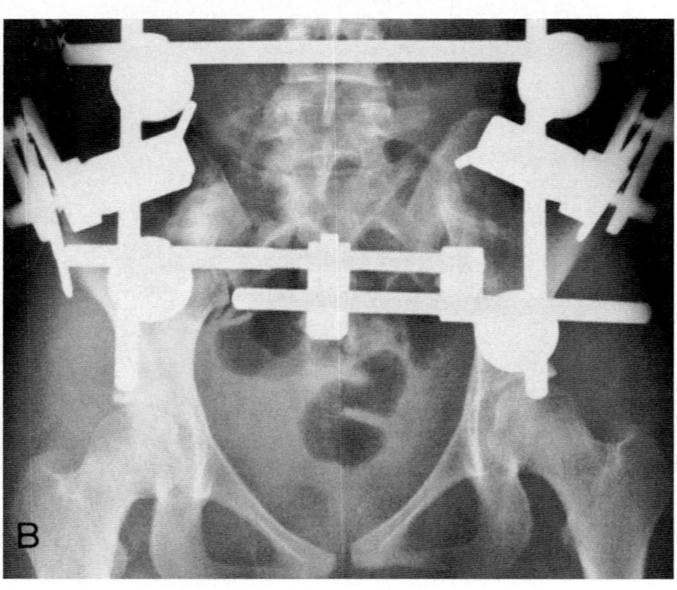

FIGURE 13-7. A: The inlet radiograph shows an open-book type fracture with an intact posterior pelvic arch and a 2.5-cm opening of the symphysis, anteriorly. This 17-year-old girl was treated with an external skeletal fixator rectangular frame, as noted in the radiograph **(B)** and photograph **(C).** Because this was a stable type of injury the patient could ambulate immediately with her external fixator.

taken. If instability remains, the fixator should be reapplied for an additional 4 to 6 weeks. It is not uncommon for the symphysis to open up slightly after frame removal.

Internal Fixation

Stable fixation of the pelvic ring also may be achieved by open reduction and internal fixation of the disrupted symphysis (see Fig. 15-3), and this is many surgeons' preferred method for the open-book injury. Open operation is not essential, because noninvasive external fixation may achieve the same end. If surgery to the pelvis is indicated for some other reason, such as an injury to the urinary tract, plate fixation may be carried out while the patient is still under anesthesia (see Fig. 15-12). Again, this restores stability to the pelvic ring. The patient may be allowed in the upright position almost immediately, but full weight bearing should be delayed 4 to 6 weeks. The major disadvantages of this technique are the necessity for an open operation, with all of its inherent problems, and for a second operation to remove the implant.

One of the major risks is the development of sepsis in the symphysis pubis, either specific or nonspecific (osteitis pubis). If fecal contamination is present, external fixation is a safer method. Also, the presence of a suprapubic tube in bladder rupture is a risk factor that is often unnecessary. At our center, the urologists use distal drainage through a Foley catheter following bladder repair, and drain the retropubic space with suction drains, a much safer method. If rami fractures are present, external fixation is the preferable choice. Posterior internal fixation is virtually never indicated in an open book type partially stable injury.

Type B2: Lateral Compression Injury: Partial Disruption of the Posterior Pelvic Arch, Intact Pelvic Floor (Internal Rotationally Unstable, Vertically Stable)

General Considerations

Lateral compression forces cause the greatest number of pelvic fractures. The force may be applied directly to the ilium, or indirectly through the femoral head. These forces may produce two distinct types of lateral compression injury.

These types have pathologic anatomy that is similar; namely, compression fractures of the posterior sacroiliac complex, a largely intact pelvic floor including the sacrospinous and sacrotuberous ligaments, and anterior injuries to the pubic rami or the symphysis. Both types may exhibit internal rotatory instability or posterior impaction in internal rotation. In fact, at the moment of impact the internal rotation may be so extreme as to allow the pubic rami to strike the opposite hemipelvis. However, vertical and posterior stability are maintained by the intact pelvic floor, by the compression fracture of the sacrum, and in some instances by an intact posterior tension band. The two types differ in their displacement. The ipsilateral kind exhibits internal rotation (see Chapter 12), whereas the contralateral (bucket-handle) injury exhibits internal plus superior rotation, through an anterior lesion displaced on the side opposite to the posterior lesion (see Chapter 12).

Management of Lateral Compression Type B2 Injuries

Ipsilateral Lateral Compression Injury

This lesion usually is produced by an indirect force through the femoral head. Many of the superior ramus injuries enter the inferior portion of the acetabulum, so this is truly an anterior column acetabular fracture.

The pathologic anatomy is as follows: First, the superior and inferior rami fracture in an oblique fashion. As the force continues, the hemipelvis rotates internally, causing a crush to the anterior aspect of the sacrum at the sacroiliac joint. The soft tissues anteriorly on the pelvic floor may be penetrated by the internally migrating rami, but the main portion of the pelvic floor remains intact. The rami may perforate the bladder. The end point is reached when the rami strike the opposite hemipelvis. In this particular type, the posterior tension band and sacroiliac ligaments usually remain intact. Therefore, elastic recoil of the soft tissues often reduces the fracture when the patient is placed in the supine position. In that instance it is only by careful physical examination and compression of the iliac crest that the surgeon may determine the degree of internal rotatory instability (see Chapter 10).

Although fractures of the superior and inferior rami are the common anterior lesions, variations of the anterior injury have been described, including a locked symphysis, and the so-called tilt fracture, in which the superior ramus fracture rotates internally until it disrupts the symphysis causing posterior displacement at the symphysis.

Ipsilateral Rami Fractures (Typical Lesion). With this injury, bed rest in the supine position usually restores the normal anatomy by elastic recoil of the tissues (Fig. 13-8). Therefore, in most instances, no other treatment is indicated. This is especially true of fractures in elderly patients, which are commonly of this type, and isolated fractures in younger persons.

However, if the patient has multiple system injuries or severe pain and is difficult to nurse, then an external skeletal frame holding the fracture reduced in external rotation restores enough stability to the pelvic ring to allow the patient to be nursed in the upright position. The patient may be ambulated as the symptoms abate, because the pelvis has sufficient stability to tolerate it.

The prognosis for this particular fracture is excellent. The fracture usually heals with minimal long-term effect; therefore, open reduction and internal fixation are virtually never

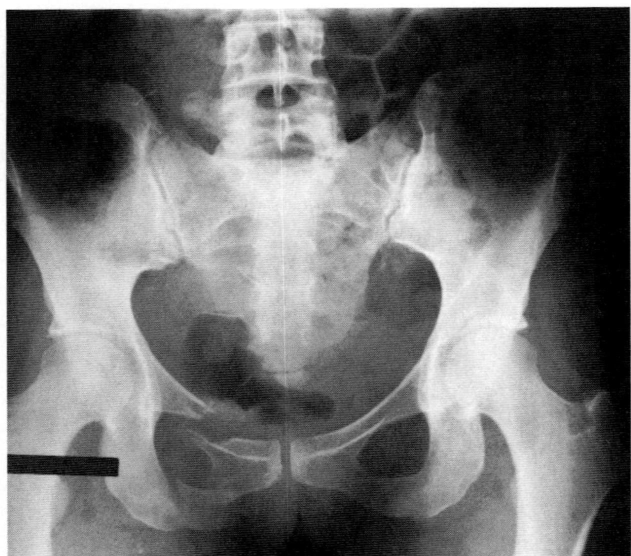

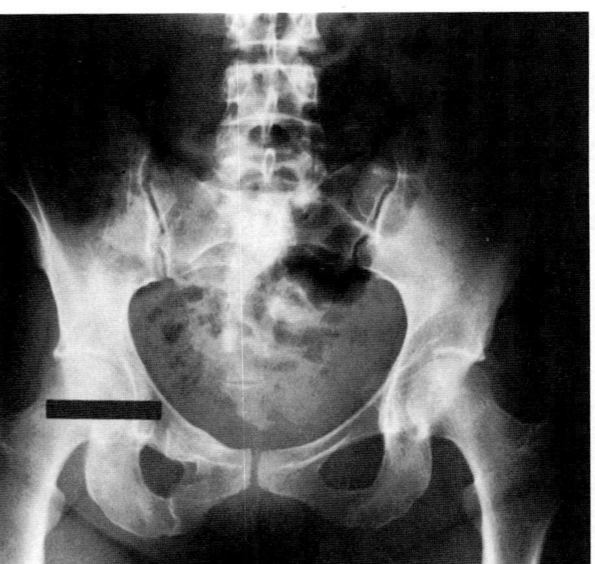

FIGURE 13-8. **A:** The anteroposterior radiograph of the pelvis shows a typical Type 1 lateral compression injury. **B:** The fracture healed in satisfactory position with bed rest alone. The patient's clinical and radiographic results were excellent.

indicated for this fracture type, except to reduce a locked symphysis or restore the symphysis in the tilt fracture. Because the rotation is internal rather than superior, leg length discrepancy does not occur. If the internal rotation is fixed, owing to posterior compression, there is usually little effect on the patient's function unless the fixed internal rotation is greater than 30 degrees. This depends on the ability of the hip joint to rotate externally and compensate for this deformity. In this particular type the patient usually can compensate for this amount of internal rotation; therefore, reduction is seldom required, a situation much different than the contralateral type, where reduction is more commonly indicated.

Locked Symphysis. A locked symphysis occasionally may be reduced closed by external rotation of the hemipelvis. The reduction force should be applied mainly to the iliac crest and not the femoral neck, which may be fractured in this maneuver (Fig. 13-9A). It may be far safer under general anesthesia, to make a small Pfannenstiel incision, insert a pointed fracture reduction clamp on each side of the symphysis, and with direct pressure on the iliac crest in external rotation reduce the locked symphysis. After reduction the symphysis can be fixed simply with a two- or four-hole plate, as described in Chapter 15, or held by an external frame if closed reduction was successful (Fig. 13-9B,C).

Tilt Fracture. In the tilt fracture, the displaced superior ramus may project posteriorly into the perineum. If such a fracture is left in the unreduced position, female patients may experience dyspareunia. Occasionally, this fracture may be reduced closed, by externally rotating the hemipelvis and applying direct pressure to the fracture (Fig. 13-10). Open reduction is indicated if closed reduction fails.

Again, through a small Pfannenstiel incision, pointed reduction forceps are applied to the superior ramus, which is derotated, and the fracture fixed internally. Because this is a stable fracture, a threaded Kirschner wire often suffices until fracture healing is complete at 6 weeks, at which time the threaded K wire across the symphysis can be removed (Fig. 13-11). The tip of the K wire must be bent to prevent migration, especially if an unthreaded wire is used. The fracture may also be fixed with a 3.5-mm reconstruction plate.

Contralateral Lateral Compression (Bucket-Handle) Injury

In this particular pattern the lateral compression force is usually applied to the iliac crest anteriorly. In that position, the main deforming force is not only internal but also superior.

The pathoanatomy is different than for the ipsilateral lesion. Anteriorly, displacement is on the side opposite the posterior lesion. The lesion may be in the two opposite rami, or a combination of all four rami or two rami plus the symphysis, but in this particular type, the *anterior displacement is on the side opposite the posterior injury.* As the hemipelvis, which now includes a portion of the opposite pelvis anteriorly, rotates upward and inward, like the handle of a bucket, the local soft tissues anteriorly may be penetrated, but the main bulk of the pelvic floor remains intact.

The posterior injury depends on the relative strength of the bone and ligaments. Usually, the sacrum crushes ante-

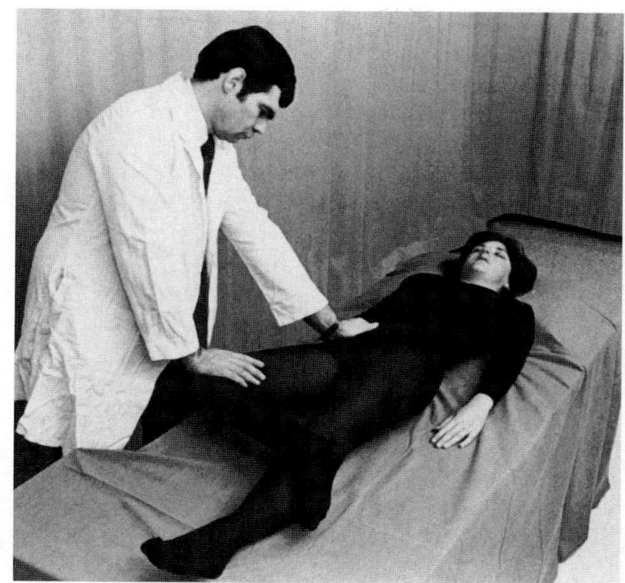

A

FIGURE 13-9. **A:** Closed reduction of a lateral compression-type injury is performed by external rotation of the hip with the knee flexed and direct pressure on the hemipelvis, as shown. Example of a patient with a locked symphysis after a fall from a height. **B:** Under general anesthesia and using the same maneuver of external rotation described in **(A)** the symphysis was unlocked. Stability was maintained with an external skeletal frame **(C)**.

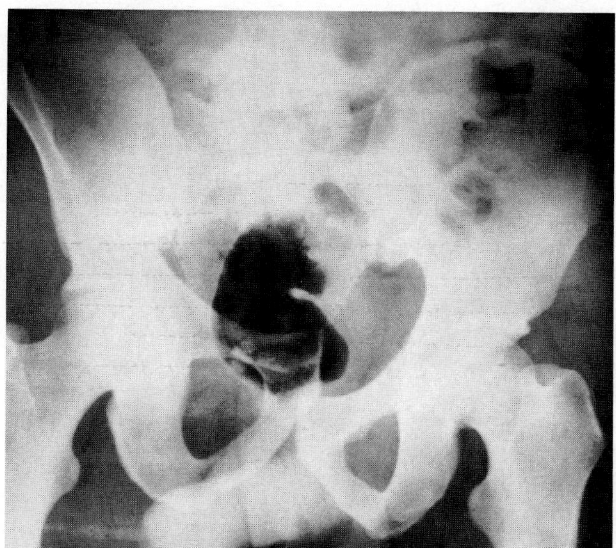

B

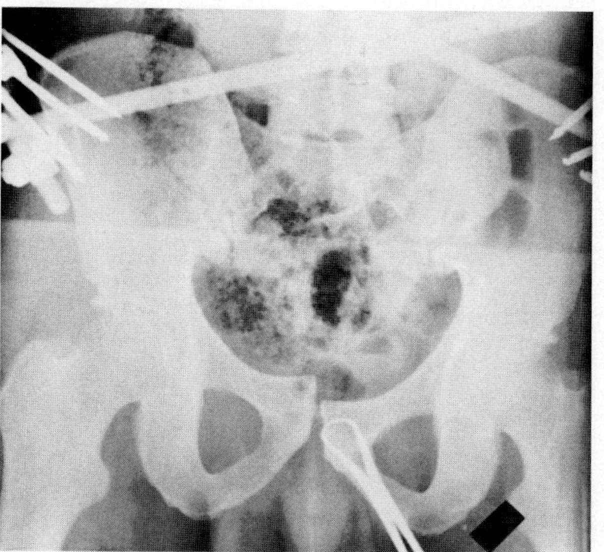

C

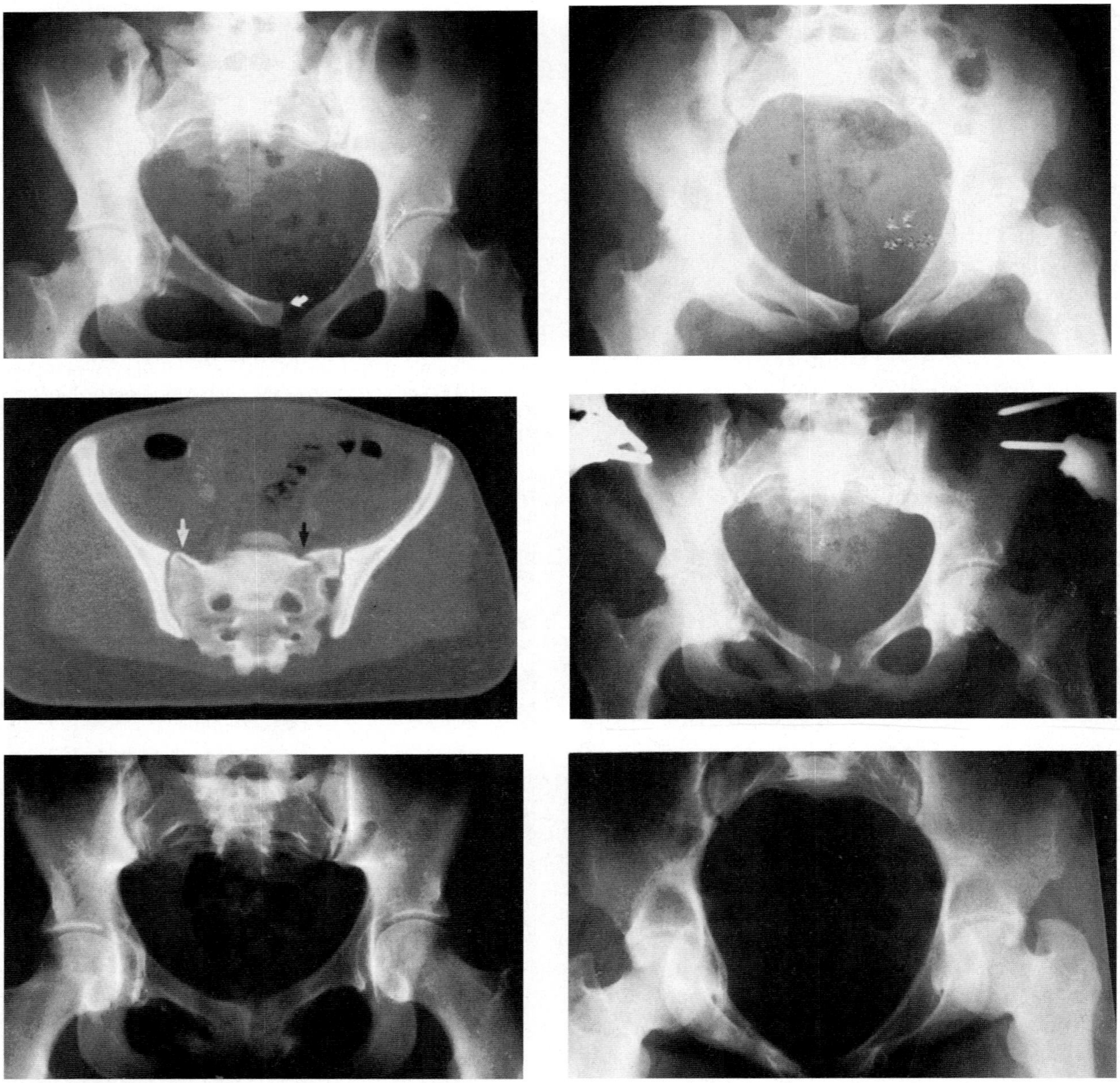

A

B

C

D

E

F

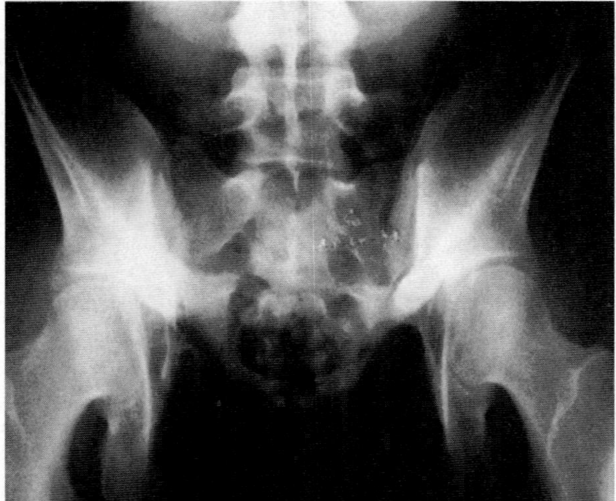

G

FIGURE 13-10. This patient was a front seat passenger in a motor vehicle hit from the right side. She sustained an unusual lateral compression injury, as noted in the anteroposterior **(A)** and the inlet radiograph **(B).** The entire superior pubic ramus was fractured laterally at the hip joint and medially through the symphysis, with the medial portion overlapped. The computed tomography **(C)** shows the left compression through the sacrum with approximately 1 cm of medial compression, as noted by the black arrow. A small compression fracture is also noted in the right sacrum *(white arrow).* Direct closed manual palpation **(D)** on the superior ramus fracture reduced it to an adequate position, obviating open reduction. An external frame with the hemipelvis in slight external rotation maintained reduction. No traction was necessary. The final result for this young woman was excellent: sound healing and no pain. In spite of the increased calcification at the symphysis noted in the anteroposterior **(E),** inlet **(F),** and outlet **(G)** radiographs taken 10 months following injury, the patient subsequently had a child through normal vaginal delivery.

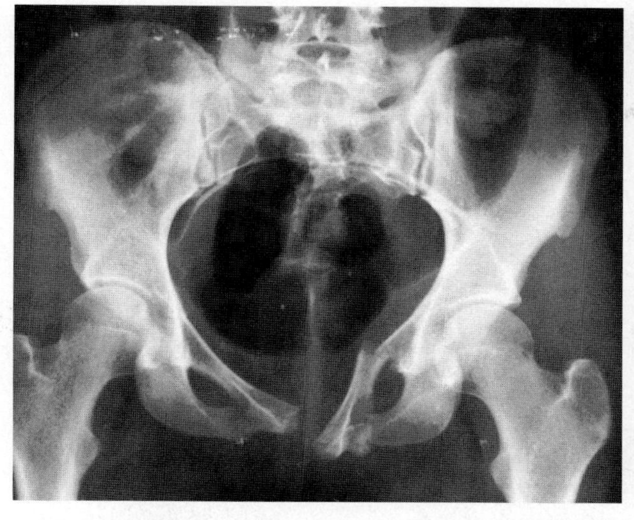

A

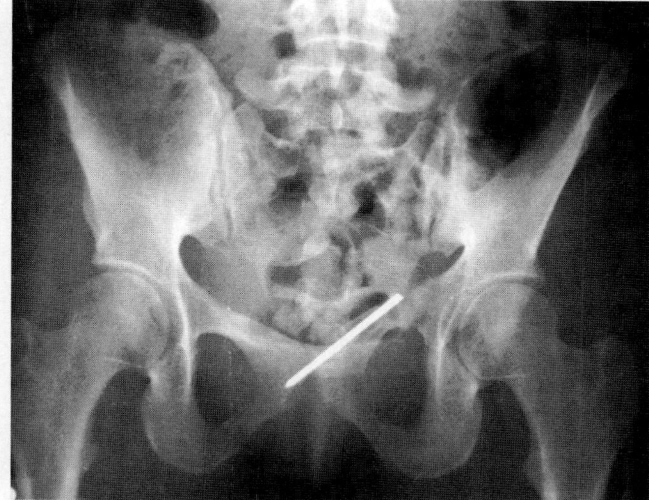

B

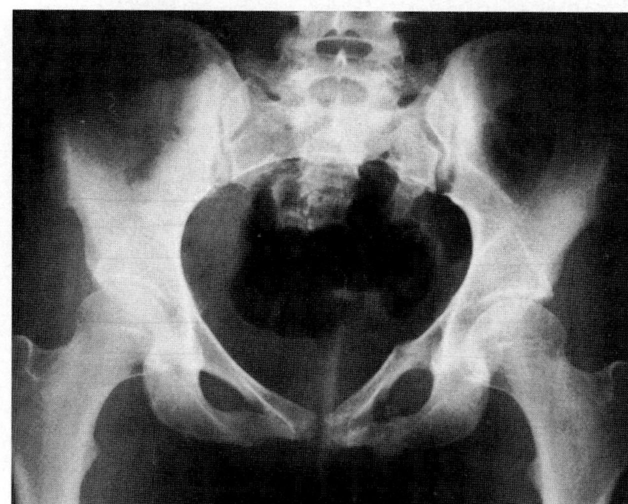

C

FIGURE 13-11. A: The original radiograph demonstrates the rotated superior ramus of the left pubis through a disrupted symphysis pubis. **B:** Because posterior complex is stable, open reduction and internal fixation with a threaded Steinmann pin restored stability. **C:** Union occurred quickly, and the pin was removed at 6 weeks.

riorly at the sacroiliac joint, occasionally through the sacrum itself. The crush of the sacrum may be so severe that the hemipelvis cannot move; that is, it is firmly impacted. This is no different than the lesion seen in a firmly impacted os calcis fracture or tibial plateau fracture (Fig. 13-12).

The posterior sacroiliac ligaments may remain intact or tear, but vertical and posterior stability is maintained by the pelvic floor. In some instances the hemipelvis can rotate internally and superiorly. In others the posterior impaction is so stable that no rotation is possible.

The management of this injury depends on many factors. As in the ipsilateral injury with minimal displacement and good posterior stability, most of these patients may be managed nonoperatively with bed rest in the supine position. To allow the patient to move, the patient may be nursed supine or prone, but never in the lateral position because that could increase the deformity.

The indications for reduction of the fracture are "significant" leg length discrepancy or an internal rotation deformity. Also, stabilization of the lateral compression injury with an external skeletal fixator is desirable in some polytrauma patients and patients with severe pain. This makes nursing difficult.

For each patient the surgeon must decide whether the degree of internal rotation and the amount of shortening warrant taking the more aggressive steps necessary to reduce the fracture. The age, general medical state, expectations of the patient, and expertise of the health care team are all factors that must be considered. The patient must be made aware of the dilemma and should share in the management decision. If a malreduced, shortened extremity is the likely outcome of the injury, the patient should be made aware of the reasons for this. In general, as much as 1 cm of leg length discrepancy is acceptable in this situation. Also up to 30 degrees of internal rotation is acceptable if the hip joint can rotate externally to compensate for the deformity. The patient should also be informed of the large bump that will remain at the posterior superior iliac spine owing to the rotated hemipelvis (Fig. 13-12F).

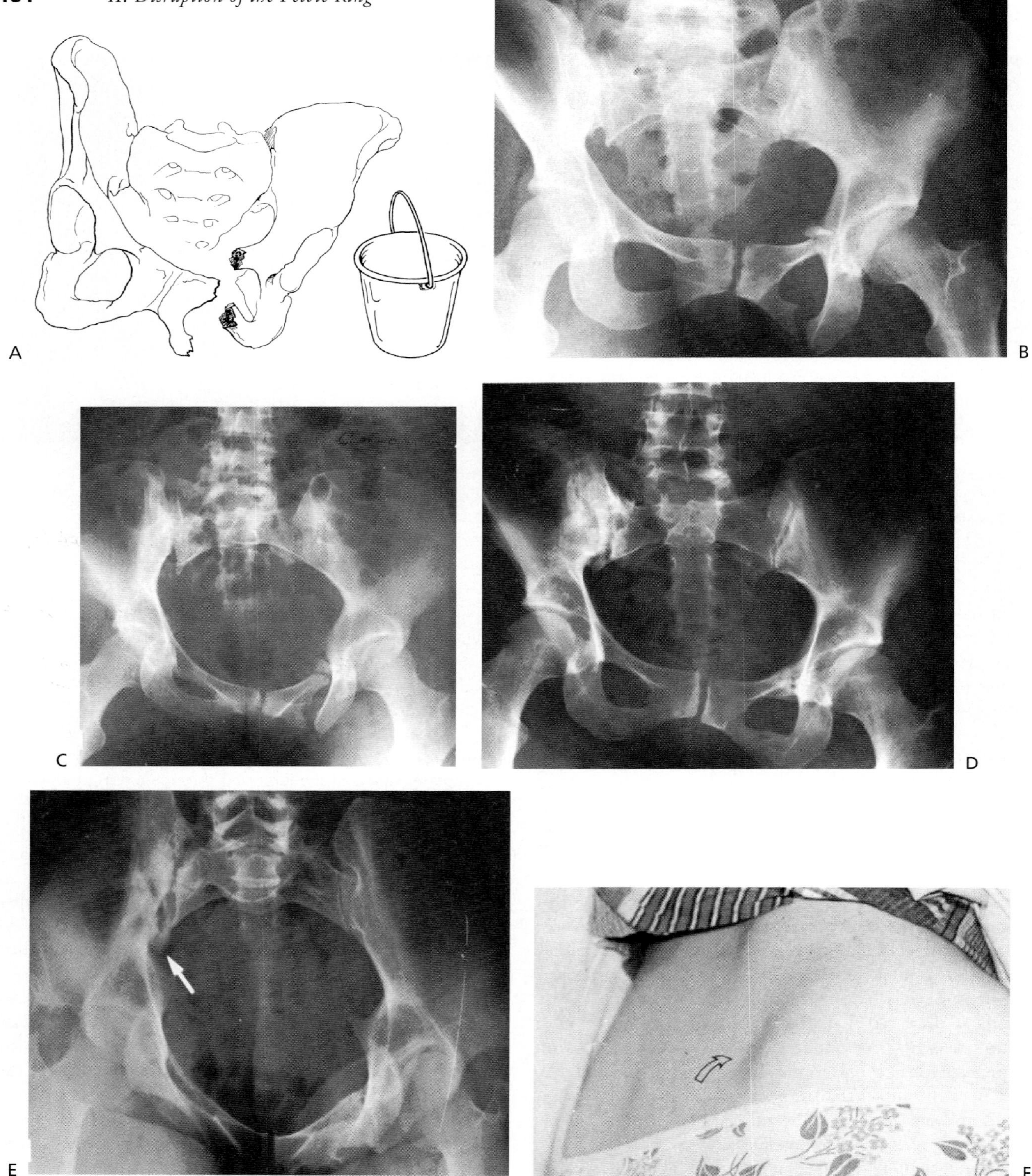

FIGURE 13-12. A: Drawing of a classic lateral compression injury of the contralateral type. The anteroposterior **(B)** and inlet **(C)** radiographs show the degree of posterior impaction, with slight posterior displacement and upward rotation of the right hemipelvis. This woman was given a general anesthetic 3 days after the injury, but the posterior impaction was so great that the hemipelvis could not be reduced. Because the displacement was not clinically significant, we elected to treat with bed rest. The final result was good. The anteroposterior **(D)** and inlet **(E)** radiographs taken 4 months posttrauma, show sound anterior progressive union at the sacral fracture. The inlet radiograph shows an anterior bony bar *(white arrow).* Healing in the rotated position shows a bony bump on the internally rotated posterior superior iliac spine *(arrow)* **(F).**

Closed Reduction and External Fixation. The first step in management is closed reduction and external fixation if the degree of shortening and malrotation is unacceptable, or in cases of polytrauma. The patient should be anesthetized and the fracture viewed on an image intensifier. Reduction may be greatly aided by inserting skeletal pins into the pelvis. By inserting the pins and applying special types of reduction clamps, each hemipelvis may be manipulated individually, and reduction obtained in this manner. The closed reduction, as illustrated in Fig. 13-9, may be further facilitated by the application of an external rotation force through the abducted flexed hip and flexed knee of the affected extremity, while applying a force to the affected anterior superior spine. The opposite anterior superior spine must be fixed by the assistant so that the entire pelvis does not rotate. The same precautions mentioned previously also apply; excessive force must not be applied to the pins or neck of the femur, lest the pins pull out or the neck of the femur breaks. Most of the reduction force should be applied to the pelvis itself at the iliac crest.

In some cases, the posterior impaction is so great that closed reduction, even with the help of external fixation pins, may prove impossible. Finally, if all attempts at closed reduction fail, as described, the pelvic compression clamp may be applied anteriorly and the affected hemipelvis externally rotated by reversing the clamp, thus helping to reduce the posterior injury. For rotational instability an external fixator is indicated for ease of nursing, especially of polytrauma patients. Reduction of pain and restoration of stability allow the patient to be moved with relative ease.

Open Reduction and Internal Fixation. If all of these attempts fail, only open reduction can restore the normal anatomy. In my opinion, open reduction for a lateral compression injury should *rarely* be performed, because it is hazardous, especially to the L5 nerve root. However, it must be considered if the patient is young or has more than 2 cm of shortening or a markedly unacceptable internal rotation deformity.

Grossly displaced rami fractures, which are unlikely to heal, or an overriding displaced symphysis also may be an indication. Some superior ramus fractures enter the anterior column of the acetabulum. In that circumstance, the surgeon is really dealing with an acetabular fracture, and the indications for open reduction and internal fixation of acetabular fractures take precedence in decision making. In almost all of these instances the intraarticular fracture is inferior, involves only a small portion of the articular surface, and can be managed nonoperatively.

After open reduction, internal or external fixation is necessary to stabilize the pelvic ring. In this particular fracture, the risks may outweigh the benefits; therefore, it is wise to proceed with extreme caution. If the fracture heals in the malreduced position and the patient has a major clinical disability, secondary reconstructive procedures may be undertaken, such as an opening wedge innominate osteotomy to restore rotation and some length to the lower extremity or closed shortening of the opposite femur.

Caution: *Lateral compression injuries are made worse if internal rotation forces are applied during the healing period. Therefore, pelvic slings are illogical, as they replicate the deforming force (Fig. 13-13). Also, the patient should not be nursed lying on one side, because this also could recreate the original deformity (Fig. 13-14).*

Type B3: Bilateral Type B Injuries

In this type of bilateral injury both lesions are Type B; that is, both have partial stability and cannot be displaced vertically. In the first subgroup, both sides may be open-book injuries. This type has already been described in the section on open-book injury (B3-1). In the second subgroup (B3-2), a lesion on one side may be B1, a unilateral open-book injury, and that on the other B2, lateral compression. A more common scenario (B3-3) is bilateral B2 lateral compression injuries, produced when the pelvis is pressed against a fixed object.

Management depends on the precise type of injury and degree of displacement. The guidelines given for unilateral Type B injuries should be followed when dealing with bilateral injuries, which usually can be managed with bed rest or an external skeletal fixator. Open reduction and internal fixation rarely are indicated.

TYPE C: UNSTABLE LESIONS COMPLETE DISRUPTION OF THE PELVIC ARCH (BY VERTICAL SHEAR)

General Principles of Management

The clinical and radiologic assessment of the patient may indicate to the surgeon that the pelvic ring is unstable. This is readily apparent on direct palpation of the ilium and confirmed by the radiographic appearance. Because high-energy shearing forces cause this injury, many associated problems that increase morbidity and mortality should be anticipated (2).

The skeletal injury may be unilateral (Type C1) or bilateral (Types C2 or C3); that is, the pelvic ring may be disrupted anteriorly through the symphysis or the pubic rami and posteriorly through one or both posterior sacroiliac complexes. The soft tissues of the pelvic floor are torn, including the sacrospinous and sacrotuberous ligaments. Obviously, a bilateral disruption with division of the pelvic ring in at least three (and occasionally four) areas is the most unstable type of pelvic injury. In the unilateral type, the stability of one hemipelvis is intact, so it can be used as a pillar against which the unstable hemipelvis is secured. If, however, both sides of the pelvic ring are unstable posteriorly, as in the bilateral types, the only area attached to the axial skeleton is the sacrum, which must be used in any direct stabilization attempt. If the sacrum, in turn, is badly shattered, complete stabilization of the pelvic ring in the bilateral types is extremely difficult.

These gross displacements, through both the sacroiliac joint and the posterior cancellous bone, have been noted by Bucholz in his cadaver study of the pathology of this injury, and at many surgical procedures (3). At surgery, all posterior soft tissues are disrupted, so the surgeon can easily put a finger or an instrument into the true pelvis. This injury should be considered an internal hemipelvectomy. Stabilization of the pelvic ring using modern techniques is desirable for many reasons.

Rationale for Stabilization

Stabilization of a grossly unstable pelvis is an important part of resuscitation and should be performed as soon as possible following injury. The objectives are these:

1. *Reduce blood loss* through tamponade by restoring the original pelvic volume. The volume of a sphere is $\frac{4}{3}\pi r^3$, so reducing the radius of the pelvis much reduces the space into which bleeding may occur. Also, blood loss may be slowed by reduction of cancellous bony surfaces.
2. *Reduce pain* to allow easier mobilization of the patient on assisted ventilation, which is helpful for nursing care.

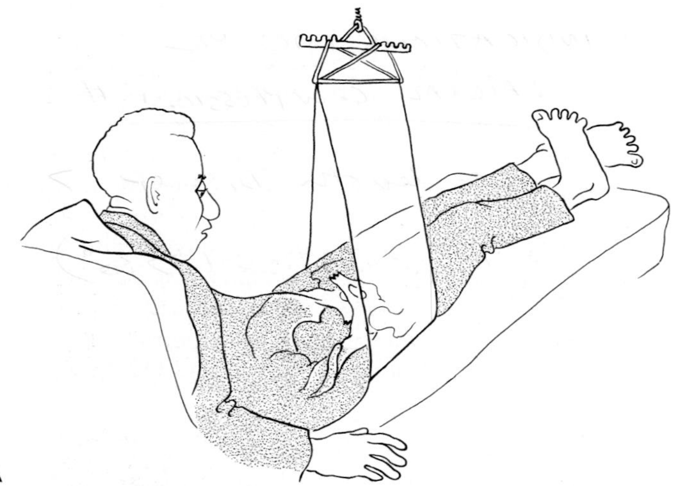
A

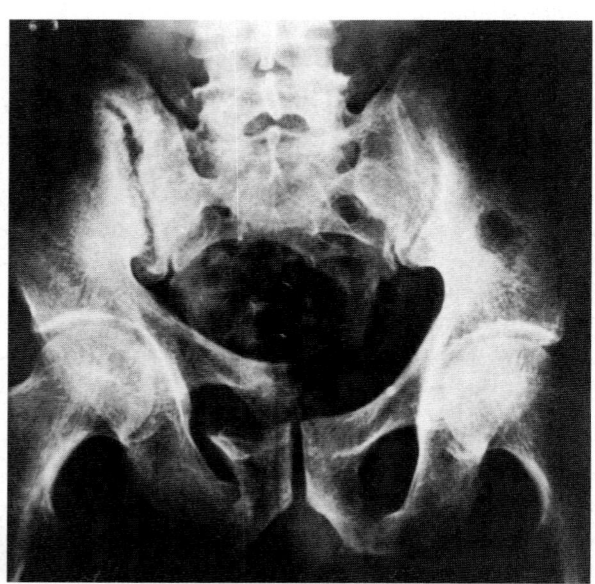
B

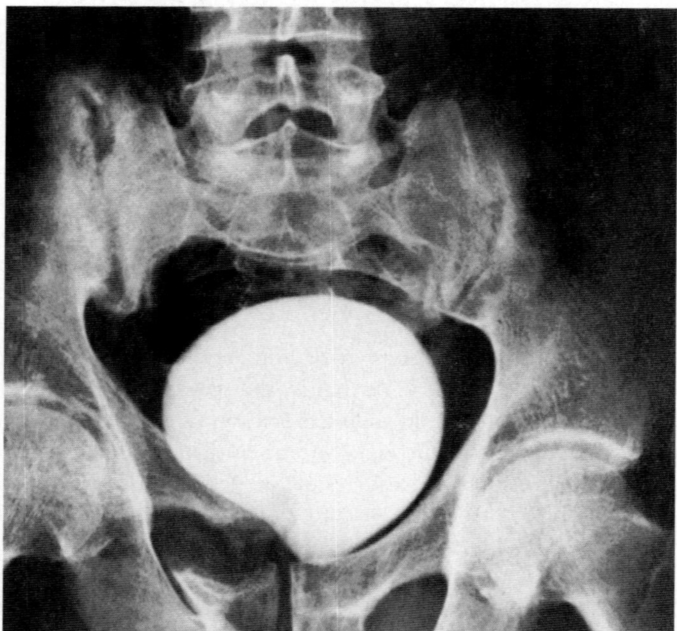
C

FIGURE 13-13. A: Pelvic slings are illogical in patients with lateral compression injuries, as they recreate the original force. Also, in unstable vertical shear injuries, the sling produces an internal rotation deformity of the pelvis. The anteroposterior radiograph **(B)** and the cystogram **(C)** show the very marked deformity resulting from the use of a sling. The patient developed urinary frequency and required excision of the bone mass. Note also that union of this fracture was grossly retarded at 1 year.

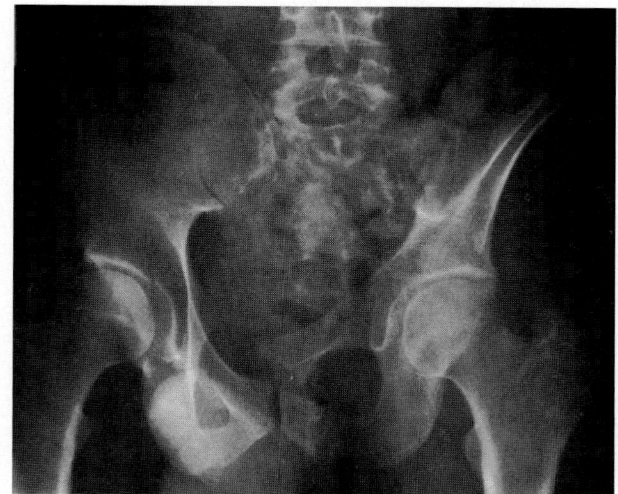

A

FIGURE 13-14. Anteroposterior **(A)** and inlet **(B)** radiographs of a 30-year-old man, 6 months after a lateral compression injury, ipsilateral type. The patient's original radiograph showed little displacement, but he was nursed on his side. The deformity on the plane radiographs **(A,B)** showed marked internal rotation of the left hemipelvis with overlap at the symphysis. The left hemipelvis is shown in an obturator oblique view, the right in straight anteroposterior projection. Computed tomography (CT) shows compression of the left hemipelvis and marked internal rotation. A fracture of the right sacrum is also noted, and healing at that time was almost complete. The CT **(D)** shows the amount of internal rotation of the left hemipelvis and the CT **(E)** shows sound union. Because the patient was able to overcome the internal rotation of the left hemipelvis through normal hip external rotation, no reconstructive surgery was required and he has been able to return to his former occupation. In this particular case the patient should not have been nursed on his side, a position that recreated the original mechanism of injury.

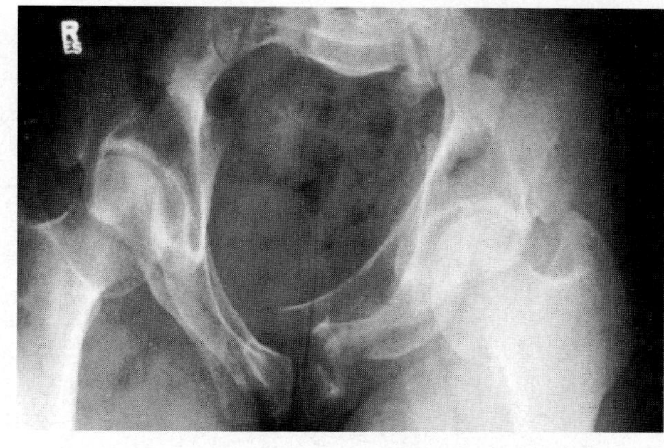

B

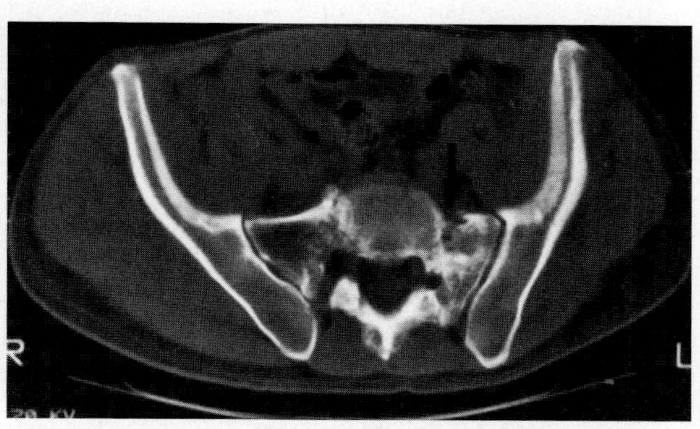

C

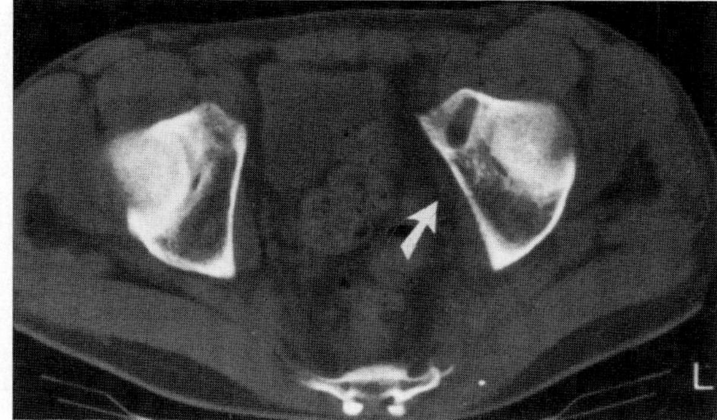

D

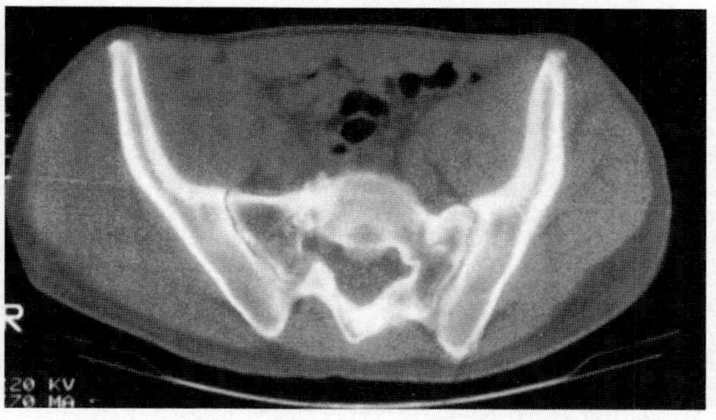

E

3. *Prevent the late sequelae of the unstable Type C injury.* The unstable posterior injury is caused by massive shearing or external rotation forces through the sacroiliac joint or the cancellous bone of the ilium or sacrum. Cancellous bone heals rapidly if compressed but poorly if not; so continued instability and displacement of the posterior complex not infrequently leads to delayed union, or even nonunion (Fig. 13-15) (4).

Also, displacement of the sacroiliac joint may result in chronic instability of that joint, with lingering pain the likely outcome (Fig. 13-16). Therefore, compression of the fractured cancellous surfaces ensures prompt union, and of the sacroiliac joint, adequate stability leading to spontaneous arthrodesis in many cases. If stabilization of the unstable pelvic ring is desirable, how can this be achieved? This is still an open question at this time, and no hard and fast answer can be given.

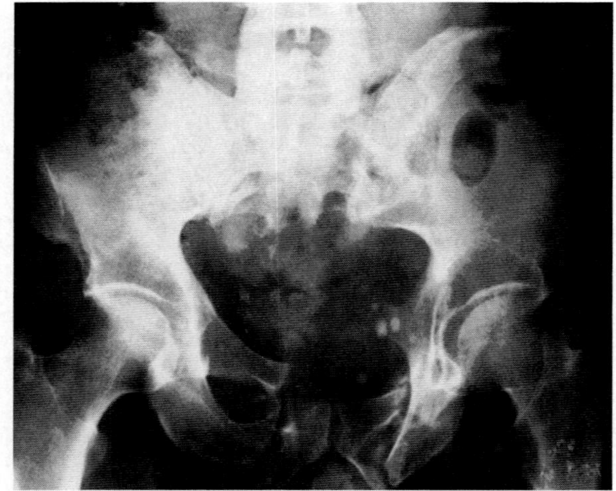

A

FIGURE 13-15. This 42-year-old man was involved in a motor vehicle accident. The anteroposterior radiograph 8 months later shows marked external rotation of the left hemipelvis and ununited fracture anteriorly. The left hemipelvis is shown in an iliac oblique view, the right in an anteroposterior view, indicating approximately 40 degrees of external rotation. This is confirmed by the computed tomography **(B)**, which shows a fracture-dislocation of the ilium with the iliac portion on the anterior border of the sacrum not united. The degree of external rotation of the left hemipelvis is noted. The patient had a lumbosacral nerve injury. Surgery consisted of surgical exposure, open reduction, and plating of the symphysis pubis and the sacroiliac dislocation through an anterior approach **(C)**.

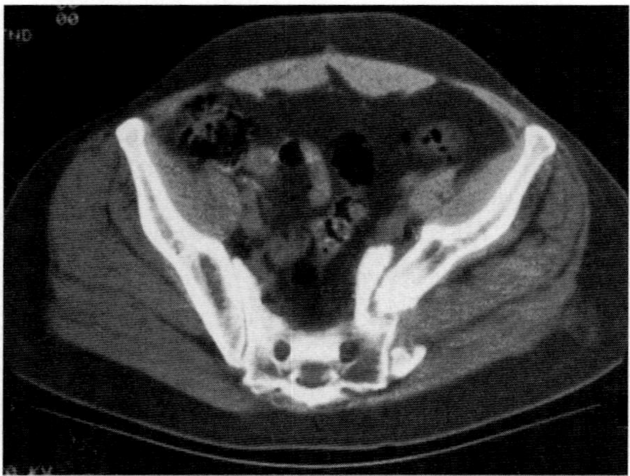

B

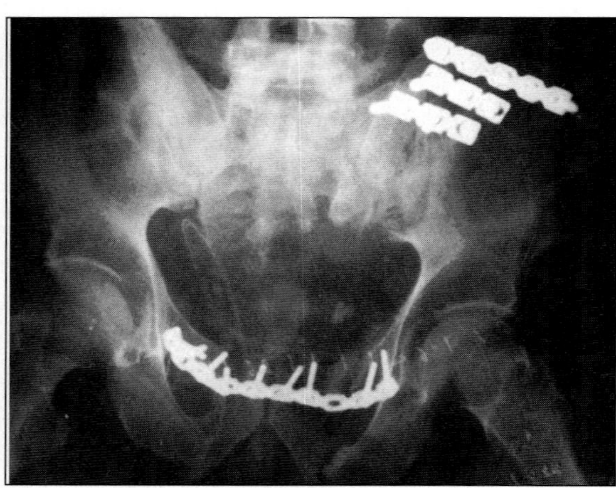

C

Methods of Stabilization

The methods available may be nonoperative or operative.

Nonoperative Methods

These consist of a double hip spica with or without skeletal traction, usually through a pin in the distal femur (Fig. 13-17). None of the nonoperative methods can compress the posterior injury, although a spica cast may reduce pain and traction may hold the fracture in the reduced position (1). Because of all the disadvantages of nursing a polytrauma patient in a hip spica, this method cannot be recommended at this time, although traction is indicated in the acute phase of treatment.

Operative Methods

These consist of the pelvic clamp, external fixation, and open reduction and internal fixation.

The Pelvic Clamp

Several groups have developed a "pelvic clamp," an approach originally suggested in our first edition. This clamp, which is akin to skull tongs for a cervical spine injury, may be applied in the emergency room for grossly unstable pelvic fractures. Some of the existing clamps are attached to the iliac crest, others just superior to the superior gluteal notch. Local anesthesia is usually preferred. Image intensification is useful for the attachment of these clamps. Applying a clamp in the emergency room, thus achieving partial stability in the unstable pelvis, is desirable for all of the reasons previously given. These clamps are temporary, and when the patient's general condition allows more definitive means of stabilization are used. These clamps are presently in the experimental stage only, but they show promise (Fig. 13-18).

External Fixation

External fixators have a major role in the early management of an unstable pelvic disruption in a polytrauma patient, es-

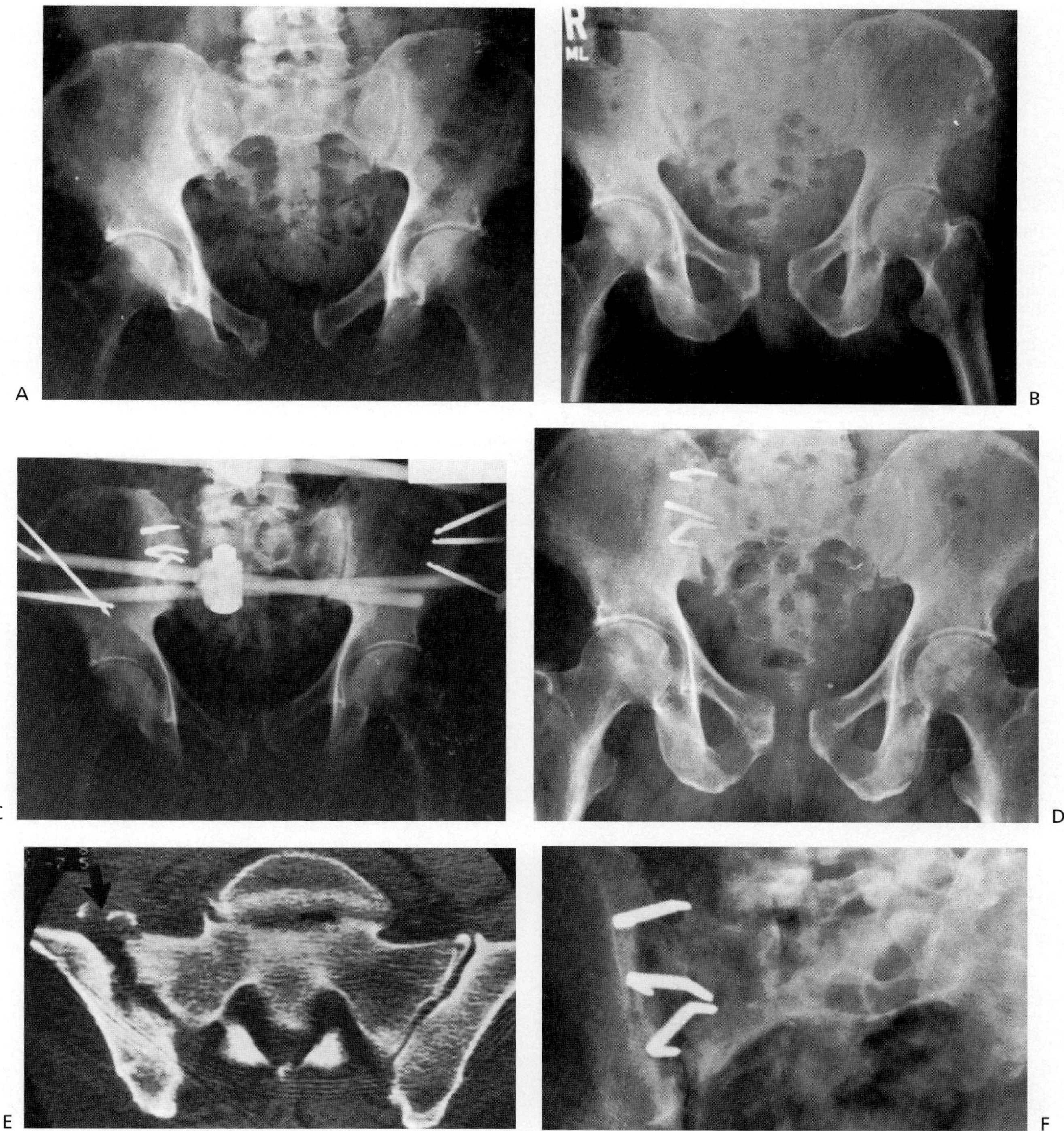

FIGURE 13-16. A: A 69-year-old man sustained an unstable shear injury to the right hemipelvis. **B:** He was treated with an external frame, but on removal of the frame at 10 weeks, he continued to exhibit motion at the symphysis pubis and complained of pain at the right sacroiliac joint. Therefore, an open bone grafting procedure was carried out anteriorly, supplemented with staples across the sacroiliac joint. **C:** External skeletal fixation was applied again. Note the displacement at the symphysis pubis, indicating that this is not a stable open-book fracture but an unstable shear injury. **D:** After removal of the pins, the nonunion was still clearly evident. This is best noted on computed tomography **(E)** and the oblique radiograph **(F).**

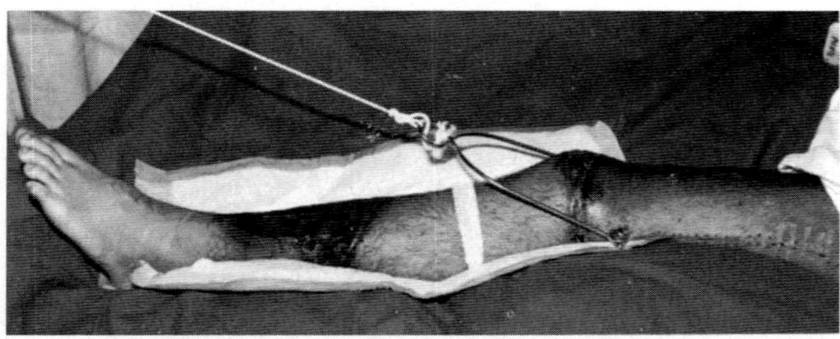

FIGURE 13-17. Skeletal traction may be maintained by a pin inserted in the supracondylar area of the femur. The pin must be inserted posteriorly, so as not to enter the knee joint through the suprapatellar pouch. Pins that perforate the pouch may result in local inflammation in the knee joint and marked limitation of flexion. This particular patient, as well as having an acetabular fracture that required traction, had an open femoral fracture, quadriceps tendon laceration, and open fracture of his tibia.

pecially one who is hemodynamically unstable, in spite of the fact that the external skeletal frame cannot fully stabilize the unstable pelvic ring disruption (Fig. 13-19A,B). By cutting the symphysis pubis and the sacrum posteriorly, these fractures have been recreated in our laboratory. Biomechanical studies, discussed in Chapter 11, have shown that the standard external fixator cannot adequately stabilize the unstable pelvic ring, allowing the patient to be fully mobilized. Therefore, attempted ambulation usually results in some loss of reduction (Fig. 13-19C,D). Some stability may be achieved by using the intact hemipelvis as a pillar in the unilateral types, but the anterior frame cannot restore posterior stability in the bilateral types.

Refinements in the external fixator (5) have slightly improved their performance, but because of their increased complexity they have little place in acute fracture management (Johnston RM, personal communication). They are difficult to apply; some require open pin insertion; the hip joint may be violated; and, most important, the minimal

A B C D

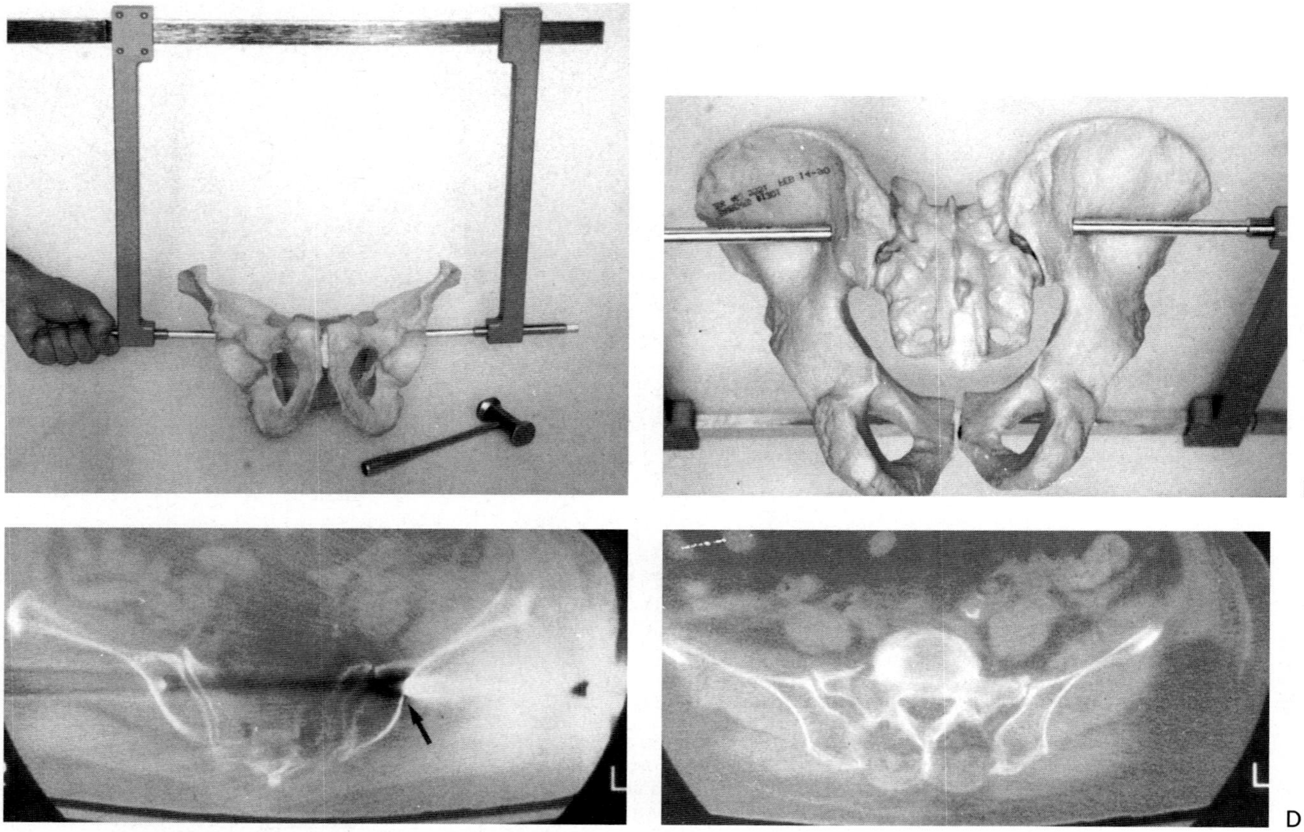

FIGURE 13-18. The AO pelvic clamp **(A)** is applied in the axis of the sacroiliac joints by hammering the spikes into the outer table of the ilium **(B).** Compression can then be obtained across the posterior lesion, stabilizing the pelvic ring, as noted in the computed tomography **(C).** This woman sustained a markedly displaced sacral fracture and had uncontrollable bleeding from the retroperineal space. Application of the clamp *(black arrow)* **(C)** allowed restoration of the posterior sacral fracture and stabilization of the patient, who survived **(D).**

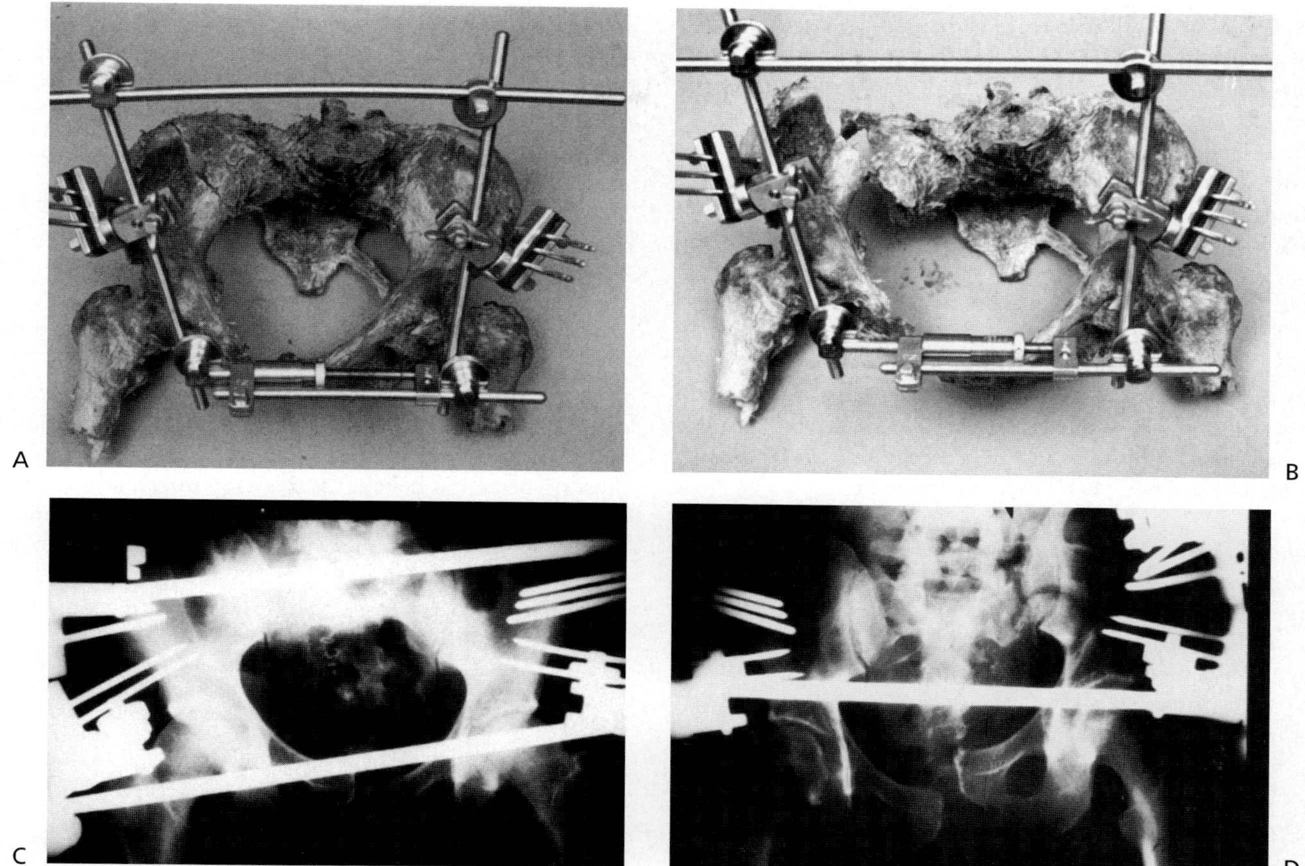

FIGURE 13-19. This cadaver specimen used in our biomechanical tests has had its symphysis pubis divided, and a fracture of the right ilium was created. The sacrotuberous and sacrospinous ligaments were also removed, creating an unstable vertical shear-type injury. **A:** It was fixed with a rectangular frame. **B:** In spite of this anterior fixation, considerable movement and displacement of the posterior lesion is seen, verifying the fact that the standard external skeletal frames cannot fully stabilize an unstable pelvic disruption (see Chapter 14). Application of an anterior external frame across an unstable pelvis does not prevent displacement if the patient is ambulated. As illustrated, the patient in **(C)** sustained a Type C unstable sacral fracture treated with a double cluster frame and no traction. The patient was allowed out of bed on the second postoperative day. Note the complete redisplacement of the left hemipelvis through the posterior fracture *(black arrow)* and the symphysis pubis **(D)**. An anterior external skeletal frame cannot stabilize a Type C pelvic disruption without additional skeletal fixation or internal fixation, as noted in the biomechanical studies and the clinical cases.

biomechanical advantage is not worth the added risk to the patient. Some modifications that improve the biomechanics of the external frame include larger skeletal pins, better placement of the pins, and better clamps.

The major advantages of the external frame in acute polytrauma are not biomechanical but biologic. Application of the frame allows some reduction of the fracture or dislocation, thus reducing the volume of the true pelvis. Blood loss is reduced by restoration of the tamponade effect of the bony pelvis. It should be applied before laparotomy if retroperitoneal hemorrhage is more likely than intraperitoneal bleeding. Because the anterior frame alone cannot stabilize the unstable pelvis, a femoral traction pin should be inserted and 30 pounds of traction applied (Fig. 13-17). This should in no way hinder early resuscitation and has the major benefit of maintaining the pelvic reduction until more definitive means of stabilization may be applied safely.

Internal Fixation

Internal fixation of fractures has been placed on a sound scientific basis. As well, stabilization of diaphyseal fractures, particularly the femur, early in the resuscitation phase, has been beneficial both for the patient and fracture (6). During the past decade, internal fixation of unstable pelvic ring disruptions has been the subject of much interest. Internal fixation of the unstable pelvis offers many advantages, but must be done by experienced surgeons to avoid complications, especially nerve and vessel injury.

Benefits of Internal Fixation. The benefits of internal fixation are considerable (see Chapter 15). Biomechanically, internal fixation of the anterior and posterior lesions can restore full pelvic ring stability. This rapidly eliminates the patient's pain and allows early mobilization. Nursing care is greatly facilitated. Also, early restoration of pelvic anatomy reduces bleeding from bone surfaces and restores the tamponade effect of the pelvic ring. As well, nonunion, malunion, and leg length discrepancy should be eliminated or greatly reduced to improve patient outcomes.

Risks of Internal Fixation. However, there may be major risks that need to be weighed against the potential benefits. These risks, which were more theoretical at the time of the early editions of this book, are now carefully documented in the literature. The risks include the following.

Hemorrhage. Bleeding has proven to be more a theoretical than practical risk, and is rarely described. Bleeding from a previously clotted superior gluteal artery is one potential hazard that has occurred. At the time of fracture the artery may be disrupted, then it clots. At the time of open reduction with dissection around the greater sciatic notch, the clot may dislodge. At that time, as a result of having the entire blood volume replaced with bank blood, the patient may have a faulty clotting mechanism that allows massive hemorrhage. If the superior gluteal artery is noted to be cut off at the time of angiography, then it must be embolized with a permanent metal coil to prevent rebleeding or intraoperative clot dislodgement.

Nerve Injury. Nerve injury, a frequent complication of internal fixation of the pelvis, occurs in different circumstances. First, reduction posteriorly of a grossly unstable sacral fracture may compress the L5 or S1 nerve root, causing permanent neurologic damage in either root. This has occurred even when the sacral foramina have been anatomically reduced. The L5 nerve root is also in jeopardy in anterior approaches to the sacroiliac joint, where they may be damaged by retractors or implants, and the sacral nerve roots, especially S1, may be damaged by screw fixation across the sacroiliac joint penetrating the sacral foramina. Also, drills, screws, and transiliac bars have been put into the cauda equina, causing neurologic catastrophes.

Injury to the Great Vessels. Drills and screws can penetrate the anterior aspect of the sacrum and damage the common iliac artery or vein.

Skin Necrosis and Sepsis. The posterior and vertical displacement of Type C unstable pelvic ring injuries usually severely damages the posterior soft tissues, and the fascia overlying the gluteus maximus may be torn, limiting the blood supply to the overlying skin even further. The posterior skin may be crushed. These two factors lead to a high incidence of skin necrosis with posterior approaches. This is now being reported in 18% to 40% of cases (7), and is especially common with crush injuries. Skin necrosis often leads to secondary sepsis.

Controversies in Internal Fixation. These risks have left many unanswered questions, and many centers are now attempting to answer them. The following issues remain.

Timing of Surgery. When is the best time for internal fixation? Two early articles have described immediate internal fixation of fractures (8,9,10). They have recommended preoperative angiography, and both reported a high complication rate, especially wound breakdown and sepsis. There was almost no perceived benefit for this early intervention. However, Routt and colleagues in a recent study recommended fixation where possible, in the first 24 hours, with no adverse side effects. With the advent of closed techniques, internal fixation should be done at the earliest possible time that the patient's general state allows.

Surgical Options

Anterior Injury

If the anterior injury is through the symphysis pubis, internal fixation across the symphysis is highly recommended, because the anterior part of the pelvic ring would be stabilized, thus simplifying the management of the patient. If the anterior strut of the pelvis is restored in this manner, an added external skeletal frame achieves compression of the posterior complex. Therefore, stabilization of the symphysis by dual plating is recommended for unstable pelvic ring disruptions associated with a symphysis disruption if posterior injury cannot be addressed surgically (Fig. 13-20).

If the anterior injury is through the pubic rami, internal fixation is also possible. If the rami fractures are medial enough to be reached through a Pfannenstiel incision, open reduction and internal fixation are desirable. However, if the fractures are lateral and require an ilioinguinal approach, management is best directed to the posterior injury, the anterior being controlled by an external frame.

In expert hands, closed reduction and closed screw fixation of the superior rami fractures under image intensification also may be done (see Chapter 15) (11).

Recent biomechanical work in our laboratory supports the importance of anterior fixation in overall pelvic stability and simplified overall patient management (see Chapter 11) (11).

Posterior Injury

The greatest number of questions remain unanswered in the management of the posterior injury.

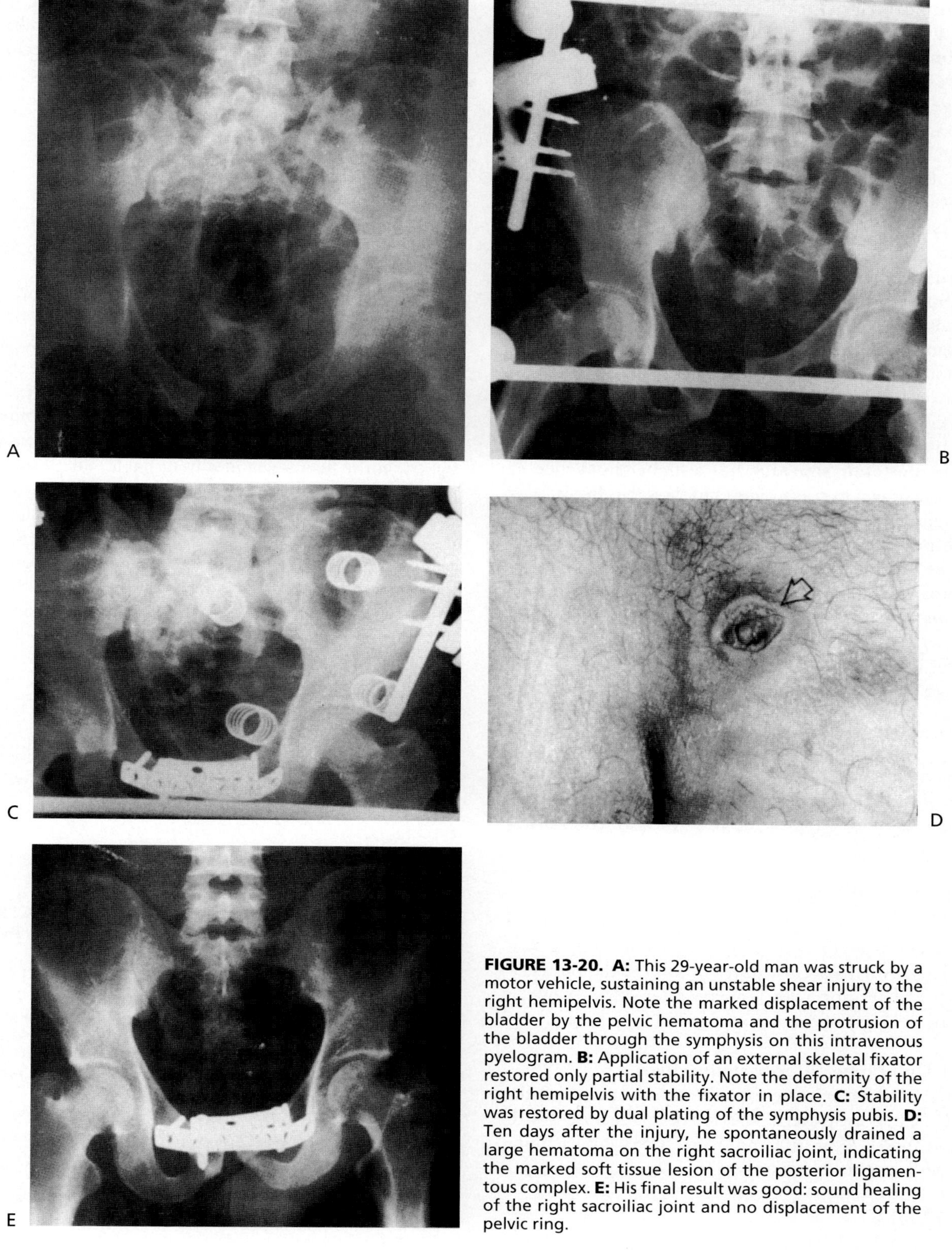

FIGURE 13-20. A: This 29-year-old man was struck by a motor vehicle, sustaining an unstable shear injury to the right hemipelvis. Note the marked displacement of the bladder by the pelvic hematoma and the protrusion of the bladder through the symphysis on this intravenous pyelogram. **B:** Application of an external skeletal fixator restored only partial stability. Note the deformity of the right hemipelvis with the fixator in place. **C:** Stability was restored by dual plating of the symphysis pubis. **D:** Ten days after the injury, he spontaneously drained a large hematoma on the right sacroiliac joint, indicating the marked soft tissue lesion of the posterior ligamentous complex. **E:** His final result was good: sound healing of the right sacroiliac joint and no displacement of the pelvic ring.

Percutaneous versus Open Techniques

During the past decade, because of the high rate of posterior wound breakdown, percutaneous techniques have been described for fixing the posterior lesion. This may be done under image intensification or CT control (12). These procedures in expert hands have produced good stabilization of sacroiliac dislocations and sacral fractures, and with almost none of the wound complications discussed in the preceding. The overall complication rate is relatively low, and the methods should be performed only in centers with much expertise in pelvic trauma. The use of cannulated screws has greatly simplified this method.

For dislocations and fracture dislocations of the sacroiliac joint, should the surgical approach be anterior or posterior? The advantage of the anterior approach relates to ease of exposure and virtually no wound breakdown. The disadvantage is the proximity to the L5 nerve root, which may be damaged.

Reduction of the dislocation may be easier through one approach or the other, depending on the exact fracture pattern. The posterior approach has a higher incidence of wound breakdown in crush injuries to the pelvis but is valuable in a fracture dislocation where the split is in the coronal plane through the posterior superior spine (crescent fracture). The potential for nerve injury is present with posterior approaches; therefore, the technique must be performed with extreme care under image intensification, as outlined in Chapter 15.

Methods of Posterior Fixation

See Chapter 15.

Iliac Fractures

Standard techniques of open reduction and internal fixation, using lag screws and/or 3.5-mm reconstruction plates are preferred.

Sacroiliac Joint Dislocations

Through an anterior approach the sacroiliac joint is fixed with a square plate or two 3.5-mm dynamic compression (DC) plates. Alternative treatment would be the posterior approach and fixation with lag screws into the ala of the sacrum or the body of the sacroiliac joint.

Fracture Dislocation of the Sacroiliac Joint

Either the anterior or posterior approach, is used, as indicated by the fracture pattern. Fixation of the fracture is with lag screws and/or reconstruction plates. The sacroiliac joint is fixed with anterior plates or posterior screws into the ala.

Sacral Fractures

See Fig. 13-25. Placing transiliac bars from one posterior superior iliac spine to the other is a safe and effective method. Alternatively, lag screws may be inserted directly across the fracture into the body of the sacrum under image intensification. Combination fixation including plating and iliosacral or transiliac screws are also effective stabilization. Recently, Pohlemann has applied direct plating techniques to the sacrum supplemented with anterior fixation.

Indications for Open Reduction and Internal Fixation of the Unstable (Type C) Pelvic Disruption

See Table 13-2.

Anterior Fixation

Symphysis Pubis Fixation

If the patient is undergoing laparotomy, and no fecal contamination is present, anterior fixation of a symphysis pubis disruption or medial rami fractures greatly simplifies further care of the patient. In the presence of fecal contamination, external fixation is preferable. In the emergency situation, if the patient is hemodynamically unstable, the posterior injury should be controlled with an external frame, after anterior internal fixation. This is a biomechanically sound construct. Anterior fixation of the disrupted symphysis pubis also is recommended, even if laparotomy is not being performed, in order to stabilize the anterior pelvis. In that situation, the timing may be delayed, at the discretion of the surgeon (Fig. 13-20).

Pubic Rami Fixation

Widely displaced pubic rami are rare indications for open reduction and internal fixation, because they may not heal in that circumstance. Other surgical indications include a ramus fracture associated with a femoral nerve or artery tear (Fig. 13-21), and/or a fractured ramus that protrudes into the vagina.

TABLE 13-2. INDICATIONS FOR OPEN REDUCTION AND INTERNAL FIXATION OF UNSTABLE (TYPE C) PELVIC DISRUPTIONS

Anterior (symphysis or rami)
To improve pelvic stability in association with laparotomy acutely (no fecal contamination or suprapubic tube) or for simplified fracture management (acute or semiacute phase)
Rami fractures associated with lesion of femoral artery or femoral nerve
Bone protruding into perineum (tilt fracture in female)
Associated anterior acetabular fracture that requires open reduction and internal fixation
Posterior
Inadequate reduction of posterior sacroiliac complex (especially sacroiliac dislocation) >1 cm displacement
Open fracture with a posterior wound (rarely for perineal wound)
Associated posterior acetabular fracture that requires open reduction and internal fixation

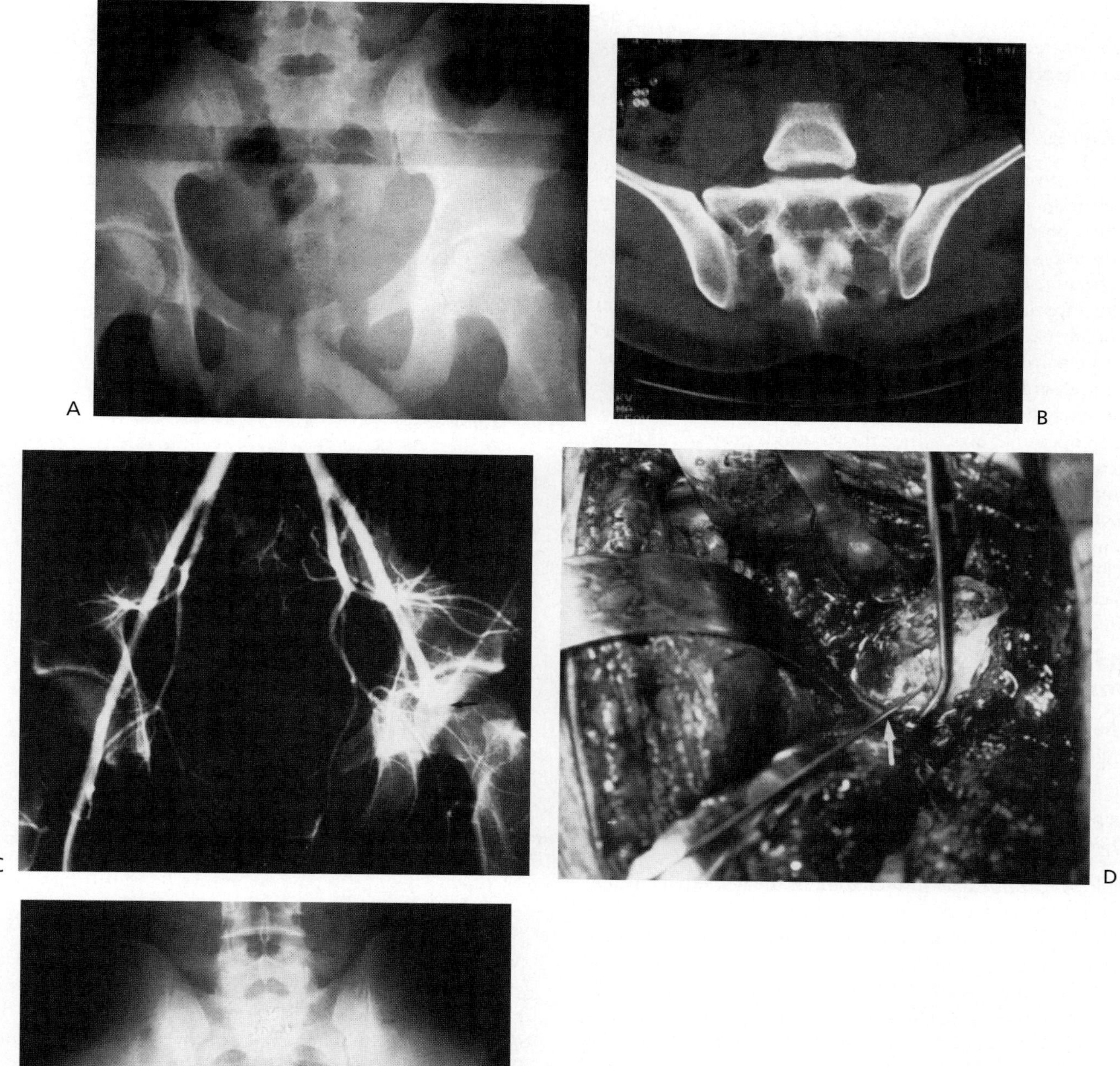

FIGURE 13-21. A: This patient sustained a direct blow to the groin, resulting in a displaced fracture through the left superior rami and inferior rami bilaterally and partial disruption of the symphysis. **B:** No posterior injury was noted on computed tomography; therefore, this is an unusual four-pillar anterior fracture from a direct blow with no posterior disruption. The patient's left leg was pulseless. **C:** Subsequent aortography shows a complete block in the external iliac artery *(black arrow)*. **D:** At surgery an intimal tear was noted in the artery. This was repaired, the fracture was reduced temporarily using a Kirschner wire *(white arrow)*. **E:** The final fixation was accomplished with a superior ramus reconstruction plate.

Finally, an unstable pelvic ring with an anterior-type acetabular fracture requiring open reduction and internal fixation should be fixed internally.

Posterior Fixation

For the posterior injury, the major indication for posterior open reduction and internal fixation is an unreduced, unstable, posterior sacroiliac complex, especially a sacroiliac dislocation. The posterior displacement should be >1 cm. Alternative treatment is an external fixator and skeletal traction, especially as emergency care for a hemodynamically unstable patient. In rare circumstances, open reduction cannot be performed because the general condition of the patient does not allow, then skeletal traction and external fixation may become definitive care.

In open fractures, where the wound is posterior over the sacroiliac joint, immediate fixation is desirable, and open wound care postoperatively. For open perineal wounds, however, internal fixation should not be used, only external frames. Posterior internal fixation also may be required for pelvic disruption associated with a posterior type acetabular fracture.

Management Protocol for Unstable Fractures

The following management protocol for unstable pelvic ring disruption is recommended (Fig. 13-22).

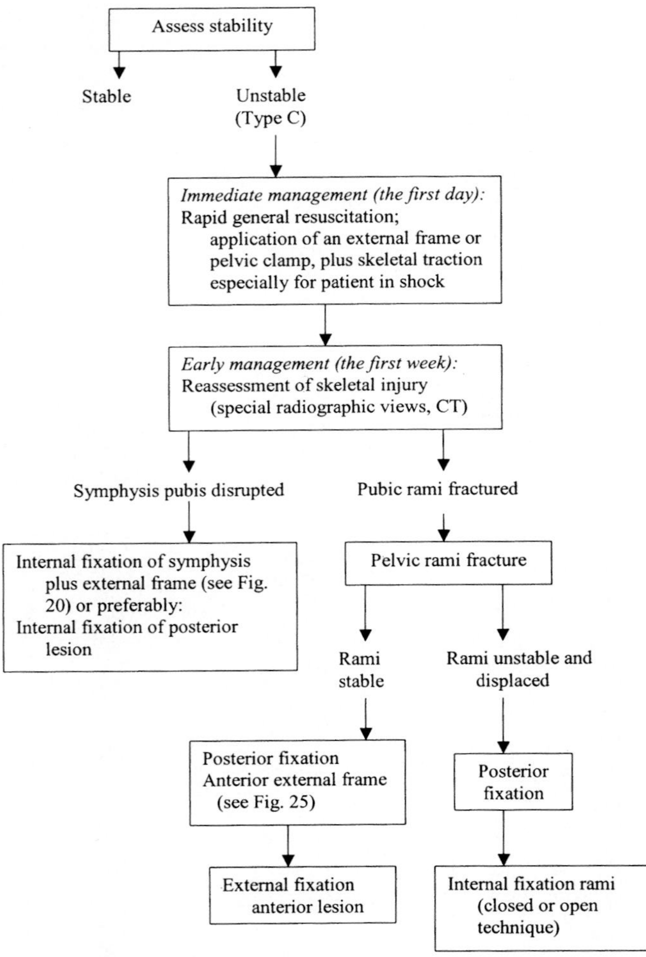

FIGURE 13-22. Algorithm showing management protocol for unstable pelvic ring disruption.

Immediate Management: The First Day: The Phase of Provisional Fixation

Following immediate resuscitation of the hemodynamically unstable patient and a careful assessment of the injury pattern, application of a simple external skeletal fixator or a pelvic clamp is recommended for the patient with an unstable pelvic ring disruption. Provisional fracture stabilization belongs in the resuscitative phase of management. Depending on the associated injury and the need for mobilization, the frame should be applied as early as is practical following the injury, usually when the patient is given an anesthetic for management of visceral injuries. Although an anterior external fixator cannot restore full stability to an unstable pelvis, it does have many advantages (already outlined). A femoral traction pin with 20- to 30-lb weights should be added to maintain reduction of the hemipelvis.

For patients undergoing laparotomy, and if there is no fecal contamination or a suprapubic tube is in place, open reduction and internal fixation of a disrupted symphysis or medial rami fractures restores some pelvic stability and anatomy and is very helpful. The addition of an external frame is biomechanically sound and may serve as definitive management for that particular injury.

If the patient is *hemodynamically stable* and the surgeon is planning anterior open reduction and internal fixation, *an external fixator is not used;* reduction is maintained with femoral traction, because operating secondarily through pin tracts may increase the risk of sepsis. In this scenario, the open reduction should be done as early as the patient's condition allows.

The unstable pelvic fracture must not be neglected during this early phase of treatment. We have learned, in the management of long bone fractures, that *what is good for the fracture is also good for the patient.* This is no less true of pelvic injury.

Early Management: The First Week: The Phase of Definitive Fixation

Following anterior skeletal fixation or skeletal traction, a careful clinical and radiographic assessment of the anterior injury should be carried out. This should be done as early as the patient's condition allows, usually within the first few days, and should include all of the standard pelvic radiographs as well as CT.

The options for definitive fixation of a completely unstable pelvis include complex external fixation, with or without skeletal traction and/or open reduction and internal fixation of the anterior or posterior pelvic ring.

Complex Frames

Complex frames have a biomechanical advantage over simple ones, but none can restore enough stability to the pelvis to allow the patient to ambulate without loss of reduction (see Chapter 14). Therefore, because the added risks of the procedure do not materially increase the benefit to the patient, they cannot be recommended.

Skeletal Traction

In the emergency situation, especially in a polytrauma patient, the combination of an anterior skeletal frame with skeletal traction affords the surgeon a safe and effective method of treatment. As much as 20 kg traction is often required through a supracondylar traction pin to maintain the posterior sacroiliac complex in the reduced position. A polytrauma patient's course is unpredictable. For example, the patient may become septic, so that further surgical intervention to the pelvis is contraindicated. The anterior frame plus skeletal traction might then become definitive treatment. This is especially true when adequate reduction of the posterior sacroiliac complex is achieved or when the posterior injury is a fracture. For traction to be successful, it must be maintained a minimum of 8 to 12 weeks and monitored carefully by radiographs (Fig. 13-23).

A long period of enforced bed rest, with its inherent risks for the polytrauma patient, is the major disadvantage of this form of treatment. Open reduction and internal fixation of

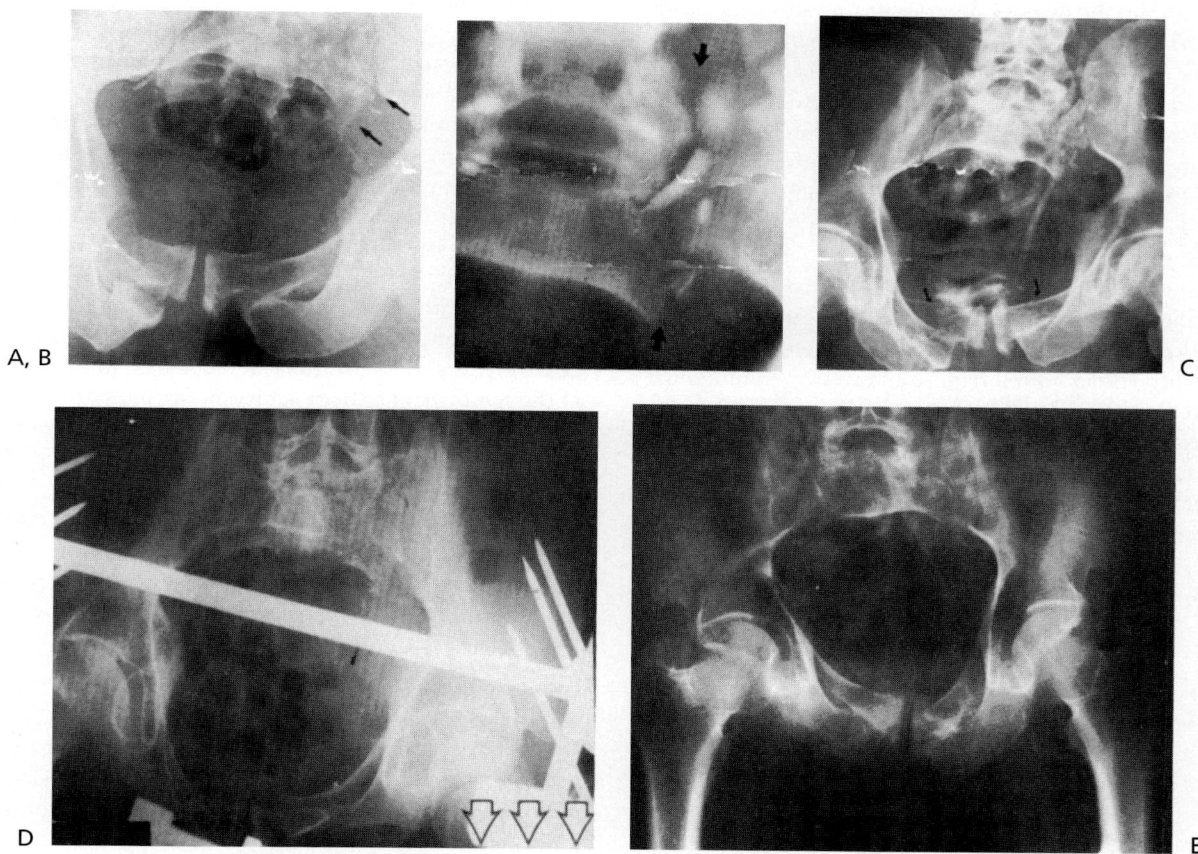

FIGURE 13-23. A 59-year-old man involved in a motor vehicle accident sustained a complex unstable fracture of hemipelvis. **A:** The two *black arrows* on the inlet view show the amount of posterior displacement of the left hemipelvis. The anterior portion of the symphysis pubis has been avulsed by the contracting rectus abdominis muscle. The remainder of the symphysis is widely displaced. **B:** A tomogram through the left sacroiliac joint shows the marked disruption through the sacrum. The upper black arrow indicates an avulsion of the transverse process of L5, always indicative of gross posterior pelvic instability. **C:** The intravenous pyelogram shows the massive left retroperitoneal hematoma. This patient also sustained a lumbosacral nerve plexus lesion. **D:** Because this was an isolated lesion, an external fixator was applied and the patient was placed in left skeletal traction, as noted in the inlet radiograph. Note the amount of distraction of the hip joint and the good posterior reduction. **E:** The patient remained in this position for 10 weeks, during which time the anterior and posterior lesions both healed in satisfactory position. He recovered his S1 root function but had a permanent L5 nerve root deficit. He has no symptoms referable to the pelvic ring disruption.

the completely unstable pelvic ring may be the preferred option in selected patients.

Open Reduction and Internal Fixation

The risks and benefits of open reduction and internal fixation were previously described under methods of stabilization.

Anterior Internal Fixation

Symphysis Disruption

If the anterior lesion is a disruption through the symphysis pubis, fixation of the symphysis pubis greatly facilitates management, especially if a patient is undergoing a surgical procedure or laparotomy, except in the presence of fecal contamination or a suprapubic tube. This procedure is recommended even if laparotomy is not performed, because it much simplifies the management of the unstable pelvis with minimal risk. Anatomic reduction and stabilization of the symphysis restores the normal anterior anatomy of the pelvis and at least partial stability to the ring, but it does not completely restore posterior stability. Adequate internal fixation of the symphysis is achieved by using methods described in Chapter 15, which restore the anterior anatomy of the ring.

Pubic Ramus Fractures

Pubic ramus fractures placed medially so that they can be reached through Pfannenstiel incision also should be fixed internally at this time. Laterally placed pubic ramus fractures are difficult and often require an extensive ilioinguinal approach. In those particular unstable situations it is more advantageous to fix the posterior lesions and control the ramus fractures with an anterior external frame.

Percutaneous screw fixation across rami fractures is another technique done to restore stability to the anterior pelvis (10). Also, using an extraperitoneal approach (Stoppa), rami fractures may be stabilized by a long plate (13).

Posterior Internal Fixation. After adequate internal fixation of the symphysis pubis or pubic rami, the posterior lesion must be assessed carefully. The posterior lesion may be unilateral or bilateral.

Management of the Posterior Lesion After Anterior Fixation

Unilateral Posterior Disruption.

Addition of External Fixation. If the unstable hemipelvis disrupts one posterior sacroiliac complex only, leaving the other one intact, the unstable hemipelvis may be fixed against the intact stable one, which acts as a strut or post. Therefore, following anterior plating of the symphysis pubis or rami, the application of an external fixator may stabilize the posterior injury, thus restoring adequate stability to the pelvic ring, provided the reduction is adequate (Fig. 13-20). A good result may be expected with this management; however, internal fixation is a much more common approach to these injuries.

Addition of Posterior Internal Fixation. Displaced, unstable posterior injuries are best managed by techniques of internal fixation, either open or closed.

Anterior approaches also may be used for iliac fractures and sacroiliac dislocations, because they can be done simultaneously with the patient in the supine position. Conventional wisdom today favors percutaneous iliosacral screw insertion under fluoroscopic guidance for most indications in either the supine or prone position. We favor fixing the anterior lesion first, especially the symphysis as it helps with the posterior reduction.

Bilateral Posterior Disruption. Anterior disruption in the pelvic ring and a bilateral posterior complex disruption represent the most unstable type of pelvic injury. As in the unilateral injury, internal fixation of the disrupted symphysis pubis much facilitates management of the patient; although posterior stability may not be adequate even with an anterior external fixator in place and adequate internal fixation of the symphysis. Although other methods are available to complete the posterior stabilization, such as plaster spica or bed rest with traction, most often open reduction posteriorly is used. The circumstances of the individual case dictate the treatment.

Nonoperative methods are rarely indicated for an isolated bilateral-type pelvic disruption and are used if further posterior surgery is contraindicated. Once internal fixation of the symphysis has been achieved, further stability may be achieved by skeletal traction, which will reduce movement at the posterior fracture site, thus reducing pain. Although imperfect with respect to complete stabilization, it nevertheless offers an alternative to open surgery in conditions that are less than ideal and for patients for whom surgery is contraindicated. At this time plaster casts have a very limited role in these cases, in civilian trauma practice.

Indications for Posterior Open Reduction and Internal Fixation

Because the posterior injury is most important for restoring pelvic ring stability, careful assessment of the posterior injury is mandatory, with or without anterior fixation (Table 13-2).

Indications for operation for posterior lesions include an unstable unreduced posterior sacroiliac complex, especially an unreduced sacroiliac dislocation with a gap >1 cm (Table 13-2). If fractures (especially through the ilium) are present posteriorly, and the gap is minimal, other methods may suffice, but if the sacroiliac joint is dislocated, open reduction and internal fixation is the preferred option.

In the rare instances when the posterior sacroiliac complex is disrupted and the posterior skin has been lacerated, immediate posterior internal fixation may be done, because the wound is already open. Internal fixation is usually contraindicated if the wound is in the perineum. Treatment should include cleansing and careful debridement of the wound followed by stabilization with an external skeletal frame and skeletal traction. Both bowel and bladder diversion are essential in order to reduce the incidence of sepsis.

If an external fixator is already in place and the anterior reduction is satisfactory at the time of posterior open reduction, it should be left in place to facilitate posterior reduction. If, however, the reduction is unsatisfactory, the fixator should be loosened.

Techniques of Posterior Internal Fixation

The type of internal fixation depends on the pathoanatomy of the injury and on whether the lesion is unilateral or bilateral. The precise methods are described in Chapter 15 but are reviewed briefly here, for completeness.

Unilateral.

1. For the *unilateral posterior disruption* the presence of the stable opposite side greatly facilitates the operative procedure, allowing it to be used as a stable post for fixation.
2. For *iliac fractures* (Type C1-1) standard methods of open reduction and internal fixation, using intrafragmental screws and reconstruction plates, are indicated. The 3.5-mm reconstruction plates are much more malleable, allowing easier contouring (Fig. 13-24).
3. For *sacroiliac dislocations* (C1-2), with or without an iliac or sacral fracture, either anterior plating or posterior

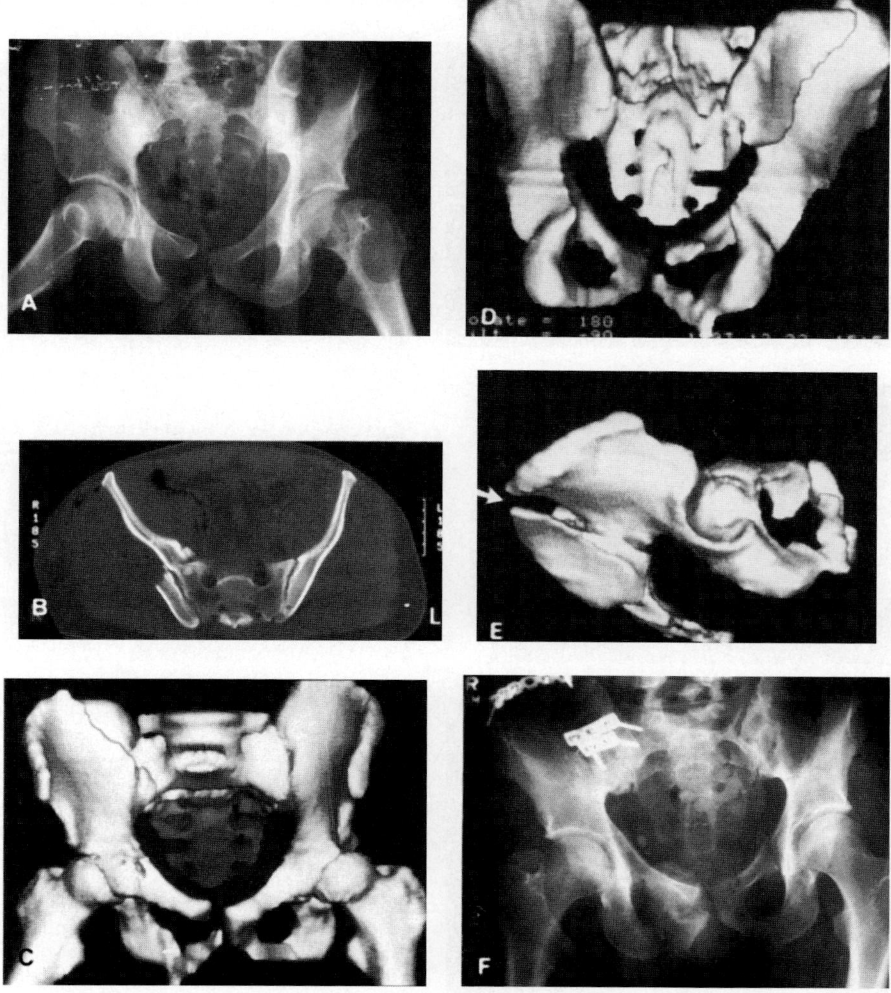

FIGURE 13-24. Unstable Type C pelvic disruption with iliac fracture. **A:** The anteroposterior radiograph shows an injury to the right sacroiliac area and a symphysis disruption with marked displacement of the inferior pubic ramus. **B:** The nature of the posterior lesion is unclear until one examines the axial computed tomography. The iliac wing has been sheared off and lies anterior to the sacrum, in this case injuring the lumbar sacral plexus. **C:** The pattern is clearly noted on the three-dimensional computed tomography, showing the right iliac fracture lying anterior to the sacrum. **D,E:** The same lesion from the posterior aspect. **E:** Note the marked displacement. **F:** The posterior injury was fixed internally through an anterior approach, as noted in the anteroposterior radiograph.

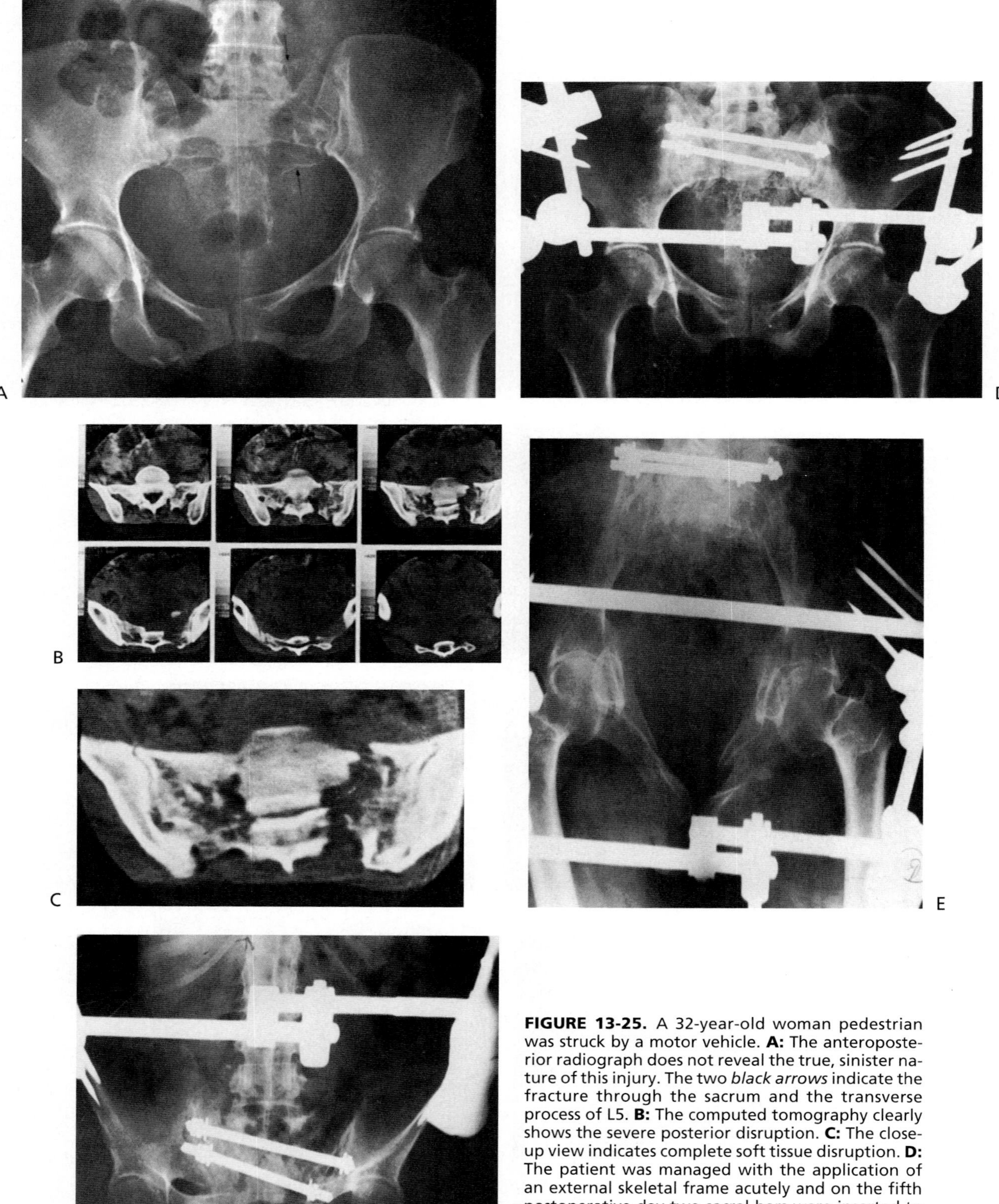

FIGURE 13-25. A 32-year-old woman pedestrian was struck by a motor vehicle. **A:** The anteroposterior radiograph does not reveal the true, sinister nature of this injury. The two *black arrows* indicate the fracture through the sacrum and the transverse process of L5. **B:** The computed tomography clearly shows the severe posterior disruption. **C:** The close-up view indicates complete soft tissue disruption. **D:** The patient was managed with the application of an external skeletal frame acutely and on the fifth postoperative day two sacral bars were inserted to stabilize the sacral fracture, as noted on the anteroposterior **(D)**, inlet **(E)**, and outlet **(F)** radiographs.

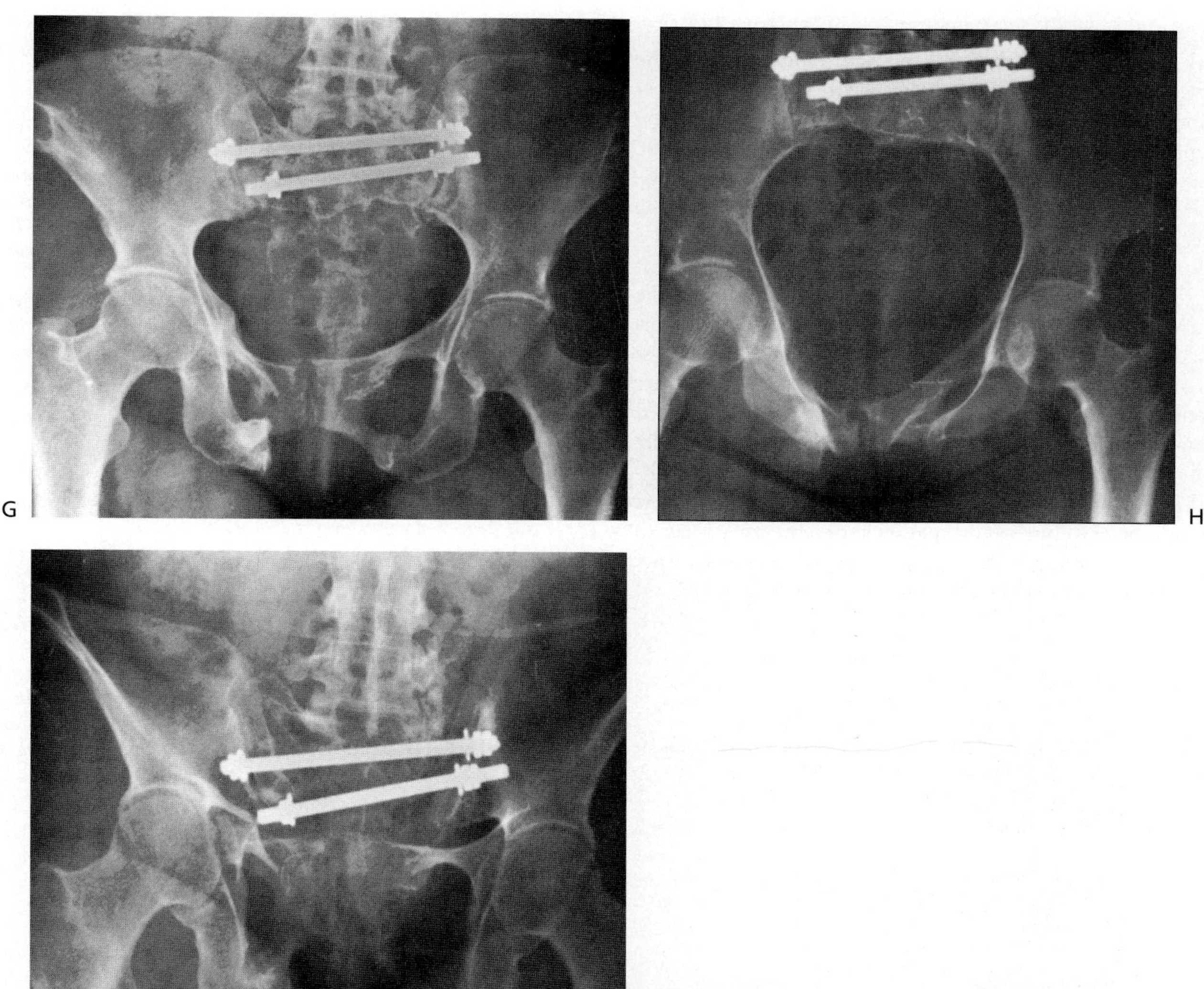

FIGURE 13-25. *(continued)* **G,H,I:** Follow-up at 8 months shows sound union on the three similar radiographic views.

screw fixation of the sacroiliac joint are acceptable depending on patient, injury and surgeon requirements (see Chapter 15). The exact method to be used depends on the configuration of the associated fracture as well. The L5 nerve root is in jeopardy as it crosses the lateral mass of the sacrum and must be protected. Posterior screw fixation provides equally good stability, and in the presence of an iliac fracture is often an easier technique (see Chapter 15). There is the added risk of skin breakdown after a posterior approach. In sacroiliac dislocations this posterior screw method is safe, because the screws need to penetrate only into the lateral mass and not into the body of the sacrum. Closed percutaneous screw fixation of the sacroiliac joint is the preferred method under image intensification.

4. For sacral fractures (Fig. 13-25), two transiliac bars from one posterior iliac spine to the other provide good stability and compression of the sacral fracture with little risk to the neural elements from direct penetration; however, the neural elements can be damaged by compression of the fracture itself. Therefore, care must be taken to avoid overcompression. Posterior screw fixation done under image intensification, either by open or closed methods, is the most frequent option. In this particular situation, because the screws must enter the body of the sacrum, there is an added risk of damage to the sacral nerve roots or cauda equina; therefore, the surgeons must have experience with this technique, and visualization on the image intensifier must be adequate.

Bilateral. In a bilateral posterior disruption (C2 or C3), the only remaining stable structure is the sacrum, so fixation to the sacrum is essential to restore stability.

Again, the methods used depend on the type of posterior injury. If the posterior lesion is a fracture of the ilium, the fracture may be fixed directly by standard techniques of stable internal fixation, usually with small dynamic compression plates or special pelvic reconstruction plates. Anatomic reduction is often possible, which allows the plates to be applied under tension, thus compressing the fracture. If the posterior injury is a sacroiliac dislocation, with or without a small iliac fracture, we favor direct fixation across the joint into the sacrum. This may be achieved by transfixing the joint with lag screws, as described. It must be done bilaterally. Alternatively, a long, heavy plate may be molded across the entire posterior sacroiliac complex bilaterally to restore the tension band in this area (5). The screw must be inserted through the plate and into the sacrum to achieve adequate stability for the axial skeleton. This fixation is again indicated if the posterior injury is a sacral fracture. A transiliac bar could be used but would require supplementary fixation with screws through a plate and across the sacral fracture. Two bars are required to eliminate rotatory instability.

REFERENCES

1. Cotter HB, LaMont JG, Hansen TS. Immediate spica casting for pelvic fractures. *J Orthop Trauma* 1988;2:222.
2. Dalal SA, Burgess AR, Siegel JH, et al. Pelvic fractures in multiple trauma: classification by mechanism is key to pattern or organ injury, resuscitative requirements and outcome. *J Trauma* 1989; 29:981.
3. Bucholz RW. The pathological anatomy of Malgaigne fracture dislocations of the pelvis. *J Bone Joint Surg* 1981;63A:400.
4. Uhthoff HK, Goto S, Cerkel PH. Influence of stable fixation on trabecular bone healing: a morphologic assessment in dogs. *J Orthop Res* 1987;5:14.
5. Mears D. *External skeletal fixation.* Baltimore: Williams & Wilkins, 1982.
6. Johnson KD, Cadambi A, Seibert GB. Incidence of adult respiratory distress syndrome in patients with multiple musculoskeletal injuries: effect of early operative stabilization of fractures. *J Trauma* 1989;25:375.
7. Kellam JF, McMurtry RY, Paley D, et al. The unstable pelvic fracture: operative treatment. *Orthop Clin North Am* 1987;18:25.
8. Ward R, Clark DG. Management of pelvic fractures. *Radiol Clin North Am* 1981;9:167.
9. Goldstein A, et al. Early open reduction and internal fixation of the disrupted pelvic ring. *J Trauma* 1986;26:325.
10. Routt ML Jr, Nork SE, Mills WJ. Percutaneous fixation of pelvic ring disruptions. *Clin Orthop* 2000;(375):15–29.
11. Ebrahim NA, et al. Percutaneous computed tomography stabilization of pelvic fractures: a preliminary report. *J Orthop Trauma* 1987;1:197.
12. Schied DK, Kellam JF, Tile M. Open reduction and internal fixation of pelvic ring fractures. *J Orthop Trauma* 1991;5:226.
13. Hirvelsalo E, Lindahl J, Bostman O. A new approach to the internal fixation of unstable pelvic fractures. *Clin Orthop* 1993 (297):28–32.

14

EXTERNAL FIXATION FOR THE INJURED PELVIC RING

POL M. ROMMENS
MARTIN H. HESSMANN

INTRODUCTION

Although the first reports of the use of external fixators as a treatment method for fractures were published more than 100 years ago, these devices were not used extensively until the 1930s and 1940s (1–3). Subsequently, recurring clinical problems caused external fixation to fall into disrepute in the 1950s and 1960s. External fixation was the object of renewed interest, especially for pelvic disruptions during the 1970s and early 1980s (4–12). However, biomechanical and practical considerations have limited its usefulness while prompting the development of a treatment philosophy and methods that incorporate indications based on musculoskeletal and associated injuries, the patient's physiologic parameters, and the appropriate timing of such treatment (11). Today, external fixation is considered an essential part of the armamentarium of the orthopedic surgeon for acute resuscitation of polytraumatized patients with unstable pelvic ring injuries and for definitive treatment of specific fractures in special circumstances (13–15). It also may be used as an adjunct to internal fixation to neutralize rotational forces in the management of completely unstable pelvic ring injuries.

BIOMECHANICS

Stability of external fixation is related to the osteoligamentous instability pattern of the pelvic ring as well as to the characteristics of the fixator itself: frame design, pin location, and size.

Gunterberg and coworkers (16) in the original biomechanical study of pelvic external fixation arrived at the following conclusions.

1. In *bilateral* injuries, stability afforded by the anterior frame does not allow early weight bearing. The same is true for a *unilateral* anterior plus complete posterior injury, such as a sacroiliac dislocation or *vertical* fracture of the ilium or sacrum.
2. *Oblique* unilateral fractures of the sacrum or ilium associated with an anterior fracture may be sufficiently stabilized by an anterior frame to allow early weight bearing.

These authors recognized the deficiency of the anterior frame and related its usefulness to the fracture pattern.

Mears and Fu studied anterior frames, acknowledged their deficiency in stabilizing the unstable pelvic ring disruption, and attempted to solve the problem with through-and-through pins connected to an anterior and posterior fixator (8,17). Stable fixation was obtained, but difficulty with nursing these patients led Mears to abandon this technique. Improvements in the stability of the anterior frame were noted by increasing the pin size to 5 mm, adding a second set of pins anteriorly, and triangulating the bars. Later work by Brown and associates (18) led to the design of a biplanar external fixator with one set of pins placed superiorly through the iliac crest and a second set placed anteriorly into the ilium, starting between the superior and inferior anterior iliac spines (19). Finally, problems in achieving stability in the most difficult cases led Mears to consider internal fixation in combination with external fixation. In his series, the stability of an anterior Slätis frame in combination with posterior transarticular sacroiliac joint screws was equivalent to an intact pelvic ring (17).

Shaw and also Brown and coworkers recognized in their studies that nonanatomic fracture reduction significantly decreased the stability of fixation. They attributed the superior stability associated with anatomic reduction to frictional and interlocking effects at the joint surfaces and fracture sites. These findings were observed with both external and internal fixation (18–20).

McBroom and Tile tested external skeletal fixation, internal fixation, and combinations of internal and external fixation constructs. The fractures tested were: (a) the external rotation open-book variety produced by division of the symphysis pubis and the sacrospinous and anterior sacroiliac ligaments; and (b) the completely unstable type (Type C) produced by dividing the symphysis pubis and the sacrotuberous and sacrospinous ligaments and dislocating the sacroiliac joint. The following types of external fixation frames were tested: for *stable external rotation open-book fractures (Type B1, B3-1),* the trapezoidal frame (Slätis), rectangular frame (several modifications), and the double frame (Mears). For *completely unstable fractures (Type C),* the same frame constructs were used (21).

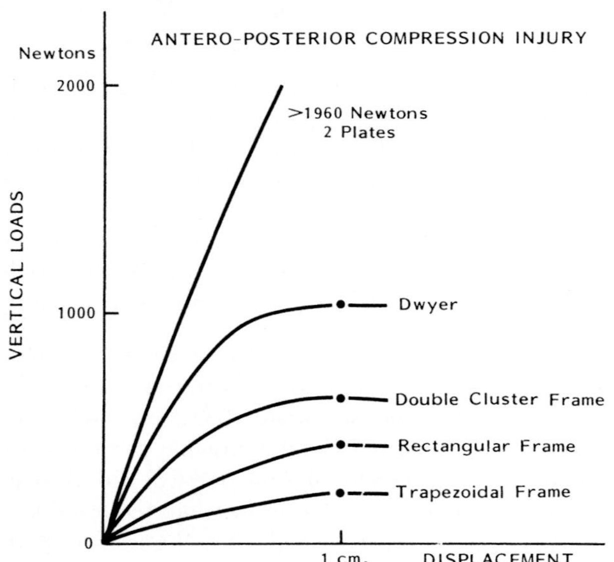

FIGURE 14-1. Results of the biomechanical tests in the typical anteroposterior (open-book) type injury produced in the laboratory by division of the symphysis pubis and anterior sacroiliac ligaments. The posterior tension band of the pelvis was intact. Of the external frames, the double-cluster frame was best, the trapezoidal the weakest. Because 1 kg equals approximately 10 N, both the rectangular and double-cluster frames gave suitable stable fixation for this type of injury.

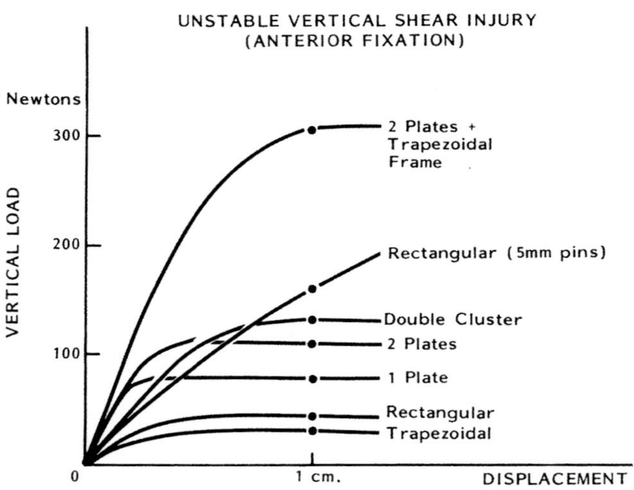

FIGURE 14-2. Graph demonstrates the biomechanical results of the unstable vertical shear injury produced by complete division of the symphysis pubis anteriorly and a fracture of the ilium posteriorly, as well as division of the sacrospinous and sacrotuberous ligaments. Note that the vertical axis is measured in hundreds of newtons, as compared with thousands in the stable configuration. A 100-N load is equal to approximately 10 kg. From this graph, one can see that all forms of anterior fixation fail under 20 kg of load when used to stabilize an unstable vertical shear type pelvic disruption. The best frame tested was one anchored on 5-mm pins with a rectangular configuration and two side bars for triangulation.

These biomechanical studies have shown that, for the rotationally unstable open-book injuries all existing external frames stabilize the pelvic ring enough to allow mobilization of the patient (Fig. 14-1). It must be remembered that the important posterior tension band of the pelvis remains intact in this injury.

In the completely unstable pelvic ring disruption produced by the division of all anterior and posterior structures, no external frame that was tested could adequately stabilize the pelvic ring. The frames were at least able to resist loads in a posterior direction. Changes in pin placement, pin size, and frame design moderately improved the stability of the frames, but not enough to stabilize the pelvis against physiologic loads (Fig. 14-2).

Pohlemann (22) compared the biomechanical properties of external fixation (simple frame with one supraacetabular screw on each side), the pelvic C-clamp according to Ganz (23), and the Browner modification of this clamp (ACE clamp) in an open book rotationally unstable injury and two different completely unstable injuries (a transforaminal sacrum fracture and a pure sacroiliac dislocation). All fixation methods withstood loading with full body weight in the open-book rotationally unstable injury (B-type) lesions. In both the completely unstable (C-type) injuries, the external fixator failed at small loads. Whereas both clamps provided acceptable stability in pure sacroiliac dislocations, no device withstood loads of more than 40 N in the transforaminal fracture model. Therefore, the author suggested enhancement of posterior clamp fixation by an anterior frame in completely unstable (C-type) injuries with transforaminal fracture.

Egbers tested the stability afforded by various AO frame assemblies and differing pin positions (24). Five-millimeter Schanz screws were inserted into the: (a) iliac crest; (b) anterior superior iliac spine; (c) ilium between the anterior superior and anterior inferior iliac spine; and (d) anterior inferior iliac spine. This biomechanical study showed that superior stability was achieved with anteroinferior pin purchase (into the supraacetabular dense bone, between the anterior superior and anterior inferior iliac spine), especially when the screws were directed 30 degrees lateromedially toward the sacroiliac joint. Highest stability was achieved with a self-constructed bow-fixator, which homogeneously distributed pressure on the unstable dorsal pelvic ring.

Kim and Tile (14) studied the effects of pin location on stability with two different external fixator models (Orthofix, Huntersville, NC; and AO tubular fixator, SynthesUSA, Paoli, PA). They found that for both the unstable external rotation open-book injury (Type B1) and the completely unstable (Type C) injuries, the anteroinferior pin location (into the supraacetabular dense bone, between the anterior superior and anterior inferior iliac spine) resulted in significantly lower sacroiliac displacement than did anterosuperior pin placement (into the iliac crest). They concluded that anteroinferior pin insertion provided increased stability of fixation.

It can be concluded from these biomechanical studies that anterior skeletal fixation provides adequate stability in the rotationally unstable (Type B) injuries, but cannot alone stabilize a completely unstable (Type C) injury sufficiently to allow mobilization unless the external fixation is supplemented with posterior internal fixation. In the laboratory, only internal fixation adequately stabilized the unstable shear fracture with sufficient strength and rigidity to safely allow early ambulation (Fig. 14-2). The biomechanical aspects of internal fixation are discussed in Chapter 11. These biomechanical studies furthermore revealed that superior stability of fixation is achieved even with simple frame constructs, when 5-mm instead of 4-mm Schanz screws are used and when these pins are placed into the dense supraacetabular bone at the level of the anterior inferior iliac spine.

Biomechanics Versus Clinical Conditions

Many of the biomechanical studies were designed in response to the clinical and practical problems associated with the inadequacy of an anterior pelvic external fixation for the management of posterior and vertical instability (12,22,24). Efforts to overcome the anterior frame's deficiency included supplemental internal fixation (21,25), new patterns of pin placement and/or new frame designs (11,26). These biomechanical studies yielded conflicting—and confusing—results, which Tile attributed to the variations in the way the investigators attached the cadaver pelves to the testing frames and the fact that most of them did not represent actual weight-bearing skeletal relationships (4). In addition, one should realize that intercurrent injuries and the necessity for timely application in a critically injured patient are frequently far more important than the exact construction of the frame. More recent investigations highlighted the clinical and biomechanical advantages of supraacetabular pin location (13,14,24,27).

In general, biomechanical tests performed on cadavers—although necessary to test frame constructs, pin size and placement, effect of adjunctive fixation, and other features—do not accurately "translate" to the clinical situation for the following reasons.

First, the laboratory situation often utilizes only dissected skeletal elements and their associated ligaments: such dissection sacrifices the stabilizing effect of the patient's soft tissues, including the abdominal, pelvic, paraspinous, and extremity muscles. Ghanayem and coworkers (28) studied the effects of abdominal wall musculature on pelvic ring stability in unilateral open-book lesions, which he created in five fresh cadaveric specimens. His results demonstrated that laparotomy further destabilized an open-book pelvic injury and increased intrapelvic volume. The pubic diastasis increased from 3.9 to 9.3 cm in a nonstabilized pelvis with the abdomen closed and then subsequently opened. He concluded that the abdominal wall provides stability to an unstable pelvic ring via a tension band effect on the iliac wings. An external fixator with one single pin inserted into each iliac wing prevented the destabilizing effects of laparotomy. For the management of the pelvic disruption associated with hemorrhagic shock, the immediate stabilization of the pelvic injury is recommended. In the circumstance where an external fixator can be applied quickly, it is an acceptable form of treatment during the resuscitation. In this role, the mechanical demands on the frame are comparable, not to those of weight bearing or resistance to significant vertical loads, but to more modest mechanical requirements of maintaining the general dimensions of the true pelvis (especially diameter) and of resisting gross movements of fracture fragments, and therefore displacement of clots. *For this reason, many completely unstable injuries are treated with frames augmented with skeletal traction to address the biomechanical limitations of the frame. In these cases, the maintenance of traction should not preclude good pulmonary toilet and wound care.*

Second, pins in the iliac wing are placed under direct vision in the laboratory, ensuring accurate positioning into the bone between its cortical tables. In the clinical situation, such perfect placement of all pins is the exception rather than the rule. Pin placement, by either percutaneous or "open" methods, is often suboptimal with regard to purchase in the ilium (i.e., between the two cortical planes of the iliac wing). In fact, in the Shock Trauma Center experience with a six-pin frame, one of the three pins placed in each crest frequently exits the iliac wing within 2 to 3 cm of its entry portal (29). Other authors recognized improper pin fixation in 18% of their cases and acknowledged that these patients were at risk for pin loosening and loss of reduction of their pelvic fracture (30). Current literature has suggested supraacetabular pin location because the supraacetabular dense bone enables strong pin purchase. Firm pin anchorage and easy orientation also in obese patients provides more effective reduction (14,27).

Third, any evaluation of biomechanical laboratory results must differentiate between frames tested on pelvic rings that are *stable posteriorly* (i.e., with intact posterior sacroiliac ligaments) and on those that are completely unstable (i.e., with both anterior and posterior ligamentous disruption, or a similar fracture pattern).

In the clinical situation, stabilizing a Type B1, B3-1 *rotationally* unstable but vertically stable pelvis requires only the simplest of frames, because the surgeon must, at most, "close the book" of a pelvis injured by external rotation forces. Even less stabilization is required for a pelvis injured by lateral compression or internal rotation forces (Type B2), in which the anterior sacroiliac, sacrotuberous, and sacrospinous ligaments are intact. Because the reduction and fixation of these external and internal rotational injuries requires little in terms of vertical stability from the frame, the simplest frame types suffice to manage such anterior injuries (13,22).

In treating the Type C, *vertically and posteriorly* unstable, disrupted ring, the biomechanical advantages of different frame types are probably not clinically important. Assuming that a frame is practical in terms of nursing and life-saving issues, unfortunately, none of the frames provide optimal mechanical stability for unstable pelvic ring disruptions. It must be noted that all frame constructs provide stability that is biomechanically inferior to that provided by direct internal fixation (screws, plates, transiliac bars, or combinations thereof) of the posterior lesion (Fig. 14-2). After stabilization of the patient's general condition, external fixation may be enhanced or replaced by internal fixation as a staged procedure. These procedures are usually done during the early secondary phase of polytrauma management (13). Retrospective analysis of a large series of 222 patients with unstable pelvic ring injuries revealed that 66% of B-type fractures and 75% of C-type fractures were initially managed by external fixation. The anterior frame was maintained for definitive fixation of the anterior pelvic ring in 52% of B-type and in 55% of C-type injuries. Seventy-three percent of C-type injuries needed additional fixation of the posterior pelvic ring in order to restore normal anatomy and provide sufficient stability for ambulation (13).

Fourth, biomechanical studies do not differentiate between using an external fixator as definitive or acute treatment. In the former situation, the fixator would be placed on a semielective basis for the management of a specific fracture configuration; in the latter, it would be placed under emergency conditions for acute reduction and stabilization of the disrupted pelvic ring in order to reduce the intrapelvic volume and control intrapelvic blood loss as part of the overall resuscitation of a polytrauma victim (31). In the acute situation, issues such as absolute vertical stability and frame design to maximize biomechanical parameters become secondary to ease and alacrity of application, maximization of pin-skeleton interface, constructs that permit access to the abdomen for management of intercurrent injuries (e.g., intraperitoneal visceral injuries), and access to open wounds.

To summarize the studies on biomechanics of external fixators: (a) Most simple type frames provide enough stability to treat Type B rotationally unstable (but vertically stable) injuries of the pelvis. (b) All external fixator frames provide only marginal stability to treat the completely unstable pelvic injuries and alone cannot ensure sufficient stability for weight bearing and ambulation. (c) Supplementation or replacement by open reduction and internal fixation provides superior stability but may not be possible in the acute management phase for clinical reasons.

INDICATIONS

Pelvic external fixation has four indications: (a) for acute-phase management of a patient with severe pelvic disruption, to control hemorrhage and provide provisional stability; (b) for early management of polytrauma patients to facilitate pulmonary toilet and appropriate nursing care and to minimize pain; (c) for definitive management of certain fracture patterns to maintain reduction and enable the patient to sit upright and ambulate (Table 14-1); and (d) for adjunctive use to enhance stability of posterior internal fixation.

In the acutely injured hypotensive patient with significant pelvic disruption, application of an external fixator is based on the results of Advanced Trauma Life Support (ATLS) primary and secondary survey response to treatment and on the evaluation of the initial anteroposterior radiograph of the pelvis (13,32). Physical examination and evaluation of this view results in a determination of the degree and type of instability, if any. Patients whose injuries demonstrate external rotational or rotational, vertical and posterior instability are deemed at high risk for significant local hemorrhage related to the fracture (33) and are candidates for emergent external fixation if in hypotensive shock (see Chapter 8). External fixation is performed before laparotomy in order to avoid deterioration of bleeding in the unstable pelvic ring injury requiring laparotomy (28).

In view of the urgency of this measure, the frame should be relatively simple and of a type that can be applied quickly. One two pins at most should be inserted into the dense supraacetabular bone of each hemipelvis. Preferen-

TABLE 14-1. PELVIC RING FIXATION

	Fixation		
Injury Type[a]	**Emergent**	**Early**	**Definitive**
A (stable)	None	None	None
B1 (open book)	Fixator[b]	Fixator Symphysis plate[c]	External fixation or open reduction and/or anterior plate fixation
B2 (lateral compression)	None	Fixator Symphysis plate[c]	To maintain reduction External fixation, occasionally anterior screw or plate fixation
C (unstable)	Fixator	Fixator	Open reduction and internal fixation (posterior and anterior), or posterior internal fixation with anterior frame

[a]According to Tile's classification.
[b]In presence of hemodynamic instability, polytrauma, or significant peripelvic soft-tissue damage.
[c]If abdomen is already open and there is no visceral contamination.

tially this should be done under fluoroscopic control in order to guarantee proper and stable pin purchase and avoid penetration of the hip joint (see Methods). The application of an external fixator should not delay subsequent laparotomy. Although the anterior inferior spine placement is ideal, in the acute situation it may be much easier to insert one pin in each crest 2 to 3 cm posterior to the anterior superior iliac spine.

The second indication for the use of external fixation of the pelvic ring is a pelvic fracture in a polytrauma patient. Although the pelvic injury might be one of the less severe types (e.g., the lateral compression injury, Type B2), which could be managed conservatively as an isolated injury, external fixation is recommended in such a patient for management of pain and pulmonary toilet as well as overall patient mobility.

External fixation also plays an important role in stabilizing unstable pelvic ring injuries with severe concomitant peripelvic soft-tissue or organ damage. Internal fixation has an increased risk for septic complications in these patients; therefore, it might be contraindicated in the initial management phase. External fixation under these circumstances is an adequate alternative for internal fixation until better soft-tissue conditions allow definitive stabilization.

In both these indications it is imperative that the reason for application is appropriately thought out, because the potential for pin tract sepsis may preclude the use of internal fixation for definitive treatment of the injury.

The third indication is for *definitive* management of an open-book or externally rotated pelvis (Type B1), an internally rotated pelvis (Type B2) or a more unstable fracture pattern (Type C). The external fixator is indicated in such cases to reduce the fracture or to reduce and maintain fixation of transpubic instability in the rotationally and/or completely unstable hemipelvis.

For patients with pure open-book lesions (Type B1) *internal* fixation (anterior plating) might be the method of choice after reduction of the pubic symphysis, but it may be precluded by other injuries, local wound conditions, or coagulopathy. In these cases, external fixation is a viable alternative, especially in symphysis disruptions that are anatomically reduced with external fixation alone. The internally rotationally unstable injury (bucket handle equivalent lateral compression injury) produces an unacceptable pelvic malunion if allowed to rotate internally. This instability can be easily controlled by placing an external fixator on the pelvis to maintain the reduced externally rotated position.

External fixation rarely may become the only definitive treatment for C-type fractures. However, external fixation plays a role for the definitive management of anterior transpubic instability in the completely unstable lesions that had been fixed internally posteriorly. Because of the complex injury profile of many of the patients with these completely unstable pelvic injuries, additional dorsal internal fixation is not always possible. In these cases the application of *traction* to the lower extremity on the affected side should be considered. Traction should not compromise pulmonary toilet or upright positioning of the patient. In effect, the traction may be applied early but the patient is nursed as if no traction were present. When and if the patient's general condition stabilizes, then a decision may be made on definitive management.

Fourth indication is as an adjunct to posterior internal fixation, especially if the anterior injury is unreduced. The application of a simple anterior frame will greatly increase the stability of the overall construct.

The indications listed in the preceding are based on the pelvic fracture type, the hemodynamic status of the patient, the local soft-tissue condition and the profile of other injuries. With regard to fracture types, injuries that are rotationally unstable but vertically and posteriorly stable (Type B) can be managed both acutely and definitively by external fixation. Injuries that have a component of vertical and posterior instability can be managed only partially by external

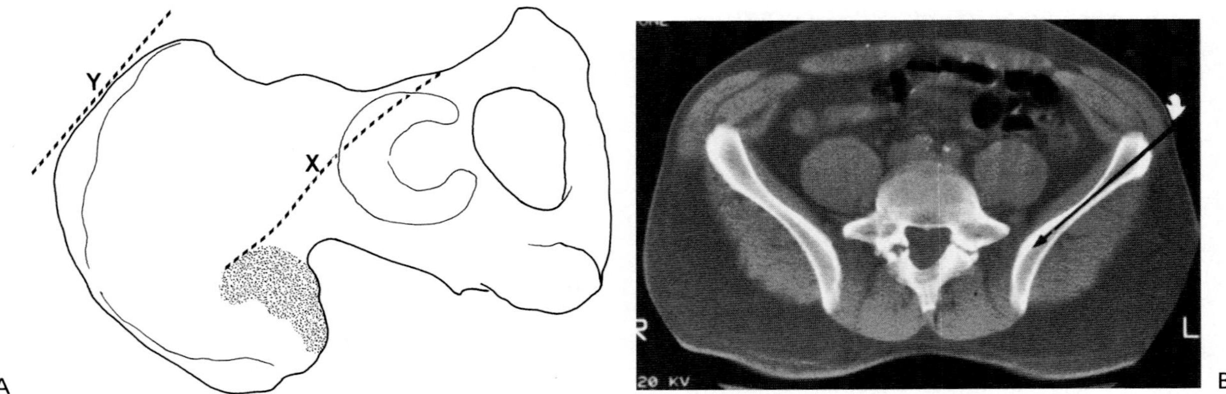

FIGURE 14-3. **A:** Position of the pelvis in the supine patient. Note the angle of the opening of the true pelvis *(x)* and the angle of the iliac crest *(y)*. **B:** The lateral-medial slant of the iliac wing is often not appreciated by clinicians. The correct angle is noted by the *black arrow* on the computed tomography scan.

fixation, although in the acute phases of resuscitation it may be all that is possible. For such completely unstable pelvic injuries, external fixation serves as a temporizing or partial management mode. Also, open reduction and internal fixation methods, such as anterior sacroiliac plating, iliosacral screws, or transiliac bars, or plating of the pubic symphysis or fixation of the pubic rami anteriorly may be required for definitive fixation (13).

METHODS

Appropriate application of an external fixator to treat a pelvic disruption is influenced by factors that relate to pelvic anatomy, type of injury, placement of fixation pins, and frame configuration.

Anatomic Considerations

For accurate pin placement and frame construction, the surgeon must appreciate and incorporate into his or her approach the following factors that affect the standard anatomic relationship among the pelvis, subcutaneous tissues, and skin.

First, the pelvis of a supine patient is not positioned at 90 degrees to either the operating table or the horizontal axis of the body. Rather, the opening of the true pelvis (Fig. 14-3a) and the lateromedial flare of the iliac wings are best seen by computed tomography (CT) (Fig. 14-3b) each present at a 45-degree angle. This lateromedial angulation is exaggerated in the unreduced, externally rotated hemipelvis. This fact is not always adequately appreciated by the surgeon. If pins are to be placed into the iliac crest between the anterior superior iliac spine and the area about the iliac tubercle, into the thick bone cephalad and cephaloposterior to the acetabulum (Fig. 14-4), the surgeon must appreciate and accommodate the obliquity of the pelvic inlet and the wide flare of the iliac bone. Failure to do so will result in incorrect pin placement. The two most frequent errors in pin positioning are pin placement at right angles to the longitudinal axis of the patient and vertical pin insertion so that they exit the ilium laterally (Fig. 14-5).

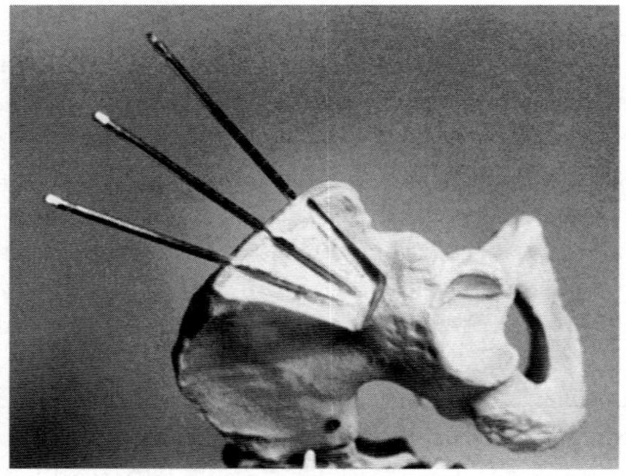

FIGURE 14-4. Cutaway model showing preferred placement of the external fixator pins. Note that the pins tend to converge in the thick column of bone cephalad to the acetabulum.

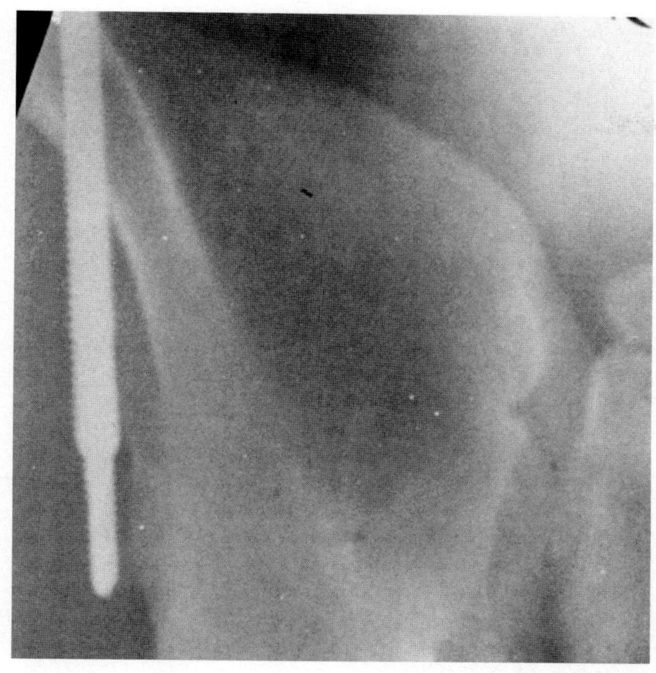

FIGURE 14-5. Radiological illustration shows the pin entering and leaving the hemipelvis almost immediately. This pin is placed too vertically and can offer no stability.

The surgeon should also realize that the iliac crest is quite curved so that straight-line placement of the pin group is contraindicated. Each pin should be placed independently of the others to optimize the anatomic relationship between pin and ilium. This also is true for a group of two or three pins (Fig. 14-4)..

If the surgeon places pins in an unreduced pelvis (preparatory to using the external fixator as a reduction tool), he or she must allow for the nonanatomic position(s) of the particular fragment(s) involved.

The surgeon also must realize that the relationship between the pelvis and soft tissues (skin and subcutaneous portions, especially in the areas covering the iliac crests) changes during the initial hours and days of treatment because of fracture reduction or changing girth secondary to edema or gain or loss of body mass.

The oblique orientation of the pelvis with respect to the normal axes of the body, curve of the natural iliac wing, and change of the ilium—soft tissue interface all ask for special recommendations for pin placement.

Fixation Pins

The application of an external fixator involves issues of pin size, number, and placement. It must be stressed that insertion of fixator pins in the emergency situation is totally different from doing the same in hemodynamically stable patients or on cadaver or skeletonized pelves in the biomechanics laboratory.

Pin Size

Clinical judgment and experimental data suggest the use of 5-mm pins. Mears and Rubash (34) established that a 5-mm pin is superior to a 4-mm pin in its contribution to overall frame strength. Personal experience has shown that a 6-mm pin is too large for use in the iliac crest of most adult pelves. However, 6-mm pins can be used if inserted in the thick supraacetabular part of the ilium bone (see the following). A variety of lengths (180, 200, and 220 mm) should be available for both pin sizes to accommodate patients of varying sizes and different amounts of subcutaneous tissue. Be aware of the small boned individual where a 5-mm pin is too large. This is only indication for 4-mm pins. This can only be determined by assessing the radiographs and appreciating the narrowness of the iliac crests.

Pin Positioning and Number

Pin positioning and number depend on the type of fixator to be used. Frame configuration (shape and hardware) and timing (emergent or definitive) will also have an important influence.

A variety of locations and numbers for pin placement have been proposed: (a) in each ilium, a single pin positioned 2 to 3 cm posterior to the anterior superior iliac spine and driven into the anterior iliac border; (b) in each iliac crest, two or three widely separated pins aimed to converge in the thick iliac bone cephalad to the acetabulum (35); (c) biplanar placement of pin pairs, one pair through the iliac crest and the second pair in the area of the anterior inferior iliac spine, traversing the ilium just cephalad to the acetabulum (36); and (d) one or two pairs of pins placed from the area of the anterior inferior iliac spine traversing the ilium just cephalad to the acetabulum (13,37).

Pin positioning depends on several factors: (a) the need for rapid placement; (b) provisional or definitive stabiliza-

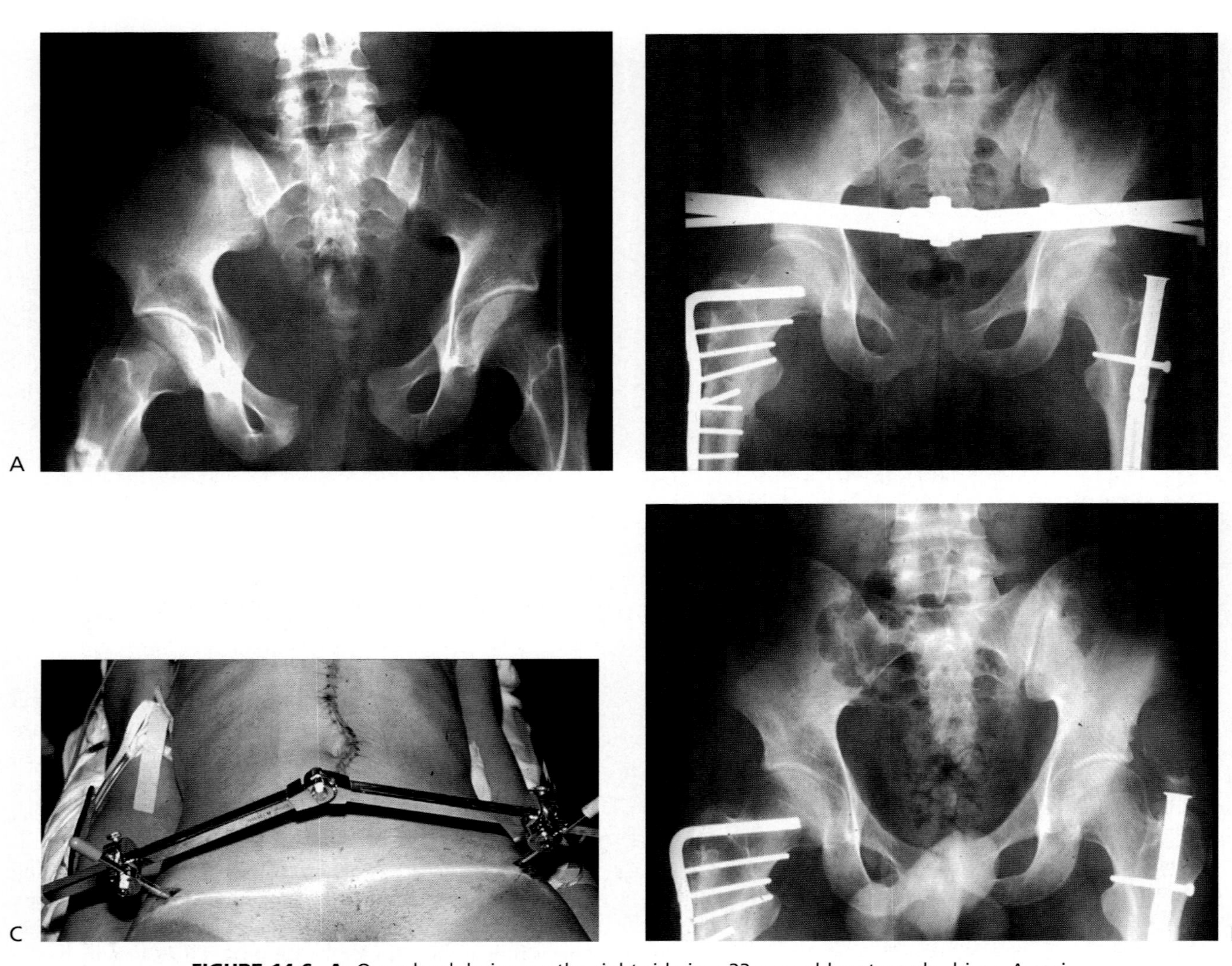

FIGURE 14-6. A: Open-book lesion on the right side in a 23-year-old motorcycle driver. Associated injuries include rupture of the spleen, diaphyseal fracture of the right femur, subtrochanteric fracture of the left femur. Hemodynamic instability. **B:** Situation after emergency reduction (close the book) and fixation of the pelvic ring with a simple external fixator. Supraacetabular pin placement. **C:** Clinical view after external fixation and laparotomy: One single bar connecting the pins provides sufficient stability under emergency conditions. **D:** Radiograph after removal of the external fixator, 10 weeks after the injury. No early secondary internal fixation was required because of the adequate reduction of the pelvic ring with the external fixator alone.

tion of the pelvic disruption; and (c) the assurance of the surgeon that accurate placement of the pins within the tables of the thickest portion of the ilium is possible. Because no frame configuration—be it simple or complicated—is able to provide sufficient stability to a completely unstable pelvic ring, and early secondary internal fixation is performed more frequently nowadays, tendency goes toward the placement of simple anterior fixators for provisional stabilization. We prefer one or two pins from the anterior inferior iliac spine area traversing the ilium just cephalad to the acetabulum in the direction if the greater sciatic notch (Fig. 14-6). Alternatively, a group of three converging pins is placed in the iliac crest. They are force-fitted into the confines of a single straight pin clamp with double-ball joints or into individual pin clamps and then to a straight bar (Fig. 14-7).

In placing the pins, the surgeon must allow for the depth of the soft tissues between the skin and iliac crest or the inferior anterior iliac spine. He or she not only considers pin length, but also the sometimes converging trajectory between the skin and iliac bone. For a thin patient whose skin overlies the iliac crest directly, skin incisions can reflect direct entry into the iliac wing. If, however, the patient is obese or edematous ($>$4.0 cm intervening tissue), the skin incisions should be a significant distance apart so that the spread, as the pins enter the crest of the ilium, is $>$1.5 cm, allowing their continued convergence in the anterior portion of the ilium, cephalad to the acetabulum.

As the distance between the skin and anterior inferior iliac spine is always larger than in the area of the anterior superior iliac spine and iliac crest, skin incisions must be situated more laterally than the anterior inferior iliac spine itself and must be large enough to allow movement of the soft tissues around the pins while movements of the hip joint take place.

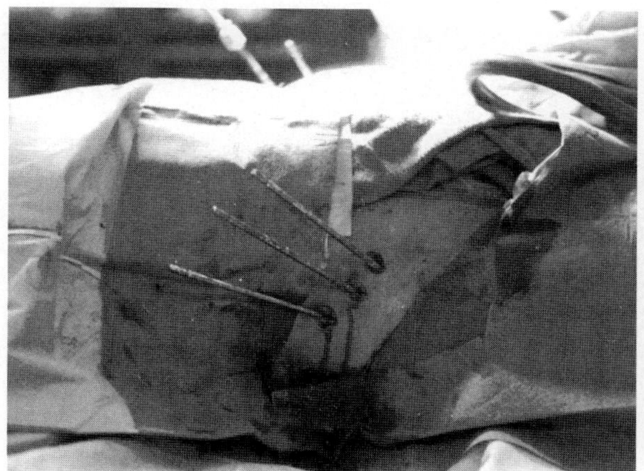

A

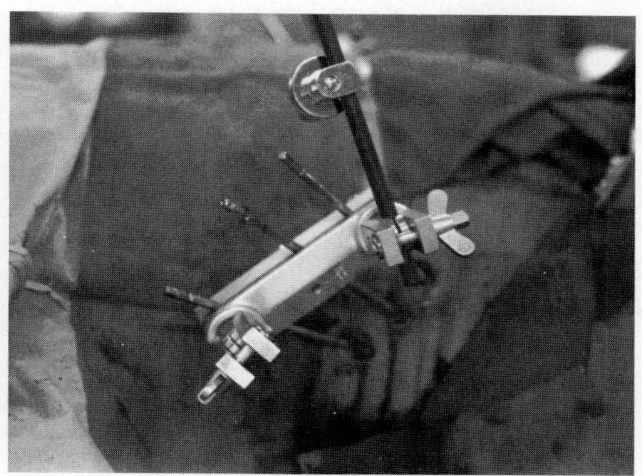

B

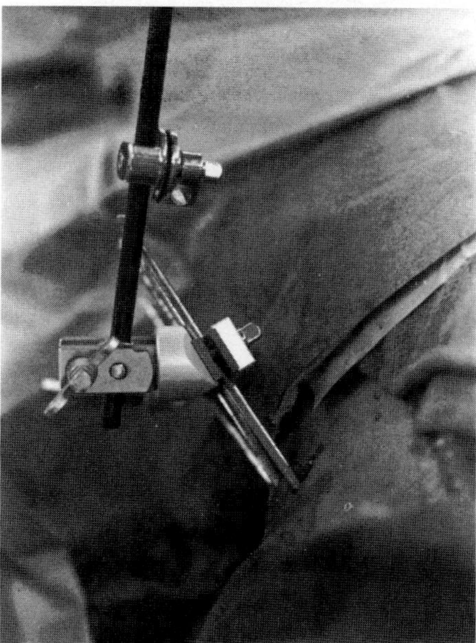

C

FIGURE 14-7. A: Three individual converging pins before application of pin clamp. (Patient's head is to the left.) **B:** Straight, double- ball-jointed pelvic pin clamp, "prestressing" the pins into a straight configuration. (Again, patient's head is to the left.) **C:** View of pin grouping from the patient's foot. Note the straight line of the pin grouping in the clamp and the angled ball joint.

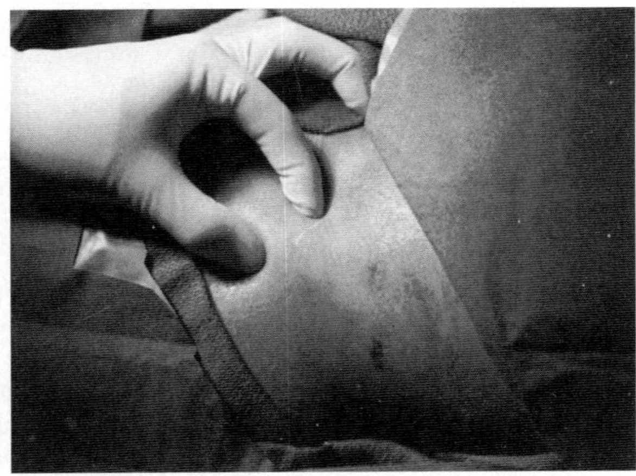

A

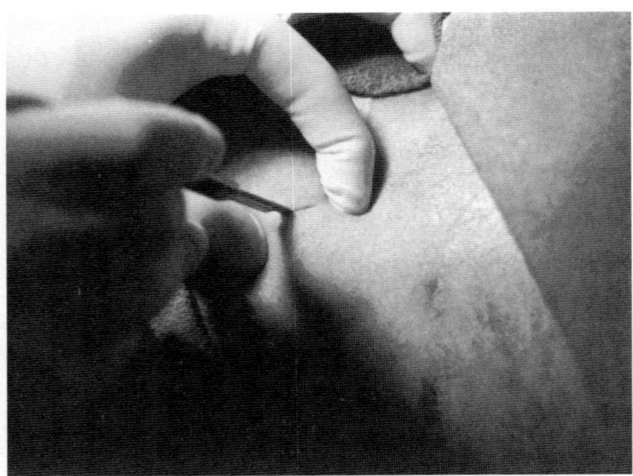

B

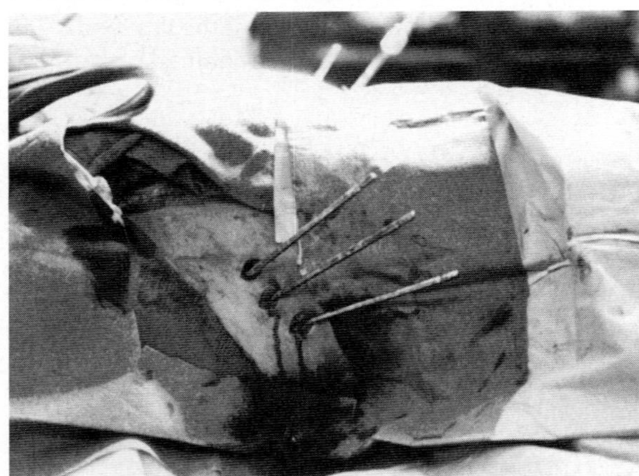

C

FIGURE 14-8. A: To begin the pin placement process, the iliac crest is localized 1 to 2 cm posterior to the anterosuperior iliac spine. **B:** The stab wound is begun directly over the crest, aiming toward the umbilicus. **C:** This clinical photograph (taken from the opposite direction after pin placement) shows the final size of the stab wounds. (The patient's head is to the right.)

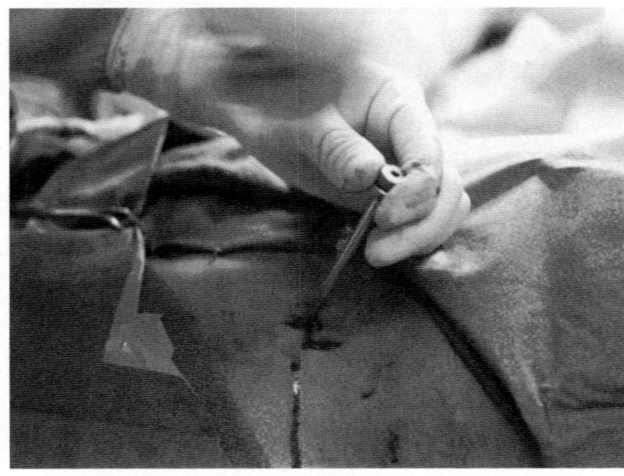

A

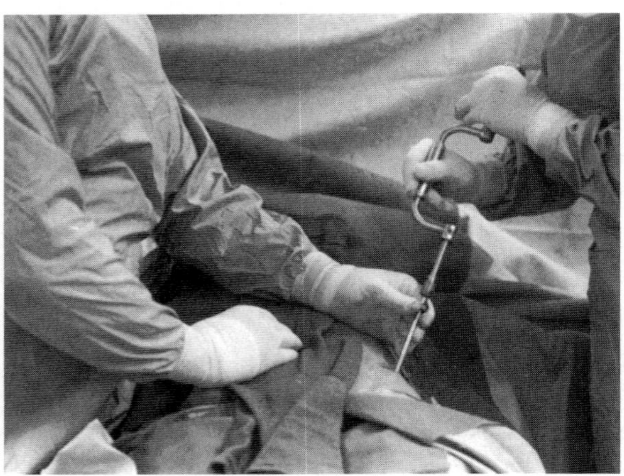

B

FIGURE 14-9. A: The sleeve-trocar system is placed through the stab wound. The trocar is removed and the sleeve system must be held firmly against the iliac crest before drilling. **B:** A 5-mm pin is placed through the external sleeve of the sleeve-trocar system. (The view is from the patient's foot.)

Pin Placement

Several authors prefer open to percutaneous pin placement in order to avoid suboptimal pin positioning, which gives low frame stability and forces subsequent frame adjustment. We prefer a minimally invasive procedure, which holds the middle between percutaneous and open procedures. Special aiming techniques also help for correct pin positioning (30).

Pin Placement in the Iliac Crest

Transverse incisions do not give the advantage of extensive visualization of the iliac crest, but avoid two important disadvantages: (a) long incisions over the iliac crest often decompress a portion of a preexisting extraperitoneal hematoma; and (b) more important, they often are at a 90-degree angle to any necessary readjustment of pin—skin interface secondary to fracture reduction maneuvers or patient girth alterations related to edema or weight change. Stab wounds are at least 1.5 cm long and are directed from the iliac crest toward the umbilicus (Fig. 14-8). The insertion of two Kirschner wires, one on the medial side and one on the lateral side of the iliac wing, provides an accurate targeting method. They identify both borders of the crest and plane of the ilium toward the acetabular roof, ensuring safe and correct placement of the pins between the two tables of the ilium. Once the 1- to 2-cm angled stab wound is made through the skin, the blade is carried down to the crest of the ilium and a surgical clamp is placed to spread the soft tissues and clear the subcutaneous fat. With the clamp spread and guided by the established Kirschner wires, a sleeve-trocar system (Fig. 14-9) is introduced in a lateral to medial 45-degree inclination on the medial side of the midline of the crest. Placing the starting point for the trocar between one third and one half the distance from the medial to lateral side allows for the lateral "overhang" (Fig. 14-10) caused by the attachment of the abductor muscles on the lateral surface of the pelvis. After the trocar system is placed, it is kept in position with firm pressure and the lateral-medial plane is checked with reference to the angulation of the iliac wing established by the Kirschner wires.

The surgeon must then ensure that the pins are placed in an appropriately cephalo-caudal direction. Pins that are to be placed through the iliac crest for simple frame management mostly require that the drill be held more cephalad than primary. Drilling from that cephalad to caudal direction while the first assistant checks for the correct lateral-medial angulation ensures that the pins will be accurately placed, both within the planes of the ilium and toward the thick bone cephalad to the acetabulum, rather than toward the thinner parts of the ilium behind and cephalad to the acetabulum. For most young patients, the iliac wing is predrilled to the appropriate size to a depth of 1 cm, the inner sleeve is then removed, and a 5-mm pin is placed, allowing the cortical walls of the ilium to guide the pin into position. The drilled hole acts only as a starting portal, ensuring—or maximizing chances for—good pin placement. The use of an image intensifier to check pin placement is useful. Most helpful are the outlet views of the pelvis, which demonstrate early exit of the pins from the iliac crest and the obturator oblique view, which is really a tangential view of the ilium and shows whether the pin is held within the tables of the ilium (Fig. 14-5).

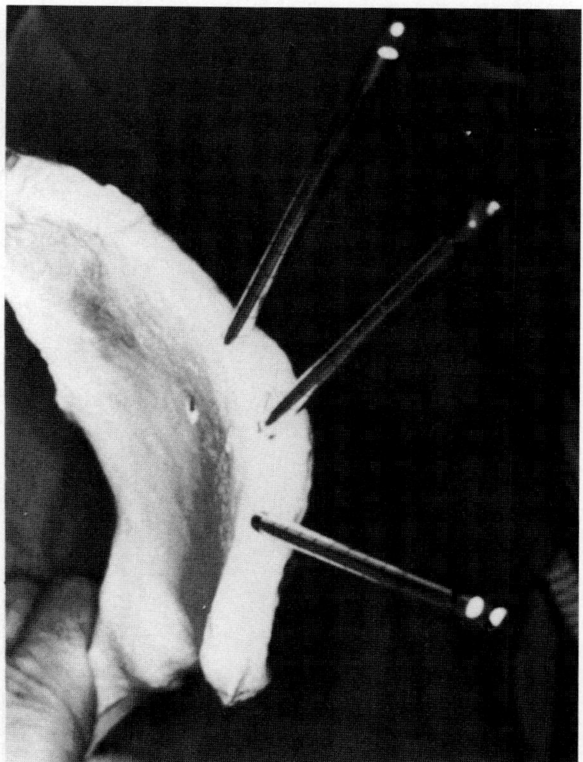

FIGURE 14-10. Iliac crest as seen from above with convergent pins placed in correct anatomic position.

Pin Placement in the Anterior Inferior Iliac Spine

The procedure is very similar to pin placement in the iliac crest. Nevertheless, the following aspects must be mentioned.

1. A transverse skin incision also is preferable with anteroinferior pin purchase. Because of the lateral toward medial direction of the pin and the longer distance between the skin and bone, the incision will be localized somewhat laterally to the anterior inferior iliac spine.
2. Care has to be taken not to injure the lateral femoral cutaneous nerve. Therefore, soft tissues below the level of the skin are split in the longitudinal and not in the transverse direction.
3. Because supraacetabular bone mass is significantly thicker, no insertion of Kirschner wires is necessary. It is recommended to insert the trocar with the drill bit *under image*

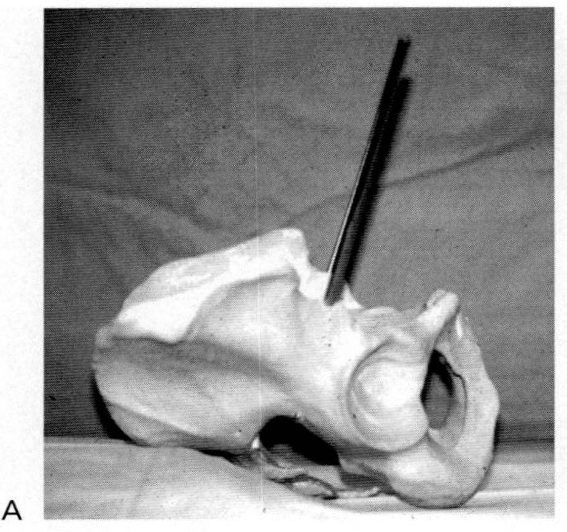

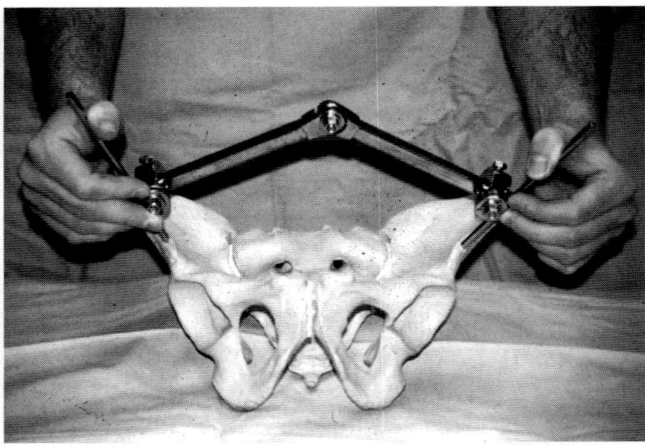

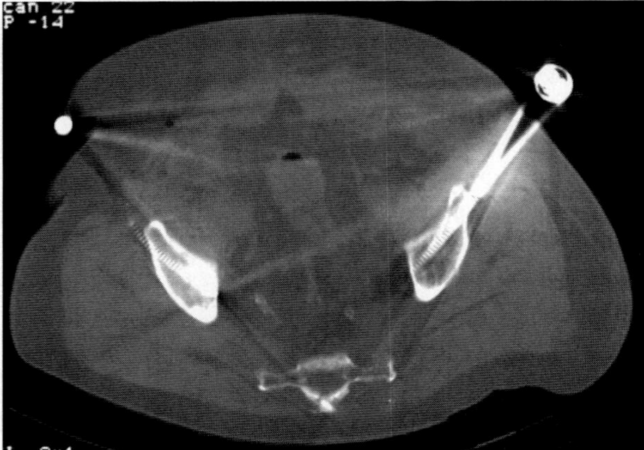

FIGURE 14-11. **A:** Supraacetabular pin placement at the level of the anterior inferior iliac spine. Note the direction of the pin toward the greater sciatic notch. **B:** Pins are directed 30 to 45 degrees toward the midline in the frontal plane. **C:** Computed tomography scan demonstrating appropriate supraacetabular pin purchase.

intensifier control in the direction of the greater sciatic notch in a 30- to 45-degree direction to the frontal or sagittal plane in the reduced hemipelvis (Fig. 14-11). The orientation of the drill bit can be perpendicular to the body axis or directed somewhat cephalad, depending on the location of the starting point in relation to the greater sciatic notch.

4. Predrilling is performed under image intensifier control, to avoid penetration into the hip joint or greater sciatic notch. The length of the trajectory is measured, so that Schanz' screws with the corresponding thread length can be inserted. Generally, pins with 50- to 70-mm thread length are appropriate.

FRAME DESIGN

Mears (17), Egbers (24), Slatis and Karaharju (38), and others described different high profile and complicated frame designs that, they hoped, would achieve some compression of unstable posterior injuries (13,15,39). A low profile and simple frame with one single bar to control the pelvic elements in a patient who (a) is hemodynamically unstable; (b) has a high risk of complete pelvic disruption (if not already diagnosed radiologically); and (c) is very likely to need a laparotomy is recommended. Positioning of the pins in the anterior inferior iliac spine permits easy access to the abdomen for laparotomy (Fig. 14-6). The fixator bar connecting the pins on both sides should, under emergency conditions, not be placed too closely to the skin, as further soft-tissue swelling because ongoing bleeding and local edema must be expected in these patients. This may decrease the original distance between the peripelvic soft tissues and the fixator frame, eventually leading to skin maceration and necrosis owing to direct pressure from the frame on the skin. A simple well-applied frame will suffice for the definitive care frame.

AFTER CARE

Care of Pins and Skin

Care of the pins and surrounding skin requires strict nursing attention. Great care must be taken to ensure that no tightly puckered skin remains around any of the pin tracts. At the end of the procedure the skin should be loose around the pin. An antibiotic spray may be applied, followed by a snug encircling bandage to stabilize the skin. These dressings should be changed, and the wounds inspected, frequently. If any tight skin remains around any of the pins, it should be incised using a local anesthetic. The pin tract sites must be kept clear of any crusting so as to allow free drainage.

Although it is not unusual for pins to become loose, a pelvic frame can remain in place 6 to 12 weeks generally. Beyond 12 weeks, the frame often loosens and must be removed. Therefore, it would be rare for a pelvic frame to remain in place longer than 12 weeks.

Care of Bone Injury

The postoperative care of the patient depends on both general and local factors, and the local factors depend on the stability of the fracture. If the fracture is vertically and posteriorly stable, such as open-book or lateral compression type, enough stability is present to allow the patient to assume the upright position as soon as this is possible. Generally, partial weight bearing on the involved side can be started after the third week.

In the open-book injury with symphysis diastasis, the frame should remain in place for a minimum of 6 weeks. At the end of that period, the frame may be loosened and the symphysis diastasis checked on the image intensifier. It is not unusual to have some loss of reduction of the symphysis pubis at this time. If the loss is minimal, the frame may be removed, but if it is excessive the frame should be left in place for another 4 weeks. Alternatively, a change of procedure to internal fixation can be considered. In case of pubic rami fracture instability, the frame usually can be removed between the fourth and sixth week. Bone consolidation at that time generally provides sufficient intrinsic stability, so that no further anterior fixation is required.

Usually, enough stability is obtained between the sixth and eight week in the lateral compression injury. Again, the frame may be loosened, the pelvis checked with the image intensifier or by plain radiographs, and at that time the frame is usually removed.

If the pelvic disruption is unstable (Type C lesion), the anterior frame cannot be used alone to ensure stability. Following primary care, further investigation, including the previously described radiographic views (AP, inlet, outlet) and a CT scan, will indicate the degree of posterior injury. Principally, the surgeon has two choices: to add posterior internal fixation, or resort to skeletal traction to prevent superior migration of the unstable pelvis. Nowadays, internal fixation should be favored whenever feasible.

CONCLUSION

In this chapter, biomechanical considerations and practical tips for the use of external fixation in the unstable pelvis are presented. Although thorough knowledge of biomechanical studies in literature is of utmost importance, practical issues (e.g., the fracture pattern, patient's other injuries, body habitus, and the need for rapid application) are more relevant to clinical management. The external fixator still has an important role in the management of pelvic ring disruptions, but is more seen as a temporary device than as a definitive treatment method.

REFERENCES

1. Gibson W. *Institutes and practice of surgery* (outlines of a course of lectures), 6th ed. Philadelphia: James Kay, Jun, and Brother, 1841.
2. Peltier LF. Joseph Francois Malgaigne and Malgaigne's fracture. *Surgery* 1958;44:777.
3. Peltier LF. Historical note: Joseph Francois Malgaigne and Malgaigne's fracture. *Clin Orthop* 1980;151:4.
4. Tile M. *Fractures of the pelvis and acetabulum,* 2nd ed. Baltimore: Williams & Wilkins, 1995.
5. Bonnel F. External fixation in fractures of the pelvis (author's translation). *Ann Chir* 1976,30:131.
6. Carabalona P, Rabichong P, Bonnel F. Apports du fixateur externes dans les dislocations du pubis et del articulation sacroiliaque. *Montpelier Chir* 1973;29.
7. Comics H. *Hoffmann's double frame external anchorage.* Paris: Gead, 1973.
8. Mears DC, Fu FH. Modern concepts of external skeletal fixation of the pelvis. *Clin Orthop* 1980;151:65.
9. Muller J, Bachmann B, Berg H. Malgaigne fracture of the pelvis: treatment with percutaneous pin fixation. Report of two cases. *J Bone Joint Surg* 1978;60A:992.
10. Muller KH, Muller-Farber J. Die Osteosynthese mit dem Fixateur externe am Becken. *Arch Orthop Trauma Surg* 1978;92:273.
11. Slätis P, Karaharju EO. External fixation of the pelvic girdle with a trapezoid compression frame. *Injury* 1975;7:53.
12. Pennal GF, Sutherland GO. *Fractures of the pelvis* (film). Park Ridge, IL: American Academy of Orthopaedic Surgeons Film Library, 1961.
13. Rommens PM, Hessmann MH. Staged reconstruction of pelvic ring disruption. Differences in morbidity, mortality and functional outcome between B1, B2/3- and C-type lesions. *J Orthop Trauma,* 2002;16:92.
14. Kim W-Y, Hearn TC, Seleem O, et al. Effect of pin location on stability of pelvic external fixation. *Clin Orthop* 1999;361:237.
15. Riemer B, Butterfield SL, Diamond DL, et al. Acute mortality associated with injuries to the pelvic ring. The role of early patient mobilization and external fixation. *J Trauma* 1993;35:671.
16. Gunterberg B, Goldie L, Slätis P. Fixation of pelvic fractures and dislocations: an experimental study on the loading of pelvic fractures and sacroiliac dislocations after external compression fixation. *Acta Orthop Scand* 1978;49:278.
17. Mears DC, Fu F. External fixation in pelvic fractures. *Orthop Clin North Am* 1980;11:465.
18. Brown TD, Stone JP, Schuster JH, et al. External fixation of unstable pelvic ring fractures: Comparative rigidity of some current frame configurations. *Med Biol Eng Comput* 1982;20:727.
19. Shaw JA, Eng M, Mino DE, et al. Posterior stabilization of pelvic ring fractures by use of threaded compression rods—case report and mechanical testing. *Clin Orthop* 1985;192:240.
20. Rubash HE, Brown TD, Nelson DD, et al. Comparative mechanical performances of some new devices for fixation of unstable pelvic ring fractures. *Med Biol Eng Comput* 1983;21:657.

21. McBroom R, Tile M. *Disruptions of the pelvic ring.* Presented at the Canadian Orthopaedic Research Society Convention. Kingston, Ontario, June, 1982.
22. Pohlemann T, Krettek C, Hoffmann R, et al. Biomechanischer Vergleich verschiedener Notfallstabilisierungsmassnahmen am Beckenring. *Unfallchirurg* 1994;97:503.
23. Ganz R, Krushell R, Jakob R, et al. The antishock pelvic clamp. *Clin Orthop* 1991;267:71.
24. Egbers H-J, Draijer F, Havemann D, et al. Stabilisierung des Beckenrings mit Fixateur externe—Biomechanische Untersuchungen und klinische Erfahrungen. *Orthopäde* 1992;21:363.
25. Browner BD, Cole JD, Graham JM, et al. Delayed posterior internal fixation of unstable pelvic fractures. *J Trauma* 1987;27: 998.
26. Slätis P, Eskola A. External fixation of the pelvic girdle as a test for assessing instability of the sacroiliac joint. *Ann Med* 1989; 21:369.
27. Rieger H. *Das instabile Becken: Diagnostik, Therapie und Prognose.* Munich: W. Zuckschwerdt Verlag, 1996.
28. Ghanayem AJ, Wilber JH, Lieberman JM, et al. The effect of laparotomy and external fixator stabilization on pelvic volume in an unstable pelvic injury. *J Trauma* 1995;38:396.
29. Burgess A. External fixation. In Tile M, ed. *Fractures of the pelvis and acetabulum,* 2nd ed. Baltimore: Williams & Wilkins, 1995.
30. Waikakul S, Kojaranon N, Vanadurongwan V, et al. An aiming device for pin fixation at the iliac crest for external fixation in unstable pelvic fracture. *Injury* 1998;29:757.
31. Burgess AR, et al. Pelvic ring disruptions: effective classification system and treatment protocols. *J Trauma* 1990;30:848.
32. Tile M, Pennal GF. Pelvic disruption: principles of management. *Clin Orthop* 1980;151:56.
33. Dalal SA, et al. Pelvic fracture in multiple trauma: classification by mechanism is key to pattern of organ injury, resuscitative requirements, and outcome. *J Trauma* 1989;29:981.
34. Mears DC, Rubash HE, Nelson DD. External fixation of the pelvic ring: the use of the Pittsburgh triangular frame. *Contemp Orthop* 1982;5:21.
35. Cepulo AJ, Dahners LF, Jacons RR, et al. A comparative study of external fixation devices for unstable pelvic fractures. *Trans Orthop Res Soc* 1984;9:273.
36. Mears DC. The management of complex pelvic fractures. In: Brooker AF Jr, Edwards CC, eds. *External fixation. The current state of the art. Proceedings of the 6th International Conference on Hoffmann External Fixation.* Baltimore: Williams & Wilkins, 1979:151–177.
37. Rommens PM, Vanderschot PM, De Boodt P, et al. Surgical management of pelvic ring disruptions: indications, techniques and functional results. *Unfallchirurg* 1992;95:455.
38. Slätis P, Karaharju EO. External fixation of unstable pelvic fractures: experiences in 22 patients treated with a trapezoid compression frame. *Clin Orthop* 1980;151:73.
39. Matta JM, Tornetta P III. Internal fixation of unstable pelvic ring injuries. *Clin Orthop* 1996;329:129.

- 5mm or 6mm pins better
- AIIS FRAME WHERE POSSIBLE
- xray 6-8/52 + LOOSEN FRAME

15

INTERNAL FIXATION FOR THE INJURED PELVIC RING

BERTON R. MOED
JAMES F. KELLAM
ALEXANDER MCLAREN
MARVIN TILE

INTRODUCTION

Many significant advances have been made in open reduction and internal fixation of pelvic ring disruptions since the previous editions of this book. The indications and contraindications, what types of pelvic fractures are best suited for open reduction and internal fixation, and the biomechanics of pelvic fixation have been clarified (1–6). Minimally invasive techniques, especially for posterior pelvic injury, have changed many facets of treatment, including the timing, methods, and overall role of internal fixation. Different implants and instruments have been developed as well (7).

RATIONALE FOR INTERNAL FIXATION OF THE PELVIS

What is the reason for the major increase of stabilization of the pelvic ring by internal devices in the past two decades? Prior to 1980, internal fixation of pelvic ring injury was

TABLE 15-1. BENEFITS OF INTERNAL FIXATION

Obtain and maintain anatomic reduction
Biomechanically more stable fixation
Safer techniques (minimally invasive, guidance systems, image intensification)
Early mobilization, shorter hospitalization, improve outcomes

rarely done; today it is commonplace. It is rarely indicated for the stable pelvic ring injury. In the unstable injury types, it has become the treatment of choice; the conventional wisdom of today (2,3,8–12).

Ultimately any discussion on rationale begs the question: Is it good for patient care? What are the benefits? What are the risks (Table 15-1)?

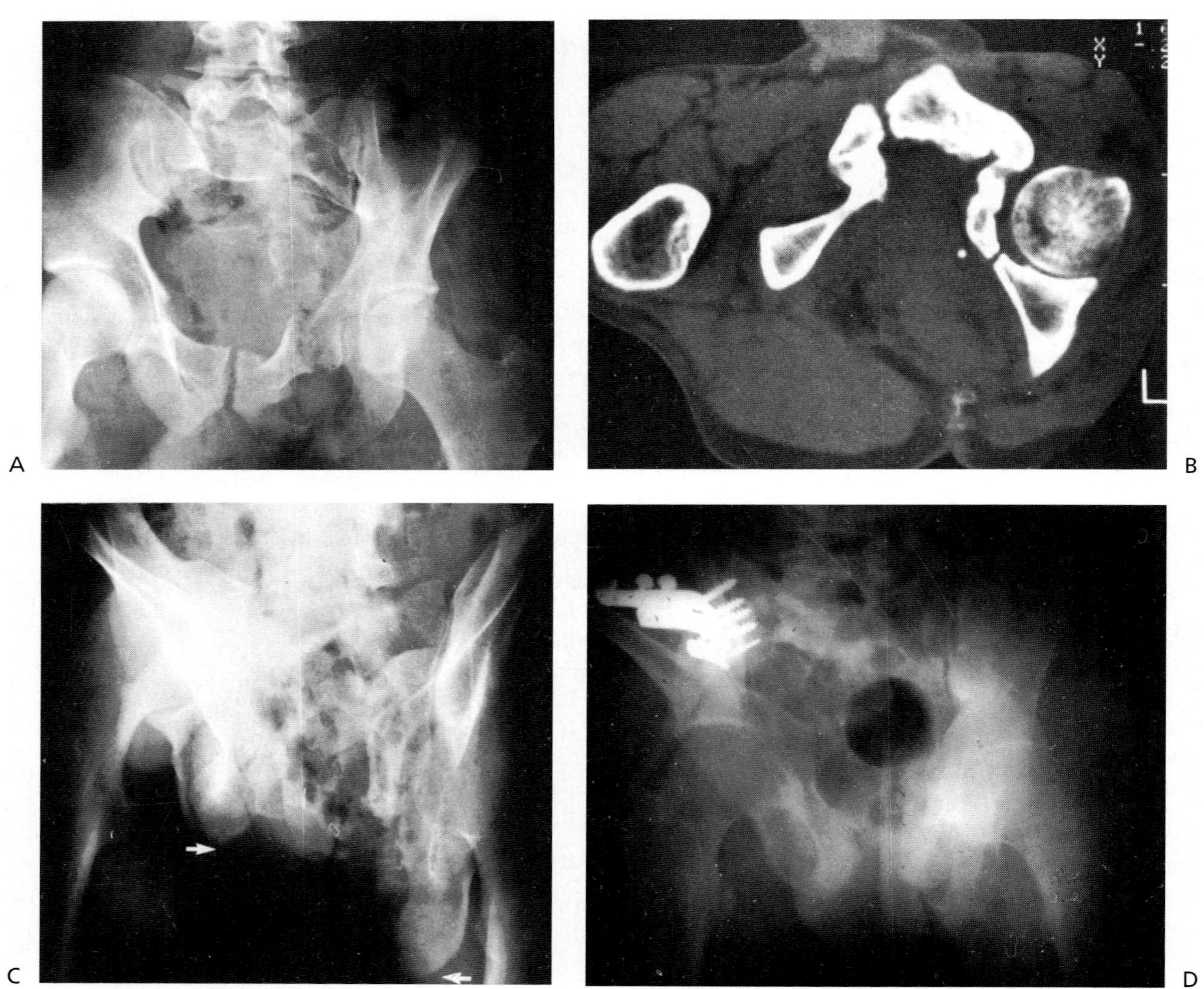

FIGURE 15-1. A: Anteroposterior radiographs of a 26-year-old man involved in a motor vehicle accident. The patient had a major soft tissue injury to his right lower extremity. The unstable nature of the right hemipelvis was unrecognized and the pelvic fracture was treated by bedrest alone, whereas attention was paid to the soft-tissue injury of the right lower extremity. The fracture healed with marked deformity, as noted by the computed tomography **(B)** and the outlet radiograph **(C)**. Note that the right lower extremity has shortened by 7 cm because of the pelvic malunion. The patient found it virtually impossible to sit because of the marked displacement of the ischial tuberosity on the right compared to the left *(arrows)*. **D:** Note the partial correction achieved by osteotomizing the right hemipelvis. The ischial tuberosities in this outlet view are almost at the same level, allowing the patient to sit comfortably. Proper original management would have prevented this malunion from occurring.

Benefits of Internal Fixation

Obtaining and Maintaining Anatomic Reduction

In surviving patients with pelvic ring injury, the outcomes are mainly dependent on residual deformity and the complications of the injury. Malunion was prevalent prior to treatment with internal fixation, leading to marked leg length discrepancy and inability to sit (Fig. 15-1) (13,14). Although many of the complications of the injury itself are beyond the control of the surgeon, obtaining and maintaining anatomic reduction by improved techniques of internal fixation is under the surgeon's control to a large degree, thereby reducing the deleterious effects of malunion, leg length discrepancy, and nonunion.

Biomechanics of Pelvic Stabilizations

In Chapter 14 it is clearly noted that external fixation provides insufficient stability to maintain reduction while allowing early ambulation for an unstable pelvic ring injury (15–18). Depending on surgeon preference, it can be used in the open book fracture (B1, B3–1), or in the lateral compression injury (B2), especially those associated with polytrauma (19). But for the unstable pelvic ring, as noted in Chapter 14, external fixators are used mainly for temporary fixation in the acute phase of treatment. When gross deformity is present in an unstable fracture, skeletal traction should supplement external fixation while waiting for the optimal timing of internal fixation (Fig. 15-2).

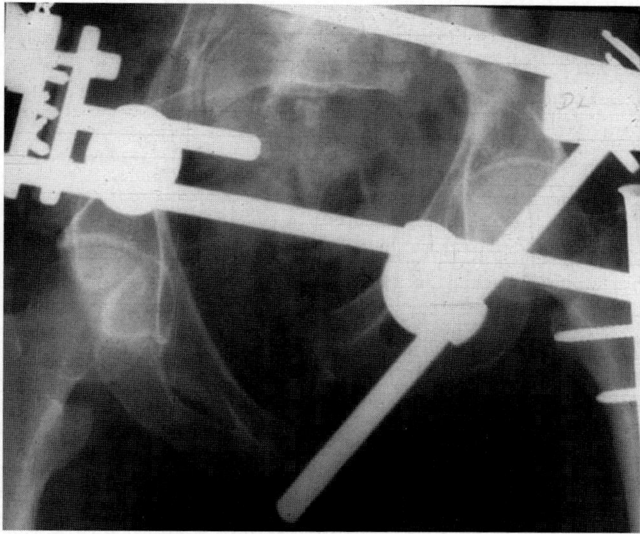

FIGURE 15-2. Unstable pelvic ring (Type C) in 19-year-old man. Note the intramedullary nail in L femur and the external fixator. Traction was not used because transfer was contemplated, but was delayed 6 weeks because of his medical state. Skeletal traction would have avoided this extreme deformity.

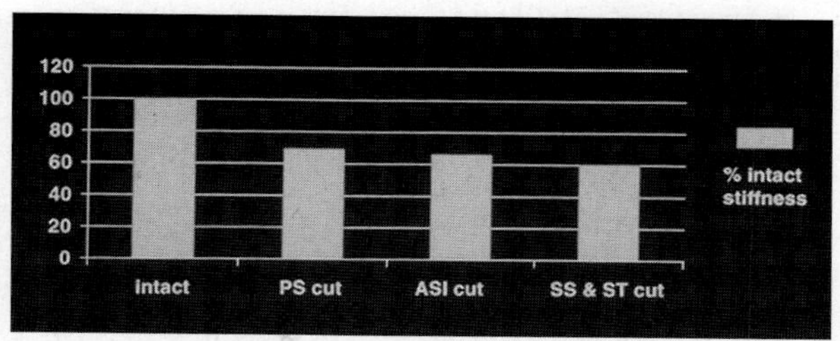

FIGURE 15-3. Graph indicating that approximately 40% of pelvic stability comes from the anterior structure and 60% from the posterior.

Safer Techniques

Minimally invasive techniques using guidance systems or real-time image intensification have made the placement of percutaneous screws across the posterior injury much safer for the patient in the hands of an experienced surgeon (7,20). Because a posterior incision is eliminated, wound breakdown is much less common, as is sepsis. These techniques are discussed in detail elsewhere in this chapter.

Early Mobilization

Early mobilization of the patient with improved techniques of internal fixation has a beneficial effect on polytrauma patients and results in shorter hospital stays (21). However, the biomechanics of stabilization must be understood to make the postoperative care logical. Loss of fixation may occur if the patient is mobilized too quickly, especially from partial to full weight bearing. Biomechanical studies have shown that 40% of the stiffness of the pelvis is from the anterior structures, and 60% from the posterior structures (Fig. 15-3) (22,23). Therefore, to mobilize a patient with an unstable pelvic ring, stable fixation must be obtained both to the anterior and posterior ring, depending on the injury type. Even then the best techniques can only stabilize 1.5 times body weight in a severe internal hemipelvectomy (Type C) injury. Therefore, protective weight bearing is essential to prevent loss of fixation (Fig. 15-4).

Risks

What are the risks of internal fixation (Table 15-2)?

General Effects of Internal Fixation

Surgical intervention in the polytrauma situation requires careful surgical judgment. In general, stabilization of unstable appendicular fractures is beneficial to the care of the patient. This is also true in the pelvis, especially when techniques of minimal internal fixation are used. It is only when anesthetic procedures become prolonged, blood loss exten-

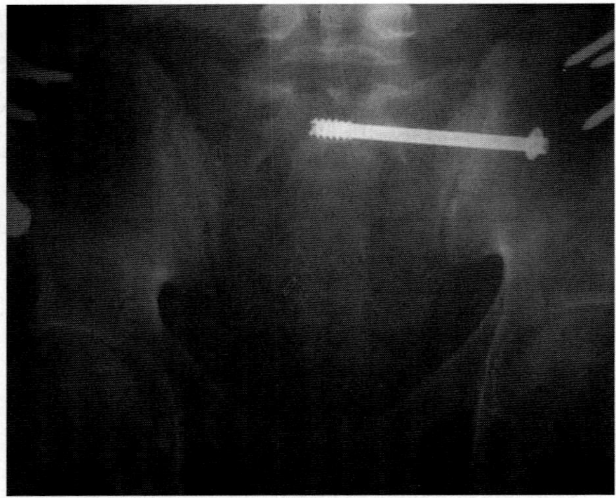

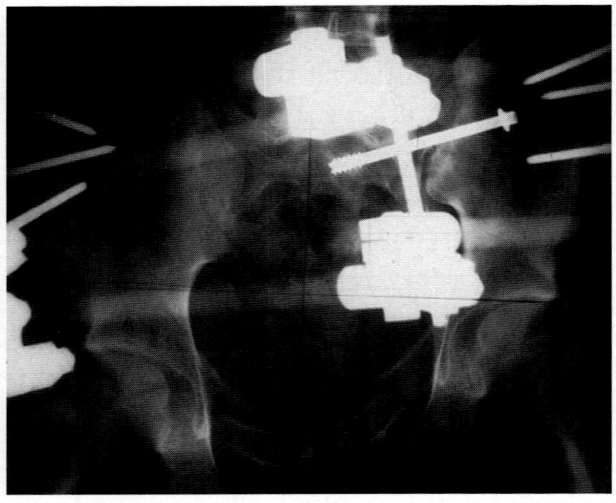

FIGURE 15-4. A: Type C pelvic injury in 40-year-old woman fixed with a single iliosacral screw and external fixator. **B:** The pelvic ring displaced to its original position within 3 days of ambulation.

sive, and complications high that the risks may be greater than the benefits in some patients.

Complications

Even in the best of circumstances in the most expert of hands, injury to nerve, vessel, and viscera are possible (Fig. 15-5). A recent study at Sunnybrook and Women's College Hospital Health Science Centre revealed only one postoperative nerve injury in 64 iliosacral screws (24).

Infection

The trend away from very large posterior wounds has helped greatly reduce the infection rate in patients with a crush injury to the pelvis. Infection still occurs with disastrous effects in some patients (Fig. 15-6).

Failure of Fixation

We have already discussed the importance of proper aftercare based on an understanding of the biomechanics of the injury and biomechanics of the fixation (Fig. 15-4).

TABLE 15-2. RISKS OF INTERNAL FIXATION

General effects of surgery
Complications to nerve, vessel, and viscera
Infection
Failure of fixation

Individual Types: Rationale

Internal fixation techniques should be used when the benefits are greater than the risks. Careful decision making is required in each individual case by the surgeon and intensive care team. In general, stable A types and partially stable B types make up 70% to 80% of the total number of pelvic ring injuries, and usually can be managed with safe simple treatment and an expected good outcome (23,25). In the open-book injury, symphyseal stabilization is indicated and greatly helps the management of the patient. In the lateral compression fracture, internal fixation techniques are rarely indicated. The greatest benefit is in the unstable (Type C, APC III, and Bucholz III) patterns. In this circumstance, if anterior and posterior stabilization are successful, they greatly benefit the outcome for the patient for reasons already stated.

Summary

Is the overall outcome of pelvic ring trauma being altered by the widespread use of internal fixation techniques? Yes, for correction of deformity, restoration of stability, ease of nursing care and earlier mobilization.

The prevention of deformity, leg length discrepancy, and surgical complications are within the control of the surgeon. Careful decision making must include the doctrine *primum non nocere* (above all, do no harm).

The outcomes have not changed with respect to biological factors, especially owing to the high incidence of nerve injury in unstable sacral fractures. However, even in those patients, if the patient is left with a poor anatomic reduction the results are much worse. Therefore, recognizing that the outcomes may be less than perfect because of other factors,

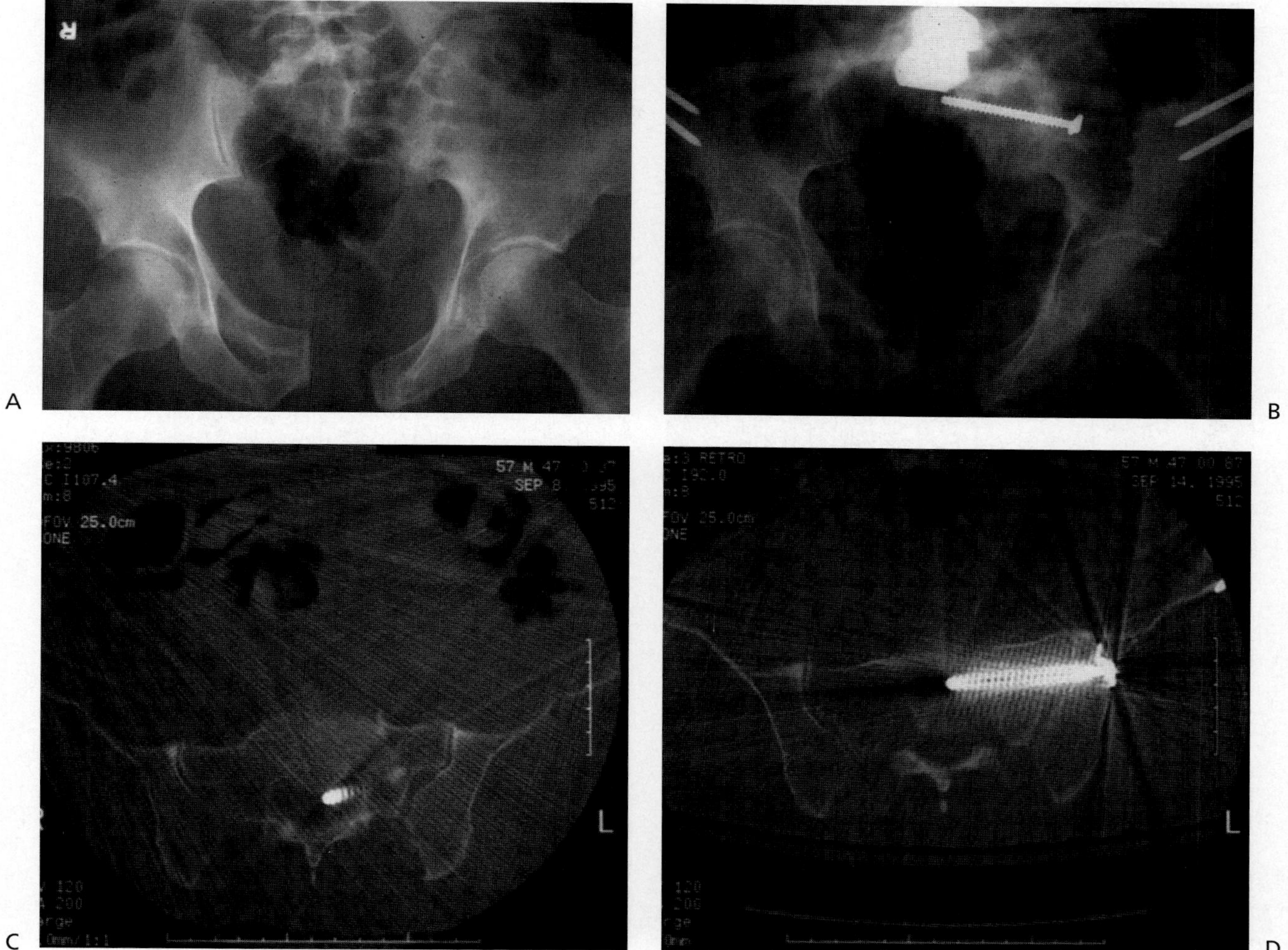

FIGURE 15-5. A: Type C pelvic fracture in a 53-year-old man. **B:** Fixation with a single iliosacral screw and external fixation. Immediately postoperatively he had intense pain in the foot and weakness in dorsiflexion (L5 syndrome). **C:** Computed tomography scan showing screw in the spinal canal. **D:** Removal of screw and replacement into proper location. Recovery of the nerve was complete.

the surgeon must still strive for restoration of the anatomy and stability to the pelvis.

BIOMECHANICS

Please see Chapter 11 for a complete discussion of the biomechanics of pelvic stabilization. We include the summary of that chapter for reference.

Summary

1. An understanding of the details of laboratory studies is necessary before the biomechanical findings of these studies are extrapolated to the treatment of patients with unstable pelvis injuries.
2. The biomechanics of each site of fixation should be considered in the context of the pelvic ring as a whole.
3. Fixation of the anterior pelvis is stronger with internal than external fixation. Both methods, when coupled with appropriate posterior internal fixation, provide adequate stability to mobilize a patient with an unstable pelvis injury.
4. Vertically or translationally unstable injuries (Type C) cannot be adequately stabilized by external fixation alone.
5. Maximal stability from internal fixation is gained by reconstituting the anterior and posterior portions of the ring through internal fixation.
6. For the unilateral sacroiliac dislocation or fracture dislocation, iliosacral compression screw fixation, transiliac bar fixation, transiliac plating, and anterior sacroil-

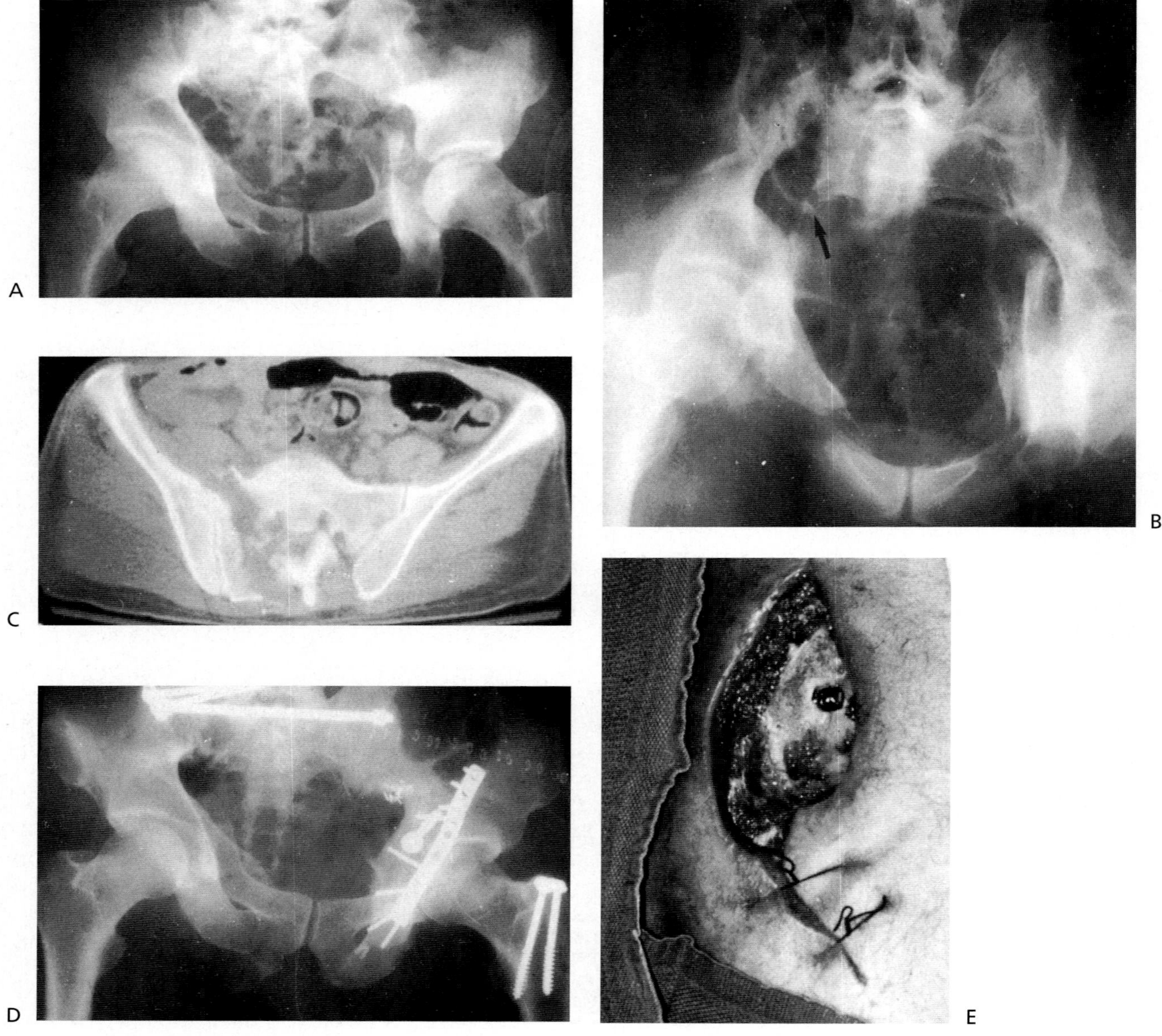

FIGURE 15-6. Anteroposterior **(A)** and inlet **(B)** radiographs of a 36-year-old man crushed by a load of steel that moved within his truck. Note the displaced fracture of the left acetabulum and the gross posterior displacement of the right hemipelvis, best seen on the inlet view **(B)** and computed tomography **(C).** The patient was not transferred for 5 weeks because of life-threatening injuries. Open reduction and internal fixation of the left acetabulum restored congruity to the joint. Full reduction of the sacral fracture was not possible because of delayed treatment. **D:** The right sacral fracture was fixed with two iliosacral screws and a transiliac bar. At the time the incision was made it was noted that the entire gluteus maximus fascia had pulled away from the iliac crest under the skin. **E:** Necrosis of the incision occurred without sepsis, and the wound dehisced. This photograph shows the granulating wound and avascular lateral aspect of the ilium. This wound eventually healed and the metal was removed.

iac plating all restore adequate stability to the posterior pelvis for patient mobilization, if the anterior pelvis is stabilized. Studies to date have shown the iliosacral screw coupled with two symphyseal plates to be the most biomechanically stable.

7. For transforaminal sacral fractures, adequate stability can be achieved with iliosacral screws, transiliac bars, transiliac plates, or direct posterior sacral exposure and internal fixation, again, only if the anterior pelvis has been stabilized.
8. With bilateral posterior pelvic injuries, at least one side of the posterior injury must be fixed to the axial spine to provide adequate stability for maintenance of the sacral reduction with patient mobilization. Combining

iliosacral screws with transiliac bars or plates provides a biomechanical advantage in resisting sacroiliac displacement bilaterally.

9. Stability of anterior external fixators can be improved by placing Schanz pins between the anterior superior and anterior inferior iliac spines through the supraacetabular bone.
10. Iliosacral screws will obtain maximal strength if long-threaded screws are placed into the sacral body.
11. In the completely unstable pelvic disruption, really considered an internal hemipelvectomy, fixation both anteriorly and posteriorly may be insufficient to allow unrestricted weight bearing. Because this fixation will only withstand 1.5 × body weight, redisplacement may occur. Postoperative regimes must take this into account.

INDICATIONS

It can be assumed that the closer the disrupted pelvic ring is reduced to its normal anatomic position, the better the overall functional result will be for the patient. Therefore, the treating surgeon should attempt to achieve an adequate reduction of the pelvic disruption. Standard orthopedic principles state that this reduction would be first performed as a closed reduction. If failure to obtain or maintain this reduction occurs, an open procedure should be performed. However, the definition of an adequate reduction remains arbitrary. Lesions with >1 cm of posterior or superior displacement at the sacroiliac complex, or rotational abnormalities of the leg that cannot be corrected past the neutral position, usually require reduction (13,15,26,27,28).

Maintenance of the reduction is the second component of the treatment algorithm. Generally speaking, this could be achieved through nonoperative means such as traction or the semiinvasive technique of external fixation. These methods have their drawbacks and generally are not suitable for all disruptions. Therefore, the use of internal fixation has played an ever-increasing role in the management of these injuries. Internal fixation now can be applied through closed percutaneous techniques as well as open methods. Consequently, when discussing indications for internal fixation, each specific lesion needs to be dealt with as an individual case.

There are certain specific situations in which open reduction and internal fixation become more imperative.

ANTERIOR FIXATION

See Table 15-3.

Acute Stabilization

Acute fixation of the disrupted symphysis pubis is indicated for pelvic disruption if laparotomy is being performed for abdominal or pelvic visceral injury. Fixation of the symphysis or parasymphyseal fractures facilitates patient management. If fecal contamination is present, external fixation is the safer and preferred method. The presence of a suprapubic cystostomy tube is also a risk factor for infection. Rami fractures associated with injury to the femoral artery or nerve should be fixed internally.

TABLE 15-3. INDICATIONS FOR ANTERIOR FIXATION OF SYMPHYSIS AND PUBIC RAMI FRACTURES

Disrupted symphysis pubis
In unstable (Type C) pelvic disruption
Symphysis open >2.5 cm
Laparotomy being performed for visceral injury
Locked symphysis
Rami fractures
Associated with femoral artery or nerve injury
Tilt fracture with ramus protruding into vagina
Marked displacement (unstable Type C disruption)

Delayed Elective Stabilization

By definition, open-book injuries are external rotationally unstable but vertically stable. The pelvic floor may be disrupted in the more severe injury, but the posterior sacroiliac osseous ligamentous complex remains intact, maintaining vertical and posterior stability (4,29). Stabilization, either internal or external, is indicated for symphyseal disruption exceeding 2.5 cm. Adequate evaluation of the posterior structures must be carried out to confirm that the posterior osseous ligamentous structures are intact, that the posterior aspect of the sacroiliac joint remains closed, and that in all three views of the pelvis there is no evidence of posterior or superior displacement. Consequently, purely anterior ring fixation may be carried out (Fig. 15-7).

The tilt fracture, especially in women, is best reduced open and fixed, to avoid bone protruding into the perineum causing dyspareunia (Fig. 15-8). As an example, one young woman was left with a large mass of bone protruding into the vagina that caused severe dyspareunia, as noted on the radiographs and computed tomography (CT) (Fig. 15-9). The bony mass, from the inferior pubic ramus, was resected through the vagina (Fig. 15-9E), which resulted in a satisfying outcome for the patient. A locked symphysis that cannot be reduced by closed means may require open reduction and internal fixation (Fig. 15-10, see also 15–51). Also, fractures associated with the anterior column of the acetabulum may require fixation. Symphyseal disruptions >2.5 cm are reduced open and stabilized with plate fixation. Pubic rami stabilization is controversial (30–32). If the pubic rami fractures are 100% displaced after the posterior lesion is reduced and stabilized, then reduction and stabilization are recommended to enhance the stability of the posterior fixation. It

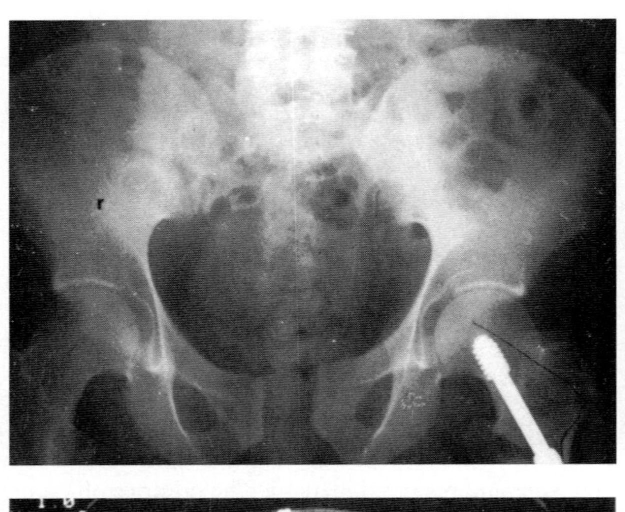

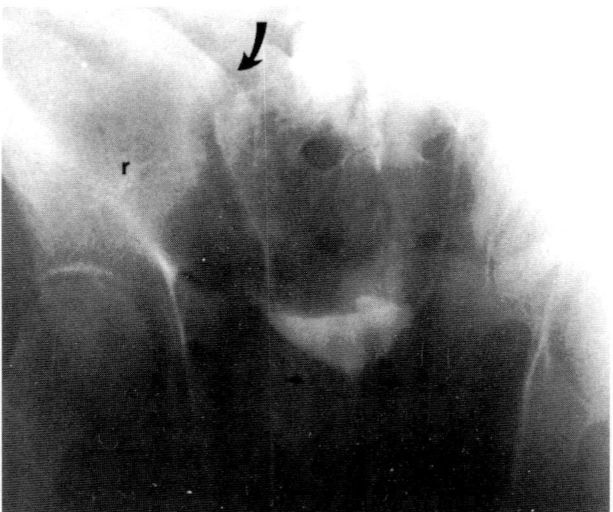

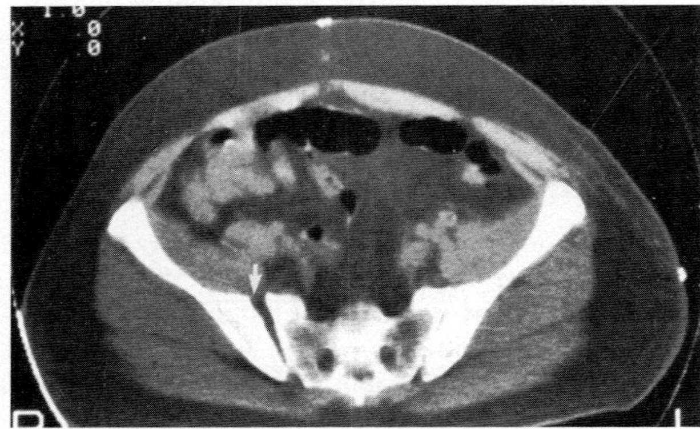

FIGURE 15-7. Anteroposterior **(A)** and outlet view **(B)** show a disrupted symphysis and an externally rotated right hemipelvis with no superior displacement *(black arrow)*. Computed tomography **(C)** shows the anterior opening of the sacroiliac joint *(white arrow)* with no posterior displacement. In this situation stabilization of the symphysis alone restores stability to the pelvic ring, as noted in the inlet **(D)** and outlet **(E)** radiographs.

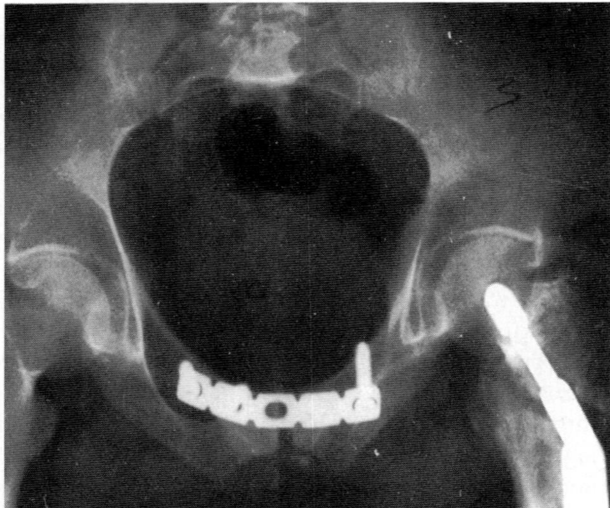

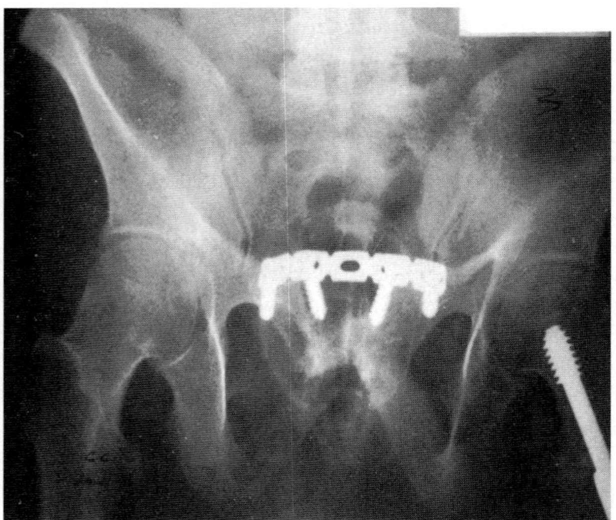

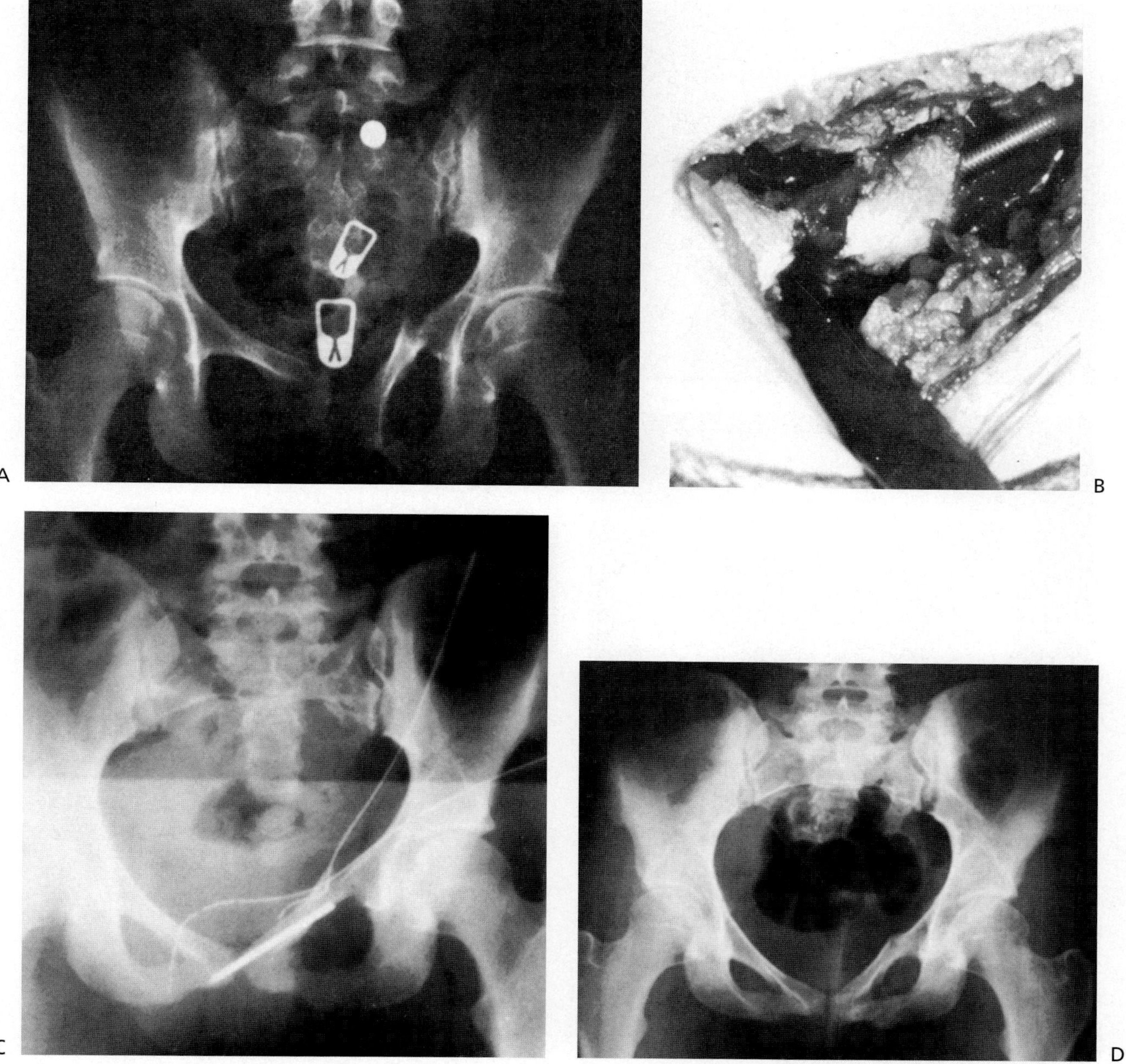

FIGURE 15-8. A: The radiograph indicates an abnormal variant of the lateral compression fracture (tilt fracture), whereby the symphysis is disrupted by the rotating superior pubic ramus on the left side. **B,C:** In this case, because the posterior fracture was stable, the anterior lesion was fixed with a threaded Steinmann pin. **D:** The Steinmann pin was removed at 6 weeks. An excellent clinical outcome was achieved for the patient, with bony healing of the ramus fracture and stability at the symphysis.

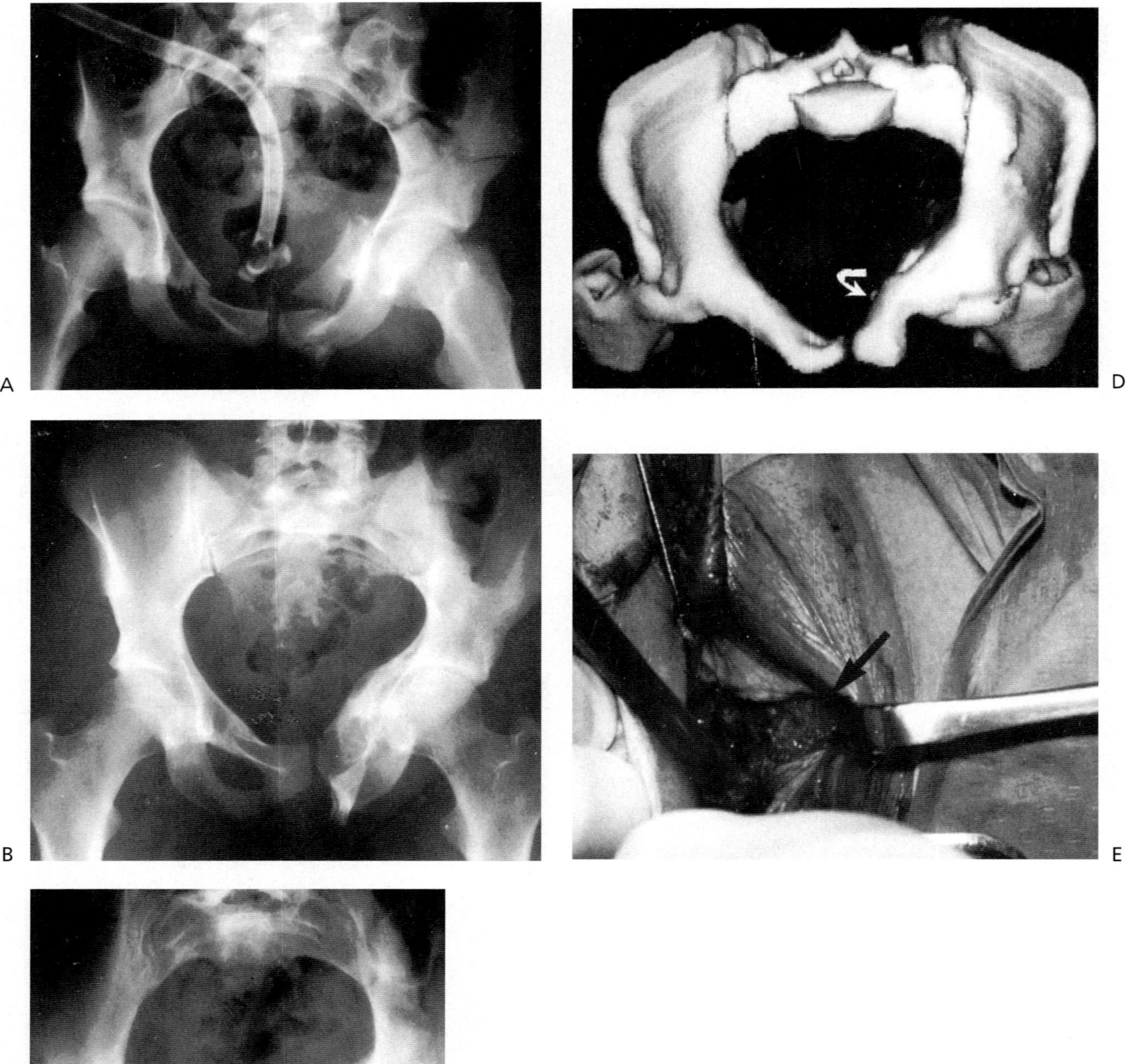

FIGURE 15-9. A: Anteroposterior radiograph of an 18-year-old woman with a lateral compression injury. Note the large spike of bone from the superior and the inferior pubic ramus. The fracture was treated nonoperatively and healed with deformity, as noted on the anteroposterior radiograph **(B)** and inlet view **(C).** On the inlet view, note the marked malunion of the inferior pubic ramus, confirmed on the three-dimensional computed tomography **D:** This large mass of bone caused dyspareunia *(white arrow).* **E:** The mass *(black arrow)* of bone protruding into the vagina was resected through the vagina, and symptoms were alleviated.

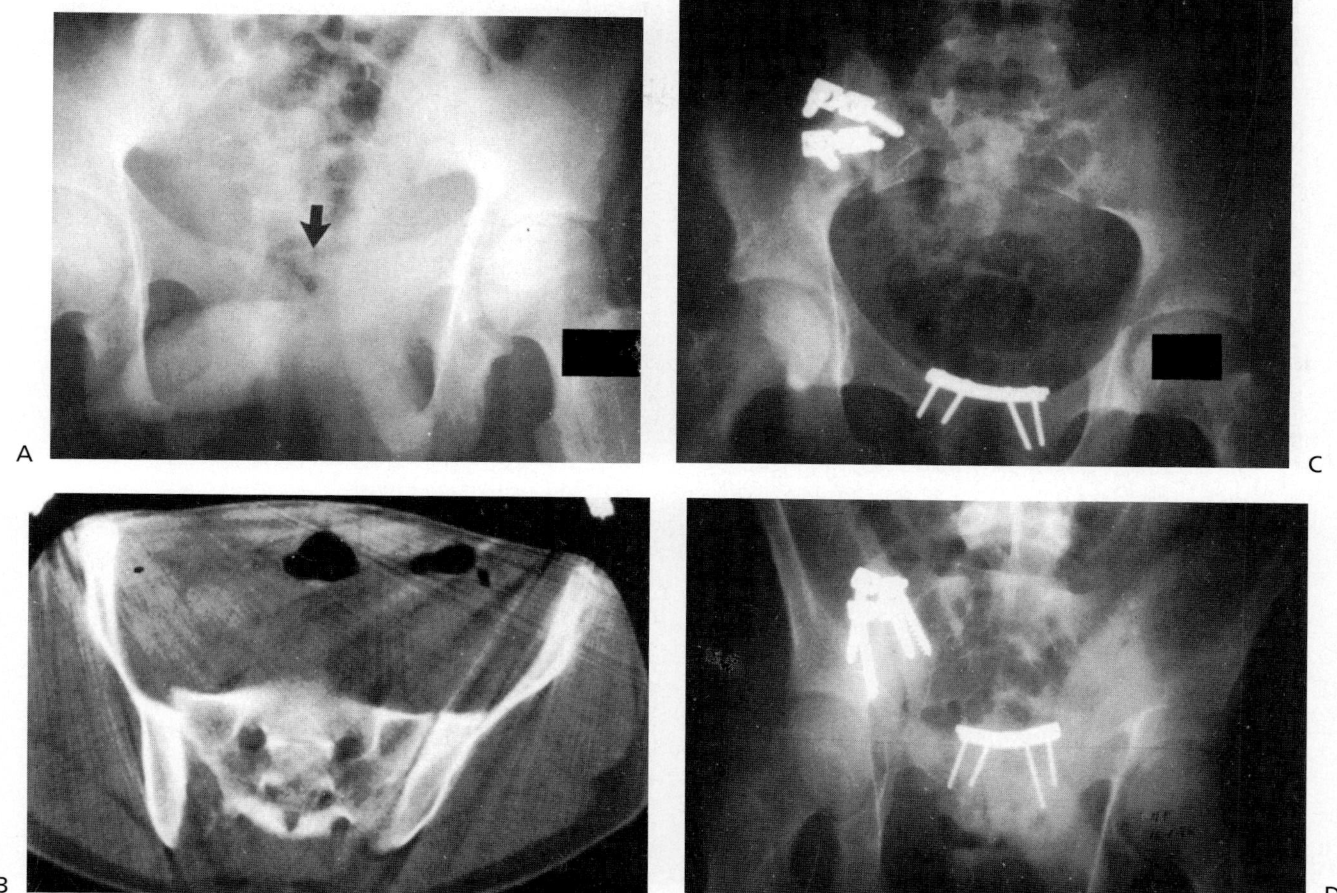

FIGURE 15-10. Anteroposterior radiograph **(A)** shows a locked symphysis *(black arrow)* and a lesion of the right sacroiliac joint as seen on computed tomography **(B).** Note on the computed tomography the marked internal rotation of the right hemipelvis and posterior displacement through the sacroiliac joint. In this case, open reduction and internal fixation were required to unlock the symphysis, which was fixed with a four-hole dynamic compression plate and cancellous screws. At the same operation, through an anterior approach, the sacroiliac joint was fixed with two short plates **(C,D).**

must be remembered that with direct plate fixation of the sacral fractures, an anterior external frame is necessary to supplement the fixation of the sacrum (33,34). Also see Chapters 11 and 16.

POSTERIOR FIXATION

See Table 15-4.

Generally, fractures that tend to open the pelvic ring (i.e., anteroposterior compression or external rotational injuries) and completely unstable injuries often require internal fixation; whereas injuries that close the pelvic ring (i.e., lateral compression injuries) rarely require any form of internal fixation (31,35).

Completely disrupted, translationally unstable posterior injuries require, at a minimum, a closed reduction and maintenance of that reduction with traction for the posterior and vertical displacement and external fixation to control rotational displacement. This treatment choice requires 6 to 12 weeks of bed rest and generally is not acceptable to most patients. It is especially undesirable in patients with multiple injuries. However, it may be required if the patient is not physiologically able to withstand surgery or wishes to avoid the risks associated with this treatment.

TABLE 15-4. INDICATIONS FOR POSTERIOR FIXATION OF PELVIC RING DISRUPTION

Unstable sacroiliac complex with more than 1 cm of displacement, especially if through the sacroiliac joint
Open fractures with posterior (not perineal) wound
Unstable posterior complex associated with acetabular fractures

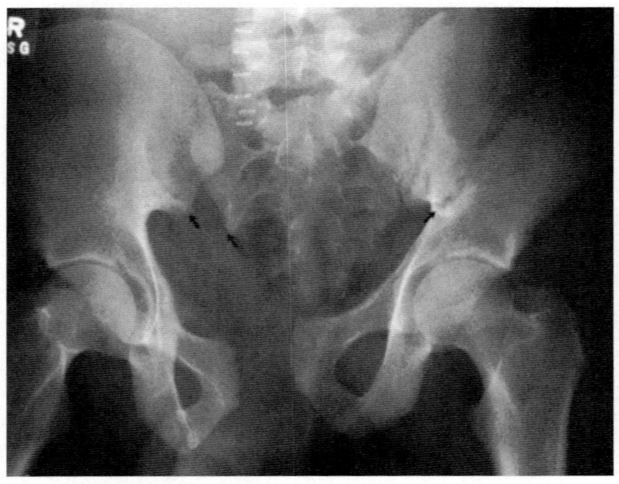

A

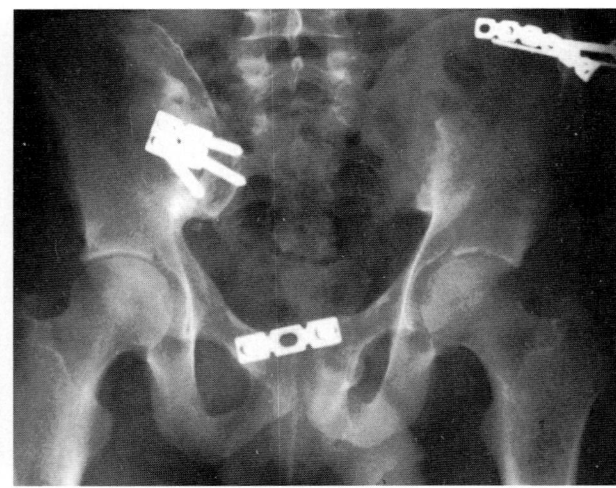

C

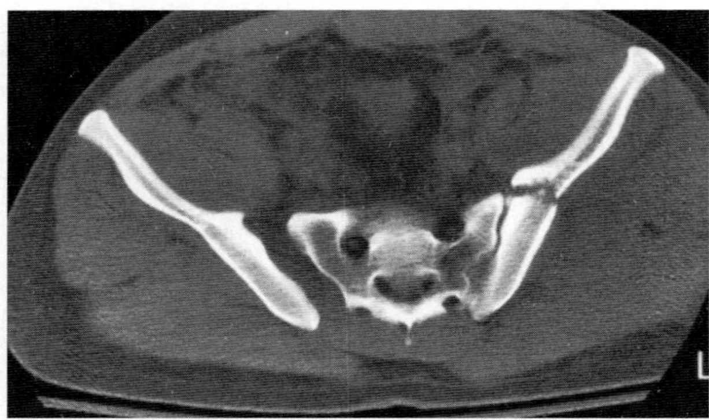

B

FIGURE 15-11. Note the marked displacement of the right sacroiliac joint on the anteroposterior radiograph **(A)** and the computed tomography **(B)**. The patient also has a disrupted symphysis and a fracture through the left ilium. In this case, the right hemipelvis is markedly unstable and the sacroiliac joint displaced >1 cm. Open reduction and internal fixation were performed through an anterior Pfannenstiel incision and bilateral anterior approaches to the sacroiliac joint on the right and the iliac crest on the left. The fixation methods are noted in the anteroposterior radiograph **(C)**. The patient has had an excellent clinical outcome.

Sacroiliac dislocations or fracture-dislocations displaced greater than 1 cm must be anatomically reduced through the articular component (Fig. 15-11). If not, this injury has a high incidence of post fracture pain and discomfort (12,15,31). Injuries that show significant displacement and gap through cancellous bone secondary to high-energy shear force may exhibit delayed union or nonunion, so internal fixation is desirable (Fig. 15-12). In patients with neurologic injuries, where it is obvious that the hemipelvic or sacral displacement may be implicated in aggravating the neurologic deficit, early open reduction and internal fixation is indicated to decompress the involved nerves. In polytrauma patients, especially those with ipsilateral or contralateral extremity injury, it is reasonable to fix the pelvis in order to facilitate postinjury mobilization and rehabilitation (Fig. 15-13) (25,36).

CONTRAINDICATIONS AND RISK FACTORS

Contraindications may be divided into patient, injury, and health-care team factors. Patient factors generally are related to the health and associated comorbidities of the patient. In the trauma situation, it is not unusual to have to delay internal fixation for weeks secondary to head injury, multiple organ failure, and sepsis. In fact, it may never be suitable to internally fix some patients; therefore, the nonoperative methods of traction and external fixation must be used to attempt to maintain the pelvic reduction. The most important injury factor preventing internal fixation is the closed, soft-tissue degloving injury that can occur with direct crush injury. This lesion may lead to increased wound problems and force a change in surgical approach. An indwelling suprapubic catheter, colostomy, or drains in the region of the surgical incisions are added risk factors. Long-term use of a suprapubic catheter may allow clinically undetected contamination of the space of Retzius and the bladder. This may increase the risk of postoperative infection if internal fixation is carried out. If possible, the anterior approach should be avoided if a suprapubic catheter or colostomy will contaminate the exposure.

Because the majority of internal fixation techniques depend on fluoroscopy, it is unwise to proceed with surgery if the bony pelvis cannot be visualized adequately by the image intensifier. This may occur with excessive bowel gas, intestinal dye from the abdominal CT scan, and poorly functioning fluoroscopy units unable to create a satisfactory image. This type of fracture surgery requires specialized

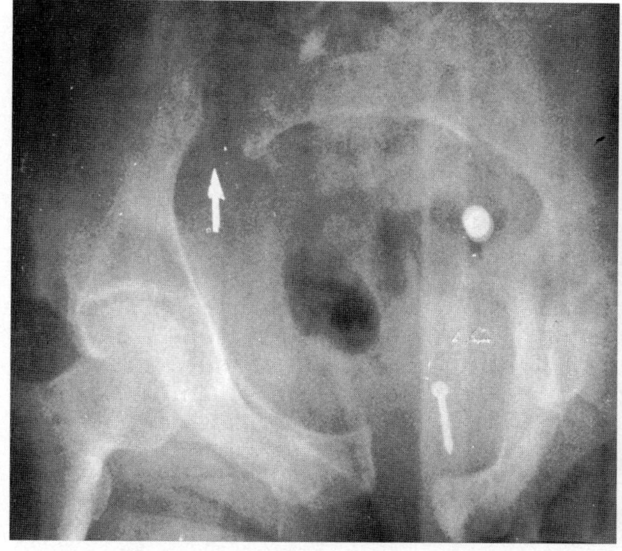
A

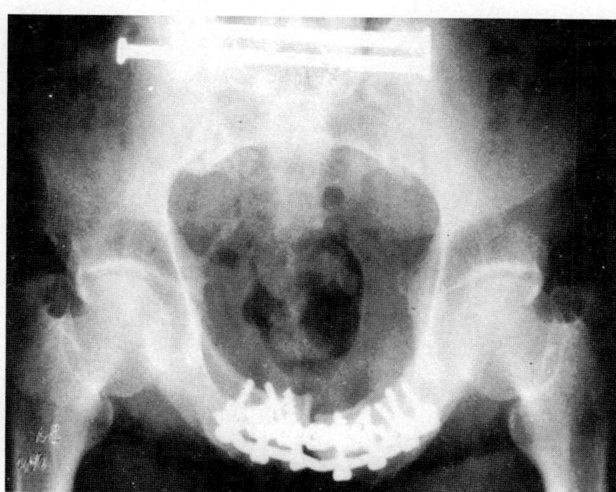
C

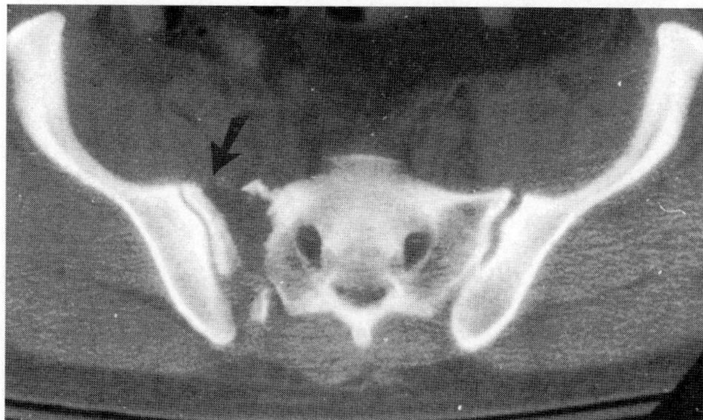
B

FIGURE 15-12. Anteroposterior radiograph **(A)** and computed tomography **(B)** show marked posterior displacement and 1-cm gap through the sacrum, secondary to a high-energy shear force in a motor vehicle accident. Treatment consisted of a double plate on the symphysis and two iliosacral bars posteriorly, resulting in a healed fracture **(C).**

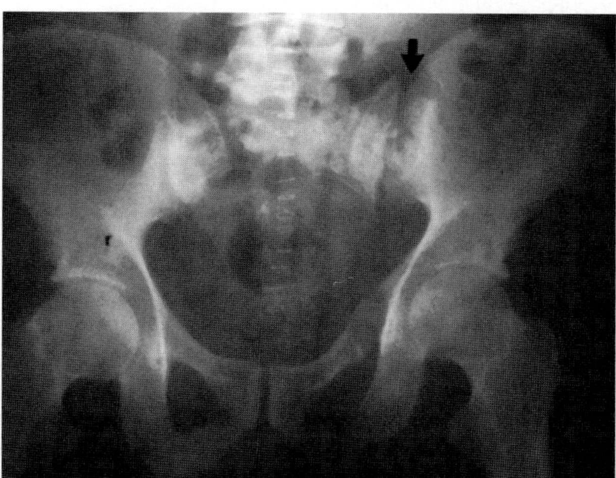
A

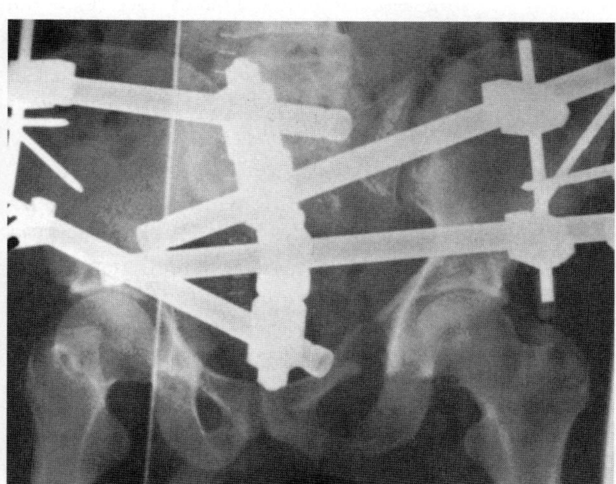
B

FIGURE 15-13. A: Anteroposterior radiograph of a patient with an open pelvic fracture. The left hemipelvis is grossly unstable with a fracture-dislocation through the sacroiliac joint. **B:** Initial treatment consisted of an external fixator.

(Figure continues)

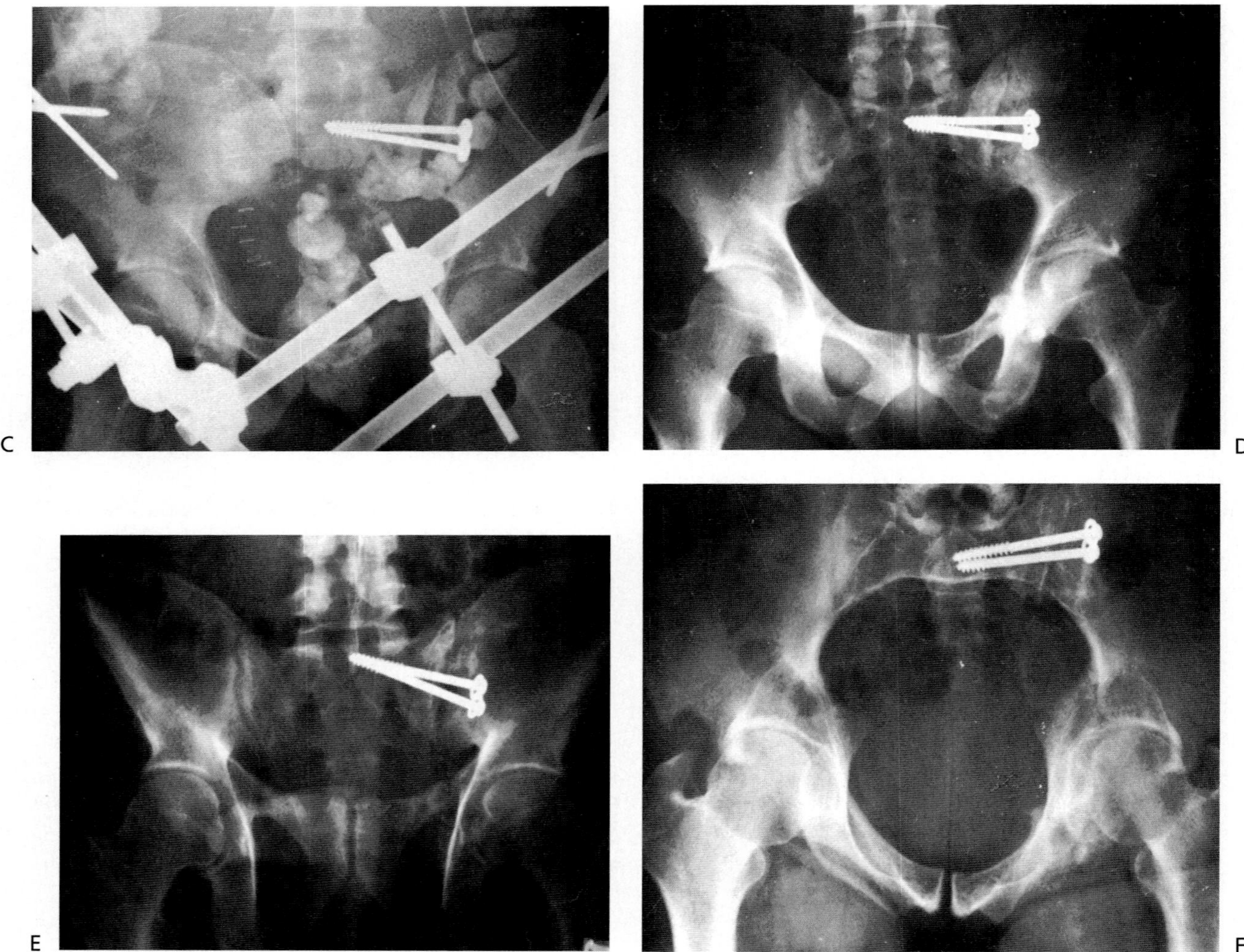

FIGURE 15-13. *(continued)* **C:** Because of the continued displacement and instability of the left hemipelvis, iliosacral screws were inserted, leading eventually to excellent healing and stability of the sacroiliac joint and ramus fractures, as noted on the anteroposterior **(D)**, inlet **(E)**, and outlet **(F)** radiographs.

instruments, knowledge, and help to be successful. These are not fractures that the general orthopedic surgeon should be treating unless the surgeon has had formal pelvic fracture operative training. Once the patient is hemodynamically stable and a decision is made that internal fixation is desirable, the patient should be transferred to a surgeon skilled in pelvic surgical techniques. A long delay owing to indecision about whether or not the fracture needs surgery only makes matters worse and compromises the end result. Therefore, it is imperative that the treating orthopedic surgeon quickly and completely evaluate the patient. Consultation with a specialist in the field should be obtained. In this way, the patient may be given adequate, quick, and definitive treatment to optimize long-term results. Finally, the hospital operating room must be supplied with the specialized instrumentation and implants to perform this surgery.

CLOSED TECHNIQUES

Preoperative Considerations

Although anterior internal fixation of the symphysis pubis often is performed in the acute phase, acute posterior internal fixation is undertaken infrequently. Most often, posterior internal fixation is delayed 3 to 5 days, or in some cases as long as 2 to 3 weeks. Because of this, some very important preoperative measures should be taken to facilitate the surgical procedure.

The completely unstable (Type C) pelvic ring disruption should be reduced and maintained by skeletal traction to achieve the appropriate leg length and position, making delayed reduction simpler. Skeletal traction through a tibial tubercle pin is safe as long as not more than 15 kg (about 30 lb) of weights are used. A femoral condylar pin is required if more than 15 kg of traction is required or there is a potential for a significant knee injury.

External fixation is commonly used with skeletal traction to control rotational abnormalities. For patients in shock the external fixator is applied for hemodynamic control. External fixators provide provisional control of pain and improve the patient's mobility (36,37). It is important that the pin site care is meticulous and surgery is performed as soon as possible. When surgery is delayed beyond 5 days, the pin sites are potentially infected. If the surgical field is compromised, removal of the frame, debridement of the pin sites, and maintenance of the reduction with skeletal traction must be undertaken before surgery.

Thromboembolic disease is a major concern in patients with pelvic disruptions, especially when a delay has occurred. When treatment has been delayed for >5 days, a greater risk of preoperative, intraoperative, or postoperative pulmonary embolus may exist. Thorough evaluation of the deep venous system is imperative to rule out venous thrombosis and its potential problems. At present there is not a definitive investigation for evaluating the internal iliac venous system of the pelvis. Magnetic resonance venography and contrast enhanced CT scanning have been proposed but both have problems with false-positive results. Prophylactic anticoagulation in the preoperative period may be used if not contraindicated by the patient's other associated injuries. A short-acting easily reversible anticoagulant such as low molecular weight heparin is suggested. If venous thrombosis is found, appropriate consultation with specialists in this disease and use of anticoagulation and venocaval filters are required if surgery is to be performed safely.

Finally, because this is major surgery with significant soft-tissue disruptions and implant usage, *prophylactic antibiotics* always should be used. Antibiotics, covering a broad spectrum of Gram-positive and -negative organisms are desirable, such as first- or second-generation cephalosporin, given either the night before or within the first several hours before the procedure and then maintained for 24 to 48 hours.

Knowledge of appropriate surgical techniques—and understanding of pelvic anatomy—are imperative for anyone who undertakes this type of treatment. Because complications are serious, any surgeon who performs this type of surgery must be aware of the problems to be faced during the perioperative period, the methods of handling them, and their follow-up care. *It always has been said that major surgery creates major complications, and any surgeon willing to undertake this type of surgery must be willing to look after these complications.*

Surgical Techniques

Posterior Iliosacral Screw Fixation: Fluoroscopic Control for Percutaneous Insertion and Reduction Techniques

When sacroiliac lag screw fixation is chosen, it is imperative that these screws are inserted with a reliable and safe technique. Fluoroscopic guidance must be used to assure the safe placement of these screws. For unstable pelvic ring disruptions, sacroiliac lag screw fixation is one choice for the posterior elements. The ilium at the sciatic buttress and the S1 vertebral body are the fixation points. Sacroiliac lag screws can be used for dislocations and fracture-dislocations of the sacroiliac joint when these key structures are intact. They are oriented perpendicular to the sacroiliac joint, allowing compression of the joint (see Fig. 15-33). The screws are used in unstable displaced sacral fractures, particularly if located at or lateral to the foramina (Denis 1, II).

Prerequisites for Use

The following criteria must be met in order that this procedure be done safely.

1. The surgeon must understand the anatomy of the posterior pelvis as well as its variations.
2. High-quality fluoroscopic images of the entire pelvis must be available intraoperatively.
3. The surgeon must completely understand the injury, including the three-dimensional anatomy of the displaced fractured pelvis.
4. The surgeon must assure himself or herself that the upper sacral anatomy is normal based on the plain radiographs and CT scan.
5. The surgeon must possess the ability to reduce this fracture, either closed or open.

Anatomy. The position of the sacroiliac lag screw is critical. It must follow the S1 pedicle mass into the body of S1, remaining completely contained within bone throughout its path.

The S1 segment is surrounded by major anatomic structures. The S1 root canal and the S1 sacral foramen limit the inferior margin of the S1 pedicle mass. Posteriorly, the cauda equina rests against the S1 vertebral body. Anterior to the sacral ala are the internal iliac vessels, L5 nerve root, and ureter. The pelvic viscera are anterior to the S1 body. The L5-S1 intervertebral disc is superior to the S1 body. Any of these structures can be injured if a screw violates the boundaries of the first sacral segment.

The S1 pedicle mass is about 1 to 1.5 cm in cross section. It is oriented slightly obliquely from medial-superior to lateral-inferior. This is the path that the screw follows. The sacral promontory is anterior to the S1 pedicle mass (Fig. 15-14), and the sacral ala is concave between the sacral promontory and the anterior aspect of the sacroiliac joint. A

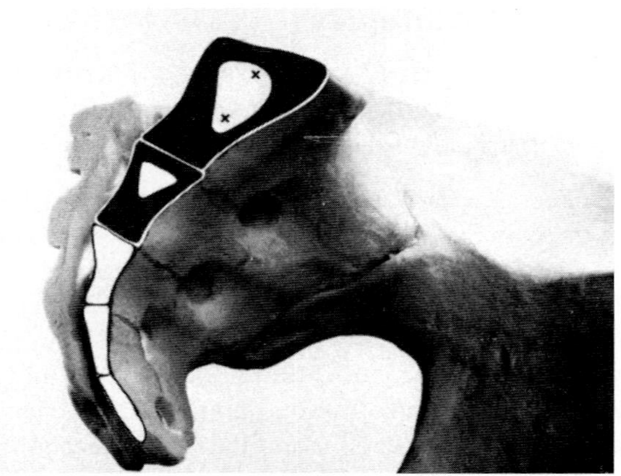

FIGURE 15-14. Model pelvis is cut sagittally in the midline to show the prominence of the sacral promontory and the concavity of the sacral ala. The white areas are safe for screw placement. The black areas must not be crossed by screws. The x's mark the best locations if two screws are used. For one screw, the safest location is between the two x's.

screw aimed at the sacral promontory has a good chance of exiting the bony mass of the S1 pedicle anteriorly, in the region of the L5 nerve root, internal iliac vessels, and ureter (Fig. 15-15). This cannot be seen on any available x-ray view. *Therefore, the sacral promontory is not an acceptable target at which to aim sacroiliac screws.*

More than half of the S1 foramen is formed by the S1 body. The S1 root canal progresses inferiorly, anteriorly, and laterally toward the S1 foramen (Fig. 15-16). If a screw is placed in the inferior half of the S1 body, it must be aimed anterior to the S1 root canal. Screws placed in the posterior half of the body will traverse the S1 root canal superior to the S1 foramen.

The ideal positions for two screws in the S1 segment are marked with x's in Fig. 15-17. One screw is placed superiorly, in the middle anterior-posterior aspect of the S1 body, near the upper S1 endplates. The second screw is placed inferiorly in the anterior portion of the anterior-posterior dimension of the S1 body. Any location in the white area is safe. When a single screw is sufficient, it could be placed in the center of the white area. In cross section the upper screw path is shown between the two dotted lines in Fig. 15-18.

It is the S1 segment that is used as a target for insertion of sacroiliac lag screws. All important nearby structures are related anatomically to the first sacral segment. The landmarks of S1 are readily identifiable, anatomically and radiographically. However, the anatomic landmarks on the ilium are important for the reduction.

Anatomic Variations. Dysmorphism of the upper sacrum makes it difficult to insert the screws safely. This abnormality occurs in up to 40% of patients and is best seen on the pelvic outlet radiograph. On this view, the upper sacrum is located at the level of the iliac crests and the upper sacral foramina are oddly shaped. The sacral ala is acutely angulated and asymmetrical and a residual disc space may be present between the upper two sacral vertebrae. On CT scan,

A

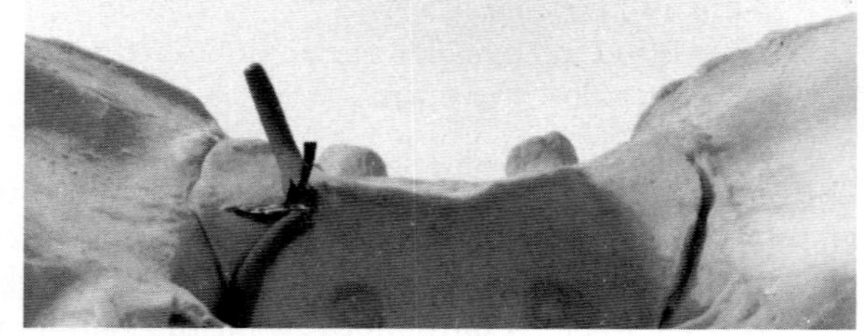

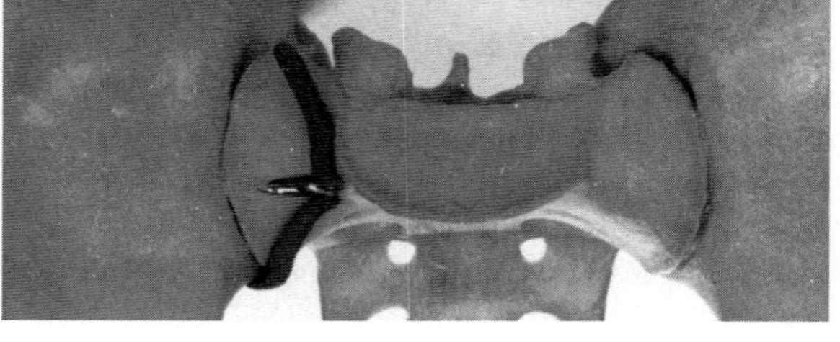

B

C

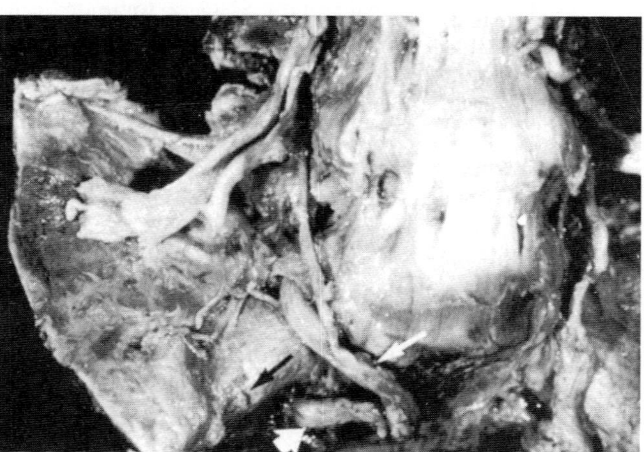

FIGURE 15-15. Model of the pelvis shows drill violating the concavity of the sacral ala within the radiographic margins of the ala in **(A)** the outlet projection, and **(B)** the inlet projection. **C:** Anatomic dissection along the anterior aspect of the sacroiliac joint. Note the proximity of the L5 nerve root *(white arrow)* to the sacroiliac joint *(black arrow).* The L5 nerve root is seen crossing the ala of the sacrum and joining with the S1 nerve root (*white arrowhead*), exiting the first sacral foramen. These nerve roots can be damaged in any anterior approach to the sacroiliac joint. The safety zone over the ala is approximately 1 cm medial to the sacroiliac joint. (From Schatzker J, Tile M. *The rationale of operative fracture care.* Heidelberg: Springer-Verlag, 1987, with permission)

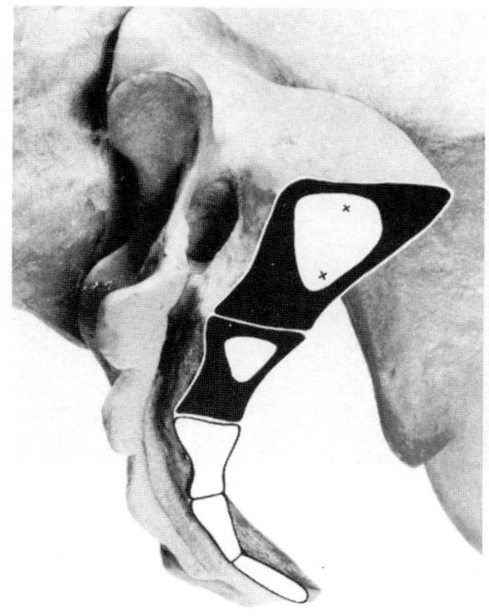

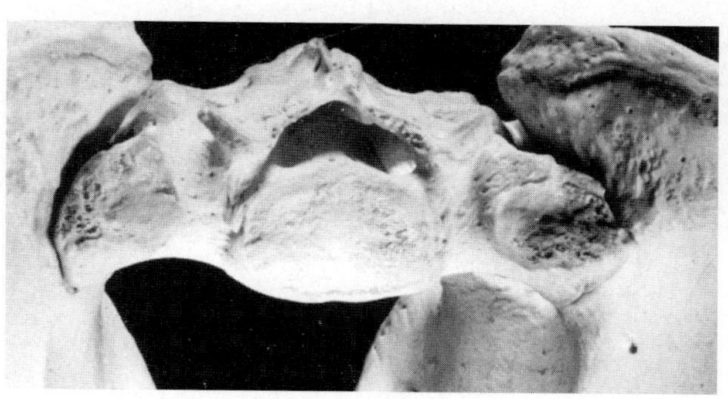

FIGURE 15-16. The course of the S1 root canal from the spinal canal progresses laterally, anteriorly, and caudally to the S1 foramen, in **(A)** the model from a posterolateral view, and **(B)** an anatomic pelvis from a superior view. The danger area in the posterior inferior triangle of the S1 vertebra is shown in black.

the sacroiliac joint demonstrates a tongue in groove appearance (Fig. 15-19) (24,38,39).

Surgical Technique

The patient and C-arm position must be set up precisely to obtain the three fluoroscopic views described (40,41). This is true for both the prone and supine positions. One can proceed only when the fluoroscopic anatomy can be seen clearly. Several important factors limit visualization of the fluoroscopic anatomy. The most important is the presence of bowel gas. Even a small bubble of bowel gas can obscure identification of the S1 foramina. The bowel is checked for gas with an abdominal radiograph. A preoperative enema may help to dispel the gas or dye.

Positioning

Supine

The patient is placed on a radiolucent operating table and a radiolucent lumbosacral support (two stacked and folded

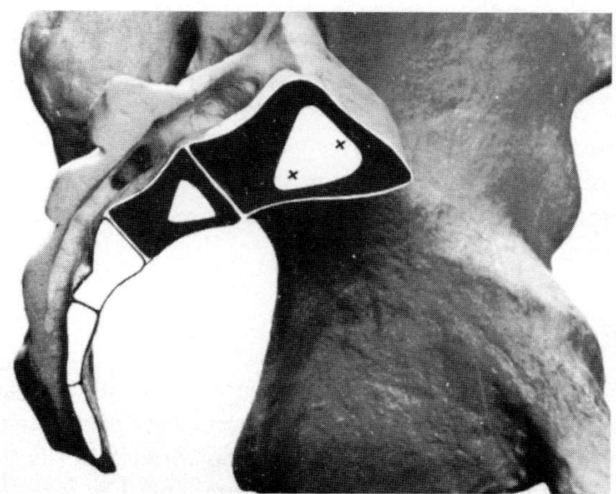

FIGURE 15-17. The lateral sacral view: anatomic model.

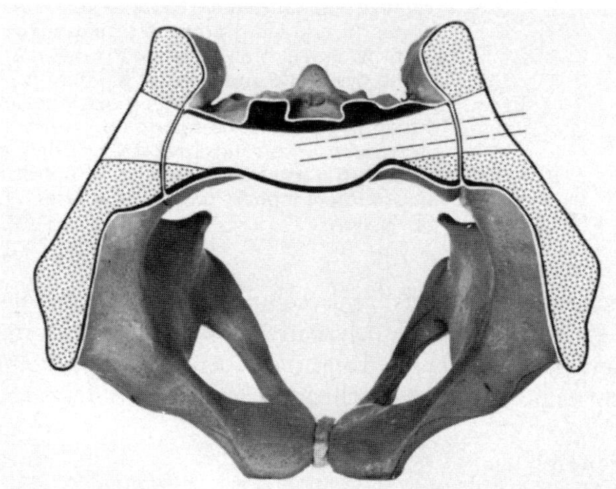

FIGURE 15-18. A cross section of the pelvis at the upper level of the S1 vertebral body shows the safest path for a screw at this level between the two dotted lines. Note the concavity of the sacral ala anteriorly. Screws should not cross any of the black boundaries, nor should they be aimed posteriorly, toward the spinal canal.

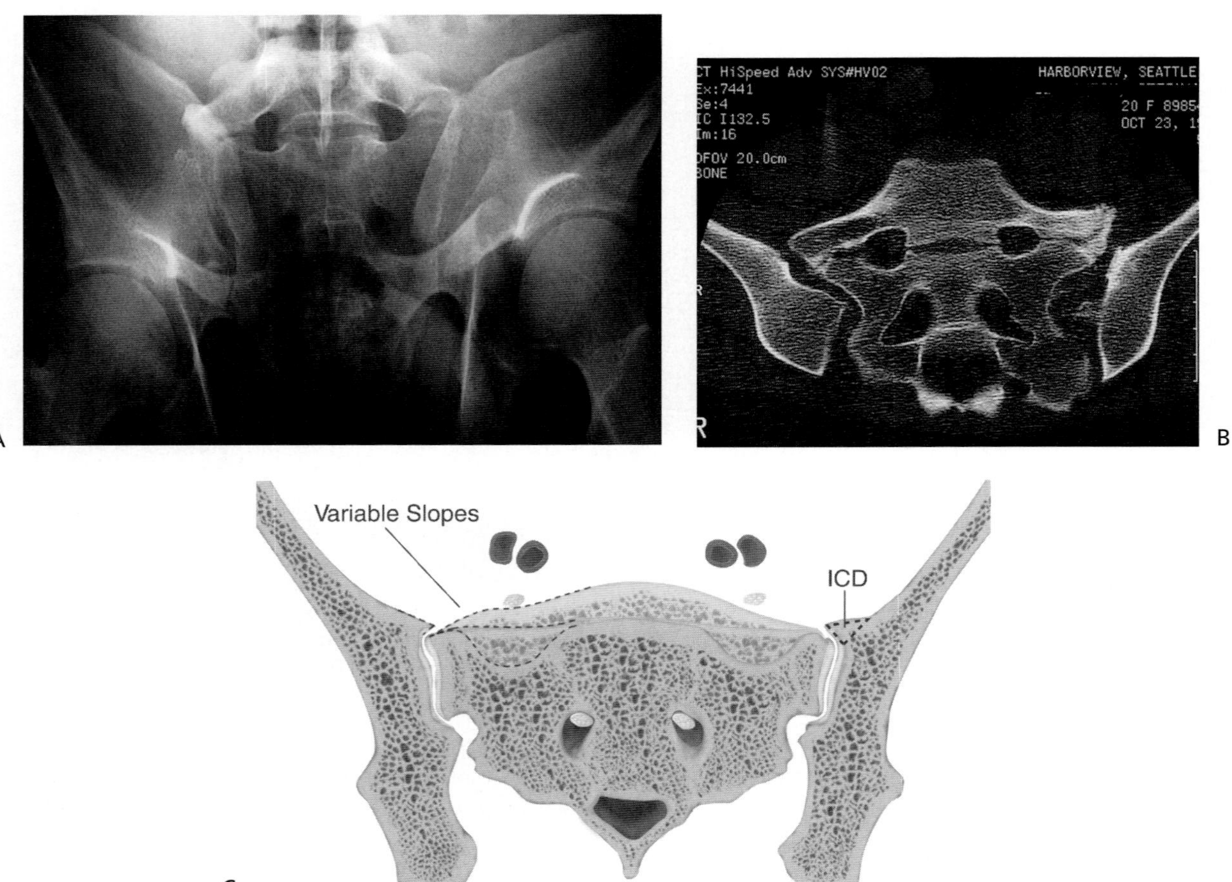

FIGURE 15-19. A: The pelvic-outlet radiograph alerts the surgeon to a potential sacral dysmorphism. The upper sacrum is located at the level of the iliac crests. The upper sacral foramina are oddly shaped. The ala are acutely angulated and often asymmetric. Mammillary processes are noted along the ala. A residual "disc space" may be present also between the upper two sacral segments. A true lateral sacral image confirms the upper sacral vertebral prominence with acutely angulated alar slopes. The alar slope is estimated based on the iliac cortical density (ICD), which is usually coplanar relative to the anterior alar surface. **B:** Computed tomography (CT) scan demonstrates "tongue-in-groove" articulations of the sacroiliac joint in sacral dysplasia. The CT scan also confirms the relation between the iliac cortical density and anterior sacral ala. The "danger zone" of the dysplastic upper sacral segment is recognized. Fluoroscopically guided iliosacral screw insertions are dangerous in these patients and are not recommended. **C:** The variable structure of the upper sacrum. The relation between the iliac cortical density and the alar slope must be understood to insert iliosacral screws safely by using fluoroscopic guidance. (From: Routt MLC, Simonian PT. Posterior pelvic-ring disruptions: iliosacral screws. In: Thompson RC Jr, ed. *Master techniques in orthopedic surgery: fractures.* Philadelphia: Lippincott Williams & Wilkins, 1998, with permission.)

operating room sheets) is placed under the midline to allow access to the posterior pelvic area. A femoral or tibial traction pin may be inserted and the patient put in traction to help reduce the fracture, which precludes a freely draped leg.

Prone

This position facilitates the open approach to the sacrum, if needed. The patient is placed on radiolucent bolsters to allow the abdomen to fall free. The chest and pelvis usually rest on the bolsters. If the pelvic bolsters impede reduction of the pelvis, they can be positioned in a more distal location (toward the thighs) to allow better access to the iliac crests.

Lateral

This position is possible but is not amenable to patients with spinal injuries and makes fluoroscopic visualization more difficult.

Fluoroscopic Views

Insertion is carried out under fluoroscopic control to ensure that sacroiliac screws are placed accurately in the first sacral segment. The fluoroscopy unit is positioned on the side opposite the injured hemipelvis. Matta described three fluoroscopic views of the pelvis—anteroposterior, inlet, and out-

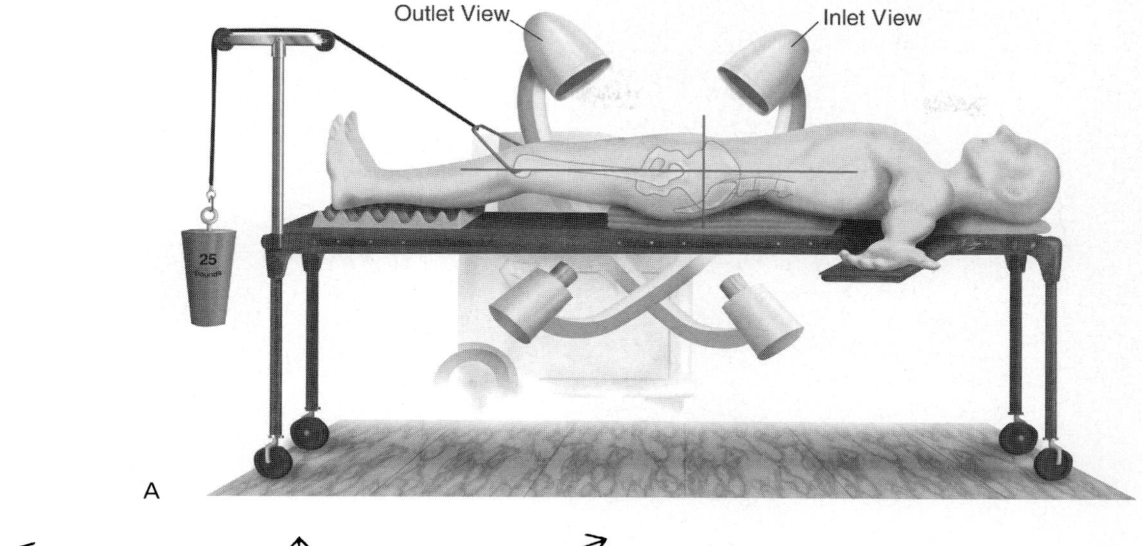

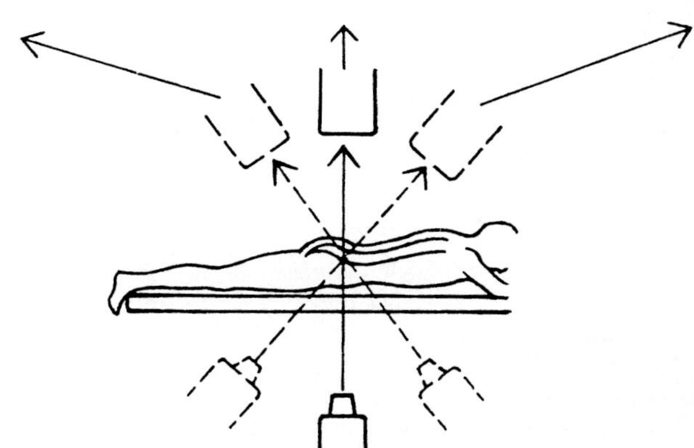

FIGURE 15-20. A: The patient is positioned supine and elevated on two folded and stacked blankets, a lumbosacral support. This operating table has no central support and allows extremes of fluoroscope rotation and therefore pelvic imaging. Distal femoral traction is possible by using a pulley system anchored to the foot of the table. (From: Routt MLC, Simonian PT. In: Thompson RC Jr, ed. *Master techniques in orthopedic surgery: fractures.* Philadelphia: Lippincott Williams & Wilkins, 1998, with permission.) **B:** Insertion of iliosacral screws requires image intensification. The C arm must be positioned to allow anteroposterior inlet and outlet views of the pelvis. (From: Muller ME. *AO manual of internal fixation,* 3rd ed. Berlin: Springer-Verlag, 1990, with permission)

let—which correspond to the views first described by Pennal and Sutherland (Fig. 15-20) (12,40,41). The starting point for screw insertion cannot be directly identified if the procedure is carried out in a percutaneous fashion. Establishing a satisfactory starting point through the very thick overlying soft tissues is difficult using these views.

The lateral sacral fluoroscopic view makes the percutaneous technique easier by allowing clear identification of the first sacral body (Fig. 15-21). Sacroiliac screw insertion is then similar to the freehand technique used for inserting locking screws through intramedullary rods. The lateral sacral view must be precisely oriented. The patient is positioned within a few degrees of pelvic rotation from the horizontal. This position can be checked by *assuring that the shadows of the femoral heads or the greater sciatic notches are superimposed.* The horizontal C arm is then coincident with the required screw path in S1 (Fig. 15-18). Anterior-to-posterior angulation must be avoided, to prevent screws from being aimed at the cauda equina. The ideal screw path tracks from inferior to superior and (depending on the fracture pattern) posterior to anterior.

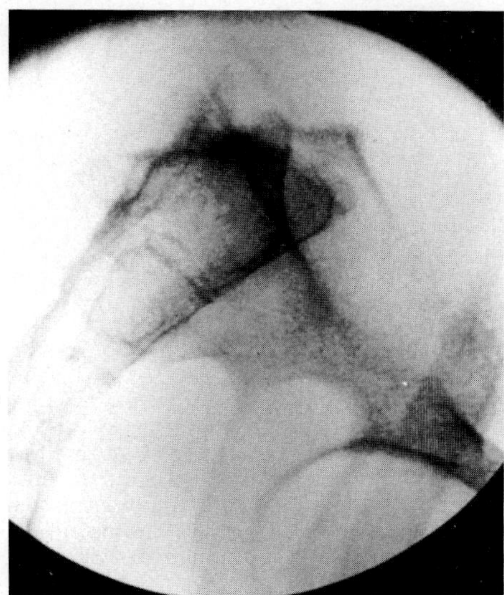

FIGURE 15-21. The lateral sacral view: fluoroscopic appearance of a bony pelvis.

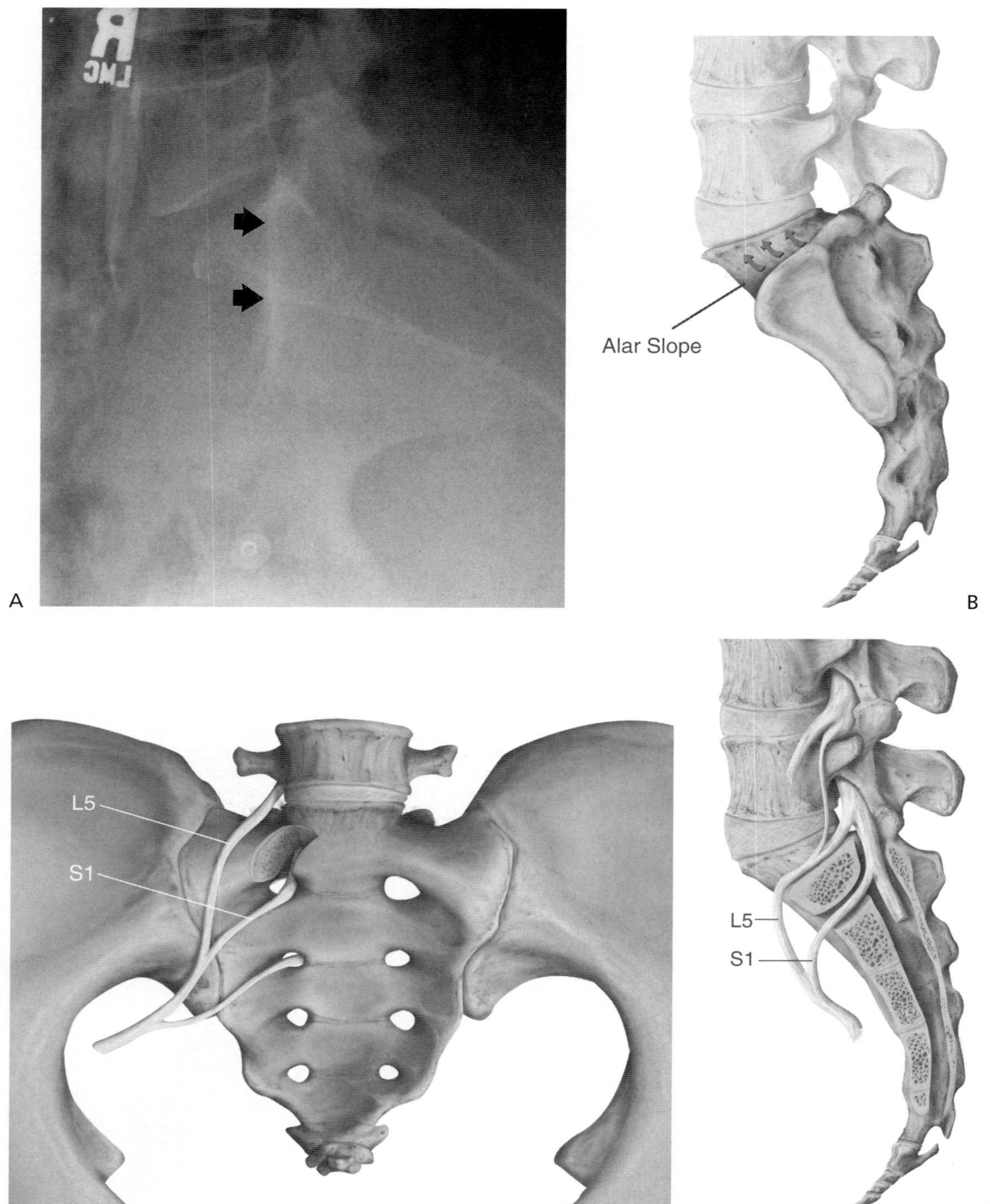

FIGURE 15-22. **A:** The true lateral sacral image is obtained only after accurate posterior pelvic reduction by superimposing the greater sciatic notches. The iliac cortical density is noted by the arrowheads. **B:** The disarticulated sacroiliac joint and the ascending sacral alar slope. **C:** The local nerve roots and their alar relations are demonstrated. **D:** Lateral sacral sagittal section indicates the changing structure of the alar zone and its neural relations. The fifth lumbar and first sacral nerve roots are highlighted. (From: Routt MLC, Simonian PT. Posterior pelvic-ring disruptions: iliosacral screws. In: Thompson RC Jr, ed. *Master techniques in orthopedic surgery: fractures.* Philadelphia: Lippincott Williams & Wilkins, 1998, with permission.)

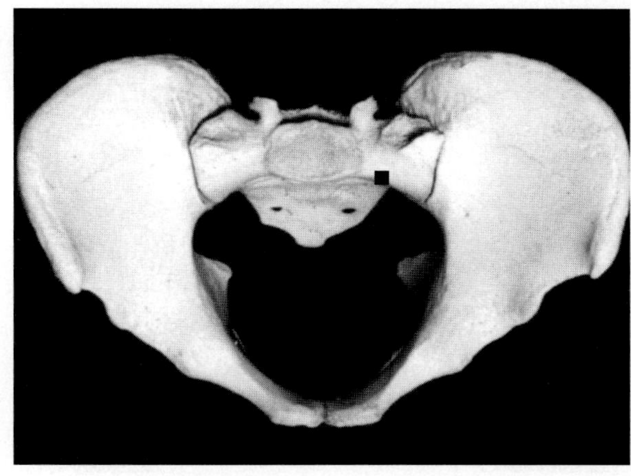
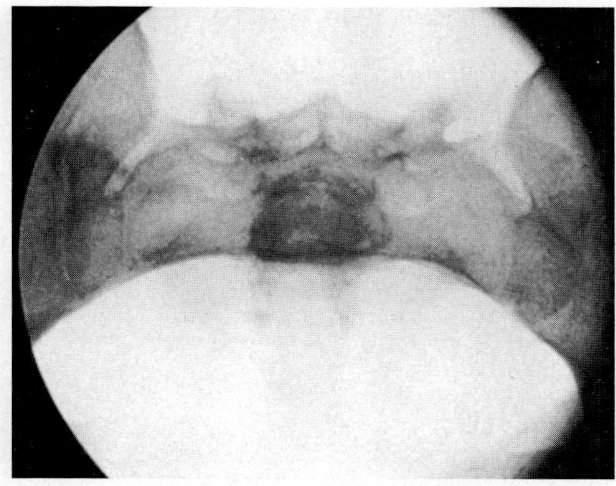

A B

FIGURE 15-23. The pelvic inlet view: **(A)** bony pelvis and **(B)** fluoroscopic appearance, showing the cortex of S1 and S2 overlapping in the correct fashion.

The C arm is first positioned so that the S1 vertebral endplates are seen in tangent. The C-arm base is then moved a few inches toward the patient's head. This aligns the C arm along the required inferior-to-superior screw path. The iliac cortical densities are identified on this view (Fig. 15-22). Significant hemipelvic deformity causes this view to be of little help. *This view is only obtainable after an accurate posterior pelvic fracture reduction is achieved.* The intensifier is brought to the anteroposterior projection and pivoted from the inlet to the outlet view.

The anteroposterior view allows assessment of the proper positioning and is helpful in determining fracture alignment and potential fluoroscopic visualization problems. The pelvic inlet view must be precisely aligned, so that the anterior cortex of S1 and that of S2 overlap as concentric circles (Fig. 15-23). If the anterior cortex of S1 overlies the coccyx, the concavity of the sacrum may not be appreciated (Fig. 15-24), and a screw could exit undetected from the anterior aspect of the S1 body. However, the posterior cortex of S1 and the spinal canal are best seen with this view.

The pelvic outlet view is obtained by pivoting the C arm until the pubic symphysis lies over the midline of the sacrum and the pubic tubercle lies just inferior to the S1 foramen over the second sacral vertebral body (Fig. 15-25). This view allows direct visualization of the entire S1 segment.

Skin Preparation and Draping

The perineum, abdomen, bilateral flanks and the involved lower extremity are prepped. The posterior lateral buttocks must be prepped down to the tabletop.

Fracture Reduction

Fracture reduction must be completed before inserting the screws. For fractures through the sacral foramina, reduction

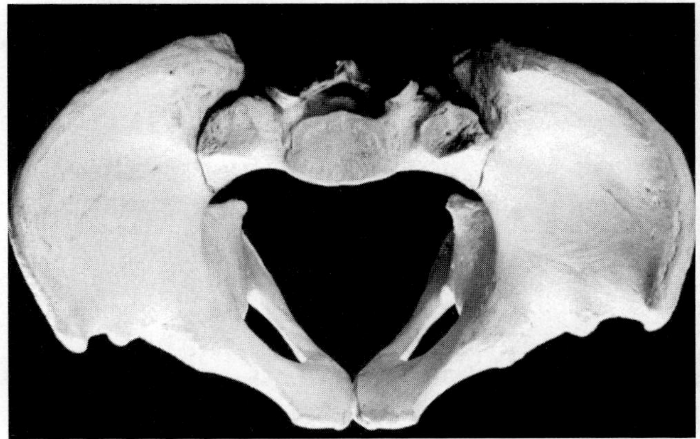
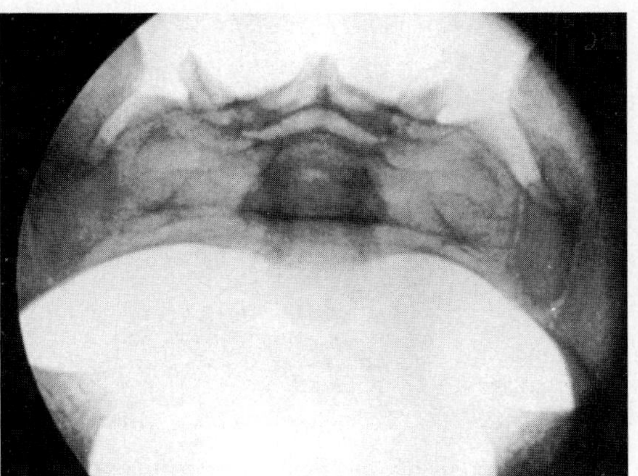

A B

FIGURE 15-24. The pelvic inlet view **(A)** of the bony pelvis and **(B)** fluoroscopic appearance show too much angle on the C arm to the anterior cortex of S2, but the posterior cortex and the spinal canal are well seen.

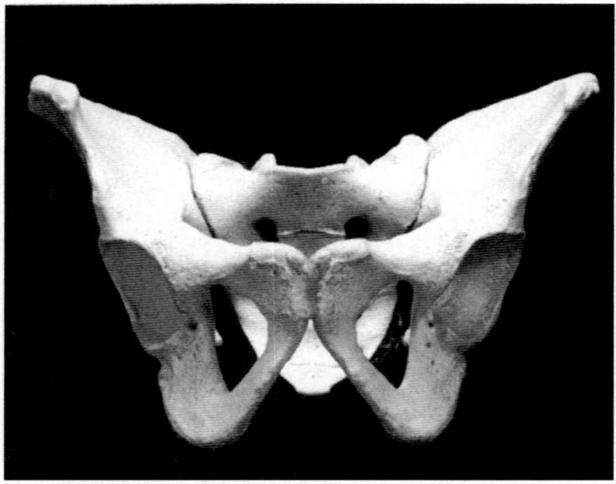
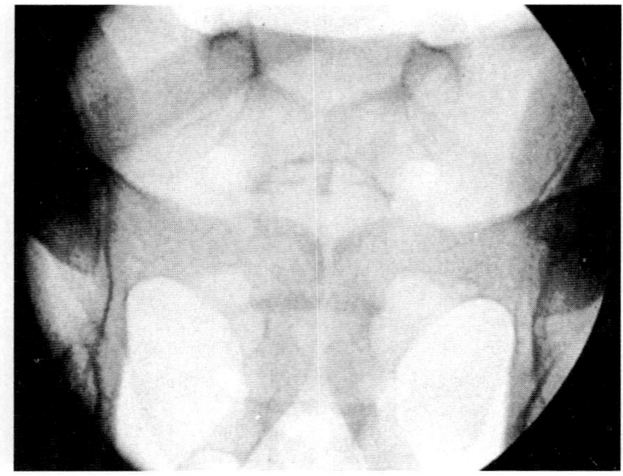

FIGURE 15-25. The pelvic outlet view **(A)** of the bony pelvis and **(B)** fluoroscopic appearance show the pubic tubercle just below the S1 foramen.

must be anatomic, to prevent injury to nerve roots contained in the displaced sacral fragments. Furthermore, when fractured, the sacral foramina can be difficult to see on fluoroscopy. If closed reduction is not anatomic, open reduction must be carried out. With open reduction, the starting point for screw insertion on the lateral aspect of the iliac wing *can* be defined under direct vision using local anatomic landmarks. However, even in open reduction cases, further dissection and reflection of the gluteal flap are not required to gain an unobstructed line of view for the screw path. Therefore, once an accurate reduction is obtained, either by open or closed means, screws are inserted percutaneously.

Because the path of the sacroiliac screws is in the midsagittal plane, they can be inserted with the patient positioned supine or prone (Fig. 15-26A,B). Closed reduction and screw insertion are performed on a radiolucent table with the patient in the supine position when other injuries dictate that position. If reduction of the sacral fracture fails, then the patient must be turned to the prone position for an open reduction. The sacroiliac screws are then inserted with the patient in the prone position. If closed reduction of the sacroiliac joints fails, then an open reduction of the sacroiliac joint may be performed, either supine or prone. When the patient has been fitted with an anterior fixator for initial management, it often has to be disassembled or removed for reduction and screw fixation posteriorly.

Closed reduction often is possible within the first few days following injury. Anatomic anterior reduction and fixation with a plate and screws of the symphysis or pubic rami often result in a satisfactory posterior reduction. The posterior sacroiliac screws then can be inserted with the patient lying supine on a radiolucent operating table.

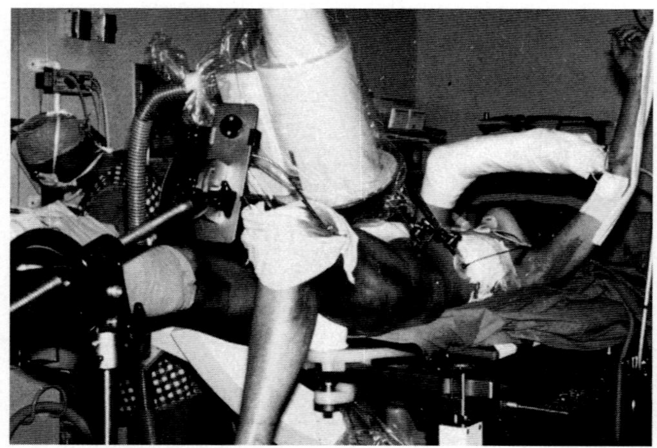
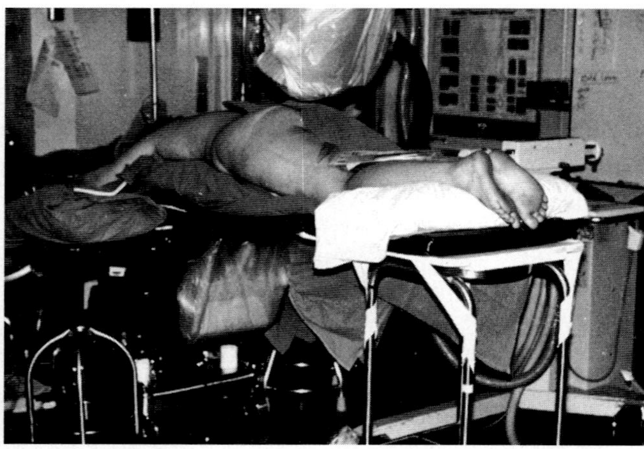

FIGURE 15-26. A: A patient lies on a radiolucent fracture table with traction applied through a femoral pin with the hip flexed. The C arm is in position for the outlet view. **B:** A patient is positioned prone on a radiolucent board. The board is 3/4-inch plywood on the operating table at the level of the head and chest, and is taped to a ring stand at the foot. This leaves enough room under the patient to pivot the C arm for the inlet and the outlet views.

If a radiolucent fracture table is available, then closed reduction maneuvers, including traction, can be carried out under fluoroscopic control. The affected hemipelvis is reduced by traction through a distal femoral pin. Traction with the hip flexed applies a reduction force in line with the direction of the posterior displacement. Subsequent abduction or adduction reduces the rotational component. In the supine position, the iliac wing may be grasped with a large bone reduction forceps and manipulated into place by correcting the translation and rotation. A Schanz screw inserted into the crest or anterior interspinous bone may be helpful, as is a large distractor. In the prone position, reduction is aided by traction and percutaneous insertion of Schanz screws into the posterior tubercles. Using a large distractor to manipulate the hemipelvis into place, a reduction may be accomplished. Ball spiked pushers are helpful to close gaps. Provisional fixation is helpful in stabilizing the reduced sacroiliac joint to facilitate percutaneous screw insertion. Large K-wires, inserted through the iliac wing into the sacral ala under fluoroscopic guidance, may be used for this purpose. If a satisfactory closed reduction cannot be obtained with the patient supine; there are a number of options: (a) if not already done, the anterior elements can be fixed, with a plate and/or screws when indicated; (b) for sacroiliac joint dislocations or fracture-dislocations without sacral involvement, open reduction using an anterior surgical approach can be performed; (c) the patient can be repositioned prone and the closed reduction (which is sometimes easier with the patient in this position) reattempted; or (d) open reduction can then be instituted if attempts at closed reduction in the prone position fail.

When the fracture involves the sacral foramina, the S1 foramen may be difficult to identify. The inferior screw cannot be placed if the S1 foramen is not clearly identified. Obesity decreases fluoroscopic detail but is usually not prohibitive.

The absolute rule for this technique is: *If you can't see it, you can't do it.* There are no exceptions (20).

Percutaneous Screw Insertion

Either cannulated or noncannulated large fragment cancellous screws are used. The procedure starts with the C arm in the lateral position, following fracture reduction. The site for skin penetration is identified with the tip of the guidewire or drill bit overlying the shadow of the S1 body (Fig. 15-27). This position is facilitated by placing the guidewire or drill bit in the posterior cephalad quadrant formed by a line drawn along the femoral shaft and intersected by a line dropped from the anterior superior iliac spine perpendicular to the operating table. The skin is then punctured with the wire. The instrument is placed through the soft tissues coincident with the x-ray beam until it abuts the outer table of the iliac wing. It is held with an instrument such as a long Kocher clamp and oriented so that it is seen end-on overlying the target area (Fig. 15-28). The guidewire or drill bit is advanced by gentle tapping for a short distance, into the posterior tubercle. The skin is incised and blunt deep dissection down to the lateral iliac wing is done. The C arm then is rotated to the anteroposterior plane. The insertion of the guidewire or drill bit is continued only after confirming a satisfactory direction on the inlet and outlet views (Fig. 15-29A,B). With the direction confirmed in both views, the guidewire is advanced by tapping or drilling, observing the progress on the pelvic inlet and outlet views. The guidewire or drill bit is halted when in the ala and the tip located just above the upper sacral foramen on the outlet view. The true lateral is obtained again. If the posterior reduction is accurate and there is no sacral dysmorphism, then the tip of the guidewire or drill bit should be caudal to the iliac cortical density and cephalad to the in-

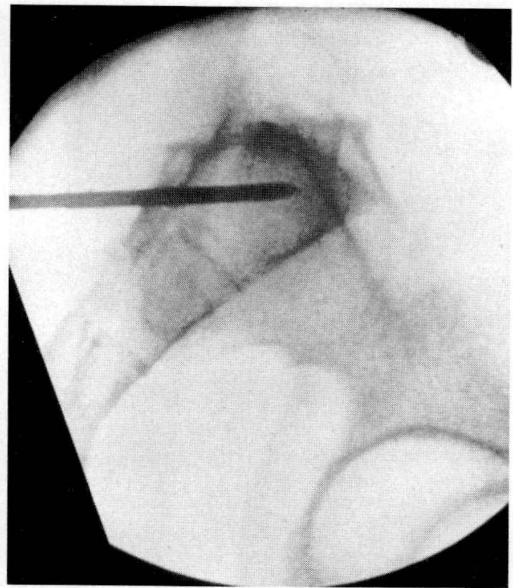

FIGURE 15-27. Guidewire positioning to locate the skin entry for the upper screw.

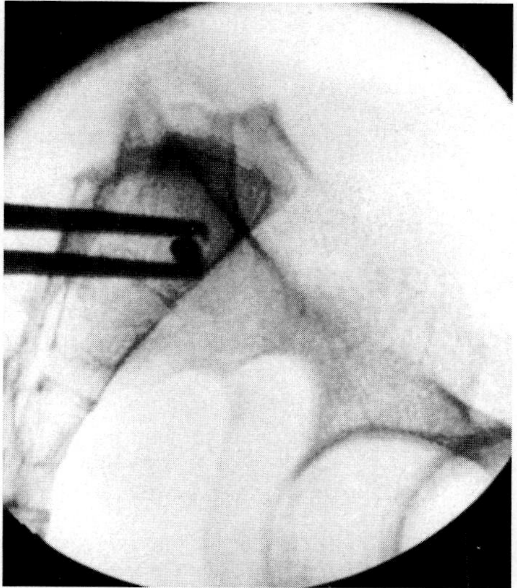

FIGURE 15-28. Guidewire positioning to locate the entry point on the ilium and to determine the path for the lower screw.

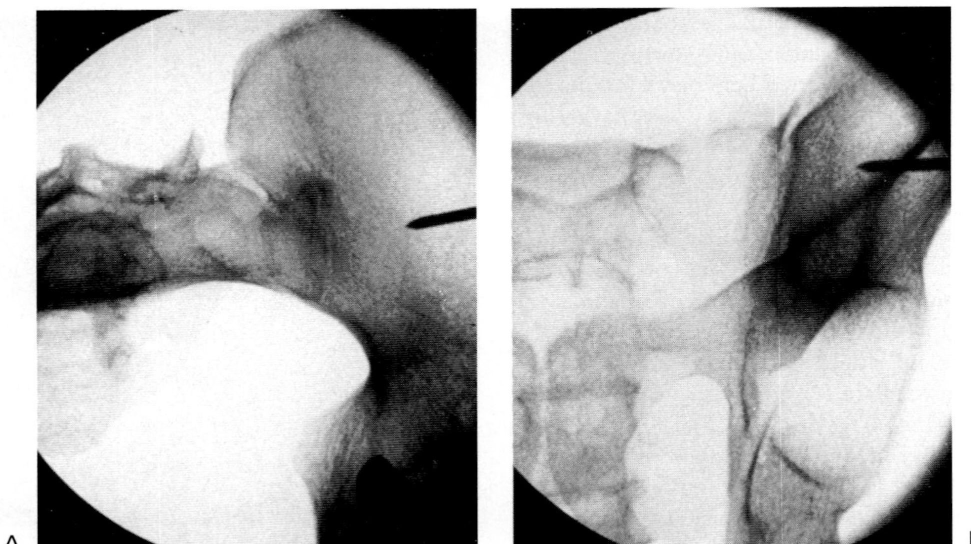

FIGURE 15-29. A: Inlet view to check the entry point and guidewire direction. **B:** Outlet view to check the entry point and the guidewire direction.

terosseous path of the upper sacral nerve root. The tip should be located within the midportion of the alar bone on the true lateral image. Now, with the C arm in the pelvic outlet view, insertion of the guidewire or drill bit is run past the S1 foramen into the body of S1 up to the midline but not past it. The C arm is then pivoted to the pelvic inlet view again. Progress of the guidewire or drill past the midline is monitored in the pelvic inlet view, to make certain it does not exit the opposite side of the S1 vertebral body anteriorly (Fig. 15-30A). The position is rechecked on the outlet view (Fig. 15-30B).

Regardless of the fracture pattern being treated, the screw must be seated into the sacral body to assure the best purchase. It bears repeating that the screw path in the upper portion of the S1 segment cannot be aimed toward the sacral promontory. It must not enter the L5-S1 disc space. It must be in the middle third of the S1 body to avoid exiting the sacral ala anteriorly (Fig. 15-18). Optimally, this guidewire

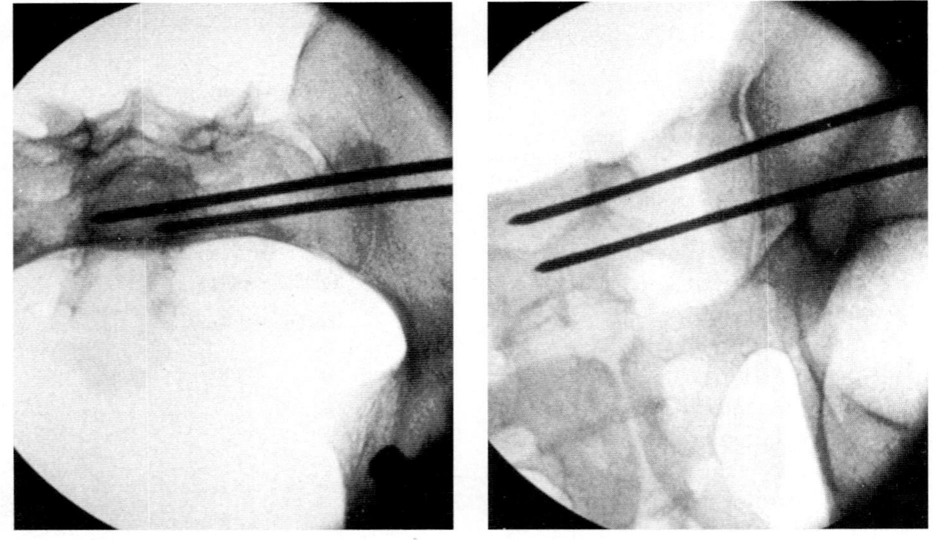

FIGURE 15-30. A: Inlet view with both guidewires in place. The tips of the guidewires are aimed slightly anterior but do not violate the anterior cortex. **B:** Outlet view with both guidewires in place. The tips of the guidewires are aimed slightly superiorly. The upper wire is the more posterior wire in Fig. 15-30A. It does not enter the L5-S1 disc. The lower wire is above the S1 foramen and is the anterior wire in Fig. 15-30A.

or drill bit is placed near the upper vertebral endplate of the S1 body, to be in the most structurally sound bone. During the insertion of the guidewire or drill, three cortical surfaces are met. They are the outer iliac table, the iliac side of sacroiliac joint, and the sacral side of the sacroiliac joint. The fourth feeling of resistance is a clue to stop inserting the guidewire or drill because it is about to perforate and leave the safety of its interosseous sacral home. The guidewire is measured using with the reverse ruler. Generally, there is no need to over-drill the bone because the self-tapping screws will penetrate the bone. Only in young individuals is it sometimes necessary to drill the path for the screw across the three cortical surfaces to allow the screw to advance easily. If using a drill, it is strongly suggested that an oscillating attachment be used to prevent damage to soft tissues. A 7.0- to 7.3-mm diameter cancellous screw with a 32-mm thread length provides the best mechanical hold in the bone. However, if the fracture line is close to the thread shaft junction, there is the potential for screw breakage. In this situation, a 16-mm thread screw should be used (34,36,42). If compression of the cancellous bone or sacroiliac joint is desired, threads must not cross the fracture line. In sacral fractures involving the foramina, the fracture must be reduced but not compressed if sacral nerve root injury is a concern. In this case, a fully threaded cancellous screw is used. A 20-degree obturator oblique fluoroscopic view can be used to show the posterior iliac crest on profile, enabling the surgeon to see that the screw head is seated onto the posterior iliac bone. A washer is desirable, especially in osteoporotic bone, to prevent the screw head from penetrating the outer table of the posterior iliac crest. The guidewire is then removed.

If there is enough space, a second screw may be inserted into the first sacral body. To avoid penetrating the S1 root canal superior and posterior to the S1 foramen, the inferior screw path must be in the anterior third of the S1 body, clearly above the level of the S1 foramen (Figs. 15-31 and 15-32).

Caution must be taken throughout all drilling and screw insertion steps in order to ensure that there is no unexpected advancement of the guidewires. This is especially true if the guidewires are threaded at the tip. During these steps, the position of the tip of the guidewire is monitored with fluoroscopy.

Screw orientation differs depending on the injury being treated. The transforaminal sacral fracture line parallels the mid-sagittal plane. Therefore, the screw is oriented more horizontally and tends to cross the chondral surface of the SI joint. The sacroiliac joint screw is angled more toward the sacral endplate to remain at right angles to the obliquely oriented joint surface. The screw starts caudal/posterior on the ilium and is directed cephalad/anterior to be perpendicular to the oblique sacroiliac joint (Fig. 15-33). This screw placement does not violate the chondral surface of the sacroiliac joint.

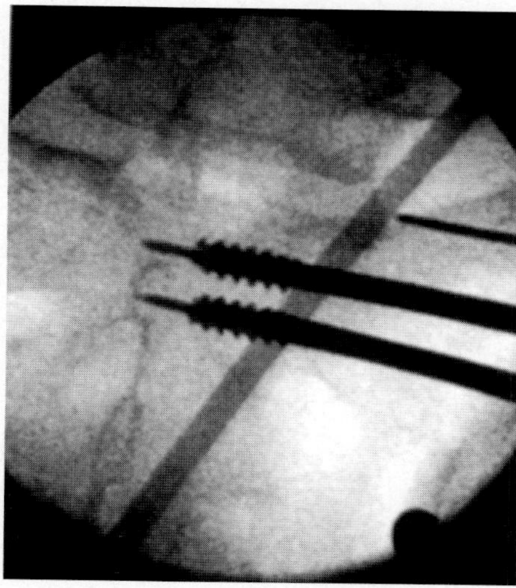

FIGURE 15-31. Fluoroscopic outlet view during a case showing the final position of the screws prior to wire removal.

The stab wounds are then closed. If not already fixed, the anterior aspect of the pelvis is stabilized with an external fixator or internal fixation, as indicated. Sacroiliac lag screw position is confirmed in the immediate postoperative period by formal anteroposterior, inlet, and outlet views of the pelvis. Bed-to-chair activity with assisted transfers and progression to featherweight–bearing ambulation is permitted by the physician, although often limited by other injuries.

A case of a left sacroiliac dislocation is shown in Fig. 15-34A. The patient was treated by external fixation of the pelvis and vascular repair on the night of the injury. Skeletal traction was used to minimize migration of the left hemipelvis, and the patient was returned to the operating room 3 days later for closed reduction and percutaneous

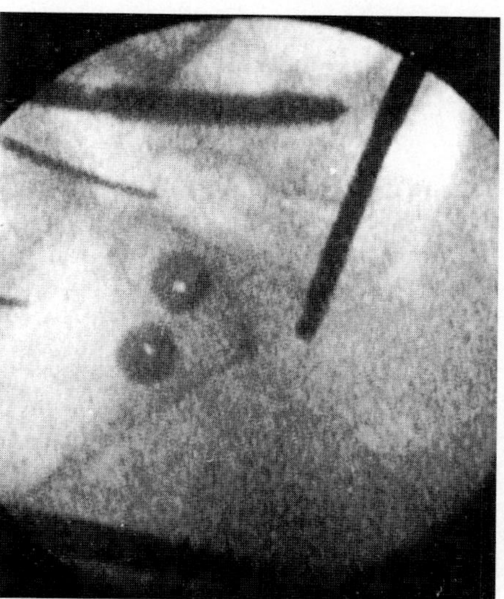

FIGURE 15-32. Fluoroscopic lateral view during a case showing the final position of the screws after wire removal. The patient is prone with the head to the right.

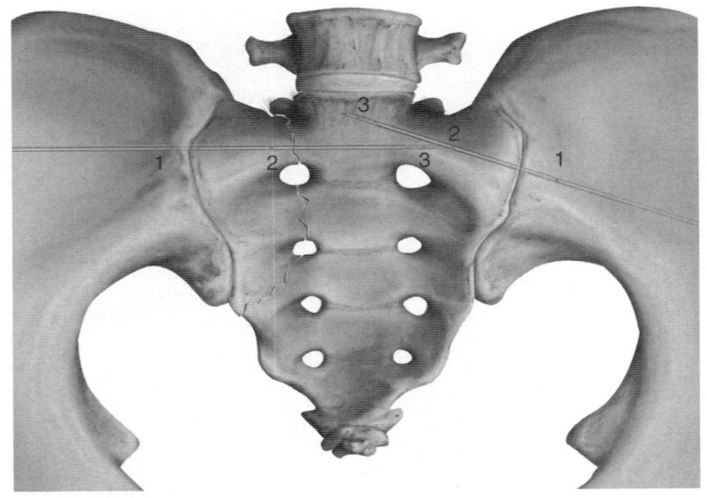

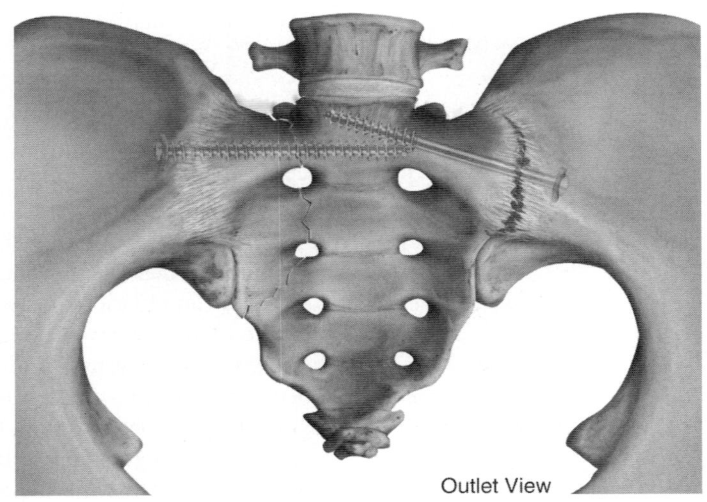

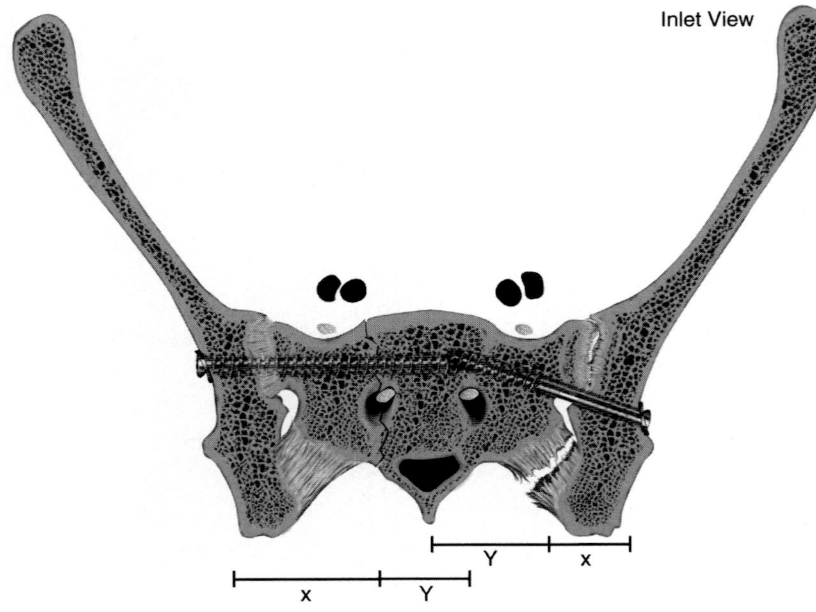

FIGURE 15-33. A: This illustration demonstrates the screw orientations for sacral fractures *(right side)* and sacroiliac joint disruptions *(left side).* Critical fluoroscopic imaging intervals are numerically labeled. **B:** The screws are oriented according to the injury. The sacroiliac joint is anatomically oblique, whereas most sacral fractures occur in a sagittal plane. Sacral fractures are medially located relative to sacroiliac-joint injuries. For these two reasons, screw orientation and length are different for each. The screws are inserted perpendicular to the injury; therefore, sacral and "SI" screws are different. "Sacral" screw orientation is more horizontal, which orients the screw perpendicular to the fracture and allows longer screw length to balance the fixation. "SI" screws are oriented obliquely to remain perpendicular to the disrupted joint surfaces. **C:** Compression screws are used for sacroiliac-joint injuries, whereas fully threaded screws stabilize transforaminal sacral fractures. "Sacral" screws are inserted through the articular surfaces of the sacroiliac joint because of their orientation, whereas "SI" screws avoid the chondral surfaces when inserted correctly. (From: Routt MLC, Simonian PT. Posterior pelvic-ring disruptions: iliosacral screws. In: Thompson RC Jr, ed. *Master techniques in orthopedic surgery: fractures.* Philadelphia: Lippincott Williams & Wilkins, 1998, with permission.)

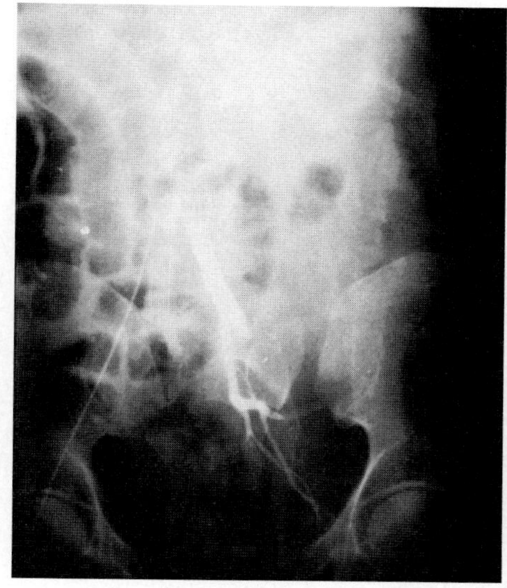

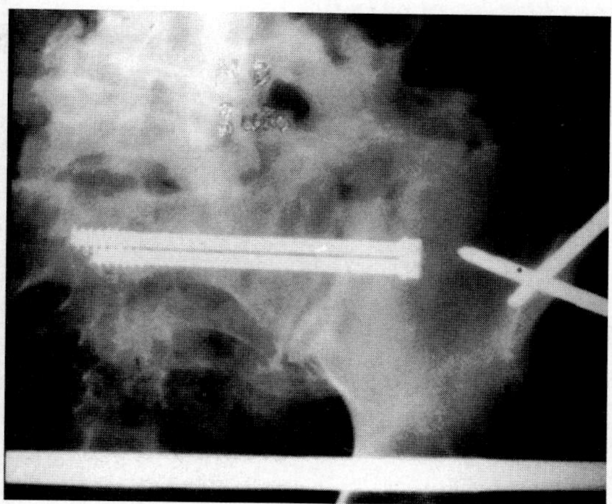

FIGURE 15-34. A: Case example: Anteroposterior pelvis radiograph showing a common iliac artery injury and an unstable left sacroiliac dislocation. **B:** Anteroposterior pelvis radiograph showing the reduced left sacroiliac dislocation with callus formation seen at the inferior margin of the S1 joint 8 weeks postinjury. The external fixator is removed when callus is seen or after 3 months if there is no callus.

sacroiliac screw fixation. A radiograph taken 8 weeks after injury is shown in Fig. 15-34B.

If a patient is stable after the resuscitative and other operative procedures are completed, then percutaneous sacroiliac fixation can be done in the same session of anesthesia, along with other long bone fracture fixation. Thus, return to the operating room is avoided. Open reduction, if required, would be delayed a few days.

Percutaneous Anterior Column Screws for Superior Rami Fractures

The patient is positioned supine on a radiolucent table with the pelvis centered on the table to allow adequate C-arm rotation (43). A lumbosacral support of approximately 3 inches elevates the patient. Low perineal access is necessary to assure the correct starting point for screw entry. With the surgeon opposite to the injury, the C arm is placed ipsilateral to the injured side, with the monitor at the foot of the table. The radiographic views required are the inlet and obturator outlet. The obturator outlet is acquired by obtaining an outlet view and then rotating the C arm to an obturator oblique view (Fig. 15-35). As with the percutaneous iliosacral screw technique, inadequate images preclude the use of this technique. The chest, abdomen, and lower extremities are prepared sterilely and draped. Reduction is accomplished with distal femoral traction as well as direct manipulation with Schanz screws placed in the gluteus medius pillar and anterior inferior iliac spine. If the reduction is unsuccessful, open reduction through a Pfannenstiel, modified Stoppa, or ilioinguinal approach is performed. To insert the screw, a stab wound is made through the skin near the base of the penis or mons pubis at the level of the pubic tubercle on the uninjured side. Blunt oblique dissection across the midline allows a drill sleeve to be placed onto the injured-side pubic tubercle, paralleling the pubic ramus. The ideal starting point is just inferior to the pubic tubercle and lateral to the symphyseal meniscus. Using a long 2.5-mm triple fluted calibrated drill-bit or guidewire on an oscillating drill, the screw is advanced as guided by the two fluoroscopic images. The drill-bit or guidewire path courses retrograde along the superior pubic ramus, across the fracture line, and exits the pelvis just above the acetabulum. The drill sleeve acts as a directional aid for the drill-bit or guidewire, whose position is checked numerous times using biplanar fluoroscopy. The depth of insertion is determined by subtracting the known drill guide sleeve length from the exposed number on the calibrated drill-bit/guidewire. The drill-bit is replaced by a 3.5- or 4.5-mm cortical screw that is inserted under biplanar fluoroscopy. The reduction aids are removed and the fracture stressed to assure stability. If the screw is misdirected, a new track must be established, which requires a new starting hole. This starting hole will be not as perfect as the first. Therefore, considerable effort should be expended to get it right the first time.

Iliac Wing Fractures

An iliac wing fracture may lend itself to percutaneous fixation if it is large and can be reduced by closed means (43,44). The method for reduction involves using Schanz pins in the fragments and relieving the muscle pull of the

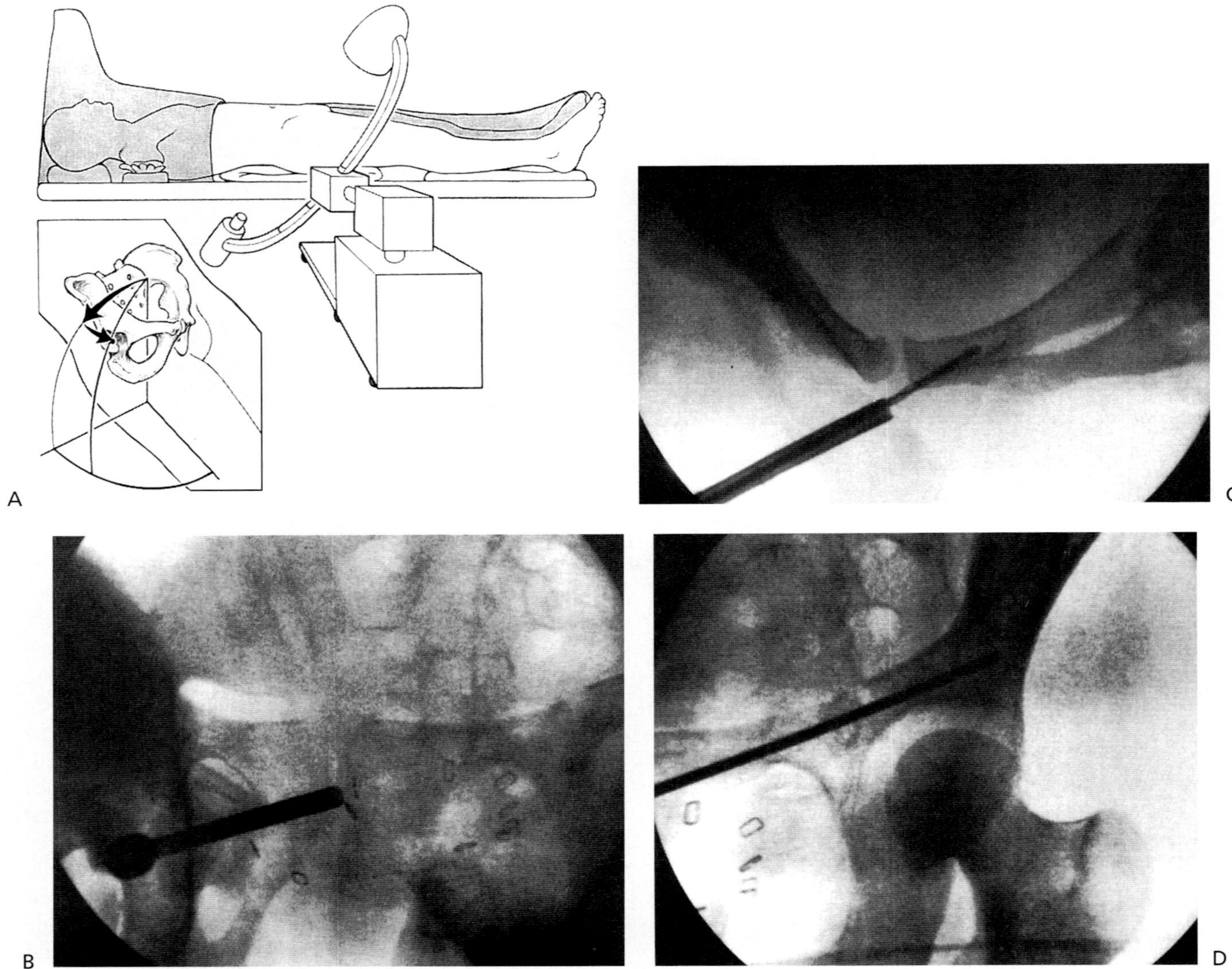

FIGURE 15-35. A: The patient is positioned supine and elevated on a soft lumbosacral support, usually a folded blanket. The contralateral thigh may obstruct screw placement in obese patients. The C-arm unit is placed on the side of injury. The obturator-outlet image is obtained by tilting the image intensifier approximately 30 degrees toward the foot of the bed *(outlet image)* and then rotating it 30 degrees toward the affected hip joint *(obturator oblique image).* This combination image demonstrates the safe zone for screw placement cephalad to the acetabulum. **B:** This intraoperative image demonstrates the ideal starting point for the retrograde medullary screw. The inlet **(C)** and obturator-outlet **(D)** images guide drilling and screw placement.

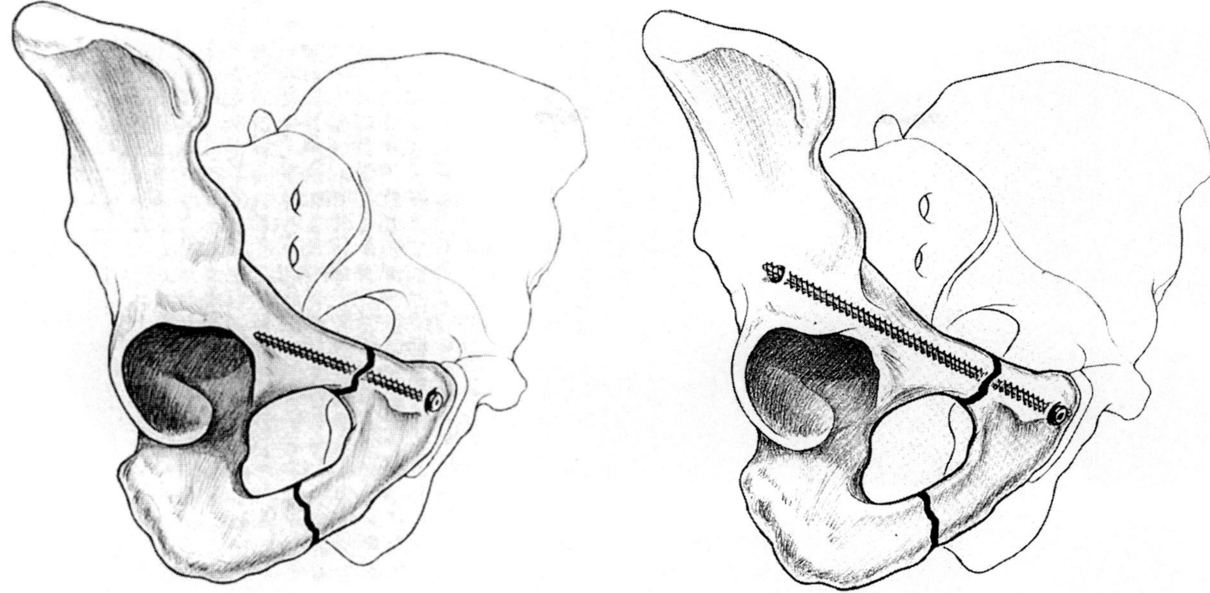

E

FIGURE 15-35. *(continued)* **E:** The retrograde ramus screw is located medial to the acetabulum or in cases of lateral ramus fracture cephalad and beyond the acetabulum, exiting the lateral iliac cortical bone. (From: Routt ML Jr, Simonian PT, Grujic L. Related articles. The retrograde medullary superior pubic ramus screw for the treatment of anterior pelvic ring disruptions: a new technique. *J Orthop Trauma* 1995;9(1):35–44, with permission.)

fragments by flexing and rotating the leg. The reduced fragments are provisionally fixed with K wires. Using the obturator oblique outlet view a 4.5-mm cortical or 6.5- to 7.3-mm cancellous screw is inserted through the anterior inferior iliac spine and aimed toward the posterior iliac tubercle region. If the fracture exits along the iliac crest, a small incision can be used to allow direct fracture reduction. A lag screw inserted percutaneously or an applied plate provides the fixation (Fig. 15-36).

Postoperative Management

If the anterior injury is treated by internal or external fixation, the stabilized hemipelvis is protected by partial weight

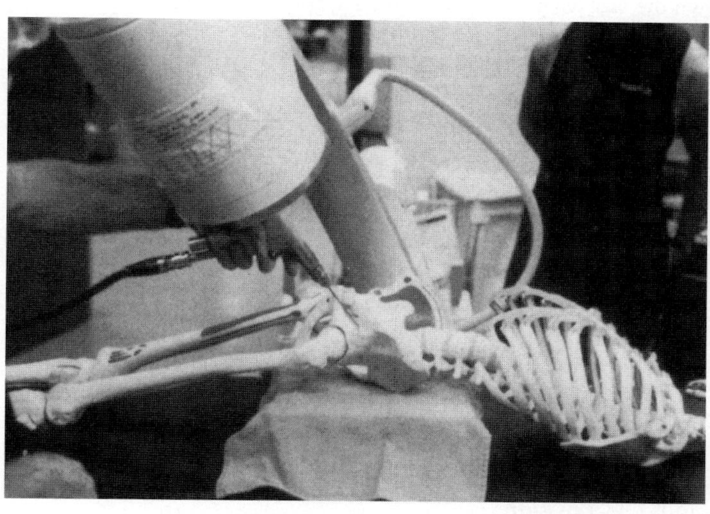

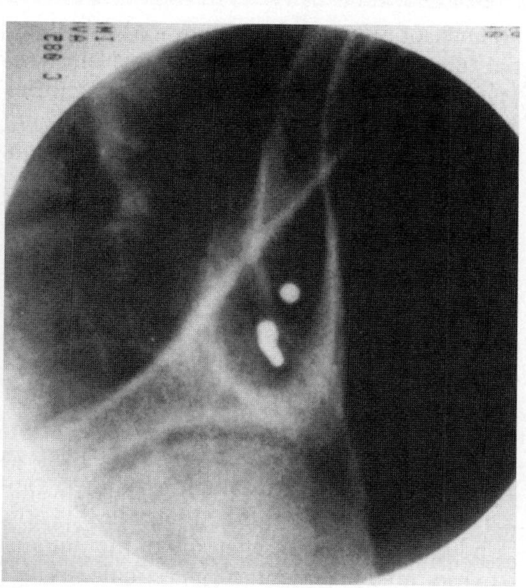

A

FIGURE 15-36. A: *Left:* Image intensifier position for the "teepee" view. To obtain this view, the C-arm is positioned to show an outlet view. It is then rotated toward the injured side, similar to the position used to obtain an obturator oblique view. *Right:* The "teepee" view. Two guidewires have been placed in the "tube" of bone that runs along the AIIS to PIIS line.

(Figure continues)

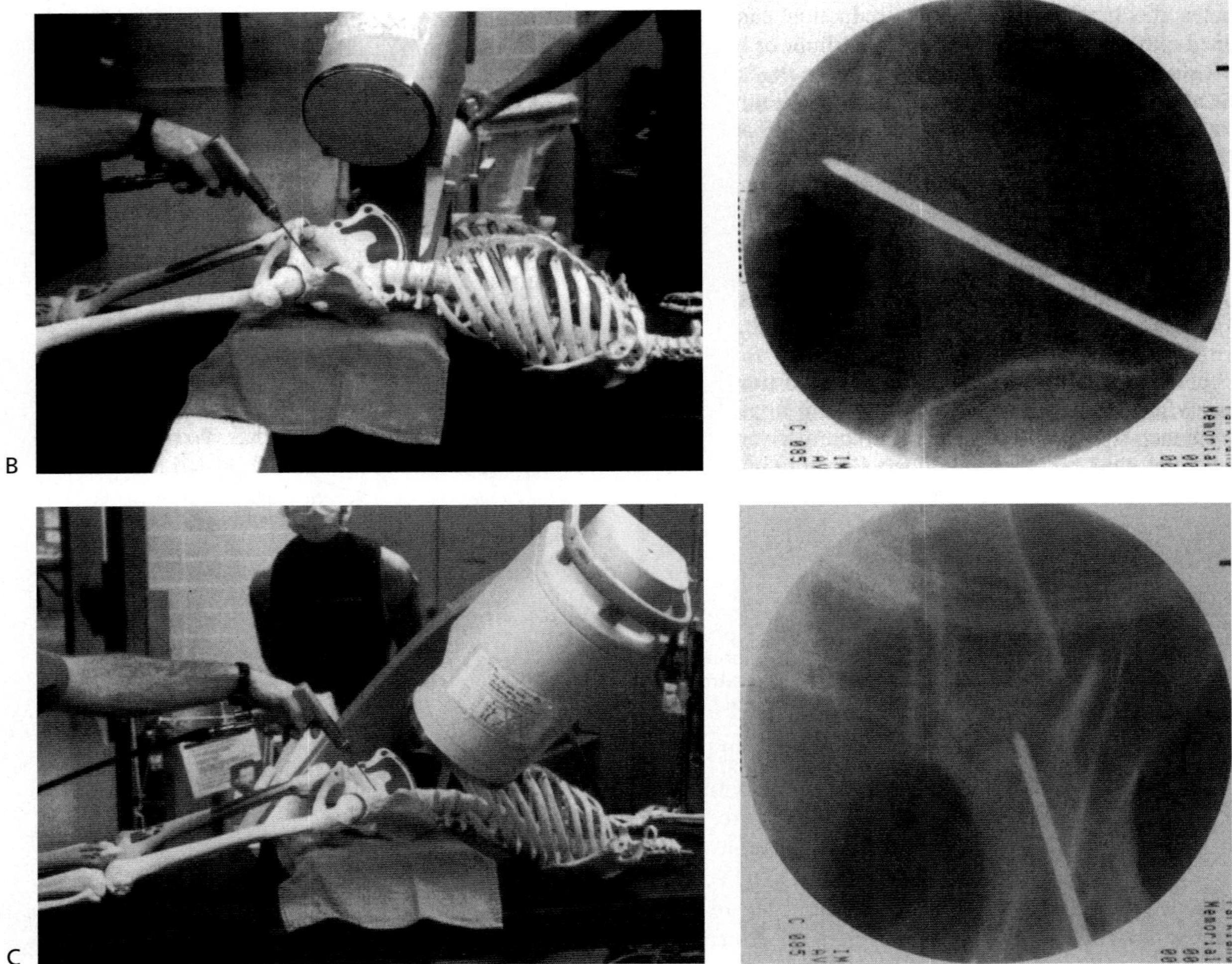

FIGURE 15-36. *(continued)* **B:** *Left:* Image intensifier position for the iliac oblique view. *Right:* Iliac oblique view showing the guidewire as it passes over the greater sciatic notch. **C:** *Left:* Image intensifier position for a view looking down the iliac wing. To obtain this view, the C-arm is positioned to show an inlet view. The C-arm is then rotated toward the injured side until the C-arm is coaxial with the ilium. *Right:* The desired view. In this example, a guidewire is passing down the center of the ilium, from the AIIS toward the PIIS. The wire tip is crossing a fracture of the ilium in this image. The sacroiliac joint is visible in the upper left quadrant of the image, as is a portion of the sacral ala. (From: Starr AJ, Walter JC, Harris RW, et al. Percutaneous screw fixation of fractures of the iliac wing and fracture-dislocations of the sacro-iliac joint. *J Orthop Trauma* 2002;16(2):116–123, with permission.)

bearing with ambulatory aids for 6 weeks if the anterior injury is treated by internal or external fixation. Otherwise, the patient is limited to bed to chair transfer using the uninjured leg to pivot. Aid-free ambulation begins at 3 to 4 months postoperatively. Radiographs (anteroposterior, inlet and outlet) are taken postoperatively, at 6 and 12 weeks and at further 6-week intervals until healed or declared a nonunion. Progressive return to full activities usually begins after 4 to 6 months.

SURGICAL APPROACHES

Anterior Ring: Symphysis and Rami

Pfannenstiel Approach

Position

The patient is placed in the supine position on the operating table. It is helpful if the table is radiolucent so that intraoperative fluoroscopy may be used. A catheter then is placed to allow bladder drainage and to define the bladder—urethra junction (10,12).

Exposure

This incision should be placed approximately one finger breadth (2 cm) superior to the superior pubic rami and *not over the bone* (Fig. 15-37A,B). It should be extended laterally on both sides to just past the external inguinal ring. Dissection is continued through the subcutaneous tissue, down to the intercrural fibers of the aponeurosis of the external oblique and anterior rectus fascia. The spermatic cord or round ligament may be identified at this time.

If the symphysis disruption is associated with bladder rupture or intraperitoneal injury requiring surgical repair, then the skin incision will most likely be a longitudinal midline one. The orthopedic surgeon must be certain that if the general or urologic surgeons do the surgical approach that the midline incision extends to the symphysis.

The linea alba between the rectus abdominis muscles is incised as it extends down onto the symphysis. Through this midline incision, the posterior rectus sheath is identified and opened, leading to the posterior aspect of the symphysis. Care must be taken in the posterior or dorsal dissection to avoid injury to the bladder or the prostatic venous plexus. This area is usually identified by a significant amount of fat surrounding the bladder. The bladder is identified and protected by malleable retractors or a lap sponge while the remainder of the exposure is done subperiosteally to expose the superior, anterior, and posterior aspects of the pubic body and symphysis. This can be carried out laterally in a similar fashion onto the rami, but at times, depending on muscle relaxation and tightness of the rectus, the lateral extent may be limited. Anteriorly it will be necessary to elevate the recti insertions from the pubic body lateral to the obturator foramen. It is quite common for a portion of the attachment of the rectus abdominis muscle to the symphysis pubis to be disrupted. What remains should be elevated carefully to allow exposure of the symphysis while maintaining as much distal fascial continuity as possible. Usually, identification of the superior medial border of the pubic bodies is all that is needed. The obturator foramina must be identified on both sides if reduction by placing bone-holding forceps in them is planned. Once the symphysis is exposed, the pubic rami can be identified laterally to the region of the iliopectineal eminence.

An alternative exposure technique uses a transverse incision through the aponeurosis of the rectus abdominis near its insertion onto the pubic rami, leaving a small cuff to which the rectus may be reattached. The subperiosteal elevation of the remainder of the aponeurosis is carried out over the superior and anterior surfaces of the proximal pubic body and rami. This method allows exposure laterally for more than 5 cm along either pubic ramus. However, the strength of the repaired rectus muscles is often suspect.

Closure

Reattachment of the rectus abdominis muscles must be done carefully. This requires that the patient be totally paralyzed, and it may require that the table be flexed slightly to allow the muscles to be reapproximated. The incision may be closed over closed-suction drains.

Modified Stoppa Approach

See also Chapter 33 (45,46). This approach is used to expose acetabular fractures, but is also helpful to reduce and

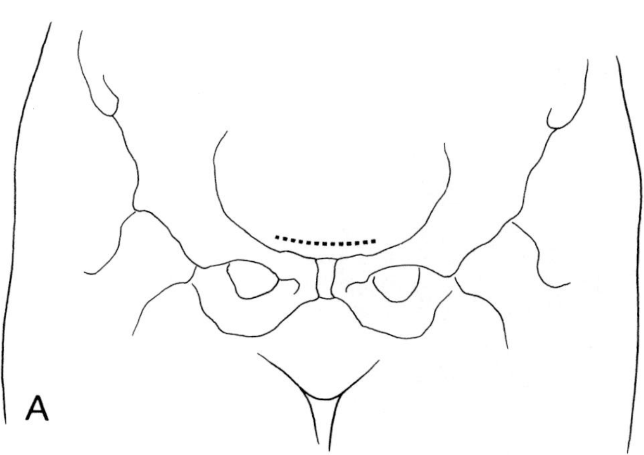

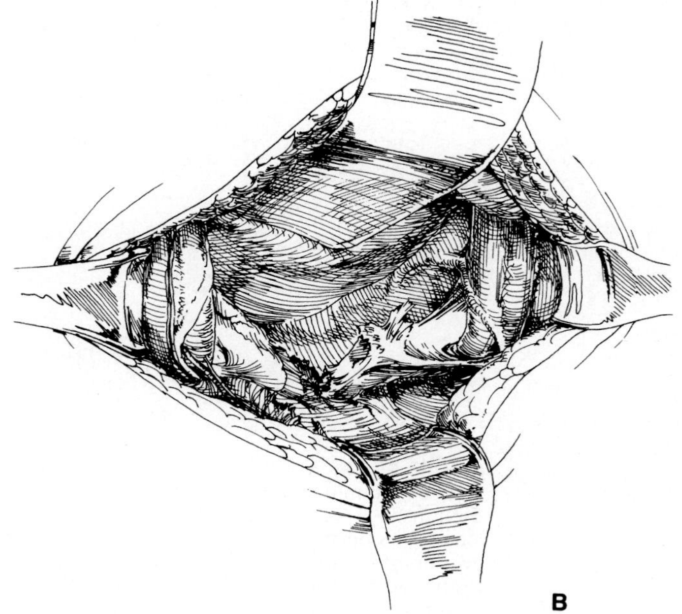

FIGURE 15-37. A: Open reduction of the symphysis pubis is done through Pfannenstiel incision. **B:** Deep dissection of the symphysis pubis. Usually, in a symphyseal disruption, the dissection is done by the injury; rarely, the rectus needs to be removed from the pubis. The bladder is retracted, as noted, and the inferior epigastric artery and the spermatic cord are protected.

stabilize lateral pubic rami fractures. It allows access to the pubic rami and quadrilateral plate, including exposure of the pelvic brim as far posterior as the sacroiliac joint.

Position

The patient is placed in the supine position on a radiolucent operating table. The entire lower abdominal pelvic region and hindquarter area of the involved side are sterilely prepped and draped. The involved lower extremity is freely draped. The surgeon operates from the side opposite the fracture.

Exposure

(Fig. 15-38.) The skin incision is 2 cm above the symphysis and runs between the external inguinal rings. The rectus abdominis muscles are split along the linea alba. The bladder is identified posterior to the symphysis and protected while the rectus muscle on the involved side is retracted upward. The pubic symphysis and rami are exposed using sharp dissection. With the rectus muscle and neurovascular structures retracted upward and laterally, the surgeon (standing on the side opposite to the fracture) is able to see the many vascular anastomoses between the obturator and epigastric vessels. These are ligated, as necessary, for the exposure. If the posterior iliacus muscle is elevated, the iliolumbar artery and its nutrient vessel branch must be controlled. The superior iliopectineal fascia and inferior obturator fascia are divided sharply exposing the lateral rami, medial wall, and pelvic brim. Various retractors (e.g. malleable, Hohman, Deaver, etc.) are very useful to achieve exposure. Flexion of the involved leg through the hip relaxes important structures crossing the pelvic brim. The obturator neurovascular structures and lumbosacral trunk are at risk of damage in this approach.

A plate can be placed from the body of the symphysis along the pelvic brim posteriorly to just in front of the sacroiliac joint. This exposure may be combined with the anterior intrapelvic approach to the sacroiliac joint to help with reduction and application of fixation implants.

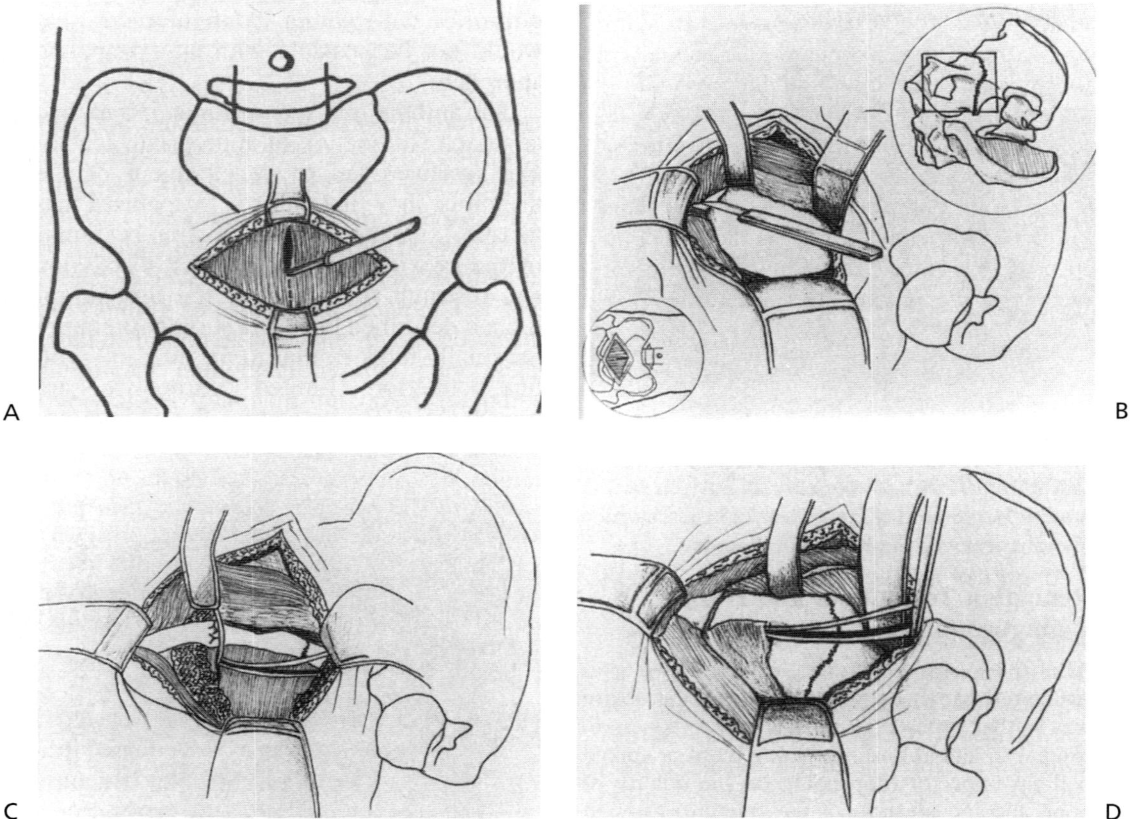

FIGURE 15-38. A: A transverse incision is made 2 cm above the symphysis. Anterior fascia is incised at the midline. **B:** Elevation of the rectus insertion on the pubis. **C:** Anastomotic branch of the inferior epigastric and obturator vessels are visualized. Retraction of the rectus and external iliac vein is performed. **D:** Elevation of the iliacus and psoas allows exposure of the iliac fossa. Elevation of the obturator internus exposes the medial wall and obturator fossa. Dissection medial to the sacroiliac joint allows exposure of the lateral sacral ala for Hohmann retractor placement. (From: Cole JD, Bolhofner BR. Acetabular fracture fixation via a modified Stoppa limited intrapelvic approach. *Clin Orthop Rel Res* 1994;305:112–123, with permission).

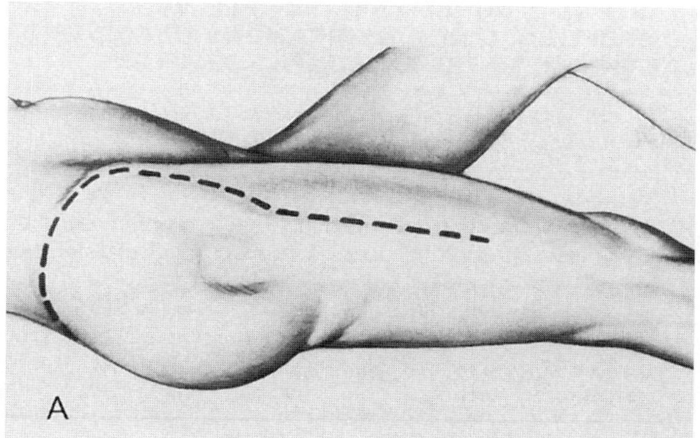

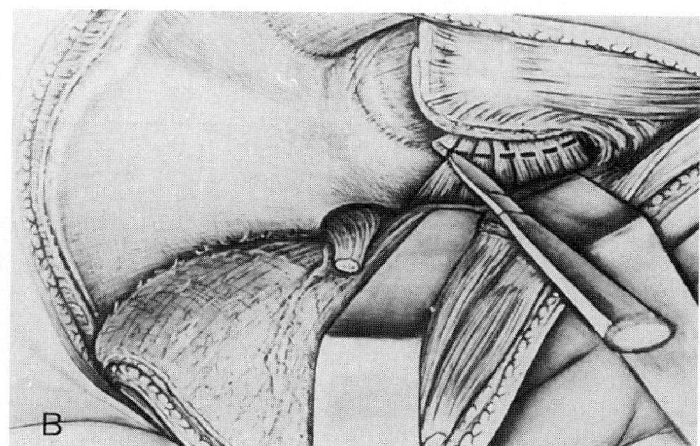

FIGURE 15-39. Extended iliofemoral approach. **A:** Diagram demonstrates the skin incision for the extended iliofemoral approach. **B:** This approach strips all the muscles from the lateral aspect of the iliac crest, divides the external fixators to completely expose the posterior column, and divides the gluteus medius and gluteus minimus tendons from the greater trochanter to allow access to the superior aspect of the acetabulum or the dome fragment. Note the position of the neurovascular bundle to the gluteus medius, exiting through the greater sciatic notch. The greater trochanter can be divided as an alternative to division of the abductor tendons. (Letournel E. Acetabular fractures: classification and management. *Clin Orthop* 151:81, 1980.)

Lateral Approach (Extrapelvic) to the Ilium

The lateral approach may be used in complex cases or for surgery for malunion (12). This approach affords a very extensive view of the ilium and is the upper portion of the extended iliofemoral approach (see Chapter 28). The soft tissues may be stripped from the intrapelvic aspect of the pelvis to allow internal visualization. Extending the incision posteriorly will allow the same visualization as the posterior extrapelvic approach (see Fig. 15-41).

Position

The patient is placed in the lateral decubitus position with the uninvolved side down.

Exposure

A curved incision is made, starting at the anterior superior spine along the iliac crest to above the most prominent portion of the crest and then down along the posterior superior spine (Fig. 15-39). This may be carried slightly farther down to the origin of the piriformis. The gluteus musculature then is reflected off the external iliac surface and turned downward to reveal its entire outer aspect of the crest. If necessary, the operator also can go inside the pelvis by taking off the abdominal musculature where it attaches to the iliac wing. This affords access both inside and outside the pelvis. Care should be taken to avoid detaching the sartorius or rectus insertions. These muscle attachments will provide some blood supply to the pelvic bone. The major risk of this approach is complete devascularization of the iliac wing or a fracture fragment, leading to complications of nonunion and infection. This exposure allows reduction of the sacroiliac joint and iliac wing fracture. It is a very extensive approach, indicated particularly for nonunion or malunion surgery and correction.

SURGICAL APPROACHES TO THE SACROILIAC COMPLEX

Advantages and Disadvantages

(See Tables 15-5 and 15-6.) For *sacroiliac injuries* the *anterior,* or intrapelvic, approach has several potential advantages (33), but it cannot be used for sacral fractures. The first major advantage is direct visualization of the sacroiliac joint. This allows the surgeon to visualize the joint during reduction of its anterior and superior portions. It must be realized, however, that a rotational abnormality may occur if the pelvis is subjected to excessive internal rotation, and this must be appreciated either through C-arm control or intraoperative radiographs. Another advantage to the anterior approach is the direct visualization of the application of the implants. A final advantage is that this is an extensile approach that allows treatment of fractures into the iliac wing or in the anterior portion of the pelvis, including pubic ramus and symphyseal disruptions. Skin breakdown is also rare with anterior approaches.

TABLE 15-5. UNSTABLE (TYPE C) PELVIC DISRUPTION: INDICATIONS FOR ANTERIOR (INTRAPELVIC) APPROACH TO THE SACROILIAC COMPLEX

Sacroiliac joint dislocation and/or fracture dislocation involving the ilium
Iliac wing fracture
Associated anterior pelvic lesions (symphysis or rami) that require surgical intervention with an iliac wing or sacroiliac joint dislocation
Posterior soft-tissue injury precluding a posterior approach

TABLE 15-6. UNSTABLE (TYPE C) PELVIC DISRUPTION: CONTRAINDICATIONS TO ANTERIOR (INTRAPELVIC) APPROACH TO THE SACROILIAC COMPLEX

Sacral fractures
- After external fixation, when there is potential for sepsis owing to chronic infected pin tracts
- Prolonged presence of a suprapubic catheter or colostomy in the vicinity of the surgical approach

The major *disadvantage* of this approach is the risk to the L5 nerve root. The L5 root lies on the sacral ala about 2 cm medial to the sacroiliac joint. As it proceeds distally to join the sacral roots and form the sciatic nerve, it crosses the sacroiliac joint (Fig. 15-15C). Therefore, it can be injured if care is not taken during medial and inferior dissection. Other potential problems include bleeding from inadvertent injury to the superior gluteal artery (as it exits through the greater sciatic notch), injury to the pelvic vascular plexus, or decompression of a retroperitoneal hematoma. In large patients, this approach is more difficult. In addition, sacral fractures cannot be fixed through this approach because of the overlying nerves and vessels.

The *posterior* approach to the posterior sacroiliac complex has the major advantage of affording application of excellent compressive forces across the sacroiliac joint (See Tables 15-7 and 15-8.). For fracture dislocations of the sacroiliac joint with fracture through the ilium, the reduction is facilitated by this approach. Iliac wing fractures can be exposed very easily by this approach, and excellent compressive interfragmentary fixation can be obtained. In addition, sacral fractures require this approach to perform an open reduction.

The major *disadvantage* of the posterior approach is the problem of wound necrosis and infection (2). When a pelvic fracture is caused by high-energy forces directly applied to the hemipelvis, significant disruption of the local skin, subcutaneous tissue, and muscle in this region often occurs. With the added insult of surgical trauma, wound healing problems, including skin necrosis and infection, may ensue.

Due to the overhanging posterior tubercle of the iliac wing, the sacroiliac joint cannot be completely visualized. The reduction can be partially confirmed by palpation through the greater sciatic notch and over the ala of the sacrum. Therefore, intraoperative fluoroscopy is needed in this approach, not only for correct placement of the implants, but to adequately evaluate the fracture and joint reduction.

TABLE 15-7. UNSTABLE (TYPE C) PELVIC DISRUPTION: INDICATIONS FOR POSTERIOR APPROACH TO THE SACROILIAC COMPLEX

Fracture/dislocation of the sacroiliac complex
Sacral fracture
Iliac wing fracture

TABLE 15-8. UNSTABLE (TYPE C) PELVIC DISRUPTION: CONTRAINDICATIONS TO POSTERIOR APPROACH TO THE SACROILIAC COMPLEX

Skin and soft-tissue compromise owing to direct high-energy crush injury and/or massive degloving injury in the surgical incision area. In this circumstance, a percutaneous technique may be used.
Associated injuries to the pelvis that would require anterior fixation if associated with an iliac fracture or sacroiliac dislocation, but not with a sacral fracture.
Any soft-tissue injury, particularly open fractures with associated communication between the perineum or ischiorectal space and the posterior sacral area exists. These are better treated with external fixation.

Decision Making: Anterior versus Posterior Approaches

A posterior sacroiliac osseous ligamentous injury may be approached either anteriorly (intrapelvic) or posteriorly (extrapelvic). The major determinants are these:

1. The type of injury (a sacroiliac dislocation or iliac wing fracture versus a sacral disruption)
2. The status of the soft tissues
3. Other associated pelvic ring injuries that require treatment
4. The surgeon's preference and experience
5. The patient's general status (e.g., the anesthetist may not wish the patient to lie prone)

Posterior Ring: Anterior (Intrapelvic) Approach to the Sacroiliac Joint

Position

For the anterior intrapelvic approach, the patient is usually positioned supine (47). A small roll is placed under the involved hemipelvis, to tilt the pelvis slightly so that it is easily manipulated. This roll must be radiolucent. It should be placed just lateral to the midline. The involved leg is draped free to allow manipulation (especially flexion to relax the iliopsoas) and facilitate the exposure.

This approach also may be used with the patient in the lateral decubitus position with the involved side superior. This allows the muscles of the anterior abdominal wall to fall medial and the hemipelvis to be manipulated more easily, which is helpful in large patients. Use of the lateral decubitus position allows the surgeon more freedom of choice during the procedure should posterior access be required. A radiolucent table is used to allow for intraoperative radiography of the pelvis to confirm reduction and implant position.

Exposure

The incision for the approach, which overlies the lower abdominal wall musculature, commences 4 to 5 cm proximal to the highest point of the iliac crest of the pelvis, where the crest begins to turn posteriorly (Fig. 15-40). This skin incision parallels the iliac crest, stopping just distal to the anterior superior iliac spine. The iliac crest is identified on completion of the skin and subcutaneous incision. The abdominal wall muscles are elevated sharply from the iliac crest in continuity with the iliacus muscle. Blunt dissection is carried out subperiosteally, along the internal iliac fossa, down to the pelvic brim, and posteriorly as far as the sacroiliac joint.

Anteriorly, the dissection extends under the iliopsoas muscle along the superior pubic ramus down to the iliopectineal eminence. At this time, adduction and flexion of the hip to about 60 degrees relaxes the psoas muscle and allows easier exposure. The muscles of the abdominal wall are then dissected bluntly in the direction of their fibers and

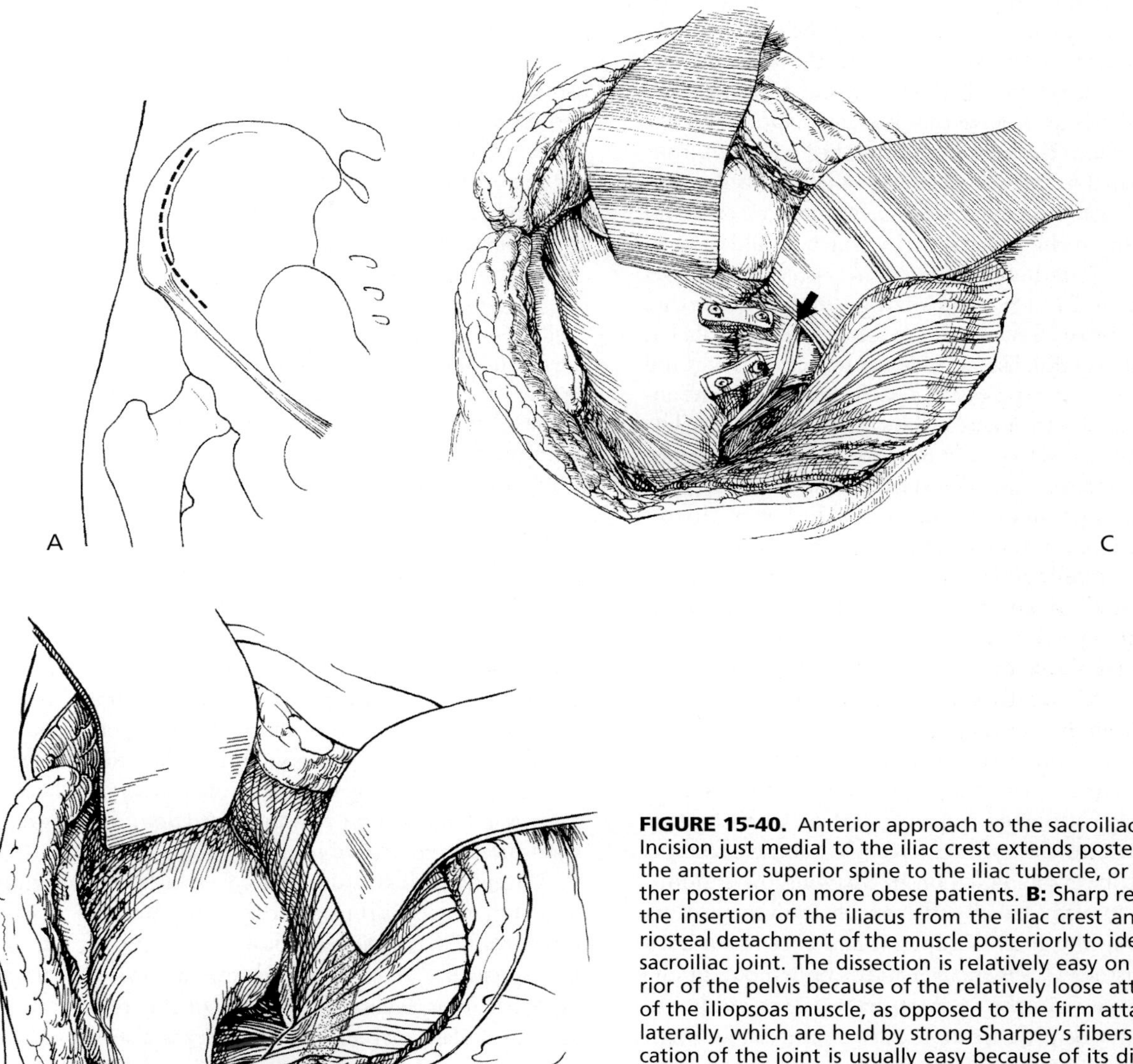

FIGURE 15-40. Anterior approach to the sacroiliac joint. **A:** Incision just medial to the iliac crest extends posterior from the anterior superior spine to the iliac tubercle, or even farther posterior on more obese patients. **B:** Sharp removal of the insertion of the iliacus from the iliac crest and subperiosteal detachment of the muscle posteriorly to identify the sacroiliac joint. The dissection is relatively easy on the interior of the pelvis because of the relatively loose attachment of the iliopsoas muscle, as opposed to the firm attachments laterally, which are held by strong Sharpey's fibers. Identification of the joint is usually easy because of its disruption. Great care must be taken when dissecting in the superior gluteal notch to avoid damage to the superior gluteal artery and nerve, which can be seen in the diagram. **C:** Following dissection, as noted in **(B),** the fracture-dislocation or fracture may be reduced. Two-plate fixation restores adequate stability to the hemipelvis. Only one screw can safely be inserted into the sacrum, because of its proximity to the L5 nerve root *(black arrow).* (From Fig. 15-40C from Schatzker J, Tile M. *The rational of operative fracture care.* Heidelberg: Springer-Verlag, 1987, with permission)

retracted medially to allow further exposure of the sacroiliac joint and sacrum. Dissection is now carried medially toward the sacroiliac joint (Fig. 15-40B). It is important to have assessed the direction of displacement preoperatively. In the majority of situations, the iliac wing component of the sacroiliac joint dislocation is displaced superiorly and posteriorly. Consequently, with dissection along the internal iliac fossa in the direction of the sacroiliac joint, one will encounter the offset sacral side of the sacroiliac joint. Therefore, it is usually easy to locate the sacral ala with blunt dissection.

The surgeon must stay close to the bone of the ala and proceed slowly with blunt dissection in a medial direction. At this point, flexion and internal rotation of the hip joint past 90 degrees improves the exposure by further relaxing the psoas muscle and allowing the muscles of the abdominal wall to fall medially. The L5 nerve root is located approximately 2 to 3 cm medial to the sacroiliac joint (Fig. 15-40C), running from medial to lateral. As the dissection continues toward the sacral ala, the surgeon must avoid placing excessive medial traction on the psoas muscle, which would tend to stretch the nerve root. It is difficult to safely isolate this nerve; consequently, one must be aware of its position and take care not to subject it to excessive traction. Once the sacral ala has been identified, careful dissection of the posterior aspect and anteriorly over the brim proceeds. It is important that the anterior aspect of the sacroiliac joint be dissected cleanly. The best way to proceed is to gently move down to the inner aspect of the pelvis and clean off part of the quadrilateral plate, then swing back into the greater sciatic notch. The risk in this area is to the superior gluteal artery and L5 root. Exposure must be done carefully and completely, so that the reduction can be evaluated adequately by palpation. The nutrient artery to the hemipelvis enters the iliac wing along the pelvic brim just distal to the sacroiliac joint and can bleed quite vigorously. Bone wax usually works well to seal this nutrient foramen and stop the bleeding.

Visualization by retraction may be obtained by careful placement of large K-wires hammered into the sacral ala (care being taken to avoid impaling L5) or by the use of long, broad retractors. It is imperative that a muscle relaxant be used to facilitate the reduction by allowing the abdominal wall to be moved medially. It is also helpful to clear the interval between the anterior superior and anterior inferior spine of soft tissue. This maneuver allows bone-holding forceps to be placed onto the anterior iliac wing to aid in the reduction. Anterior plate fixation can be done safely when exposure is complete (Fig. 15-40C).

Posterior Ring: Posterior (Extrapelvic) Approach to the Sacroiliac Joint

Position

The standard patient position for this approach is prone (48,49). This usually means placing the patient on bolsters so that the abdomen and chest are supported and the iliac wing is free. The other option is to place the patient in the lateral decubitus position with the involved side up. Adequate radiographic visualization throughout the case is mandatory. Prior to beginning the surgery, the patient should be evaluated with the C-arm to ensure that satisfactory anteroposterior, inlet, and outlet views of the pelvis are obtainable. This is important for the placement of posterior screw fixation into the sacrum (Fig. 15-20B).

Exposure

The surgical incision for this approach is a straight incision that begins either medial or lateral to the posterior superior iliac spine (Fig. 15-41A). The incision should not be placed directly over the spine, otherwise breakdown of the wound would result in exposure of the underlying bone. Whether the incision is placed medial or lateral to the spine depends on the fracture configuration. With an iliac wing fracture or a sacroiliac joint dislocation, a more laterally placed incision is suitable; for a sacral fracture, a more medial approach is preferable. The incision extends from the level of the maximal height of the iliac crest to the posterior inferior spine and ends just past the greater sciatic notch. The gluteus maximus and abductor muscles are stripped from the outer aspect of the iliac crest as far forward as the iliac tubercle (Fig. 15-41B). Inferiorly, the gluteus maximus origin blends with the midline spinal muscles; therefore, sharp dissection is required to expose the lower half of the sacroiliac joint and the origin of the piriformis. The surgeon must be very wary of the superior gluteal artery as it exits through the greater sciatic notch. Once the origin of the piriformis has been identified, it should be sharply divided and retracted to allow access to the inner aspect of the pelvis through the greater sciatic notch.

If a sacral fracture is present, dissection should be carried across the medial aspect of the posterior superior spine onto the posterior aspect of the sacrum to identify the fracture. The posterior sacral neural foramina can serve as landmarks for screw fixation and fracture reduction. Therefore, their exposure can be helpful in this regard.

With unstable fracture patterns, there is often significant local soft-tissue disruption; therefore, much of the dissection already may have been done by the injury itself. A laminar spreader should be placed carefully into the dislocated sacroiliac joint to clear debris and possibly remove the damaged articular surface. Sacral fractures also should be exposed, debrided as necessary, and reduced. It is important at this point to identify the posterior aspect of the sacrum, the posterior iliac spine, the ala of the sacrum, the L5 transverse process, and, through the piriformis origin to introduce into the pelvis a palpating finger and identify the anterior aspect of the sacrum, the sacroiliac joint, the iliac wing, and the anterior sacral roots (Fig. 15-41C). These landmarks guide the reduction and insertion of implants.

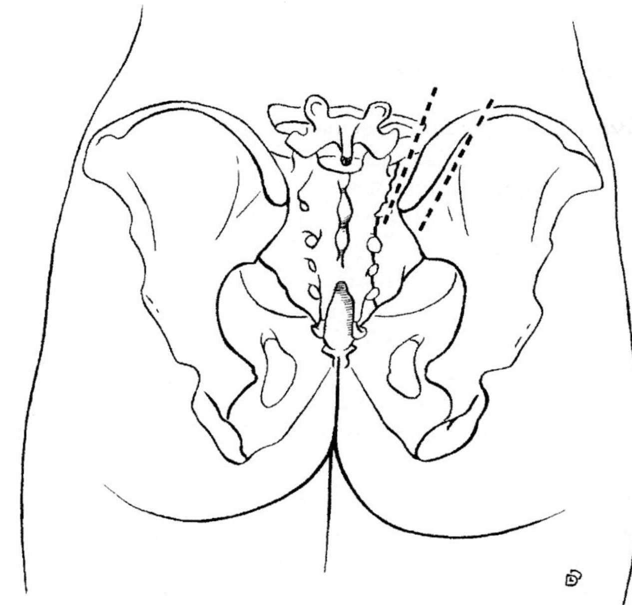

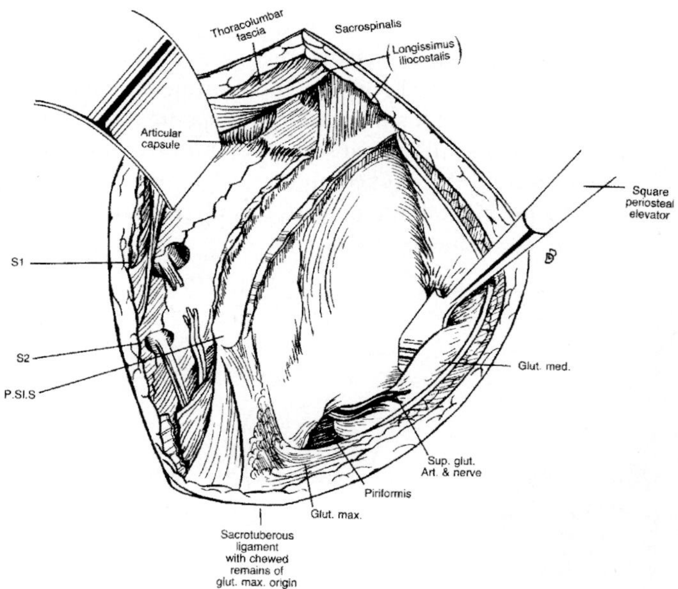

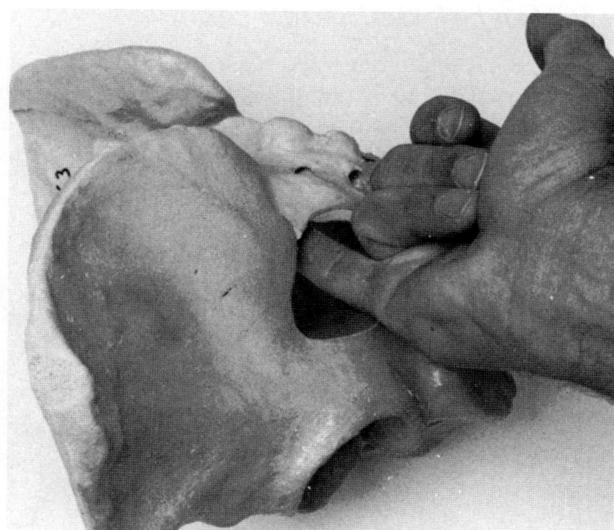

FIGURE 15-41. The posterior approach to the sacroiliac complex. Note that the surgical incision should be made either 1 cm medial or lateral to the posterior iliac spine and not directly over the subcutaneous border **(A).** Depending on the amount of exposure required posteriorly, the insertion of the gluteus maximus may be dissected from the lateral aspect of the ilium into the greater sciatic notch with an elevator, as noted in the diagram **(B).** Note also that the superior gluteal artery and nerve exit from the greater sciatic notch, and great care must be taken when dissecting in that area. If exposure to the posterior aspect of the sacrum is required because of sacral fracture, note the medial dissection and the sacral fracture. Exposure of the posterior foramina may help with reduction **(B).** Dissection should allow the palpating finger to explore the anterior aspect of the joint, to confirm anatomic reduction **(C).**

Posterior Ring: Posterior Approach to the Sacrum

Position

The patient is positioned prone on a regular radiolucent operating table (50). Intraoperative fluoroscopic control with inlet and outlet views should be possible, but is not mandatory for the procedure. Draping is performed with access to following landmarks: both posterior iliac crests, the spinous process of L4, and the upper end of the rima ani. The exact position of the skin incision is varied according to the fracture pattern (Fig. 15-42).

Exposure

Transforaminal and trans-alar sacrum fractures: A longitudinal incision in the midline between the posterior iliac crest and the medial sacral crest is performed. The lumbosacral fascia is incised close to its origin at the spinous process of L4 and L5 and the medial sacral crest (Fig. 15-43). The muscle is elevated from the sacrum with a sharp dissector or a cautery knife. If a more extensile exposure of the lateral sacral region ("ala") is necessary, then the complete muscle mass can be elevated by dissecting its lateral attachment to the posterior iliac crest. Care has to be taken to keep the soft tissues moist during the entire procedure.

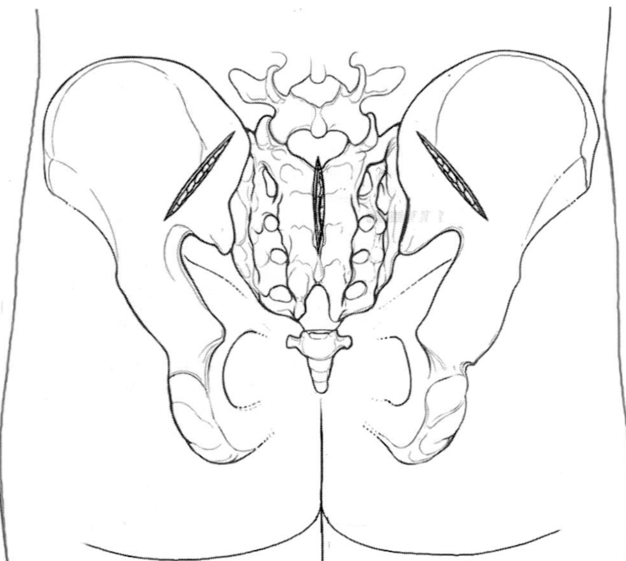

FIGURE 15-42. Incisions for posterior sacral plating can be as mentioned previously or as described by Albert, with oblique incisions starting at the posterior tubercle and a midline incision to allow reduction and plate passage.

Central and Bilateral Sacrum Fractures

A longitudinal midline incision close to the central sacral crest is used. The previously described deep dissection can be extended to both sides of the sacrum. In this way, the complete posterior aspect of the sacrum can be exposed using a single incision.

OPEN REDUCTION TECHNIQUES

General Comments

Preoperative planning, including the reduction maneuvers, is essential for the successful operative management of pelvic ring injuries. A detailed study of all the radiographs and CT scans is mandatory in order that the plan can be formalized. It is best to draw the plan on paper or, better yet, a plastic pelvis, as well as preparing a surgical tactic. This exercise assures the surgeon that the appropriate instruments, exposure, and fixation construct will be available and achievable.

Adequate intraoperative radiographic confirmation of the reduction and placement of fixation are mandatory. Consequently, no matter what the surgical approach, the patient should be lying on a radiolucent operating table in such a way that visualization is easily achieved using a C-arm or plain radiography. It is necessary to ensure that the three pelvic radiographic views (anterior-posterior, inlet, and outlet) as well as a true lateral of the sacrum are obtainable.

Antibiotics are routinely used in all pelvic surgery. Neurologic monitoring of the lower extremity may be used. Sensory or motor evoked potential monitoring is accurate in expert hands, though still considered experimental. It is not readily available in most institutions and therefore not routinely used. Motor-evoked potentials have the disadvantage of not allowing full intraoperative paralysis, which may hinder fracture reduction (51).

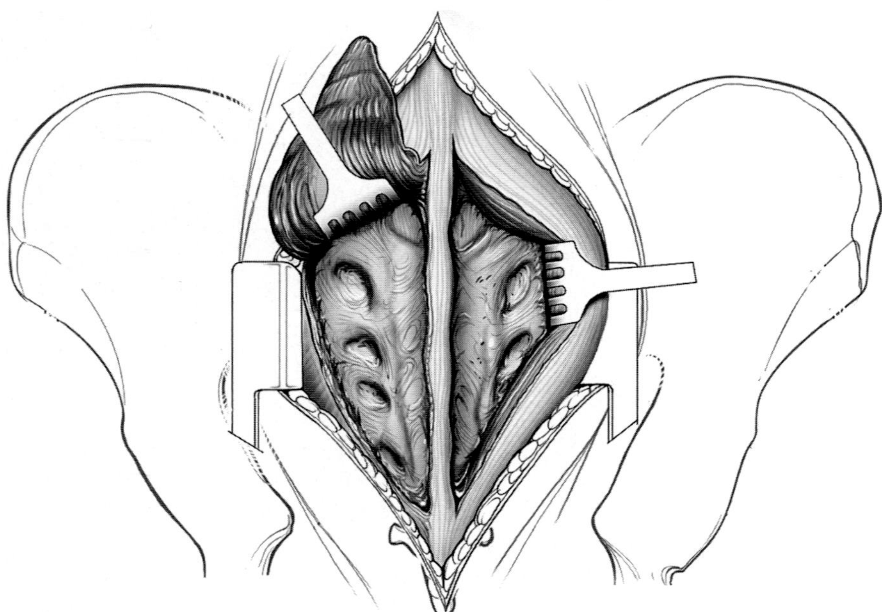

FIGURE 15-43. Deep exposure through a midline incision allows elevation of the lumbosacral musculature to expose the posterior aspect of the sacrum. This allows an extensile approach to the posterior aspect. A limited incision allows removal of the lumbosacral fascia from the medial sacral crest and lateral displacement of the muscle.

With the patient positioned lateral or supine, the involved extremity should be "free draped," allowing an assistant to manipulate the extremity in a sterile environment.

For this type of surgery, specialized equipment is mandatory. An array of large bone forceps is required for the reduction maneuvers, along with a large distractor, which is used to apply traction (Fig. 15-44). A critical reduction tool is the large pointed reduction forceps, which can hold the fragments while allowing rotational manipulation. Other reduction forceps can be screwed into the bone or used with special spike washers, which stabilize the forceps position, as well as prevent crushing of the underlying bone. If there is a delay in treatment and the fracture has shortened, a traction device attached to operating table (though not a common surgical tactic) may be used to provide the force required to reduce a completely unstable injury. Implants are specially designed to allow for contouring in bending and rotation, including extra-long screws of 3.5 and 4.5 mm (upwards of 130 mm) to accommodate the size of the pelvis.

Anterior Ring: Disruption of the Symphysis Pubis

We now turn to the open-book injury (Type B1 unilateral, Type B3 bilateral.

Exposure: Pfannenstiel

Reduction Techniques

Open reduction of a symphyseal disruption can be facilitated by use of bone-holding forceps such as a Farabeuf or Lane clamp, or specially designed pelvic reduction clamps attached to the pubis with prominent screws as pulling posts, or a large, pointed reduction clamp (Fig. 15-45) (12,30). To reduce the disruption, the jaws of the tenaculum clamp or pointed reduction clamps are placed into the obturator foramina and closed. Occasionally, the inferior portion of the posterior sacroiliac joint ligaments is also disrupted, allowing one hemipelvis to have a tendency to malrotate at the time of reduction. To control this, a second pointed reduction forceps (applied through 3.2-mm drill holes) is placed on one superior surface of the symphysis and angled into the inferior portion of the obturator foramen on the opposite side. These two reduction forceps usually are applied simultaneously to effect the reduction.

The use of a pelvic reduction clamp attached by 4.5-mm screws can be very helpful. This clamp can be applied to either the superior or anterior aspect of the pubic body, well out of the way of plate fixation. Reduction is facilitated by the excellent control (especially of rotation) that the clamp affords. Manual reduction using the clamp is assisted by internal rotation of the leg or pushing on the iliac wings. If external fixation pins are in place, it is not advisable to grasp these and use them as handles. These pins may pull out and

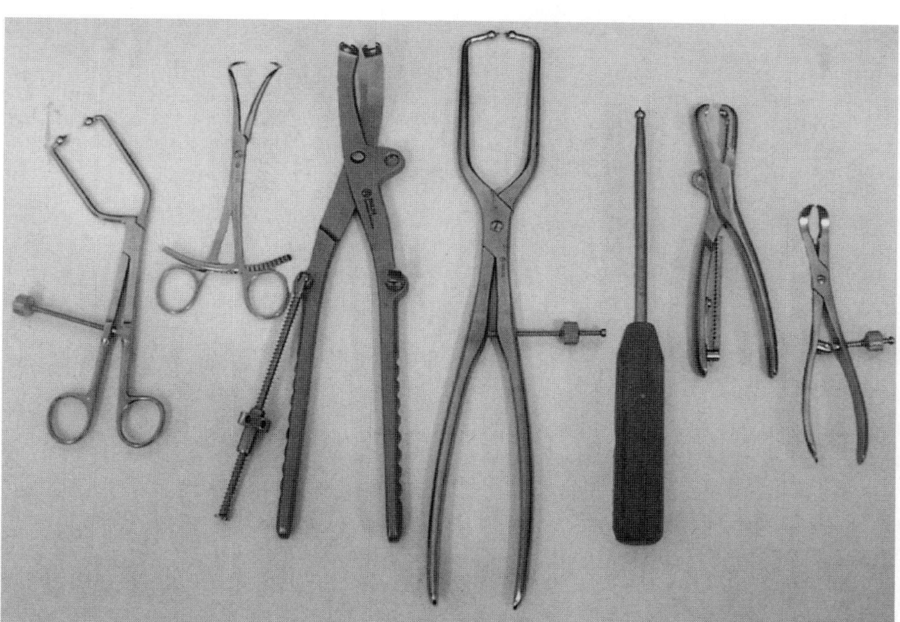

FIGURE 15-44. Example of various reduction clamps (Synthes USA, Paoli, PA). From left to right: oblique reduction forceps with pointed-ball tips; large reduction forceps with points; pelvic reduction clamp; large pelvic reduction forceps with pointed-ball tips; straight ball spike; Farabeuf reduction forceps; and serrated reduction forceps.

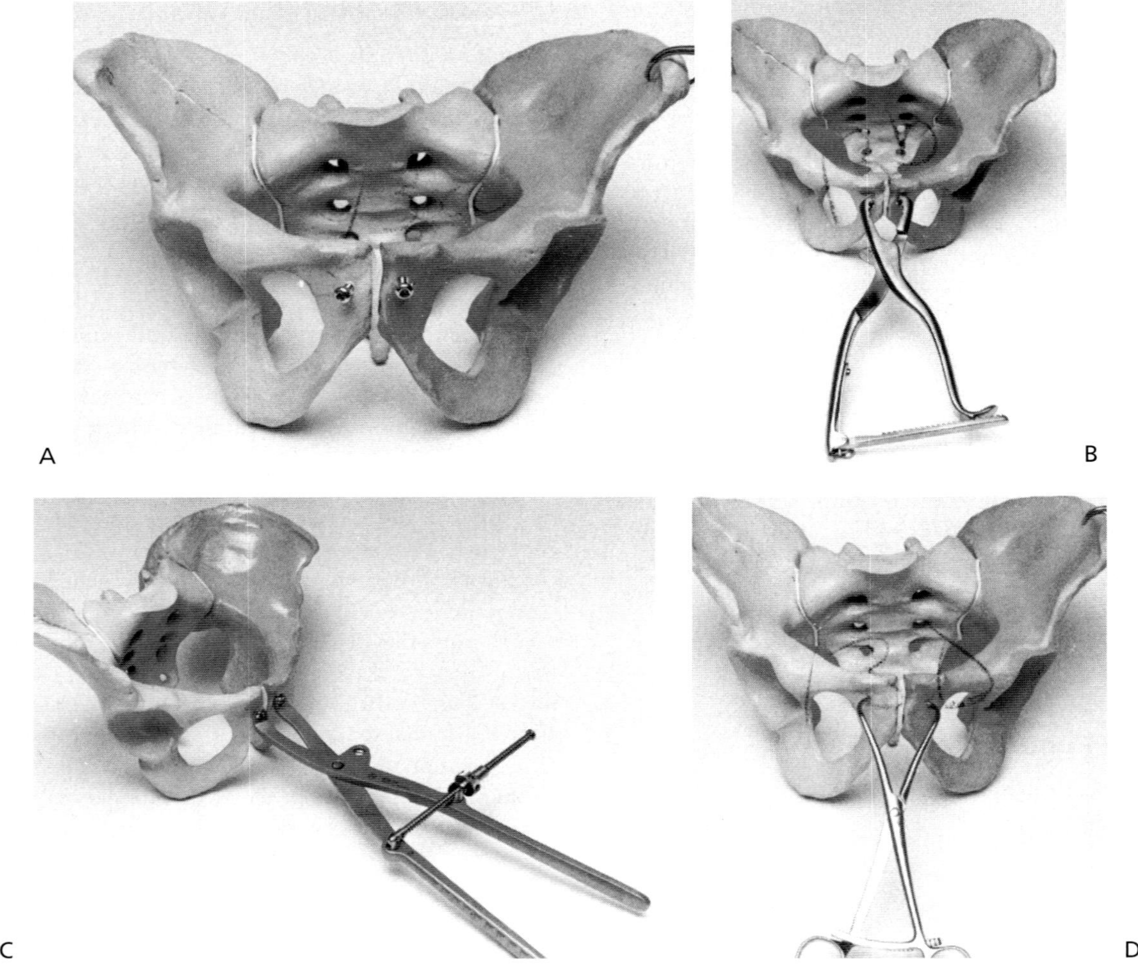

FIGURE 15-45. Reduction techniques for the symphysis pubis. Reduction of the symphysis pubis may be achieved by inserting two screws anteriorly **(A)** and placing a Farabeuf-type clamp **(B)** or a special pelvic reduction clamp **(C)** over the screws to achieve reduction. In most cases symphysis reduction can be achieved by using the pointed reduction clamp **(D)**, either directly into the cancellous bone or through two screw holes.

lose their purchase or, as a worst-case scenario, cause fracture of the iliac wing.

Another method of reduction is placing a 3.5-mm screw into each of the pubic rami and then putting a figure-of-eight wire about them; tightening the wire reduces the symphysis. A plate is then applied. Alternatively, a Farabeuf clamp may be used instead of the wire. It is also possible to precontour a plate so that there are three holes on each side of the symphysis. This precontoured plate is fixed to one side and then the pubic rami and body of the opposite side are reduced to the plate.

Reduction is confirmed by palpation of the symphysis from the space of Retzius as well as radiographic confirmation. The Foley catheter must be palpated in the bladder and continued urine output noted to assure that the bladder or bladder neck has not been entrapped in the reduction.

Types of Fixation

In the stable open-book fracture, where the posterior structures are intact, a single plate is all that is required (3,12,14). During activity there is some rotational motion through the symphysis, which has created a controversy over whether a two-hole, four-hole, or longer plate is more desirable. It was felt that a two-hole plate allows some rotation to occur and is strong enough to withstand major displacement (Fig. 15-46A). A four-hole plate was felt to be necessary to control the rotation and thus not loosen the screws; however, plate breakage may occur (Fig. 15-46B). Review of studies has shown that there is no significant difference between the two. Most pelvic surgeons use a four-hole, 3.5-mm or 4.5-mm dynamic compression (DC) plate or reconstruction plate, depending on the size of the patient, using the appropriate fully threaded cancel-

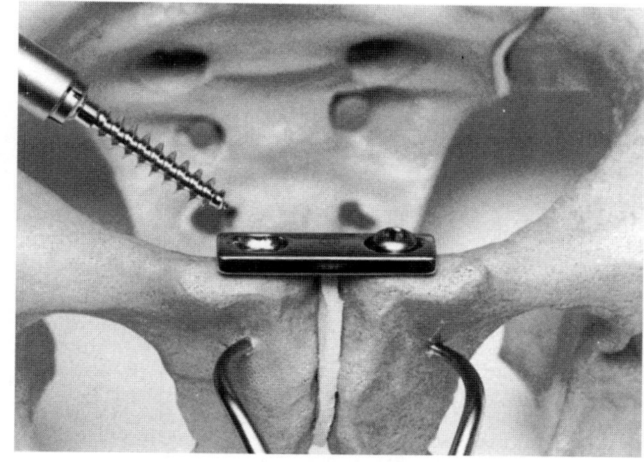

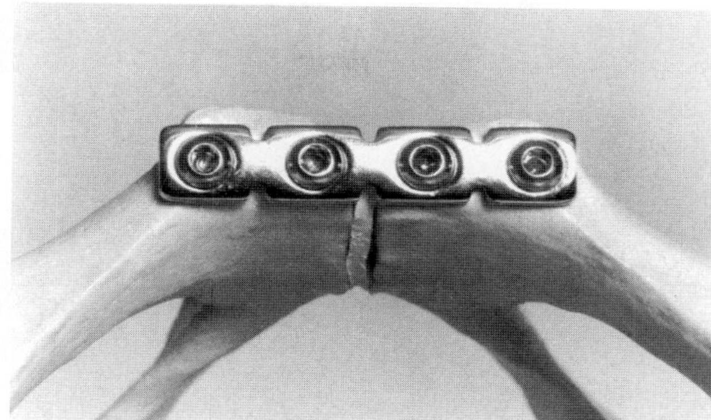

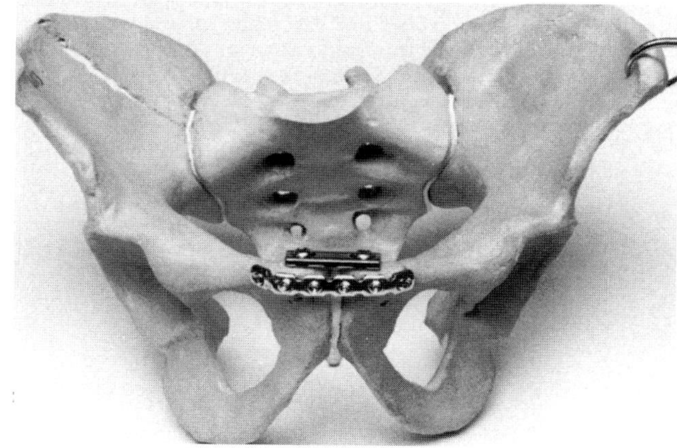

FIGURE 15-46. Symphyseal stabilization in open-book fractures. A two-hole DC plate next to the superior surface of the symphysis with fully threaded cancellous screws **(A)** is advocated for fixation of open-book fractures. Our preference is a four-hole plate stabilized with fully threaded cancellous screws on the superior surface, which increases the stability and prevents redisplacement **(B).** Biomechanically, the most stability is obtained by using two plates—a two- or four-hole, 3.5 or 4.5-mm DC plate to the superior surface and a four- to six-hole anterior 3.5-mm DC plate **(C).** This is rarely required for a stable open-book fracture (B1).

lous screws for fixation. The plate must be positioned so that there is no screw hole over the symphysis because this is a weak point in the plate and predisposes the plate to failure. The best mechanical stability is achieved by using two plates, a two-hole 3.5- or 4.5-mm DC plate applied to the superior surface and a four- to six-hole 3.5-mm DC placed anteriorly (Fig. 15-46C); however, this is rarely required in the open-book (B1) type fracture. Double-plating is used for osteoporotic bone (52).

Postoperative Care

In the stable injury, the patient may be mobilized as soon as comfortable. The patient may be up in a chair, and after 3 to 10 days mobilized onto crutches, bearing full weight on the uninvolved side. In women of childbearing age, consideration should be given to removing the plate when healing is complete (not sooner than 1 year postinjury), to allow for the natural diastasis of the symphysis during pregnancy and delivery.

Symphyseal Disruption in Type C (Unstable) Fractures

Stabilization of a symphysis disruption associated with an unstable pelvic injury is desirable and greatly simplifies management of the patient. In this particular injury, two plates placed at right angles to each other are desirable to restore pelvic stability *if no posterior stabilization is contemplated.* In severely traumatized patients, the clinical course may be very unpredictable, owing to sepsis and other complications; therefore, the surgeon can never be sure that he or she will be able to surgically approach the posterior injury safely. Thus, the two-plate method should be used to be certain of maximum obtainable stability, which may become definitive treatment (Fig. 15-47). If that method is combined with an external skeletal fixator, then reasonable stability in an unstable Type C injury may be obtained, as shown in biomechanical studies (2,17,18,53). One plate is placed across the superior surface of the symphysis, usually a four-hole plate, and a four- or six-hole plate is then

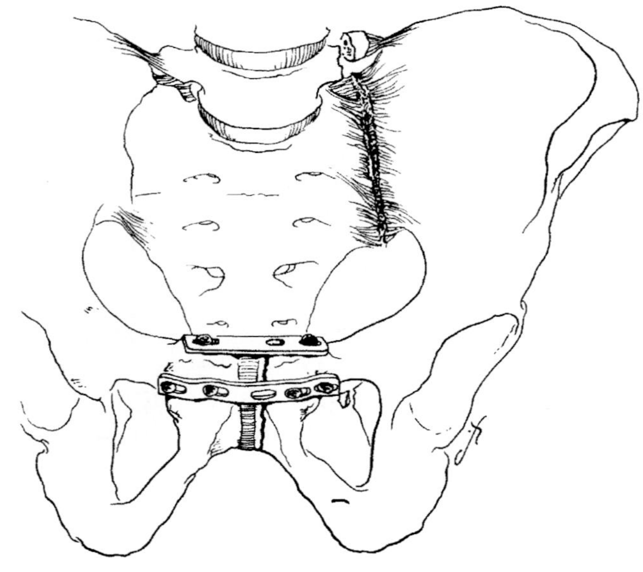

A

FIGURE 15-47. For symphyseal stabilization of an unstable pelvic fracture two DC plates at right angles to each other are preferred **(A).** Anteroposterior radiograph **(B)** and inlet view **(C)** show marked disruption of the symphysis pubis in a dislocation of the left sacroiliac joint. Management consisted of immediate application of an external frame to minimize hemorrhage **(D)** and anterior fixation using two plates at right angles to each other **(D).** Because of extremely poor skin, fixation of the posterior lesion was not carried out. In spite of this, using anterior plating and external fixation, a satisfactory outcome was achieved **(E).**

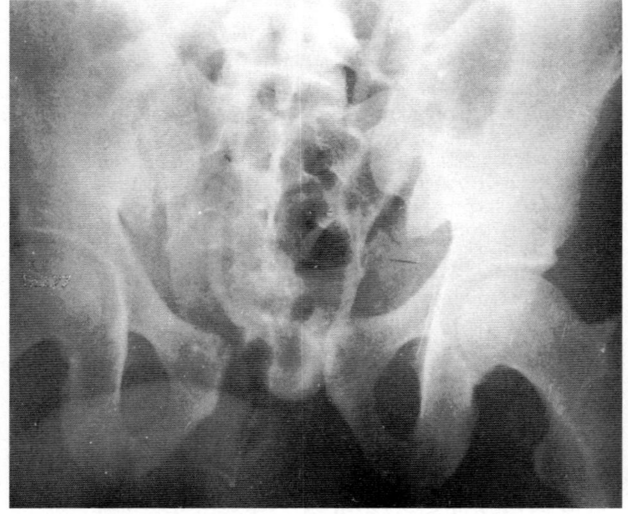

B

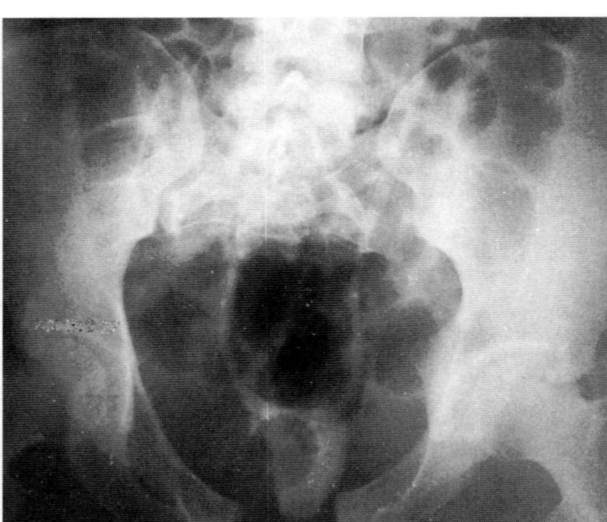

C

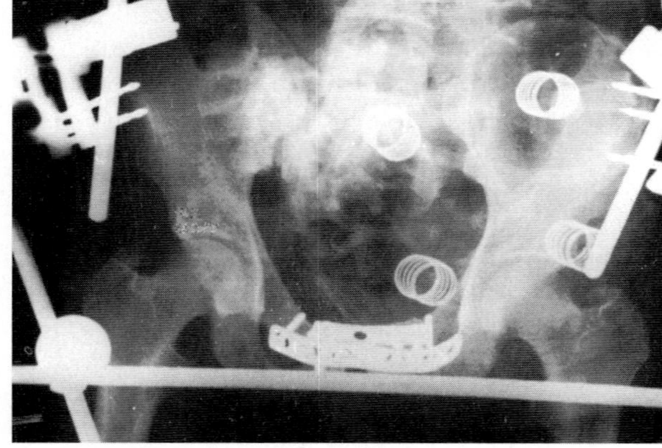

D

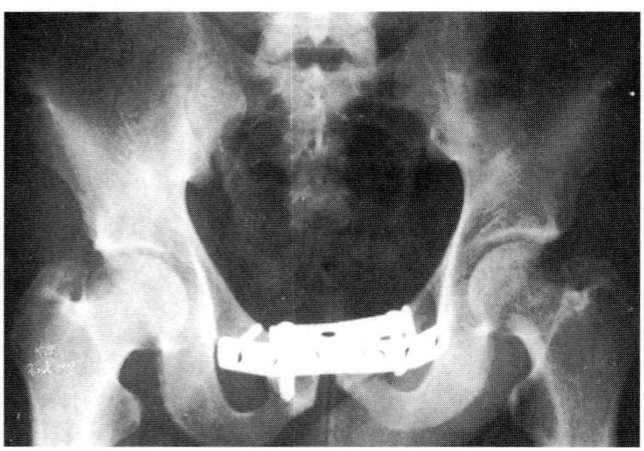

E

placed across the anterior aspect of the symphysis. It must be remembered that anterior fixation alone in the unstable pelvis is a compromise for fixation. It must be supplemented by an external fixator, which much improves the biomechanical strength of the construct. It is not stable enough to allow the patient to be up and bearing weight on the uninvolved side; it is simply a method of reducing the pelvic ring disruption and restoring some stability, which may be helpful in allowing mobilization of the patient from bed to chair.

Anterior Ring in the Lateral Compression Injury

Open reduction and internal fixation are rarely required for a lateral compression injury. However, there are some specific indications. The most common reason is an unacceptable deformity, either leg length discrepancy or internal malrotation. In the contralateral (bucket-handle) injury, the hemipelvis on the involved side rotates inward and upward, resulting in leg length discrepancy. Also, the affected leg may be incapable of external rotation beyond the neutral position. If the leg cannot be externally rotated past neutral, then serious consideration should be given to realigning the pelvis.

How much leg length discrepancy is acceptable is debatable; however, serious consideration should be given to reduction of the pelvic fracture for any leg length discrepancy >2 cm. In the acute situation, it may be difficult to determine the true leg length discrepancy. An antero-posterior pelvic x-ray, scanogram, or CT examining the differential between the height of the two acetabula or hips may be very helpful in this regard.

A special situation exists when a lateral compression injury is associated with an iliac wing fracture (crescent fracture). These injuries are very difficult to manage nonoperatively due to the internal rotation injury in combination with the posteriorly applied impaction force. Conversely, the surgical treatment is straightforward.

Other indications for open reduction and internal fixation in lateral compression injuries include the irreducible locked symphysis and tilt fractures that cannot be reduced by closed means, especially in a female patient as has been described previously.

Approach

The symphysis and medial pubic rami may be approached in most cases using a Pfannenstiel approach (Fig. 15-37A,B). Alternatively, a midline longitudinal approach is used if an abdominal or pelvic visceral exploration is contemplated. Bilateral ilioinguinal approaches may be used in fractures involving all four rami (the bucket-handle fracture). The use of the Stoppa approach as modified by Bolhofner and Cole is a less demanding alternative.

Reduction Techniques

These injuries are caused by internal rotation forces, and the hemipelvis is malrotated internally. Therefore, external rotation of the hemipelvis is required for reduction. This can be accomplished manually by placing the involved leg in a figure-of-four position and applying the rotationally directed force across the knee by pushing down on the knee, which externally rotates the hemipelvis through the femoral head (Fig. 15-48A). However, especially in older persons, care must be taken to avoid fracturing the neck of the femur by this maneuver. Therefore, manual pressure over the iliac wing and anterior superior spine is the preferred method. In many cases, closed reduction achieves satisfactory position and may obviate more invasive treatment, as seen in Fig. 15-49. This 19-year-old woman sustained a lateral compression fracture (B2), tilt variety, as well as other fractures and general injuries (head, chest). An excellent closed reduction was obtained using general anesthesia and manual pressure over the iliac wing, resulting in a satisfactory outcome.

Direct force may be applied to the displaced hemipelvis through external fixation pins placed into the iliac wing (Fig. 15-48B,C). A handle then can be placed on the pins, and a gentle external rotation force can be applied. Using femoral distraction or external fixation with pins in the opposite iliac crest and into the ilium just above the acetabulum may allow gentle derotation (Fig. 15-50). Care must be taken to see that the pins are accurately placed, lest they tear out of the bone or fracture the ilium and render the reduction useless. Finally, the use of a pelvic reduction clamp, which can be fixed across the symphysis pubis to unlock the symphysis, may be helpful. In this particular situation, the pelvic reduction clamp is used in the distraction mode.

Fixation Techniques

Fixation techniques are identical to those already described (Fig. 15-46A–C). In this relatively stable injury, stability may be achieved by the use of a single four- to six-hole anterior plate (Fig. 15-51). Longer plates may be required for fixation of ramus fractures. In fixation of ramus fractures, great care must be taken to ensure that the lateral screw does not enter the hip joint. In the stable "tilt fracture," either a plate or threaded Kirschner wires may be used, which are removed at 6 to 8 weeks (Fig. 15-52). A screw inserted retrograde from the pubis to the iliac wing along the pubic ramus, as previously described, is another ramus fracture fixation alternative. Anterior fixation of a lateral compression injury usually restores stability to the pelvic ring because this particular injury already is partially stable, owing to the intact pelvic floor and posterior ligamentous structures.

Postoperative Care

The majority of these injuries are stable once fixed, owing to the configuration of the fracture. Therefore, it is safe to mo-

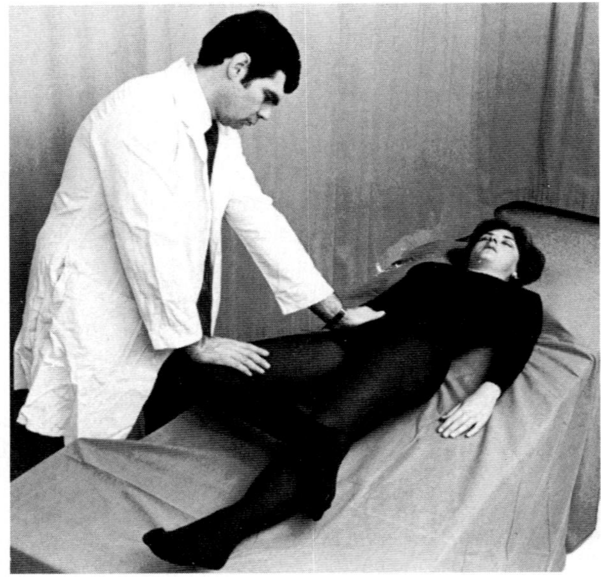

FIGURE 15-48. **A:** Closed reduction of a lateral compression injury is performed by external rotation of the hip with the knee flexed and direct pressure on the hemipelvis. **B:** The photograph demonstrates the type of leverage one can obtain by placing handles on the crossbars of the external fixation device to allow both internal and external rotation of the unstable hemipelvis. **C:** The diagram on a computed tomography scan indicates the type of direct leverage one can obtain on the affected hemipelvis; though great care must be taken when putting any type of direct leverage on the pin, as it could pull out of the bone. It is far better to use the maneuver in **(A)** to achieve reduction than to risk pulling out the pins.

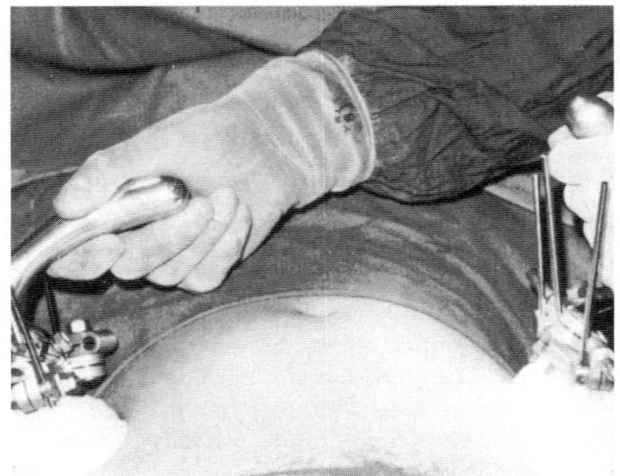

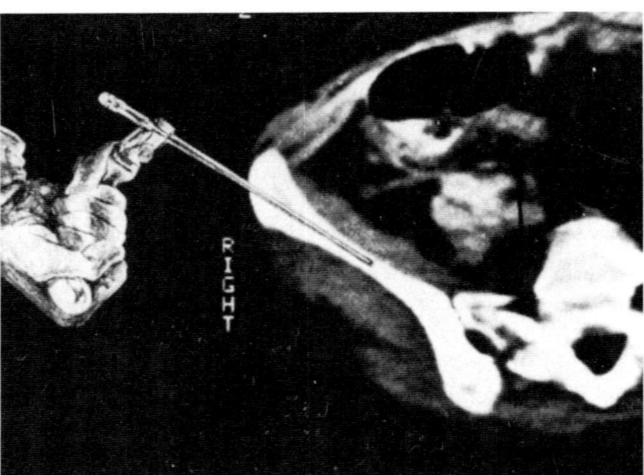

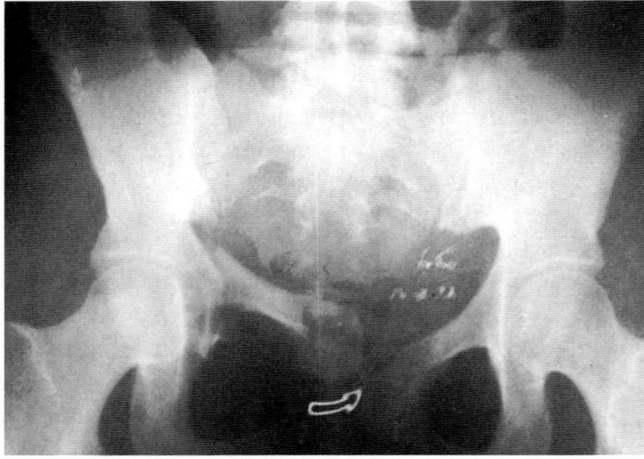

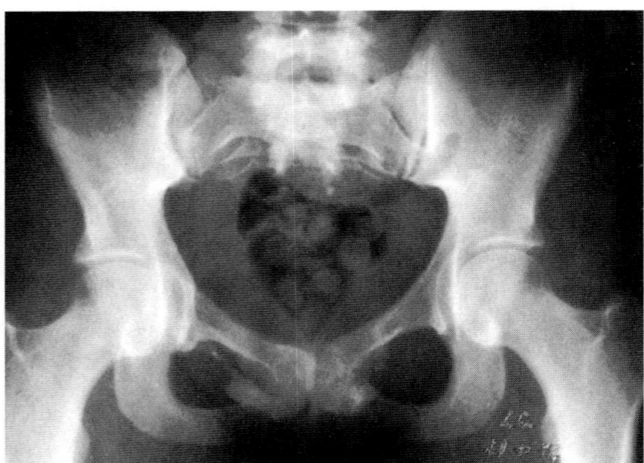

FIGURE 15-49. Closed reduction for overlapped symphysis. **A:** Anteroposterior radiograph of a 19-year-old woman who sustained a lateral compression type (B2-1) injury to her pelvis in a motor vehicle accident. Note the internal rotation of the right hemipelvis, the fracture through the right superior ramus, and the superior portion of the symphysis fractured and overriding the left hemipelvis *(white arrow).* **B:** The patient was taken to the operating room with the intent of doing open reduction; however, under image intensification closed reduction was achieved by direct pressure over the right iliac crest, which externally rotated the hemipelvis, and direct pressure on the superior fragment. The fracture was reduced virtually to anatomic position, without need for open reduction. Note the anatomic healing of the superior ramus and the calcification at the symphysis. The final outcome was excellent.

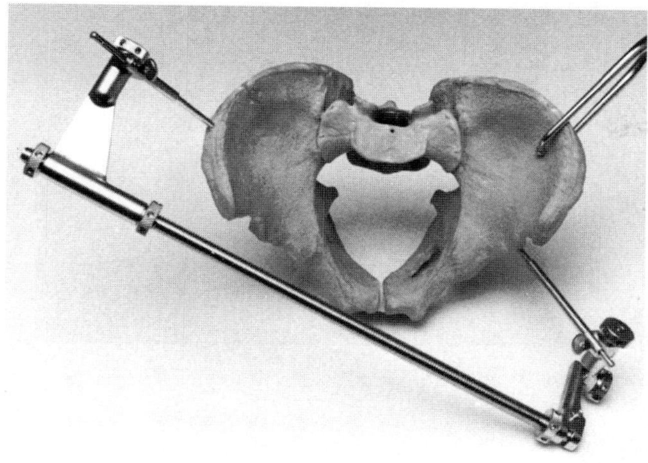

FIGURE 15-50. A femoral type distractor may be used to externally rotate the pelvis when necessary. One pin is placed in the iliac crest, the other just proximal to the hip joint in the region of the anterior inferior spine. This allows gentle external rotation through the distraction device.

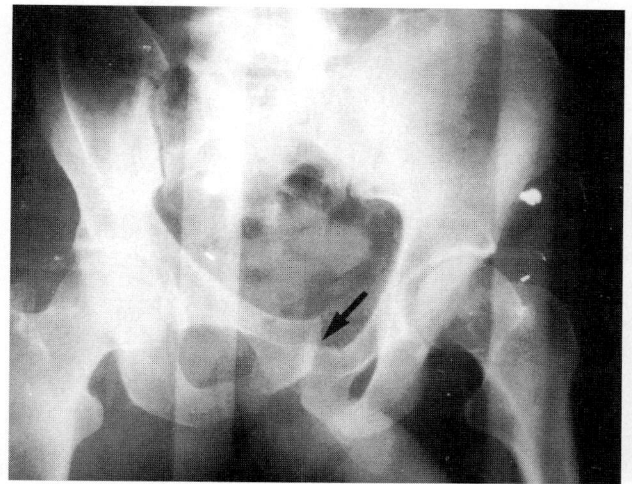

A

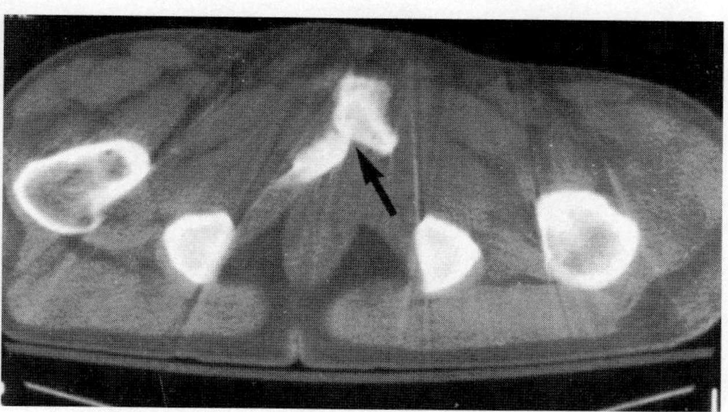

B

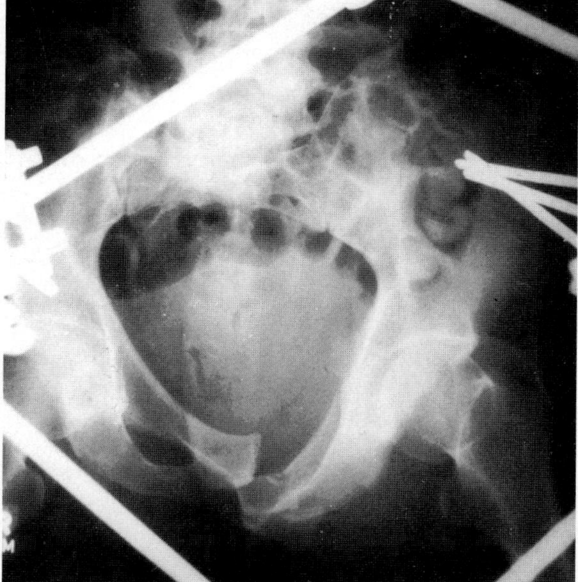

C

FIGURE 15-51. Anteroposterior radiograph shows a locked symphysis **(A)** in a lateral compression injury, confirmed on computed tomography **(B).** Initial treatment with an external fixator and an attempt at closed reduction failed to reduce the locked symphysis **(C).** Open reduction and internal fixation using a six-hole reconstruction plate shows good reduction on the postoperative radiograph **(D)** and a good surgical outcome, as noted in the inlet **(E)** and outlet **(F)** views.

(Figure continues)

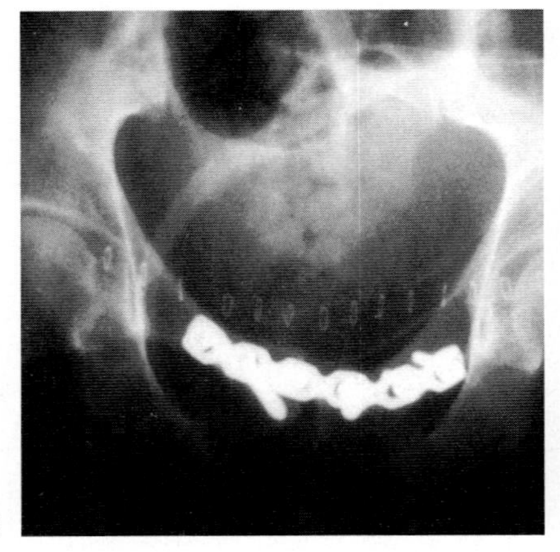

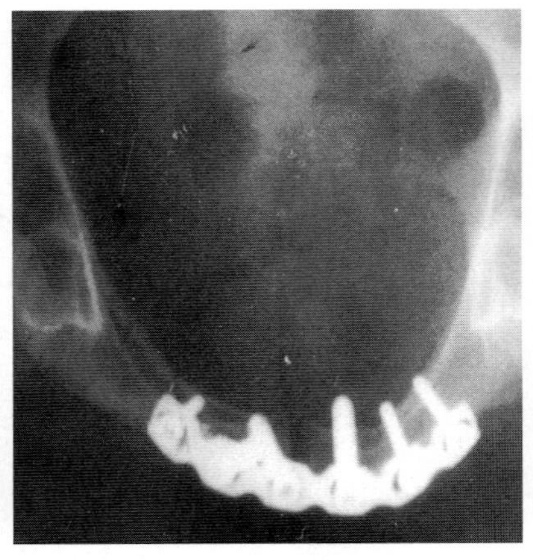

D, E

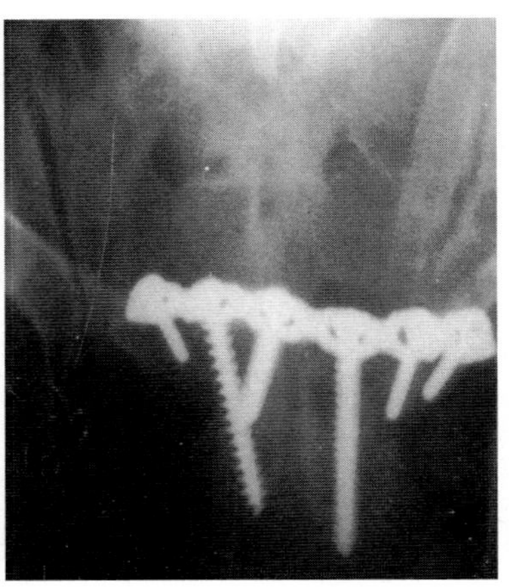

F

FIGURE 15-51. *(continued)*

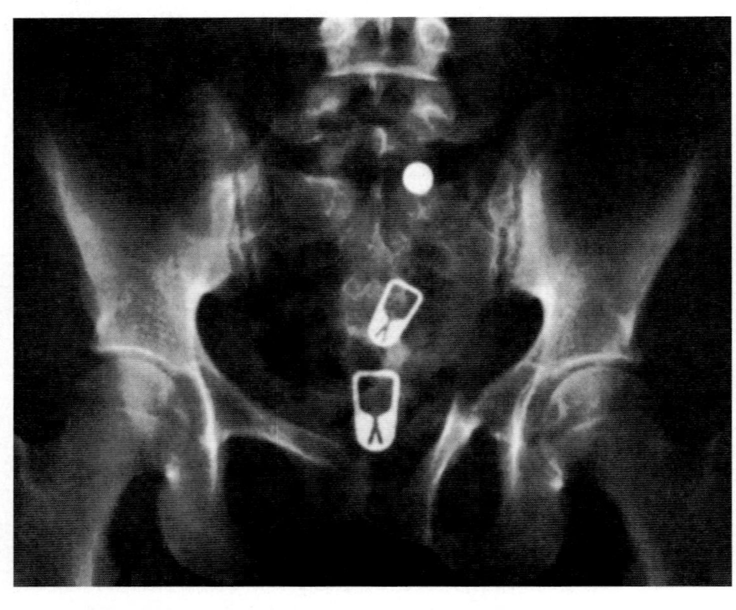

A

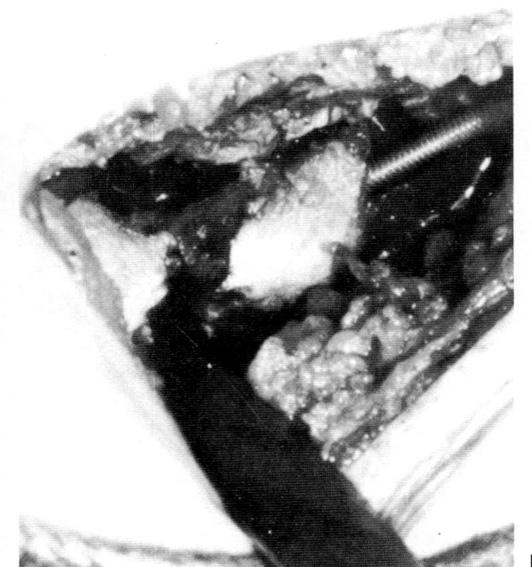

B

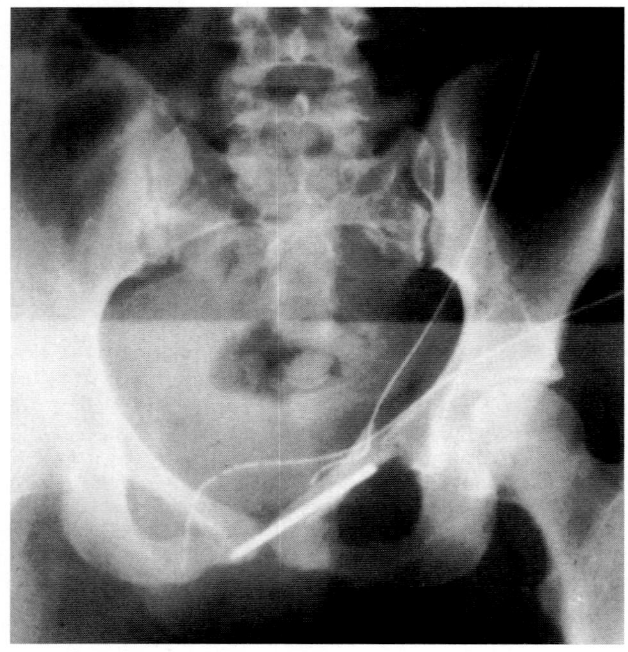

C

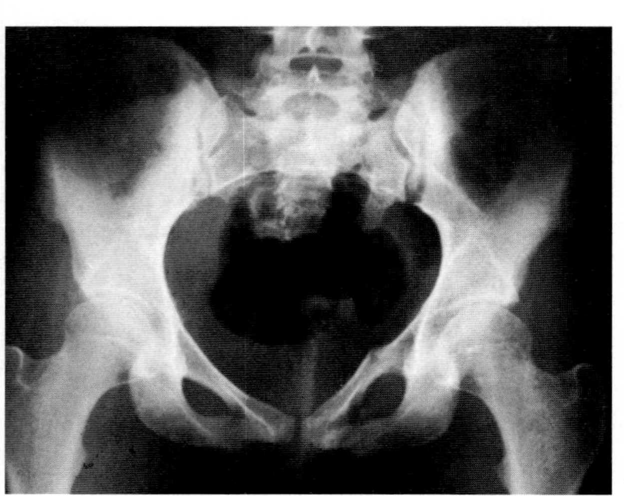

D

bilize patients by allowing full weight bearing (as tolerated) on the uninvolved side. Partial weight bearing on the involved side may begin after 6 to 8 weeks. As healing progresses, the patient may progress to full weight bearing within 3 months.

POSTERIOR RING

Introduction

As has been discussed in previous chapters, the biomechanical stability of the pelvis depends on an intact posterior sacroiliac complex. Therefore, internal fixation of a disrupted posterior sacroiliac complex is necessary to regain stability. The pelvis is a ring structure. Consequently, an injury to the ilium or sacroiliac joint cannot occur in isolation, but must be accompanied by a second injury elsewhere in the ring (1,2). The location of this second area of injury usually is somewhere in the anterior ring. The anterior structures act as a strut to prevent anterior collapse during weight bearing and resist rotational forces. Despite the fact that these anterior structures play a much more minor role in the pelvic stability equation, operative fixation of the anterior ring can be an important adjunct to internal fixation of a posterior injury (27,32). Therefore, the techniques demonstrated in the previous section for fixation of the anterior ring often find application in conjunction with internal fixation of iliac fractures and sacroiliac joint injuries.

Although all these injuries have a commonality, resulting in disruption of the posterior sacroiliac complex, each has its own particular personality. The surgical tactic often is dictated by these differing characteristics. This variability requires a number of reduction clamps of different shapes and sizes (Fig. 15-44). The sacroiliac fracture-dislocation behaves like an iliac fracture or a sacroiliac dislocation, depending on the amount of ilium that remains attached to the posterior sacroiliac ligamentous structures (Fig. 15-53). Therefore, selection of the particular method for internal fixation of these fractures is mainly dependent on the relationship of the iliac fracture line to the sacroiliac joint.

Iliac Wing Fractures

Isolated fractures of the iliac wing (Duverney) that do not involve the major weight bearing area of the pelvis are biomechanically stable injuries and usually respond well to

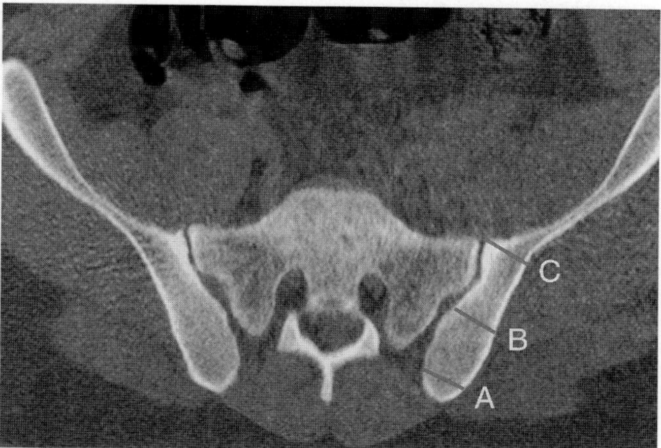

FIGURE 15-53. Zones of fracture through the posterior ilium. Fractures in the region marked by line A are avulsion injuries and behave like pure sacroiliac joint dislocations. Fractures anterior to line C are extraarticular fractures. Fractures in the region of line B are classic crescent fractures. These fracture-dislocations, as well as those in the region between lines B and C, behave more like an extraarticular fracture. As the fracture line moves posteriorly from B toward A, the personality of the injury, as well as the treatment methods, transition from that of an iliac fracture to that of a sacroiliac dislocation.

nonoperative management. However, they may require open reduction and interrnal fixation to prevent deformity. Iliac fractures violating the weight-bearing arch of the pelvis are unstable, usually resulting in a rotationally unstable hemipelvis (54). These unstable fractures of the posterior aspect of the ilium may be completely extraarticular or involve the sacroiliac joint to a varying degree. In the context of fracture fixation, the extraarticular fractures and fractures that extend from the midportion of the sacroiliac joint in which the posterior superior iliac spine remains firmly attached to the sacrum by an intact posterior ligamentous complex (crescent fracture) should be grouped together (54). An important feature of the crescent fracture pattern is an associated impaction fracture of the ipsilateral anterior sacrum (Fig. 15-54) as lateral compression is the deforming force responsible for this injury. In all of these fractures, stable internal fixation can be achieved using extraarticular internal fixation techniques. Fracture-dislocations located more posteriorly through the sacroiliac joint, having a small or compromised residual attachment of the posterior superior iliac spine to the sacrum, should be grouped with sacroiliac dislocations, as transarticular internal fixation is required.

FIGURE 15-52. The radiograph **(A)** indicates an abnormal variant of the lateral compression fracture (tilt fracture), whereby the symphysis is disrupted by the rotating superior pubic ramus on the left side. In this case, because the posterior fracture was stable, the anterior lesion was fixed with a threaded Steinmann pin **(B,C)**. The Steinmann pin was removed at 6 weeks. An excellent clinical outcome was achieved for the patient, with bony healing of the ramus fracture and stability at the symphysis **(D)**.

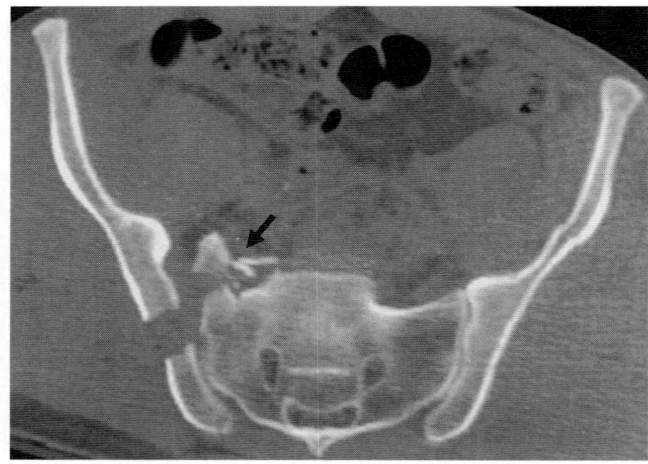

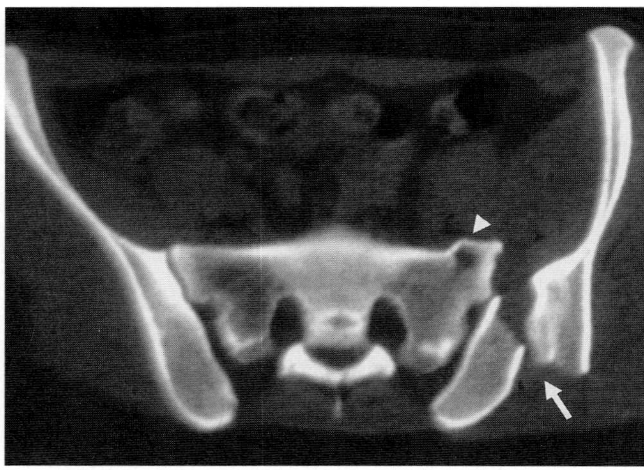

FIGURE 15-54. Computed tomography scan examples of the crescent fracture. **A:** Severe impaction fracture of the ipsilateral sacrum *(arrow)* is shown, which is caused by the lateral compression deforming force. **B:** A case with less severe sacral impaction *(arrowhead)* also showing the oblique orientation of the fracture *(arrow)* and internal malrotation of the ilium.

Stable Extraarticular Iliac Fractures

Approach

These fractures may be approached from the anterior intrapelvic route or the posterior extrapelvic method. However, the anterior route involves less surgical damage to the soft tissues and is, therefore, preferred. Duverney fractures that extend into the sacroiliac joint may be adequately addressed via the anterior approach. The joint reduction is straightforward and both the wing fracture and sacroiliac joint can be assessed simultaneously.

Reduction Techniques

Reduction is accomplished using a Schanz screw in the anterior superior spine as a joystick to pull the fragment up and rotate it into position.

Fixation Techniques

Fixation usually is accomplished with a lag screw along the iliac brim and neutralized by a plate (one third tubular or 3.5-mm reconstruction) below the iliac crest and/or along the sciatic buttress.

A posterior approach may be used if the fracture is an extraarticular iliac wing. The gluteal muscle is stripped from the outer crest, the fracture is reduced and provisionally fixed with 2-mm K wires. Definitive stabilization is performed with either 3.5- or 6.5/7.3-mm cancellous screws in a lag fashion. Because there are usually two large surfaces of cancellous bone to interdigitate, these fractures generally require no further internal fixation. If concern about stability exists, then a neutralization plate may be added along the iliac crest.

Unstable Extraarticular Iliac Fractures

Approach

Extraarticular iliac fractures can be addressed using the superior portion of the iliofemoral incision (Fig. 15-40) (55). With the patient in the supine position and the leg draped free, it is usually not necessary to release the sartorius muscle and inguinal ligament origins from the anterior superior spine. However, release of these structures will increase the exposure of the internal iliac fossa, if needed. Intraoperative fluoroscopic imaging is helpful in these cases (Fig. 15-55). Therefore, the use of a radiolucent table is advisable.

Reduction Techniques

The extraarticular iliac fracture patterns are commonly in an oblique orientation, similar in nature to the supraacetabular fracture line (spur sign) of the both-column acetabular fracture (Fig. 15-56). Therefore, an initial reduction technique often includes placing a straight ball spike at the level of the pelvic brim (Fig. 15-57A). Perhaps a more effective method involves inserting a reduction clamp over the iliac crest, across this oblique fracture line (Fig. 15-57B). Only minimal stripping of the muscles on the external iliac surface (just along the fracture line) should be needed for clamp positioning. A Farabeuf clamp placed in the notch between the anterior superior and inferior iliac spine is helpful to assist in the reduction. To complete the reduction, a clamp also is positioned across the fracture line at the level of the iliac crest.

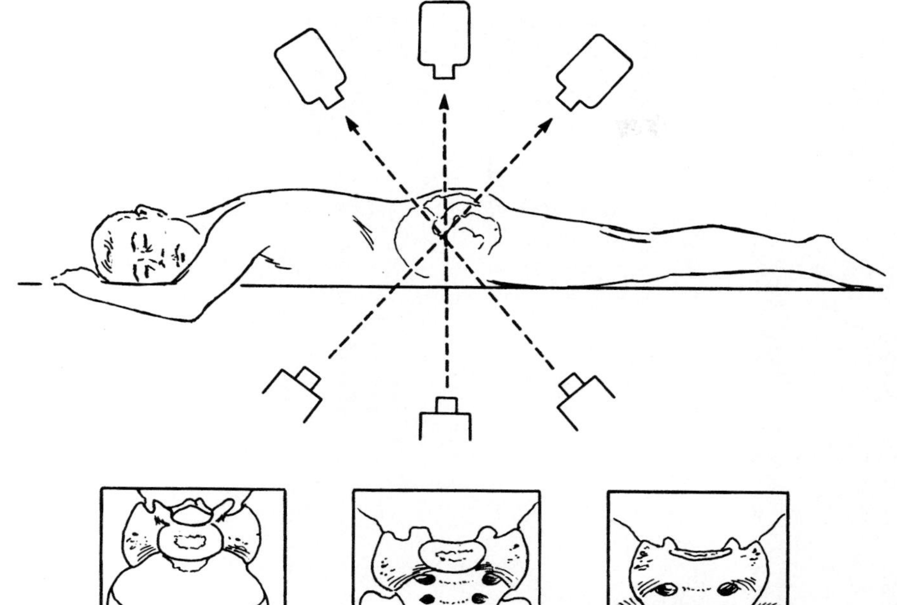

FIGURE 15-55. Patient position and fluoroscopic visualization of the posterior sacroiliac complex. (Modified from Matta JM, Saucedo T. Internal fixation of pelvic ring fractures. *Clin Orthop* 1989;242:83–97, with permission)

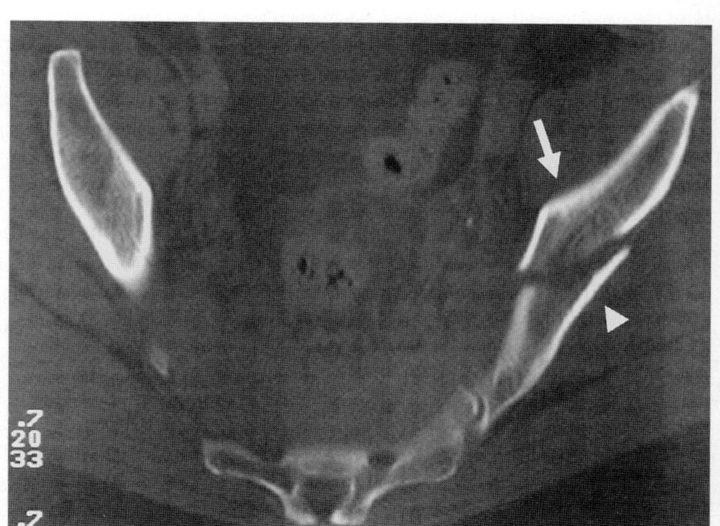

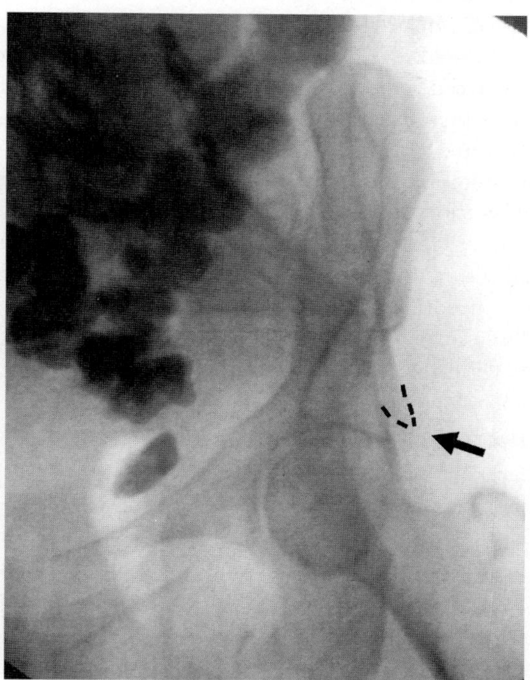

FIGURE 15-56. Example of an extraarticular fracture. **A:** Computed tomography section showing the fracture obliquity, which is similar to the supraacetabular fracture line in a both-column acetabular fracture. The arrow shows the location to place a straight ball spike for fracture reduction. If a bone clamp is used for fracture reduction, the position for each forceps tine is shown on the inner table *(arrow)* and external surface *(arrowhead)* of the ilium. **B:** Internal oblique fluoroscopic view showing the iliac fracture *(arrow)* with a similar appearance *(dashed lines)* as the both-column acetabular spur sign.

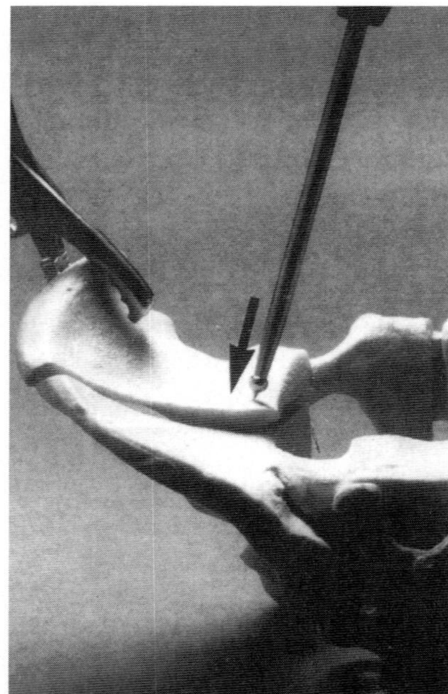

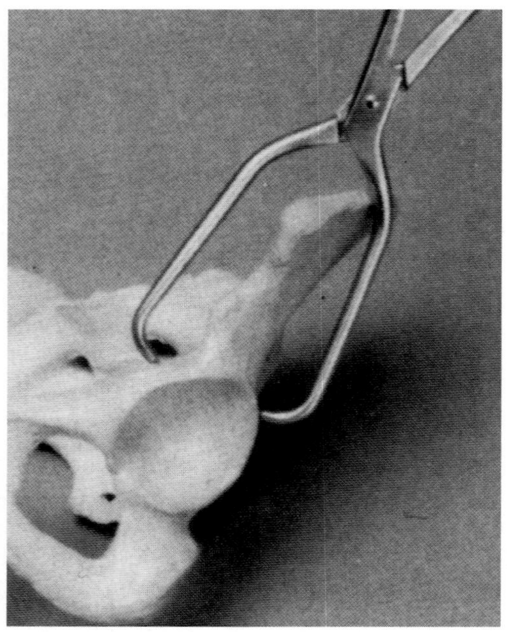

FIGURE 15-57. Reduction techniques. **A:** Use of the ball spike. A Farabeuf clamp is shown placed at the anterior superior iliac spine to assist in the reduction. (Modified from Tornetta P III, Riina J. Acetabular reduction techniques via the anterior approach. *Op Tech Orthop* 1997;7:184–195, permission pending.) **B:** Position of a large reduction forceps.

The type of clamp used at the iliac crest level depends on the fracture orientation. A transverse fracture orientation at the crest level can be reduced using a pointed reduction clamp (Fig. 15-58A). With an oblique fracture pattern, a serrated clamp placed across the fracture usually is all that is needed. These reduction methods are highly desirable because they do not interfere with subsequent screw placement. When these methods prove ineffective, either owing to fracture comminution or the need for additional force in mobilizing the fracture fragment, a pelvic reduction clamp or Farabeuf clamp inserted over screws may be required (Fig. 15-58B). Care is needed to ensure that these screws inserted for reduction clamp purposes do not compromise the positioning of the definitive internal fixation plates and screws.

Fixation Techniques

After fracture reduction, fixation is accomplished using lag screws supplemented by a buttress plate. Ideally, lag screws are placed at the level of the iliac crest, pelvic brim and anterior inferior iliac spine where bone stock is best (Fig. 15-59) (55). The exact screw placement is dictated by the specific fracture pattern. The lag screws used are usually 3.5-mm in diameter with washers. However, the anterior inferior iliac spine will accommodate up to a 7.3-mm screw. A contoured plate (3.5-mm pelvic reconstruction type) is placed along the inner aspect of the iliac crest (Fig. 15-60). Alternative plate placement, along the superior surface of the iliac crest, provides excellent fixation, but usually precludes use of a lag screw at this level and often becomes symptomatic. After the completion of internal fixation, for this operative procedure as well as for all those with descriptions to follow, the final reduction and hardware position should be confirmed intraoperatively by anteroposterior, inlet, and outlet radiographic imaging.

Intraarticular Iliac Fractures

Approach

Selection of the surgical approach for these fractures is mainly dependent on the relationship of the iliac fracture line to the sacroiliac joint. A posterior approach is used with the prototypical crescent fracture (35,54). Although surgery can be performed with the patient in the prone position, lateral patient positioning is more helpful in facilitating fracture reduction. With the patient lateral on a radiolucent table, the leg is draped free and available to apply manual traction, if needed. The anterior aspect of the iliac crest is also available for clamp application, secondary incisions, and reduction maneuvers (Fig. 15-61). If the lateral position is used, care must be taken to have the surgical field include the midline posteriorly. In addition, the patient should be tilted slightly forward from the lateral position and placed at the near edge of the table to facilitate access to the posterior crest (Fig. 15-61). Table rotation can be used to improve access (forward rotation). Fluoroscopic imaging with the pelvic fracture patient in the lateral position has some idiosyncrasies. Similar views can be obtained with the patient supine. However, allowances must be made for the approximate 20 degrees of forward flexion normally associated with lateral positioning. In addition, most C-arm fluo-

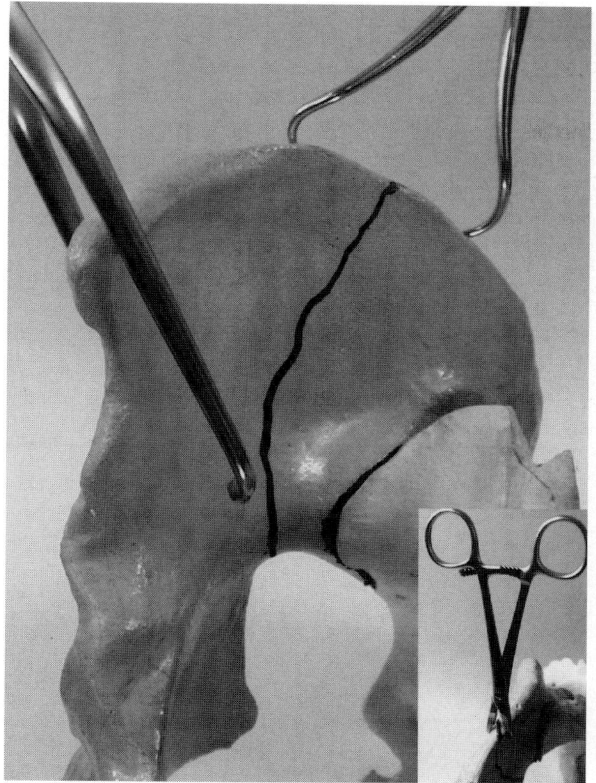

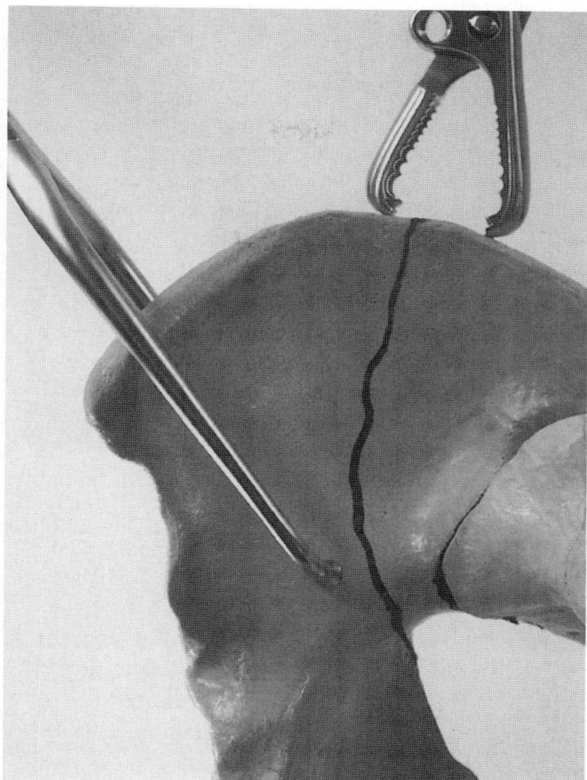

FIGURE 15-58. A: Reduction technique adding a pointed clamp at the crest level. A serrated clamp works well if the fracture line is oblique *(inset)*. **B:** Reduction technique adding a Farabeuf clamp at the crest level.

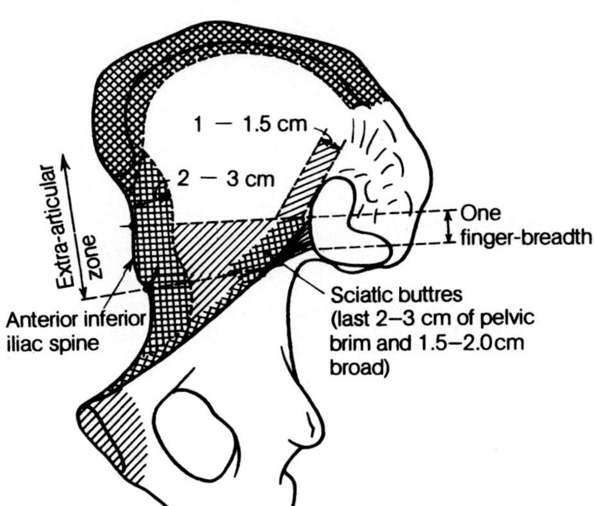

FIGURE 15-59. The most solid areas of the innominate bone. (From: Letournel E, Judet R. *Fractures of the acetabulum,* 2nd ed. New York: Springer-Verlag 1993:403, permission pending.)

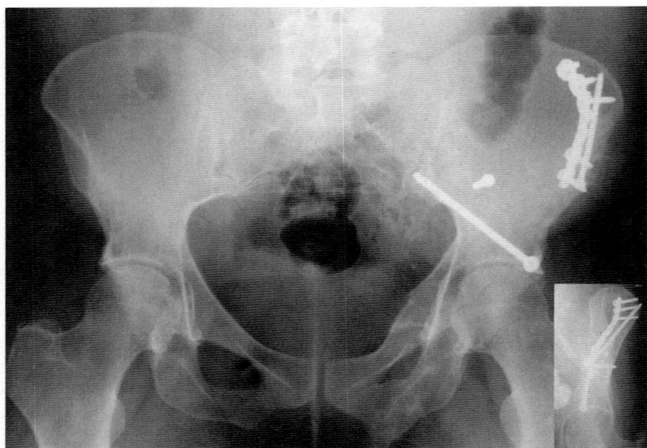

FIGURE 15-60. Postoperative radiographs from the patient shown in Fig. 15-9. The anteroposterior radiograph at fracture healing and an immediate postoperative oblique view *(inset)* show the fixation construct and correction of the malrotation.

roscopy units cannot rotate past a horizontal position. Therefore, with the C-arm placed opposite to the surgical field, (anterior to the patient) backward rotation of the operating room table often is required to obtain an adequate anteroposterior imaging. Patient position satisfactory to allow adequate fluoroscopic imaging should be checked prior to preparation and draping of the surgical area. Whatever the patient position, however, the basic posterior surgical approach is the same (Figs. 15-41 and 15-61).

The anterior extent of the posterior approach at the level of the greater sciatic notch is limited by the superior gluteal neurovascular bundle. Therefore, fracture-dislocations involving only the anterior portion of the sacroiliac joint can be more easily (and safely) fixed using the anterior approach described in the preceding. As the iliac fracture line moves more anteriorly at the posterior crest level, access using the posterior approach may result in an extensive release of the gluteus maximus muscle and more than desirable involvement of the gluteus medius origin, as well as traction on the superior gluteal neurovascular bundle. With the patient in the lateral position on the operating table, intraoperative adjustment can be made to minimize this problem by making secondary incisions located more anteriorly at the crest level fracture line. Relative indications for the anterior approach include patients with conditions that weigh against prone or lateral intraoperative positioning, such as those with multiple injuries and those with bilateral hip/pelvic injuries (Fig. 15-62). A crescent fracture pattern in conjunction with medial translation of the main iliac fragment into a position anterior to the sacral ala (Fig. 15-63) presents an uncommon indication for the anterior approach. In these circumstances in which the crescent fracture is treated using an anterior surgical approach, the operative management may require combination of techniques (see Special Considerations).

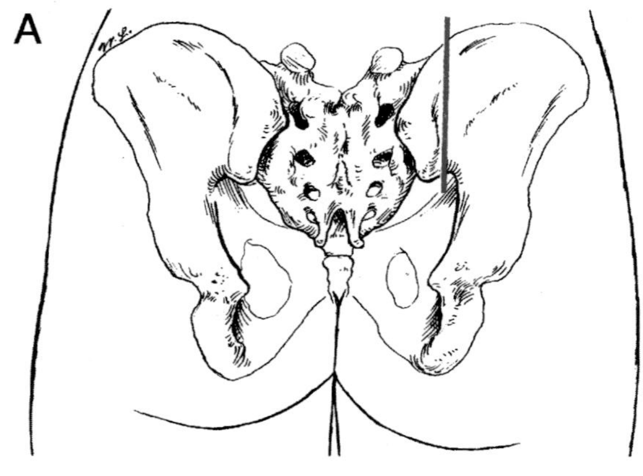

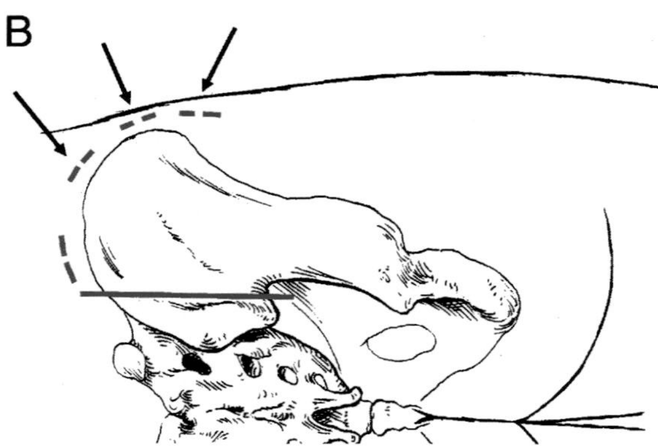

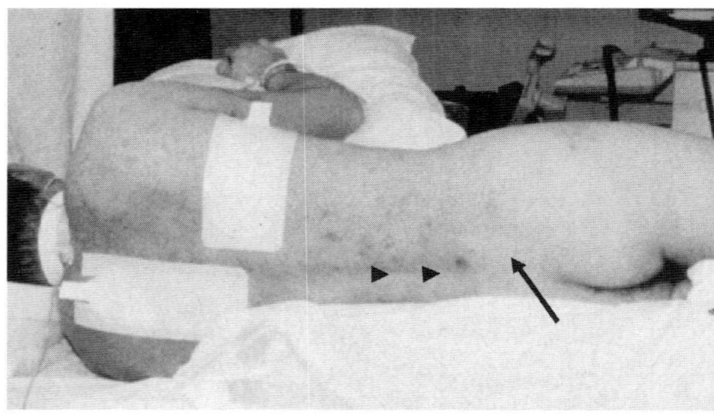

FIGURE 15-61. A: Vertical incision for the posterior approach to the pelvis with the patient prone. Potentially, there is access to the posterior aspect of both ilia and the entire sacrum. **B:** With the patient lateral, posterior contralateral access is limited to just past the midline. However, this patient position allows additional access for reduction clamp application and fracture fixation via secondary small incisions *(dashed lines)*. In addition, manual traction can be applied through the ipsilateral leg that has been draped free. **C:** Patient in the lateral position on a radiolucent table. The patient is rolled slightly forward to improve access to the posterior crest and the angulation needed for insertion of screws *(arrow)*. The sterile field should include the midline *(arrowheads)*.

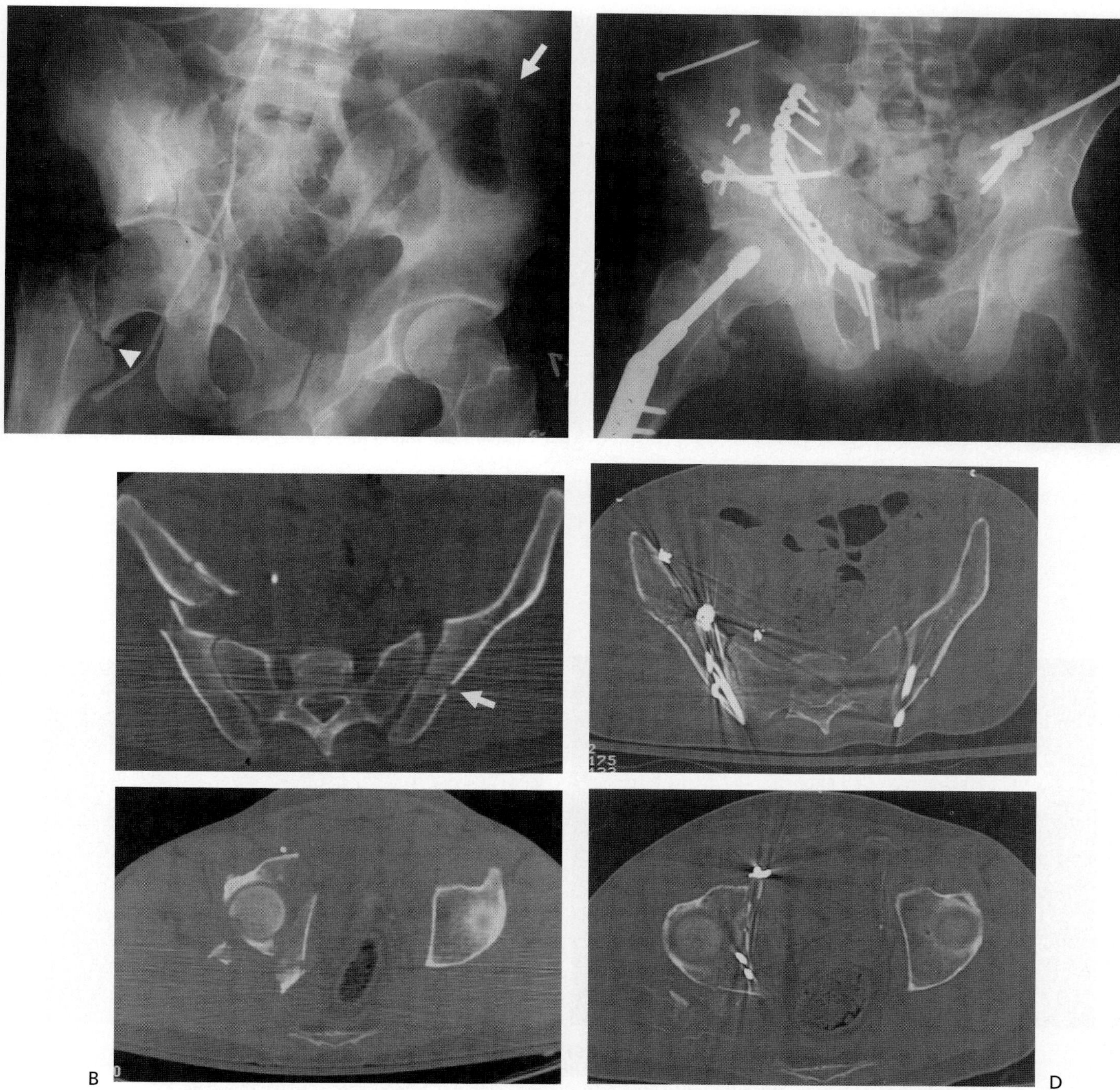

FIGURE 15-62. Anteroposterior radiograph **(A)** of a 26-year-old man involved in a motor vehicle accident who sustained multiple injuries, including a right both-column acetabular fracture, right femoral neck fracture *(arrowhead),* and left iliac fracture *(arrow).* **B:** Computed tomography sections further delineate the acetabular fracture and crescent fracture *(arrow).* These fractures were treated with the patient supine on a radiolucent operating room table. Postoperative anteroposterior **(C)** and computed tomography sections **(D)**. Lag screws alone were used owing to the patient's excellent bone quality.

(Figure continues)

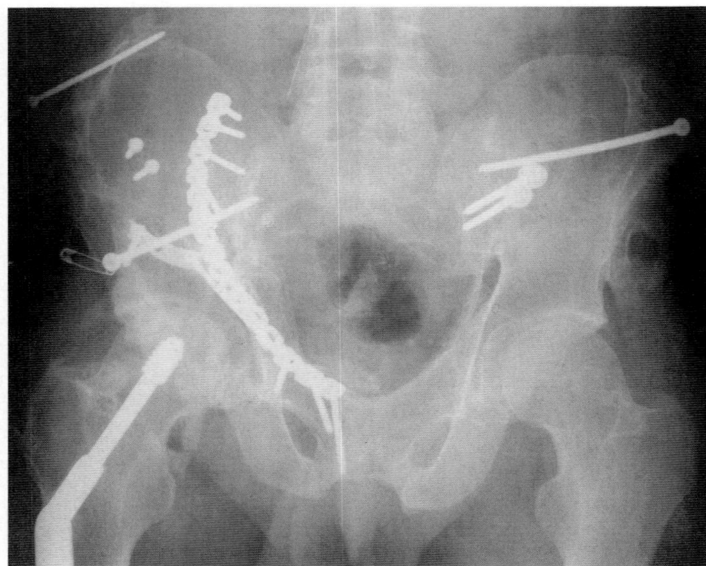

FIGURE 15-62. *(continued)* **E:** At follow-up 3 years later the patient was found to be doing well and had returned to full activities.

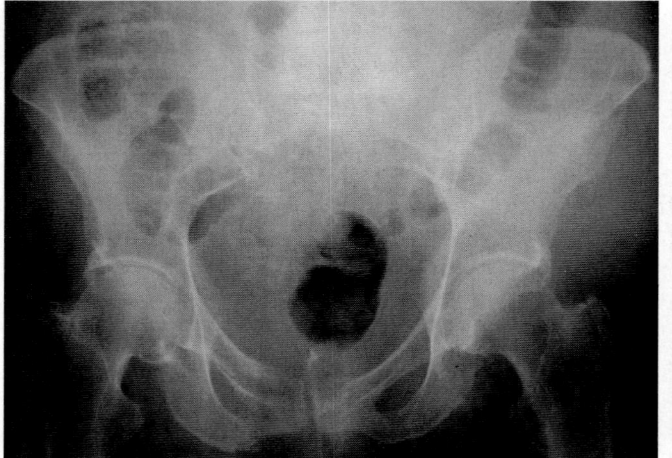

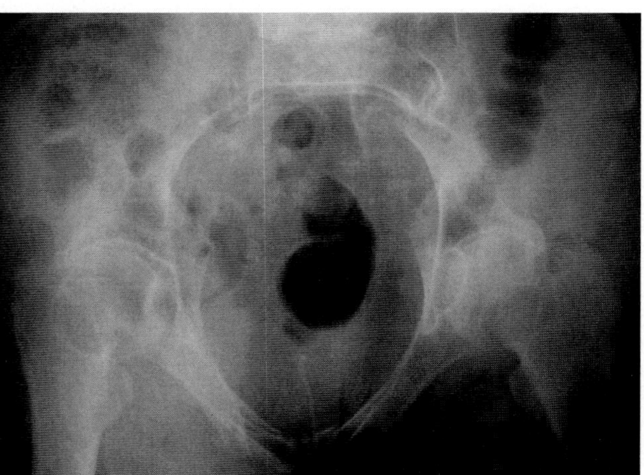

FIGURE 15-63. Anteroposterior **(A)**, inlet **(B)**, and outlet **(C)** radiographs of a 78-year-old woman involved in a motor vehicle accident. Although at first glance the radiographs do not appear that impressive, the outlet view *(dashed lines)* and computed tomography scan **(D)** show the severe medial fracture displacement anterior to the ala of the sacrum. Postoperative anteroposterior **(E)**, inlet **(F)**, outlet **(G)**, and computed tomography sections **(H1, H2)**. Using a ball spike and Farabeuf clamp, the major displacement was partially corrected, putting the reduction in close proximity. Final reduction was accomplished using a Farabeuf clamp across the joint as shown in Fig. 15-81E. Anterior plates were applied as a buttress in this 78-year-old patient.

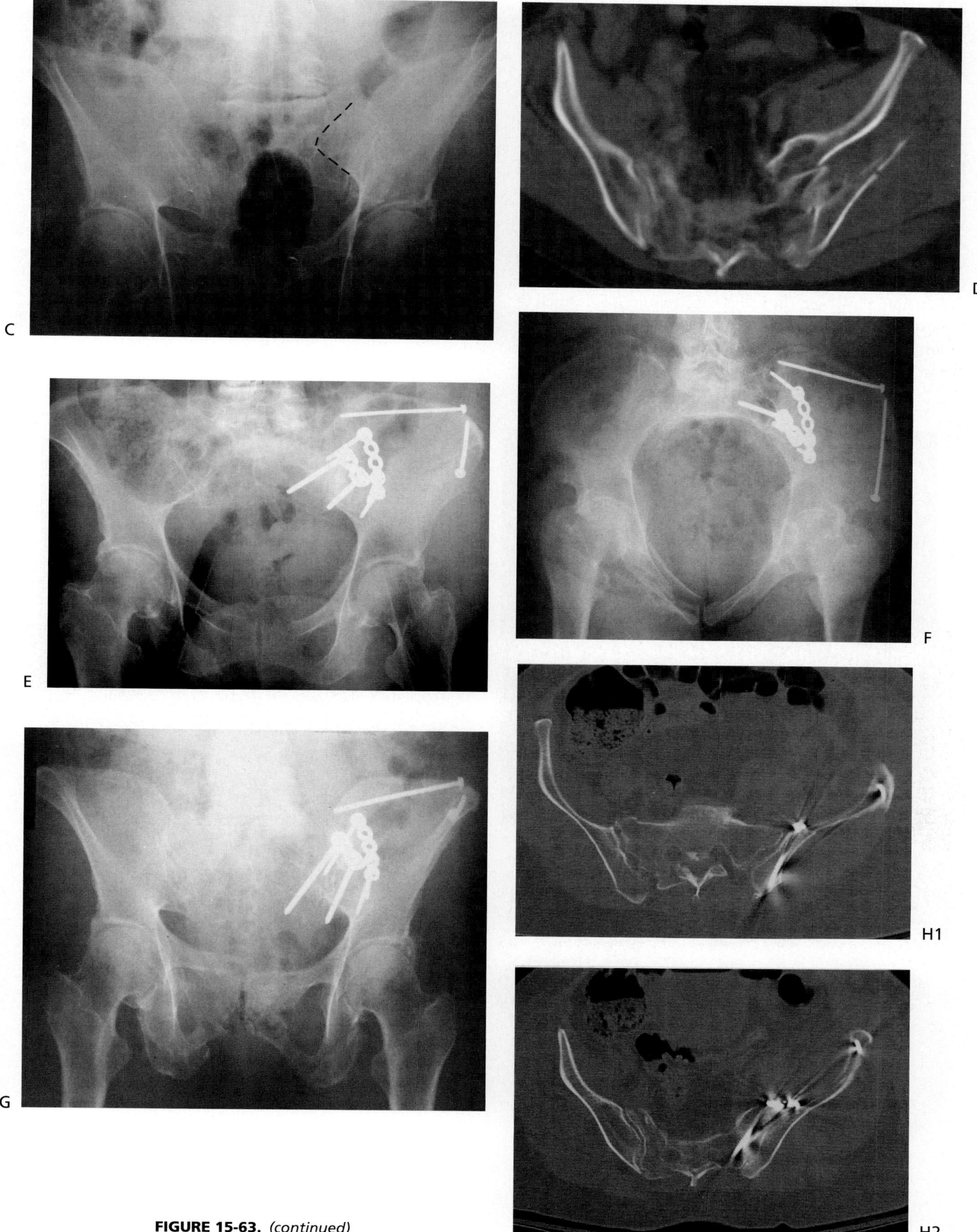

FIGURE 15-63. *(continued)*

Reduction Techniques

The crescent fracture often has an oblique configuration, angling from posterolateral to anteromedial while the hemipelvis is internally malrotated and often translated posteriorly (Fig. 15-54B) (45). The inferior aspect of the injury is a dislocation of the sacroiliac joint. One way to reduce this fracture-dislocation consists of initially placing a serrated clamp in the greater sciatic notch in a position similar to that for reducing a pure dislocation (Fig. 15-64). This is an excellent way to achieve complete reduction of the fracture-dislocation. However, the use of this technique is limited by the extent of the associated compression fracture of the anterior sacrum that may be present (Fig. 15-54B). Alternatively, a pelvic reduction clamp is inserted over screws placed on either side of the fracture site. The pelvic reduction clamp is preferable to the Farabeuf clamp owing to the internal malrotation and posterior translation, which often requires great force (initially combined with distraction) to reduce effect. To complete the reduction, a second clamp is positioned across the fracture line at the level of the iliac crest, as in the extraarticular fracture reduction techniques described in the preceding pages (Fig. 15-65). Sometimes placing a serrated clamp anterior to the fracture line through a secondary incision along the iliac crest, as noted in the preceding, is helpful in applying traction and reducing the malrotation.

After fracture reduction, fixation is accomplished using lag screws supplemented by a 3.5-mm pelvic reconstruction buttress plate placed near the level of the posterior superior

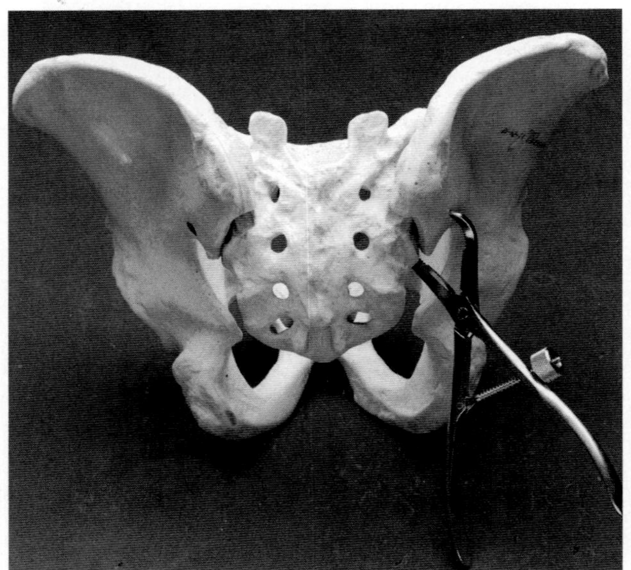
A

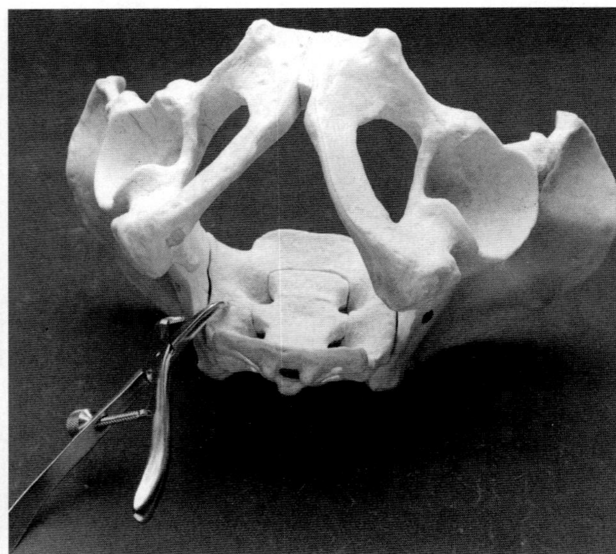
B

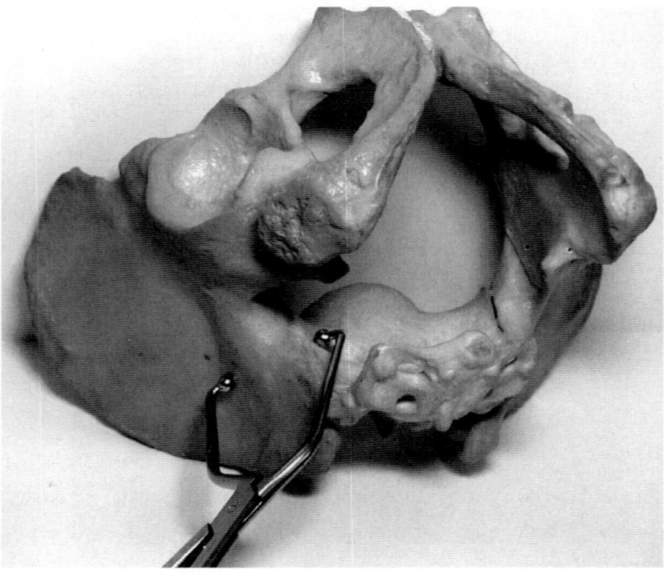
C

FIGURE 15-64. Application of a serrated bone forceps through the greater notch. **A:** Posterior view. **B:** Anterior view, which shows the inner jaw of the clamp just lateral to the sacral foramina at the S1-S2 level. **C:** An angled reduction clamp also can be used. Comminution of the sacrum in this area precludes the use of this reduction method.

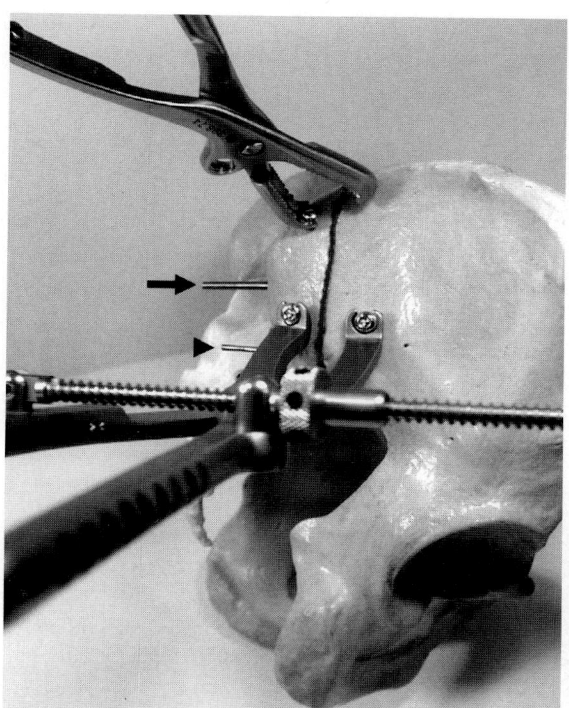

FIGURE 15-65. Application of a pelvic reduction clamp across a simulated crescent fracture *(line)* with a Farabeuf clamp at the crest level. It is important to ensure that the anterior screw for the pelvic reduction clamp is not too long. Otherwise, it may impinge on the sacral side of the sacroiliac joint during reduction maneuvers and impede the reduction. K-wires have been inserted at the posterior superior *(arrow)* and posterior inferior *(arrowhead)* iliac spines. After reduction, lag screws can be inserted at these points without obstruction from the clamps. The clamps then are removed and a buttress plate applied.

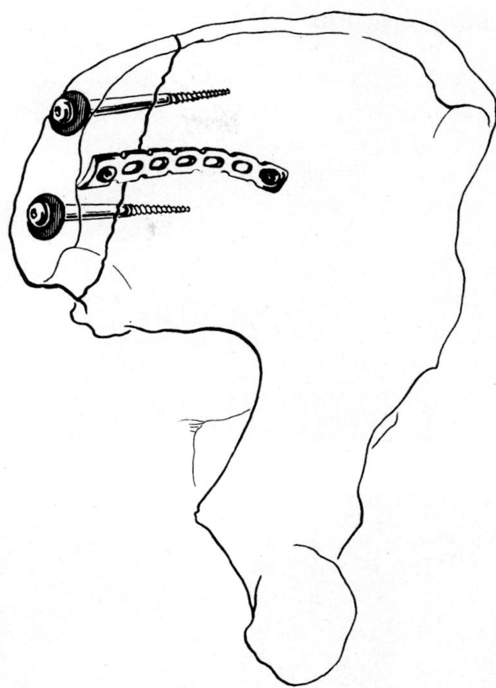

FIGURE 15-66. Example of typical screw and plate construct for crescent fracture fixation.

iliac spine, the posterior inferior iliac spine and/or the iliac crest (Fig. 15-66). The lag screws used are usually 3.5-mm in diameter with washers. However, the posterior inferior iliac spine accommodates a 4.5-mm screw. The exact screw and plate placement, and combination thereof, is dictated by the specific fracture pattern (Fig. 15-67). Care is needed to ensure that any screws inserted for reduction clamp purposes do not compromise the positioning of the definitive internal fixation. One method is to place the reduction screws in the area planned for plate application. The pelvic clamp can be removed after lag screw insertion, which is then followed by application of the plate. As noted, fracture lines that propagate anteriorly at the crest can be accessed and fixed using a secondary crest incision.

Fixation of the anterior ring may be an important adjunct to fixation of the crescent fracture, mainly depending on the extent of the impaction fracture of the anterior sacrum. Without reconstitution of the strut that the anterior ring provides, the hemipelvis will rotate inward until it abuts the fractured sacrum, approximating the malrotation caused by the initial lateral compression injury pattern. This occurs despite satisfactory extraarticular crescent fracture fixation. A plate should be used in cases with the anterior disruption through the pubic symphysis. An external fixator applied until anterior fracture healing (usually 6 weeks time) is all that is required in cases with the anterior disruption through the rami (Fig. 15–67).

Sacroiliac Dislocation and Fracture Dislocation

Displaced fracture-dislocations with a small fracture component involving the ilium or sacrum behave like pure dislocations. All are biomechanically unstable Type C injuries and require transarticular internal fixation. In the context of fracture fixation, fracture-dislocations involving the ilium located more posteriorly through the sacroiliac joint and pure dislocations can be fixed using either an anteriorly applied sacroiliac joint plate or iliosacral screws. In fracture-dislocations with sacral involvement, the sacral fracture component usually precludes anterior sacroiliac joint plating (56).

Indications for adjunctive fixation of the associated anterior ring injury consist of symphysis pubis disruption >10 mm and widely displaced rami fractures (>20 mm) (29). Biomechanical study has shown that anterior plating is better than external fixation, but both provide adequate stabilization when combined with internal fixation of the

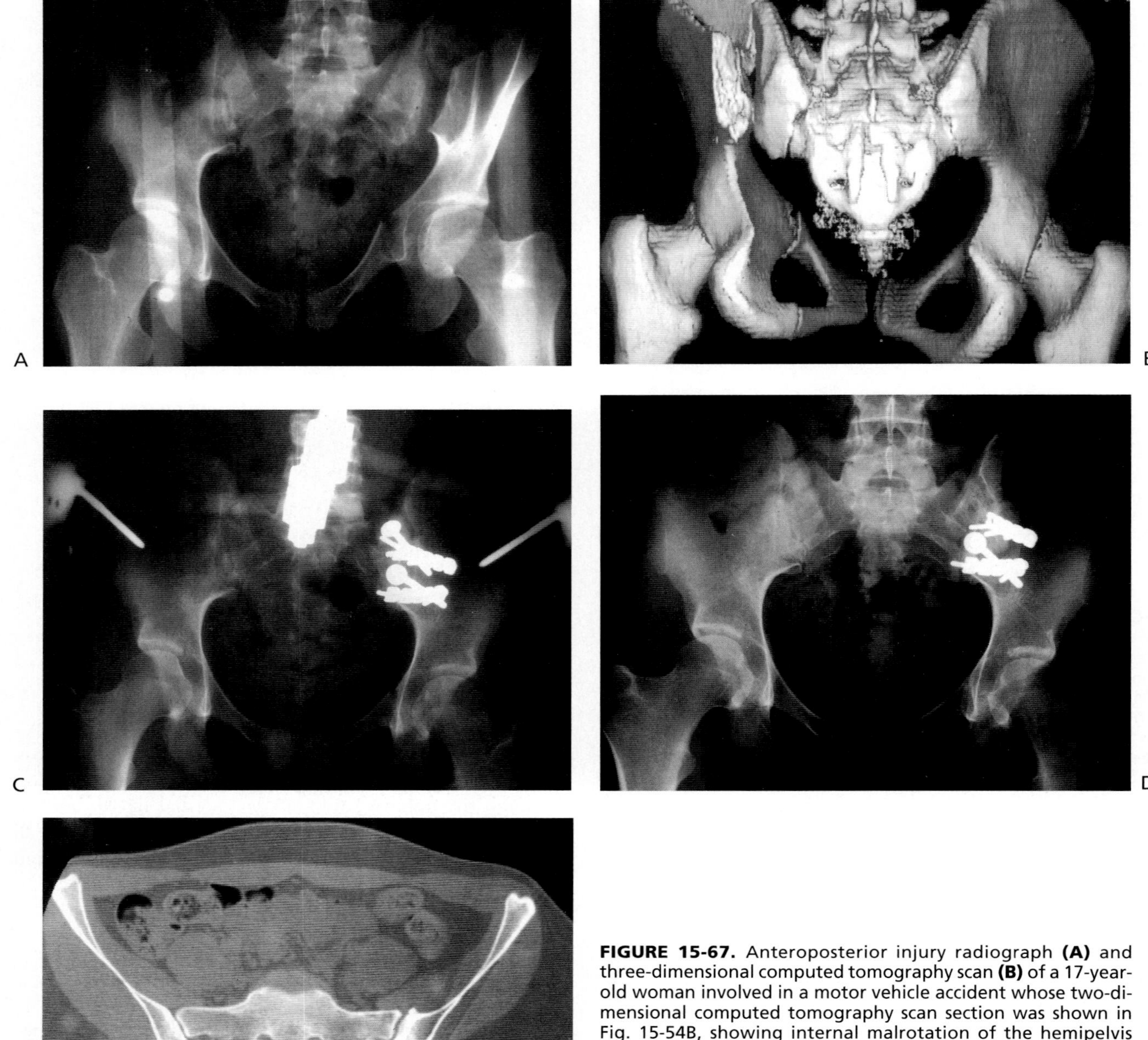

FIGURE 15-67. Anteroposterior injury radiograph **(A)** and three-dimensional computed tomography scan **(B)** of a 17-year-old woman involved in a motor vehicle accident whose two-dimensional computed tomography scan section was shown in Fig. 15-54B, showing internal malrotation of the hemipelvis with lateral and posterior translation at the fracture site. Postoperative anteroposterior radiograph **(C)** showing a two lag screw/two plate construct in combination with an anterior external fixator. Followup anteroposterior radiograph **(D)** and computed tomography section **(E)** after fracture union and return to full activities. The external fixator had been removed 6 weeks postoperatively after healing of the fractures in the anterior ring.

posterior ring injuries (30). As a general rule in these situations, the posterior ring injury is fixed first. However, if the symphysis pubis is disrupted and both innominate bones are intact (i.e., no fracture of the rami, acetabuli, or ilia), the symphysis is addressed first (31). Reduction of the symphysis usually results in improved position of the posterior injury (Fig. 15-68). Reduction of the anterior ring injury may actually result in a near complete reduction of the posterior displacement, especially within 5 days of injury (7). In this case, as described elsewhere in this text, a percutaneous rather than an open fixation technique is indicated.

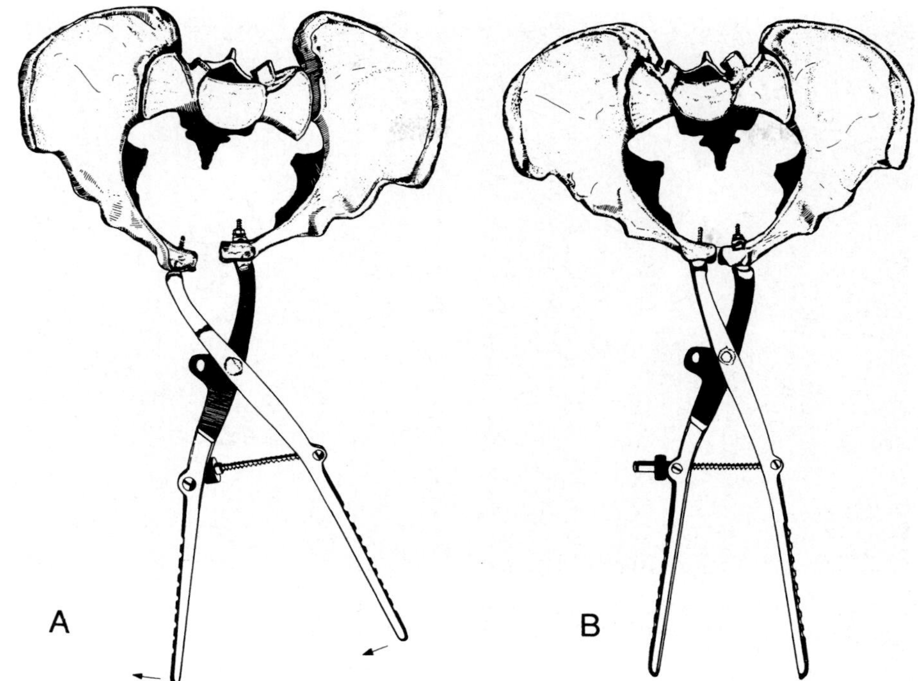

FIGURE 15-68. A: Method for using strong anterior force to reduce a pubic symphysis disruption *(arrows)*. The risk of screw pullout is avoided by placing nuts on the screw. **B:** With the innominate bone intact, reduction of the symphysis improves the position of the posterior injury. (From: Matta JM, Tornetta P III. Internal fixation of unstable pelvic ring injuries. *Clin Orthop* 1996;329: 129–140, with permission.)

Reduction and Fixation Through the Posterior Approach

Approach

The patient is placed in the prone position. A radiolucent operating room table that allows C-arm fluoroscopic visualization for anteroposterior, inlet, and outlet views of the pelvis is mandatory for the use of iliosacral screws (Fig. 15-55). The posterior approach to the sacroiliac joint is used (as previously described). Clearing of the greater sciatic notch region is extremely important. Only its posterior inferior aspect can be visualized after a disrupted sacroiliac joint has been reduced. Greater notch dissection allows direct palpation of the anterior aspect of the joint to further assess the status of the dislocation and provides access for the insertion of reduction clamps (Figs. 15-41 and 15-64).

Reduction Techniques

A reduction clamp placed across the sacroiliac joint through the greater sciatic notch is in excellent position to reduce the dislocation, because it is nearly perpendicular to the obliquity of the joint line. There is a slight propensity for the joint to gap at its most superior aspect. Care must be taken when positioning this clamp. The anterior aspect of the sacrum lateral to the foramina is cleared of soft tissue by blunt, finger dissection through the greater sciatic notch. One jaw of the clamp comes to lie in proximity to the exiting nerve roots, lateral to the foramina at the S1/S2 level (Fig. 15-64). The specific reduction instrument that can access this area is dependent on the size of the patient, and some trial and error is required. One of the most useful instruments is the small, 170-mm long, serrated bone forceps (Synthes USA, Paoli, PA). As delivered from the manufacturer, this clamp often does not open widely enough to be inserted and placed across the sacroiliac joint. However, the stop on the locking speed nut can be easily removed with pliers, allowing wider opening of the jaws of the clamp. The speed nut can be reapplied to lock the jaws in place after application of the clamp (Fig. 15-69).

A fairly standard and less demanding method for reduction of a sacroiliac joint dislocation involves the use of a pointed reduction clamp with one tine located in the ilium and the other in a sacral spinous process (Fig. 15-70). This technique frequently is successful. However, the line of reduction force is such that there may be residual anterior gapping or posterior subluxation of the joint. A combination of techniques often is the best solution (Fig. 15-71). Other reduction aids include Schanz screws inserted in the iliac crest as a manipulative tool (joystick), as well as bone screws placed in the ilium and the lateral crest, ala and pedi-

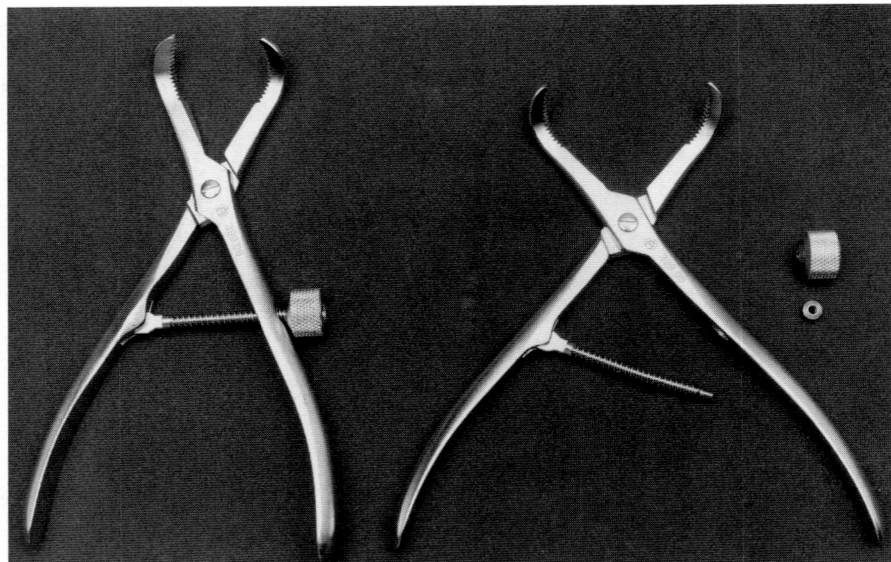

FIGURE 15-69. The small, 170-mm long, serrated bone forceps *(left).* Removal of the stop on the locking speed allows increased opening of the jaws of the clamp *(right).*

cles of the sacrum, serving as anchoring points for clamp application (Fig. 15-72).

Fixation Techniques

When treating sacroiliac dislocations through the posterior approach, it is important to realize that it is the reduction of the dislocation that requires an open approach. The fixation with iliosacral screws is similar, if not identical, to the percutaneous method. The technique for inserting iliosacral lag screws into the body of S1 has been well described (26,40,41). The best purchase is obtained by using a 6.5- or 7-mm cancellous screw with a long (32-mm) thread length placed over a washer into the S1 body rather than into the sacral ala. Intraoperative anteroposterior, 40-degree oblique fluoroscopic, and true lateral views of the pelvis are required. Preoperative radiographs should be obtained to ensure that there is nothing to obscure these views. Two points of posterior fixation are needed to provide stable fixation (57). Therefore, two fixation screws are desirable, with their starting points on either side of the midpoint of a line running from the iliac crest to the greater sciatic notch approximately 15 mm anterior to and paralleling the crista glutea and oriented at a right angle to the surface of the ilium (Fig. 15-73). These general guidelines assume an anatomic reduction in all planes, an accurate distance measurement along the external surface of the ilium, and minimal patient to patient anatomic variability. The optimal distance from the crista glutea for this starting point ("a" in Fig. 15-73) has been described as 15 and 20 mm. Use of the lateral fluoroscopic view to locate the starting point followed by insertion of the screws in a manner similar to that described for the percutaneous technique allow the surgeon to deal more effectively with these concerns (Fig. 15-74).

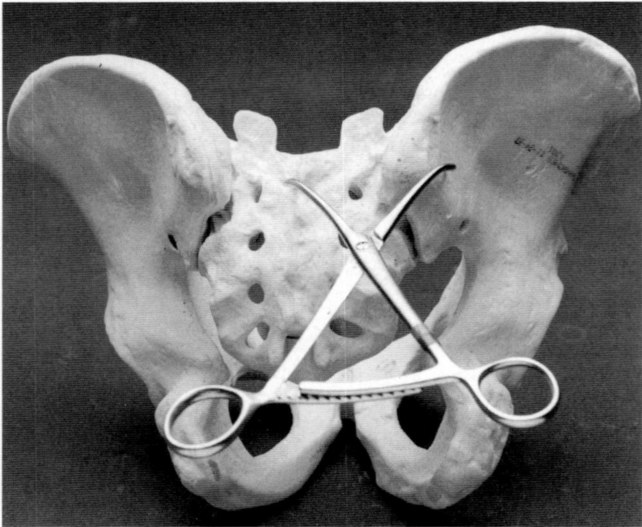

FIGURE 15-70. Application of the large reduction forceps with points spanning the sacroiliac joint from the S1 spinous process to the ilium. (From: Moed BR, Karges DE. Techniques for reduction and fixation of pelvic ring disruptions through the posterior approach. *Clin Orthop* 1996;329:102–114, with permission).

Adequate space for the insertion of two screws into the S1 body is another concern (20,38,39). Alternatives to a second screw in the S1 body include placing a second screw in the S2 body (Fig. 15-75), a transiliac plate, and a transiliac bar. The S2 body is one alternative for patients in whom adequate space is shown to be available on the preoperative CT scan. Insertion of the screws requires the inlet and outlet flu-

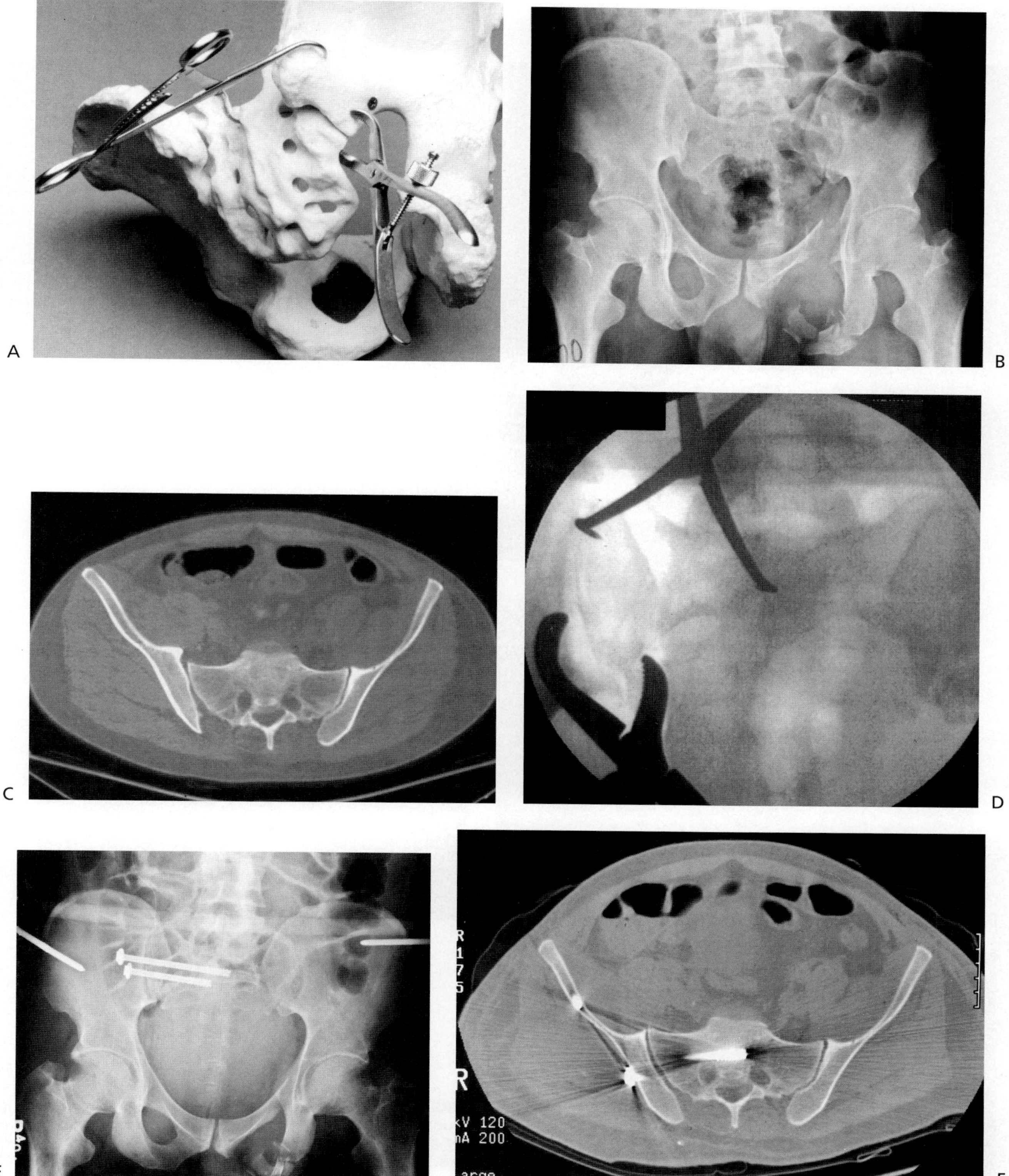

FIGURE 15-71. Illustration of the combined use of the serrated bone forceps in the greater sciatic notch and the large reduction forceps with points spanning the sacroiliac joint from the S1 spinous process to the ilium. **A:** Bone model. **B:** Anteroposterior radiograph. **C:** Computed tomography scan section through the S1 body of a clinical case of a 32-year-old man involved in a motor vehicle accident. **D:** Fluoroscopic intraoperative anteroposterior view illustrating the clamp application as shown in **(A)**. **E,F:** Postoperative radiograph and computed tomography scan section show the reduction and fixation. (From: Moed BR, Karges DE. Techniques for reduction and fixation of pelvic ring disruptions through the posterior approach. *Clin Orthop* 1996;329:102–114, with permission.)

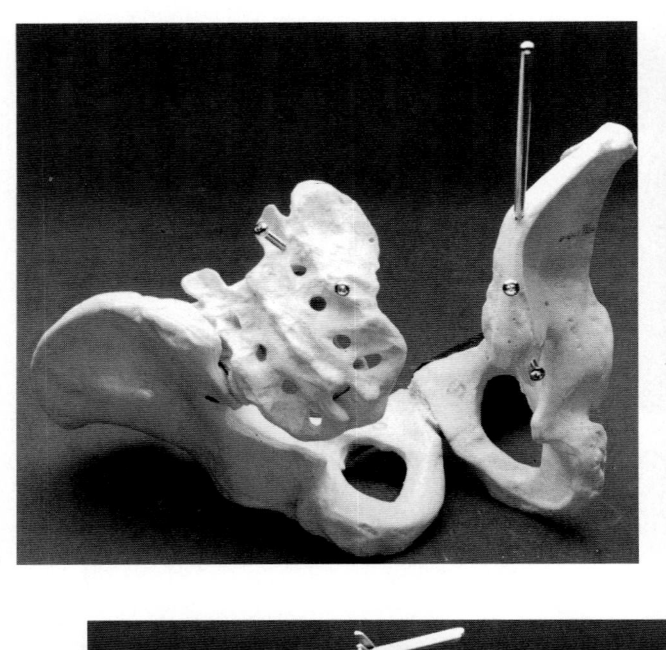
A

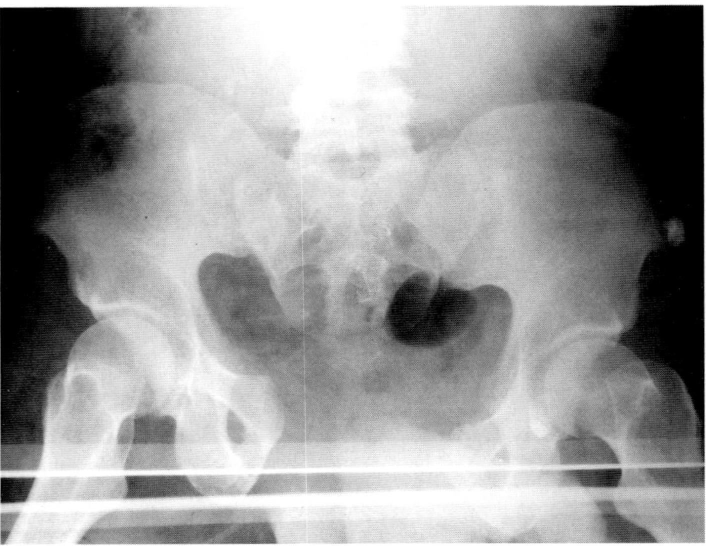
C

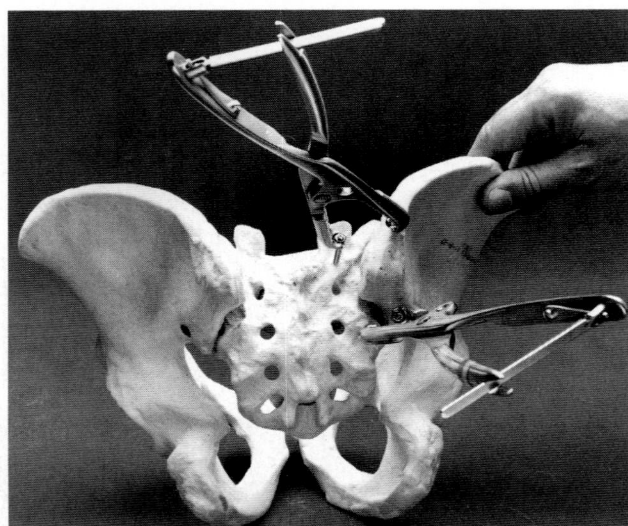
B

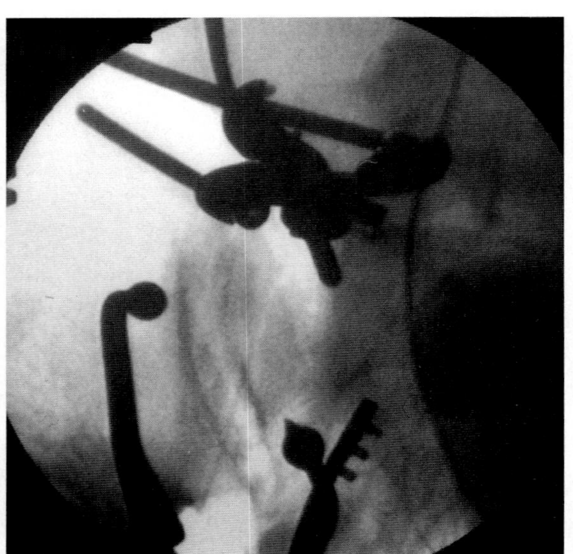
D

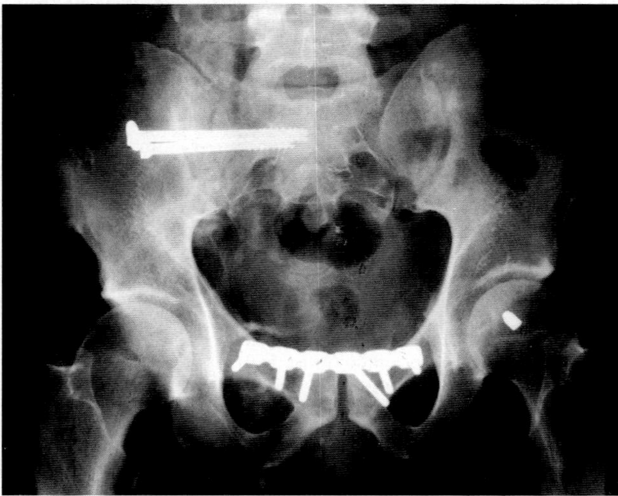
E

FIGURE 15-72. Demonstration of the use of screws to anchor reduction clamps. **A:** Bone model with screws inserted and a Schanz screw as a joy stick for reduction. **B:** Application of Farabeuf clamps. **C:** Anteroposterior radiograph of a clinical case with disruption through the right sacroiliac joint and the pubic symphysis. **D:** Intraoperative anteroposterior fluoroscopic view of the reduction using an angled oblique reduction forceps with pointed ball tips through the greater sciatic notch (Fig. 15-64C) and a Farabeuf clamp attached to screws in the ilium and S1 pedicle. **E:** Postoperative anteroposterior radiograph. (From: Moed BR, Karges DE. Techniques for reduction and fixation of pelvic ring disruptions through the posterior approach. *Clin Orthop* 1996;329:102–114, with permission.)

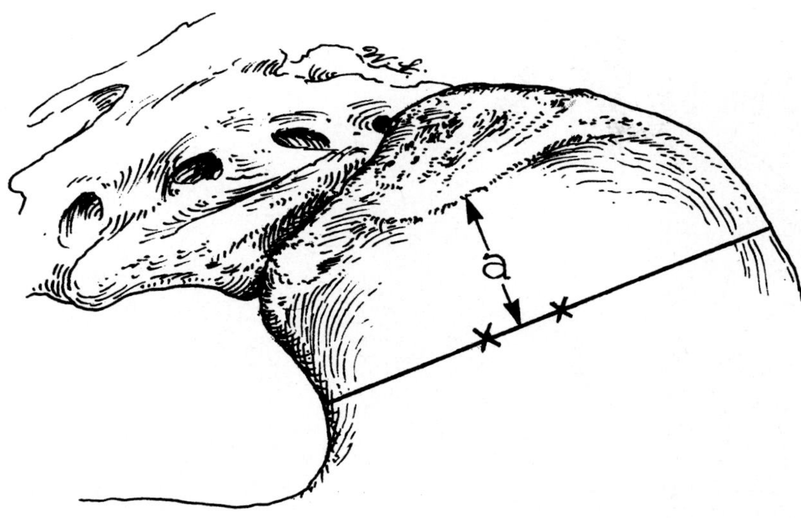

FIGURE 15-73. The line paralleling the crista glutea *(uppermost arrow tip)* running from the iliac crest to the greater sciatic notch. The optimal distance (*a*) between this line and the cristae glutea is approximately 15 mm. Insertion points for screws (x) are on either side of the midpoint of this line.

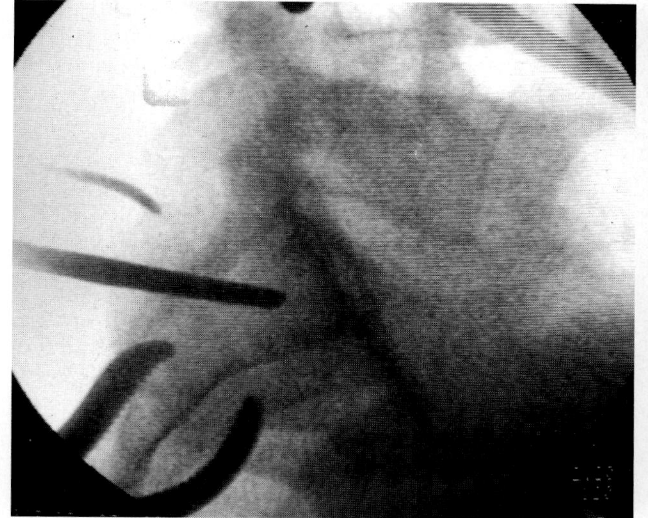

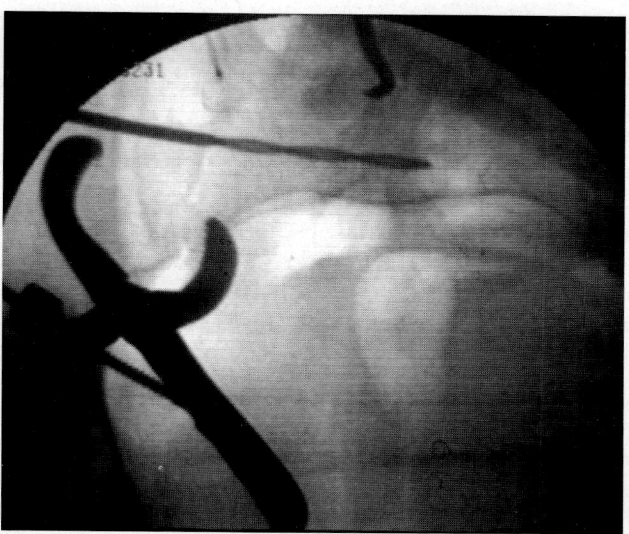

FIGURE 15-74. Intraoperative fluoroscopic views from the case shown in Fig. 15-71. **A:** The lateral fluoroscopic view after reduction. The starting point has been targeted posterior to the sacral promontory and inferior to the line of the iliac cortical density (15). **B,C,D:** Inlet, outlet, and lateral views showing drill bit insertion. The reduction clamps can be seen on all views.

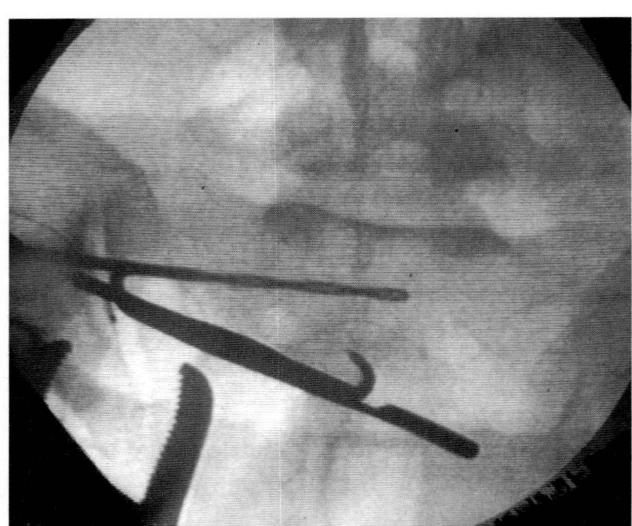
C

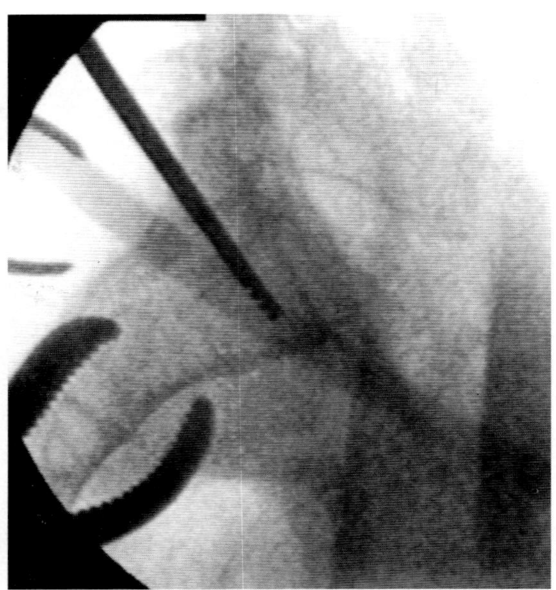
D

FIGURE 15-74. *(continued)*

oroscopic views, as in the percutaneous technique. The appropriate starting point can be located by using the lateral fluoroscopic view and the orientation for S2 screw insertion is essentially perpendicular to the sagittal and transverse planes, which facilitates the procedure (Fig. 15-76). However, insertion of the a screw into the S2 body is more demanding than for S1 (20). Although the angle for screw insertion is somewhat more straightforward, the space available (safe zone) for screw insertion leaves little margin for error (20) (Figs. 15-17 and 15-77). In addition, the bone stock for screw purchase may be deficient in S2, especially in the elderly.

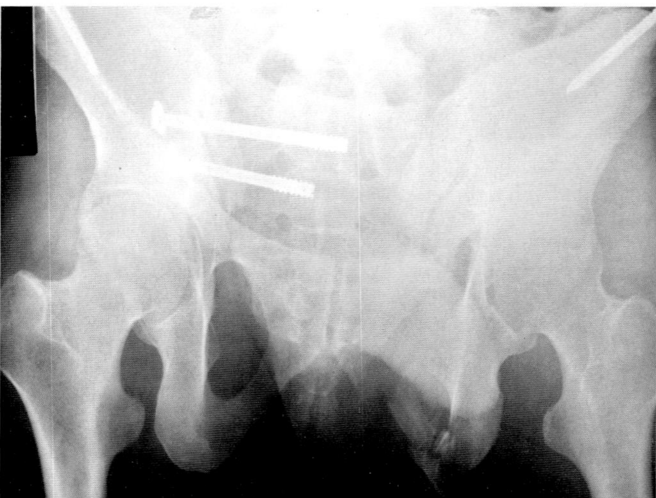

FIGURE 15-75. Postoperative outlet radiograph from the case shown in Figs. 15-71 and 15-74 illustrating the use of an S2 screw.

As opposed to the situation with fractures of the sacrum, transiliac devices are not satisfactory as stand-alone fixation for sacroiliac joint dislocations. A transiliac plate or transiliac bar in combination with an iliosacral screw are satisfactory and similar in effectiveness, although less so than two

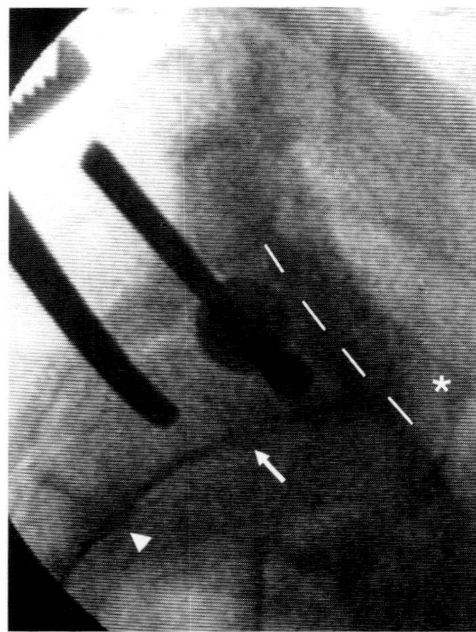

FIGURE 15-76. Intraoperative lateral fluoroscopic view from the case shown in Fig. 15-71. The starting point for an S2 screw has been targeted. A cannulated screw with guidewire previously inserted into the body of S1 is present. The sacral promontory *(asterisk)*, iliac cortical density *(dashed lines)*, S1/S2 segmentation line *(arrow)*, and S2/S3 segmentation line *(arrowhead)* are shown.

A

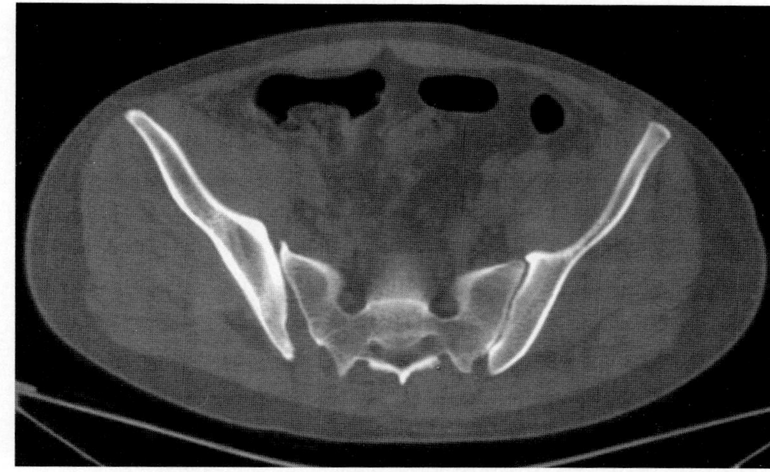

B

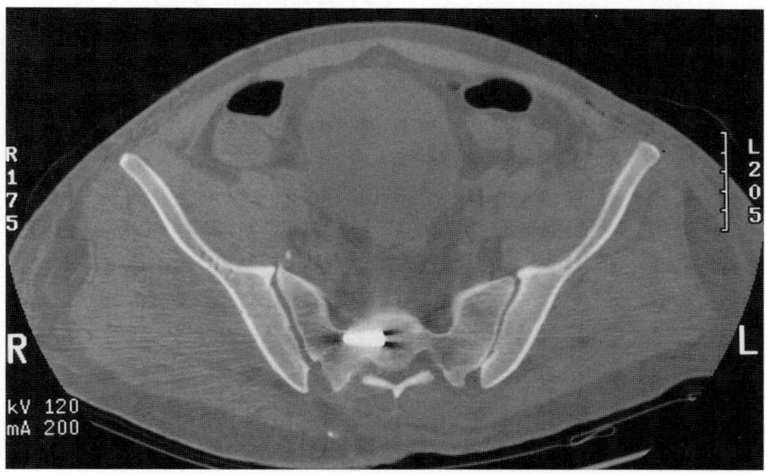

FIGURE 15-77. A,B: Preoperative and postoperative computed tomography scan sections through the body of S2 from the case shown in Fig. 15-71 showing the narrow window available for safe screw insertion.

S1 screws (57). Both have the disadvantage of requiring a second incision over the contralateral posterior ilium (Fig. 15-78). This additional dissection is much greater for plate insertion. The least invasive, and perhaps safest, second point of posterior fixation can be provided by a cannulated, self-locking transiliac screw (Fig.15-79). At the completion of fixation, the final reduction and hardware position should be confirmed by anteroposterior, inlet, and outlet radiographic imaging.

Reduction and Fixation Through the Anterior Approach

Approach

The anterior approach to the sacroiliac joint is similar to that described in the preceding for extraarticular iliac fractures and can be addressed using the superior portion of the iliofemoral incision (55). The patient is in the supine position on a radiolucent operating room table with the leg draped free. If iliosacral screws are to be considered as a possible part of the fixation construct, a soft support should be placed under the lumbosacral spine to slightly elevate the pelvis from the table. A bump is placed under the knee as a compromise position to relax both the femoral nerve and the L5 nerve root. It may not be necessary to release the sartorius muscle and inguinal ligament origin from the anterior superior spine. However, release of these structures will increase the exposure. Again, intraoperative fluoroscopic imaging is important in these cases.

Because the dissection is carried posteriorly along the internal iliac fossa with a periosteal elevator, the sacral side of the sacroiliac joint is usually encountered owing to its anterior position relative to the ilium. Dissection over the sacral ala should be cautious, because the L5 nerve root lies approximately 2 to 3 cm from the joint line (Figs. 15-15C and 15-40).

Reduction Techniques

Because the majority of the displacement is posterior and superior, one very simple, but effective, technique consists of flexing the hip and applying manual in-line traction to the leg. A bone clamp is used to grip the iliac wing and manip-

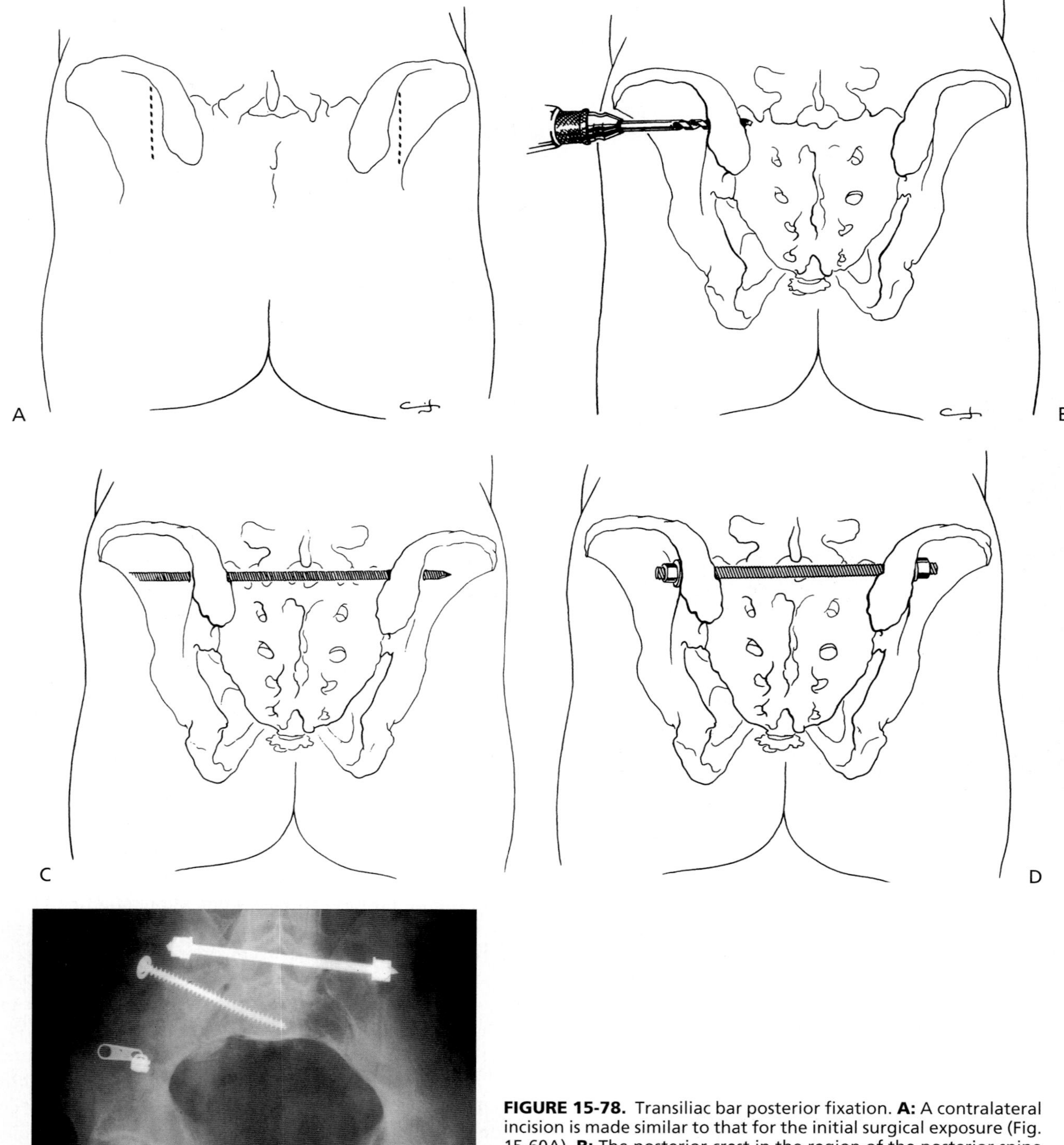

FIGURE 15-78. Transiliac bar posterior fixation. **A:** A contralateral incision is made similar to that for the initial surgical exposure (Fig. 15-60A). **B:** The posterior crest in the region of the posterior spine is predrilled with a 6.4-mm (0.25-inch) drill bit to provide a gliding hole. **C:** The sacral bar is then inserted posterior to the sacrum and the sharp trocar point driven through the opposite ilium. Blunt elevation of the erector spinae and multifidus muscles and palpation of the posterior sacrum may be necessary to ensure that the bar does not compromise the sacral canal. **D:** Washers and nuts are applied with the nuts tightened to compress the sacroiliac joint. The bar is cut to size using a bolt cutter. **E:** Inlet radiographic view of a clinical case showing a sacral bar in proper position used as a second point of posterior fixation.

ulate the wing into position. Once reduced, the sacroiliac joint is temporarily held in position by driving a wide step staple across the superior aspect of the joint (Fig. 15-80) (58–59). The iliac wing should be predrilled to seat the staple. Otherwise, the staple will displace the iliac wing posteriorly when it is impacted into place. If done within 14 days of injury, this method has been reported to be successful in 85% to 95% of cases (58). The provisional staple is removed after plate application but prior to applying compression through the plate.

Reduction techniques are noted in Fig. 15-81A–F. One reduction option is to use bone-holding forceps, such as a Farabeuf, Lane, or pointed reduction-type clamp, placed on the anterior pelvis between the anterior inferior and superior

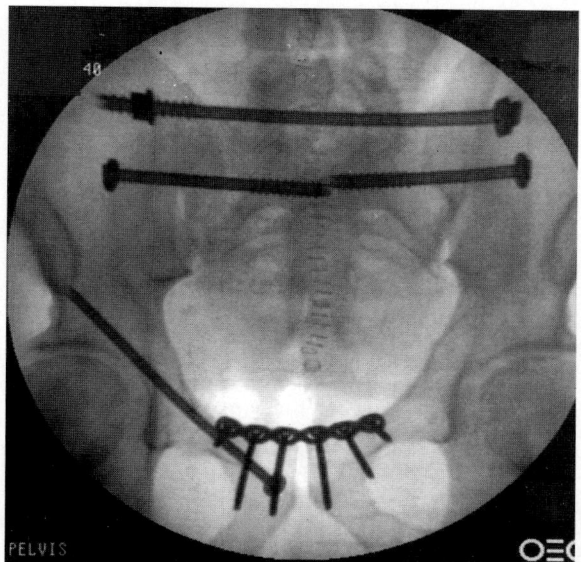

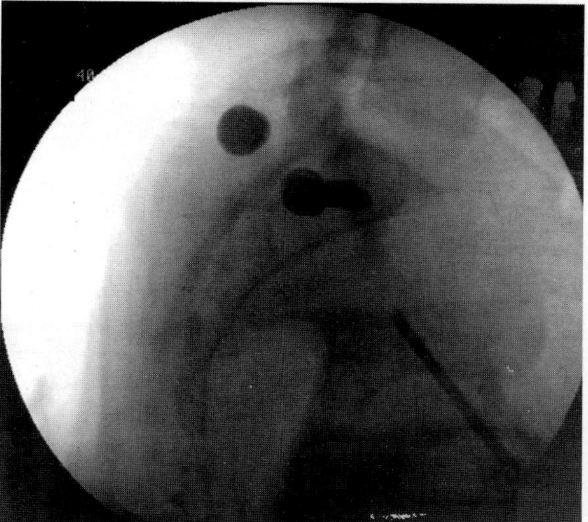

FIGURE 15-79. Clinical example of a cannulated, self-locking transiliac screw (patent pending) as the second point of fixation in a 29-year-old man with bilateral posterior injury. Anteroposterior *(top)* and lateral *(bottom)* fluoroscopic views obtained at the completion of the surgical procedure.

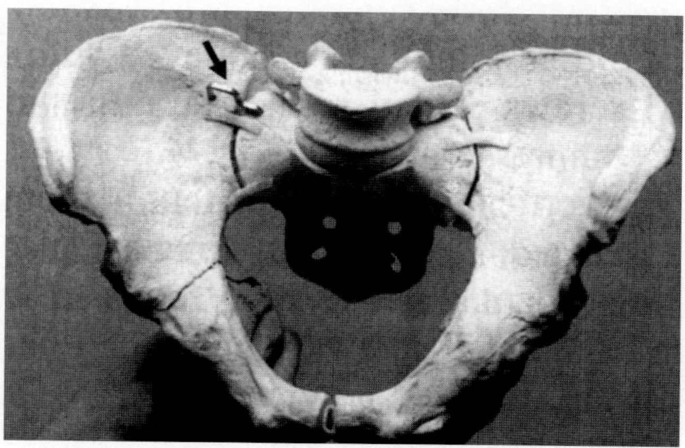

FIGURE 15-80. Bone model showing the use of a wide step staple *(arrow)* for provisional joint stabilization. This type of staple allows easy removal following definitive fixation. (Modified from Leighton RK, Waddell JP. Techniques for reduction and posterior fixation through the anterior approach. *Clin Orthop* 1996;329: 115–120, with permission.)

spine (Fig. 15-81A). The pelvis may be lifted forward and rotated to obtain the appropriate reduction with this and a Schanz screw in the iliac wing about the level of the iliac wing tubercle (Fig. 15-81B). The maneuver is necessary to lift the hemipelvis upward, correct posterior displacement, and obtain the correct amount of rotation. Once the fracture-dislocation is reduced, insertion of a pointed reduction clamp (Fig. 15-81C) may hold the dislocation. Insertion of one screw on either side of the sacroiliac joint (Fig. 15-81D) also helps achieve and hold the reduction by the use of the Farabeuf clamp (Fig. 15-81E), or the pelvic reduction clamp (Fig. 15-81F). A cerclage wire around the screws is another alternative. The reduction should be confirmed by C-arm fluoroscopy, as it is not uncommon for the well-visualized superior sacroiliac joint to be reduced leaving a residual gap in its inferior aspect, which is not in the surgical field. Additional provisional fixation may be obtained by percutaneous insertion of a 3.2-mm Kirschner wire (or guide pin for a cannulated screw), which is inserted into the iliac side of the sacroiliac joint under direct vision prior to joint reduction (Fig. 15-82). After the dislocation is reduced, the wire is advanced into the ala. This allows accurate placement of the wire. Alternatively, C-arm fluoroscopy can be used to place the Kirschner wire after joint reduction. In either case, position of the wire in the ala must be confirmed by fluoroscopy.

Fixation Techniques

There are two possible methods of fixation or combinations thereof once joint reduction is achieved: anterior sacroiliac joint plating and percutaneous posterior sacroiliac joint fixation with cannulated screws.

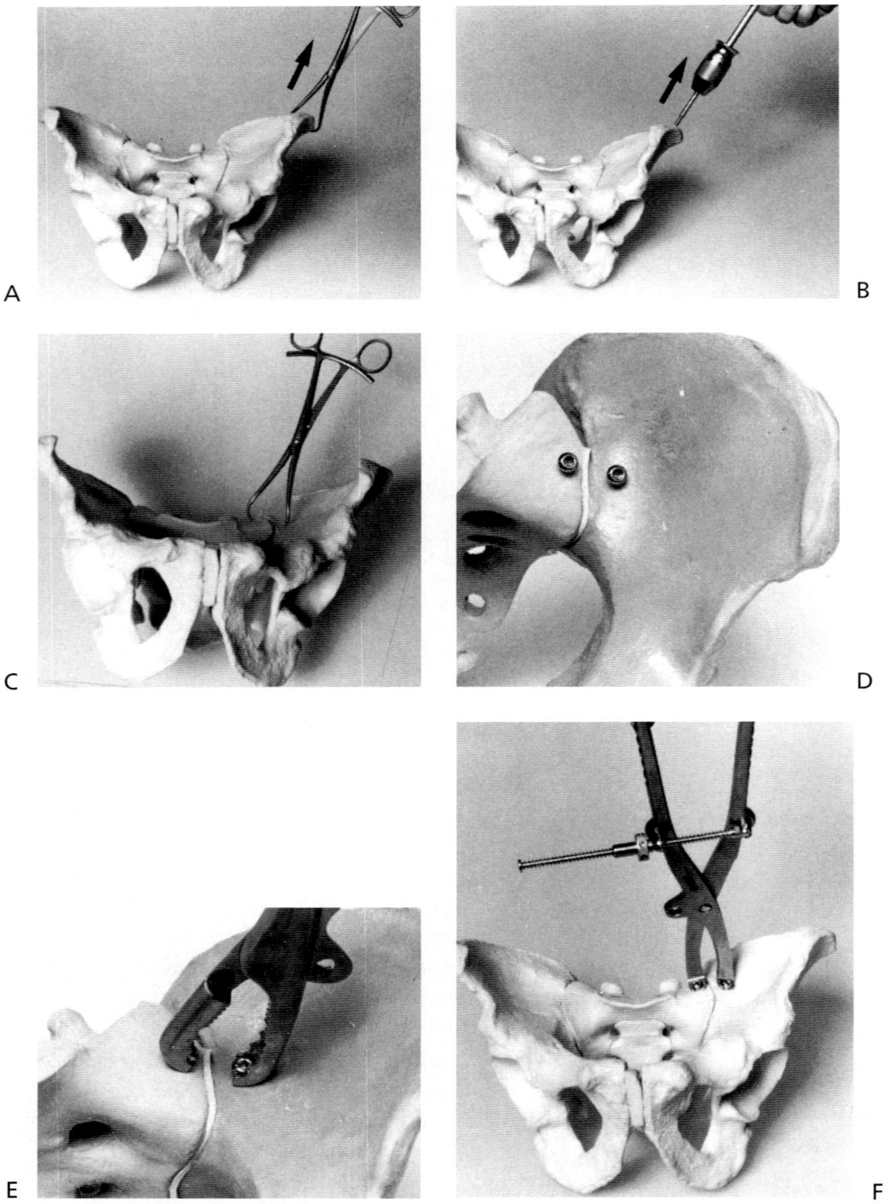

FIGURE 15-81. A–F: Reduction techniques for sacroiliac joint dislocation, anterior approach. To reduce the unstable hemipelvis, and with the patient in the supine position, various methods may be used, including insertion of a pointed reduction clamp into the iliac crest **(A).** Other types of clamps may be used in this area, or a Schanz screw on a "T" handle **(B).** Once the reduction has been obtained, it may be held with a pointed reduction clamp **(C).** Another method involves inserting a screw on either side of the sacroiliac joint **(D).** These screws may be held using a Farabeuf clamp **(E)** or a pelvic reduction clamp **(F).**

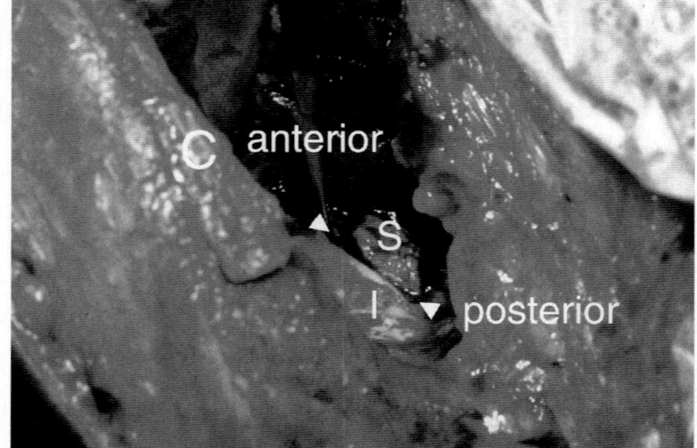

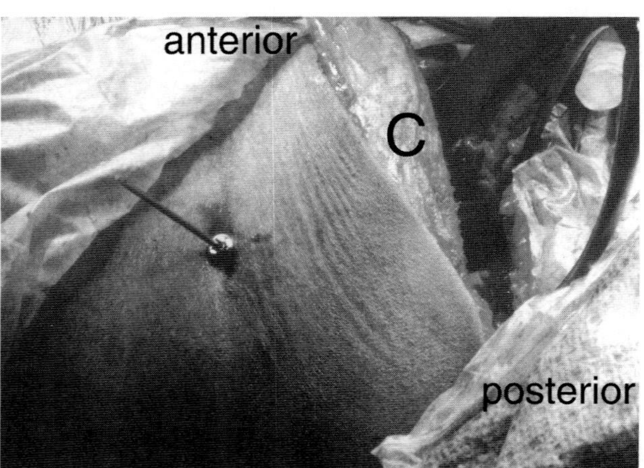

FIGURE 15-82. Clinical example of percutaneous insertion of an iliosacral screw after open reduction of the sacroiliac joint through the anterior approach. **A:** View of the sacroiliac joint *(between the arrowheads)* after reduction and temporary K-wire stabilization. The iliac crest **(C),** Sacral ala (s), and iliac side of the joint (i) are shown. **B:** The screw is being inserted over the K-wire.

Two anterior DC or pelvic reconstruction plates constitute the usual fixation construct for the anterior plating of pure sacroiliac dislocations (Fig. 15-40C). These plates usually have two or three holes, one on the sacral side and one or two on the iliac wing side. The operator must be mindful that the iliac wing rapidly thins out as one progresses laterally from the sacroiliac joint. The best bone lies within the first 3 cm lateral to the sacroiliac joint. This is the cancellous bone that extends posteriorly as the posterior superior iliac spine. Consequently, plates that extend farther laterally onto the iliac wing tend to gain no more purchase because of the thin iliac wing. At least two plates are necessary to control the rotation. These should be placed under compression through the dynamic compression holes. The plates used are either 3.5- or 4.5-mm plates, or a combination thereof, depending on the size of the patient. They are fixed to the pelvis by appropriate-sized, fully threaded 6.5-mm cancellous or 4.5- and 3.5-mm cortical bone screws, usually 50 to 75 mm in length in the sacrum (Fig. 15-83). Such plates are placed onto the iliac wing at a diverging angle with its apex on the sacral side of the joint.

The initial fixation plate may help with reduction by using a flat plate, which is overbent relative to the slightly concave contour of the sacroiliac joint at this location. The idea is that the joint is then reduced to the plate, compressing the directly underlying superior aspect without gapping the in-

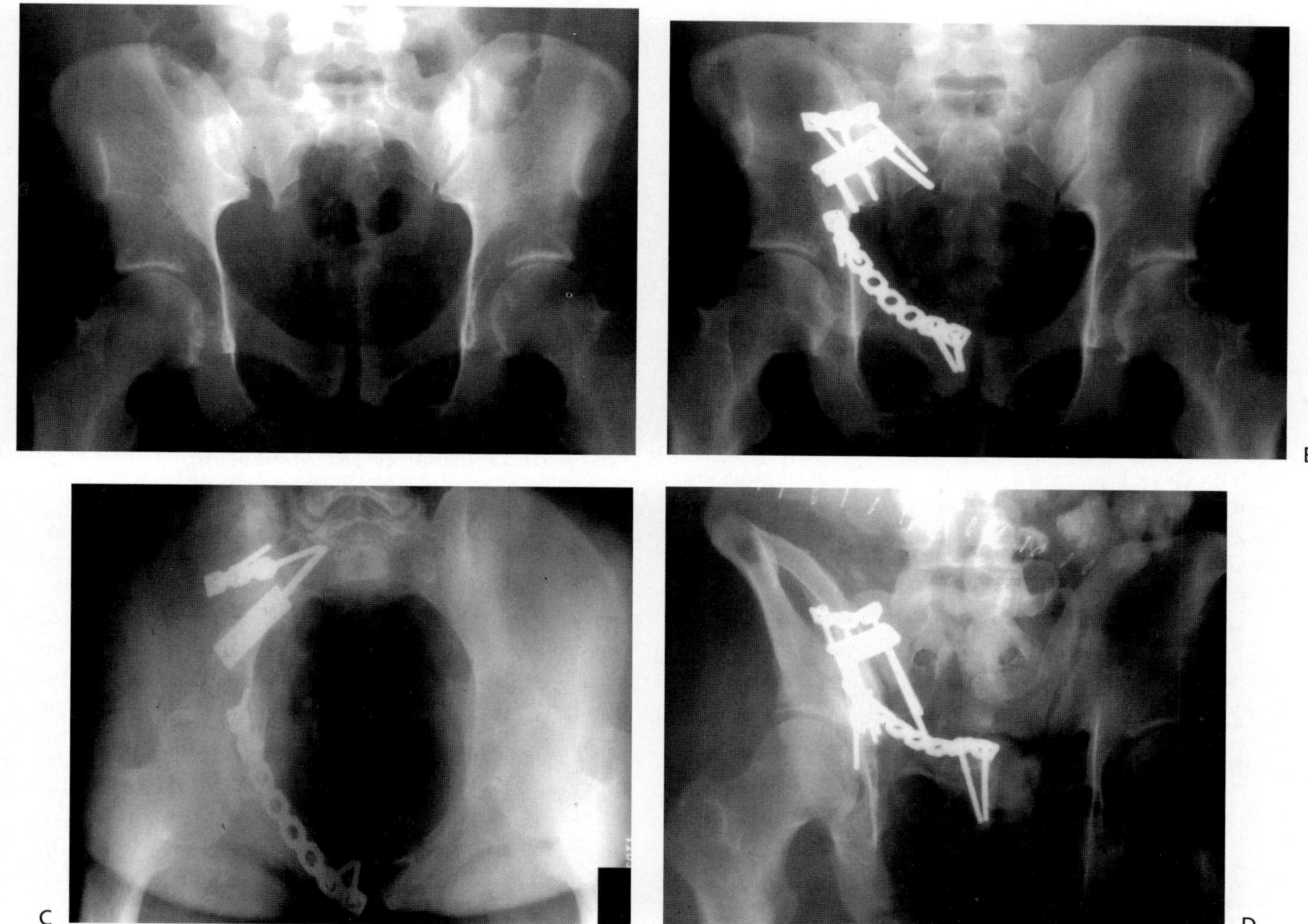

FIGURE 15-83. Anteroposterior radiograph **(A)** of a 28-year-old man with a right sacroiliac joint disruption in combination with rami fractures. Postoperative anteroposterior **(B)**, inlet **(C)**, and outlet **(D)** radiographs showing the fixation construct. An ilioinguinal surgical approach was used.

ferior aspect of the joint (Fig. 15-84). This technique is similar in theory to slightly overbending a compression plate applied to a long bone fracture so that the near cortex compression does not result in gapping on the far cortex. Unfortunately, this technique is not as successful when applied to pelvic ring injuries. Often, rather than achieving the desired result, the region directly underlying the plate is compressed; the ilium is translated; and a gap remains inferiorly (Fig. 15-85). Two alternative plating methods have been describe to avoid this problem.

A special four-hole plate designed specifically for sacroiliac joint dislocations is touted as preventing gapping without causing translation by providing additional compression capability (58,59). Excellent results have been reported (58). Alternatively, one of the two usually applied plates can be extended to the crest by increasing its length to five or more holes, as needed (Fig. 15-86). With this lengthened plate, the overbending technique, as described in the preceding, appears to function as intended (60).

Once the fracture has been reduced via the anterior approach, fixation can also be provided by inserting percutaneous iliosacral screws, either alone or in combination with an anterior plate. Two anterior plates combined with an iliosacral screw has been shown to be one of the most stable fixation constructs (57). The 3.2-mm wire, percutaneously inserted as additional provisional fixation (as described in the previous section), can serve as the guide for a cannulated iliosacral screw. Alternatively, the standard percutaneous iliosacral screw insertion method with the patient supine (as previously discussed) can be used (40).

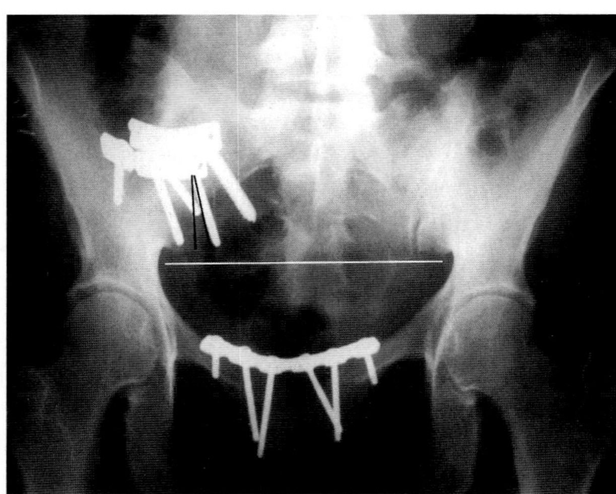

FIGURE 15-85. Clinical example of incomplete reduction *(white line as reference)* and inferior gapping *(black lines show either side of the sacroiliac joint)* after open reduction and internal plate fixation via the anterior approach.

Special Considerations

Crescent fracture type sacroiliac fracture/dislocations that for reasons other than fracture location (see Figs. 15-62 and 15-63) may be best treated through an anterior surgical approach merit additional mention. The surgical approach usually requires dissection to the sacral ala. Reduction may require any number of maneuvers. However, use of the ball spike and Farabeuf (Fig. 15-57A) in combination with a clamp across the sacroiliac joint (Fig. 15-81) is often successful. If screws are placed as anchor points (Fig. 15-81D-F), care must be taken to ensure that the iliac screw does not cross the fracture site. Fixation is dependent upon the size of the crescent fracture remnant attached to the posterior ligaments and the patient's bone quality. Intertable lag screws alone may be successful (Fig. 15-62). When supplemental buttress fixation is deemed necessary, this can be accomplished by applying an anterior plate across the sacroiliac joint (Fig. 15-63).

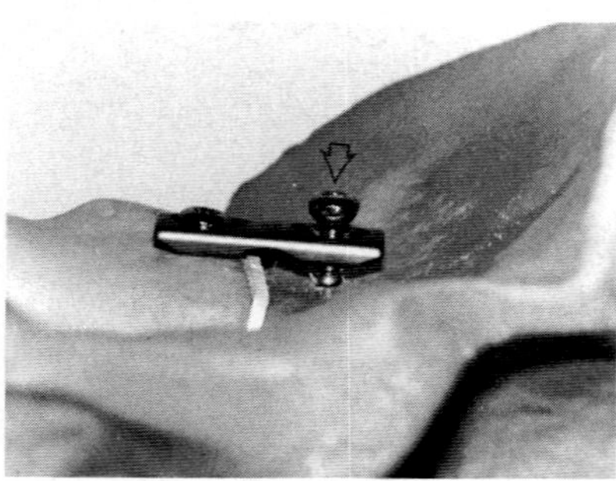

FIGURE 15-84. Bone model showing the use of a flat plate to aid the reduction of the ilium. In theory, when the screw is tightened *(arrow)*, the ilium will be brought in toward the plate.

Other Techniques of Posterior Sacroiliac or Sacral Fixation

Transiliac Bars

Posterior fixation can be safely and effectively accomplished by using transiliac bars or rods. The bars are placed posterior to the sacrum, to avoid having to penetrate the sacrum directly (Fig. 15-87). The bars must be inserted proximally, to avoid entering the sacral canal and damaging the cauda equina. The bars are placed between the two intact posterior tubercles of the iliac wing. This technique is most useful for unilateral unstable sacral fractures, but if combined with a posterior screw into the ala it may be useful for sacroiliac dislocations or bilateral disruptions (Figs. 15-78E and 15-79). On the side of the injury, the exposure is the same as for iliosacral screws (Fig. 15-78). On the opposite side, a smaller exposure is made just lateral to the posterior tubercle, to expose the lateral aspect of the iliac wing anterior to the posterior spine. The fracture is then reduced. Drill holes are placed through the posterior tubercles just dorsal to the sacral lamina. Care must be taken not to go through the sacral lamina into the roots

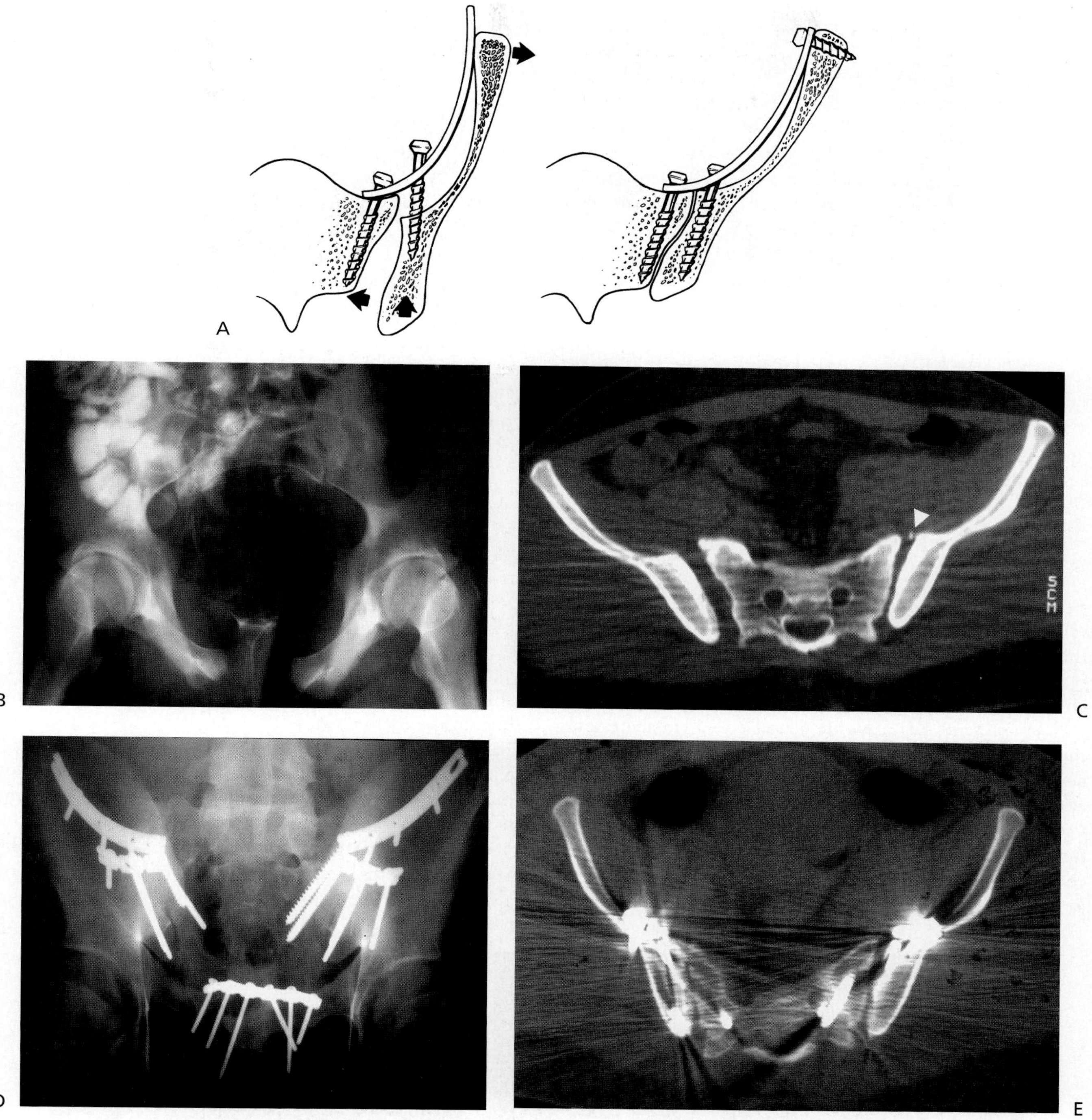

FIGURE 15-86. Method using a longer "overbent" plate. Illustration of the technique **(A)** (courtesy of Fred Behrens, MD). Clinical example showing the injury radiograph **(B)** and computed tomography scan section **(C).** Gross disruption of the right sacroiliac joint and pubic symphysis were evident. An occult injury to the left sacroiliac joint, suggested on the computed tomography scan **(C)** *(arrowhead),* was found on physical examination. Postoperative outlet radiograph **(D)** and computed tomography scan section through the inferior aspect of the sacroiliac joints **(E)** show the reduction and fixation.

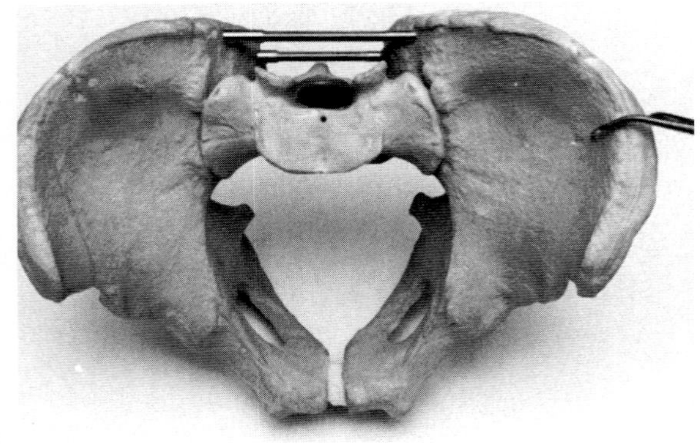

A

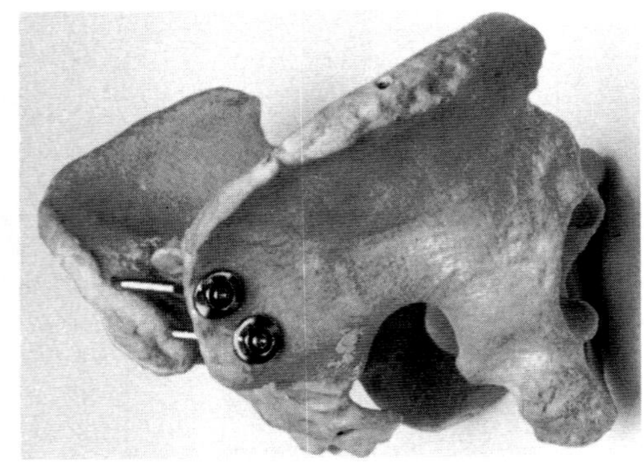

C

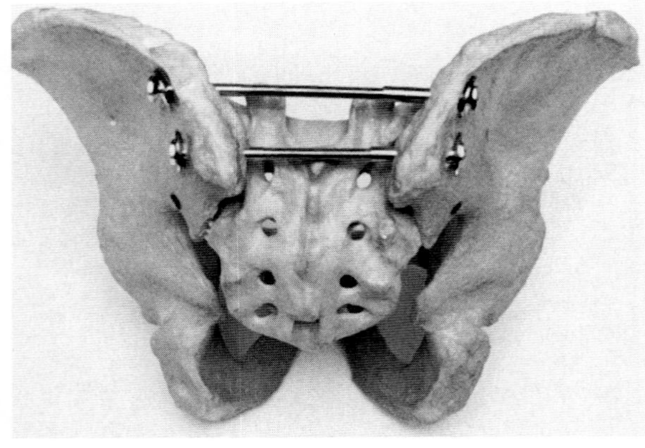

B

FIGURE 15-87. Transiliac bars. Note the placement of the rods posterior to the sacrum, obviating the need to penetrate the sacrum directly, as seen on the inlet view **(A)** and the posterior aspect of the pelvis **(B).** The bars must be inserted proximally to avoid entering the sacral canal and damaging the cauda equina, taking into account the normal lumbar lordosis **(C).**

and to avoid entering into fractures of the sacral lamina, if such are present. Two rods are placed 2 to 4 cm apart, and then nuts with washers are added to compress the system and improve stability. The advantage of this system is that the fixation is posterior to the sacrum and lessens the potential for problems with nerve roots; however, nerve injury may occur if a rod enters the spinal canal, or, more commonly, if the nerve root is compressed in the foramen as the rods are tightened. Nerve monitoring may be valuable in this technique. The first rod should be placed proximal to the S1 foramen at the level of the L5-S1 disc space and the second one just distal to that foramen. At least 2 cm of bone should be between the two rods. Again, care must be taken when tightening not to overcompress the sacrum if there is a foramen fracture.

Correct placement of the bars may be seen in Fig. 15-88. Specialized cannulated transiliac bars (Fig. 15-87) now are available. The technique is similar, but the rods are con-

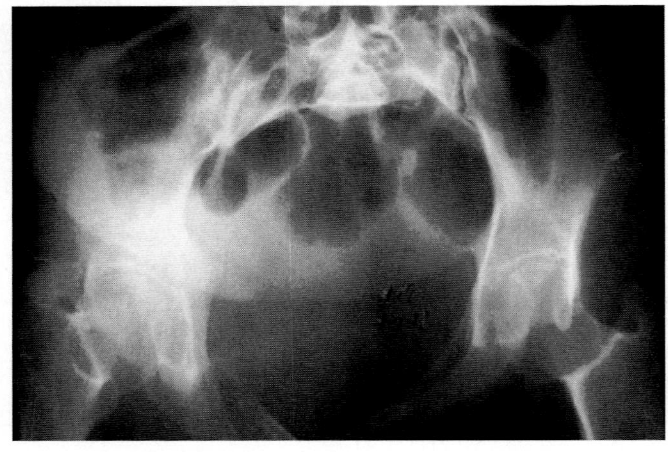

A

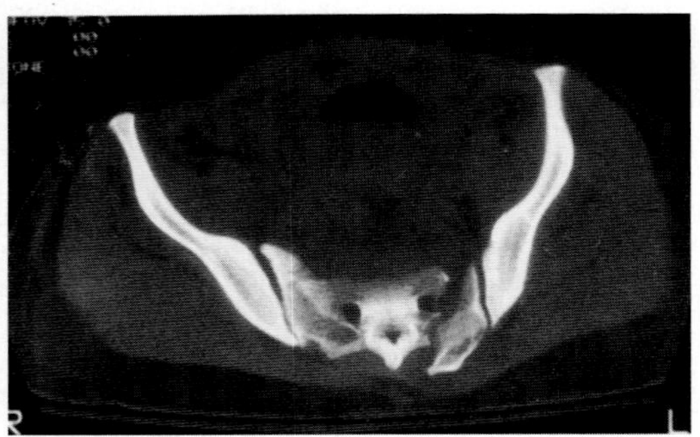

B

FIGURE 15-88. Anteroposterior radiograph **(A)** and computed tomography **(B)** of a polytraumatized 25-year-old woman with an unstable left hemipelvis owing to a sacral fracture and an open-book type injury on the right hemipelvis. *(continued)*

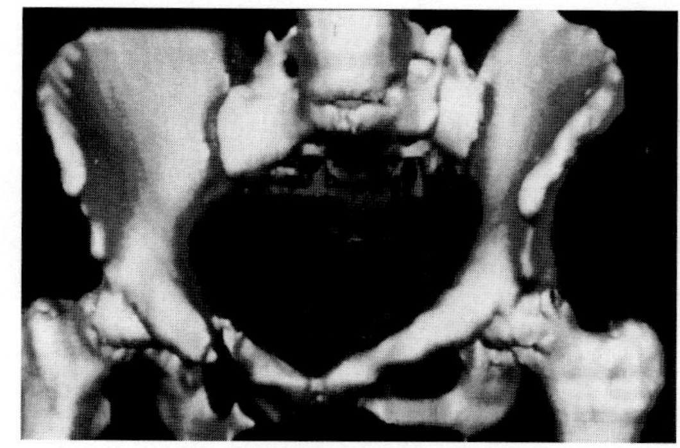

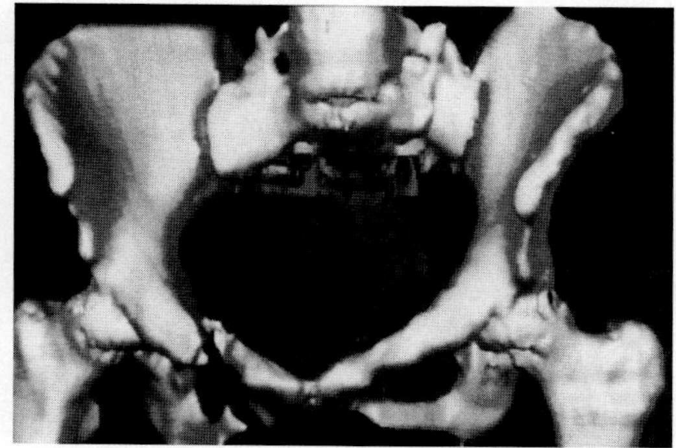

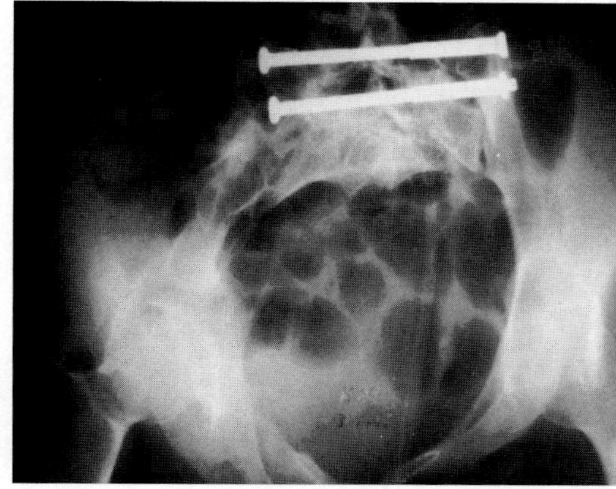

FIGURE 15-88. (Continued). **C,D:** The three-dimensional computed tomography further show the lesion. **E:** Treatment with two cannulated transiliac bars led to sound healing of the sacral fracture and a good clinical outcome.

nected medial to the superior iliac spine and locked with a spinal locking nut (Fig. 15-79). Cannulated cancellous screws may be used as transiliac bars because they can be inserted over a guidewire (Fig. 15-79).

For bilateral unstable fractures this technique should be combined with screw fixation in the body of the sacrum. In that situation, the bars act as a neutralizing force to restore the posterior tension band of the pelvis (Figs. 15-79 and 15-89).

Plating Techniques

Other techniques of posterior fixation include the use of 4.5- or 3.5-mm plates, which can be contoured to go across the posterior aspect of the sacrum and down the iliac wing (Fig. 15-90). Mears and associates described the use of a double cobra plate, but we feel this implant is too massive to be used for acute trauma (61). A 4.5-mm plate, con-

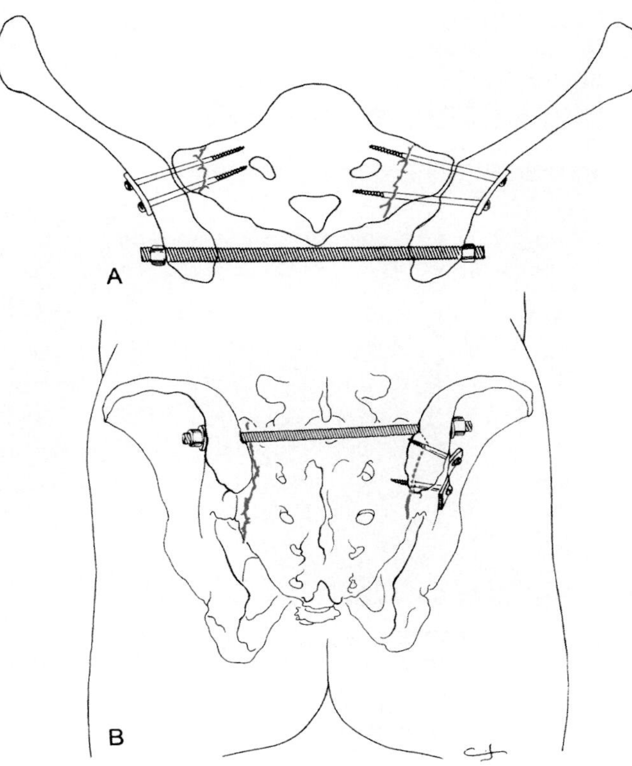

FIGURE 15-89. Bilateral posterior fixation. If the posterior lesion is bilateral and internal fixation is desirable, then the fixation must be secured into the sacrum, the only remaining portion of the pelvic ring remaining attached to the axial skeleton. **A:** In the cross-sectional view, the bilateral sacral fracture has been fixed with two plates used as a washer for lag screw fixation into the sacrum. The posterior tension band is completely stabilized with one or two sacral bars. **B:** The anatomic view is depicted, a case of a dislocation on the right side and a fractured sacrum on the left. Fixation devices similar to those in **(A)** are used.

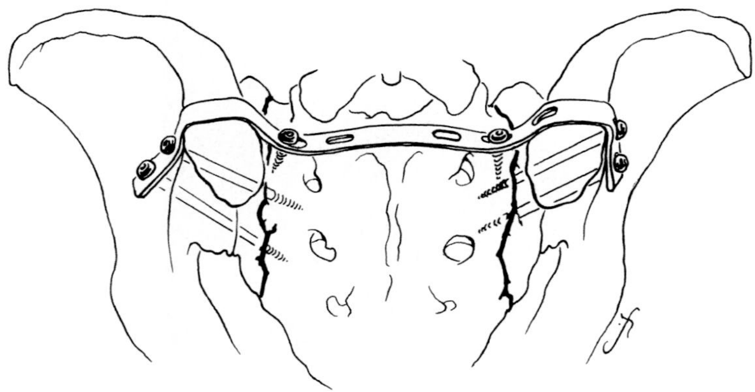

FIGURE 15-90. An alternative method is posterior fixation with a long, prebent plate with fixation across the bilateral fractures into the main body of the sacrum.

toured to go across the back of the sacrum and down the iliac wings, passing through an osteotomy and creating a tunnel in both posterior spines and underneath the posterior midline musculature, is preferable (Fig. 15-91). This is done through two vertical incisions. A transverse incision should not be undertaken in this region in the acute case, but it could be useful in reconstruction of a nonunion.

Another technique for the use of plate fixation is to run the plate below the posterior superior spine, across the region of the S3 foramen of the sacrum, and fix it to both il-

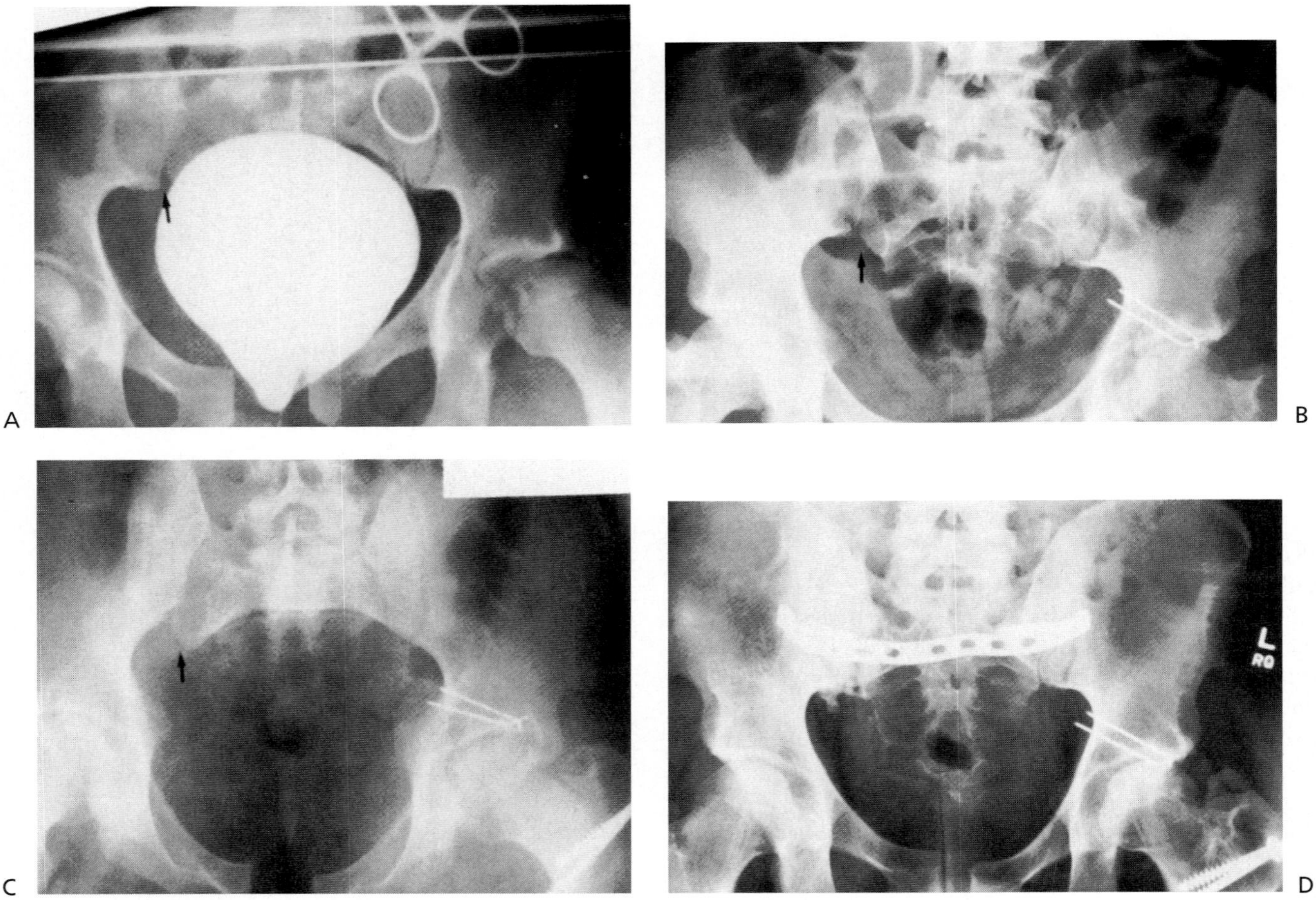

FIGURE 15-91. A: Cystogram **(A)** of the pelvis demonstrates a bilateral posterior lesion, as with symphysis disruption. The left hip has an acetabular fracture and is dislocated posteriorly. The hip required reduction to remove the small bone fragments that blocked reduction. Following open reduction, the anteroposterior radiograph **(B),** and especially the inlet view **(C),** demonstrate marked posterior displacement of the sacroiliac joint. Stable fixation of the pelvic ring was achieved with a long plate across both sacroiliac joints **(D).**

iac wings. This is almost like a U plate, which acts as a tension band plate. It is only useful for a unilateral fracture unless, in a bilateral injury, one side has been fixed to the sacral body.

Pohlemann and coworkers (see Chapter 16) have described direct open reduction of sacral fractures with plate fixation of the posterior sacrum (33,50). Small fragment plates are used between the posterior neural foramina to stabilize the sacrum directly. This new technique has yet to be evaluated. Other techniques include tension band wires, either directly from the posterior spine to posterior spine or around screws inserted into these posterior spines. Ebraheim and coworkers described fixation of the posterior sacroiliac complex under CT monitoring (62).

Intraoperative Complications

The intraoperative complications from this approach usually stem from hemorrhage owing to disruption of the superior gluteal artery. Other complications, usually noted later postoperatively, are discussed elsewhere.

Closure

Closure of the posterior wound requires that great care be taken with assessment and handling of the soft tissues. In addition, postoperative suction drains may be considered-.

Postoperative Care

Postoperative care is like that used with the anterior approach. If stability has been restored to the unstable injury by internal and/or external fixation, the patient may be mobilized from bed to chair within 3 to 5 days, but each case must be judged individually, depending on stability and bone quality. With unilateral unstable disruption, as the patient's comfort improves, consideration could be given to crutches on the uninvolved side. In bilateral unstable fractures (bilateral Type C2 or C3), patients may be mobilized from bed to chair if stability is good, but ambulation must be delayed until signs of healing are observed.

CONCLUSION

At this particular time, conventional wisdom states that open reduction and internal fixation of pelvic ring disruption has come of age. Careful patient selection is imperative, and the surgery must only be done by experienced surgeons who can operate *safely* in an appropriate environment, with staff capable of looking after these patients. This environment must include excellent critical care facilities as well as an expert operative team and the resources to provide neurophysiologic monitoring.

The rationale is clear: Internal fixation allows the surgeon to obtain and maintain a satisfactory reduction and obtain better pelvic stability. As well, percutaneous methods using image guidance have reduced the risks of wound problems and visceral complications, and allowed earlier ambulation and reduced hospital stays. However, there are still many risks; therefore, the surgery should only be done when the benefits clearly outweigh the risks by a well-trained surgical team.

Early *anterior fixation* of the symphysis much simplifies management of symphysis disruption. This is true for virtually all types of disruption: the open-book fracture, the locked symphysis in the lateral compression injury, and especially the unstable pelvic ring.

The role of ramus fixation is less clear because of the more difficult surgical approach; however, internal fixation may be beneficial in grossly unstable rami fractures. Plating using the extraperitoneal approach (Stoppa) and percutaneous techniques may be used. Both improve the stability of the pelvis more than external fixation. The majority of rami fractures do not require fixation internally because they have inherent stability. External fixation is a better option in those circumstances.

The roles and methods of *posterior fixation* are still controversial, but less so than when the last edition of this book was published. With few exceptions, posterior fixation should be limited to unstable (Type C) pelvic disruption.

For *iliac wing fractures,* standard techniques of open reduction and internal fixation, using lag screws and/or reconstruction plates suffice. For *pure sacroiliac dislocation,* anterior plates are safe, as are posterior iliosacral lag screws, which may be percutaneously inserted under image intensification after either closed reduction or open reduction. If an *iliac fracture is associated with sacroiliac dislocation,* open anatomic reduction of the iliac fracture is a great help in achieving anatomic reduction of the sacroiliac joint. Unstable sacral fractures may be managed by transiliac bars, direct plate fixation, or iliosacral lag screws inserted under image intensification percutaneously, following closed or open reduction of the fracture.

REFERENCES

1. Pennal GF, Tile M, Waddell JP, et al. Pelvic disruption: assessment and classification. *Clin Orthop* 1980;151:12.
2. McBroom R, Tile M. Disruption of the pelvic ring. *Orthop Trans* 1982;6:493.
3. Webb LX, Caldwell K. Disruption of the pelvic ring caused by vertical shear. *South Med J* 1981;10:1217.
4. Bucholz RW. Pathological anatomy of Malgaigne fracture dislocation. *J Bone Joint Surg* 1981;63A:400.
5. Matta J. *Pelvic ring injuries: orthopedic knowledge update 2.* Park Ridge, IL: American Academy of Orthopedic Surgeons, 1987.
6. Pennal GF, Sutherland GO. *Fractures of the pelvis* (motion picture). Park Ridge, IL: AAOS Film Library, 1961.
7. Routt MLC Jr, Simonian PT. Closed reduction and percutaneous skeletal fixation of sacral fractures. *Clin Orthop* 1996; 329:121–128.
8. McGowan S, Kellam JF, Tile M. Unstable pelvic ring disruptions-results of open reduction and internal fixation, *Orthop Trans* 1987;11:478.
9. Goldstein A, et al. Early open reduction and internal fixation of the disrupted pelvic ring. *J Trauma* 1986;26:325.

10. Mears DC, Rubash HE. *Pelvic and acetabular fractures.* Thorofare, NJ: Slack, 1986.
11. Schied DK, Kellam JF, Tile M. Open reduction and internal fixation of pelvic ring fractures. *J Orthop Trauma* 1991;5:226.
12. Tile M. *Fractures of the pelvis and acetabulum.* Baltimore: Williams & Wilkins, 1984.
13. Holdsworth FW. Dislocation and fracture dislocation of the pelvis. *J Bone Joint Surg* 1948;30B:461.
14. Letournel E, Judet R. *Fractures of the acetabulum.* New York: Springer-Verlag, 1981.
15. Karaharju RO, Slatis P. External fixation of double vertical fractures with a trapezoidal compression frame. *Injury* 1978;10:142.
16. Mears DC, Fu FH. Modern concepts of external skeletal fixation of the pelvis. *Clin Orthop* 1980;151:65.
17. Dahners LE, et al. A study of external fixation systems for unstable pelvic fractures. *J Trauma* 1984;24:876.
18. Kellam JF, Boyer M, Dean R, et al. *Results of external fixation of the pelvis.* Presented at the 12th International Congress on Hoffman Fixation. Garmisch Partenkirchen Murnau, Germany, Oct. 9–10, 1986.
19. Wild JJ, Hanson GW, Tullos HS. Unstable fractures of the pelvis treated by external fixation. *J Bone Joint Surg* 1982;64:1010.
20. Routt MLC Jr, Simonian PT, Inaba J. Iliosacral screw complications. *Oper Tech Orthop* 1997;3:206–220.
21. Bone LB, Johnson KJ, Weigelt JA, et al. Early versus delayed stabilization of femoral fractures. *J Bone Joint Surg* 1989;71A:336.
22. Hearn TC, et al. *The effects of ligament sectioning and internal fixation on bending stiffness of the pelvic ring.* Proceedings of the 13th International Conference on Biomechanics. Perth, Australia, Dec. 9–13, 1991.
23. McMurtry RY, Walton D, Dickenson D, et al. Pelvic disruption in the polytraumatized patient: a management protocol. *Clin Orthop Relat Res* 1980;151:22–30.
24. Cogley D, Stephen DJG, Kreder HJ. *Functional outcomes of pelvic fractures treated by ilio-sacral screw fixation.* Presented at the Canadian Orthopedic Association Annual Meeting. Ottawa, Canada, June 1998.
25. Pohlemann T, Gansslen A, Schellwald O, et al. Outcome after pelvic ring injuries. *Injury* 1996;27(Suppl 2):SB31–SB38.
26. Matta JM, Saucedo T. Internal fixation of pelvic ring fractures. *Clin Orthop* 1989;242:83.
27. Stocks GW, Gabel GT, Noble PC, et al. Anterior and posterior internal fixation of vertical shear fractures of the pelvis. *J Orthop Res* 1991;9:237.
28. Ward EF, Tomasin J, Vander Griend RA. Open reduction and internal fixation of vertical shear pelvic fractures. *J Trauma* 1987;27:291.
29. Matta JM. Indications for anterior fixation of pelvic fractures. *Clin Orthop* 1996;329:88–96.
30. Schopfer HT, DiAngelo D, Tile M. Biomechanical comparison of internal fixation in vertically unstable disruptions of the pelvic ring. *Orthop Trans* 1992–1993;16:659.
31. Matta JM, Tornetta P III. Internal fixation of unstable pelvic ring injuries. *Clin Orthop* 1996;329:129–140.
32. Gorczyca JT, Watt P, Goltz, et al. *A mechanical comparison of anterior internal fixation vs external fixation for unstable pelvic injuries with iliosacral screws.* Presented at the Orthopedic Trauma Association 16th Annual Meeting. San Antonio, TX, October 12–14, 2000.
33. Pohlemann T, Angst M, Schneider E, et al. Fixation of transforaminal sacrum fractures: a biomechanical study. *J Orthop Trauma* 1993;7:107.
34. Kellam JF, McMurtry RY, Paley D, et al. The unstable pelvic fracture: operative treatment. *Orthop Clin North Am* 1987;18:25–41.
35. Moed BR, Karges DE. Techniques for reduction and fixation of pelvic ring disruptions through the posterior approach. *Clin Orthop* 1996;329:102–114.
36. Delal SA, et al. Pelvic fractures in multiple trauma. Classification by mechanism is key to pattern of organ injury. Resuscitative requirements and outcome. *J Trauma* 1989;29:981.
37. Evers MB, Cryer HM, Miller FB. Pelvic fracture hemorrhage. *Arch Surg* 1989;124:422.
38. Routt MLC Jr, Simonian PT, Agnew SG, et al. Radiographic recognition of the sacral alar slope for optimal placement of iliosacral screws: a cadaveric and clinical study. *J Orthop Trauma* 1996;10:171–177.
39. Templeman D, Schmidt A, Freese J, et al. Proximity of iliosacral screws to neurovascular structures after internal fixation. *Clin Orthop* 1996;329:194–198.
40. Routt MLC Jr, Meier MC, Kregor PJ, et al. Percutaneous iliosacral screws with the patient supine. *Op Tech Orthop* 1993;7:35–45.
41. Routt ML, Simonian P. Posterior pelvic ring disruptions: iliosacral screws. In Wiss D, ed. *Master techniques in orthopedic surgery: fractures.* Philadelphia: Lippincott-Raven, 1998.
42. Routt ML, Simonian PT, Grujic L. The retrograde medullary superior pubic ramus screw for the treatment of anterior pelvic ring disruptions: a new technique. *J Orthop Trauma* 1995;9:35–44.
43. Routt ML, Nork SE, Mills WJ. Percutaneous fixation of pelvic ring disruptions. *Clin Orthop* 2000;375:15–29.
44. Starr AJ, Walter JW, Harris RW, et al. Percutaneous screw fixation of fractures of the iliac wing and fracture-dislocations of the sacro-iliac joint (OTA Types 61-B2-2 and 61-B2-3 or Young-Burgess "lateral compression Type II" pelvic fractures). *J Orthop Trauma* 2002;16:116–123.
45. Hirvensalo S, Lindahl J, Partio E. *Technique for internal fixation of pelvic fractures.* Presented at the SICOT Meeting. Seoul, Korea, August 28–September 3, 1993.
46. Cole JD, Bolhofer BR. Acetabular fracture fixation via a modified Stoppa limited intrapelvic approach. *Clin Orthop* 1991;305:112–123.
47. Simpson LA, et al. Anterior approach and stabilization of the disrupted sacroiliac joint. *J Trauma* 1987;12:1332.
48. Ruedi T, von Hochstetter AHC, Schlumpf R. *Surgical approaches for internal fixation.* Berlin: Springer-Verlag, 1984.
49. Mears DC, Capito CP, Deleeuw H. Posterior pelvic disruptions managed by the use of the double cobra plate. *AAOS, Instructional Course Lectures* 1988;37:143.
50. Pohlemann T, Tscherne H. Fixation of sacral fractures. *Tech Orthop* 1995;9:315.
51. Webb LX, de Araujo W, Donofrio P, et al. Electromyography monitoring for percutaneous placement of iliosacral screws. *J Orthop Trauma* 2000;14(4):245–254.
52. Varga E, Hearn T, Powell J, et al. Effects of method of internal fixation of symphyseal disruptions on stability of the pelvic ring. *Injury* 1995;26:75–80.
53. Templeman D, Schmidt A, Freese J, et al. Proximity of iliosacral screws to neurovascular structures after internal fixation. *Clin Orthop* 1996;329:194–198.
54. Borrelli J, Koval KJ, Helfet DL. The crescent fracture: a posterior fracture dislocation of the sacroiliac joint. *J Orthop Trauma* 1996;10:165–170.
55. Letournel E, Judet R. *Fractures of the acetabulum,* 2nd ed. New York: Springer-Verlag 1993:373–375, 403.
56. Leighton RK, Waddell JP. Techniques for reduction and posterior fixation through the anterior approach. *Clin Orthop* 1996;329:115–120.
57. Yinger K, Scalise JJ, Bay, BK, et al. *Biomechanical comparison of relative stability of pelvic ring fixation constructs.* Presented at the

American Academy of Orthopedic Surgeons 68th Annual Meeting. San Francisco, CA, February 28–March 4, 2001.
58. Leighton R, Waddell J. Open reduction and internal fixation of vertical fractures of the pelvis using the sacroiliac joint plate. *J Orthop Trauma* 1991;5:225.
59. Ragnarsson B, Olerud C, Olerud S. Anterior square plate fixation of sacroiliac disruption: 2–8 years followup of 23 consecutive cases. *Acta Orthop Scand* 1993;64:138.
60. Behrens F, Comfort T. *Anterior fixation of dislocations and fracture dislocations of the sacroiliac joint.* Presented at the Orthopedic Trauma Association 2nd Annual Meeting. San Francisco, CA, November 20–22, 1986.
61. Mears DC, Capito CP, Deleeuw H. Posterior pelvic disruptions managed by the use of the double cobra plate. *AAOS, Instructional Course Lectures* 1988;37:143.
62. Ebraheim NA, Coombs R, Hoeflinger MJ, et al. Anatomic and radiological considerations in compressive bar technique for posterior pelvic disruptions. *J Orthop Trauma*1991;5:434–438.

16

SACRAL FRACTURES

TIMOTHY POHLEMANN
AXEL GÄNSSLEN
HARALD TSCHERNE

INTRODUCTION

There is controversy about the diagnosis and treatment of sacral fractures (1–13). The majority of patients suffer from polytrauma; therefore, significant injuries to other body regions usually dominate the primary diagnostic and therapeutic regimen. The typical clinical signs of the injury are usually missing, plain radiographs are difficult to interpret, and neurologic deficits are not always obvious on the primary examination. Consequently, these injuries frequently are overlooked, misdiagnosed, or even neglected.

The significance of sacral fractures relates to a high rate of concomitant neurologic injuries as well as their importance as part of posterior pelvic ring instability (6,14–17). Over the last few years, several methods for external or internal stabilization of the unstable posterior pelvic ring have been described (13,20–29), but a specific protocol for sacrum fractures as part of this management plan is missing.

ANATOMY

The sacrum is a median triangular bone, connecting the two hemipelves to the spinal column. It consists of five fused sacral vertebrae and the rudimentary coccygeal bones. Additionally, it acts as an important stabilizing part of the pelvis by its ligamentous attachments.

The sagittal contour has a slight kyphosis with an average anterior inclination of 47 degrees. Spine orientation changes from a more horizontal to a vertical shape at the third sacral.

Osseous Structure

(See Fig. 16-1.) The ventral, pelvic sacral surface forms the posterior wall of the true pelvis with a close relationship to the rectum. Two rows of sacral foramina are present, normally four on each side for the exiting S1 to S4 anterior motor nerve roots. The foramina are connected with the central canal via the intervertebral foramina. The anterior foramina are larger in diameter than the corresponding posterior foramina.

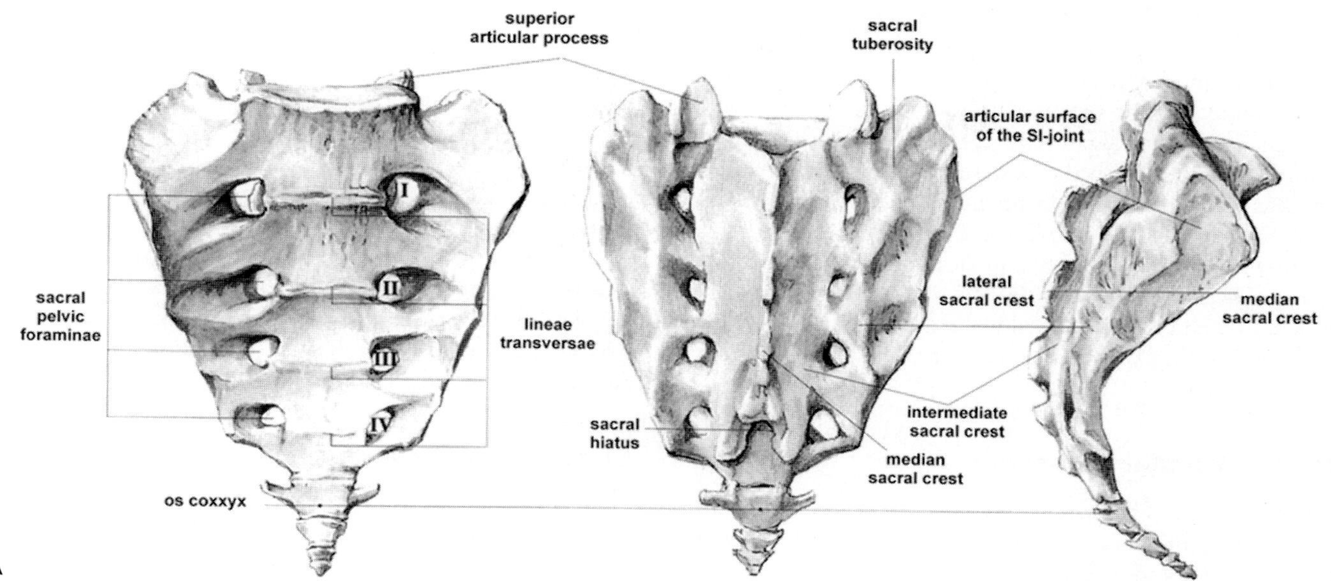

FIGURE 16-1. A,B: Osseous anatomy of the sacrum. Anterior, posterior, and lateral views. The sacrum is roughly and irregularly formed and marked with three major vertically orientated crests. On the lateral side the articular surface of the SI joint is visible. (From: Tscherne H, Pohlemann T, eds. *Unfallchirurgie Becken und Acetabulum*. Heidelberg: Springer-Verlag, 1998, with permission.)

The thin dorsal cortical surface is rough and marked by three major vertically oriented crests. The rudimentarily visible former spinal processes are fused within the median sacral crest. The smaller intermediate sacral crest is visible medial to the neuroforamina, representing the former facet joints of the sacral spines. The lateral sacral crest is formed by the fused transverse processes. The dorsal rami of the nerve roots exit through the posterior sacral neuroforamina. The sacral hiatus takes up the dural sac at the S1 vertebra.

The lateral surface of the upper three sacral vertebrae forms the kidney-shaped articular surface, which corresponds to the articular surface of the iliac wing. The upper sacrum is formed by the superior surface of the S1 body. In the midline the S1 vertebral body forms the sacral promontory. Laterally, the sacral ala slopes from posterior-superior to anterior-inferior in direct association with the common iliac vessels and lumbosacral trunk.

Ligaments

(See Fig. 16-2.) Anteriorly, the sacrum is connected to the articular surface of the ilium by the weak anterior sacroiliac ligaments (SI joint). The stronger sacroiliac interosseous lig-

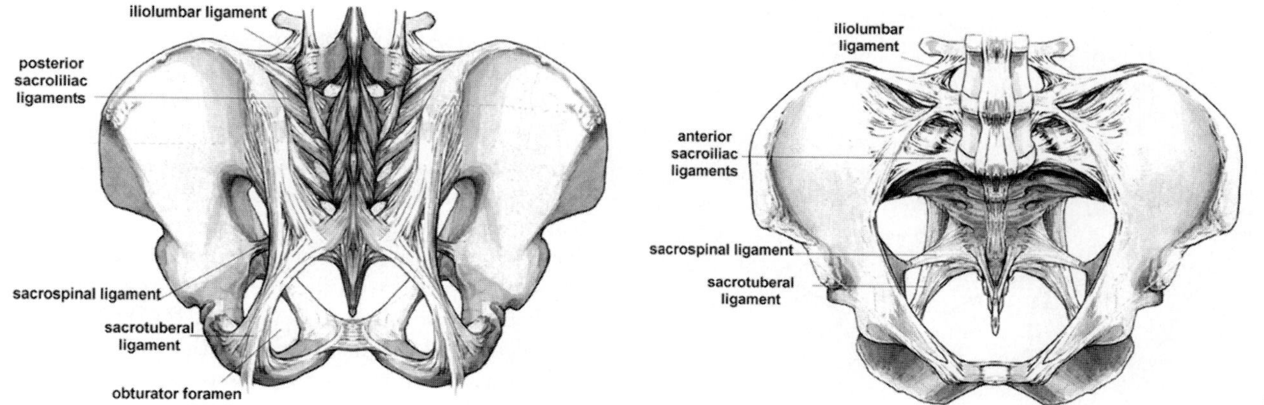

FIGURE 16-2. Ligaments around the sacrum. **A:** Posteriorly, the strong sacroiliac interosseous ligaments stabilize the sacrum within the pelvic girdle. **B:** In contrast, the anterior sacroiliac ligaments are much weaker. (From: Tscherne H, Pohlemann T, eds. *Unfallchirurgie Becken und Acetabulum.* Heidelberg: Springer-Verlag, 1998, with permission.)

aments stabilize the sacrum within the pelvic girdle posterior to the SI joint. The strong posterior sacral ligaments arise from the dorsal sacral interforaminal and lateral surfaces, connecting the sacrum with the iliac bone.

The iliolumbar ligaments connect the fifth lumbar transverse process with the posterior part of the iliac crest, whereas the lumbosacral ligaments connect the L5 transverse process with the sacral ala. Thus, displaced fractures of the fifth lumbar transverse process may indicate an unstable posterior pelvic ring lesion. Additionally, the sacrospinal and sacrotuberal ligaments act as pelvic stabilizers by limiting anterior rotation of the sacrum around a horizontal axis.

Neurovascular Anatomy

(See Fig. 16-3.) The sacral canal contains the spinal nerves of the sacral and coccygeal plexus, which leave the sacrum through the anterior sacral foramina. The S1 root exits to join the L4 and L5 roots in front of the sacroiliac joint. The S2 through S4 roots exit and join the sciatic nerve in front of the pyriformis muscle. All of these nerve roots are invested in a fascia. In addition to the nerve roots forming the sciatic plexus, the pelvic floor also contains pelvic splanchnic nerves, which are mixed parasympathetic nerves that control involuntary sphincter muscle action of the rectum and bladder, and the nervi erigentes, which supply the penis and clitoris and are important for sexual function.

The dural sac ends at the level of S2 in 84% of patients. The diameter of the S1 and S2 nerve roots are about one third to one fourth of the diameter of the surrounding foramina, decreasing to one sixth at the level of S3 and S4. The cross section of the roots S2 to S5 amounts to 80%, 60%, 20%, and 15% of the cross section of S1, respectively (14). Therefore, the S1 or S2 nerve roots are more endangered for injury by fractures involving these neuroforamina than at lower levels. The lumbosacral trunk (L4-5 nerve root) is closely related to the lateral upper sacral alar surface. Therefore, fractures in this area or cranial displacement of the hemipelvis can be associated with a stretch injury of the L5 nerve roots.

The major pelvic vessels (internal iliac artery and vein) follow the course of the lumbosacral trunk. The median sacral artery and sympathetic component of the autonomic nervous system are closely related to the anterior sacral surface in the area of the promontory.

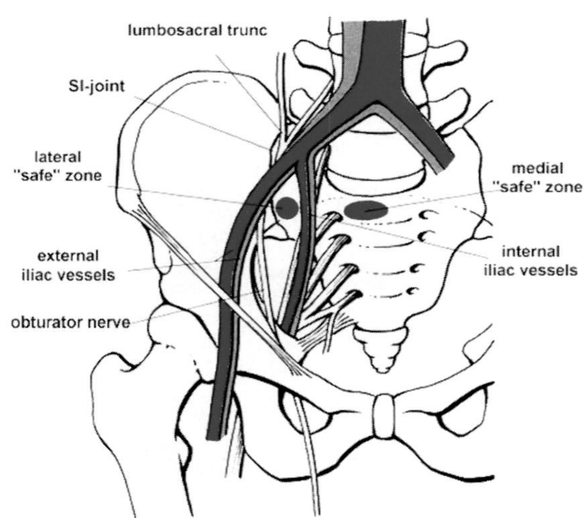

FIGURE 16-3. Lumbosacral plexus from anteriorly. (From: Tscherne H, Pohlemann T, eds. *Unfallchirurgie Becken und Acetabulum.* Heidelberg: Springer-Verlag, 1998, with permission.)

Clinical Importance of the Sacral Anatomy

The sacral foramina, particularly at the level of S1 and S2, tend to weaken the junction between the body of the sacrum and its ala. A significant number of sacral fractures are known to extend through the sacral foramina and up to the groove at the L5 articular process. Because of the sacral roots' fascial investment, they tend to maintain the relationship with the medial or midline portion of the sacrum during fractures. If there is significant vertical or posterior displacement, the sacral roots, which are fixed at the sacral canal and the greater sciatic notch of the pelvis, come under tension, causing traction injuries and even nerve root avulsion. Lateral compression injuries of the sacrum involve the sacral foramina. The fracture may cause buckling of bone in the foramen, which compresses the roots, leading to neurologic injury and/or causalgic pain.

Sacral Biomechanics

The load transfer from the lower extremities to the spine takes place through the posterior column of the hip joint to the SI joint and the sacrum. In the upright stance the body weight is divided into a dorsocranial and a ventrocranial component, which is represented by the structure of the interosseous ligaments (30). The specific anatomy of the posterior pelvis produces translational and rotational forces to the sacrum.

This movements leads to a tightening of the dorsal sacroiliac ligaments under load, whereby the iliac bones are compressed and the sacrum is stabilized (31–33). The resulting torsion of the sacrum (nutation) is limited by the strong pelvic floor ligaments (sacrotuberal and sacrospinal ligaments) together with the inserting muscles (gluteus maximus muscle, piriformis muscle) (Fig. 16-4) (34,35).

Analyses indicate that motion of the sacroiliac joint is of complex nature and cannot be described with a single horizontal axis. An approximated transverse rotational axis can be projected posteriorly to the SI joint between the first and the second sacral body with moving position under load (36–41).

In summary, a combined motion range with 2 to 12

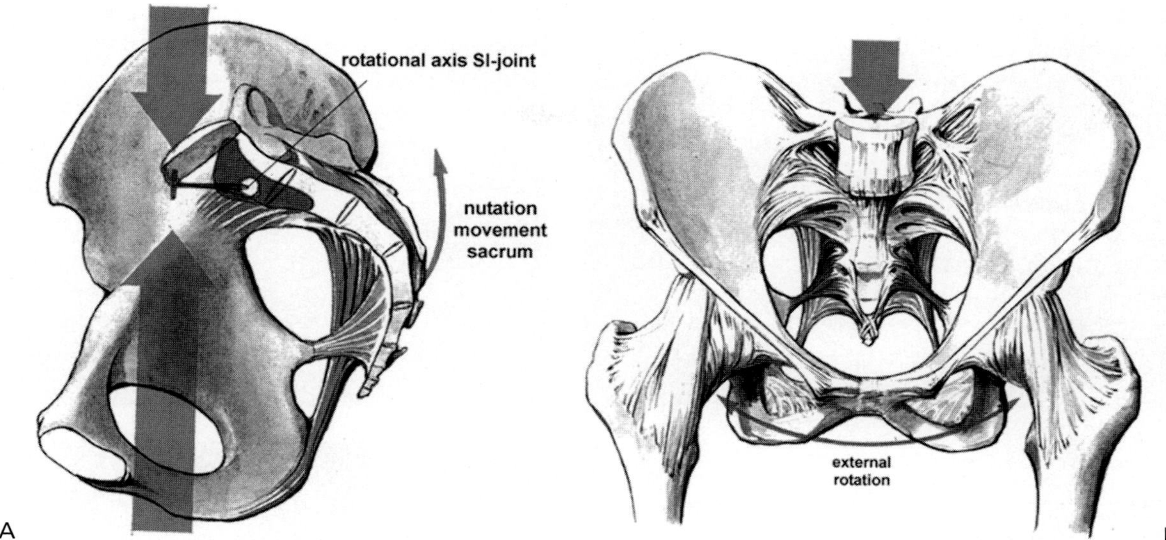

FIGURE 16-4. A,B: Sacral biomechanics. Axial load leads to a tightening of the dorsal sacroiliac ligaments; thereby, the iliac bones are compressed and the sacrum is stabilized. The resulting torsion movement of the sacrum is limited by the sacrotuberal and sacrospinal ligaments. (From: Tscherne H, Pohlemann T, eds. *Unfallchirurgie Becken und Acetabulum.* Heidelberg: Springer-Verlag, 1998, with permission.)

degrees of rotation and 2 to 26 mm of translation is to be expected (38,42). The amount of movement depends on age and gender. In women, the range of motion is larger and increases during pregnancy. Mobility decreases with increasing age. Men >50 years old have an observed ankylosis rate of 75% (43).

INCIDENCE

In 1847 Malgaigne reported only one isolated sacrum fracture in an analysis of 2,358 fractures observed in all body regions (Table 16-1) (44). In 1929 Wakeley reported a 4% and in 1930 Noland reported a 2.4% incidence of sacrum fractures after pelvic fractures (45,46). The first detailed analysis of sacrum fractures that included a classification was published in 1945 by Bonin. It estimated a 45.5% incidence after pelvic fractures (47). In 1972 Huittinen and colleagues reported 14% sacrum fractures in a series of 407 pelvic fractures (48). In 1988 Denis and colleagues analyzed 776 pelvic fractures, reporting an incidence of 30.4% sacrum fractures (14). The Hannover experience and the results of the German Multicenter Pelvic Study Group found a rate of 18% to 30% (49).

TABLE 16-1. INCIDENCE OF SACRUM FRACTURES

Author (Ref)	Year	Number of Patients	Sacrum Fracture (%)
Wakeley (46)	1930	100	4.0
Noland (45)	1933	60	11.7
Medelman (64)	1939	50	44.0
Furey (65)	1942	94	74.0
Bonnin (47)	1945	44	45.5
Huittinen (66)	1972	407	14.0
Laasonen (67)	1977	156	33.3
Melton III (68)	1981	204	13.7
Denis (14)	1988	776	30.4
Gibbons (6)	1990	253	17.4
Isler (16)	1990	193	69.4
Pohlemann (15)	1992	1,350	27.8
German Pelvic Study (49)	1998	1,076	17.3
	TOTAL	5,409	22.8

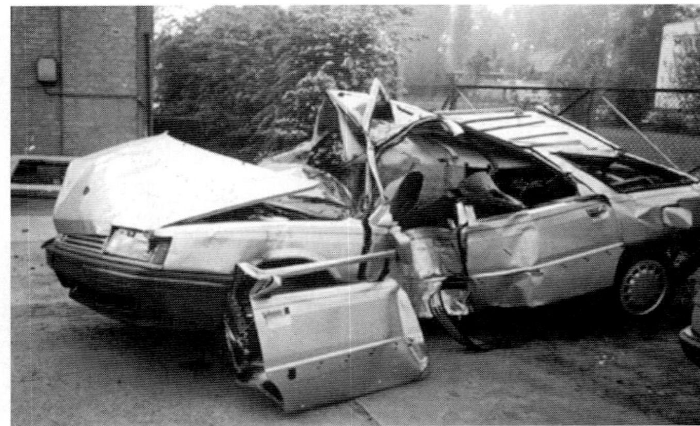
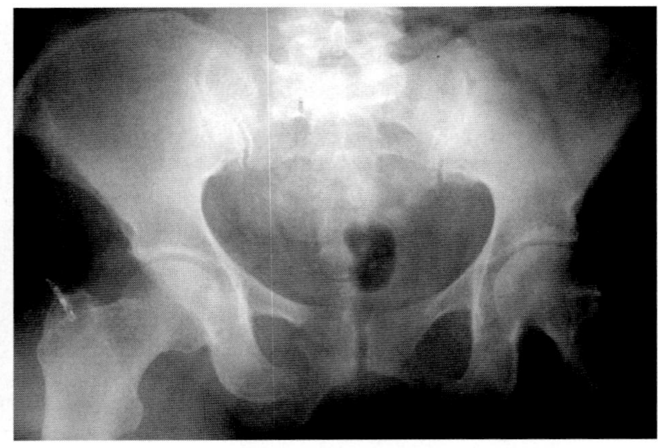
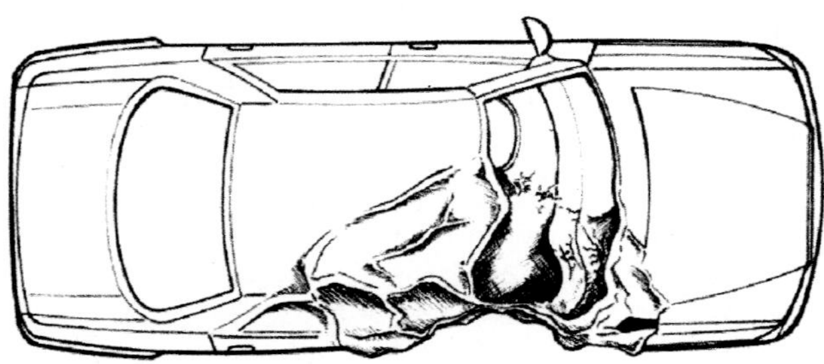
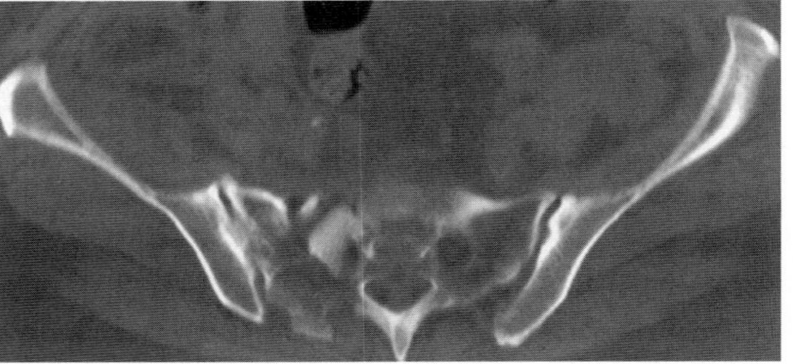

FIGURE 16-5. A: Trauma mechanism and sacral fracture. **B:** Typical lateral compression injury mechanism. The reconstruction of the car deformation shows the extended impression zone near the front seat. The x-rays **(C)** and computed tomography **(D)** reveal the complete transforaminal compression fracture of the sacrum (Type C). (From: Tscherne H, Pohlemann T, eds. *Unfallchirurgie Becken und Acetabulum.* Heidelberg: Springer-Verlag, 1998, with permission.)

Trauma Mechanism

Several injury mechanisms are accompanied with sacral fractures. The main type of accident producing a sacral fracture is high-energy trauma after a motor vehicle accident or fall from a great height.

Although normally a significant correlation between the injury mechanism and the severity of the pelvic fracture is present in pelvic ring fractures, no correlation between the sacral fracture pattern and mechanism of injury is present in sacral fractures. Only the rare transverse sacral fracture normally is associated with a simple fall. Additionally, a lateral impact is associated with acetabular or sacral fracture (Fig. 16-5), whereas frontal collisions in the majority lead to acetabular fractures. Rare mechanisms are indirect dislocation mechanisms, such as severe hyperflexion injuries (suicidal jumper's fracture) (50).

DIAGNOSIS

Beside the standard clinical examination of the patients, radiologic diagnostics includes at least an anterior-posterior view of the pelvis (8,50–52). The diagnosis of a sacral fracture can be evaluated in 88% to 94% of cases with the standard anterior-posterior pelvis; however, the amount and direction of displacement cannot be judged. Therefore, if an injury to the posterior pelvic ring is suspected, then the standard pelvic anterior-posterior radiograph has to be complemented by oblique (inlet/outlet) views and computed tomography (CT) scan (Fig. 16-6), as described in Chapter 10 (54). The inlet view allows analysis of an anterior-posterior displacement and rotation, whereas the outlet view shows craniocaudal displacements and superior rotation.

The true lateral view of the sacrum is indicated in displaced transverse fractures as well as in suicidal jumper's fractures for analyzing the amount of displacement in the sagittal plane.

The CT scan provides definitive information to detect even minor injuries to the sacrum (50,51,54). In many cases of sacral fractures only the detailed analysis of the CT scan allows the distinction of the posterior pelvic injuries to the rotational group (Tile Type B, partial posterior stability) and the translational group (Tile Type C, no posterior stability) (55). The CT scan allows the analysis of the detailed fracture pattern, the detection of fragments compromising neurologic structures, and zones of fragmentation. The size of the sacral fragments can be evaluated for planning of the internal fixation. A CT scan, especially with frontal and sagittal reformations, thus is recommended in every sacrum fracture. The three-dimensional CT reconstruction gives a summary of the radiologic diagnostics.

Important markers that may indicate the presence of sacrum fractures are the interruptions of the arcuate lines of the sacrum, a fractured transverse process of L5, and avulsion fractures of the sacrospinal and sacrotuberous ligaments (Fig. 16-7) (8,50).

The diagnosis has to be completed by a neurologic examination as early as possible. The quality of clinical examination often is reduced in the early phase because of the polytrauma situation. Thus, the risk of neurologic damage can be predicted only indirectly by the grade of pelvic instability, fracture pattern, and nature of the fracture line (fragmentation, fragments close to nerve roots) (15).

CLASSIFICATION

Sacrum fractures must be classified into: (a) fracture types not involving the pelvic ring; and (b) fracture patterns involving the ring and normally leading to at least some amount of pelvic ring instability.

Generally, sacral fractures are part of a pelvic ring fracture (56). According to the Müller-AO/OTA-classification, sacral Type A fractures consist of coccyx fractures or sacrococcygeal dislocations (Müller-AO/OTA: 61-A 3.1), nondisplaced transverse fractures of the sacrum below the level of S2, not involving the pelvic girdle (Müller-AO/OTA: 61-A 3.2) and displaced transverse fractures of the sacrum below the level of S2, not involving the pelvic girdle (Müller-AO/OTA: 61-A3.3).

Sacral Type B fractures consist of unilateral or bilateral "open-book" sacral fractures (Müller-AO/OTA: 61-B1.2 or 61-B3.1), unilateral (Müller-AO/OTA: 61-B2.1), or bilateral lateral compression injuries (Müller-AO/OTA: 61-B3.3).

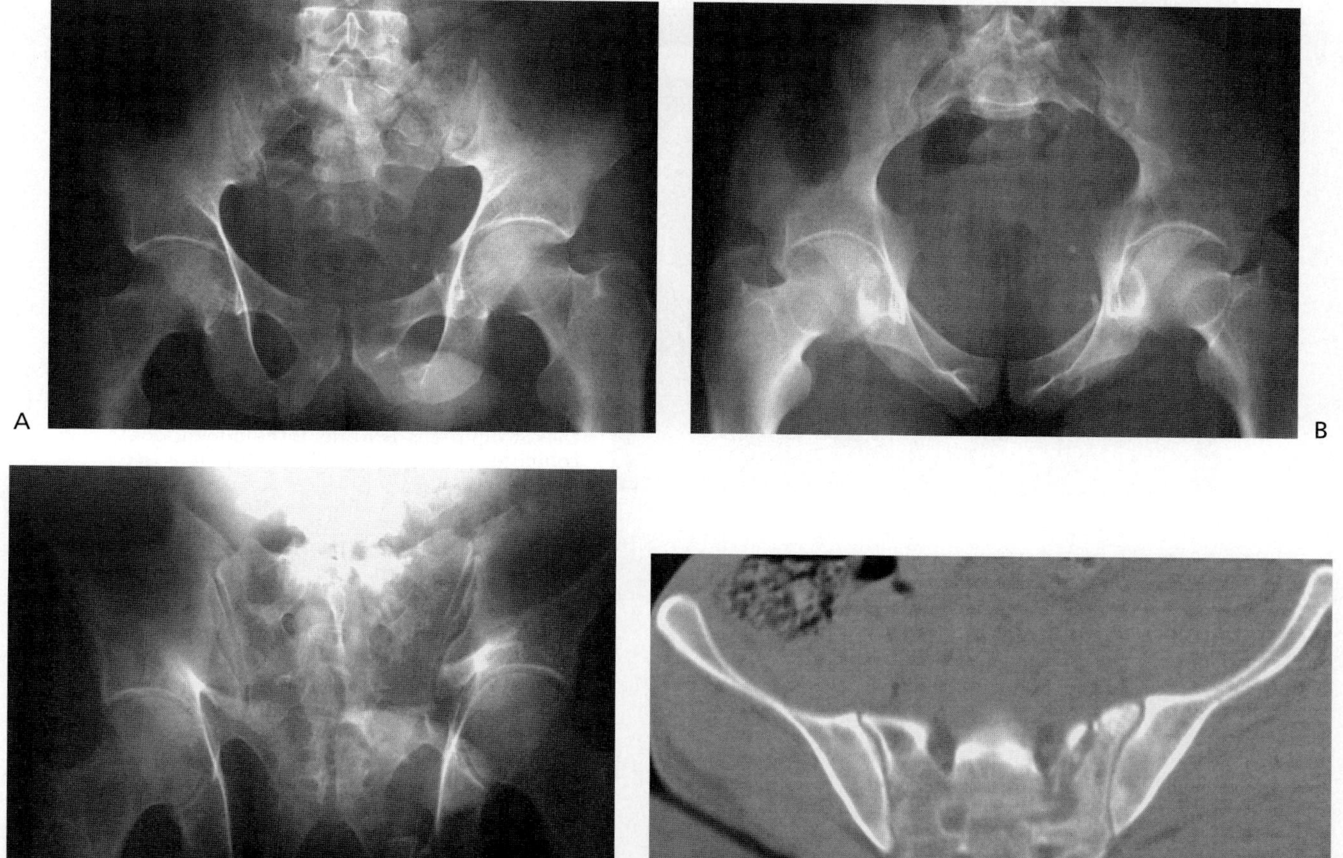

FIGURE 16-6. Radiologic diagnostics in suspected sacral fractures. The pelvic anterior-posterior radiograph is useful in the polytrauma situation, but added views are needed. The oblique views (inlet **(B)**/outlet views **(C)**) and the two-dimensional computed tomography scan **(D)** are the standard views.
(*Figure continues*)

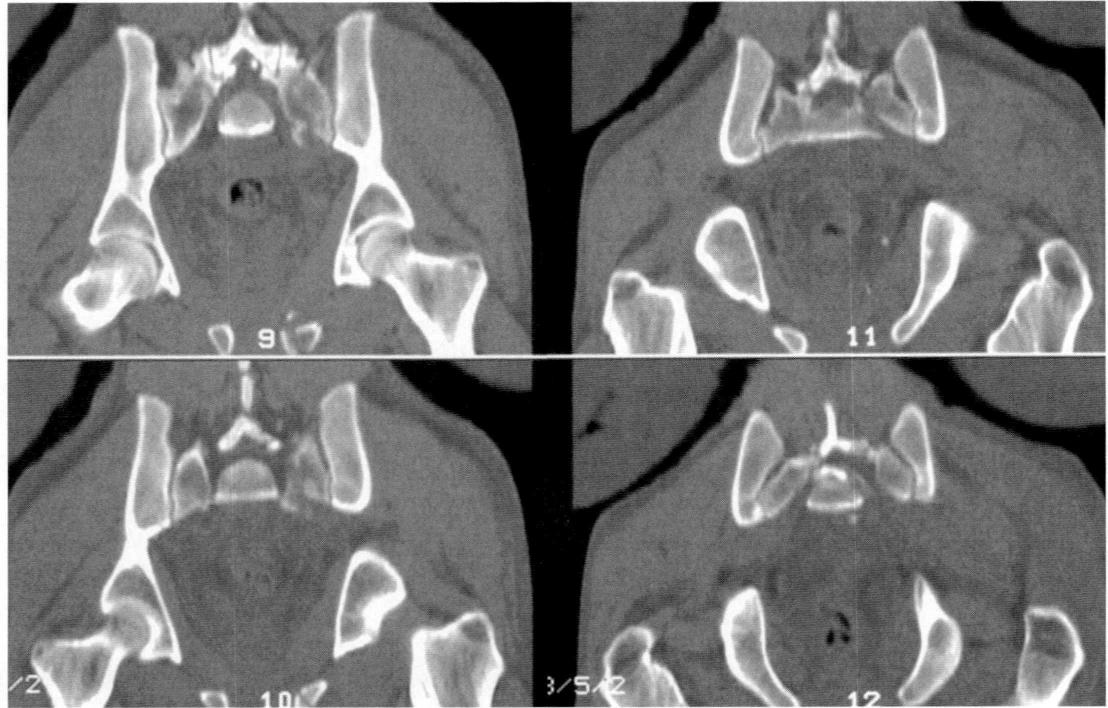

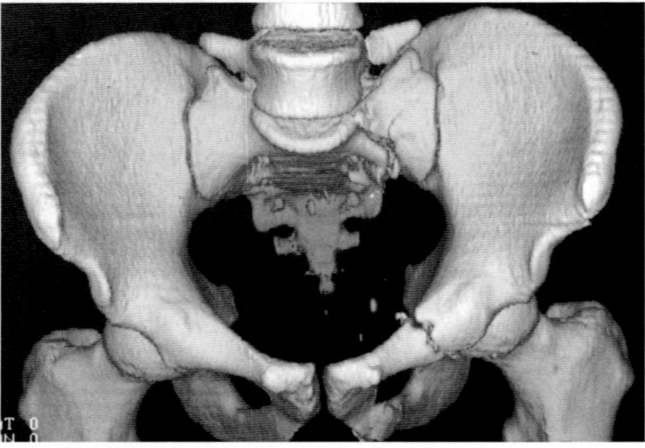

FIGURE 16-6. ***(continued)*** Frontal and sagittal reformations **(E)** and three-dimensional computed tomography **(F)** are desirable (see Chapter 10).

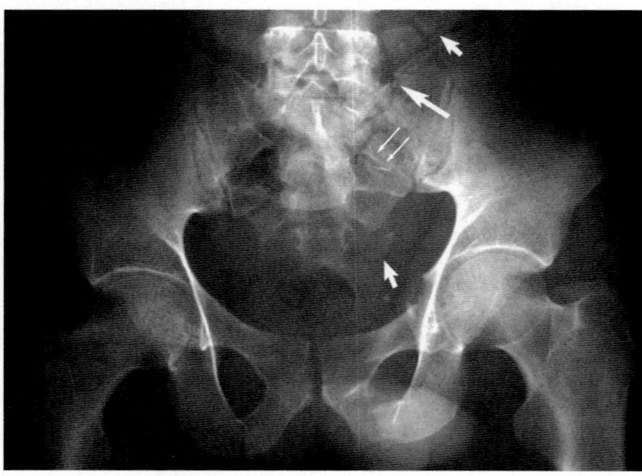

FIGURE 16-7. Typical signs indicating a sacrum fracture a fractured transverse process of L5 *(top arrow);* interruptions of the arcuate lines of the sacrum *(middle large and two smaller arrows);* and avulsion fracture of the sacrospinal and/or sacrotuberous ligaments *(bottom arrow).*

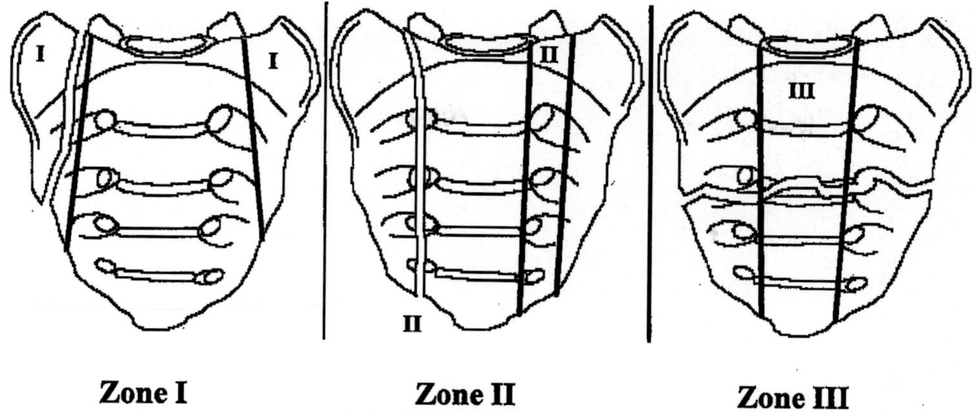

FIGURE 16-8. Classification of sacral fractures according to Denis (14). Denis' classification of sacrum fractures is based on three zones with transalar, transforaminal, and central fractures.

Sacral Type C fractures are unilateral unstable sacral fractures (Müller-AO/OTA: C1.3) or unilateral sacral fractures together with a contralateral posterior Type B pelvic ring injury (Müller-AO/OTA: C2.3). Additionally, bilateral sacral fractures (Müller-AO/OTA: C3.3) often are suicidal jumper's fractures.

In 1988 Denis and colleagues published a widely used classification based on three zones of the sacrum (14). The lateral part of the sacrum represents zone I (transalar fractures); zone II, the region of the foramen (transforaminal fractures); and zone III, the region medial to the foramen (central fractures) (Fig. 16-8). The most medial part of the fracture line defines the classification group in fracture lines crossing the zones. After an analysis of 236 sacrum fractures, the authors found a close relation between the anatomic fracture pattern and rate of neurologic deficits. The rate of neurologic injuries was 5.9% in zone I, 28.4% in zone II, and 56.7% in zone III. Pohlemann's review of 377 sacrum fractures confirmed these results. However, the main prognostic criterion for outcome of a sacral fracture in related nerve injury was the grade of instability of the pelvic ring injury (15). The Hannover group described a more complete sacral fracture classification involving four different types with nine typical fracture lines (Table 16-2).

The practical clinical significance of these descriptions is to help focus the surgeon so that any potential injury or complication is not missed or allowed to occur. The pelvis is first assessed and classified because the majority of sacral fractures are associated with a pelvic ring injury. If a sacral fracture exists at this time, then it is further explained using one of the described classification systems and appended to the pelvic ring description.

ASSOCIATED NEUROLOGIC INJURIES

Concomitant nerve injuries are of high importance because of their frequency and functional disabilities. The nerve damage normally is caused by direct compression by fragments or results from overstretching. Therefore, nerve structures can be damaged at a higher or lower level than the fracture. Generally, all muscles and skin areas below the knee are innervated by the L4 to S2 nerve roots. The damage of S3-5 nerve roots needs special attention. Clinically, they present as disturbances of the genitourinary system and sexual function or as sensory disturbances in the perineal region.

The incidence of accompanying nerve damage is reported to be as high as 21% to 60%, depending on the sacral fracture type, in large series of sacral fractures (14,15). The analyses of our own series showed some differences from Denis' observations. The rate of neurologic damage was primarily related to the amount of pelvic ring instability (Müller-AO/OTA classification of pelvic fractures) (56), and secondarily to the specific fracture pattern in the sacrum (zones I to III) (15). Stable Type A pelvic fractures normally did not show neurologic failures, whereas in rotationally unstable Type B fractures nerve damage was observed in <10% in each sacral fracture zone (DENIS I, II, and III). Completely unstable (Type C) fractures showed the highest rates of additional nerve injury, with an increase of 32.6% in zone I (lateral), 42.9% in zone 2 (foraminal), and 63.6% in zone III (central). Bilateral sacral fractures showed the highest rates of nerve damage.

Additionally, the type of neurologic deficit depends on the specific pattern of the fracture line. Unilateral vertical fractures may involve the sacral roots of one side and preserve normal bladder and bowel function unless the S1 root is involved. Minimal sensory loss normally is difficult to detect.

Vertical displacement, which often is indicated by a fracture of the L5 transverse process, can lead to injuries to the L5 root ("far out syndrome," usually leading to a footdrop).

The neurologic disturbances in the central fracture pattern include bowel, bladder, and sexual dysfunction. The amount of dysfunction depends on the involvement of the different sacral roots. The preservation of at least one of the two S2 and S3 roots might result in the absence of functional incontinence.

TABLE 16-2.

Type 0 (avulsion fracture)

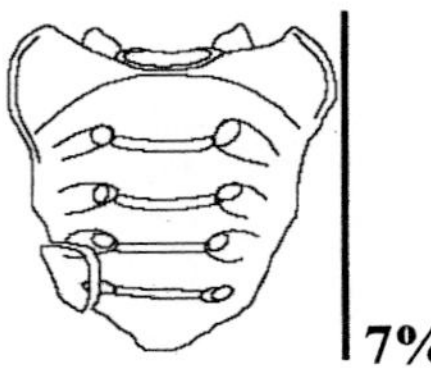

transalar fracture

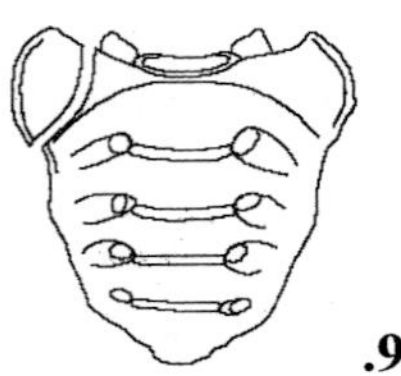

Ia avulsion fracture

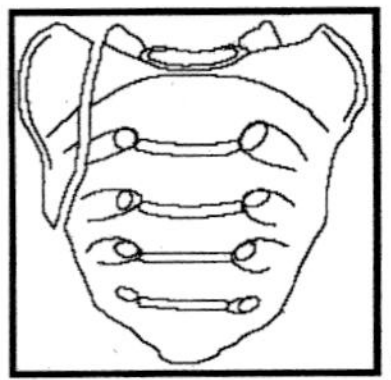

Ib complete transalar fracture

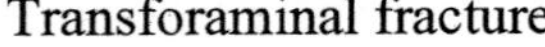

Transforaminal fracture

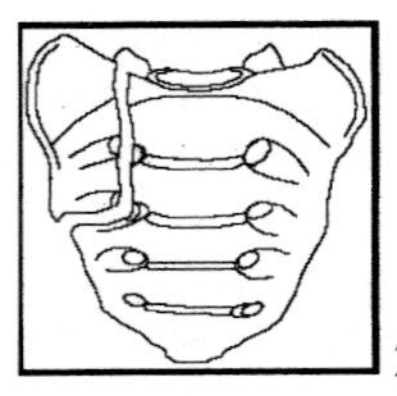

IIa fracture above S2

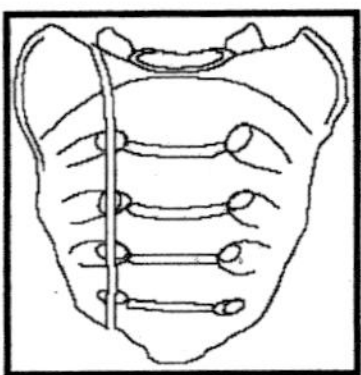

IIb vertical fracture below S2

Sacrum central fracture

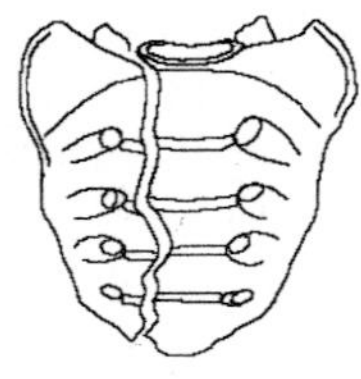

IIIa vertical fracture

4%

IIIb transverse fracture

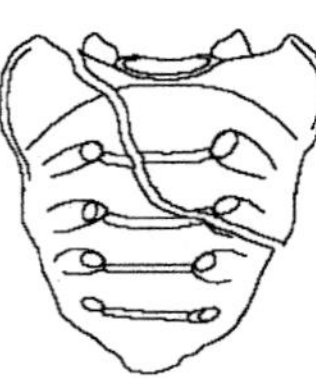

IIIc oblique fracture

bilateral sacrum fracture

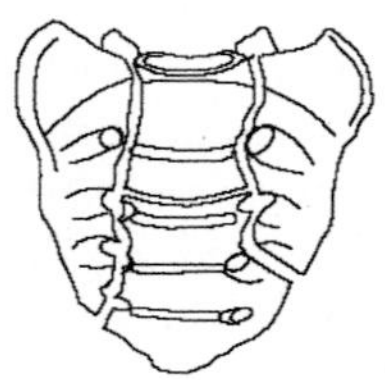

Even if the malfunction is discrete and often stays undiagnosed in the initial and early evaluation it can lead to a significant reduction of the patient's quality of life.

The following observations were made in a recent analysis of 600 sacral fractures in the Hannover series (57).

- Patients with coccyx fractures, sacrococcygeal dislocations, or nondisplaced transverse fractures of the sacrum below the level of S2 showed no nerve injuries.
- Two of seven patients with displaced transverse sacral fractures below the level of S2 had sacral fracture–related nerve injuries. Both required open reduction and sacral nerve root decompression, with no complete recovery of their nerve deficit.
- Four of 307 patients with a Type B fracture had a sacral fracture–related lesion of the lumbosacral plexus; all after a transforaminal fracture.
- Sacral fracture–related nerve injury was present in 36.5% of neurologically evaluated patients after Type C sacral fractures.
- The incidence of a nerve deficit was 11.1% after transalar, 28.9% after transforaminal, and 53.8% after central fractures in Type C injuries.
- Bilateral Type C fractures had the highest incidence of nerve deficits (79.2%).
- There was a significant correlation of sacral fracture displacement and the presence of a lumbosacral plexus injury in Type C fractures (threshold: 5 mm, 22% versus 38%).
- A fractured L5 transverse process in Type C fractures was a significant indicator for a lumbosacral plexus lesion (25% versus 39%).

INDICATIONS

The indication for operative treatment is based on the grade of instability of the pelvis, the fracture displacement, and the probable additional sacral fracture–related nerve injury.

Type A fractures of the sacrum (e.g., transverse fractures below the level of S2 or injuries of the coccyx) are predominantly treated nonoperatively because they are normally nondisplaced. Indications for operative treatment are severe displacement disturbing the rectum or anal region, and lesions of the lower sacral nerve roots in displaced transverse fractures. Nonoperative treatment consists of pain-dependent weight bearing and analgesics.

Specific stabilization of the sacrum usually is not performed if the sacrum fracture represents the posterior part of a rotational injury (Type B), most frequently a lateral compression type injury. A distracting external fixator sometimes is indicated in the presence of a narrowing of the plane of the pelvic brim by lateral compression or internal rotation. For the anterior-posterior/open-book injury, the anatomy of the pelvic ring is sufficiently restored by anterior internal (e.g., symphysis plate) or external fixation. A decompression of the central canal is indicated in the rare case of concomitant neurologic injury caused by nerve root compression from fragments. The specific fracture pattern can be analyzed clearly on the CT scan.

Internal fixation of the sacrum is indicated if the sacral fracture represents the posterior part of a completely unstable injury (Type C pelvic instability). A minimally displaced sacral fracture line associated with a fracture of the L5 transverse process and/or an avulsion of the sacrotuberous or sacrospinal ligaments is highly suspicious for Type C pelvic instability. The risk of a secondary displacement of the fracture under functional treatment is high if a complete anterior-posterior sacral fracture line exits through DENIS zone II and III injuries, because no posterior pelvic ligaments are crossing this specific anatomic region. Unstable Type C fractures of the sacrum should be posteriorly stabilized by open or closed techniques, especially when combined with lesions of the lumbosacral plexus or fragments compromising the lumbosacral nerve roots. Nerve root decompression becomes mandatory because early results show at least a partial recovery (58).

A special fracture type is the "suicidal jumper's fracture," with a U- or H-shaped fracture of the upper sacrum and transverse fracture line, normally at the level of S1 or S2, without an anterior pelvic ring lesion in the majority of cases. These fracture types generally show an anterior rotational deformity with the first sacral spine anterior to the lower sacrum and have a high incidence of additional lumbosacral plexus lesions. Therefore, reduction and nerve root decompression may be indicated.

Poor general health and severe osteoporosis of the bony pelvis are contraindications for operative treatment.

TREATMENT

The type of treatment depends on the instability of the complete pelvis, sacral fracture type, and perhaps additional lumbosacral nerve injury.

Sacrococcygeal Injuries (A3.1 Injuries)

Injury to the os coccyx presents as a fracture or a sacrococcygeal dislocation (Fig. 16-9). Conservative, functional treatment with pain medication and pain-dependent mobilization is the treatment of choice.

A closed digital reduction may be indicated if displaced fractures are present with disturbances of the anal region. Persistent disturbing instabilities can be treated with coccygectomy or rarely open reduction with suturing by a median approach.

Undisplaced Sacral Transverse Fractures (A3.2 Fractures)

Nondisplaced transverse fractures of the sacrum below the S2 level (Fig. 16-10), that do not involve the pelvic girdle

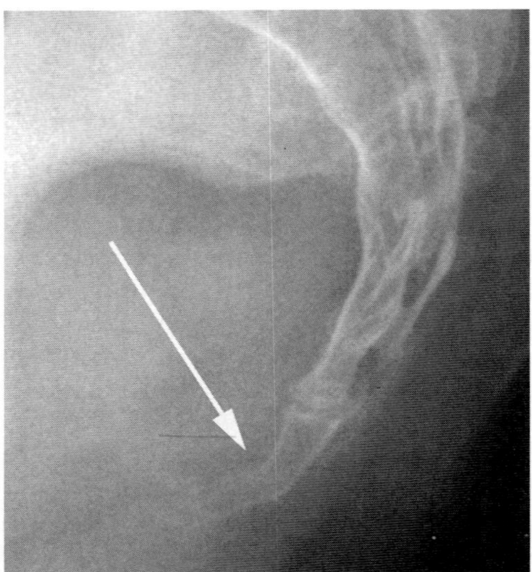

FIGURE 16-9. Example of an A 3.1 sacrum injury (e.g., a coccyx-fracture or sacrococcygeal dislocation).

should be treated with analgesics and pain-dependent mobilization directly after trauma, because nerve injuries normally are not present.

Displaced Sacral Transverse Fractures (A3.3 Fractures)

Displaced transverse sacral fractures below the S2 level (Fig. 16-11) are rare, but sacral plexus lesions are not uncommon. A sacral laminectomy with nerve root decompression and plate stabilization in the latter cases is recommended (technique: see Type C Fractures). The rate of neurologic recovery is unknown.

Rotationally Unstable Sacral Fractures (Type B Fractures)

Vertical fractures of the sacrum normally present as interruption of one or more sacral arcuate lines with no or only minor displacement. The pelvic girdle is completely stable with no instability of the anterior region in the majority of patients. Thus, conservative treatment of the pelvis is recommended, which consists of partial weight bearing of 3 to 6 weeks, dependent on the posterior pelvic pain. Follow-up x-rays after starting ambulation are highly important to detect possible secondary displacement in an unsuspected completely unstable (Type C) fracture.

Sometimes a fracture reduction by external rotation and anterior stabilization is performed in the presence of a malalignment of the pelvic ring (normally moderate internal rotation deformity). Anterior stabilization depends on the anterior pathology and consists of symphyseal plating, transpubic lag screws, or a simple supraacetabular anterior external fixator, which provides sufficient stability for anatomic healing under early ambulation (Fig. 16-12). An open reduction and internal stabilization of the sacrum normally is not necessary. Operative intervention in the sacrum region is only necessary when a neurologic deficit is present and bony fragments compromising neural structures are detected in the CT scan.

The treatment of an external rotation injury of the sacrum (OTA B1.2) is not clear, because the authors never saw such an injury within 600 sacral fractures at the Hannover series. However, if this is associated with >2.5 cm of symphyseal displacement, reduction of the anterior pelvic injury is required either by external fixation or internal plate stabilization.

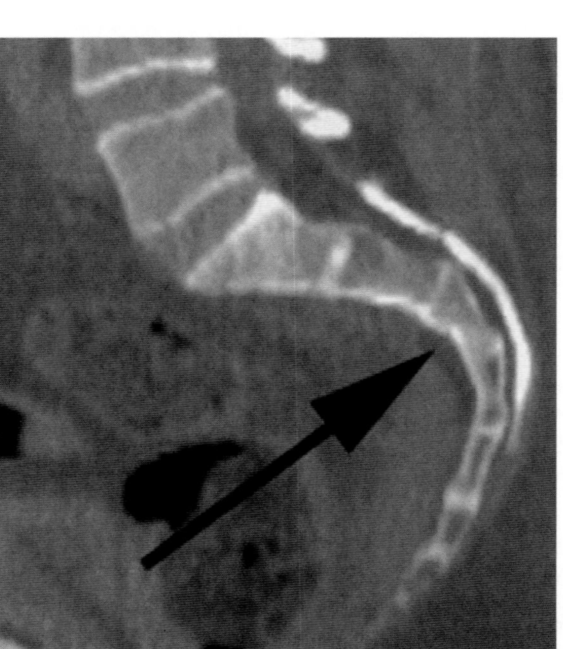

FIGURE 16-10. Example of an A 3.2 sacrum fracture, a nondisplaced transverse fracture of the sacrum below the level of S2, not involving the pelvic girdle.

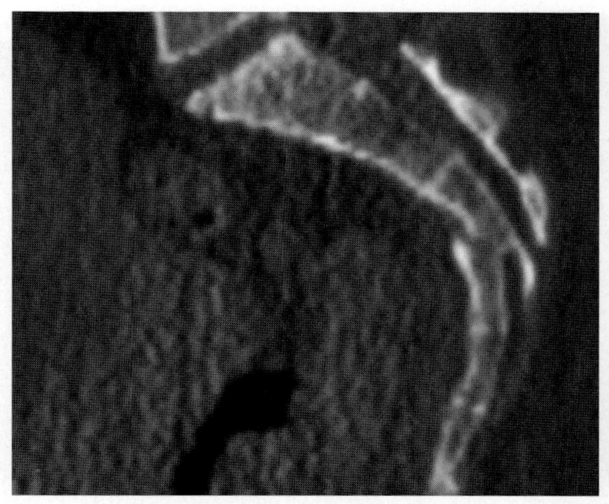

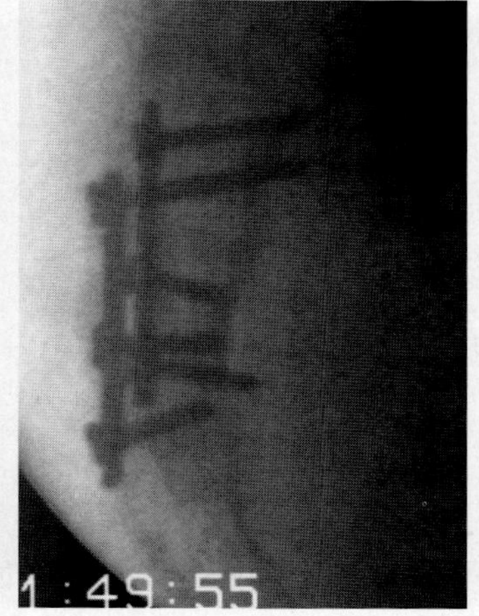

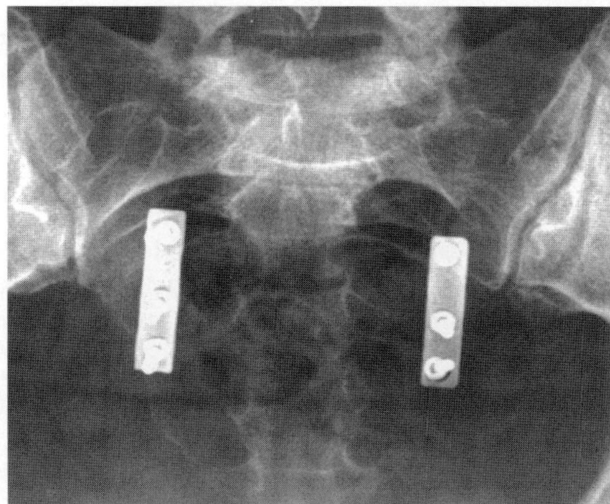

FIGURE 16-11. A: Example of displaced transverse sacral fractures below the level of S2 (A3.3 sacrum fracture). **B,C:** Sacral laminectomy with nerve root decompression and plate stabilization was performed because of a sacral plexus lesion.

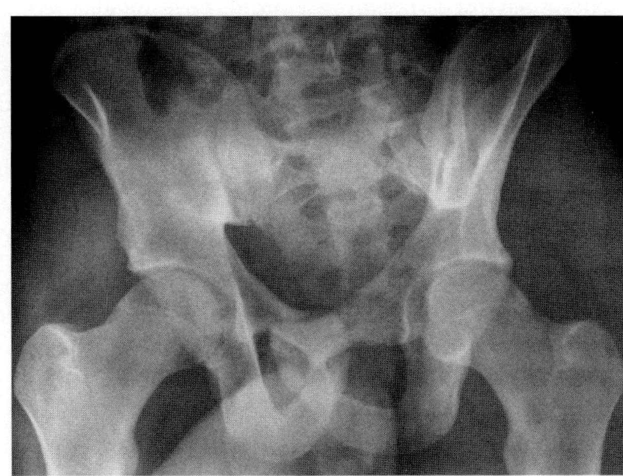

FIGURE 16-12. A: Lateral compression injury of the left sacrum together with a "locked" pubic symphysis with an internal rotation deformity after motor vehicle accident. (*Figure continues*)

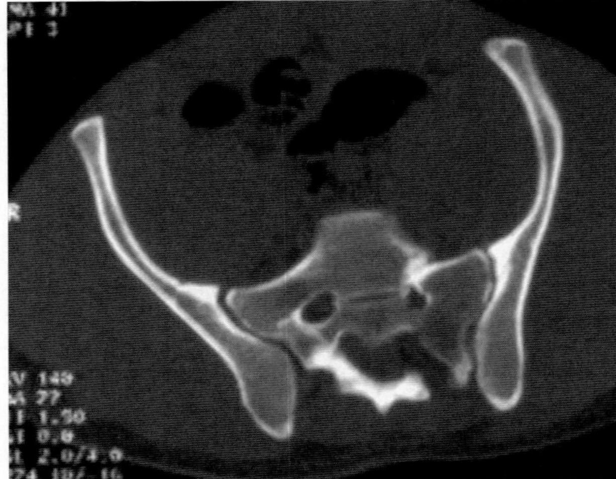
B

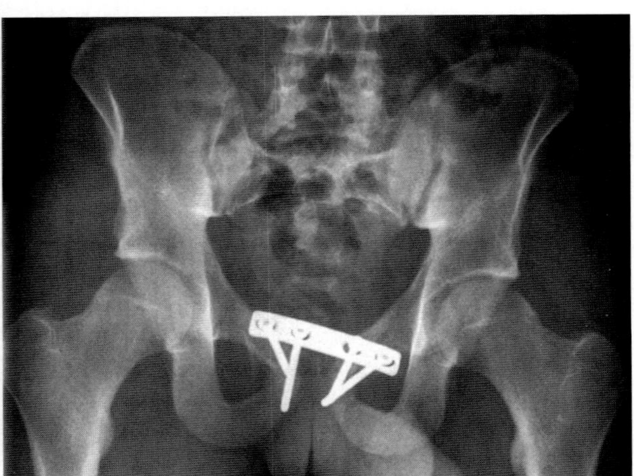
C

FIGURE 16-12. ***(continued)*** **B:** Computed tomography scan. **C:** Anterior reduction and plate fixation of the pubic symphysis led to an anatomic reconstruction of the pelvic girdle.

Completely Unstable Pelvic Ring Injury (Type C) with Potential Displacement and without Neurologic Deficit

These fractures can be treated sufficiently by percutaneous transiliosacral screw fixation techniques in order to minimize operative trauma.

The patient is placed either in the supine or prone position. Preoperatively, standard fluoroscopic views (anterior-posterior pelvis, inlet view, outlet view, and lateral sacral view) are mandatory. The lateral sacral view identifies the safe area of the S1 body and shows the sacral alar slope (Fig. 16-13).

A stab incision of about 1.5 to 2 cm in length is performed at the recommended entry point (crossing a line parallel to the axis of the femur with a line reaching from the anterior superior iliac spine to the posterior superior iliac spine). Further dissection is made by the use of a blunt instrument (e.g., clamp or hemostat). The outer cortex of the innominate bone is reached after spreading the fibers of the gluteus maximus and medius.

A 2-mm threaded K-wire is directed and drilled 10 mm into the S1 body under fluoroscopic control. The orientation of the K-wire is then evaluated in all four radiologic pelvic planes and corrected if necessary. The optimal position is reached with further drilling, when the fracture is overdrilled at least 20 mm. The pin depth is measured using a reverse ruler. The pin is overdrilled with a cannulated drill and a cannulated 7.3-mm screw with a 16-mm thread usually is inserted over a washer (Fig. 16-14). Matta recommended 16-mm threaded screws because of screw breakage in larger threads (63). An additional screw can be inserted into the S1 body, if necessary.

A screw insertion into the S2 body should be used only if it is ascertained that the pedicle diameter is adequate.

Completely Unstable Pelvic Ring Injury (Type C) with Major Displacement and/or a Neurologic Deficit

Open reduction, posterior sacral laminectomy with decompression of the sacral nerve roots, and stable internal fixation are recommended in these cases. The authors' preferred technique in stabilizing sacrum fractures is described in the following.

Surgical Approach

The patient is positioned prone on a regular radiolucent operating table. Intraoperative fluoroscopic control with inlet and outlet views should be possible, but are not mandatory for the procedure. Draping is performed with access to following landmarks: the posterior iliac crests, the spinal process of L4, and the upper end of the rima ani. The exact position of the skin incision is varied according to the fracture pattern (Fig. 16-15).

1. *Transforaminal and transalar sacrum fractures.* A longitudinal incision in the midline between the posterior iliac crest and the medial sacral crest is performed. The lumbosacral fascia is incised close to its origin at the spinal process L4 and L5 and the medial sacral crest (Fig. 16-16). The muscle is elevated from the sacrum with a sharp dissector or cautery knife (Fig. 16-17). If a more extensile exposure of the lateral sacral region ("ala") is necessary, then the complete muscle mass can be elevated by dissecting its lateral attachment to the posterior iliac crest. Take care to keep the soft tissues moist during the whole procedure.

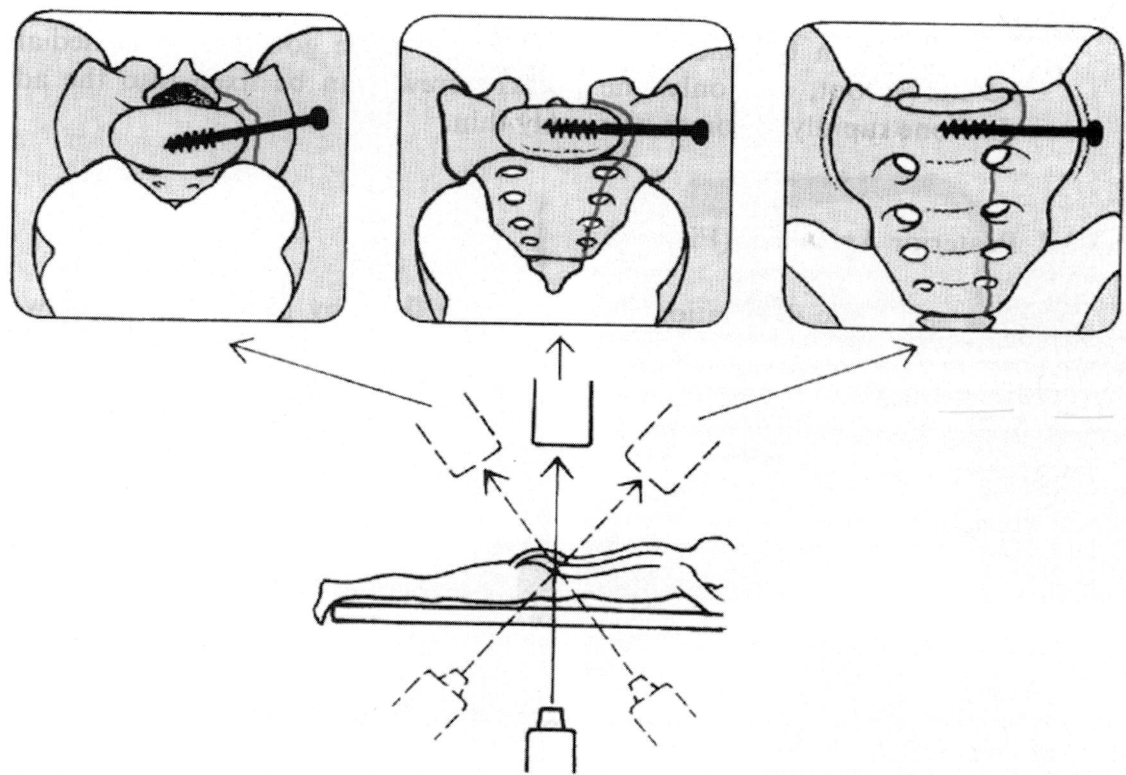

FIGURE 16-13. Standard fluoroscopic views intraoperatively. The technique of Matta (63) together with the true lateral view of the sacrum is used for transiliosacral screw fixation of sacrum fractures with fluoroscopic control of the screw insertion. (From: Matta J, Saucedo T. Internal fixation of pelvic ring fractures. *Clin Orthop* 1989;242:83–97, with permission.)

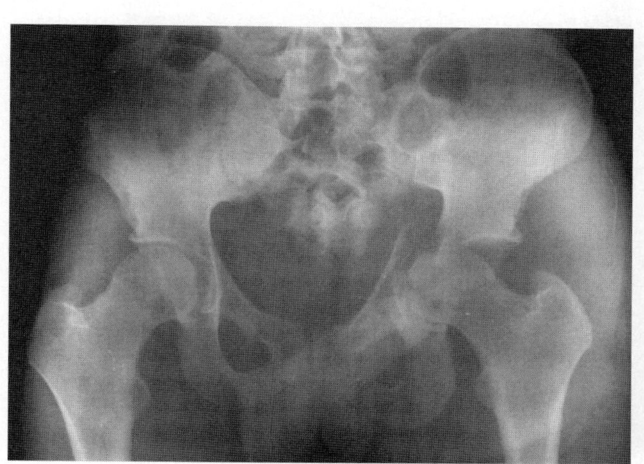

A

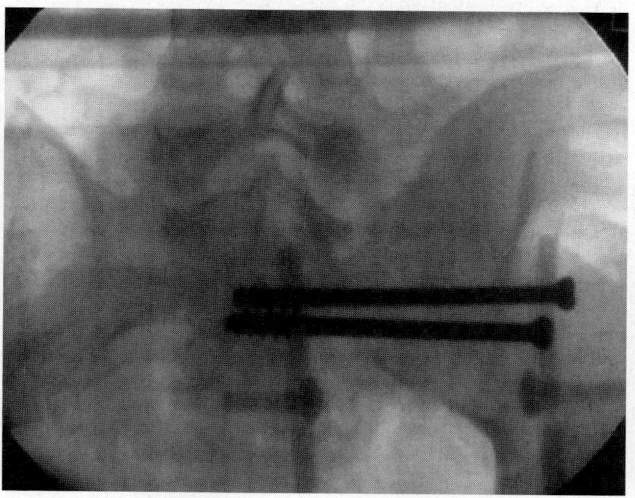

B

FIGURE 16-14. Example of a transiliosacral screw fixation in a transforaminal sacrum fracture with only minor displacement. The pelvic anterior-posterior x-ray shows the transforaminal fracture on the left side. Additionally, an ipsilateral T-type acetabular fracture is present **(A).** Under fluoroscopic control **(B–E)** two screws were inserted into the S1 and S2 body, because the S2 body had an adequate pedicle diameter. The postoperative x-ray shows anatomic reconstruction of the sacrum **(F).**

(Figure continues)

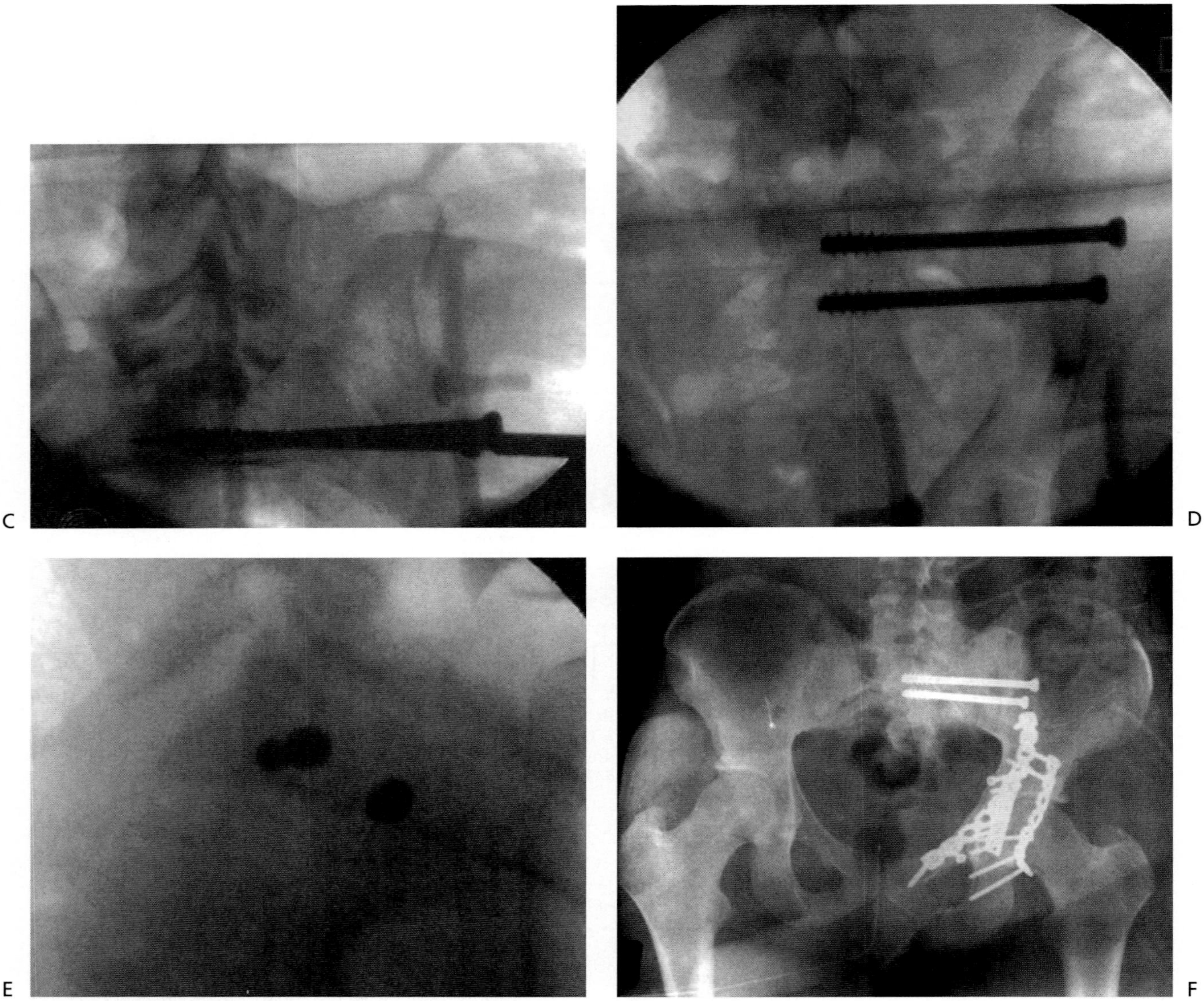

FIGURE 16-14. ***(continued)***

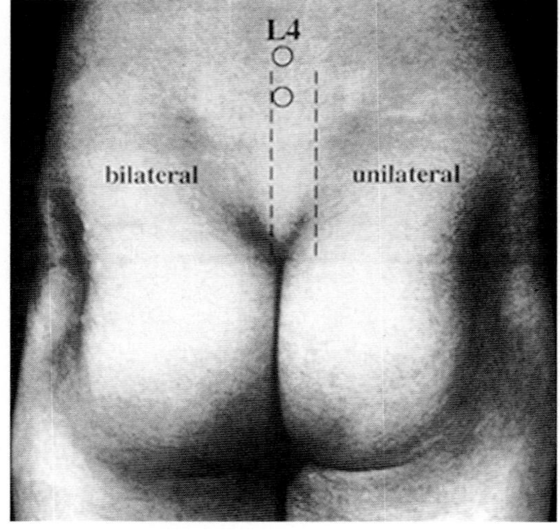

FIGURE 16-15. Landmarks for skin incision. In the prone position the following landmarks should be accessible after draping: the spinal process L4 and L5, posterior iliac crest, and upper border of the rima ani. If only the hemisacrum has to be exposed (transforaminal and transalar fracture pattern), then a longitudinal incision is performed in the midline between the medial sacral crest and posterior iliac crest. If a bilateral exposure of the sacrum is required (central fracture pattern, bilateral fractures), then a midline incision is performed.

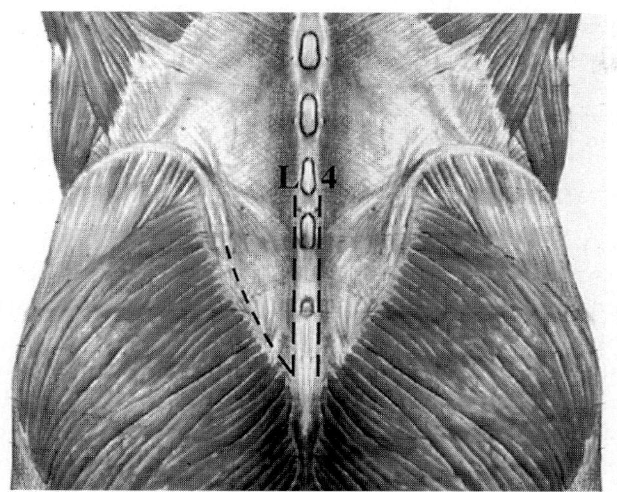

FIGURE 16-16. Deep exposure I. The lumbosacral fascial is incised close to its attachment at the median sacral crest and along the posterior iliac crest.

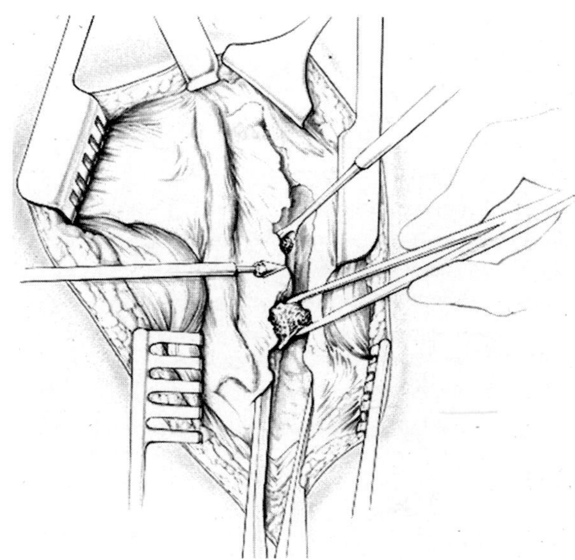

FIGURE 16-18. Sacral nerve root decompression I. The complete fracture line is inspected by using a lamina spreader. (From Tscherne H, Pohlemann T, eds. *Unfallchirurgie Becken und Acetabulum.* Heidelberg: Springer-Verlag, 1998, with permission.)

2. *Central and bilateral sacrum fractures.* A longitudinal midline incision close to the central sacral crest is used. The described deep preparation can be extended to both sides of the sacrum. The complete posterior aspect of the sacrum can be exposed using a single incision using this technique.

Reduction Techniques and Decompression

The complete fracture line has to be cleaned out completely and inspected. The overview is enhanced using a lamina spreader (Fig. 16-18). Fragments that may compromise the sacral nerve roots are extracted (Fig. 16-19). Their exact position preferably should be checked prior to operation by

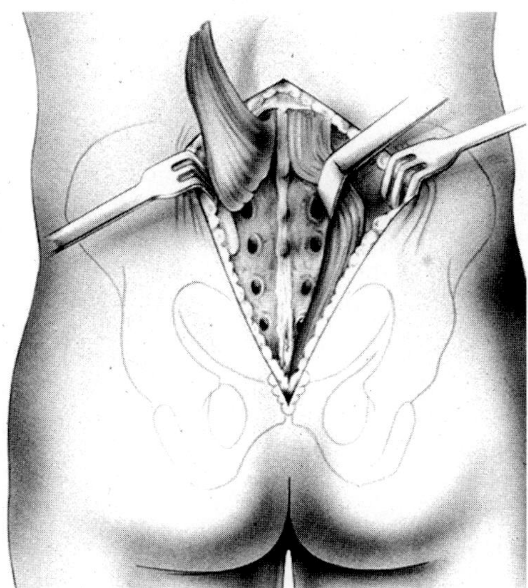

FIGURE 16-17. Deep exposure II. The posterior aspect of the sacrum is exposed by elevation of the lumbosacral muscles.

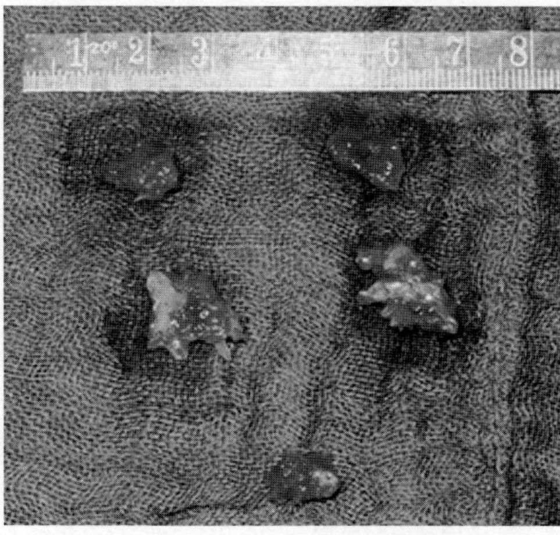

FIGURE 16-19. Sacral nerve root decompression II. Fragments that may compromise the sacral nerve roots are extracted.

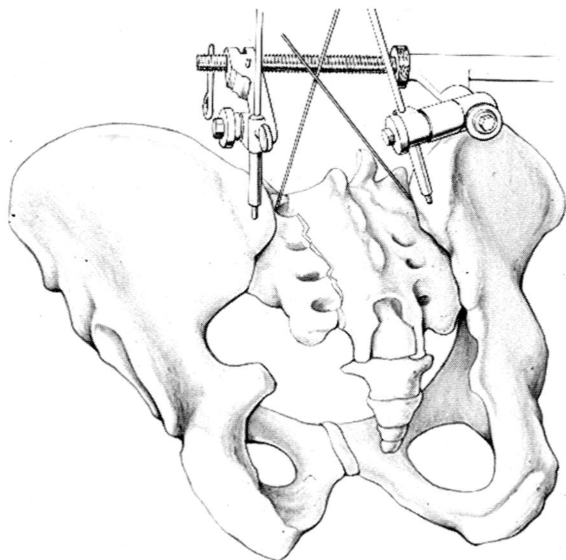

FIGURE 16-20. Reduction technique I. If a significant craniocaudal displacement of the main fragments is present, then a standard AO distractor is applied to both posterior iliac crests as a reduction aid. The reduction is achieved by slight manual elevation of the patient using the distractor.

analysis of the preoperative CT scan. A standard AO distractor is applied to both posterior iliac crests as a reduction aid if a significant craniocaudal displacement of the main fragments is present (Fig. 16-20). The fracture line can be exposed completely by distraction and the sacral nerve roots usually can be inspected down to the level of the ventral sacral foramen. Care has to be taken to avoid an iatrogenic injury to the presacral venous plexus. The reduction is achieved by slight manual elevation of the patient using the distractor. By torsion of the connecting bar of the distractor the vertical displacement is reduced and the compression is applied. The final anatomic reduction is realized and preliminarily fixed with pointed reduction forceps (Fig. 16-21). The orientation for reduction control is detected easily by inspecting the specific fracture pattern at the interforaminal region.

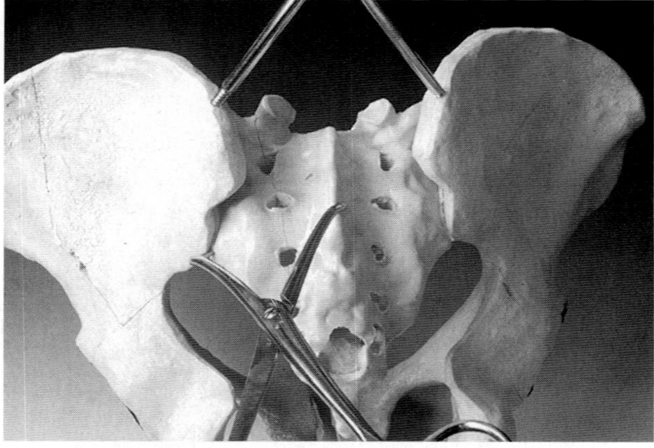

FIGURE 16-21. Reduction technique II. The final anatomic reduction is realized and preliminarily fixed with pointed reduction forceps.

Fixation

The implant fixation in the sacrum is complicated by the central sacral canal, the sacral foramina, and neurovascular structures close to the anterior sacrum lamina. Some "safe zones" have been identified in anatomic studies (Matta J, personal communication, 1992). The density of the sacral lamina is different in the various anatomic locations of the sacrum. Dense bone always can be expected at the region of the pelvic brim, close to the SI joints, and at the interforaminal regions. The potential for iatrogenic damage of nerve roots in the distal central canal is low because at that level the central canal is >70% filled with fat and connecting tissue (60). The use of a three-fluted drill together with the oscillating drill is generally recommended in the sacrum for increased safety.

1. *Lateral screw position (Fig. 16-22).* Screws can be placed lateral to the zone of the foramina without danger of perforating the foramina or central canal if the direction of the drill is strictly parallel to the plane of the SI joint. This plane can be identified easily by insertion of a Kirschner wire into the SI joint through the posterior sacroiliac ligaments. Care has to be taken when perforating the ventral lamina with the drill in order to avoid overpenetration, because neurovascular structures are in a close anatomic relation to the ventral aspect of the sacrum (as well as internal iliac vessels and lumbosacral trunk).

   The lateral screws have to be additionally orientated to the cranial lamina of the sacrum at the level of S1. This plane can be palpated by inserting a fingertip between the L5 transverse process and the sacrum.
2. *Medial screw position at S1.* At the level of S1 the medial entry point is directly underneath the distal rim of the L5-S1 facet joint. According to the larger anatomic dimensions at this level, usually two 3.5-mm screws can be placed from this position. The orientation of the drill is varied according to the specific fracture pattern.
   a. *Transalar (lateral) fracture line.* The drill is orientated perpendicular to the posterior sacral lamina, parallel to the orientation of the plane of the cranial sacral lamina and strictly in the sagittal plane (Fig. 16-22).
   b. *Transforaminal fracture line.* The direction of the drill for the medial screw can be angulated up to 20 degrees in the horizontal plane using the same inser-

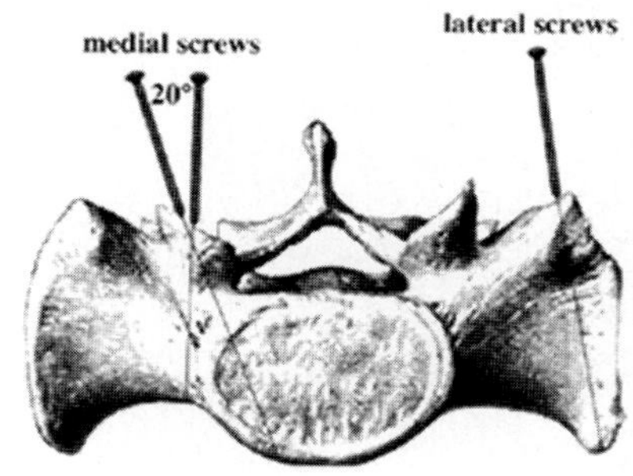

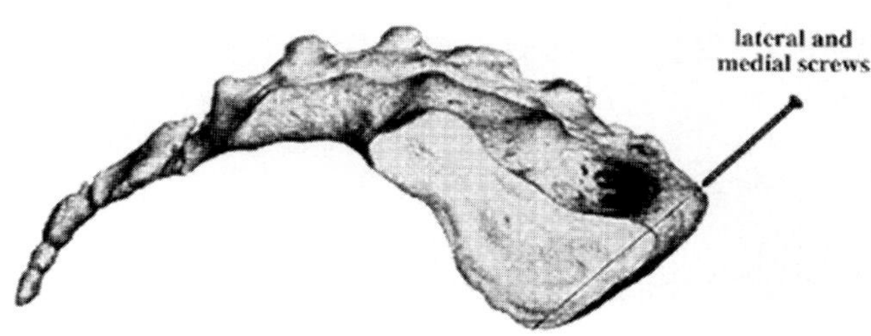

FIGURE 16-22. The lateral screws (alar screws) are positioned parallel to the plane of the SI joint. The medial screws are inserted perpendicular to the posterior aspect of the sacrum. Two orientations are possible at the level of S1. If a lateral fracture line is present, the screw is oriented in the sagittal plane and parallel to the cranial sacral lamina. In the transforaminal fracture line, the direction is inclined 20 degrees to the lateral side in order to realize a "transpeduncular" screw placement.

tion points, as described in the preceding (Fig. 16-22). The direction of the drill is parallel to the plane of the cranial sacral lamina in the sagittal and frontal plane. The screws are placed "transpeduncular" in this direction. At least two 3.5-mm screws should be used. Directed toward the sacral promontory an average screw length of 50 to 80 mm can be realized providing excellent stability.

3. *Medial screw position S2 to S4 (Fig. 16-22).* The entry points for the standard medial screws are identified by an imaginary vertical line through the foramina. The exact location is in the middle of the distance between two foramina. The direction of the drill has to be oriented perpendicular to the posterior sacral lamina. The implant fixation must be extended to the contralateral side if the fracture line is running into the intended fixation area. The more medial screw placement described poses a significant danger of perforating the central canal.

Fracture Stabilization and Choice of Implants

Implants for stabilization are standard AO small fragment DC plates, H plates that are cut to the required length, and flattened one-third tubular plates. The fracture line has to be crossed by at least two implants, preferably at the S1 and S3 or S4 level. The position of the implants is determined by the specific fracture pattern.

1. *Transalar fractures (zone I).* If the lateral sacral fragment is of sufficient size for screw placement, then the fracture is plated using H plates at the level of S1 and additionally at S3 and/or S4. If a zone of fragmentation is close to the SI joint and prevents secure screw placement, then the lateral fixation has to include the ilium. An H plate or reconstruction plate is contoured to the posterior aspect of the sacrum at the S1 level, extending from the medial insertion point beneath the L5-S1 facet joint to the medial aspect of the posterior iliac crest, and ending at the posterior superior iliac spine (Fig. 16-23). The lateral 3.5-mm screws (up to 80 to 100 mm) are inserted between the iliac cortices. The distal fracture line is stabilized by standard H plates or one-third tubular plates (Fig. 16-24). In cases where a medial screw fixation cannot be realized, the midline has to be crossed and LCDC plates are used as described for central and bilateral fractures.
2. *Transforaminal fractures (zone II).* The fracture line is stabilized using standard or modified small fragment plates (AO H plates, flat one-third tubular plates). A recently developed prototype sacrum plate (25) has the advantage of increased stiffness and optimized positions for medial screw placement at the S1 level (34,35). The distal fracture line is stabilized by additional H plates or one-third tubular plates at the level S3 and/or S4 (Figs. 16-25 and 16-26).
3. *Central fractures (zone III) and bilateral fractures (Figs. 16-27 and 16-28).* The fracture is stabilized by two LCDC plates that are positioned parallel to each other at the S1 and S3 levels. A lateral screw is placed at each end of the plates. Stability can be increased by additional

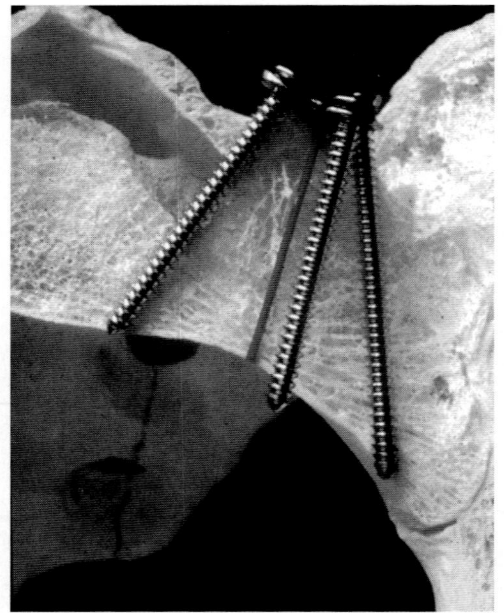

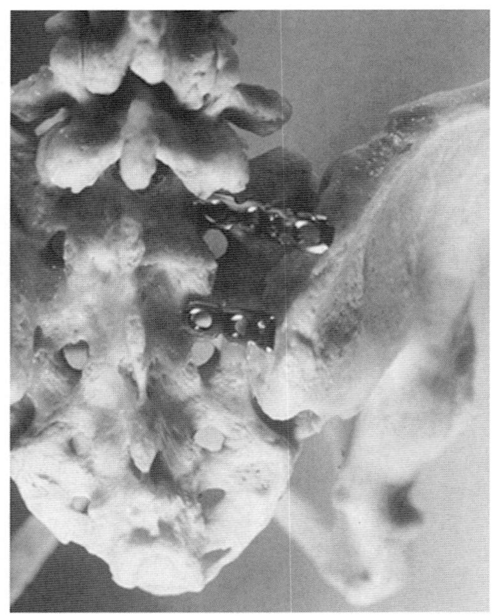

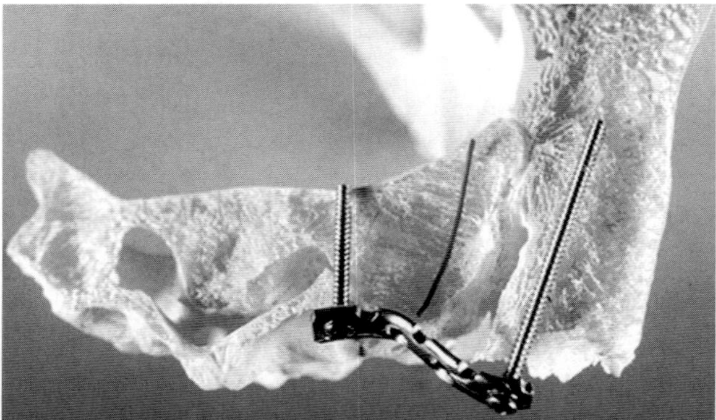

FIGURE 16-23. Stabilization technique in transalar fractures. If the lateral sacral fragment is of sufficient size for screw placement, then the fracture is plated using H plates at the level of S1 **(A).** If a comminution zone in the lateral part of the sacrum prevents safe screw positioning in the sacrum, then the lateral fixation has to be extended to the ilium. Reconstruction plates, or H plates, are applied as demonstrated. **B:** The implant position is shown on the posterior view. **C:** The screw position is demonstrated with a specimen cut horizontally at the level of S1.

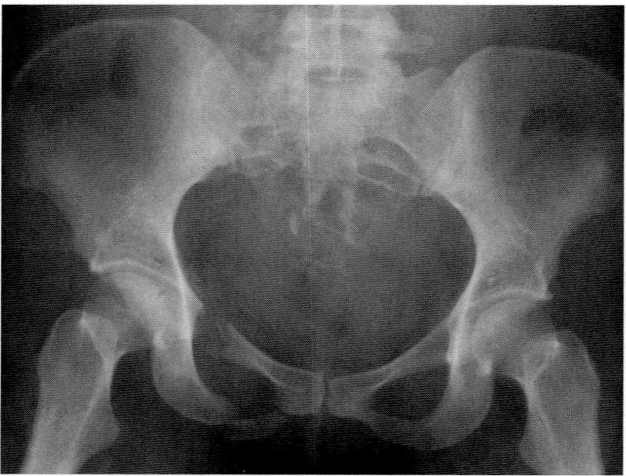

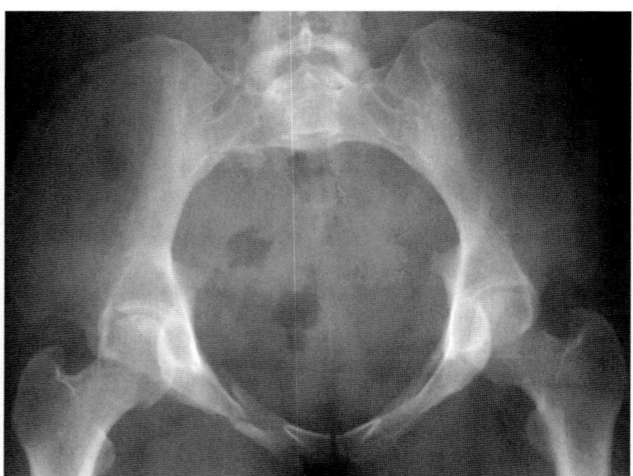

FIGURE 16-24. Example of an iliosacral plate fixation in a transalar fracture. The pelvic anterior-posterior view **(A),** inlet **(B),** and outlet view **(C)** show the fracture line on the right. The computed tomography reveals the comminution zone within the transalar region **(D).**

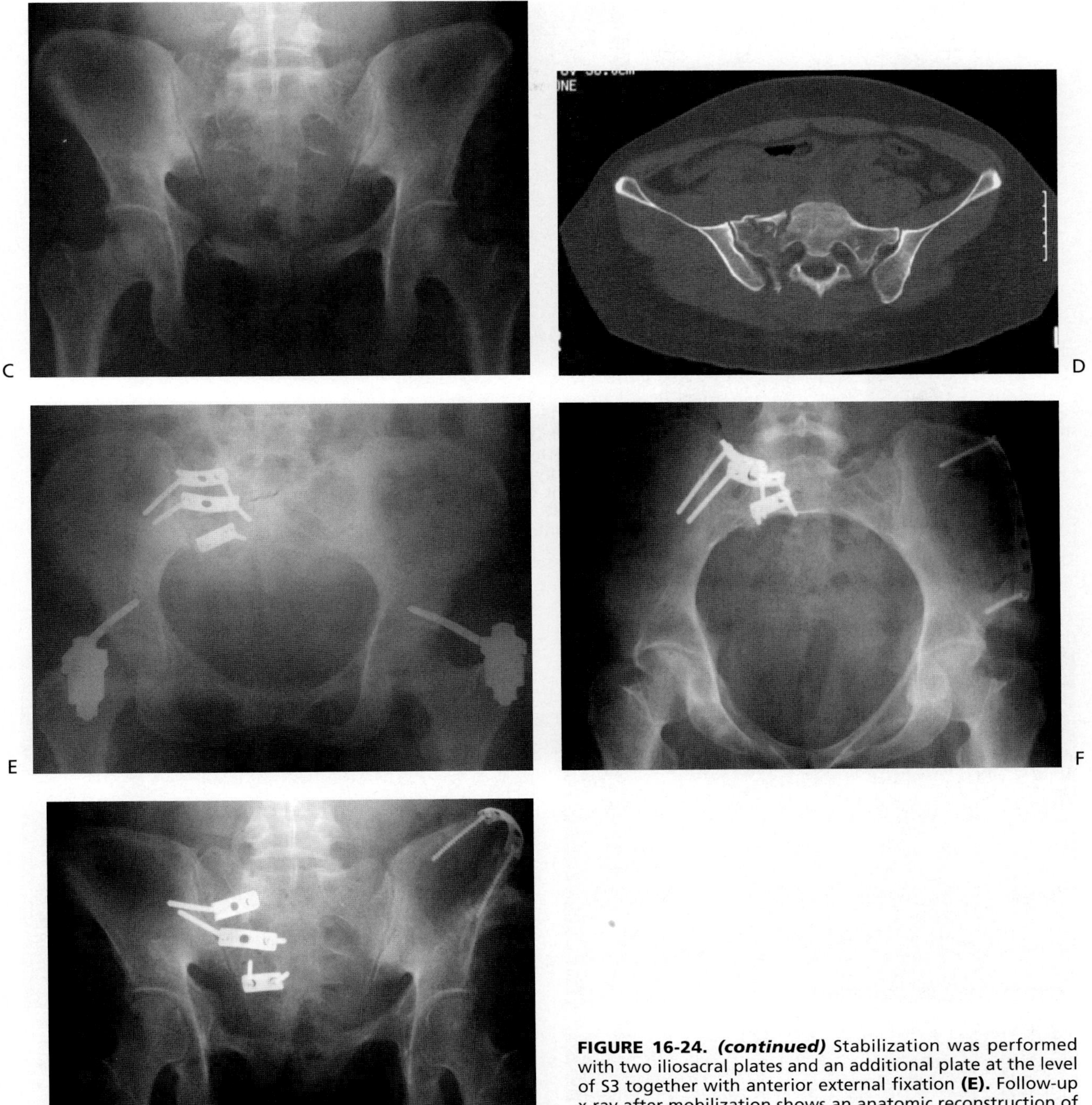

FIGURE 16-24. ***(continued)*** Stabilization was performed with two iliosacral plates and an additional plate at the level of S3 together with anterior external fixation **(E).** Follow-up x-ray after mobilization shows an anatomic reconstruction of the pelvic girdle **(F–G).**

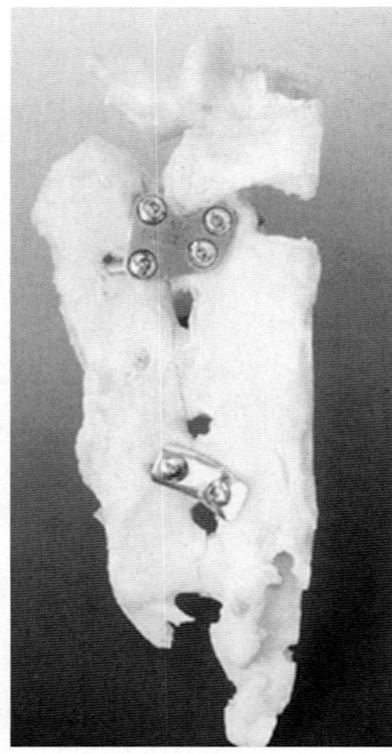

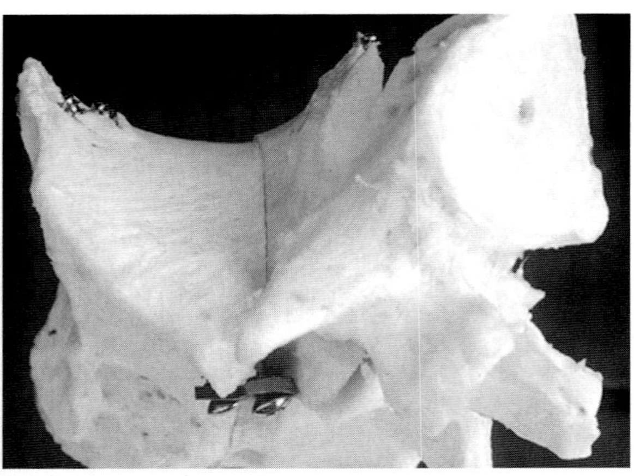

FIGURE 16-25. Stabilization technique in transforaminal fractures: The implant position for transforaminal fractures is demonstrated in a posterior **(A)** and cranial view **(B)** of a dry sacrum. A prototype sacrum plate allows the placement of two lateral and two medial screws at the level of S1. A flat two-hole one-third tubular plate provides additional stability at the level of S4.

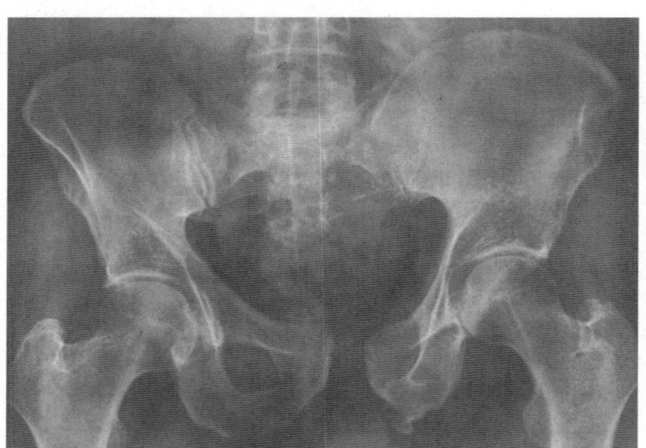

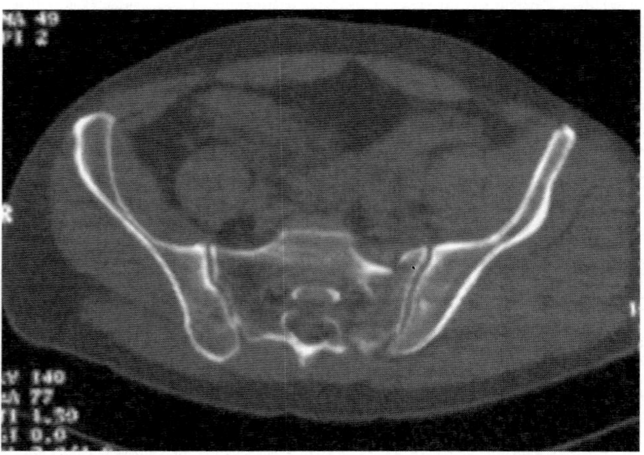

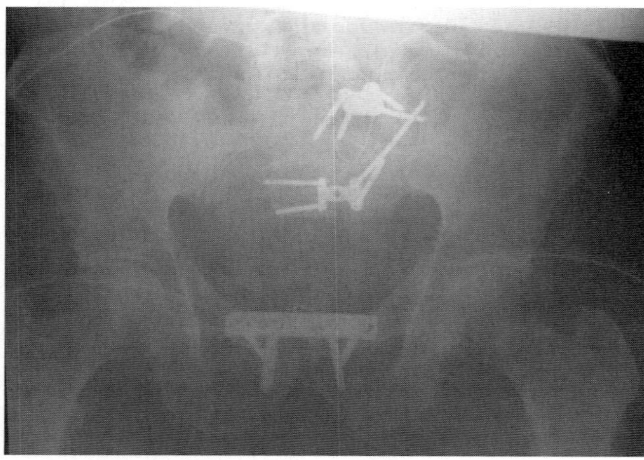

FIGURE 16-26. Example of a typical "localized" plate fixation in a transforaminal fracture. The pelvic anterior-posterior view **(A)** shows the fracture line on the left. The computed tomography reveals the typical transforaminal fracture **(B).** Stabilization was performed with a prototype sacrum plate at the level of S1 and an additional flat H plate at the level of S3. The pubic symphysis was fixed with a four-hole DC plate **(C).**

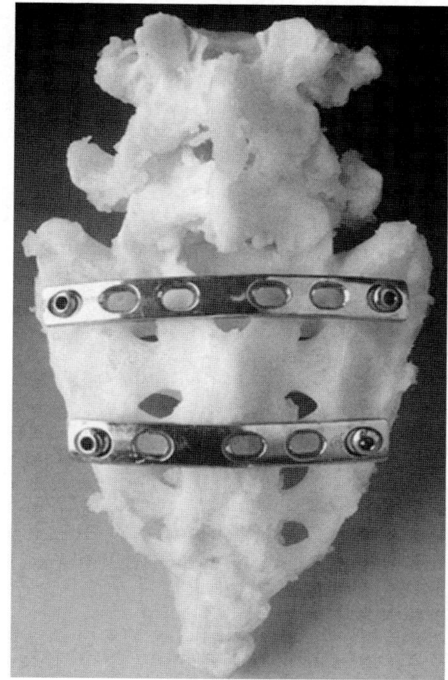

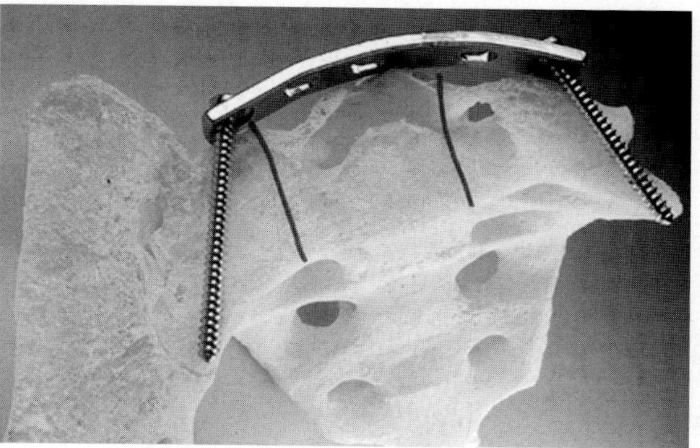

FIGURE 16-27. Stabilization technique in central and/or bilateral sacrum fractures: Two 3.5-mm DC plates are contoured to the posterior aspect of the sacrum **(A)** and are fixed in the left and right alar region of the sacrum **(B).**

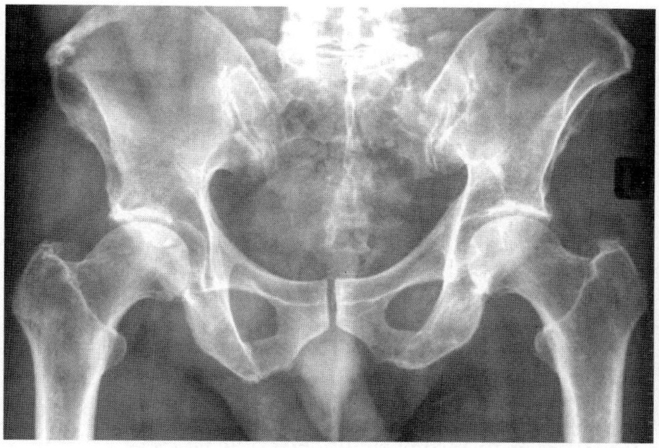

FIGURE 16-28. Example of a plate fixation in a central fracture. The pelvic anterior-posterior view **(A)** shows a transforaminal fracture line on the left. The computed tomography reveals the transforaminal component **(B).** Sagittal reconstruction shows the transverse component of the central fracture **(C).**Stabilization was performed with four plates contoured to the posterior aspect of the sacrum. Both cranial plates were fixed within the iliac bone because of a lateral extension of the fracture into the transalar region **(D).**

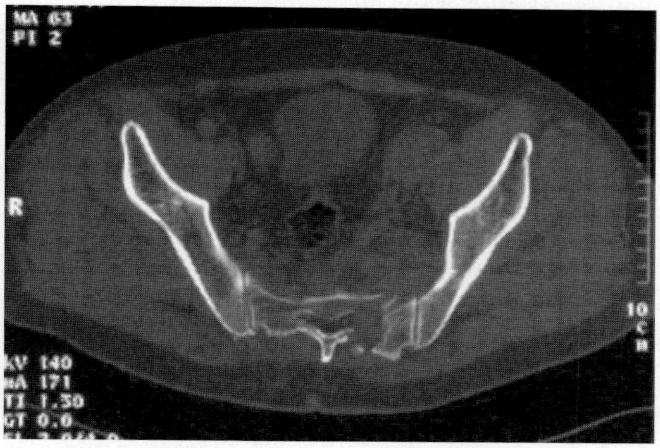

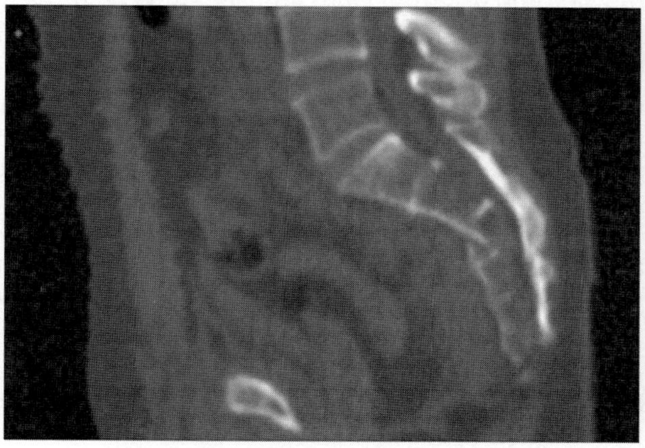

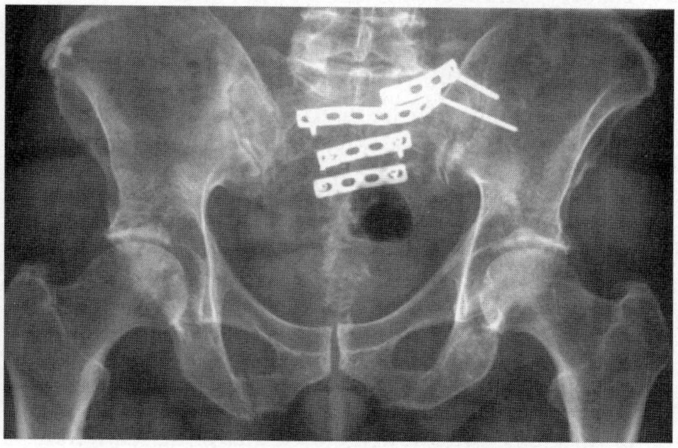

medial screws if the described anatomic requirements can be met. The stabilization can be increased by additional H plates or one-third tubular plates according to the fracture pattern. If a zone of fragmentation about a foramen is present, overcompression of the foramen must be avoided so that the nerve root is not injured. However, the fracture must be reduced, and bone grafting the nonforaminal areas is necessary to assure union if gaps are left. The LCDC plates have to act as "neutralization" plates.

Stabilization of the anterior pelvic ring is necessary after the posterior stabilization of the sacrum is finished, because the posterior implants can only act as "tension band" types of stabilization; therefore, they need additional anterior fixation for sufficient stability (closure of the anterior pelvic ring).

The following standard methods are recommended.

- At least a four-hole plate is used for disruptions of the symphysis pubis plate fixation. The procedure is performed using a Pfannenstiel incision.
- An anterior external fixator is applied if an unilateral or bilateral fracture of the pubic rami is present. A simple two-pin frame is sufficient, with one pin in each supraacetabular region. The frame is removed after 3 weeks, because a rapid callus formation provides early stability.
- The pubic fractures can be stabilized easily by additional transpubic lag screws after plating of the symphysis if the disruption of the symphysis pubis is combined with transpubic instabilities. The Pfannenstiel incision must not be extended for this additional procedure. The direction of the 3.5-mm lag screws corresponds to an anterior column screw frequently used in acetabular surgery, which is inserted in the opposite direction. Another option is plating the symphysis. If the pubic rami fractures reduce, then neutralize them with an anterior external fixator.

After stabilization of the fracture, one deep and one epifascial suction drainage may be inserted. The fascia and skin are closed as per surgeon's protocol.

Completely Unstable Pelvic Ring Injury (Type C) with Major Displacement and without Neurologic Deficit

This complete unstable pelvic ring injury (Type C) with major displacement and without neurologic deficit can be treated in different ways. When closed anatomic reduction is possible percutaneous transiliosacral screw fixation in the prone or supine position is feasible.

Open reduction and internal sacral fixation as described or spino-pelvic fixation techniques (see Suicidal Jumper's Fracture) are possible with persistent displacement.

Suicidal Jumper's Fracture

The criteria of a suicidal jumper's fracture are a U-shaped or H-type fracture of the upper sacrum with a transverse fracture line, normally at the level of S1 or S2.

According to the Roy-Camille classification for suicidal jumper's fractures (50), a flexion fracture with anterior bending (Type 1), a flexion fracture with posterior displacement (Type 2), and an extension fracture (Type 3) can be distinguished.

These fractures are accompanied by a high rate of lumbosacral plexus lesions. Roy-Camille recommended sacral decompression with lumbosacral or lumboiliac plate stabilization for this specific fractures type (50).

Stabilization of H-Type Fractures/Displaced U-Shaped Fractures

Our concept of open reduction, posterior decompression of the central canal and the sacral nerve roots in combination with posterior spinopelvic fixation showed an encouraging rate of adequate reductions and an acceptable rate of neurologic recovery (62).

Reduction is preoperatively performed by hyperextension of the hip joints with simultaneous extension in the prone position (raising the extended legs under lateral fluoroscopic control of the sacrum). A closed percutaneous transiliosacral screw fixation can be performed in case of successful reduction. Open reduction is necessary in all other cases. Nerve root decompression is performed as described after dorsal laminectomy.

A longitudinal midline incision is performed from L3 to the rima ani. The deep preparation elevates both erector spinae muscles from the lumbar spine and sacrum. Laminectomy and nerve root decompressions sometimes have to be extended to the lumbar nerve roots because avulsions can be present up to the L1 nerve roots. After adequate reduction, the posterior iliac crest is prepared bilaterally from the midline approach for insertion of the pedicle screws.

Stabilization is performed by spinopelvic fixation from the lumbar spine to the posterior iliac bone. A standard internal fixator system is used, with transpeduncular anchorage within the L4 and L5 pedicles and pedicle screw insertion in the posterior ilium. One or two transverse stabilizers are attached to the system to avoid rotational deformity (Fig. 16-29).

A careful mobilization under avoidance of lumbosacral flexion movements is recommended because of substantial

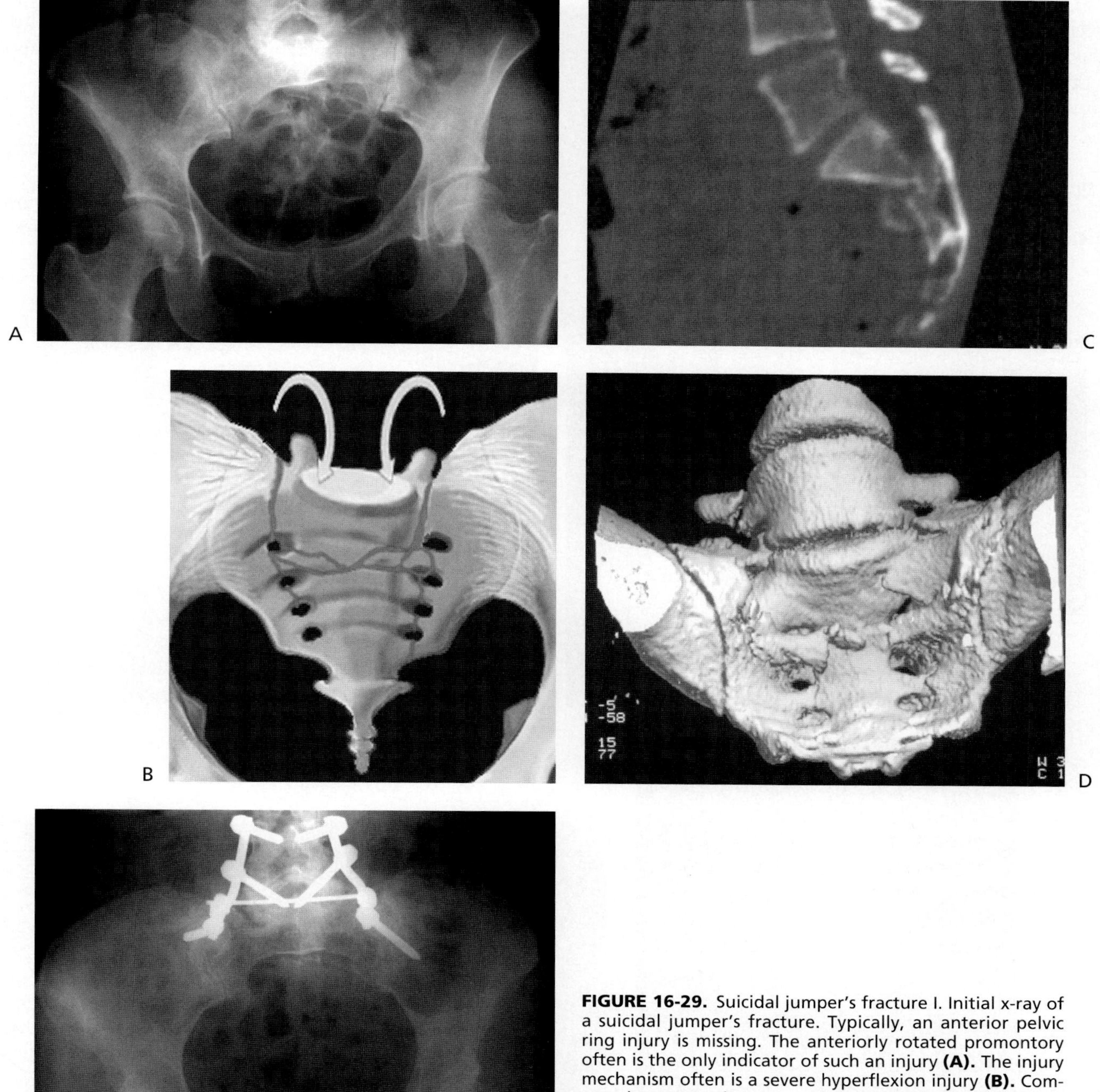

FIGURE 16-29. Suicidal jumper's fracture I. Initial x-ray of a suicidal jumper's fracture. Typically, an anterior pelvic ring injury is missing. The anteriorly rotated promontory often is the only indicator of such an injury **(A).** The injury mechanism often is a severe hyperflexion injury **(B).** Computed tomography scan and sagittal reformation shows the anteriorly displaced S1 and S2 bodies **(C).** Three-dimensional computed tomography shows the direction of displacement and the typical H-type fracture **(D).**The postoperative view after spinopelvic fixation shows a good reduction of the promontory **(E).**

lever forces. Partial weight bearing of the predominantly affected leg is allowed for 12 weeks postoperatively. A careful prophylaxis for decubital ulcers is recommended because of the superficial implants. Thus, implant removal is performed 6 to 9 months after the injury.

Stabilization of Undisplaced U-Shaped Fractures

Undisplaced U-shaped fractures have the advantage of persistent stability of the sacrum within the pelvic girdle as both vertical fractures do not leave the sacrum. Thus, no stabilization of the sacrum itself is needed. Reduction can be held with bilateral transiliosacral screw fixation of the U-shaped fragment in these cases (Fig. 16-30).

PERIOPERATIVE AND POSTOPERATIVE CARE

If the patient is in an adequate general condition early ambulation with partial weight bearing is allowed after removal

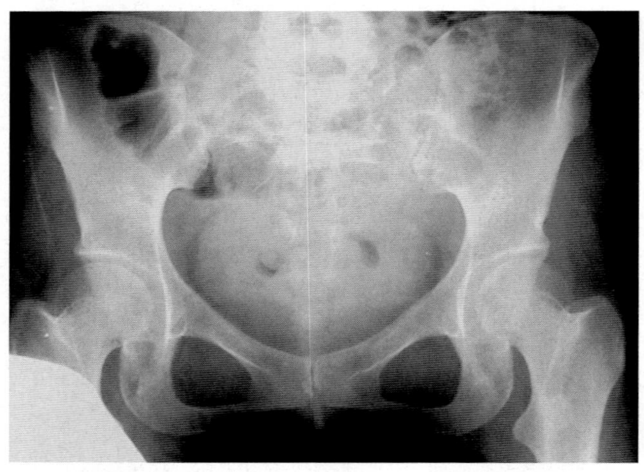
A

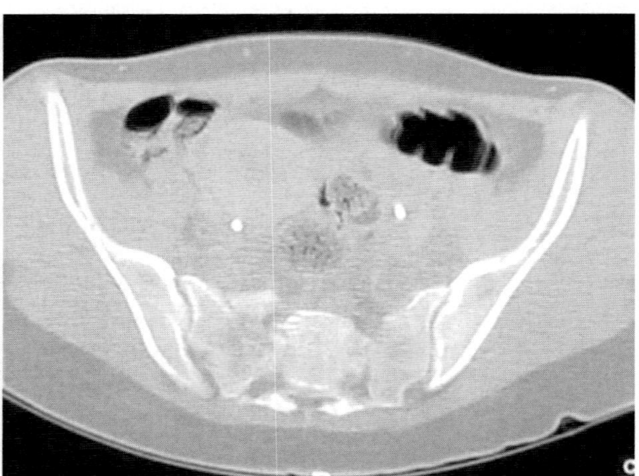
C

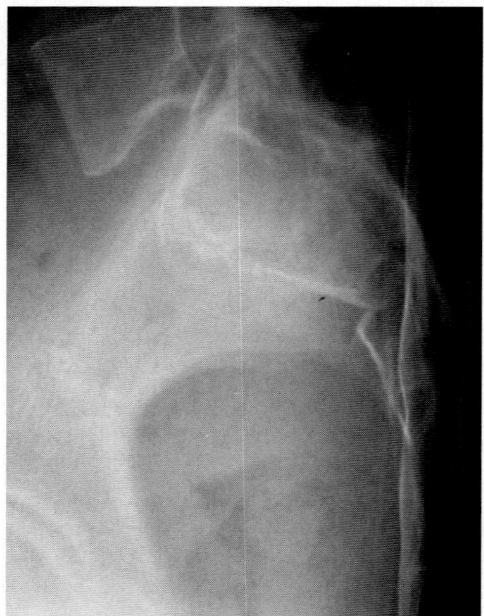
B

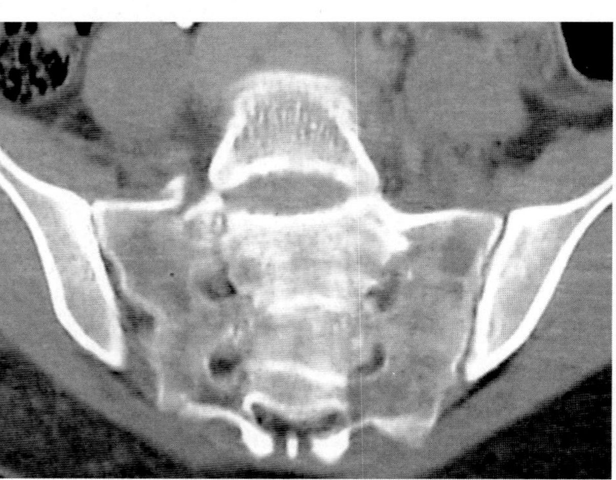
D

FIGURE 16-30. Suicidal jumper's fracture II. Undisplaced U-shaped fractures can sufficiently be stabilized by transiliosacral screw fixation in the absence of an additional nerve injury. Initial x-ray of a suicidal jumper's fracture without injury to the anterior pelvic ring **(A).** The true lateral view shows the transverse fracture line at the level of S1-2 **(B).** Axial computed tomography scan **(C),**frontal reformation **(D),** and sagittal reformation **(E)** show the nearly undisplaced S1 and S2 bodies. The postoperative x-rays after bilateral transiliosacral screw fixation show an anatomic reconstructed posterior pelvic ring **(F)** and a safe screw position within S1 **(G).**

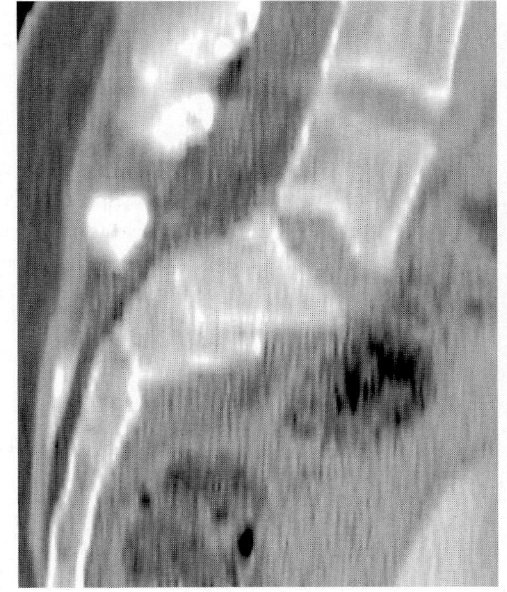
E

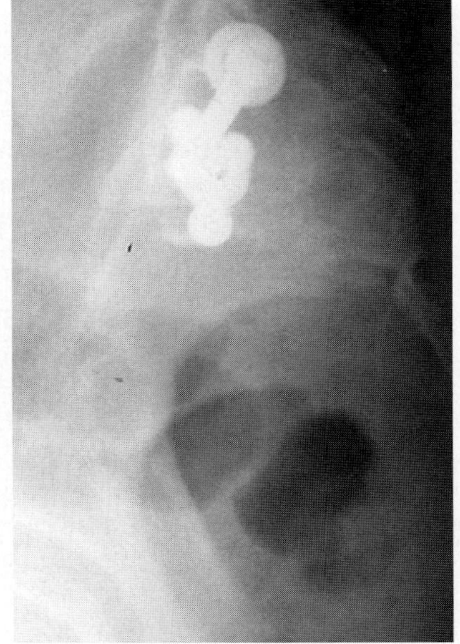
G

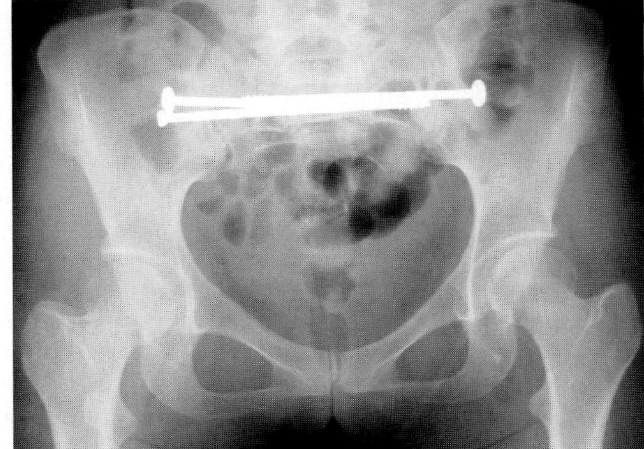
F

FIGURE 16-30. ***(continued)***

of the suction drainages. Complete healing can be expected after 6 weeks. Implants may be removed 12 month after the injury if symptomatic.

RESULTS OF TREATMENT

Open Reduction and Internal Fixation of Sacral Fractures: Completely Unstable Pelvic Ring Injuries (Type C)

Between 1989 and 1998, 101 patients with completely unstable (Type C) sacral fractures were treated within the Hannover series. Fifty-six patients were treated operatively. Six patients had sacral stabilization with sacral bars, three had transiliosacral leg screw fixation, two had iliosacral plate fixation, one had a lumbo-iliosacral internal fixator (spinopelvic fixation), and one had a combination of different stabilization techniques. Forty-three patients were stabilized with the preferred, previously described "localized" sacral stabilization techniques.

Thirty-five patients had unilateral sacral fractures (61-C1.3). In six patients the sacral fracture was part of the posterior Type C instability in combination with a contralateral Type B injury (61-C2.3). Two patients had bilateral translational unstable pelvic ring injuries: The sacral fracture was accompanied by an SI-dislocation and an ilium fracture. According to Denis, 35 patients had a zone II transforaminal fracture, two had a zone I injury (transalar fracture), and six had a central sacral fracture (zone III).

The average preoperative sacral displacement was 14.4 mm (2- to 35-mm). The average direction of displacement was 11.9 mm in the cranial, 6.4 mm in the lateral, and 6.8 mm in the dorsal direction.

A sacral nerve root decompression (e.g., laminectomy, fragment removal) of the central sacral canal was performed during stabilization in 34 patients. No nerve deficit was found preoperatively and postoperatively in the nine patients without decompression.

The quality of reduction was completely anatomic in 37 cases (86%). In five cases cranial displacement up to 5 mm was accepted. A persistent 26-mm distraction of the fracture side was accepted in one case of a comminuted transforaminal fracture during pregnancy.

Postoperative secondary displacement was observed in two cases. A suboptimal screw-hold was noted in all cases.

The 41 survivors were mobilized an average of 5 days (range, 4 to 6 days) after internal stabilization. In all cases, the patient had partial weight bearing for 6 weeks.

Twenty-five of the surviving 41 patients had no signs of a sacral fracture–related nerve deficit at primary and postoperative evaluation. Primary neurologic examination was impossible in two patients because of artificial unconsciousness—one patient had no nerve injury postoperatively, and the other had a sensory and motor nerve deficit of the L3, L4, L5, and S1 nerve roots. Three patients had incomplete paraplegia at the level of their spinal injury.

Primary neurologic evaluation revealed lesions of the lumbosacral plexus in the remaining 11 patients. The S1 root was involved in the majority ($n = 7$); five had lesions of the L4, L5, or S3-5 roots. One patient had an insufficiency of the rectal sphincter preoperatively.

Of 11 patients with preoperative sacral fracture–related nerve deficit, three patients had complete recovery and three patients had partial recovery postoperatively. No change from the preoperative nerve deficit was found in five patients.

One iatrogenic nerve injury was seen (motor deficit L3-S1), with complete recovery 8 weeks postoperatively.

Suicidal Jumper's Fracture

Sixteen patients with a suicidal jumper's fracture were treated within the Hannover series between 1977 and 1999.

According to the OTA classification, 15 patients had a complete suicidal jumper's fracture (61-C3.3) and one patient an incomplete suicidal jumper's fracture (61-C2.3). The anterior pelvic ring injury was involved in five of the cases.

According to Roy-Camille, four patients had a flexion fracture with anterior bending (Type 1), five had flexion fracture with posterior displacement (Type 2), and seven had an extension fracture (Type 3).

The type of treatment was nonoperatively in five patients and operatively in 11 patients. In the nonoperative group four patients had closed reduction and were treated with bed rest for 3 to 12 weeks. In one patient with a minimally displaced sacral fracture (20 degrees angulation) no reduction was performed, bed rest was done for 3 weeks.

Of the 11 patients treated operatively, a posterior sacral decompression without sacral stabilization was performed in two patients. The remaining nine patients were treated with open reduction, posterior decompression, and spinopelvic stabilization. Postoperative mobilization was started 4 days after operation, dependent of additional lower leg injuries. Full weight bearing was allowed after 12 weeks.

The postoperative angulation was decreased to a mean angle of 16 degrees (10 to 35 degrees) compared to a preoperative mean angular deformity of 35 degrees (10 to 67 degrees).

Perioperative local wound complications were observed in three operatively treated patients. One patient developed deep infection, which healed after surgical revision. Two seromas were observed, requiring single revision. No deep vein thrombosis was observed.

All but one patient had a primary neurologic deficit with involvement of the sacral plexus. In 14 of 16 patients there was a sensory deficit at the perineum (S3-5 nerve roots), 11 patients had an S2 sensory involvement, and 10 had an S1 sensory injury. The lumbar levels L3-5 were uncommon for sensory deficits.

Motor dysfunction was present in 11 cases for the S1 root and eight cases for the L5 root. In the nonoperative group one patient had a partial recovery and one had a complete recovery of the initial nerve deficit.

Decompression of the central sacral canal and/or spinopelvic stabilization of the sacral fracture resulted in two partial recoveries of the preoperative sacral fracture–related nerve deficit, as well as two complete recoveries. No change to the preoperative nerve deficit was found in seven patients.

REFERENCES

1. Asher M, Strippgen W. Anthropometric studies of the human sacrum related to dorsal transsacral implant design. *Clin Orthop* 1985;203:58–62.
2. Brown T, Stone J, Schuster J, et al. External fixation of unstable pelvic ring fractures: comparative rigidity of some current frame configurations. *Med Biol Eng Comput* 1982;20:727–733.
3. Dowling T, Epstein JA, Epstein NE. S1-S2 sacral fracture involving neural elements of the cauda equina. A case report and review of the literature. *Spine* 1985;10(9):851–853.
4. Duwelius P, et al. Computed tomography-guided fixation of unstable posterior pelvic ring disruptions. *J Orthop Trauma* 1992;6(4):420–426.
5. Ecke H, Hofmann D. Indikation und Technik der Osteosyn-

these bei Beckenringverletzungen: Zuggurtung. *Hefte Unfallheilkunde* 1986;181:581–582.
6. Gibbons K, Soloniuk D, Razack N. Neurologic injury and patterns of sacral fractures. *J Neurosurg* 1990;72:889–893.
7. Goodell C. Neurologic deficits associated with pelvic fractures. *J Neurosurg* 1966:837–842.
8. Jackson H, Kam J, Harris J. The sacral arcuate lines in upper sacral fractures. *Radiology* 1982;145:35–39.
9. Kellam JF, McMurtry RY, Paley D, et al. The unstable pelvic fracture: operative treatment. *Orthop Clin North Am* 1987;18(1): 25–41.
10. Mears D, Fu F. Modern concepts of external skeletal fixation of the pelvis. *Clin Orthop* 1980;151:65–72.
11. Mears D, Rubash H. External and internal fixation of the pelvic ring. *AAOS Instr Course Lect* 1984;33:144–158.
12. Mears D, Capito C, Deleeuw H. Posterior pelvic disruptions managed by the use of the double cobra plate. *AAOS Instr Course Lect* 1988;37:143–150.
13. Nelson D, Duwelius P. CT-guided fixation of sacral fractures and sacroiliacal joint disruptions. *Radiology* 1991;180:527–532.
14. Denis F, Steven D, Comfort T. Sacral fractures: an important problem, retrospective analysis of 236 cases. *Clin Orthop* 1988; 227:67–81.
15. Pohlemann T, Gänsslen A, Tscherne H. Die Problematik der Sakrumfraktur, klinische Analyse von 377 Fällen. *Orthopäde* 1992;21:400–412.
16. Isler B. Lumbosacral lesions associated with pelvic ring injuries. *J Orthop Trauma* 1990;4(1):1–6.
17. Schmidek H, Schmith D, Kristiansen D. Sacral fractures. *Neurosurgery* 1984;15:735–746.
18. Sabiston C, Wing P. Sacral fractures: classification and neurologic implications. *J Trauma* 1986;26(12):1113–1115.
19. Wörsdörfer O, Magerl F. Sacrumfrakturen. *Hefte Unfallheilk* 1980;149:203–214.
20. Egbers H, et al. Stabilisierung des Beckenrings mit Fixatuer Externe: Biomechanische Untersuchungen und klinische Erfahrungen. *Orthopäde* 1992;21:363–372.
21. Josten C, Schildhauer T, Muhr G. Therapie instabiler Sacrumfrakturen bei Beckenringbrüchen. *Chirurg* 1994;65:970–975.
22. Käch K, Trentz O. Distraktionsspondylodese des Sakrums bei "Vertical-shear-Läsionen" des Beckens. *Unfall Chirurg* 1994; 97(1):28–38.
23. Levine A. Fixation of fractures of the sacrum. *Op Tech Orthop* 1997;7(3):221–231.
24. Norris B, et al. Pelvic fractures: sacral fixation. In: Wiss DA, ed. *Master techniques in orthopaedics: fractures.* Philadelphia: Lippincott Williams & Wilkins, 1998:613–630.
25. Pohlemann T, et al. Fixation of transforaminal sacrum fractures: a biomechanical study. *J Orthop Trauma* 1993;7(2): 107–117.
26. Pohlemann T, Tscherne H. Fixation of sacral fractures. *Tech Orthop* 1995;9(4):315–326.
27. Routt M, Simonian P. Closed reduction and percutaneous skeletal fixation of sacral fractures. *Clin Orthop* 1996; 329:121–128.
28. Schildhauer T, Josten C, Muhr G. Triangular osteosynthesis of vertically unstable sacrum fractures: a new concept allowing early weight bearing. *J Orthop Trauma* 1998;12(5):307–314.
29. Templeman D, et al. Internal fixation of displaced fractures of the sacrum. *Clin Orthop* 1996;329:180–185.
30. Weisl H. The movements of the sacro-iliac joint. *Acta Anatom* 1955;23:80–91.
31. Albee F. A study of the anatomy and the clinical importance of the sacroiliac joint. *JAMA* 1909;53:1273–1276.
32. Meyer G. Der Mechanismus der Symphysis sacro-iliaca. *Archiv Anat Physiol* 1878;2:1–19.
33. Rauber A, Kopsch F. *Lehrbuch und Atlas der Anatomie des Menschen.* Leipzig: Georg Thieme, 1940.
34. Berner W. *Biomechanische Untersuchungen am Sakroiliakalgelenk, Topographie, Beanspruchung und operative Stabilisierung.* Hannover: Habilitationsschrift, 1986.
35. Kapandji I. *Funktionelle Anatomie der Gelenke.* Bd. III: Enke: Rumpf und Wirbelsäule, 1985.
36. Borell U, Fernström I. The movements at the sacro-iliac joints and their importance to changes in the pelvic dimensions during parturition. *Acta Obstet Gynecol Scand* 1957;36:42–57.
37. Colachis SJ, et al. Movement of the sacro-iliac joint in the adult male: a preliminary report. *Arch Phys Med Rehab* 1963;44: 490–498.
38. Egund N, et al. Movements in the sacroiliac joints demonstrated with roentgen stereophotometry. *Acta Radiol Diag* 1978;19: 833–846.
39. Frigerio N, Stowe R, Howe J. Movement of the sacroiliac joint. *Clin Orthop* 1974;100:370–377.
40. von Schubert E. Röntgenuntersuchung des knöchernen Beckens im Profilbild. Exakte Messung der Beckenneigung beim Lebenden. *Zentralblatt f. Gynäkol* 1929;53:1064–1068.
41. Weisl H. The ligaments of the sacro-iliac joint examined with particular reference to their function. *Acta Anat* 1954;20: 201–213.
42. Lavignolle B, et al. An approach to the functional anatomy of the sacroiliac joints in vivo. *Anat Clin* 1983;5:169–176.
43. Brooke R. The sacro-iliac joint. *J Anat Physiol* 1924; 58:299–305.
44. Malgaigne J. *Traites des fractures et des luxations.* Paris: JB Balliere, 1847.
45. Noland L, Conwell H. Fractures of the pelvis. *Surg Gynecol Obstet* 1933;56:522–525.
46. Wakeley C. Fractures of the pelvis: an analysis of 100 cases. *Br J Surg* 1930:22–29.
47. Bonnin J. Sacral fractures and injuries to the cauda equina. *J Bone Joint Surg* 1945;27:113–127.
48. Huittinen V, Slätis P. Fractures of the pelvis: trauma mechanism, types of injury and principles of treatment. *Acta Chir Scand* 1972;138:563–569.
49. Pohlemann T, et al. Beckenverletzungen. Hefte zu "Der Unfallchirurg." *Heft* 1998:266.
50. Edeiken-Monroe B, Browner BD, Jackson H. The role of standard roentgenograms in the evaluation of instability of pelvic ring disruption. *Clin Orthop* 1989;240:63–76.
51. Montana MA, et al. CT of sacral injury. *Radiology* 1986; 161(2):499–503.
52. Rommens P, et al. Diagnosis and treatment of unstable fractures of the pelvic ring. *Acta Chir Belg* 1986;86(6):352–359.
53. Tile M, Pennal G. Pelvic disruptions: principles of management. *Clin Orthop* 1980;151:56–64.
54. Civil ID, et al. Routine pelvic radiography in severe blunt trauma: is it necessary? *Ann Emerg Med* 1988;17(5):488–490.
55. Pohlemann T, et al. Indikationsstellung und Osteosynthesetechniken am Beckenring. *Unfall Chirurg* 1992;95:197–209.
56. Tile M. Pelvic ring fractures: should they be fixed? *J Bone Joint Surg* 1988;70-B:1–12.
57. Gänsslen A, et al. *Clinical experience with 600 sacral fractures.* Abstract. Orthopaedic Trauma Association. San Antonio, TX, October, 2000.
58. Gänsslen A, et al. *Early results of ORIF of unstable sacral fractures.* Orthopaedic Trauma Association, 14th Annual Meeting. Vancouver, October 8–10, 1998.

59. Roy-Camille R, et al. Transverse fracture of the upper sacrum: suicidal jumper's fracture. *Spine* 1985;10(9):838–845.
60. Fardon D. Displaced transverse fracture of the sacrum with nerve root injury: report of a case with successful operative management. *J Trauma* 1979;192:119.
61. Mirkovic S, et al. Anatomic consideration for sacral screw placement. *Spine* 1991;16(6):289–294.
62. Gänsslen A, et al. *Suicidal jumper's fractures. Analysis of treatment in 17 cases.* Orthopaedic Trauma Association. Louisville, KY, 1999.
63. Matta J, Saucedo T. Internal fixation of pelvic ring fractures. *Clin Orthop* 1989;242:83–97.
64. Medelman J. Fractures of the sacrum: their incidence in fractures of the pelvis. *Am J Roentgenol* 1939;152:100–103.
65. Furey W. Fractures of the pelvis with special reference to associated fractures of the sacrum. *Am J Roentgenol* 1942;157: 89.
66. Huittinen V. Lumbosacral nerve injury in fracture of the pelvis. *Acta Chir Scand* 1972;(Suppl 429):1–43.
67. Laasonen E. Missed sacral fractures. *Ann Clin Res* 1977;9:84–87.
68. Melton L, et al. Epidemiologic features of pelvic fractures. *Clin Orthop* 1981;155:43–47.

17

OPEN PELVIC FRACTURES

JORGE BARLA
JAMES N. POWELL

INTRODUCTION

This section on the open pelvic fracture historically might well have been entitled the lethal pelvic fracture. For patients with this particular injury, a mortality rate of near 50% was reported. This was significantly higher than the 10% to 15% rates for closed pelvic fractures (1,2). Reports published in the 1990s showed improved survival rates, with an average mortality of 25% to 30%, obviously still a very high figure (3,4). Long-term follow-up using specific validated outcome measures as well as generic outcome measures has led to an improved understanding of morbidity in the survivors. In the worst-case scenario for survivors, many patients become severely disabled and have a long and difficult course, battling pelvic sepsis to survive.

By definition, an open pelvic fracture is a fracture that communicates with the rectum or vagina or with the environment through a break in the skin. Contamination of the fracture by an infected urinary tract or by gastrointestinal tract contents is common. An isolated bladder rupture is not considered an open fracture. The soft-tissue injury often is accompanied by a significant disruption of the pelvic ring. Raffa and Christensen suggested that this injury is often the first stage of a traumatic hemipelvectomy (5). The mechanism of the injury is either violent external rotation of the lower extremity of the affected hemipelvis or vertical shear. The pelvic floor is disrupted. This leads to loss of tamponade and greater difficulty controlling hemorrhage.

The powerful forces that cause these injuries are reflected by the high injury severity score. Particular attention to the ABCs of resuscitation is necessary because normally these patients are multiply injured.

CLINICAL PICTURE

Any patient with a laceration in the region of the perineum or gluteal area associated with the clinical signs and symptoms of a pelvic fracture should be considered to have an open pelvic fracture until proven otherwise (Figs. 17-1, 17-2, and 17-3). Usually an anterior laceration communicating with a pelvic fracture is obvious.

The diagnosis may be delayed if the open injury is hidden in either the vagina or rectum. Spicules of bone may perforate vaginal or rectal mucosa. Hemorrhage from the introitus and blood on the examining finger following a vaginal or rectal examination, in the presence of a pelvic fracture, demands further examination. A speculum examination is mandatory with vaginal bleeding, and a proctoscopic and sigmoidoscopic examination is prudent to investigate the cause of rectal bleeding, if a rectal tear is not obvious.

As in all patients with pelvic fractures, the posterior soft tissues must be examined carefully. Attention should be paid to evidence of both a shear injury of the soft tissues and lacerations. It is important to log roll all patients with pelvic fractures and examine the posterior soft tissues carefully. Although all open pelvic fractures are serious and even potentially lethal, patients with open injuries into the peroneum face a much poorer outcome than those with a skin lesion in the iliac crest region (6).

MANAGEMENT

General Management, Resuscitation, and Hemorrhage Control

Immediate resuscitation measures must be instituted rapidly. We follow the general principles of resuscitation as outlined

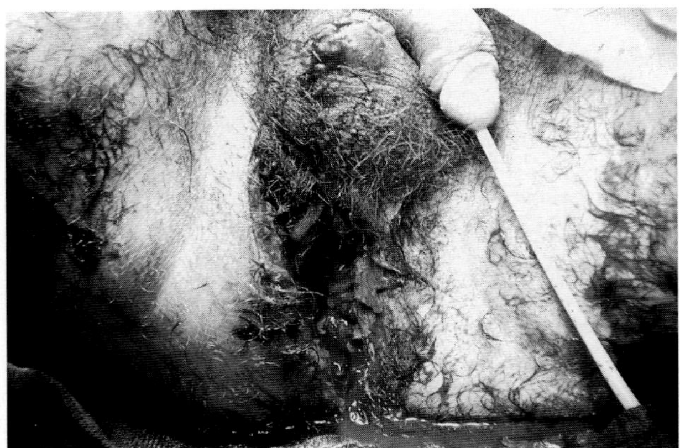

FIGURE 17-1. This patient had an open pelvic fracture after being run over by a tractor-trailer. The open laceration that you see in his perineum communicated directly with the presacral space. His initial management included immediate packing of the wound.

in the Advanced Trauma Life Support (ATLS) protocols (7). After an airway has been secured and the patient's ventilatory status is determined to be satisfactory, attention is paid to hemodynamic parameters. Two large-bore intravenous lines are established and if the patient is hypotensive, packed red cells are generally given immediately. Un–cross-matched Type O-positive blood is given in the case of life-threatening hemorrhage when time does not permit a full cross-matching. Type O-negative blood is given to girls and women of childbearing age. A Foley catheter is inserted early in the resuscitative phase of the patient's care, after the integrity of the genitourinary tract has been established by clinical and if necessary radiologic criteria. A urethrogram is important in the radiologic investigation of all male patients. A cystogram should be performed on any patient who sustains a high-

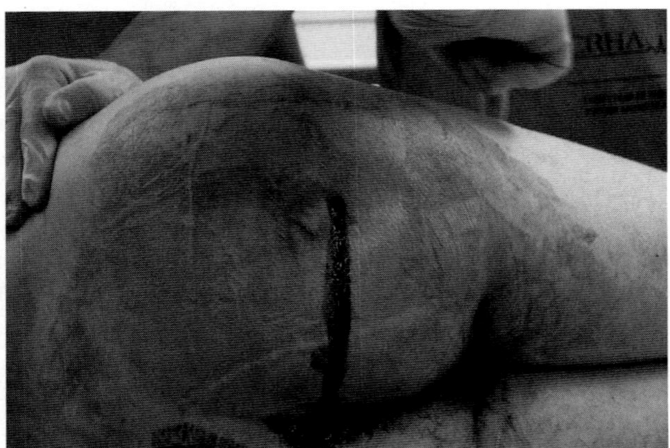

FIGURE 17-2. This patient was injured when thrown off a tire tube, which was being pulled by a snowmobile. He had a small puncture wound in his buttock, which communicated with a severe unstable fracture of his sacrum (Type C1, Denis Type 2) as well as a fracture of his right acetabulum.

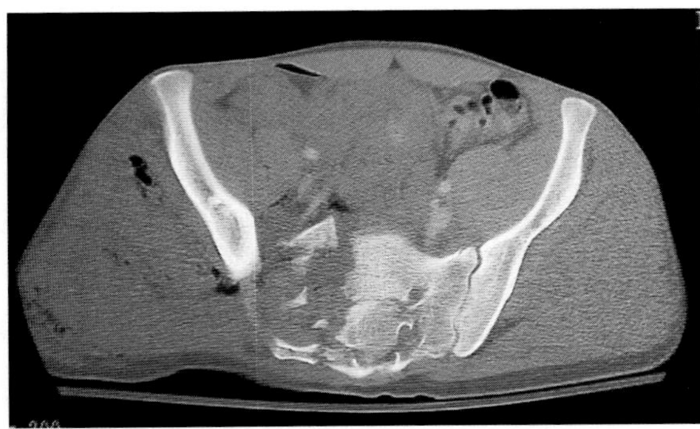

FIGURE 17-3. This is the computed tomography scan of the patient in Fig. 17-2.

energy pelvic injury with hematuria to rule out a bladder rupture. Historically, contraindications to Foley catheter placement on a clinical basis include a high-riding prostate, scrotal hematoma, and blood at the tip of the urethral meatus of the penis. However, a scrotal hematoma is a virtually universal feature of a significant pelvic fracture; if the patient is seen more than 4 hours after the fracture, then a hematoma is quite common. Our current practice is now to make one gentle attempt to pass the catheter through the urethra into the bladder.

The principles of hemorrhage control follow.

1. Packing of open pelvic wounds using pressure dressings. This should be done in the emergency department. The wound should be packed very tightly.
2. Reduction of a displaced hemipelvis, if vertically displaced, by the application of traction to the limb through a femoral or tibial traction pin.
3. Further measures to reduce the volume of the pelvis, including rotational reduction and application of a pelvic clamp or application of an external fixator. Several commercially available clamps are available and were designed for application in an emergency room (ER) setting. An external fixator can be applied in an ER setting but is more often applied in the operating room. The goal of both devices is to maintain a provisional reduction and assist with securing tamponade.
4. Immediate laparotomy where necessary when there is evidence of intraabdominal injury. Most trauma units now are able to perform fairly rapid abdominal imaging using either ultrasound or spiral computed tomography (CT). The trauma team leader may elect to proceed rapidly to a formal laparotomy and possible pelvic packing if the patient is critically ill (see Chapter 8).
5. Previously, angiography only was used in many centers as a last resort. It now plays an earlier role in our management protocol. Once the pelvic wounds have been packed, the pelvis reduced and provisionally stabilized, and intraabdominal injuries ruled out or dealt with surgically, we frequently send the patient for an an-

giogram if the blood requirement has been >4 to 6 units of pack red blood cells (Fig. 17-4).

Early definitive management of pelvic ring fractures, which are open, and with significant hemorrhage requires a team approach. A trauma team leader and orthopedic surgeon need to work cooperatively, both during the early management and later beyond the resuscitation phase. In the operating room at the time of laparotomy, one frequent scenario is that there is either no major intraabdominal injury or a large retroperitoneal hematoma is evident after definitive management of intraabdominal injuries. In the older literature, exploration of retroperitoneal hematoma was eventually universally lethal. However, this tactic is being reassessed in several European trauma centers. We are more frequently packing the true pelvis through the lower end of the laparotomy incision and empirically have found this to be of significant benefit in some patients. The problem of hemorrhage control, of course, is much greater with an open injury because of the difficulty in achieving tamponade when the retroperitoneal hematoma initially has been decompressed by the open wound. Many of the initial laparotomies that are now performed are so-called "damage control" laparotomies, where major sources of hemorrhage are dealt with rapidly; however, other injuries, such as bowel wounds, are dealt with on a delayed basis.

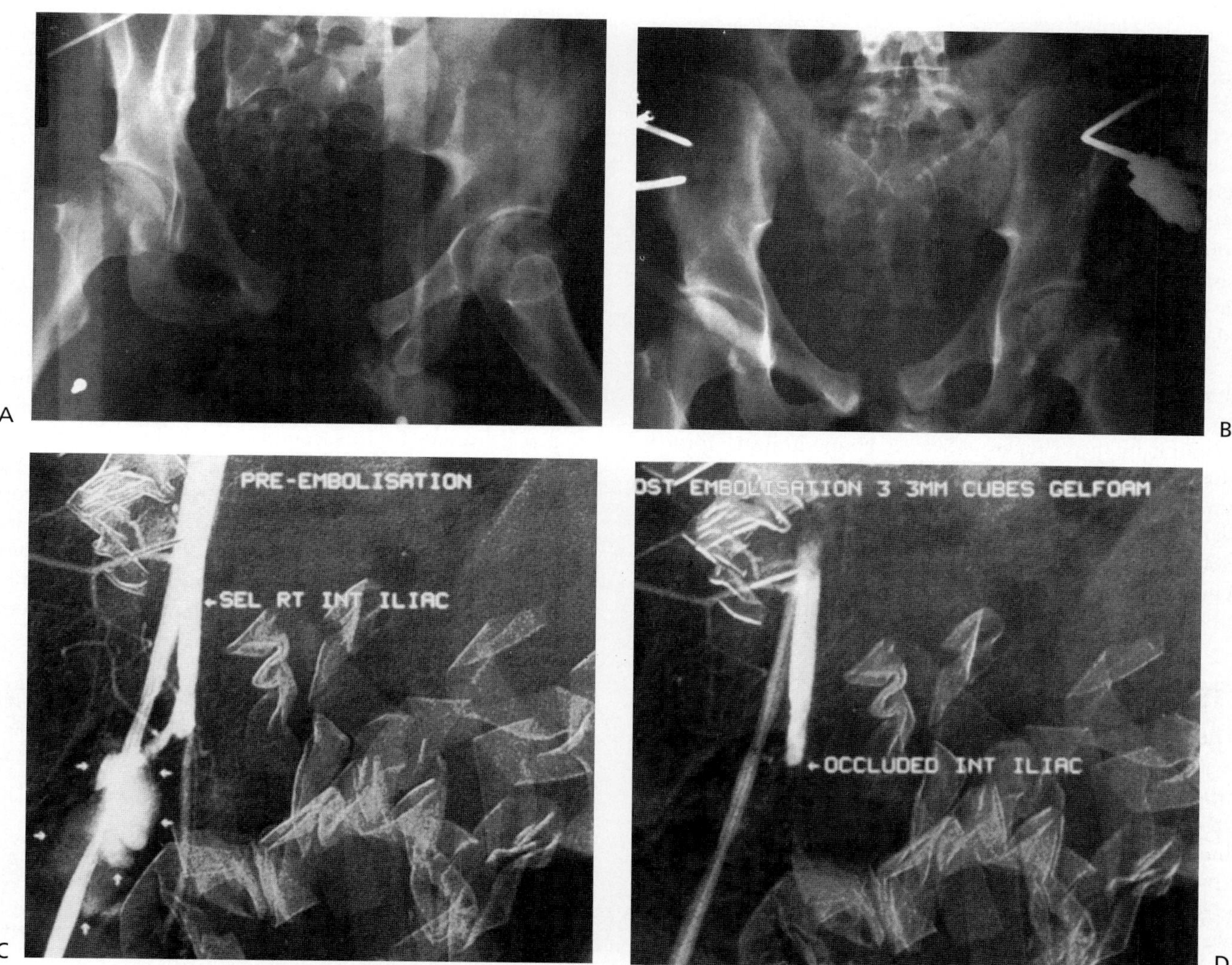

FIGURE 17-4. A: The anteroposterior pelvic radiograph of a pedestrian run over by a motor vehicle. The patient's wound was packed and sutured in the emergency department. **B:** Radiograph demonstrates the pelvis reduced and stabilized. Laparotomy showed no intraabdominal injury, and the pelvis was packed. The patient went to the angiography suite, because he remained hemodynamically unstable (by this point in his resuscitation he had received >60 units of red cells). **C:** An oblique view of the pelvis at the time of angiography shows dye leaking from a major branch of the internal iliac artery. The tapes of the sponges used to pack the pelvis also are evident. **D:** The patient's hemodynamics stabilized rapidly after arterial embolization. Unfortunately, he died of sepsis 2 weeks after the injury.

Richardson and colleagues reported on two patients who underwent hemipelvectomy in desperate circumstances to control hemorrhage (8). Both survived.

Tetanus prophylaxis and broad-spectrum antibiotics are recommended, particularly if bowel contamination has occurred. A triple antibiotic regimen for a minimum of 48 hours is appropriate.

Control of Sepsis

Principles of open fracture management used in extremity fracture apply in the pelvis as well. The wound requires meticulous debridement and irrigation, instituted once the patient's hemodynamics are stable. All wounds are packed open to prevent the development of gas gangrene.

The presence of a rectal laceration is an absolute indication for an immediate diverting colostomy. When perineal wounds occur, each must be judged by location for the potential to contaminate the fracture and retroperitoneal hematoma. Generally, it is appropriate to perform a colostomy whenever a perineal wound is present; therefore, consultation with the general surgical service should be obtained. Most centers now accept that a distal loop washout is appropriate as soon as practical. The morbidity and mortality rise if the colostomy is delayed beyond 48 hours.

Urethral injuries generally are managed conservatively, either by primary realignment or suprapubic catheter insertion. The treatment of intraperitoneal bladder ruptures is operative by direct repair, whereas extraperitoneal ruptures often are managed by urethral catheter drainage alone. The use of suprapubic tubes must be discouraged if surgery is planned for an anterior pelvic ring injury or an acetabular fracture. Anterior fixation following direct formal open repair of the bladder, in our experience, has not led to a problem with pelvic sepsis.

Fracture Management

The hemodynamic status of the patient, location of the soft-tissue injury, and degree of contamination are important factors in the decision-making process concerning fracture stabilization. The role of external fixation and clamps is outlined in this chapter with regard to their use in resuscitation. Application of an external fixator can be undertaken and achieved rapidly in an emergency situation. Generally, one pin is inserted in each iliac crest, starting 2 cm posterior to the anterior superior iliac spine. A simple frame is constructed and generally turned down, permitting the general surgical team to perform a laparotomy.

External fixation can be used definitively in situations where the soft-tissue injury or degree of contamination preclude internal fixation or if the fracture pattern is not amenable to internal fixation. An example of such a fracture pattern is bilateral displaced superior and inferior pubic rami fractures, which we prefer to handle with anterior external fixation in most situations.

If an external fixator is used definitively, we favor use of a minimum of two pins in each hemipelvis. One supraacetabular pin shown in Fig. 17-5 has led to an improved purchase with our external fixator pins. This construct has proven quite satisfactory in management of patients for a 6-week time interval. In unstable fracture patterns (Type C), skeletal traction must supplement the external fixator, in order to prevent shortening or malrotation of the hemipelvis.

Internal fixation is the preferred method of management of most open pelvic ring injuries now. A disrupted pubic symphysis is best managed by an open plating technique. A plate can be easily and rapidly applied at the time of a laparotomy if one is undertaken as part of the initial care of the patient. A simple two-hole plate is adequate as a tension band fixation. Packing of the space of Retzius assists with hemorrhage control. If the patient is hemodynamically stable, then we favor stabilization using a 3.5-mm curved pelvic reconstruction plate. Again, stabilization can be undertaken in the presence of a bladder rupture as long as the rupture is repaired and drainage achieved by Foley catheter insertion. Plating the anterior pelvis in the presence of a rectal laceration is more controversial.

Internal fixation of the posterior pelvic ring now is accepted in the management of the translationally unstable pelvic ring. Early internal fixation of a posterior ring injury can be accomplished in several circumstances. If the wound is along the iliac crest, posteriorly, then open reduction may follow debridement and wound care. As in other types of open fractures, the method chosen depends on the assessment of the wound and fracture; however, percutaneous methods are favored posteriorly. The wounds should be left open, with early follow-up care as indicated. If the patient is hemodynamically stable enough to remain in the operating room, then closed reduction and percutaneous stabilization

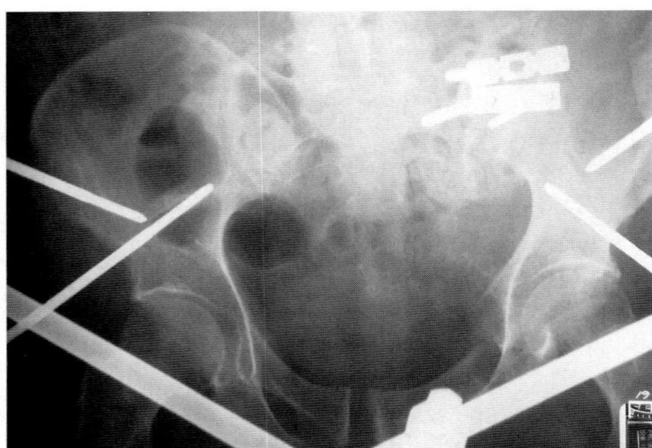

FIGURE 17-5. This radiograph shows the placement of one pin in the iliac crest and a second supraacetabular pin placed in bone above the dome of the acetabulum. The purchase of the supraacetabular pins is excellent.

in fact may well help with the ultimate resuscitation of the patient by helping to secure tamponade. If a satisfactory closed reduction cannot be obtained, then a posterior fixation technique is contraindicated and provisional stabilization with a pelvic clamp is preferred until the patient is more hemodynamically stable.

If the wound is in the perineum, the general state of the patient will dictate the timing and method of posterior fixation. Percutaneous techniques are ideal in this situation (iliosacral screws). These may be inserted early if the general state of the patient allows; if not, external fixation and skeletal traction are used until the patient's state allows internal fixation.

Biomechanically, iliosacral lag screw fixation has been shown to be one of the strongest methods of fixation of the posterior pelvic ring (9,10). The benefits of early stable internal fixation include patient comfort, facilitation of nursing care, and maintenance of a reduction of the pelvic ring disruption with the elimination of traction. Two screws can be solidly and safely placed into the ala of the sacrum or preferably the body of S1, dependent on the actual posterior injury (10). In those posterior ring injuries where a Denis Type II or III central sacral fracture occurred, we prefer to use fully threaded iliosacral screws as opposed to lag fixation to minimize the risk of iatrogenic neurologic injury. Neurologic monitoring has been shown to be a useful adjunct with the use of posterior pelvic ring stabilization. These screws are technically demanding and only should be placed by surgeons with special training in these techniques because they are potentially dangerous.

Recent biomechanical studies have shown that stabilization of the anterior pelvis in unstable C fractures is important, if the patient is to be mobilized and fracture reduction maintained (see Chapter 11). Preferably, internal fixation is used in symphysis disruption and external fixation for rami fractures. Percutaneous fixation of rami fractures also is used when indicated.

After Care

The after care of these injuries varies depending on the specific soft-tissue injury complex. Patients require repeated examination of the wound in the operating room and frequently return each 24 hours until definitive wound management has been established and definitive internal fixation accomplished. Aggressive wound management is necessary if an infection ensues. Development of a clinical picture of infection mandates a search for pelvic sepsis. We have found CT scanning of the abdomen and pelvis very useful in helping to determine the exact site of the infection. If wound closure is attempted, then attempts must be made to eliminate dead space and the use of suction drains is recommended. However, much more commonly, these wounds are left to granulate and may take a prolonged period of time. Many of the soft-tissue defects are so large that free flap application of a latissimus dorsi flap does not permit complete elimination of the dead space. We have been reluctant to consider use of a latissimus dorsi flap in several patients because the potential donor site morbidity might be too great. In the patient with a severe neurologic injury, which is very common in this high-energy trauma group, we have noted that our patients rely more heavily on their upper extremities for locomotion. As such we have been reluctant to consider the use of an upper extremity free flap.

Outcome

Raffa and Christensen described 26 patients with open pelvic fractures (5). Of these, 16 had injuries caused by blunt, high-energy trauma, and eight died (mortality rate of 50%). In seven cases, the death was directly related to the sepsis. In the eighth, death occurred as a result of massive hemorrhage. The high-energy nature of these injuries is reflected by the presence of genitourinary injuries in 12 of 16 and gastrointestinal lesions in seven of 16 patients.

In this series, 13 of 16 soft-tissue injuries were either perineal or gluteal, two were into the rectum, and one into the vagina. Aside from sepsis, massive hemorrhage, often uncontrollable, was common: Nine of 16 patients required more than 20 units of blood. The authors related the high-energy rate from sepsis to the delayed colostomy or no colostomy at all. In the 14 patients managed by immediate fecal diversion, only one death occurred, whereas among those who had delayed diversion or none, seven of 12 patients died.

Perry and colleagues reported on 31 patients with open pelvic fractures (2). The mortality rate for those with open pelvic fractures was 42%, as compared with 10.3% for the remaining 707 patients with closed pelvic fractures. The major causes of death from open pelvic fractures were again noted to be hemorrhage and sepsis.

Hanson and coauthors reported the experience in Sacramento from 1984 to 1988 (3). Their series report retrospectively on 43 patients. They noted 3.1 additional injuries per patient, and only two isolated open pelvic injuries. The average injury severity score for those who died was 40. An attempt to classify the fractures using mechanistic classifications proved difficult, because 13 of 43 patients had a fracture pattern that did not fit the classification. The patients generally were treated by the principles outlined in the preceding section. Two patients required hip disarticulation, two a hemipelvectomy, and one a gracilis flap for coverage.

The two important factors in mortality were age and the mechanism of injury. The most significant factor was the age of the patient: Those older than 40 years of age had a 78% mortality rate, as compared with 18% for younger persons. The mortality rate for the series overall was 30%. They found no significant correlation between fracture pattern and wound type or location.

A combined report, including patients treated in three trauma centers, including Sunnybrook Health Science Center in Toronto (4), report on 39 patients with open pelvic fracture. Their average injury severity score was 29.

Treatment was generally by the established ATLS protocols, with irrigation and debridement of wounds and identification and treatment of associated injuries. Diverting colostomy was performed in each of nine patients with rectal lacerations, although only five patients in this series underwent diverting colostomy within 48 hours. One of the five whose diverting colostomy was performed in the initial 48 hours died, whereas three of the four whose colostomy was delayed died of sepsis. A total of ten patients were treated by open reduction and internal fixation. The anterior stabilization was performed in the acute phase in four patients. The six posterior stabilizations were performed on a delayed basis. One of the patients in the posterior fixation group developed an infection.

Ten of 39 (25%) of the patients in this series died. All who died sustained unstable Tile Type B or C pelvic fractures, and all who died from sepsis had an associated rectal tear. In this series, instability of the pelvic fracture had a statistically significant association with mortality.

Brenneman and associates (6) reported on 44 open pelvic fractures. They published a mortality rate of 25%. Hemorrhage was the cause of death in six patients, multiple organ failure in three, and head injury in the remaining two. Forty-five percent of the fractures were classified as unstable Tile C.

Davidson reported a very low mortality rate of 5% after reviewing 25 cases of open pelvic fractures (11). He suggested early fracture stabilization and angiographic embolization to control bleeding and reduce transfusion requirements. Furthermore, he mentioned the important role of associated injuries in morbidity and mortality.

There is a lack of information in the literature referring to the long-term outcome of patients after an open pelvic fracture. Using validated outcome measures in the series of 44 patients, Brenneman and coworkers (6) presented their findings after an average follow-up of 4 years. Twenty-seven of 33 survivors were available. Three were incontinent of feces, two incontinent of urine, and three had nonhealed fractures. Four of the men were impotent. Only 13 of the 27 had no clinical sequelae from their open pelvic fracture and virtually all of these had soft-tissue lesions on the posterior skin, as opposed to those with perineal wounds, whose results were much worse. Among the half of those who were previously employed, 14 of 22 returned to work. The average self-rated general health was 73% of good health. The SF-36 suggested some differences between closed and open pelvic fractures. Long-term survivors scored significantly worse on physical functioning scale and physical role scale than did patients with closed pelvic fractures, as published in other reports. Both open and closed pelvis fractures score below population norms on long-term follow-up using generic outcome measures. We do not know if these altered scores reflect the outcome of the pelvic fracture or other system injury. Long-term survivors require prolonged periods in rehabilitation settings after open pelvic fractures (12). The trauma surgeon needs to be aware of the long-term sequelae and potential poorer outcome to support the patient during recovery.

REFERENCES

1. Tile M. *Fractures of the pelvis and acetabulum.* Baltimore: Williams & Wilkins, 1984.
2. Perry JF. Pelvic open fractures. *Clin Orthop* 1980;151:41.
3. Hanson P, Milne J, Chapman M. Open fractures of the pelvis. *J Bone Joint Surg* 1991;73B:325.
4. Jones A, et al. *Open pelvic fracture.* Presentation. American Academy of Orthopaedic Surgeons. New Orleans, LA, February 13, 1990.
5. Raffa J, Christensen NM. Compound fractures of the pelvis. *Am J Surg* 1976;132:282.
6. Brenneman DF, Katyal D, Boulanger BR, et al. Long-term outcomes in open pelvic fractures. *J Trauma Injury Infect Crit Care* 1997;42:773.
7. *Advanced Trauma Life Support Instructor Manual.* Chicago: American College of Surgeons, 1989.
8. Richardson JD, et al. Open pelvic fractures. *J Trauma* 1982; 22:533.
9. Hearn TC, et al. Mechanics of the pelvic ring in relation to ligamentous loading and the stability of internal fixation. Presentation. Combined Orthopaedic Societies of the English-Speaking World. Toronto, June 9, 1992.
10. Kraemer W, Hearn TC, Tile M, et al. The effects of thread length and location on extraction strength of iliosacral lag screws. *Injury* 1994;25:5.
11. Davidson BS, Simmons GT, Williamson PR, et al. Pelvic fractures associated with open perineal wounds: a survivable injury. *J Trauma* 1993;35:36.
12. Woods RK, O'Keefe G, Rhee P, et al. Open pelvic fracture and fecal diversion. *Arch Surg* 1998;133:281.

18

PELVIC RING DISRUPTION IN WOMEN: GENITOURINARY AND OBSTETRIC IMPLICATIONS

CAROL E. COPELAND

INTRODUCTION

Traumatic injuries to the female genitourinary tract are relatively rare, but the long-term implications are of great concern to the patients (1–3). Frequently asked questions include: Will I be able to have children? Will I need to have a cesarean section? When can I start having sex again? Patients report having a high level of concern but rarely ask their orthopedist about these issues (3).

THE NONPREGNANT FEMALE PATIENT

Incidence of Associated Genitourinary Trauma

Early recognition of trauma to the female genitourinary tract is important because of the potential for severe complications. The incidence of injuries to the female genitourinary tract associated with pelvic fracture is reported to be 7% to 14.5% (2,4,5). Early complications include sepsis and necrotizing fasciitis, particularly in unrecognized injuries (6,7). Late sequelae include incontinence, dyspareunia, dysmenorrhea and menstrual irregularities, swelling in the labia during voiding, fistulae, vaginal or urethral stricture, and infertility (4,7–14).

In one series, bladder injuries were reported in two of 123 women with pelvic fractures (2%) (3). Other studies have reported vaginal lacerations to occur in 1% to 7% of women with pelvic fractures (3,5,6). Urethral injuries in women, once thought to be extremely rare, are now being recognized in 4.6% of women with pelvic fractures (7). Most urethral injuries (75% to 100%) are found in combination with vaginal injuries (9,11,15–17). In patients with known bladder neck or urethral injury, careful examination should be performed for vaginal injury as well. Vaginal laceration in the presence of pelvic fracture should trigger a search for urethral or bladder neck injury if hematuria, vulvar swelling, or inability to void are present (7,14).

Urethral lacerations are frequently missed, with potential disastrous consequences (9). Perry and Husmann (7) reported on six patients with urethral injuries and pelvic fractures; there were three initially missed urethral injuries, all in patients who had not had a careful vaginal inspection. Two of the patients with missed injuries developed life-threatening sepsis secondary to necrotizing fasciitis. Missed injuries also can be associated with late development of urethrovaginal fistulae and incontinence (9).

Perry and Husmann (7) also reported that blood at the vaginal introitus was present in 80% of their cases with vaginal and urethral injuries. Difficulty with voiding, hematuria, and vulvar edema also are frequently found. Blood at the vaginal introitus in a patient with a pelvic fracture should trigger a careful search for vaginal lacerations as well as urethral tears (7,18). Because abduction of the lower extremities causes severe pain in the fractured pelvis, adequate examination of the vagina is best performed under anesthesia. To minimize the chance of fracture displacement or exacerbation of hemorrhage, vaginal examination in the hemodynamically unstable patient may be deferred until provisional stabilization with external fixation or other methods has been obtained. The orthopedic surgeon should take an active role in ensuring that the vaginal examination is performed during acute treatment of the pelvic fracture.

The principles of open fracture management used in extremity fractures apply to the pelvis as well. Open fractures, whether through the vagina or perineum, should be debrided meticulously. Early stabilization should be followed by frequent reexamination and repeat debridement of the wounds as necessary. Vaginal wounds may be packed open after debridement and irrigation. In certain instances, primary closure can be accomplished. For example, in the case of a lower energy lateral compression (LC) injury, the fracture can be carefully reintroduced into the vagina for debridement and irrigation. Distraction external fixation then is used to stabilize the fracture in the reduced position and facilitate vaginal healing by prevention of repetitive trauma from normal patient movement in bed (Andrew R. Burgess, personal communication, 2001).

Although severe gynecologic injury is fairly uncommon, the literature does record case reports of injuries to the uterus, ovaries, and fallopian tubes in association with pelvic fracture (10,18). Ovarian injury may occur in up to 2% of pelvic fractures (5) and in up to 11% of pelvic fractures associated with large retroperitoneal hematoma (19). The incidence of infertility after blunt ovarian injury has not been reported.

Genitourinary Outcome

Urinary System

In 1997, Copeland and coworkers (3) performed a retrospective review of 255 female trauma patients, interviewing women who had sustained pelvic fractures (subjects, n = 123) and comparing them with women who had sustained upper or lower extremity fractures (controls, n = 118). Urinary complaints occurred significantly more frequently in patients with pelvic fractures than in controls (21% versus 7%, p = 0.003). Most women complained of more than one problem. In particular, nocturia (p = 0.04), stress incontinence (p = 0.007), and frequency (p = 0.02) were reported significantly more often in subjects than in controls. Only one of the 26 subjects with urinary tract complaints had sustained acute trauma to the genitourinary tract (a vaginal laceration requiring repair); she complained of frequency and recurrent urinary tract infections. Patients with moderate and severe pelvic fractures (equivalent to Tile B and C injuries) were significantly more likely to have urinary complaints (30%, 36%, and 14%, respectively; p = 0.037) than patients with minor (Tile A) fractures (3). In addition, direction of displacement correlated with the frequency of urinary complaints. Patients with fractures that were displaced laterally (anterior-posterior compression, AP) or vertically (vertical shear, VS) or with combined AP and VS injuries were much more likely to have late urinary tract complaints (60%, 67%, and 21%, respectively; p = 0.04) than patients with medially displaced fractures.

Injury to the pudendal nerve and pelvic floor has been documented to contribute to incontinence (20,21). It is postulated that tearing of the pelvic floor musculature contributes to the urinary tract complaints in the open-book (B1) and vertical shearing (C) injuries. In contrast, in lateral compression (B2) injuries (medially displaced fractures), the pelvic floor becomes redundant and does not tear (Fig. 18-1).

Pelvic floor (Kegel) exercises have been shown to improve stress incontinence (22–24) and protect against perineal tears caused by childbirth (25). Based on this information, clinicians at the R. Adams Cowley Shock Trauma Center now include instruction in pelvic floor exercises as a physiotherapy component for women at risk for adverse urinary outcomes (displaced APC or VS injuries) (unstable rotation and shear injuries (C) after pelvic fracture). In addition to isometric exercises, progressively increased weighted vaginal cones may be used for muscular training.

Fertility

Infertility after pelvic fracture is uncommon. Infertility, defined as the inability to conceive despite 1 year of unprotected intercourse, was found to be similar in subjects and controls (6% in both) (3). Massive trauma to the genitourinary tract, in association with pelvic fracture, can result in infertility. Donner and coworkers (10) reported a case of primary amenorrhea related to pelvic fracture. A 12-year-old girl was crushed underneath a boat-style swing, sustaining an AP injury with bilateral sacroiliac joint and ramus fractures. Traumatic separation and scarring between the uterine corpus and cervix resulted in primary amenorrhea, requiring reconstruction at age 18. At age 32, the same patient presented with primary infertility from scarring at this region and the adnexa; she was treated successfully with *in vitro* fertilization and cesarean section (C section) delivery.

Pregnancy After Pelvic Fracture

Dystocia caused by pelvic deformity has been reported in the literature (5,26–29), and many authors have stressed the importance of restoring the anatomy of the pelvis in women of childbearing years (26,28). However, vaginal delivery is possible even after displaced pelvic ring disruption (1,26–30). The literature does not provide much guidance on the issue of delivery after pelvic fracture because the incidence and risk factors for cephalopelvic disproportion are unknown.

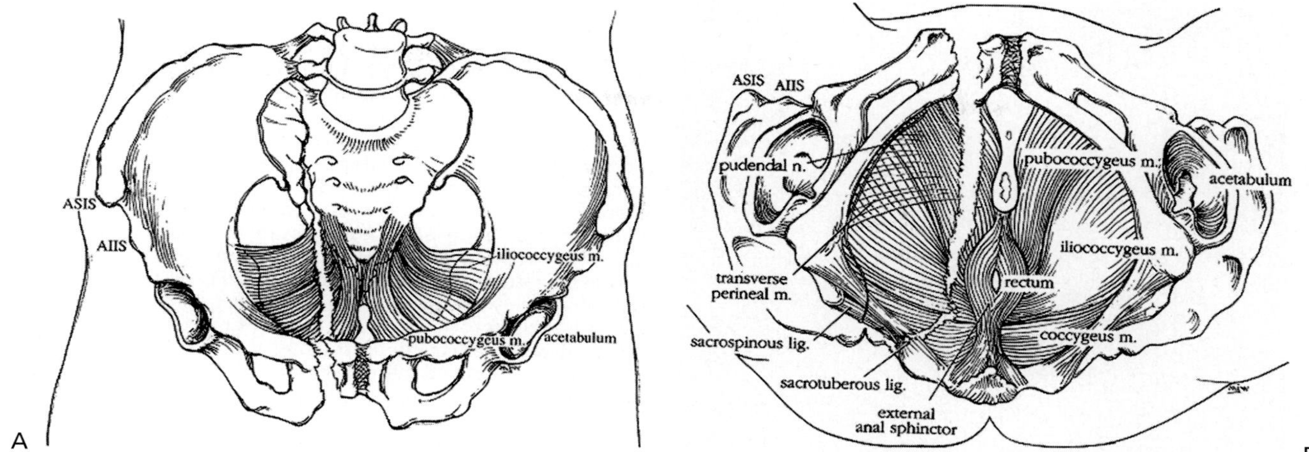

FIGURE 18-1. Open book (B1, APC-11) pelvic ring disruption with disruption of the pelvic floor and lateral displacement of the hemipelvis. **A:** Anterior-posterior view. **B:** Inferosuperior view. AIIS, anterior inferior iliac spine; ASIS, anterior superior iliac spine. (From: Copeland CE, Bosse MJ, McCarthy ML, et al. Effect of trauma and pelvic fracture on female genitourinary, sexual, and reproductive function. *J Orthop Trauma* 1997;11:79, with permission.)

Speer and Peltier (29) summarized 20 reported cases of women who became pregnant after pelvic fractures; they also reported on five patients of their own. Fetal death occurred in 10%. Vaginal delivery was successful in 53.5%, and C section was necessary in 36.5%. Zhou (5) reported that of 75 women sustaining displaced fracture-dislocations of the pelvis, 45 (60%) experienced dystocia and 30 (40%) required C section. This population appears to have sustained very high-energy trauma, as evidenced by the high incidence of urogenital trauma (14.5%). Madsen and coworkers (1) reported on 17 women with displaced fractures of the pelvis who gave birth; in only one was cesarean section carried out for a suspicion of cephalopelvic disproportion. This patient had a lateral compression (Tile B2) injury with a decrease in the diameter of the hemipelvis and superior displacement of the right superior pubic ramus. Three of the patients in that series (1) delivered vaginally after having both pelvic ring fractures and C section for complicated pregnancies (uterine inertia requiring vacuum extraction in two patients, symphysiolysis in one).

The study by Copeland and coworkers (3) of young women sustaining pelvic fractures showed that the C section per term pregnancy rate was significantly higher ($p <$ 0.0001) postinjury than preinjury after pelvic fracture. In the subject group (pelvic fracture), C section was performed in 48% (11 of 23 initial pregnancies after trauma). For purposes of comparison, the rate of C section delivery in 1995 was reported to be 21% in the United States and 16% in Great Britain (31). A follow-up study was performed to determine the reason for this high C section rate (32). Of 23 women giving birth after pelvic fracture, 11 underwent C section; seven of 11 had no trial of labor. Of the seven, five (no previous history of C section) underwent elective C section for history of pelvic fracture, and two underwent elective C section for history of previous C section. Four patients underwent C section after unsuccessful labor trials. Two of these four experienced inefficient uterine action similar to preinjury pregnancies delivered by C section. In the remaining two patients undergoing C section, dystocia secondary to the injury was a possible, but not definite, explanation for the C section. In one, the decision to perform a C section came immediately after a change in physician coverage. Both of these patients had minimally displaced lateral compression (B types) (B2) fractures with mildly decreased radius of the affected hemipelvis (Fig. 18-2).

It was concluded that physician bias and a desire to avoid childbirth complications, as opposed to dystocia due to the pelvic fracture, contributed to the high C section rate. The decision to perform elective C section may have been inappropriate because four patients were subsequently able to deliver vaginally despite the history of both pelvic fractures and C section.

No patient in that series (32) had fixation crossing either the symphysis or sacroiliac joint. External fixation of the pelvis and open reduction of the iliac wing have been found to be compatible with subsequent vaginal delivery (1,32,33). In the literature, there are no reports of vaginal delivery with indwelling transarticular (symphyseal or sacroiliac) hardware or vaginal delivery after arthrodesis of the sacroiliac or symphyseal joints. Madsen and coworkers (1) performed elective removal of symphyseal plates before planned conception in two patients; resymphysiolysis was a complication in both. One delivered vaginally despite the resymphysiolysis. The second patient delivered by elective C section and subsequently had a successful vaginal delivery. Resymphysiolysis also can occur after nonoperatively treated pelvic fractures (34). Resymphysiolysis does not preclude uncomplicated vaginal delivery in subsequent pregnancies (1,34).

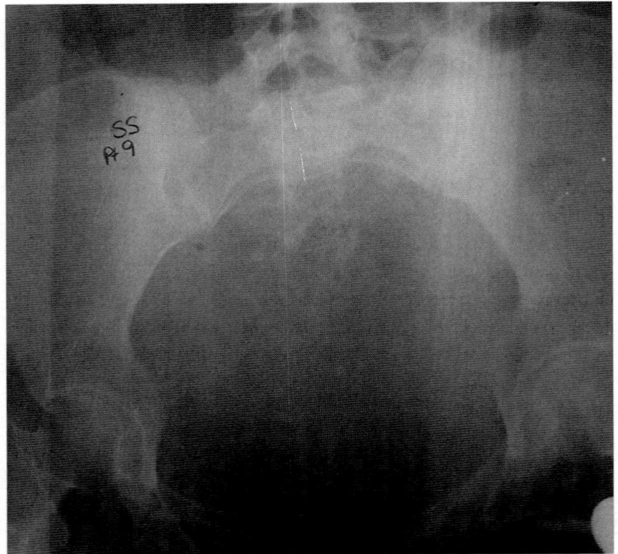

A

FIGURE 18-2. A: Admission AP radiograph of multiple trauma patient, 22 weeks pregnant at time of motor vehicle accident. Her open-book (B1, AP-II) injury was treated conservatively. The fetus did not survive. She required cesarian section (C section) in one preinjury pregnancy. Her first postinjury pregnancy was complicated by failure to progress and C section was performed. Two later pregnancies ended in uncomplicated spontaneous vaginal delivery. **B:** Two-year radiographic follow-up of primiparous woman (history of previous C section) sustaining lateral compression (B2, LC-III) pelvic ring disruption in a motor vehicle accident. She was treated with external fixation. The symphysis has healed in an overreduced position. Nine years after her injury she was admitted in early labor. Her obstetrician decided at that time to avoid an attempt at vaginal delivery on the basis of both the history of previous C section and her pelvic fracture. **C:** Anteroposterior radiograph of a minimally displaced lateral compression (B2, LC-I) fracture with mildly decreased radius of the affected hemipelvis, treated conservatively. Developmental hip changes are incidentally noted. The patient had no previous pregnancies. She was given a trial of labor, and underwent C section for uterine inertia with suspicion of dystocia. A second child was delivered by elective C section.

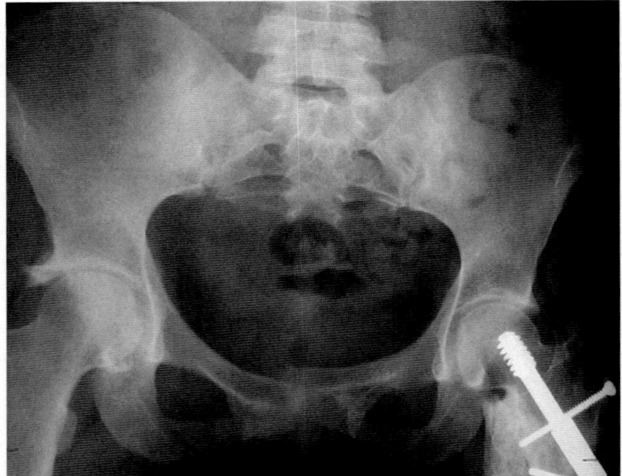

B

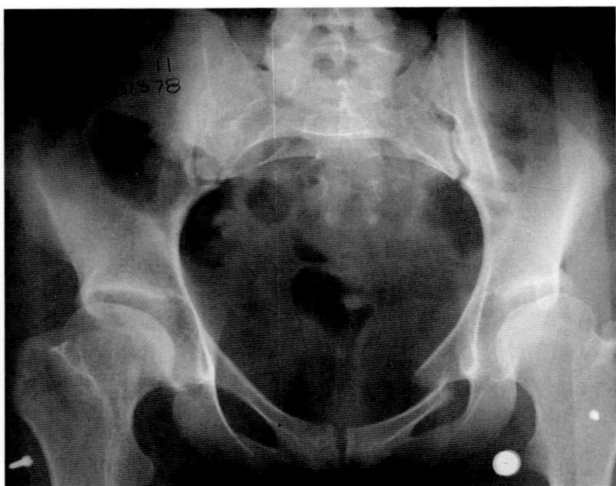

C

Vaginal delivery is possible in women with a fused symphysis. In Fig. 18-3 an overlapped symphysis (lateral compression type B1) in this 19-year-old patient was treated by closed manipulation and external fixation, resulting in an acute fusion of the symphysis. She was able to deliver two children vaginally with little difficulty.

The author's current recommendation is to provide clear information to the patient and obstetrician regarding the anatomic location and displacement of fractures, the presence of hardware, and the perceived ability of the symphysis and sacroiliac joints to relax. The distinction between acetabular and pelvic fracture also should be made clear to the patient and obstetrician. Acetabular fractures, even when operatively fixed, do not preclude vaginal delivery unless the screw enters the pelvis (Fig. 18-4) (29,32). Acetabular fractures with limited hip range of motion may preclude the lithotomy position; however, this information can be determined by physical examination. Vaginal delivery is recommended in the absence of gross deformity (specifically, narrowing of the true pelvis), bridging callus formation, or hardware across the sacroiliac or symphyseal joints. If fusion of the symphysis or sacroiliac joints has occurred, it is presumed that the pelvic outlet will be less compliant; in such a case, it is probably in the patient's best interests to deliver by elective C section.

Medicolegal concerns have long been a concern for obstetricians (30). Elective C section, although perhaps safer than attempted vaginal delivery through a grossly scarred and deformed outlet, is not without risks (31). The orthopedist's role is to proactively counsel the patient regarding the specifics of their injury. Supplying patients with diagrams of their injury and fixation, postoperative radiographs, or follow-up computed tomography scans for pelvimetry might decrease the rate of unnecessary C section after pelvic fracture.

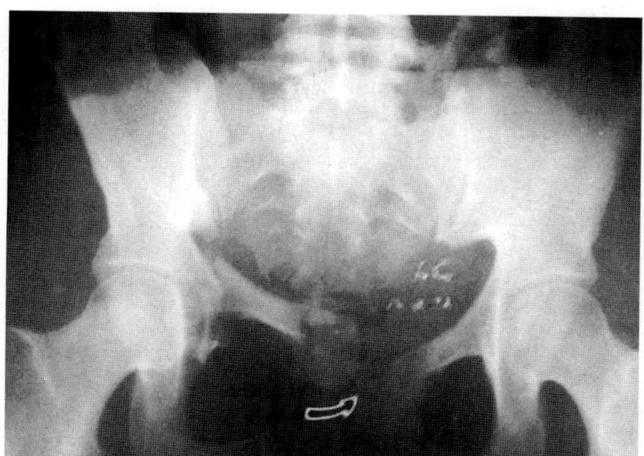

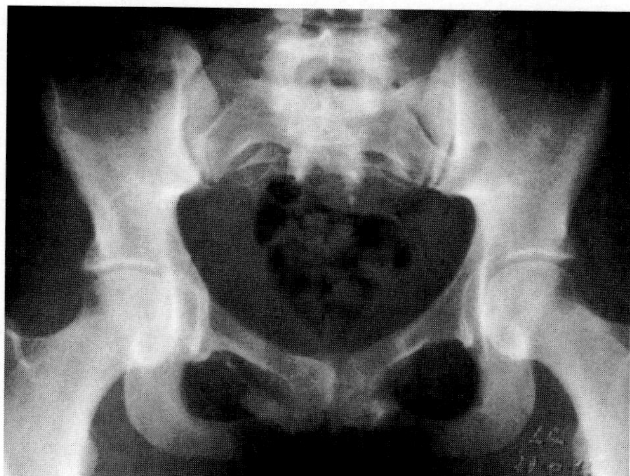

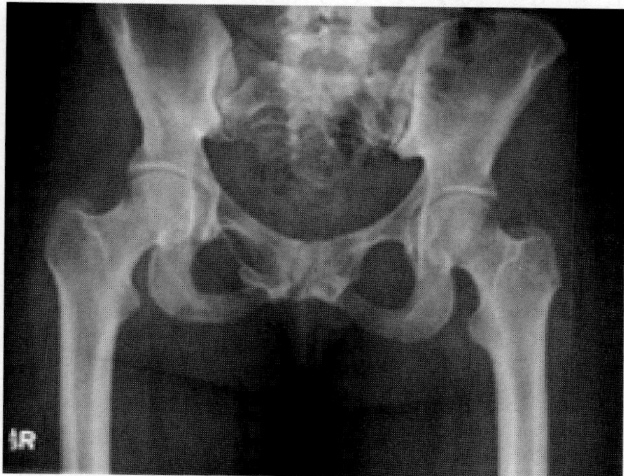

FIGURE 18-3. Closed reduction for overlapped symphysis. **A:** Anteroposterior radiograph of a 19-year-old woman who sustained a lateral compression type (B2-1) injury to her pelvis in a motor vehicle accident. Note the internal rotation of the right hemipelvis, the fracture through the right superior ramus, and the superior portion of the symphysis fractured and overriding the left hemipelvis *(white arrow)*. **B:** The patient was taken to the operating room with the intent of doing open reduction; however, under image intensification closed reduction was achieved by direct pressure over the right iliac crest, which externally rotated the hemipelvis, and direct pressure on the superior fragment. The fracture was reduced virtually to anatomic position, without need for open reduction. Note the anatomic healing of the superior ramus and the calcification at the symphysis. The final outcome was excellent. **C:** In spite of a solid fusion of the symphysis the patient was able to deliver two children vaginally; weight 6 lb 13 oz and 6 lb 7 oz.

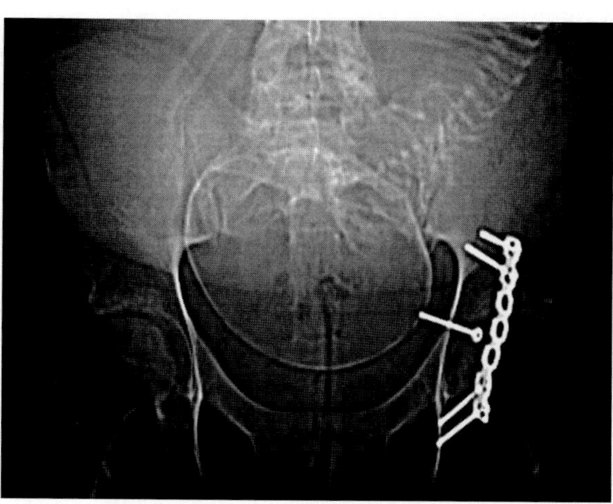

FIGURE 18-4. Note the screw used for previous fixation of the acetabular fracture impinging on the fetal head

Sexual Function

Sexual function can be affected by trauma in general and pelvic fracture in specific. Miranda and coworkers (35) found that only 60 of 80 patients (75%, both genders) returned to their premorbid sexual function after pelvic fracture. McCarthy and coworkers (2) reported a negative impact on sexual function after pelvic fracture, specifically with respect to body image, and frequency of and pleasure derived from sexual activity.

Physiologic components of normal sexual function in the female include arousal (lubrication and lengthening of the vagina) and orgasm. Copeland and coworkers (3) reported that physiologic problems with sexual function were uncommon (between 3% and 6%) and did not correlate with pelvic fracture. No significant differences between subjects and controls were found with respect to arousal and orgasm.

Sexual problems may be related to the severity of fracture (2). Tornetta and Matta (36) reported unspecified sexual problems in six out of 46 patients (13%, both genders) with unstable posterior pelvic ring injuries. Rotationally unstable injuries treated at the same center (37) were not found to be associated with sexual problems of any kind. Cole and coworkers (38) reported sexual difficulties in 15 of 64 patients (29%, both genders) with unstable posterior pelvic ring injuries. Pohlemann and coworkers (39) found no instances of sexual problems in women with Tile A or B injuries; sexual problems were reported in only one of 11 women with Tile C injuries.

Dyspareunia

Dyspareunia, or pain during sexual intercourse, after pelvic fracture has been described by many authors (2–5,38,40). Bony spicules from, or displacement of, the pubis can cause dyspareunia (Fig. 18-5) (4,5,39). Vaginal stricture may also contribute to dyspareunia (5). Fallat and coworkers (40) reported dyspareunia in two of five women with pelvic fractures associated with reproductive tract injuries. Both had open fractures with vaginal lacerations. Cole and coworkers (38) reported dyspareunia in four of 28 women (19%) treated operatively for unstable posterior pelvic ring injuries. Two of these four patients had received an open anterior approach to the pelvis. Pohlemann and coworkers (39) reported dyspareunia in one of 11 women with Tile C injuries. This woman had residual posterior displacement of the symphysis after treatment in an external fixator.

Copeland and coworkers (3) distinguished between musculoskeletal pain affecting sexual function and pain specifically in the reproductive tract. The incidence of musculoskeletal discomfort during intercourse was not found to be different between subjects and controls (30% and 21%, respectively; $p > 0.05$). However, subjects reported pain in the reproductive tract significantly more frequently than did controls (19% and 9.5%, respectively; $p = 0.045$). Of subjects with residual displacement >5 mm, 43% reported discomfort during intercourse, significantly more than subjects with nondisplaced pelvic fractures (25%, $p = 0.04$). Fracture type and fracture severity did not correlate with dyspareunia. Thirteen of the 123 subjects had severe residual anterior pathology (displaced ramus fractures, overriding rami, exuberant callous, heterotopic ossification) but did not have an increased risk of dyspareunia.

THE PREGNANT TRAUMA PATIENT

Physiologic Issues

Basic resuscitation rules apply during the emergency department evaluation of the pregnant trauma patient (41–43). However, pregnancy alters maternal physiology in several ways that alter the response to blood loss after trauma and that may complicate the diagnosis of hemodynamic instability.

During pregnancy, women experience an increase in the circulating blood volume, mostly because of an increase in the plasma volume. Therefore, the hematocrit decreases to an average of 32% by the 34th week of gestation. The heart rate increases by 10 to 15 beats per minute by the third trimester. The cardiac output is increased by 30% to 40%. Blood pressure drops in the second trimester, returning to normal at term. Because of the relative hypervolemia, the mother may lose 1,200 to 1,500 mL of blood before exhibiting the signs and symptoms of hypovolemia, whereas the fetus may show distress (bradycardia) at this amount of hemorrhage (42,43). The fetus may be in shock while the mother appears stable. Early crystalloid resuscitation, and type-specific blood transfusion is indicated to recreate the relative hypervolemic state. Hypotensive resuscitation is contraindicated in the pregnant patient. Because of the sensitivity of the placental circulation to catecholamines, they have no role in resuscitation of the pregnant trauma patient (42,43).

Pregnant patients should be placed in the left lateral decubitus position to improve venous return through the inferior vena cava (41–43). The supine position may decrease cardiac output by 30% and lead to hypotension in some women. This position may be achieved temporarily while the patient is on a backboard in cases with suspected spinal cord injury or unstable pelvic fracture. Early external fixation of the pelvis may be necessary to facilitate safe positioning.

Diaphragm elevation decreases the functional residual capacity, increasing the minute ventilation leading to a compensated respiratory alkalosis, which in turn decreases the maternal capacity to buffer acidosis from shock. Small increases in maternal oxygen saturation are protective of the fetus, because of the difference in the fetal hemoglobin oxygen dissociation curve (42).

Pregnancy is associated with a hypercoagulable state because of increased circulating clotting factors. The placenta and amniotic fluid have high contents of tissue thromboplastin (42). Abruptio placenta and amniotic fluid embolization increase the risk of disseminated intravascular coagulation. Skeletal stabilization, and replacement of platelets, fibrinogen, and clotting factors are adjuncts to treatment of the underlying obstetric injury.

Diagnostic Workup

Fetal ultrasound may miss severe placental abruptions (42), but it is useful for determining gestational age and fetal viability as well as certain intraabdominal maternal injuries (41). Cardiotocographic monitoring (the most sensitive test for placental abruptions) should be implemented in all pregnancies beyond 20 to 24 weeks (42–44). Helical computed tomography, useful for diagnosing maternal injuries, also can detect placental infarct or abruption (45).

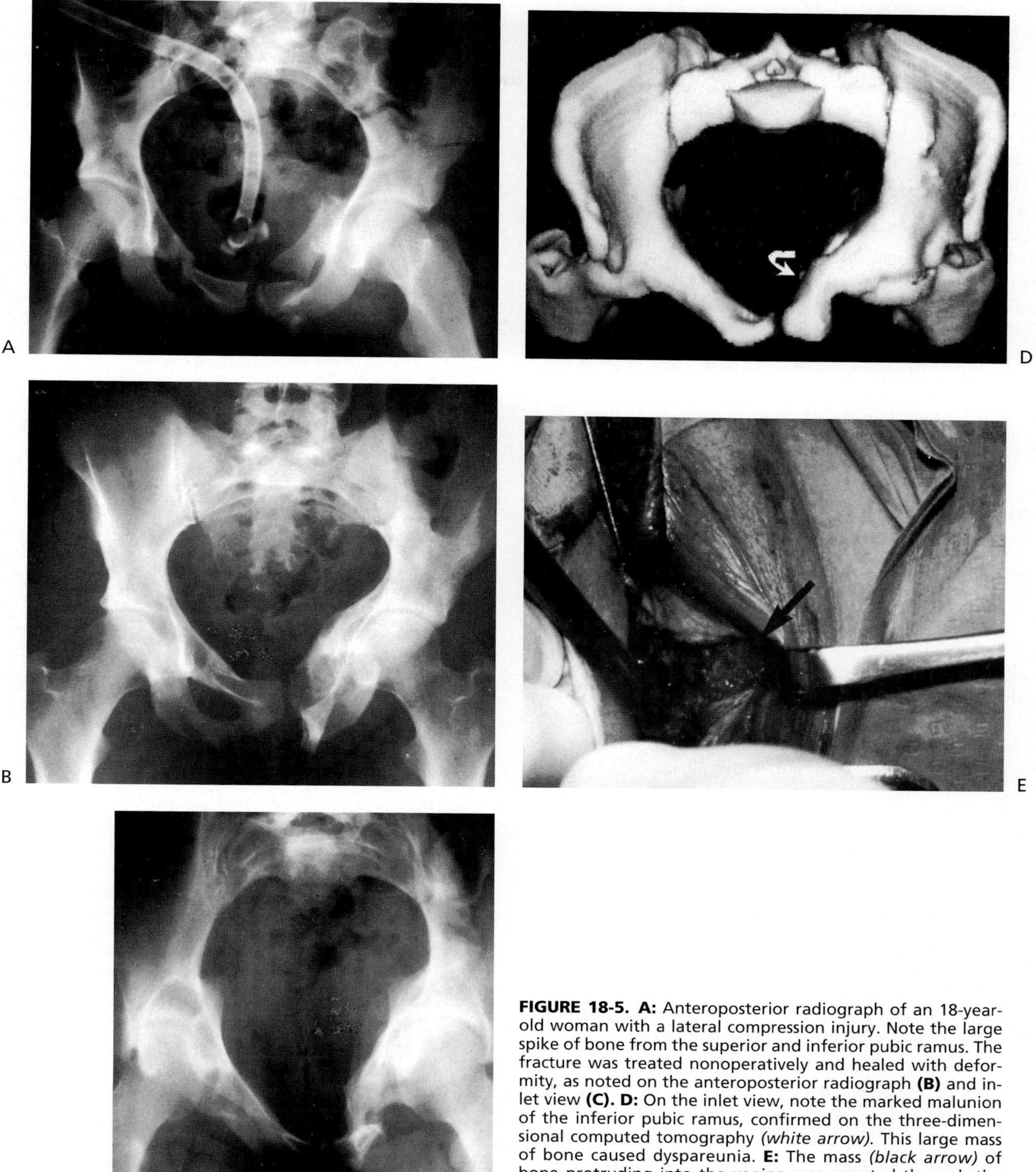

FIGURE 18-5. A: Anteroposterior radiograph of an 18-year-old woman with a lateral compression injury. Note the large spike of bone from the superior and inferior pubic ramus. The fracture was treated nonoperatively and healed with deformity, as noted on the anteroposterior radiograph **(B)** and inlet view **(C)**. **D:** On the inlet view, note the marked malunion of the inferior pubic ramus, confirmed on the three-dimensional computed tomography *(white arrow)*. This large mass of bone caused dyspareunia. **E:** The mass *(black arrow)* of bone protruding into the vagina was resected through the vagina, and symptoms were alleviated.

Because maternal survival is the most important factor in fetal survival, most authors advocate pursuing the necessary radiographic workup to diagnose any maternal injuries (41–43,46–50). Peak kilovoltage and fluoroscopy time should be minimized without compromising the quality of the examination. Shielding should be undertaken whenever possible, and unnecessary films should be avoided.

Fetal radiation risk can grossly be lumped into low (<10 mGy), intermediate (10 to 250 mGy), and high (>250 mGy) risk levels of exposure. Fetuses between 2 and 15 weeks gestational age have a small additional risk of somatic deformities when exposed to intermediate and high doses of radiation (probable threshold, 100 mGy). Rough estimates of radiation exposure are 2 mGy for a conventional pelvic radiograph, 5 mGy per slice of abdominal or pelvic computed tomography, or 10 mGy per minute of pelvic fluoroscopy (41,46,51). Formal radiation dose assessment is recommended in the first trimester if fetal exposure is believed to approach 10 mGy, or if it is requested by the patient or her family (51).

Injury Patterns

Pregnant women are more likely than nonpregnant women to sustain abdominal trauma as a result of blunt trauma (50). Fetal vulnerability to trauma is related to gestational age. Up to 12 weeks of gestation, the fetus is entirely contained within the pelvis and is relatively protected. By the third trimester, however, the fetus becomes much more vulnerable because of its extrapelvic position, the decrease in the volume of amniotic fluid, and the thinning of the uterine walls. The head is engaged, and the torso is exposed. Trauma to the fetal head (subdural and subarachnoid hemorrhage, skull fracture, and decapitation) have all been reported with maternal pelvic fracture (30,33,47,52).

Outcomes

As in nonpregnant trauma patients, death in pregnant trauma patients is related to the Injury Severity Score, blood hemoglobin, and shock. Mortality for pregnant trauma patients has been reported to range between 3.8% and 17.5% (49,53). In the presence of a pelvic fracture, maternal mortality ranges from 6% to 28% (30,33,54).

Preterm labor occurs in up to 11% of pregnant trauma patients, whereas preterm delivery occurs in up to 25% (55). Fetal death is most often related to maternal death, prolonged maternal shock, placental abruption, uterine rupture, or direct fetal trauma in association with any of the preceding (47,54). Fetal death can occur in up to 80% of pelvic fractures (3,46,53).

Ali and coworkers (47) reported on 68 pregnant trauma patients and found that Injury Severity Score, hemoglobin, blood transfusion, and disseminated intravascular coagulation were predictors of fetal mortality. Maternal abdominal and pelvic trauma were found to be nonpredictive of fetal outcome in this and other studies (47,52), but several studies have shown a trend toward higher fetal mortality in the presence of a pelvic fracture (3,54). Nonsurviving fetuses are usually nonviable at presentation (33,55).

Prevention

Failure to use seat belts is associated with a trend toward higher maternal death rates, particularly if ejection occurs (48,52,54). Inappropriate use of seat belts (i.e., worn over the most protuberant portion of the abdomen) has been related to uterine rupture (56). Seat belts should be worn with the lap portion below the protuberance of the abdomen. Three-point restraints with appropriate placement of the lap and shoulder portions of the belt have been shown to decrease fetal mortality (44,57).

Orthopedic Treatment Modification

Orthopedic management in the pregnant trauma patient should be directed at minimizing ongoing hemorrhage, managing pain, avoiding bed rest, and facilitating the left lateral decubitus position whenever possible. External fixation is extremely valuable in achieving these goals. In the near-term patient with a viable fetus, particularly if preterm labor begins, nonoperative care or minimally invasive provisional stabilization (traction or external fixation) usually is indicated (Fig. 18-6). The orthopedist's role is to manage pain and facilitate positioning of the limbs for delivery. After delivery has occurred and the patient's coagulation profile has stabilized, operative stabilization can be addressed.

Pape and coworkers (33) reported on seven pregnant patients with pelvic (five) or acetabular (two) fractures. Five women survived. In all five, modified goals of pain management and provisional stabilization were achieved. Treatment included external fixation (two), traction (two), and modified open reduction and internal fixation (one). In the last patient, full reduction (which would have required aggressive anterior and posterior fixation) was not achieved. Posterior *in situ* fixation of the sacrum was supplemented by anterior external fixation. No adverse orthopedic outcomes were detected at short-term follow-up in these patients.

PELVIC TRAUMA SECONDARY TO PREGNANCY

Incidence

The symphysis normally widens 1 to 1.5 mm and vertically translates up to 2 mm in nonpregnant patients (58,59). In normal pregnancy, mobility of the sacroiliac joints and the symphysis increases (34). Ligamentous relaxation from circulating estrogen, progesterone, and relaxin can lead to a physiologic widening of the symphysis 3 to 7 mm (43,60). In most cases, physiologic widening at the symphysis resolves spontaneously (34).

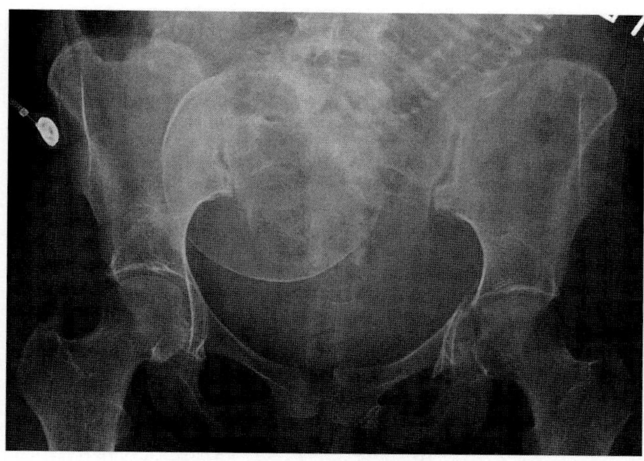

A

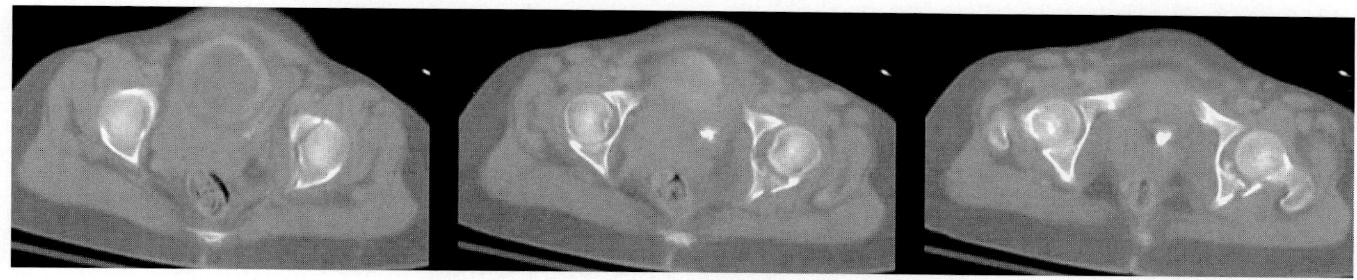

B

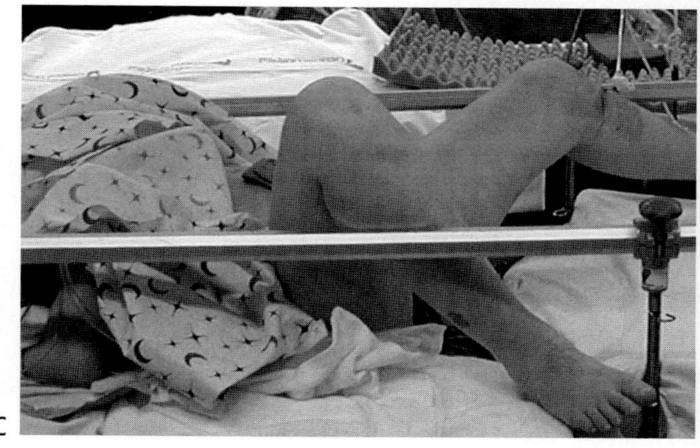

C

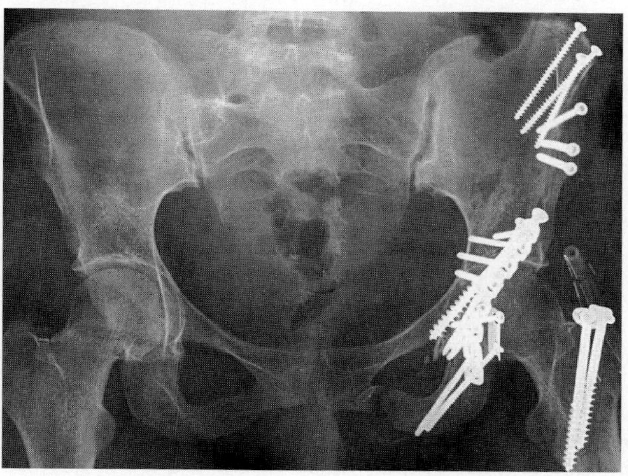

D

FIGURE 18-6. Provisional stabilization with traction used in a patient, 36 weeks pregnant, with an acetabular fracture dislocation. **A:** Pelvic radiograph, showing T type acetabular fracture. **B:** Computed tomography scan of pelvis. **C:** Temporary traction placed to assist in positioning, prevent hip subluxation, and minimize discomfort during vaginal delivery. **D:** Postoperative radiographs showing fixation performed in the immediate postpartum period. (Pictures courtesy of Alan Jones.)

Postpartum rupture of the symphysis pubis has been reported to have an incidence of 1:600 to 1:20,000 deliveries (60,61). The widespread use of C section may have decreased the incidence over time. Estrogen and relaxin are thought to play roles in the development of symphysiolysis (62,63), and elevated serum relaxin levels have been shown in patients with pelvic diastasis during pregnancy (62). In one study, members of a Norwegian support group for sufferers of postpartum pelvic pain and pelvic joint instability differed significantly from the population norms with respect to postterm deliveries, birth weight >4,000 g, female birth, and congenital hip dysplasia, all factors thought to correlate with elevated estrogen and relaxin levels (63).

The clinical findings of symphyseal rupture are tenderness, crepitus, a palpable defect at the symphysis, and difficulty with ambulation. A waddling gait is often noted (61,63–65). In most cases, onset of symptoms usually occurs within the first postpartum day, but it can occur as late as postpartum day 5 (60,61). Taylor and Sonson (60) reported 11 cases of symphysiolysis in a 5-year period, all of which occurred after spontaneous vaginal delivery. A common finding in all patients was rapid descent of the presenting part during the second stage of labor (second stage of labor lasting less than 30 minutes). Parity, maternal age, fetal size, and pelvimetry did not correlate with symphysiolysis. Rapid descent, or "violent" labor, also has been implicated in the pathogenesis of symphysiolysis by other authors (Fig. 18-7) (61).

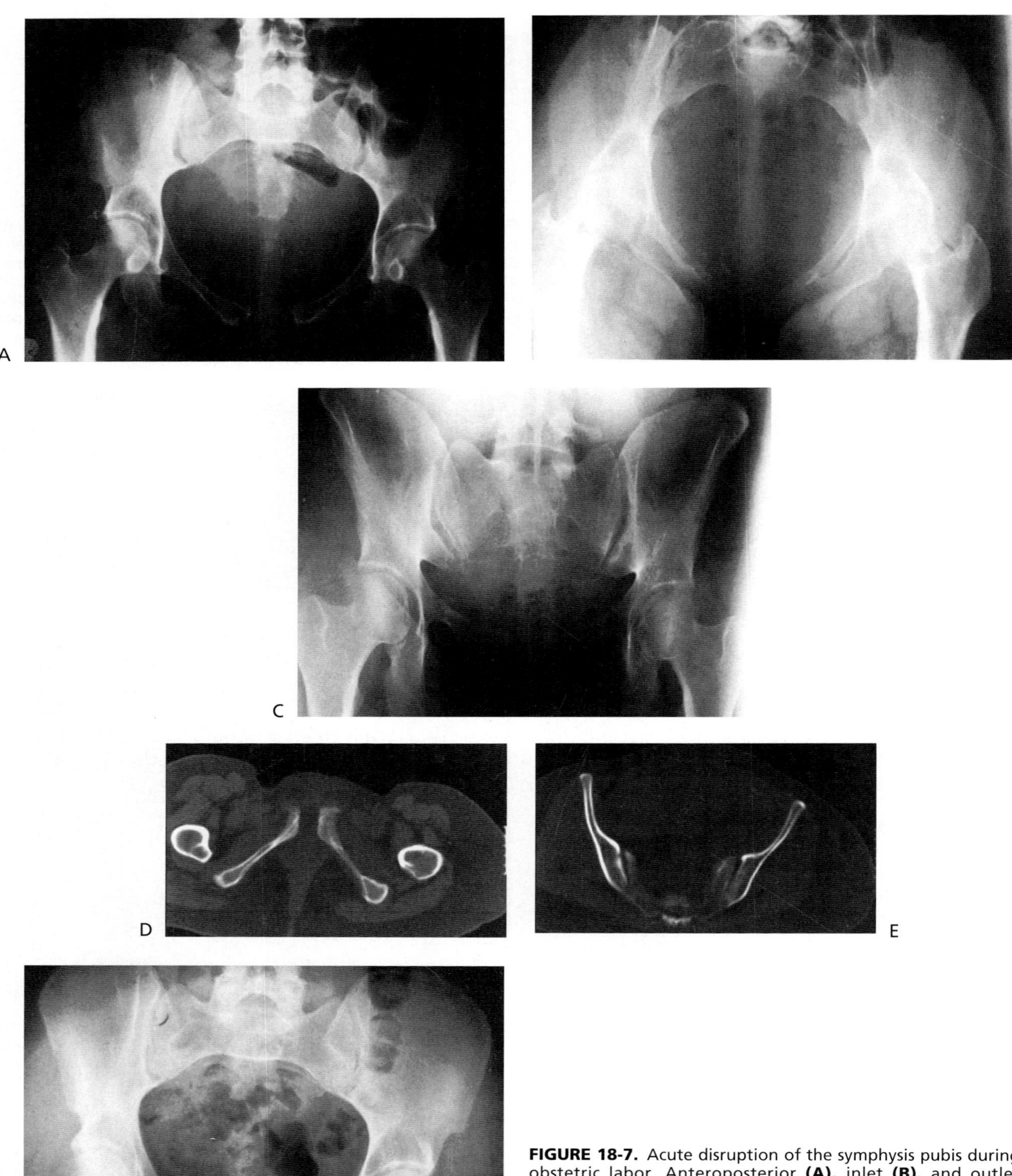

FIGURE 18-7. Acute disruption of the symphysis pubis during obstetric labor. Anteroposterior **(A),** inlet **(B),** and outlet **(C)** radiographs of the pelvis show disruption of the symphysis pubis and anterior opening of the sacroiliac joints during a difficult labor. The patient, anesthetist, and obstetrician all heard a loud crack during the delivery. The lesion was confirmed on computed tomography **(D,E).** Nonoperative symptomatic care resulted in the symphysis stabilizing, albeit in a slightly widened position **(F).** (Courtesy of S. Cartan.)

Acute Treatment

Taylor and Sonson (60) treated their patients with symphysiolysis with a brief period of bed rest (24 to 48 hours), followed by a pelvic binder (not tolerated by one patient) and mobilization. Symptoms generally resolve within 4 months. Only one patient had persistent low back pain at 1 year. Diastasis was 38 mm at delivery but had diminished to 8 mm at 1-year follow-up without evidence of degenerative changes.

Pelvic binders may be used in most cases of symphysiolysis. Pelvic slings have been used in the past but have the major disadvantage of requiring bed rest for several weeks. Prolonged bed rest is undesirable for medical reasons (thromboembolism, pulmonary toilet issues) as well as psychosocial reasons (care of and bonding with the neonate). Nonoperative care is effective in most cases (60,61,64,65).

Indications for surgical intervention include inadequate reduction, recurrent diastasis, intractable symptoms, and open rupture (65–67) Pennig and coworkers (67) successfully treated a patient with symphysiolysis (whose course was complicated by intractable postpartum pain and difficulty in ambulating) with closed reduction and anterior external fixation.

Open rupture of the symphysis owing to childbirth, with associated vaginal tear, also has been reported (61,66). In 1932, Reis and coworkers (61) reviewed the literature and found a 10.4% incidence of abscess formation and a 36% incidence of bladder trauma. Five deaths occurred, three of which were related to sepsis from abscess formation. Blum and Orovano (66) successfully treated a patient with open rupture of the symphysis by operative stabilization of the diastasis and vaginal debridement and repair.

Late Musculoskeletal Complications

Although symptoms of symphysiolysis improve with time in most cases, nonoperative treatment is not always successful

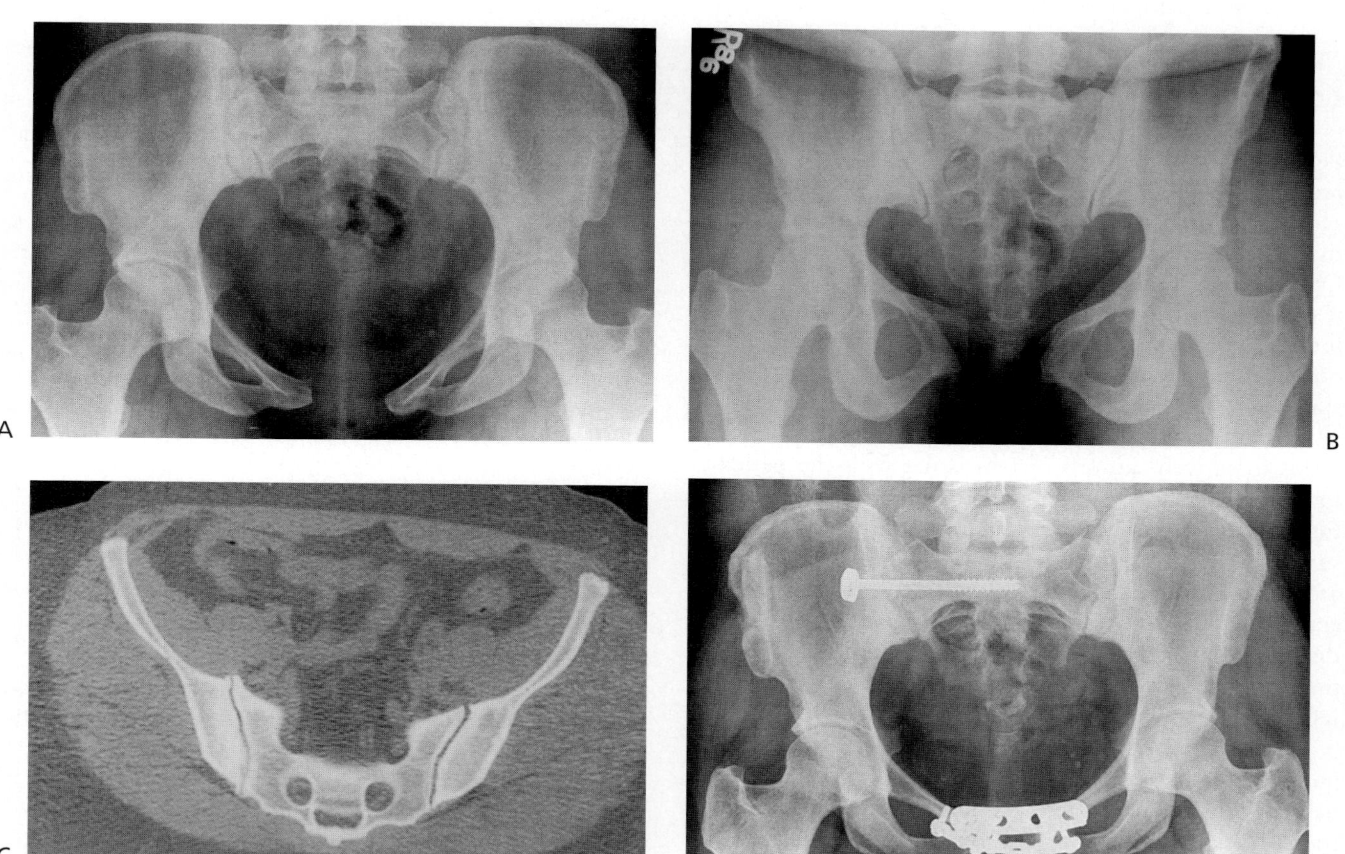

FIGURE 18-8. Postpartum pelvic instability: 30-year-old woman who presented 3 years after vaginal delivery, during which she felt a violent "pop" and immediate pain in the right sacroiliac joint and symphysis. A urethral tear was treated by prolonged catheterization. She presented with chronic right sacroiliac pain and symphyseal pain. The left sacroiliac joint was not symptomatic. **A:** Anterior-posterior pelvis radiograph at presentation. **B:** Outlet radiograph at presentation. **C:** Computed tomography scan at presentation. Right sacroiliac fusion combined with symphyseal plating was performed. **D:** Postoperative anterior-posterior radiograph at 18-month follow-up. The sacroiliac joint is asymptomatic, and the patient has resumed full activities. She continues to have mild pain in the symphyseal region.

(Fig. 18-8). Taylor and Sonson (60) reported that one of 11 patients had chronic pain more than 1 year postpartum. Grace and coworkers (68) reported on wedge resection of the symphysis pubis in 10 women with chronic pain from osteitis pubis. Nine of the women were parous. Despite substantial improvements in pain levels, 30% were not satisfied at 7-year follow-up. Rommens (69) reported three patients for whom nonoperative treatment failed to resolve pain and instability. All had residual widening of the symphysis of at least 15 mm, with degenerative changes, and a qualitative vertical shift of the pubis on single-stance radiographs. Open reduction and internal fixation of the symphysis was performed for all three patients and was supplemented by transiliac bars in one patient. All healed, improved, and had implants removed. Shuler and Gruen (70) reported a case of chronic postpartum pain in both the sacroiliac joints and the symphysis, which began immediately after a high forceps delivery. The patient had an excellent clinical result after open reduction of the symphysis and percutaneous fixation of both sacroiliac joints.

CONCLUSION

Pelvic fracture in the female patient of childbearing age represents a unique situation for orthopedic surgeons. In the acute situation, the orthopedic surgeon needs to be proactive in recognition and care of associated soft-tissue injuries. Open injuries to the genitourinary tract can be catastrophic if unrecognized. Insuring that a pelvic examination is performed, and that gynecologic or urologic consultations are obtained is often the responsibility of the orthopedic surgeon.

In the later postinjury period, the orthopedic surgeon needs to actively address certain issues with the patient. Female patients report high levels of anxiety regarding future sexual activity and reproductive ability. Simple reassurance and education about the complexity of the injury are helpful. Inquiring about urinary function in the postoperative period is important, especially in patients at risk for disruption of the pelvic floor external rotation or AP compression injuries. Pelvic floor muscle retraining and early referral to urologic specialists can be helpful.

When a former trauma patient becomes pregnant, the question is always whether she will be able to deliver vaginally or require a C section. Although dystocia after pelvic fracture is very rare, the current medicolegal climate favors elective C section in this patient population. Many obstetricians are hampered in their decision making by a poor understanding of the pelvic injury and are given inadequate information regarding the location and extent of the pelvic injury. The orthopedist may decrease the number of unnecessary cesarean sections by providing clear information, radiographs, or diagrams to the patient (and/or her obstetrician) at the time of her discharge from follow-up care. Education and communication are among the most important responsibilities in this specific patient population.

REFERENCES

1. Madsen LV, Jensen J, Christensen ST. Parturition and pelvic fracture. Follow-up of 34 obstetric patients with a history of pelvic fracture. *Acta Obstet Gynecol Scand* 1983;62:617–620.
2. McCarthy ML, MacKenzie EJ, Bosse MJ, et al. Functional status following orthopedic trauma in young women. *J Trauma* 1995;39:828–837.
3. Copeland CE, Bosse MJ, McCarthy ML, et al. Effect of trauma and pelvic fracture on female genitourinary, sexual, and reproductive function. *J Orthop Trauma* 1997;11:73–81.
4. Patil U, Nesbitt R, Meyer R. Genitourinary tract injuries due to fracture of the pelvis in females: sequelae and their management. *Br J Urol* 1982;54:32–38.
5. Zhou SR. [Fracture-dislocation of pelvis in the adult female: clinical analysis of 105 cases]. *Chung Hua Wai Ko Tsa Chih* 1989; 27:479–481, 509–510.
6. Niemi TA, Norton LW. Vaginal injuries in patients with pelvic fractures. *J Trauma* 1985;25:547–551.
7. Perry MO, Husmann DA. Urethral injuries in female subjects following pelvic fractures. *J Urol* 1992;147:139–143.
8. Parkhurst JD, Coker JE, Halverstadt DB. Traumatic avulsion of the lower urinary tract in the female child. *J Urol* 1981;126: 265–267.
9. Pode D, Shapiro A. Traumatic avulsion of the female urethra: case report. *J Trauma* 1990;30:235–237.
10. Donner GG, Pel M, Lammes FB. Primary amenorrhea caused by crushing trauma of the pelvis. *Am J Obstet Gynecol* 2000;183: 500–501.
11. Casselman RC, Schillinger JF. Fractured pelvis with avulsion of the female urethra. *J Urol* 1977;117:385–386.
12. Webster GD, Sihelnik SA, Stone AR. Urethrovaginal fistula: a review of the surgical management. *J Urol* 1984;132:460–462.
13. Williams DI. Rupture of the female urethra in childhood. *Eur Urol* 1975;1:129–130.
14. Barach E, Martin G, Tomlanovich M, et al. Blunt pelvic trauma with urethral injury in the female: a case report and review of the literature. *J Emerg Med* 1984;2:101–105.
15. Netto NR Jr, Ikari O, Zuppo VP. Traumatic rupture of the female urethra. *Urology* 1983;22:601–603.
16. Gourlay N. Accidental rupture of the female urethra. *J Obstet Gynecol Br Emp* 1960;67:991–993.
17. Bredael JJ, Kramer SA, Cleeve LK, et al. Traumatic rupture of the female urethra. *J Urol* 1979;122:560–561.
18. Doman AN, Hoekstra DV. Pelvic fracture associated with severe intra-abdominal gynecologic injury. *J Trauma* 1988;28:118–120.
19. Goins WA, Rodriguez A, Lewis J, et al. Retroperitoneal hematoma after blunt trauma. *Surg Gynecol Obstet* 1992;174: 281–290.
20. Smith AR, Hosker GL, Warrell DW. The role of pudendal nerve damage in the aetiology of genuine stress incontinence in women. *Br J Obstet Gynaecol* 1989;96:29–32.
21. Smith AR, Hosker GL, Warrell DW. The role of partial denervation of the pelvic floor in the aetiology of genitourinary prolapse and stress incontinence of urine. A neurophysiological study. *Br J Obstet Gynaecol* 1989;96:24–28.
22. Wilson PD, Al Samarrai T, Deakin M, et al. An objective assessment of physiotherapy for female genuine stress incontinence. *Br J Obstet Gynaecol* 1987;94:575–582.

23. Nielsen CA, Sigsgaard I, Olsen M, et al. Trainability of the pelvic floor. A prospective study during pregnancy and after delivery. *Acta Obstet Gynecol Scand* 1988;67:437–440.
24. Hahn I, Milsom I, Fall M, et al. Long-term results of pelvic floor training in female stress urinary incontinence. *Br J Urol* 1993; 72:421–427.
25. Klein MC, Janssen PA, MacWilliam L, et al. Determinants of vaginal-perineal integrity and pelvic floor functioning in childbirth. *Am J Obstet Gynecol* 1997;176:401–410.
26. Voegelin AW, McCall ML. Some acquired bony abnormalities influencing the conduit of labor. With reports of recent cases. *Am J Obstet Gynecol* 1944;48:361–370.
27. Schuman W. Fractured pelvis in obstetrics (with report of cases). *Am J Obstet Gynecol* 1932;23:103–107.
28. Mulla N. Fractures of the pelvis in pregnancy. *Am J Obstet Gynecol* 1957;74:246–250.
29. Speer DP, Peltier LF. Pelvic fractures and pregnancy. *J Trauma* 1972;12:474–480.
30. Dyer I, Barclay DL. Accidental trauma complicating pregnancy and delivery. *Am J Obstet Gynecol* 1962;83:907–929.
31. Sachs BP, Kobelin C, Castro MA, et al. The risks of lowering the cesarean-delivery rate. *N Engl J Med* 1999;340:54–57.
32. Clasper JC, Copeland CE, McCarthy ML, et al. *Vaginal delivery and cesarean section after pelvic fracture.* Presented at the 64th Annual Meeting of the American Academy of Orthopaedic Surgeons, San Francisco, February 15, 1997.
33. Pape HC, Pohlemann T, Gansslen A, et al. Pelvic fractures in pregnant multiple trauma patients. *J Orthop Trauma* 2000;14: 238–244.
34. Ekas WL. Traumatic separation of the symphysis pubis. *Am J Obstet Gynecol* 1931;21:680–689.
35. Miranda MA, Riemer BL, Butterfield SL, et al. Pelvic ring injuries. A long term functional outcome study. *Clin Orthop* 1996;Aug:152–159.
36. Tornetta P III, Matta JM. Outcome of operatively treated unstable posterior pelvic ring disruptions. *Clin Orthop* 1996;Aug: 186–193.
37. Tornetta P, Dickson K, Matta JM. Outcome of rotationally unstable pelvic ring injuries treated operatively. *Clin Orthop* 1996;Aug:147–151.
38. Cole JD, Blum DA, Ansel LJ. Outcome after fixation of unstable posterior pelvic ring injuries. *Clin Orthop* 1996;Aug:160–179.
39. Pohlemann T, Bosch U, Gansslen A, et al. The Hannover experience in management of pelvic fractures. *Clin Orthop* 1994; Aug:69–80.
40. Fallat ME, Weaver JM, Hertweck SP, et al. Late follow-up and functional outcome after traumatic reproductive tract injuries in women. *Am Surg* 1998;64:858–861.
41. Goldman SM, Wagner LK. Radiologic ABCs of maternal and fetal survival after trauma: when minutes may count. *Radiographics* 1999;19:1349–1357.
42. Maull KI. Maternal-fetal trauma. *Semin Pediatr Surg* 2001;10: 32–34.
43. American College of Surgeons. *Advanced trauma life support program for doctors,* 6th ed. Chicago: American College of Surgeons, 1997:315–321.
44. Stone IK. Trauma in the obstetric patient. *Obstet Gynecol Clin North Am* 1999;26:459–467, viii.
45. Lowdermilk C, Gavant ML, Qaisi W, et al. Screening helical CT for evaluation of blunt traumatic injury in the pregnant patient. *Radiographics* 1999;19:S243–255;discussion S256–8:S243–S255.
46. Drost TF, Rosemurgy AS, Sherman HF, et al. Major trauma in pregnant women: maternal/fetal outcome. *J Trauma* 1990;30: 574–578.
47. Ali J, Yeo A, Gana TJ, et al. Predictors of fetal mortality in pregnant trauma patients. *J Trauma* 1997;42:782–785.
48. Curet MJ, Schermer CR, Demarest GB, et al. Predictors of outcome in trauma during pregnancy: identification of patients who can be monitored for less than 6 hours. *J Trauma* 2000;49: 18–24.
49. Rogers FB, Rozycki GS, Osler TM, et al. A multi-institutional study of factors associated with fetal death in injured pregnant patients. *Arch Surg* 1999;134:1274–1277.
50. Shah KH, Simons RK, Holbrook T, et al. Trauma in pregnancy: maternal and fetal outcomes. *J Trauma* 1998;45:83–86.
51. Mann FA, Nathens A, Langer SG, et al. Communicating with the family: the risks of medical radiation to conceptuses in victims of major blunt-force torso trauma. *J Trauma* 2000;48:354–357.
52. Baerga-Varela Y, Zietlow SP, Bannon MP, et al. Trauma in pregnancy. *Mayo Clin Proc* 2000;75:1243–1248.
53. Esposito TJ, Gens DR, Smith LG, et al. Evaluation of blunt abdominal trauma occurring during pregnancy. *J Trauma* 1989;29: 1628–1632.
54. Corsi PR, Rasslan S, de Oliveira LB, et al. Trauma in pregnant women: analysis of maternal and fetal mortality. *Injury* 1999;30:239–243.
55. Connolly AM, Katz VL, Bash KL, et al. Trauma and pregnancy. *Am J Perinatol* 1997;14:331–336.
56. Astarita DC, Feldman B. Seat belt placement resulting in uterine rupture. *J Trauma* 1997;42:738–740.
57. Pearlman MD, Phillips ME. Safety belt use during pregnancy. *Obstet Gynecol* 1996;88:1026–1029.
58. Walheim G, Olerud S, Ribbe T. Mobility of the pubic symphysis: measurements by an electromechanical method. *Acta Orthop Scand* 1984;55:203–208.
59. Walheim GG, Selvik G. Mobility of the pubic symphysis: in vivo measurements with an electromechanical method and a roentgen stereophotogrammetric method. *Clin Orthop* 1984; Dec:129–135.
60. Taylor RN, Sonson RD. Separation of the pubic symphysis. An underrecognized peripartum complication. *J Reprod Med* 1986; 31:203–206.
61. Reis RA, Baer JL, Arens RA, et al. Traumatic separation of the symphysis pubis during spontaneous labor: with a clinical and x-ray study of the normal symphysis pubis during pregnancy and the puerperium. *Surg Gynecol Obstet* 1932;55:336–338.
62. Crim MW, Moss SW. Pelvic diastasis in pregnancy. *Am Fam Phys* 1987;35:185–186.
63. Saugstad LF. Persistent pelvic pain and pelvic joint instability. *J Obstet Gynecol Reprod Biol* 1991;41:197–201.
64. Dhar S, Anderton JM. Rupture of the symphysis pubis during labor. *Clin Orthop* 1992;Oct: 252–257.
65. Lindsey RW, Leggon RE, Wright DG, et al. Separation of the symphysis pubis in association with childbearing. A case report. *J Bone Joint Surg* 1988;70A:289–292.
66. Blum M, Orovano N. Open rupture of the symphysis pubis during spontaneous delivery. *Acta Obstet Gynecol Scand* 1976;55: 77–79.
67. Pennig D, Gladbach B, Majchrowski W. Disruption of the pelvic ring during spontaneous childbirth. A case report. *J Bone Joint Surg* 1997;79B:438–440.
68. Grace JN, Sim FH, Shives TC, et al. Wedge resection of the symphysis pubis for the treatment of osteitis pubis. *J Bone Joint Surg* 1989;71A:358–364.
69. Rommens PM. Internal fixation in postpartum symphysis pubis rupture: report of three cases. *J Orthop Trauma* 1997;11:273–276.
70. Shuler TE, Gruen GS. Chronic postpartum pelvic pain treated by surgical stabilization. *Orthopedics* 1996;19:687–689.

19

INSUFFICIENCY FRACTURES OF THE PELVIS

KENNETH A. EGOL
KENNETH J. KOVAL

INTRODUCTION

The insidious onset and progression of groin or low back pain in an elderly patient can pose a diagnostic dilemma. Often the symptoms are attributed to mechanical back pain, degenerative disc disease, muscle spasm, osteoarthritis, or malignancy. In addition, pelvic stress fractures can simulate loosening following total hip arthroplasty (1,2). Insufficiency fractures occur in elderly, mainly female individuals during normal activities of daily living. This occurs because in the elderly bone fatigue strength has been lowered secondary to osteoporosis, osteomalacia, or other disease states, thus allowing lower loads (normal activities) or fewer loading cycles to result in osseous failure. Stress fractures also may occur through areas of the pelvis weakened by bone grafting, especially at the donor site of the posterior iliac crest.

The treatment and healing of most stress fractures is straightforward and uneventful. The principles of treatment are to give the bone time to catch up to and heal the microdamage. Stress fracture healing parallels the healing of all frank fractures where different bones and different areas within the bones generally heal at various rates. A small number of cases may heal more rapidly than average, but some are slow to heal and may produce hideous deformities with major disabilities from malunion and nonunion (Fig. 19-1). These cases are difficult to treat surgically because the internal fixation devices may not hold in the severely osteoporotic bone (Fig. 19-2).

BIOMECHANICS

The mechanics of stress fracture in long bones is better understood. Tension stress fractures, as their name implies, occur on the tension side of the bone (i.e., superior femoral neck, anterior tibial cortex, etc.). Tension fractures occur because of a total strain in tension that causes debonding of osteons, eventually leading to a transverse fracture line. These fractures, however, do not incite a biologic response that would produce callus and healing. These "cracks" may persist for a long period of time before bridging callus is formed or complete displacement occurs. The presence of a tension crack acts as a stress riser. Continued exercise or loading makes it more likely that completion will occur and displacement will follow (3). This mechanism may be responsible for stress fractures of the pubic rami.

Compression fractures usually are oblique fractures and are caused by a completely different process than tension fractures. Instead of debonding osteons, the bone fails through the formation of oblique cracks. These oblique cracks isolate areas of bone, which receive no nutrients and are devascularized. The result is a process of creeping substitution with an osteoclastic response. This is a slower process that usually does not result in a displaced fracture. Completion may occur if activity continues as shear cracks coalesce leading to an oblique fracture. Most compression type stress fractures heal with rest, external supports, or immobilization (3). This may be responsible for the sacral fractures.

The biomechanics of pelvic stress fractures are not as well understood. The common thread of all involves repetitive

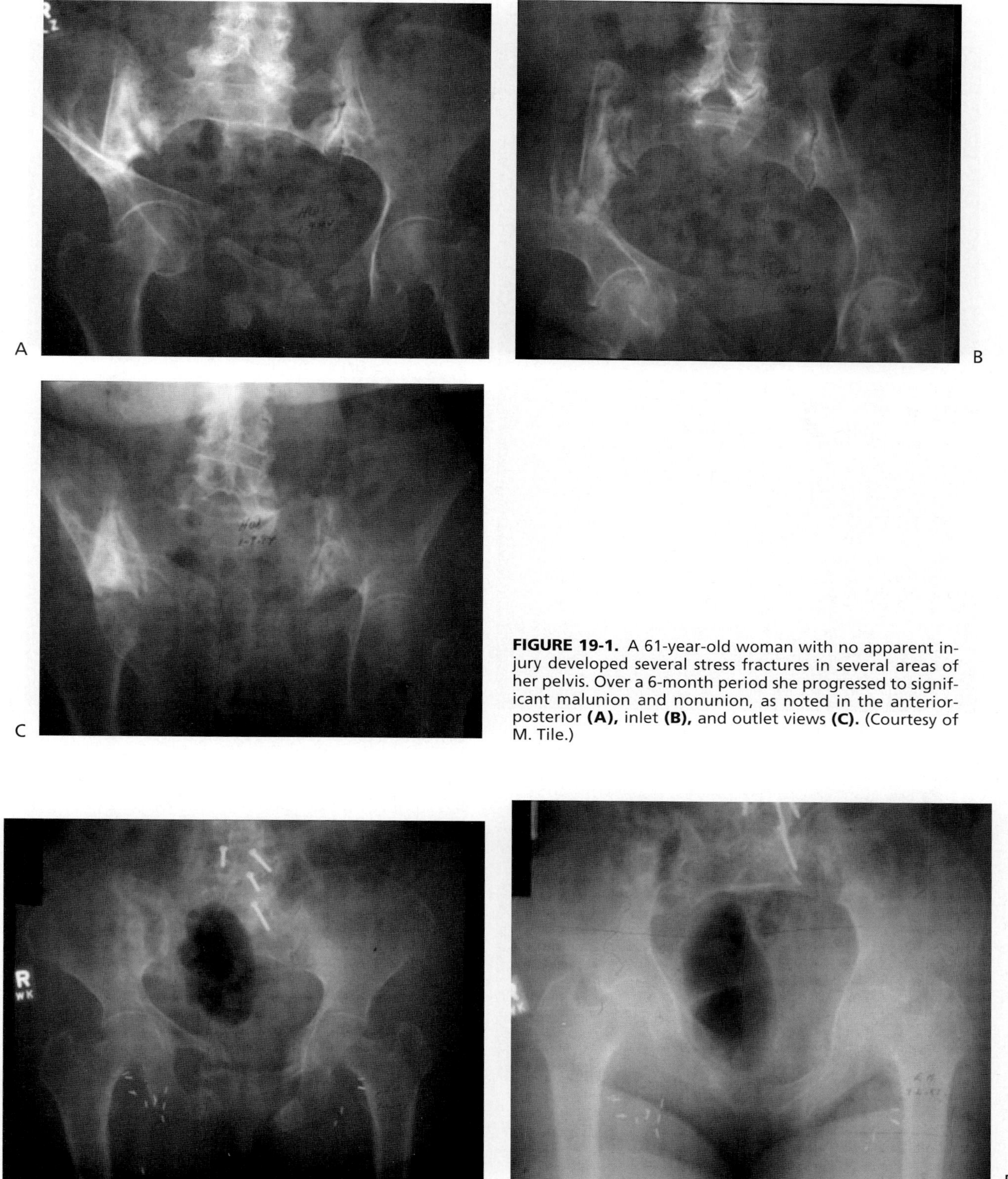

FIGURE 19-1. A 61-year-old woman with no apparent injury developed several stress fractures in several areas of her pelvis. Over a 6-month period she progressed to significant malunion and nonunion, as noted in the anterior-posterior **(A)**, inlet **(B)**, and outlet views **(C)**. (Courtesy of M. Tile.)

FIGURE 19-2. A 67-year-old woman with a severe insufficiency fracture caused by osteoporosis with no trauma as noted in the anterior-posterior **(A)**, inlet **(B)**, and outlet views **(C)**. Computed tomography (CT) scan shows the nonunion posteriorly in the CT **(D)** and anteriorly in the CT scan **(E)**. Attempts at surgical correction proved extremely difficult, because virtually all of the screws began to turn in the osteoporotic bone and fixation was tenuous at best. *(Figure continues)*

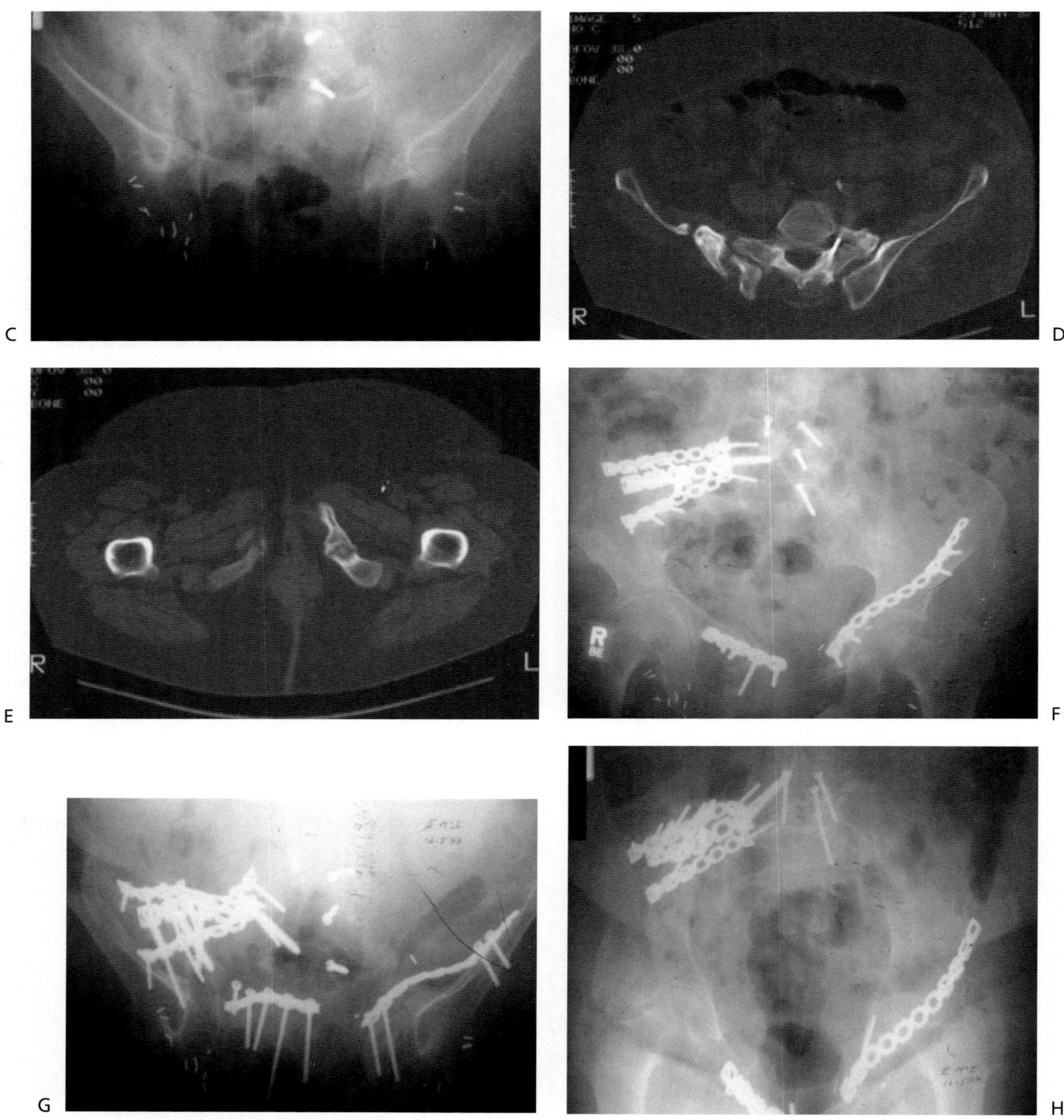

FIGURE 19-2. ***(continued)*** Ultimately, many of the screws pulled out, as noted on the three views, and the fixation failed **(F,G,H).** (Courtesy M. Tile.)

and abnormal loading, which lead to muscle fatigue. In addition to tension and compression, the pelvis is subjected to shear, bending, and rotational forces.

CLINICAL EVALUATION

Although the true incidence of insufficiency fracture of the pelvis is unknown, a prospective study of 2,366 patients presenting with low back pain found an incidence of 0.9% of insufficiency fracture of the sacrum. This number increased to 1.8% when women over 55 were evaluated (4). There are several predisposing factors that may lead to a pelvic insufficiency fracture, with osteopenia as a common pathway. These include prolonged corticosteroid treatment, rheumatoid arthritis, renal insufficiency, hyperparathyroidism, fibrous dysplasia, previous irradiation, and alcoholism (4–7). In addition, old anterior arch disruptions such as postpartum symphyseal widening, may lead to insufficiency fracture of the posterior ring over time (8).

Patient history is key in the diagnosis of pelvic insufficiency fracture. Commonly, patients with insufficiency fractures of the pelvis present with no history or some minor history of trauma. If the fracture involves the pubis, then they complain of a dull aching groin pain (9). Patients with sacral insufficiency fractures present with low back pain, with or without radiation into the buttock (4,6,10–12). Typically there are no neurologic defects.

The diagnosis of pelvic stress fracture often is one of exclusion. The physical examination of suspected pelvic stress fracture consists of direct palpation of the inferior and superior pubic rami. A bilateral examination is necessary because this region is ordinarily sensitive and comparison to the unaffected side may elucidate subtle tenderness. For evaluation of the sacrum, direct finger palpation may elicit tenderness. In addition, if there is SI joint involvement, a flexion, abduction, and external rotation maneuver (FABER) or Patrick's test with the affected hip elicits pain (13). Pain with axial loading, such as a heel strike maneuver, may signify an anterior fracture (14).

RADIOGRAPHIC EVALUATION

Diagnosis of pelvic insufficiency fractures on plain radiograph is variable and often not appreciated until late in the course when healing has begun. Many areas about the pelvis can be involved. Typical sites include: pubic rami, parasymphyseal regions, the sacral ala, and the iliac wing (5,15–18). Early on these stress fractures may be faint radiolucent lines, which may be obscured by bowel gas. If plain films are obtained during the healing phase, then a more aggressive appearance with significant lysis and callus formation may be seen and may be confused with a neoplastic process. Three views of the pelvis, the anterior-posterior, inlet and outlet, as well as computed tomography, anteriorly and posteriorly, outline the deformity and the presence or absence of nonunion (Fig. 19-3).

Until recently, bone scintography with technetium-99 methylene diphosphonate has been the gold standard as an early and reliable method for the detection of occult fractures (5,11,19–21). Scintigraphic images may be obtained at 2 hours postinjection (21). Multiple views must be attained to adequately assess affected areas. Standard views for assessing the pelvis consist of anterior and posterior views with the addition of an outlet or squat view to visualize the pubis if there is residual contrast in the bladder. There is a characteristic H-shaped appearance to the uptake pattern with sacral insufficiency fractures. This modality is widely available and multiple studies have attested to its sensitivity for detection of occult fractures.

Computed tomography (CT) has become an important adjunct to plain radiography. CT has been used to confirm the diagnosis in selected cases and is of importance in the sacrum where the fractures may occur in the sagittal plane. Many feel that CT scanning is most accurate because areas of sclerosis representing the reparative process are well seen and may show occult fracture lines not visible on plain radiograph (5,11,20,22).

Magnetic resonance imaging (MRI) has emerged as a very sensitive technique in the diagnosis of musculoskeletal pathology. Recent studies have shown MRI to be more sensitive than radionuclide imaging for the detection of occult hip fractures. Others have found MRI to be quite sensitive, but not specific with regard to the detection of occult sacral or iliac wing fractures (Fig. 19-4) (5,20,22,23).

A combination of T1-weighted images that optimize anatomic detail and depict bone marrow edema is essential. Sequences are usually performed in multiple orthogonal planes, depending on the region of interest. Two MRI patterns of stress fracture have been described. The most common, a bandlike fracture line that is low signal on all pulse sequences, surrounded by a larger, ill-defined zone of edema. The second, although less common pattern on MRI is an amorphous alteration of the marrow signal without a clear fracture line. This pattern is characterized by low signal intensity on T1-weighted images, with increased signal on T2-weighted images, and is considered a stress response to injury (23). Advantages of MRI include rapidity in obtaining results compared to radionuclide imaging and its lack of ionizing radiation. Disadvantages include increased cost when compared to radionuclide scanning and the absence of a total body image, which may lead the treating physician to miss asymptomatic stress fractures or multiple site stress fractures.

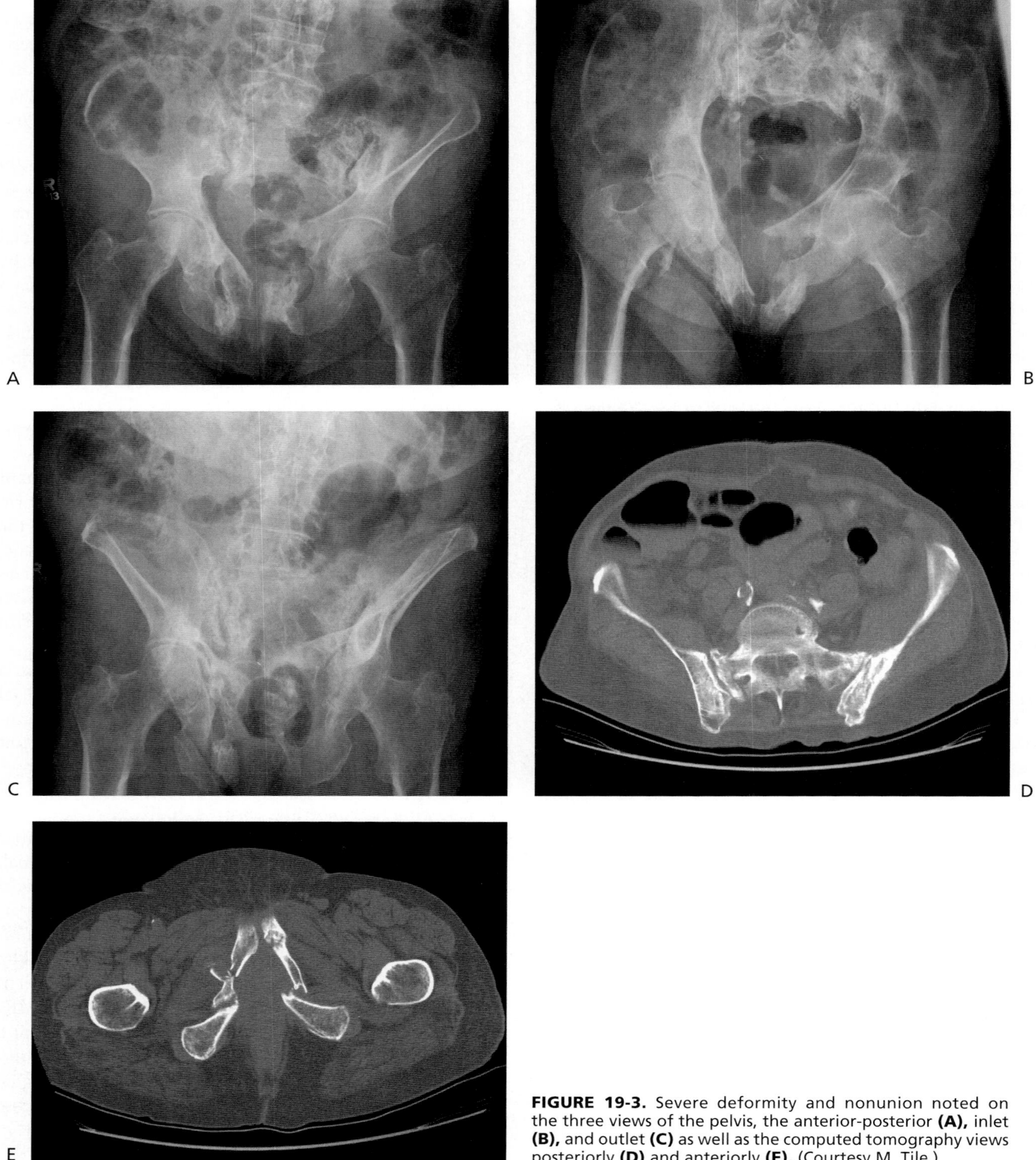

FIGURE 19-3. Severe deformity and nonunion noted on the three views of the pelvis, the anterior-posterior **(A),** inlet **(B),** and outlet **(C)** as well as the computed tomography views posteriorly **(D)** and anteriorly **(E).** (Courtesy M. Tile.)

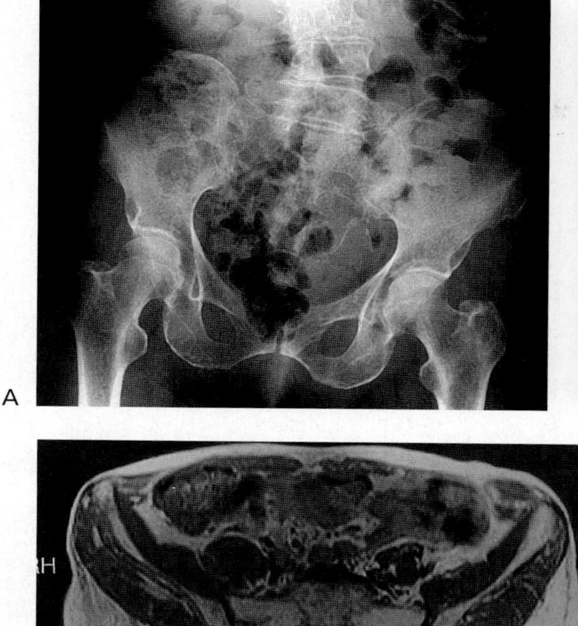

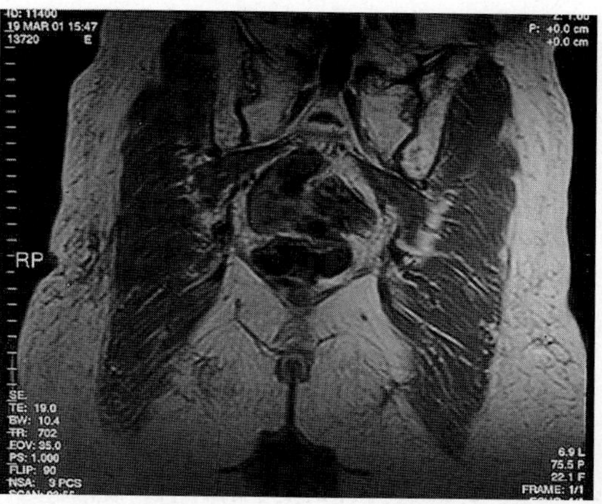

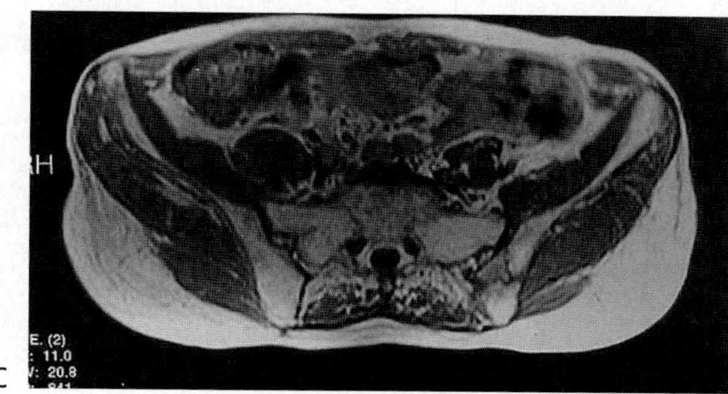

FIGURE 19-4. The case of a 77-year-old woman with a history of atraumatic onset of left hip and back pain. **A:** Plain radiographs of the pelvis are negative. A T1-weighted magnetic resonance image in both the coronal **(B)** and axial **(C)** planes reveal an insufficiency fracture of the left iliac wing. The patient was treated with rest and nonsteroidal antiinflammatory drugs and was symptom-free at 6 weeks.

MANAGEMENT

The common thread in the treatment algorithm for all stress fractures is a decreased level of activity. Management plan should be based on the concept of imbalance between bone resorption and remodeling. Pain free motion is a healthy indicator that the bone is progressing toward healing. Cessation of the stress allows the repair process to dominate over bone resorption. Most stress fractures heal with rest followed by mobilization (6,19,22).

The majority of patients become asymptomatic by 12 months with conservative treatment. Analgesics are a mainstay of therapy and usually include acetaminophen or nonsteroidal antiinflammatory drugs. Some have recommended calcitonin injections 100 IU s.c., which seem to be beneficial in controlling pain (4). Although adjunctive methods of treatment, such as pulsed electromagnetic fields and low-intensity ultrasound, have been used with success with other stress fracture sites, currently there is no literature to support their use about the pelvis.

Fortunately, pelvic insufficiency fractures are stable. Rarely, these fractures go on to pseudarthrosis. Surgical treatment of pelvic insufficiency fracture should be considered only after a long course of conservative therapy. Surgical treatment is aimed at repair of the nonunion (Fig. 19-5).

A further example is noted in Fig. 19-6. WB is a 42-year-old white female with a past medical history significant for Crohn's disease maintained on chronic oral steroids. The patient had a history of 2 years of dull aching groin pain, which is worse on the right than the left side. She had been to several physicians regarding her pain over the past 2 years, including a general surgeon who performed an inguinal hernia repair. The patient began to experience severe left-sided back pain over the 6 months prior to presentation.

On physical examination the patient was a thin, white female. She ambulated with an antalgic gait. There was a 1-cm leg length discrepancy, left shorter than right. There was pain with palpation of the pubic rami bilaterally and pain

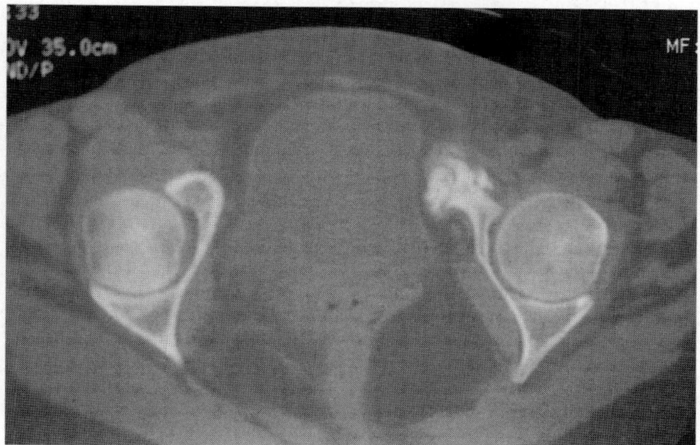

FIGURE 19-5. Computed tomography scan showing a hypertrophic nonunion of the superior pubic ramus following stress fracture.

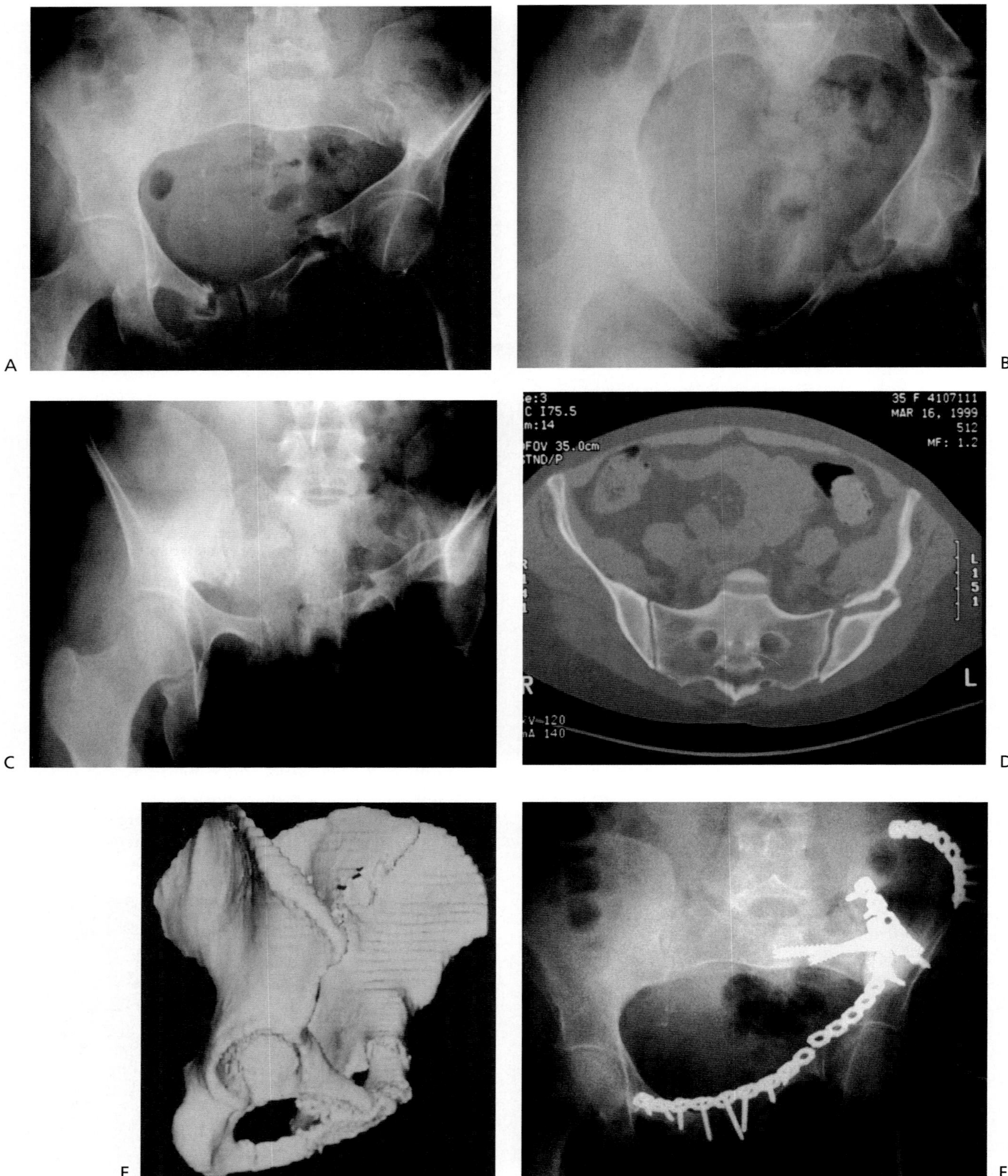

FIGURE 19-6. A: Initial presenting series of radiographs that demonstrate bilateral pubic rami stress fractures with an insufficiency fracture-dislocation of the sacroiliac joint. Anterior-posterior (AP) of the pelvis. **B:** Inlet view of the pelvis. **C:** Outlet view of the pelvis. **D:** Computed tomography scan confirms the lesion of the SI joint. **E:** Three-dimensional reconstruction of the pelvis. **F:** Radiographs at 2 years postoperative and include an AP

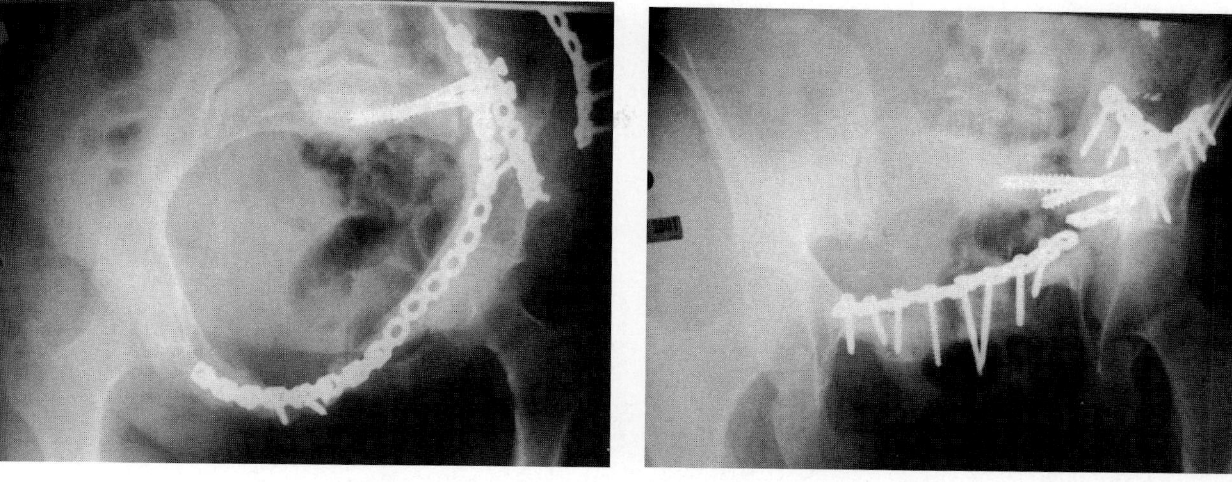

FIGURE 19-6. ***(continued)*** **(G)**, inlet, and outlet views **(H)**.

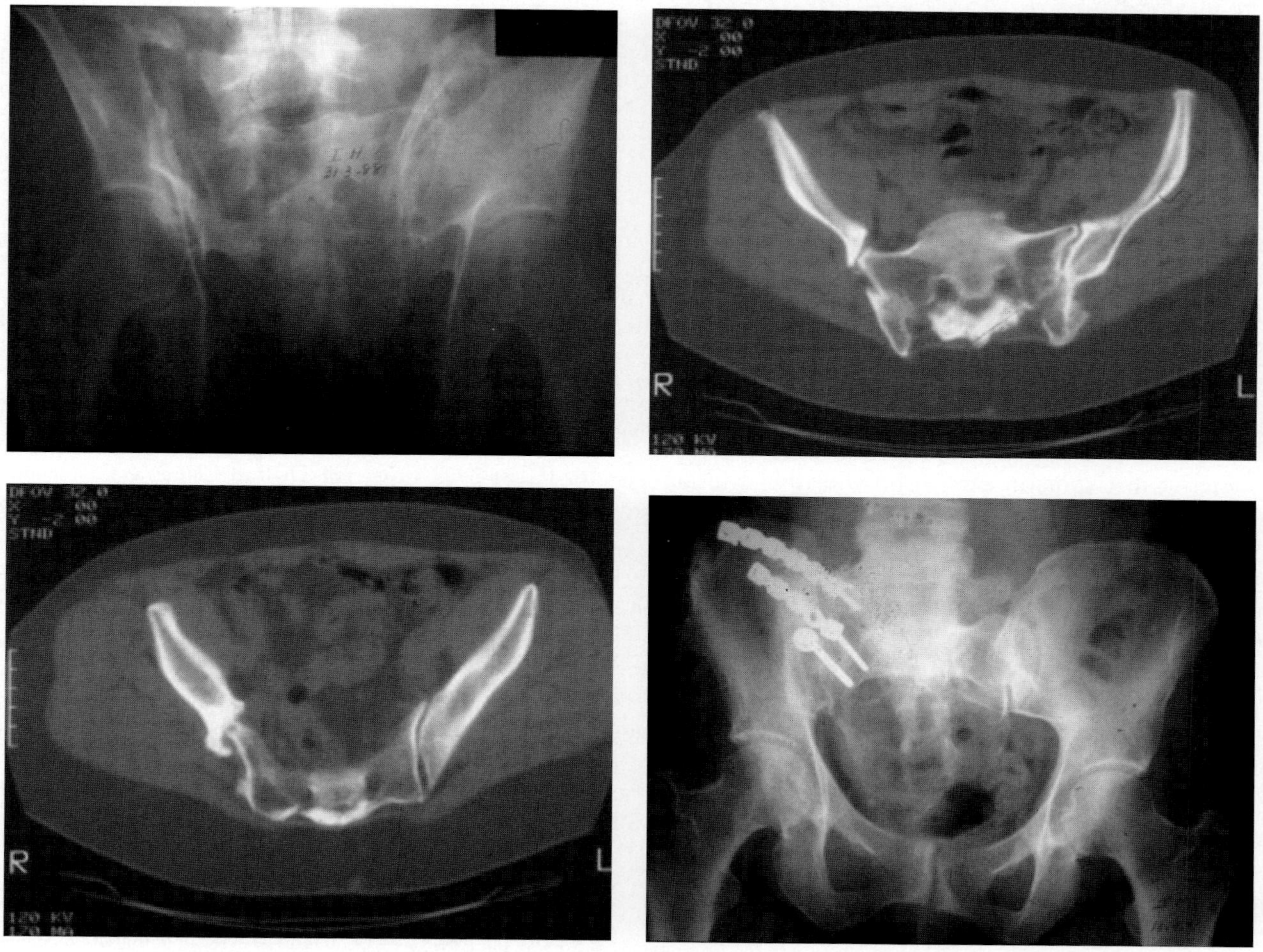

FIGURE 19-7. A 50-year-old woman who suffered from low back pain and sciatica. Six months prior to this x-ray she had a laminectomy and spinal fusion with bone taken from both posterior iliac crests. The anterior-posterior x-ray shows the nonunion through the bone graft site, which is seen much more clearly on the computed tomography (CT) scan **(B,C)**. Note that there is almost no bone in the posterior spine on the CT. Therefore, a surgical solution becomes extremely difficult. In this case, the nonunion through this bone graft donor site insufficiency fracture was treated by anterior SI plating **(D)**, which was technically very demanding. (Courtesy M. Tile.)

with flexion, abduction, and external rotation of the left leg. Radiographs, including an anterior-posterior, inlet, and outlet view of the pelvis were obtained (Fig. 19-6) and revealed bilateral pubic rami insufficiency fracture nonunions with an insufficiency fracture-dislocation of the sacroiliac joint. A CT scan was obtained (Fig. 19-6), which confirmed hypertrophic nonunions of the pubic rami and iliac wing insufficiency fractures.

The patient underwent repair of the multiple pelvic ring stress fracture nonunions with a fusion of the left sacroiliac joint through an anterior ilioinguinal approach. The patient's postoperative course was complicated by the development of a Crohn's fistula with the operative wound. The wound healed following colostomy placement and irrigation and debridement. The rest of the patient's postoperative course was unremarkable. The colostomy was reversed 6 months postoperatively. All of the nonunion sites healed.

The patient was seen for latest follow-up at 2 years postoperatively. She was doing well: Her groin pain had resolved but she still had pain over both SI joints, for which she took no medication. Radiographically there was evidence of solid union of the pelvic ring, even with hardware breakage over the symphysis and anterior column (Fig. 19-3). Clinically, the patient had a 0.5-cm leg length discrepancy, for which she used a 3/8-in. shoe lift. Range of motion of the left hip was full. There were no long-term consequences of her colostomy.

STRESS FRACTURE AT PELVIC BONE GRAFT DONOR SITES

Donor site stress fractures are not uncommon, especially at the posterior iliac spine in association with spinal fusion procedures. In fact, it may become the most devastating complication of that procedure. The principles of treatment are the same, but may end in failure, because internal fixation is difficult if too much bone has been removed at the time of surgery. In some cases, we have seen an almost complete collapse of the pelvis, where cancellous bone was taken from multiple sites of the pelvis (Fig. 19-7). Hu and coworkers (24,25) have done a biomechanical study recommending guidelines for prevention of this potentially difficult complication.

CONCLUSION

Orthopedists will begin to see more and more pelvic insufficiency fractures as the population ages. It is important to recognize the presence of a stress fracture by maintaining a high index of suspicion and implementing the proper treatment protocol.

REFERENCES

1. Launder WJ, Hungerford DS. Stress fracture of the pubis after total hip arthroplasty. *Clin Orthop Rel Res* 1981;159:183–185.
2. Marmor L. Stress fracture of the pubic ramus simulating a loose total hip replacement. *Clin Orthop Rel Res* 1976;Nov-Dec: 103–104.
3. Egol KA, Koval KJ, Kummer F, et al. Stress fractures of the femoral neck. *Clin Orthop* 1998;348:72–78.
4. Weber M, Hasler P, Gerber H. Insufficiency fractures of the sacrum: twenty cases and review of the literature. *Spine* 1993; 18(16):2507–2512.
5. Peh WCG, Khongg PL, Yin Y, et al. Imaging of pelvic insufficiency fractures. *Radiographics* 1996;16(2):335–348.
6. Schapira D, Militeanu D, Israel O, et al. Insufficiency fractures of the pubic ramus. *Semin Arthritis Rheum* 1996;25(6):373–382.
7. Tauber C, Geltner D, Noff M, et al. Disruption of the symphysis pubis and fatigue fractures of the pelvis in a patient with rheumatoid arthritis: a case report. *Clin Orthop Rel Res* 1987;215: 105–108.
8. Albertson AB, Egund N, Jurik AG. Fatigue fracture of the sacral bone associated with septic arthritis of the symphysis pubis. *Skeletal Radiol* 1995;24:605–607.
9. Noakes TD, Smith JA, Lindenberg G, et al. Pelvic stress fractures in long distance runners. *Am J Sports Med* 1985;13(2):120–123.
10. Carter SR. Stress fracture of the sacrum: brief report. *J Bone Joint Surg* 1987;69-B(5):843–844.
11. Davies AM, Evans NS, Struthers GR. Parasymphyseal and associated insufficiency fractures of the pelvis and sacrum. *Br J Radiol* 1988;61(722):103–108.
12. Stroebel RJ, Ginsburg WW, McLeod RA. Sacral insufficiency fractures: an often unsuspected cause of low back pain. *J Rheumatol* 1998;18:117–119.
13. Eckenman I. Physical diagnosis of stress fractures. In: Burr DB, Milgrom C, eds. *Musculoskeletal fatigue and stress fractures.* Boca Raton, FL: CRC Press, 2001.
14. Rawlings CE III, Wilkins RH, Martinez S, et al. Osteoporotic sacral fractures: a clinical study. *Neurology* 1988;22(1):72–76.
15. Hill F, Chaterji S, Chambers D, et al. Stress fracture of the pubic ramus in female recruits. *J Bone Joint Surg* 1996,78B:383–386.
16. Hoang TA, Nguyen TH, Draffner RH, et al. Case report 491. *Skeletal Radiol* 1988;17:364–367.
17. Kerr R. Stress fracture of the inferior pubic ramus. *Radiol Case Study* 1987;10:1466–1467.
18. Nishizawa Y, Kudo H, Iwano K, et al. Stress fracture of the pubic ramus in rheumatoid arthritis: a report of three cases *Ryumachi* 1984;24:189.
19. Cotty PH, Fouquet B, Mezenge C, et al. Insufficiency fractures of the sacrum: ten cases and a review of the literature. *J Neuroradiol* 1989;16:160–171.
20. Deutch AL, Coel MN, Mink JH. Imaging of stress injury to bone. *Clin Sports Med* 1997;16:275–290.
21. Schneider R, Yacovone J, Ghelman B. Unsuspected sacral fractures: detection by radionuclide bone scanning. *Am J Radiol* 1985;144:337–341.
22. Newhouse KE, Elkhoury GY, Buckwalter JA. Occult sacral fractures in osteopenic patients. *J Bone Joint Surg* 1992;74A: 1472–1477.
23. Lee JK, Yao L. Stress fractures: MR imaging. *Radiology* 1988; 169:217–220.
24. Hu R, Hearn T, Yang J. Bone graft harvest site as a determinant of iliac crest strength. *Clin Orthop Rel Res* 1995;310:252–256.
25. Hu RW, Bohlman HH. Fracture at the iliac bone graft harvest site after fusion of the spine. *Clin Orthop Rel Res* 1994;309: 208–213.

20

INJURY TO THE PELVIS AND ACETABULUM IN THE PEDIATRIC PATIENT (THE IMMATURE SKELETON)

JOHN A. OGDEN

INTRODUCTION

The child's pelvis includes multiple growth regions that are the equivalents of the epiphyses and apophyses of the long bones. Fractures at these chondro-osseous interfaces create growth plate injuries that may be difficult to detect because of the late appearance of secondary ossification centers (1). The developing pelvic bones, especially the ilium, are quite flexible, a factor that allows considerable temporary elastic or plastic deformation without an obvious fracture. This injury pattern is the equivalent of a greenstick or torus injury in an extremity bone. Rebound to "normal" anatomy following deformation may create a false sense of security when evaluating the extent of any injury. Such deformations put the contained soft-tissue structures at risk for injury. The potential for urethral, genitourinary, rectal, and abdominal injuries must be assessed carefully, even when the radiologic appearance of the pelvis does not suggest severe injury.

ANATOMY

Prenatally each hemipelvis forms from three primary centers of ossification for the ischium, pubis, and ilium. These primary ossification centers converge within the acetabulum to form the triradiate cartilage. Such chondro-osseous interrelations allow continual integrated growth and hemispheric expansion of the acetabulum commensurate with the progressive spherical growth of the capital femoral epiphysis (1). During adolescence multiple secondary centers of ossification develop within the triradiate cartilage as well as peripherally (Fig. 20-1). These centers should not be misconstrued as fracture fragments during the evaluation of any potential pelvic injury in a child or adolescent. The triradiate cartilage normally undergoes physiologic epiphysiodesis at 12 to 14 years in girls and 14 to 16 years in boys.

The ischium and pubis also have an interposed bipolar growth cartilage within the inferior pelvic ramus. Fusion of this particular region normally occurs between 4 and 7

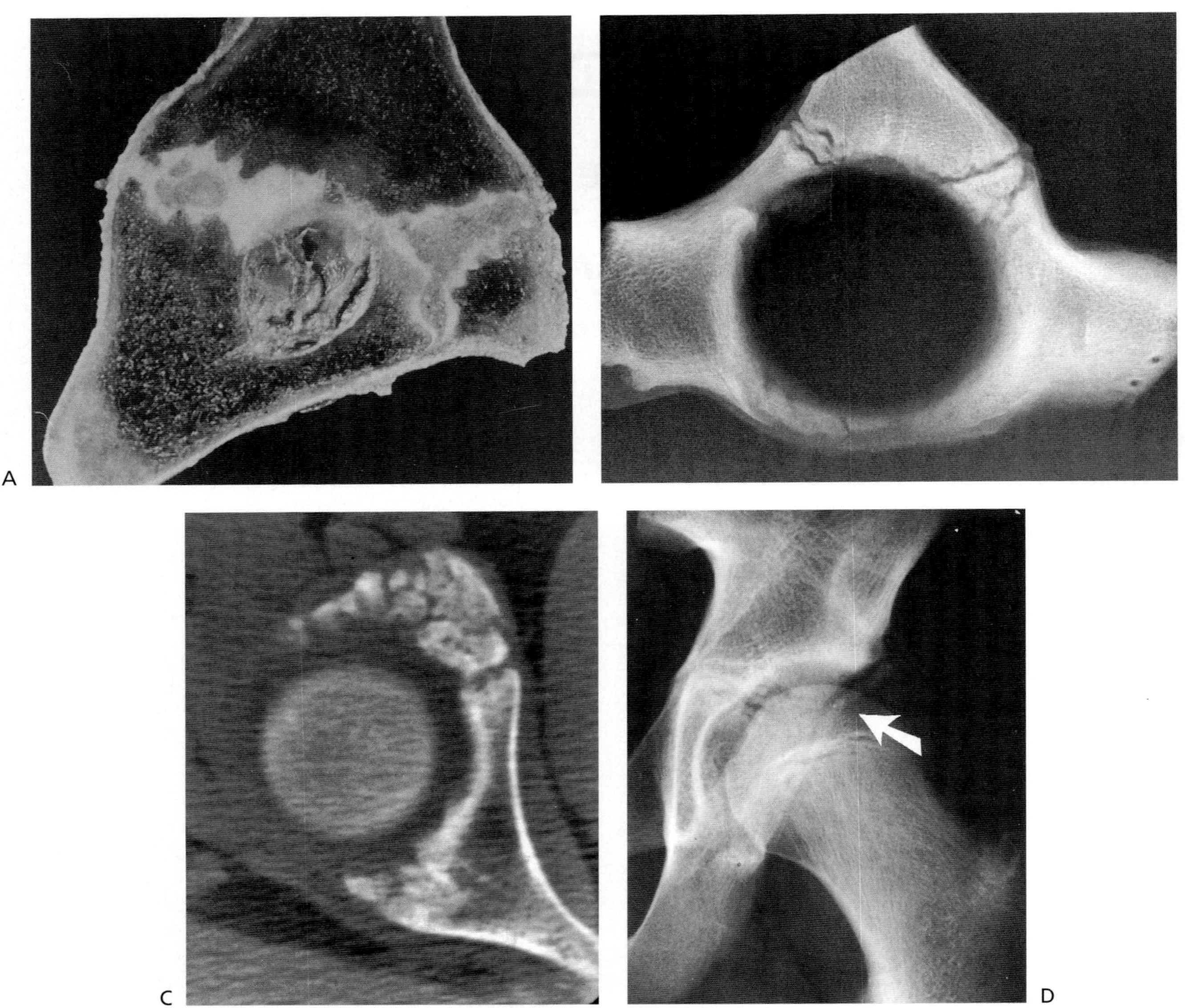

FIGURE 20-1. A: Slab section of the acetabulum from a 12-year-old boy showing the secondary ossification centers within the triradiate cartilage. The ilium is superior, the ischium to the left and a small portion of the pubis to the right. **B:** Radiograph of another slab section from the same post mortem study shows secondary ossification in two arms of the triradiate cartilage. **C:** Computed tomography scan in a 12-year-old patient being evaluated for multiple trauma. This shows multifocal secondary ossification superiorly in the arms of the triradiate cartilage, and similar secondary ossification in the peripheral posterior acetabulum (inferiorly). These are normal ossification patterns rather than fractures. **D:** Radiograph from a 15-year-old boy demonstrates secondary ossification along the posterior rim *(arrow).* This is not a peripheral fracture, as would be likely in an adult.

years. Fusiform enlargement of the ischiopubic junction during physiologic closure often is preceded by irregularity of ossification. The latter is most frequent between the ages of 5 and 8 years and may be asymmetric in 22% of normal patients. Such enlargement of the ischiopubic junction has been described, variably, as normal, an osteochondrosis, a stress fracture, infection, or malignancy (1). In children in the 6- to 10-year range, irregularity of this area should be considered a normal variation of skeletal maturation. It should not be misinterpreted as a healing fracture, even though the radiographic appearance may be suggestive of callus formation or reactive new bone. In the older child increased bone formation in the ischiopubic junction should be considered a possible stress fracture, infection, or neoplasia.

The normal, maturing ischial tuberosity often is irregular and may be mistaken for a fracture, infection, or tumor, especially if the patient presents with excessive reactive bone formation after a defined injury. Because secondary ossification is not present until adolescence, the only indication of a traction injury, with or without displacement, may be cystic change or osseous irregularity in the metaphyseal equivalent region.

The iliac crest and spines are cartilaginous until adolescence. Secondary centers of ossification appear along the anterolateral iliac crest when a child is approximately 13 to 15 years old. Posterior advancement continues until the posterior iliac spine is reached. Fusion of crest secondary ossification to the rest of the ilium occurs by 15 to 17 years, although complete fusion may be delayed until 25 years. Alternatively, after the ossification center first appears, separate ossification may proceed from a posterior center, with the central portion being ossified at a later date as the centers grow toward each other.

The symphysis pubis is a growth region connecting the two hemipelves anteriorly. The normal endochondral ossification process may be associated with an irregular, undulated appearance that should not be confused with that owing to trauma (1). Radiographic "widening" of the symphyseal region is highly variable and depends on the extent of maturation of chondral into osseous tissue. Adult width measurements of the symphysis are inapplicable, especially prior to ten years of age, when attempting to diagnose a traumatic diastasis.

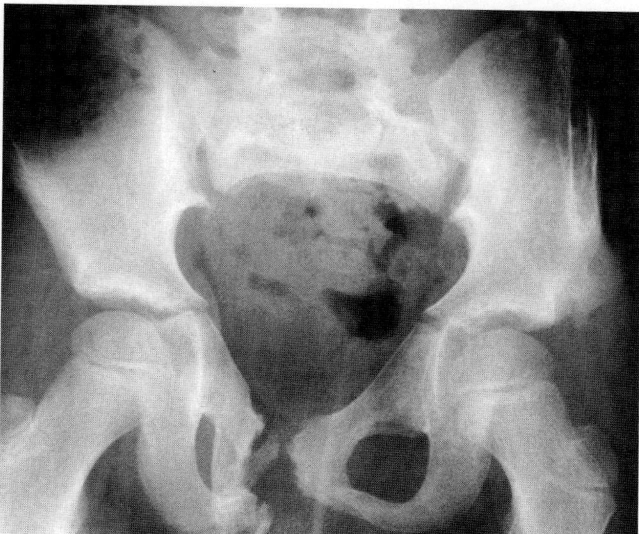

FIGURE 20-2. This 11-year-old boy was involved in a bicycle-auto injury 5 months prior to this radiograph. The left ilium was plastically deformed, the left anterior inferior iliac spine had been avulsed and now appears as an exostosis because of bone formation in the traumatic gap (comparable to chondrodiastasis). On the right side an apparent pubic diastasis has now begun to form bone within the intact periosteal sleeves.

GENERAL CONSIDERATIONS

The pelvis of the child differs from that of the adult in that the bone, cartilage, and joints (sacroiliac, symphysis pubis, triradiate, ischiopubic) are more pliant and susceptible to separations (fractures) at the chondro-osseous interfaces (Fig. 20-2). This greater volume of cartilage and the less brittle bone provide a significant buffer for energy absorption, much like the developing skull. Accordingly, pelvic osseous fractures, especially complex, comminuted ones, are less common than in adults. When fractures do occur, the contiguous radiolucent cartilage may be damaged, usually following Type 1 or 2 physeal injury mechanism patterns (1). As an example, the triradiate cartilage may be microscopically injured (i.e., not readily radiologically evident), leading to acetabular maldevelopment and a morphologic situation similar to developmental hip dysplasia. A displaced fracture of the ischiopubic ring (essentially reversing an innominate or similar pelvic osteotomy) may lead to uncovering of the femoral head with subsequent capital femoral subluxation. The presence of growth cartilage along several pelvic margins allows avulsion fractures to occur. These fractures are comparable to epiphyseal-physeal injuries in a long bone and are subject to all the potential acute and long-term complications. Leg length discrepancy may be a problem when a hemipelvis is shifted superiorly and may lead to scoliosis during the adolescent period owing to the post-traumatic pelvic obliquity and the relative leg length discrepancy. Patients with hemipelvic displacement of more than 1 to 2 cm may have minimal problems as children, but frequently develop pain and discomfort during adolescence and in their early adult years when they are followed for an extended period of time (Fig. 20-3). The leg length

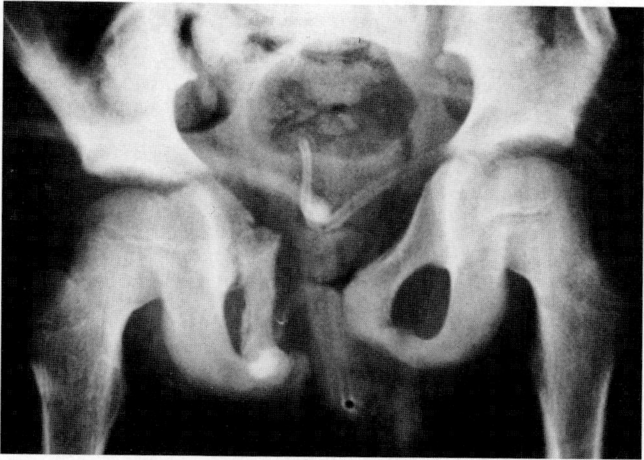

FIGURE 20-3. Upward shift of the left hemipelvis. This created an acute and subsequently chronic leg length discrepancy. This should be corrected by traction or intraoperative manipulation, if possible, when the child is hemodynamically stable. This child developed a mild scoliosis in adolescence and back pain in his twenties. The child also had a complete separation of the bladder (central gas-filled viscus) from the urethra that required surgical intervention, as evident by the catheters suprapubically and within the urethra.

inequality often requires treatment. Back pain becomes a significant problem with further growth and increasing physical demands.

The developing chondro-osseous pelvis is more resilient and affords less rigid protection to the contained viscera, which may be damaged more easily than comparable adult organs because of immature fibrous capsules and stroma. The juvenile pelvis may undergo considerable elastic and plastic distortion without readily evident fracture. Organ damage may occur with little subsequent roentgenographic evidence of the severity of the maximum degree of chondro-osseous trauma. The identification of a pelvic fracture in a child, particularly if displaced, thus assumes even more clinical significance.

Reed reviewed 84 children with pelvic fractures, with more than 80% resulting from vehicular injuries (2). Sixteen patients had associated visceral injuries. Eighteen had transient microhematuria, but none had significant injuries to the genitourinary tract. Eleven had gross hematuria, and all had major injuries to the lower urinary tract or the kidney. Two patients had severe intracranial injuries. One third of the patients sustained fractures of other bones, the most common being the femur and skull (Fig. 20-4). Four children had acetabular fractures through the triradiate cartilage, a pattern that must be closely sought, because it is probably more common than realized. Other studies also have emphasized the importance of concomitant skeletal and organ injuries as major factors in long-term outcome in these children (3–6).

Fractures of the pelvic components should be placed in proper perspective. During the initial phase the orthopedist must be acutely aware of potential injury to the intrapelvic and intraabdominal visceral and vascular contents, rather than the obvious osseous injuries. Osseous damage assumes secondary importance until internal tissue injuries are completely evaluated and treated as necessary. Massive retroperitoneal bleeding following pelvic fracture produces high morbidity and mortality in victims of blunt trauma, *no matter what their age.* Although less common in children, hemorrhage still represents a significant potential complication.

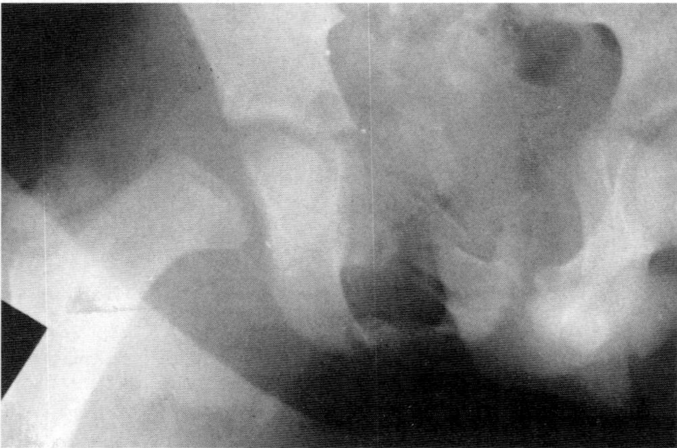

FIGURE 20-4. Seven-year-old boy with ramus fractures. He also has sustained a Type 1 physeal fracture of the proximal femur that was treated by closed reduction and percutaneous pinning.

Quinby reported 20 pediatric patients with fractures of the pelvis (7). The patients were divided into three treatment groups. Group 1 (six patients) did not require laparotomy; the pelvic fractures were relatively mild, undisplaced (including one mild separation of the sacroiliac joint); and none showed clinical shock or required blood transfusion. Group 2 (nine patients) all underwent laparotomy for visceral injuries (organ lacerations) accompanying the pelvic fractures. One child died. Group 3 (five patients) all had massive retroperitoneal and pelvic hemorrhage with severe pelvic fractures and disruption of the sacroiliac joint. All were in clinical shock, with four of five eventually dying. Death remains a significant problem in the pediatric population, although the percentage is decreasing. Ismail and coworkers found a 5% mortality rate in children, as compared to 17% in adults (8). Diagnostic methods (computed tomography, CT; magnetic resonance imaging, MRI) and minimally invasive laparoscopy now allow better comprehension of the extent of soft-tissue injury (1).

Garvin and coworkers reviewed 36 pediatric patients who were classified using both the Torode and Zieg system and the Modified Injury Severity Score (MISS) (5,9). Associated injuries occurred in 67% of the patients, with a long-term morbidity or mortality of 30%. They stressed the high probability of minimal bony injury being associated with life-threatening visceral injuries and morbidity. The most common concomitant organ system involved was musculoskeletal, with 18 long bone fractures in 11 patients. The abdomen was the second most common site of injury. Six injuries involved the prostatic urethra; two patients with prostatic urethral injuries were still incontinent. One patient died of sepsis. Two patients had permanent neurologic sequelae. There were organ lacerations or severe contusions in nine patients. Three patients sustained closed head injuries; none had permanent damage from the associated injury. They found that all patients with long-term morbidity had an original fracture that would be classified as ring disruption.

DIAGNOSIS

Examination

The accurate diagnosis of pediatric pelvic injuries may be difficult only on the basis of clinical findings. Children tend to be at the extremes, having either a relatively simple pelvic injury (usually an avulsion or ramus fracture) or extensive trauma with pelvic disruption. Variable levels of consciousness may limit the response to pain. Physical examination should include pelvic compression, which may cause pain. The absence of pain, however, does not effectively rule out injury because of possible lumbosacral plexus or spinal cord injury. Posterior subluxation of the ilium at the sacroiliac joint generally is missed because the patient is usually supine, especially if severely injured. The region may not be examined with sufficient care when there are multiple injuries. Soft-tissue injuries—abrasions, lacerations, ecchymoses—should increase the index of suspicion. The perineum should be examined carefully.

As reasonable a neurologic examination as possible should be undertaken initially, depending on the level of consciousness of the patient. Sacral sensation should be tested. Many nerve injuries are missed when the initial neurologic examination is neglected or cursory, especially in the child with life-threatening injury. Remember that a hinged Type 1 or 2 growth mechanism injury of the posterior ilium contiguous with the sacroiliac joint may spring back after injurious forces dissipate, creating a seemingly innocuous injury. However, at maximum positional deformation considerable attenuation of adjacent neurovascular and muscular tissues may occur. The lumbosacral plexus is closely related to the sacroiliac joint; there may be some neural damage when the joint is dislocated or separated. The lumbosacral trunk, superior gluteal nerve, and obturator nerve may be stretched or even disrupted. Intrathecal rupture of the roots of the cauda equina may be produced by traction.

Imaging Studies

Adequate radiographic examination is critical. However, the static radiographic appearance may not indicate the maximum deformity that was attained when the injury was actually occurring. A gonad shield should not be used during the initial screening, because it may obliterate areas that need to be critically evaluated. The anteroposterior view of the pelvis that adequately demonstrates the pelvic ring is not always acceptable for determining fracture details because of the normal lumbar lordosis. The best view in the anterior-posterior (AP) position may be oblique, depending on how much curvature there is in the spine. An inlet or down shot view is obtained 60 degrees off the vertical, with the cone aimed distally to demonstrate bursting of the ring. Other projections (e.g., Judet views) may provide important information about fragment displacement, especially in the adolescent. Lordosis changes as the child develops, which affects the standard AP appearance.

CT offers the best method for detecting subtle injuries and defining the specific fracture anatomy more precisely (10). For example, apparent sacroiliac disruption actually may be a chondro-osseous disruption comparable to a Type 1 or 2 growth mechanism injury of a long bone (Fig. 20-5). CT scanning also is useful for detecting inward or outward winging that is hinged at the sacroiliac joint, as well as diagnosing posterior displacement of an ilium. Silber and coworkers showed that the use of CT scans in addition to standard radiography led to a change in fracture classification in nine children and a change in management in two children in a series of 103 young patients with pelvic injury (10).

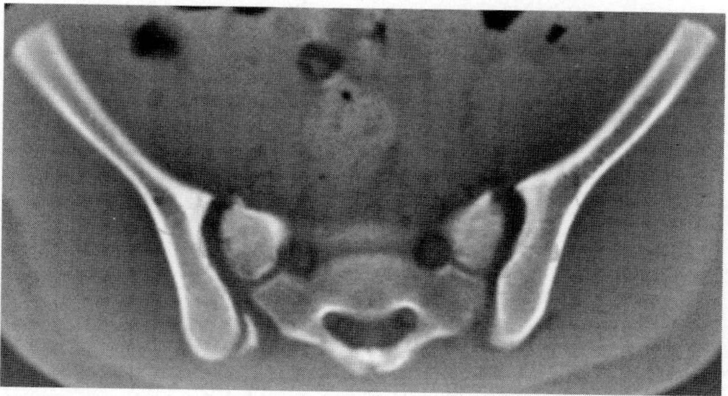

FIGURE 20-5. Pelvic fracture in an 11-year-old girl. This patient was struck by an automobile directly against the right pelvis. A small bone fragment is evident posteriorly. This is a Thurstan Holland equivalent metaphyseal piece from the ilium, typical of a Type 2 growth mechanism injury in a long bone. Anteriorly a small piece of the sacrum sustained a torus deformation. Most likely the right ilium was hinged inwardly by the impact of injury, and spontaneously reduced as the child was thrown away from the car.

Magid and coworkers discussed the role of two-dimensional CT (2DCT) and three-dimensional CT (3DCT) imaging in the evaluation of acetabular and pelvis fractures in pediatric patients (11). Using standard technology the acquired images may be rotated through multiple positions in any 360-degree sequence until the best view is obtained. This capability is important, because conventional films may not provide the optimum view or the injured young patient may be unable or unwilling to comply with positioning maneuvers. Furthermore, excessive gastric air (air swallowing is common in injured children), colonic air, and solid intestinal content may obscure the posterior pelvic ring. Much of the recent trend toward more conservative, less invasive management of pediatric patients with abdominal or thoracic trauma is related to the ability to adequately document the extent of injury by CT, rather than resorting to exploratory laparotomy or laparoscopy.

Although CT imaging provides additional information for evaluating traumatized patients, not every pediatric patient with pelvic trauma requires such a study. Particularly, patients with simple, stable injuries to the symphysis or anterior ring that are readily evident on routine films probably do not require scanning. 2DCT and 3DCT images are most useful in pediatric patients with complex injuries in whom the full definition of injury is essential to determine whether external fixation or operation may be necessary. Contrast in the bladder or intravenous pyelography does not interfere with the CT scan and, further, may delineate any extravasation. Scanning by CT also is useful for follow-up of disruptive pelvic injuries. It allows evaluation of the extent of healing and residual anatomic deformity.

MRI probably has limited use in pediatric pelvic fractures, because osseous detail is better visualized in a CT scan (12). However, intraabdominal and intrapelvic soft-tissue injury and hematoma accumulation may be discerned and documented. Furthermore, cartilaginous damage (e.g., avulsion of an unossified anteroinferior iliac spine) may become evident.

GENERAL MANAGEMENT GUIDELINES

The Pelvic Injury

Silber and Flynn used the status of the triradiate cartilage to determine the likely severity of pelvic injury and basic approach to management (13). Patients with an open triradiate cartilage tended to have isolated pubic rami or iliac wing fractures. In contrast, adolescent patients with closure of the triradiate cartilage had a greater likelihood of adult pattern acetabular fractures or sacroiliac disruption. They felt adolescent pelvic fracture classifications and management principles should follow adult guidelines in these situations (14,15). In contrast, management of the usual fractures of the pelvis when the triradiate cartilage is open should focus on associated injuries. The exception is involvement of the triradiate cartilage in the injury, a pattern unique to the young child that is discussed later. Most pelvic fractures prior to triradiate closure may be treated with immobilization or protected weight-bearing contingent on other musculoskeletal injuries (1,13,16).

Function is minimally impaired with stable injuries. Usually the basic pelvic ring is undisplaced or minimally displaced. Comfort, the primary treatment goal, is attained most effectively by bed rest (frequently mandated by accompanying injuries). Reduction, either closed or open, rarely is necessary, particularly in the young child, because of the extent of remodeling that will occur and the possibility of damaging intrapelvic structures.

Lacheretz and Herbaux questioned whether unstable ring fractures in children should ever be treated surgically (17). They reviewed 126 cases, 10 of whom had acetabular involvement. There were 80 stable fractures (Type A), 29 unstable transverse fractures (Type B), and seven unstable transverse and vertical fractures (Type C). They found that all Type A and B fractures healed by conservative means. Only in Type C fractures was there a need to consider closed reduction with external fixation or surgical intervention.

However, given the inherent instability of posterior disruption of the pelvis, closed reduction and minimal external fixation are recommended when displacement is evident. Fixation frames allow easier nursing care and access to management of soft-tissue damage and catheters. External fixation must be used carefully in the young child, because placement of threaded pins or screws through apophyseal regions (e.g., iliac crest) may cause localized physeal damage. Because the chondro-osseous nature of these fractures allows relatively rapid healing, fixators do not have to remain in place in a child as long as they would in an adult. It may be necessary to use limited internal fixation.

An infrequent complication is leg length inequality secondary to a shifted hemipelvis (Fig. 20-3). Vigorous manipulation in the child to reduce the superior shift anatomically may not be appropriate because it may cause recurrent bleeding or genitourinary damage. Remodeling, as in long bones, may alter such relations in a positive way. Nonunion and delayed union are uncommon complications of childhood pelvic injuries. Limb lengthening may be corrected at a later date. Because the discrepancy is usually <2 cm, most children may be treated effectively with a lift and, if indicated, an appropriately timed epiphysiodesis. Pelvic osteotomy also may be used to address leg length inequality (1).

Other Skeletal Injuries

Pelvic fractures may be accompanied by other skeletal injuries. Because many pelvic injuries are caused by direct blows and vehicular trauma, adjacent fractures of the proximal femur, hip dislocation, and spinal fractures may occur. Such injuries should not be overlooked during the initial evaluation. Associated musculoskeletal injuries may require much more treatment than the pelvic fracture itself.

Vasquez and Garcia found that children with pelvic fractures who also had an additional nonpelvic fracture had a high incidence of head and abdominal injury (6). They felt this constellation of injuries could be treated best by early transfer to a regional pediatric trauma facility. Closed head injury is a significant cause of morbidity and mortality in children (1,6). Patients in the additional fracture group generally require more transfusions and must be hospitalized for longer periods of time. In the study by Silber and coworkers, 50% of 166 children with pelvic fractures had additional skeletal injuries, and 60% had multisystem injuries, including head trauma (38%), chest trauma (19%), and abdominal/visceral injuries (20%) (10). The associated fractures are shown in Table 20-1. Because Silber and coworkers specifically excluded skull and facial bone fractures, the actual incidence of nonpelvic skeletal injury probably is even higher than 40%.

Vascular Injuries

Despite having a distribution of pelvic fracture sites similar to that of adults, only five of 372 children in four separate investigations died as a result of massive hemorrhage (7,18–20). Possible explanations for reduced bleeding from pelvic fractures in children have anatomic bases. First, the periosteal tissues appear to be more adherent to the underlying bone in the child, which may limit the displacement and thus lessen the likelihood of disruption of major vessels that course over and around the pelvis. Second, children's vessels are much more vasoconstrictive, which limits hemorrhage from smaller vessels.

TABLE 20-1. CONCOMITANT NONPELVIC FRACTURES

Fracture Site	Number	Percentage[a]
Femur	39	23.5
Tibia/fibula	24	14.5
Clavicle	18	10.8
Radius/ulna	14	8.4
Humerus	10	6.0
Rib	9	5.4
Foot/hand/spine[b]	21	12.0

[a] Percentage of 166 patients; many patients had multiple nonpelvic fractures.
[b] Spine injuries included nine sacral fractures (no root injuries), one T1 fracture (neurologically intact), and one T12/L1 burst fracture associated with T12 paraplegia.
Source: Silber JS, Flynn JM, Katz MA, et al. Role of computed tomography in the classification and management of pediatric pelvic fractures. *J Pediatr Orthop* 1992;12:621–625.

Shock may accompany severe pelvic fractures and usually is hemorrhagic (see Chapter 8). Appropriate volume replacement, transfusion, and temporary postponement of laparotomy or laparoscopy until the circulatory status is stable is recommended. A delay in the repair of visceral or arterial injuries probably is less serious than the crisis of cardiac arrest during an exploratory operation performed while the general circulation is in a tenuous state. The sacroiliac region of the child and adolescent seems to be the point where the vessels and nerves are most susceptible to significant injury. If this area is disrupted, there should be concern for laceration of vessels up to the size of the iliac artery. Shock that is poorly responsive to volume replacement and pressor agents in the presence of a rapidly enlarging abdomen, with absence of one or both femoral pulses, should be cause for immediate surgical exploration (laparoscopy). It is a good surgical principle not to disturb stable retroperitoneal hematomas, regardless of their size, but rather to control the specific visceral or vascular lacerations. CT and MRI scans may be more efficacious than abdominal taps for identifying large hematomas. In addition to being a method of repair, limited laparoscopy may be helpful for diagnosis.

Sources of external hemorrhage should be sought around the urethral meatus, vagina, and anus. Abdominal and rectal examinations are essential. Pulses in the lower extremities must be assessed carefully by palpation. Doppler studies should be obtained if a pulse cannot be felt.

When the sacroiliac joint is separated and pulses in one leg are diminished or absent, a major branch of the internal iliac artery has probably been disrupted. The child generally is in profound shock and requires rapid transfusion of blood in massive quantities. This type of injury is associated with high mortality, even in children. The importance of concealed hemorrhage owing to fractures of the pelvis cannot be overstated. The possible consequences of allowing continued rapid retroperitoneal blood loss, such as intraperitoneal rupture with exsanguination, prolonged jaundice, renal failure, coagulopathy, and prolonged ileus, should be avoided.

Angiographic evaluation of bleeding associated with pelvic fracture and treatment by selective embolization of clotted blood to sites in the vicinity of the fractures (usually branches from the obturator artery along the pubic rami) have been described in adults and more recently in children (18). This technique may be considered a nonoperative approach to massive pelvic hematomas, when contrasted with the hazards of surgical exploration. The technique involves arterial catheterization on the side opposite the trauma. A flush aortogram is performed with the catheter at the level of the renal arteries, with the urinary tract visualized as well. Selective celiac axis arteriography then follows to evaluate the liver and spleen. For embolization, the catheter is advanced proximally to the obturator artery, and pieces of Gelfoam (mixed with contrast material) or autologous clot may be injected into the obturator artery under fluoroscopic control.

Abdominal Organ Injuries

Injury to the bowel is an uncommon complication of childhood pelvic fracture and probably occurs in fewer than 3% of cases (21). In contrast, a reactive ileus and gastric dilatation (air swallowing) are extremely common in children. A nasogastric tube may be used if such complications are present. Children have a propensity to swallow air when injured. Accordingly, gastric dilatation, per se, does not indicate a definite bowel injury.

Entrapment of bowel between osseous fragments of the pelvis has been reported (22). Nimityongskul and coworkers reported an 8-year-old who had small bowel incarceration associated with a central fracture dislocation of the hip (23). The bowel was entrapped when the temporarily widened fracture spontaneously reduced, progressively leading to perforation of the bowel, infection of the hip joint, separation of the capital femoral epiphysis, and osteomyelitis of the femoral shaft.

The liver is the second most commonly injured intraabdominal organ in pediatric patients. The need for operative intervention for liver lacerations in children is controversial (21). Splenic injury requiring complete splenectomy requires appropriate medical follow-up and vaccination (1,21). Splenic regeneration may occur in some children.

Perineal avulsion may be associated with genitourinary and rectal injury. Stabilization of the pelvic injury may contribute substantially to the necessary reconstruction of these tissues and organs. Perineal trauma is associated with mortality rates of 30% to 60%, which are improved by control of hemorrhage and sepsis.

Neurologic Injuries

Neurologic injury may occur at several levels, particularly when the sacroiliac region is disrupted. The nerve roots may be stretched or avulsed at the spinal foramina. Injury to the sciatic nerve as it courses past the acetabulum is unusual, primarily because these injuries usually leave an intact periosteum that protects the nerve. Some degree of function may be permanently lost if the sciatic nerve is injured.

Children with residual nerve damage, no matter what the final level, may have major problems with stress fractures, recurrent fractures, epiphyseolyses, Charcot-like joints, soft-tissue contractures, and decubiti. Relative osteoporosis may significantly weaken the metaphyseal areas (Fig. 20-6), predisposing to subsequent growth mechanism and metaphyseal fractures.

Incomplete injuries to the lumbosacral plexus, especially stretch injuries, may be overlooked when evaluating more life-threatening aspects of a traumatized child. Lesions around the areas of the sacral roots may be painless. Because of overlap of sensory fields it may not be easy to detect discrete sensory loss, and there may be subtle motor damage that results in problems around the hip region and distally. Repetitive examinations should detect these neurologic injuries, especially if head injury recovery allows more cooperation.

Head injury is of major concern, and usually correlates well with the various trauma scoring systems such as the Glasgow Coma Scale (1,10). In the study of Silber and coworkers, four children died from massive head injury and one died from head and myocardial injury out of 166 patients (10). In distinct contrast to adults, children with head injury are much more likely to have significant to complete recovery from coma (1). Thus, proper management of concomitant axial, extremity, and pelvic fractures is paramount.

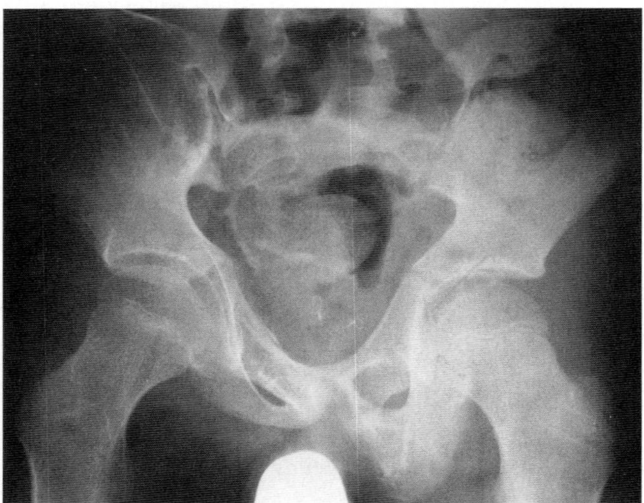

FIGURE 20-6. Two years after a pelvic fracture there is osteoporosis evident in the right hemipelvis and femur. This child has a significant sciatic disruption associated with the hemipelvic fracture-separation. Note the distorted pelvic anatomy in this 14-year-old boy. Comparable anatomy in a girl could lead to subsequent obstetrical difficulty.

Urologic Injuries

Disruption of the symphysis or displaced fractures of the pubic rami may cause injury to the bladder and urethra (24–28). This is of most concern in the "straddle" injury involving bilateral rami injuries from an anteriorly directed force. As many as 10% of children with such an injury pattern have some type of urologic injury (1,2,10). Complete urologic evaluation with urethrography, cystography, or an intravenous pyelogram may be required. The urinary tract is second only to the central nervous system in terms of the frequency of injury.

About 10% to 25% of bladder injuries are caused by penetrating trauma from a displaced osseous fragment, especially when the bladder is full at the time of injury; 17% of pelvic fractures are associated with rupture of the bladder or urethra. The degree of bladder trauma may be classified into four groups: (a) contusion; (b) extraperitoneal rupture; (c) intraperitoneal rupture; and (d) combined extraperitoneal and intraperitoneal rupture.

Suprapubic tenderness may be associated with a contusion or tear of the bladder wall. A catheter should be placed through the urethra; if it proves difficult, then a tear of the urethra should be suspected (Fig. 20-3). If the catheter enters the bladder without difficulty, then a major urethral injury usually can be excluded. If the urine is bloodstained, then cystography may be performed by injecting dye into the bladder through the catheter and looking for extravasation of the dye beyond the bladder outline. Detailed management of major urinary tract injuries—bladder or urethral tears—should be left to the discretion of the urologic surgeon. If it is necessary to make a suprapubic approach to the urethra to place a stent, then it may be possible to perform concomitantly, a better reduction of a fracture fragment (Fig. 20-7). However, metallic internal or external fixation should be used cautiously, because there is a risk of bladder infection during the early postinjury course. Osteomyelitis by hematogenous or direct spread is a complication that may occur.

Urethral trauma is infrequent in children, but may be caused by blunt or penetrating trauma. Boys are more likely to be injured than girls. Tears are more common than complete severance of the urethra. The most significant injury is disruption of the urethra close to the apex of the prostate. The puboprostatic ligament is ruptured, and the bladder is displaced upward and posteriorly. In a rupture below the urogenital diaphragm, the extravasation of dye is often contained within Buck's fascia. Urethral injury always should be suspected and ruled out in any child with a pelvic fracture. There is usually an inability to void, and frequently blood is seen at the urethral meatus. A retrograde urethrogram should be obtained, because it can demonstrate the area of tear or severance with extravasation of contrast. Multiple projections may be required. Impotence may complicate urethral injury in the male patient.

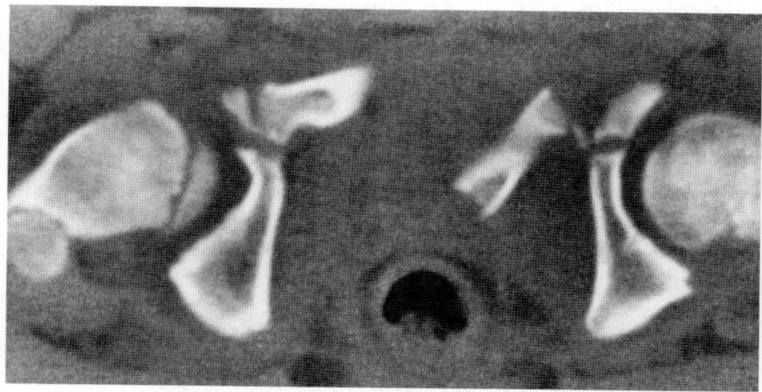
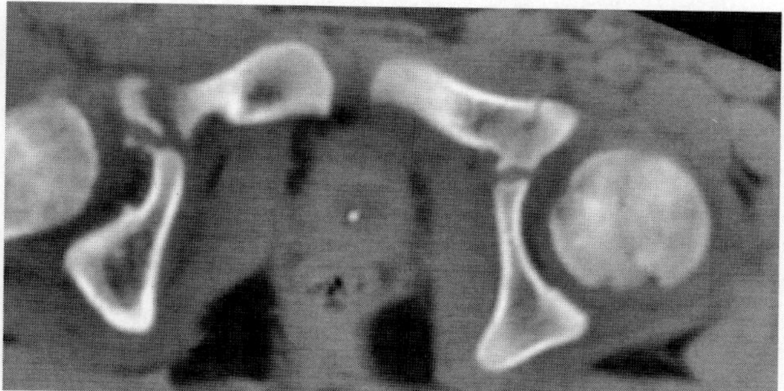

FIGURE 20-7. A: Bilateral pubic ramus fractures with inward displacement of the left side. This was associated with a bladder injury. **B:** During urologic surgery the displaced pubic ramus was relatively simply reduced into the torn periosteal sleeve, which was then repaired with sutures. No metallic fixation was necessary.

Obstetric and Gynecologic Injuries

There is a possibility of future obstetric problems if the pelvic outlet is significantly narrowed or distorted owing to a displaced fracture (Fig. 20-6). Again, long-term studies in immature girls who sustain pelvic fractures have not been conducted to ascertain whether there is a significant risk of such a complication and increased need for cesarean section. Heinrich and coworkers noted the association of an open pelvic fracture coupled with vaginal laceration and pelvic diaphragmatic rupture in a 4-year-old child (29).

TYPES OF PELVIC FRACTURE

Fractures of the skeletally immature pelvis may be classified into four basic groups: (a) stable fractures with continuity of the pelvic ring; (b) unstable fractures with disruption of the pelvic ring anteriorly, posteriorly, or both; (c) fractures of the acetabulum especially involving the triradiate cartilage; and (d) avulsion (apophyseal) fractures, often resulting from muscular avulsion during athletics, rather than direct violence. The most common pelvic ring osseous fracture in children, constituting almost 50%, is a ramus fracture, with most being unilateral and primarily involving the superior (pubic) ramus. However, avulsion fractures, which rarely are included in most series concentrating on significant pediatric pelvic injuries, are not usually included statistically. Realistically these constitute the majority of childhood injuries. If they were included, the combination of avulsion and ramus injuries would comprise 75% to 80% of pediatric pelvic injuries.

In Reed's review of pelvic fractures in children, 39% were unstable (2). The most frequent type was the diametric fracture, in which there was a fracture of the ilium or sacrum or sacroiliac separation, combined with a pubic fracture anteriorly on either the same or the opposite side. However, many diametric fractures in children are stable, because the posterior fractures often are undisplaced or incomplete epiphyseal separations through the sacroiliac region, with a considerable degree of retained periosteal and ligamentous continuity and stability.

The changing anatomy and radiographic appearances and nonadult fracture patterns has made an ideal classification system difficult, especially if the purpose of such is to appropriately predict management that will be most likely to lead to a successful outcome. As previously discussed Quinby ignored the pelvic fracture, per se, and classified the injured children by whether or not they required laparotomy or had vascular injury (7). Similarly the classification of Torode and Zeig originally concentrated on the spectrum of injury rather than the specifics of the pelvic fracture or fractures (5). Recently, Silber and coworkers modified the Torode and Zeig system (Table 20-2).

In contrast to adult pelvic disruption, pelvic fractures in children are less likely to be significantly displaced. Most pediatric pelvic fractures are stable, including diametric fractures in which the posterior fractures tend to be incomplete. This stability is the result of the relatively thick periosteum

TABLE 20-2. CLASSIFICATION OF PEDIATRIC PELVIC FRACTURES

Type	Anatomic Pattern
1	Chondro-osseous region (ischial tuberosity, anterior iliac spines, etc.)
2	Iliac wing
3	Simple ring fractures
	Isolated fractures
	Anterior disruption of symphysis pubis; no posterior sacroiliac injury
	Acetabular involvement (including triradiate cartilage)
4	Ring disruption fractures
	Fracture or diastasis of both anterior and posterior structures
	Pelvic fracture combined with acetabular fracture
	Straddle fracture—bilateral superior and inferior pubic rami fractures

Source: Silber JS, Flynn JM, Katz MA, et al. Role of computed tomography in the classification and management of pediatric pelvic fractures. *J Pediatr Orthop* 1992;12:621–625.

and the frequent involvement of the chondro-osseous regions. The majority of these injuries are analogous to physeal-metaphyseal injuries. Fractures also are likely to be incomplete (i.e., greenstick) because of the resilient nature of the immature bone.

Stable Pelvic Ring Fractures

Wing of the Ilium

The wing of the ilium may be displaced outward, inward, upward, or downward. The pull of muscles on this fragment may be reduced by abduction and flexion. This type of fracture, which is not common in children, is a result of direct force against the pelvis, causing disruption of the iliac apophysis or an infolding of the pliable wing of the ilium (Figs. 20-2 and 20-8). The infolding may cause a splitting injury of the iliac crest apophysis along the rim or at the iliac spines. Such disruption may lead to subsequent growth distortion of the iliac wing or elongation (prominence of an iliac spine). These injuries usually are treated conservatively.

Ischiopubic Rami

If one ramus is fractured (Fig. 20-9), or both rami on the same side (Fig. 20-10), the patient usually may be treated symptomatically. If only one ramus is fractured, always look carefully for concomitant injury completing the fracture somewhere within the pelvic ring (Fig. 20-11). Particularly, the possibility of a "physeal" fracture at the junction of the involved ramus with the triradiate (Fig. 20-11) or symphyseal cartilage should be assessed. Confirmation of a concomitant chondro-osseous injury may not adversely affect the intrinsic fracture stability or principles of management, although it may affect subsequent growth and maturation of the involved pelvic chondro-osseous region. These injuries are relatively stable, because a portion of the periosteal sleeve usually is intact. However, separation that allows angulation may render the ramus fracture unstable. Significant displacement may require manipulative (closed) reduction (Fig. 20-7). Open reduction may be necessary if the osseous fragment is angulated inward and impinges on structures such as the bladder. The intact periosteal tube allows new bone formation, which fills the displacement gap (Fig. 20-2), again lessening the need for operative reduction. Evaluation is also particularly important at the sacroiliac joint. A fracture may occur but spontaneously reduce, making radiographic diagnosis difficult. CT scanning may be the only way to determine such injury (Fig. 20-5). However, because the pelvic components are resilient in the child, a solitary ramus fracture is possible, whereas in the adult a fracture is invariably completed through contraposed portions of the ring. Even multiple fractures of three or four rami may be reasonably stable in a child because of the dense ligamentous, periosteal, and cartilaginous continuities.

Separation of the Symphysis

The changing size and irregular undulation of the symphysis region during growth always must be borne in mind. Frequently, an injury to this area must be diagnosed by physical examination (e.g., pain, overlying ecchymosis), because there may be little radiographic evidence. These separations are physeal injuries with separation of the ramus metaphysis

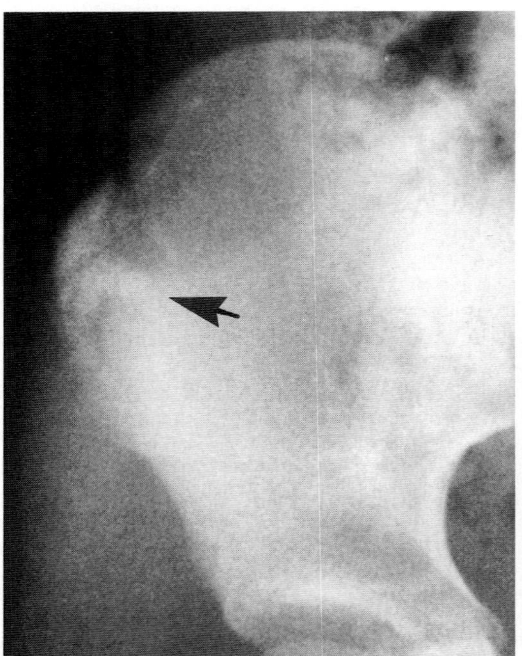
A

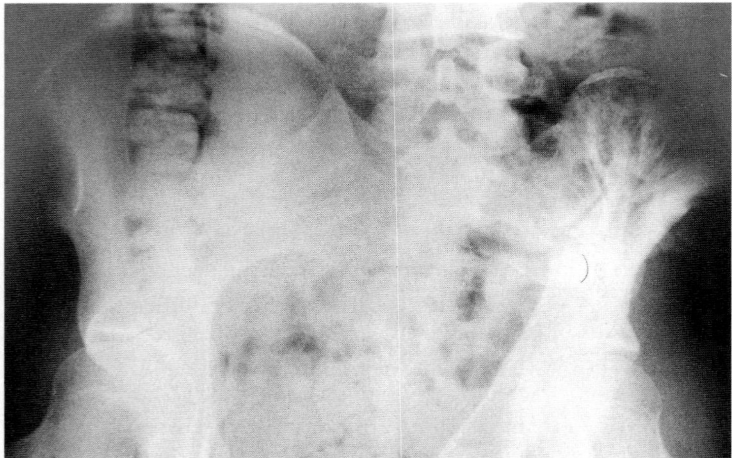
B

FIGURE 20-8. A: Fracture of the lateral margin of the ilium *(arrow)* owing to a direct blow. **B:** Pattern of altered iliac growth consequent to damage to the physis of the iliac crest. This 17-year-old-boy had been struck by a car when he was 6 years of age.

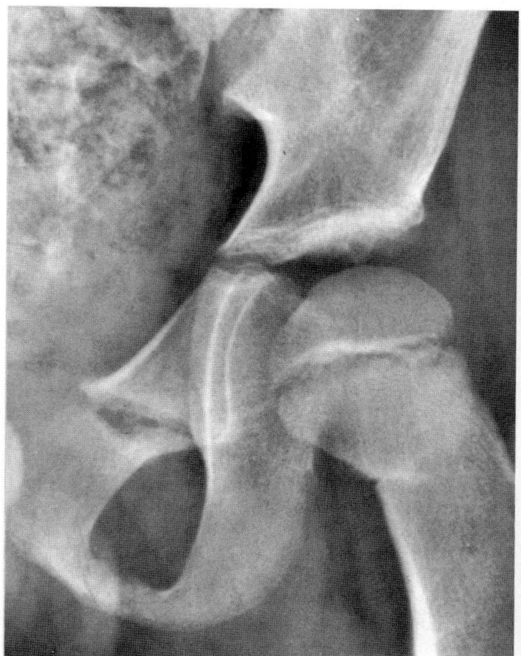

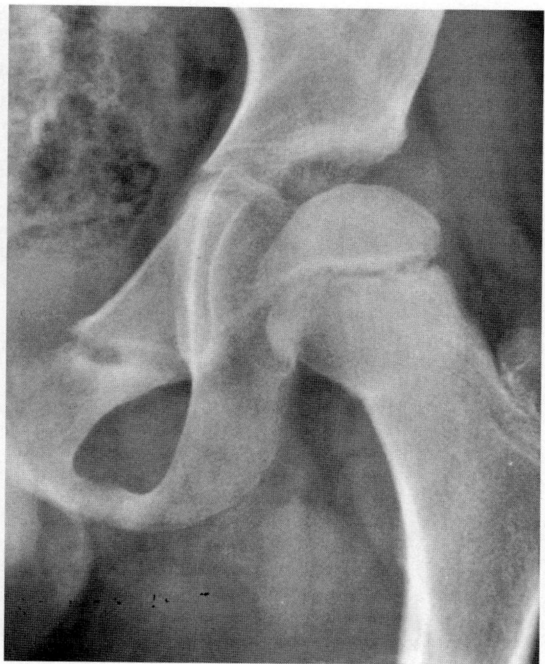

FIGURE 20-9. A: Fracture of pubic ramus. While no other pelvic injuries were readily evident (radiographically), there is a subtle, concomitant fracture of the inferior femoral neck. **B:** Five weeks later both fractures are healing.

from the epiphyseal and fibrocartilage of the symphysis (Fig. 20-12). In children, diastasis of the pubic symphysis usually occurs by separation of the bone–cartilage junction on one or both sides, rather than by disruption of the fibrous joint, as in the adult.

Radiographic diastasis of the pubic symphysis may occur in children without resultant instability of the sacroiliac joints posteriorly, presumably because of the elasticity of the bony pelvis, partial disruption of the anterior sacroiliac joint, or triradiate fracture. The sacroiliac joint in the young child may split anteriorly at the bone–cartilage interface of either the posterior ilium or sacrum. More importantly, a displaced ramus with separation at the pubic symphysis is more likely to fail additionally within the triradiate cartilage (i.e., the other end of this developing bone), rather than posteriorly at the sacroiliac joint (Fig. 20-13). *This difference between ramus fractures in adults and children is extremely important.*

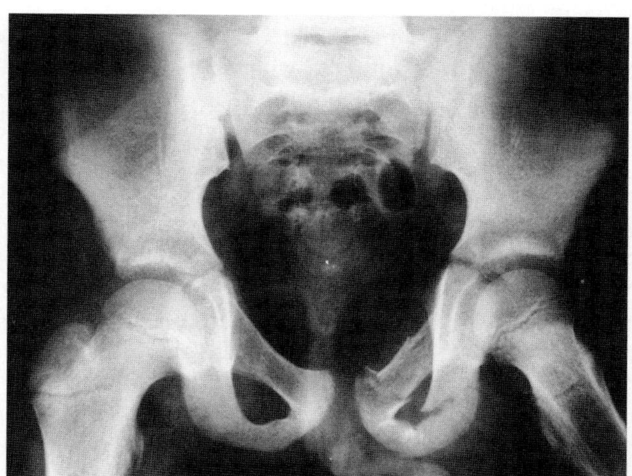

FIGURE 20-10. Ipsilateral fractures of the pubic and ischial rami. A small, additional greenstick fracture is evident within the midportion of the pubic ramus. There is a questionable widening of the contralateral sacroiliac joint. The differing appearances of the triradiate cartilages should be evaluated with computed tomography scanning.

A fixation plate may be used for traumatic diastasis of the symphysis pubis (Fig. 20-13). However, the need to use such fixation in a child is unlikely, particularly as the sym-

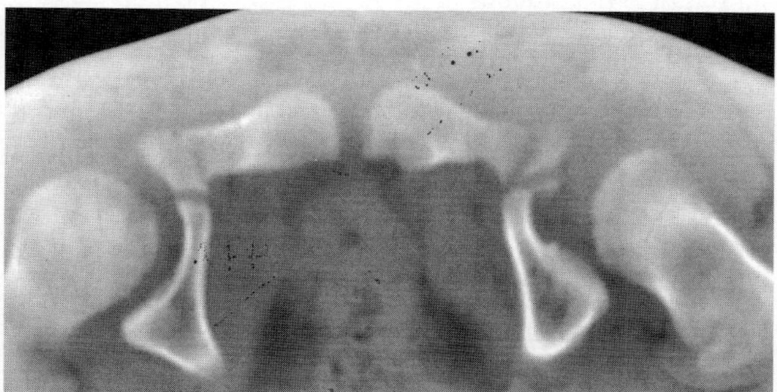

FIGURE 20-11. Computed tomographic scan of bilateral pubic ramus fractures. The left side involves the triradiate cartilage, whereas the right side is a greenstick injury that does not involve the triradiate cartilage.

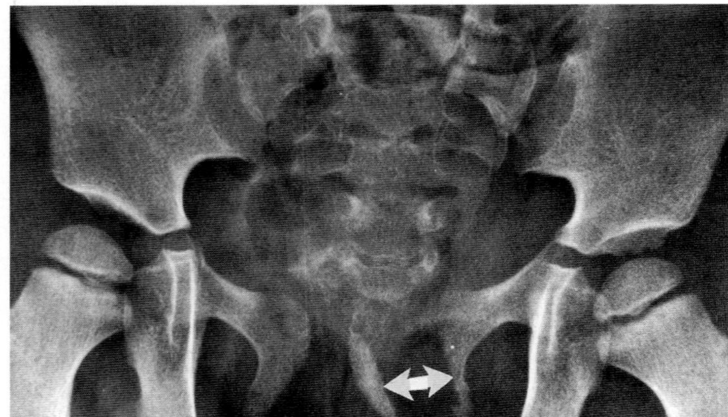

A

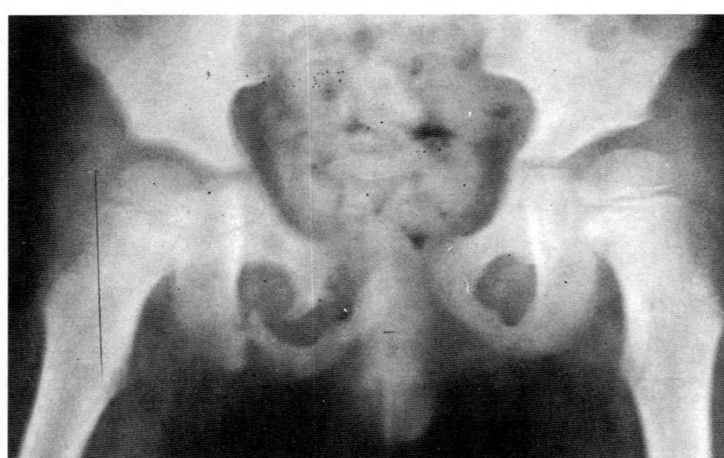

B

FIGURE 20-12. Apparent symphyseal separations. **A:** Ten weeks after multiple trauma new bone has formed at the intact periosteal sleeve and true symphysis. The gap *(arrows)* is filled with fibrocartilage. This region remained radiolucent. However, the patient was asymptomatic. **B:** This patient sustained a "separation" of the symphysis pubis. However, follow-up demonstrated new pubic and ischial ramus bone within the intact periosteal sleeves.

physis, per se, is not disrupted but, rather, is a "physeal fracture analogue." Early application of plate fixation restores the disrupted anterior pelvic ring, contributes to early immobilization of the patients, and makes reduction of the concomitantly disrupted sacroiliac joint easier. A child is more likely to have a concomitant injury at the triradiate cartilage than at the sacroiliac joint. Open reduction back into the periosteal sleeve, with repair of periosteum, with or without temporary fixation, may be considered. The pin should be percutaneous, bent at 90° and removed at 2 to 3 weeks to avoid the risk of breakage or migration. An external fixator applied to the ilia can close the anterior chondro-osseous fracture (not diastasis) as effectively as a plate. Because the fracture is a growth mechanism, injury is usually stabilizes within a few weeks.

Unstable Pelvic Ring Fractures

Separation of the Symphysis Pubis, with Partial Disruption at the Sacroiliac Joint

With separation of the symphysis pubis, the ring is disrupted and opened anteriorly at the symphysis. The posterior separation at the sacroiliac joint may be owing to disruption of the anterior capsule of the joint or an epiphyseal iliac fracture (Fig. 20-14). Comparable epiphyseal separation at the sacrum may occur, but is less likely because of developmental patterns of the sacrum.

The supine position aggravates the deformity, and the child may be more comfortable lying on his or her side. Frequently, placement of a pelvic sling relieves symptoms. This sling may allow some control of the pelvic diastasis, because the straps may be crossed to increase compression. Compression immobilization with a sling or spica should be maintained for 6 to 8 weeks, depending on the age of the child, to ensure adequate ligamentous or chondro-osseous union at the symphysis and prevent late spreading. An external fixator may be used (Fig. 20-15). However, the threaded pins may lead to iliac crest apophyseal damage in the young child. Smooth pins should be used whenever possible. The relatively rapid rate of healing allows early removal of the fixator. Alternatively, posterior internal fixation may be used (Fig. 20-16).

Fractures of the Anterior Arch

Crush injuries in the anteroposterior direction may cause fractures of both rami bilaterally to give a floating segment

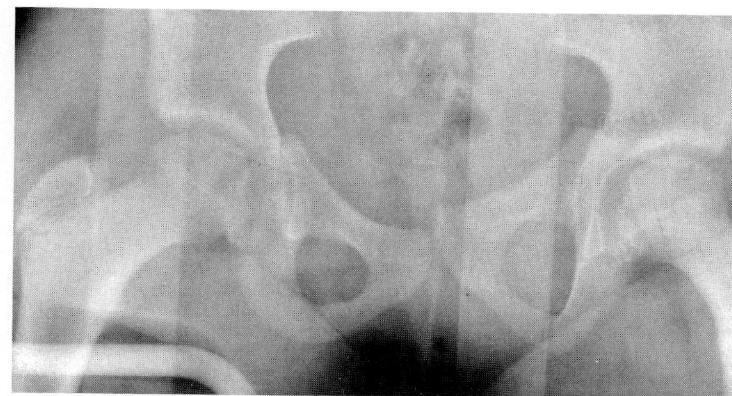

A

FIGURE 20-13. A: Bilateral pubic ramus fractures in a 14-year-old boy that involved closing the triradiate cartilages. The symphysis also was displaced. B: Computed tomographic scan of the injuries. C: Internal fixation was used to stabilize the fractures.

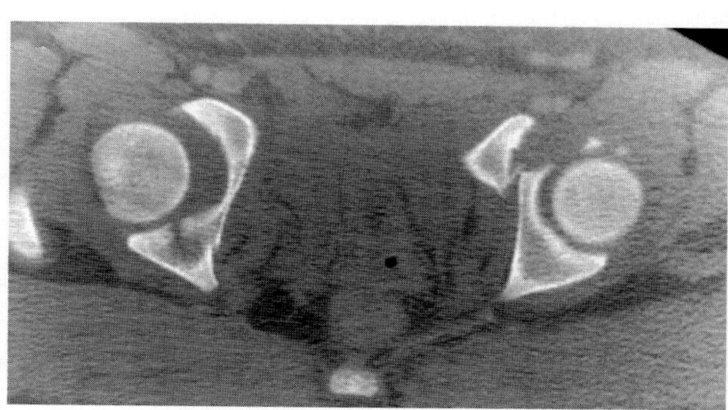

B

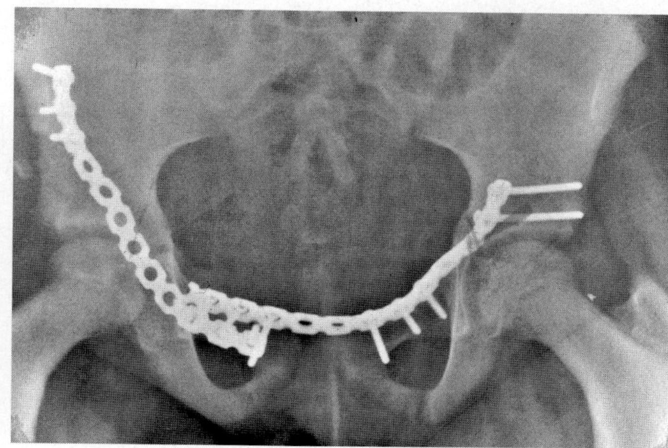

C

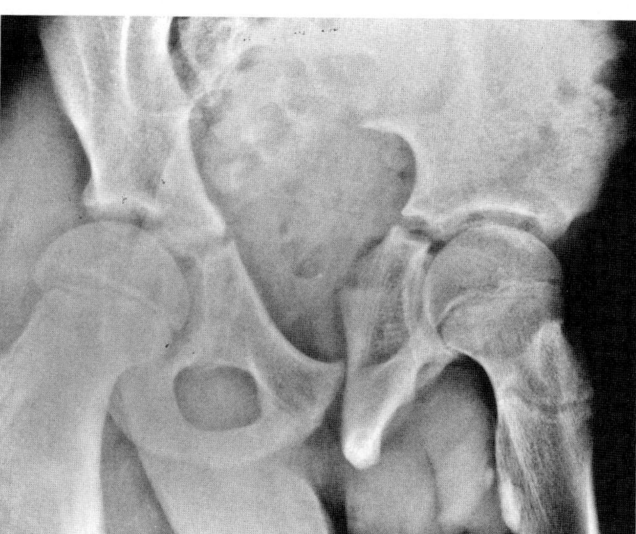

FIGURE 20-14. Hemipelvic disruption of the sacroiliac joint and the symphysis. There was additional triradiate injury in the left acetabulum.

(straddle injury). In the child, a variation of this injury involves fractures of both rami along with an ipsilateral separation of the bone from the symphyseal cartilage or the triradiate cartilage. The fragment may be displaced posteriorly to cause bladder displacement or damage. Disruption of the symphysis pubis usually is associated with separation of the bone (metaphysis) away from the cartilage and thick periosteal sleeve. The separation gap subsequently may be filled in by endochondral bone formation. The segment may be displaced posteriorly (usually by impact), superiorly because of the rectus abdominis muscles, or inferiorly because of the adductors and hamstrings.

A pelvic sling should not be used in this situation, because it may cause inward compression of an unstable ramus. Children with this injury should be rested supine and placed in a semi-Fowler's position to relax the abdominal and adductor muscles. Treatment is maintained for 2 to 3 weeks, depending on the degree of displacement. Disruption of this region must be carefully assessed, particularly with regard to urethral and bladder injuries. Thickened periosteum may not be damaged completely; therefore, major fragment displacement is not common in children. External fixation may be considered. If the fragment is displaced into the pelvis, injuring or potentially injuring the bladder, consider using some type of stabilization.

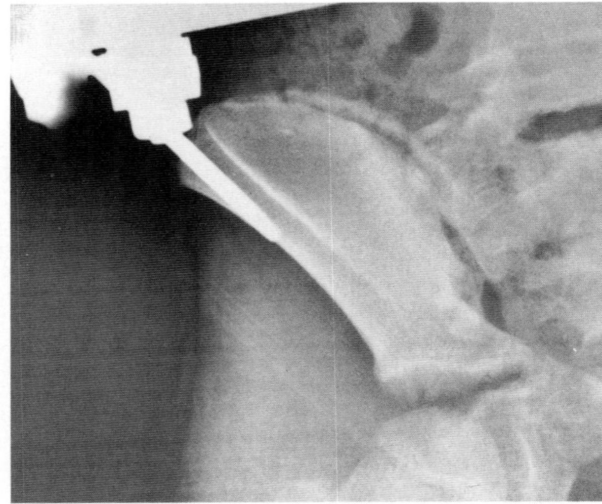

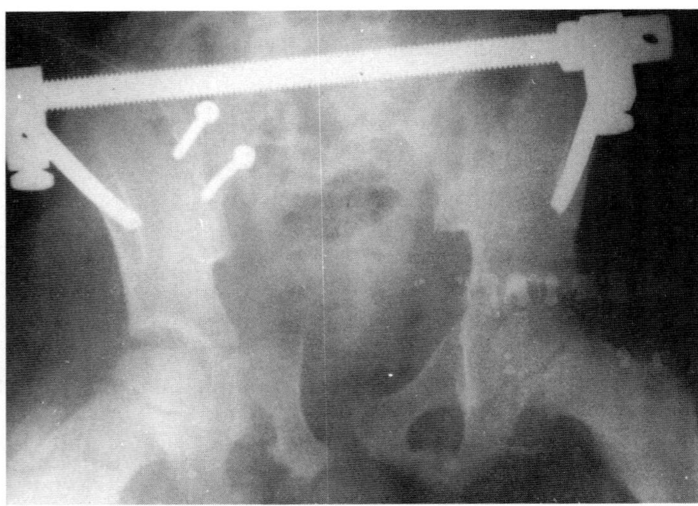

A B

FIGURE 20-15. A: This adolescent had an outward disruption of the ilium along the iliac crest and sacroiliac "joint." There also was disruption at the superior arms of the triradiate cartilage. This was reduced and stabilized with an external fixator. **B:** This patient had a fracture of the ischial ramus, the triradiate cartilage and the "SI joint." A combination of internal and external fixation was used to stabilize the fractures.

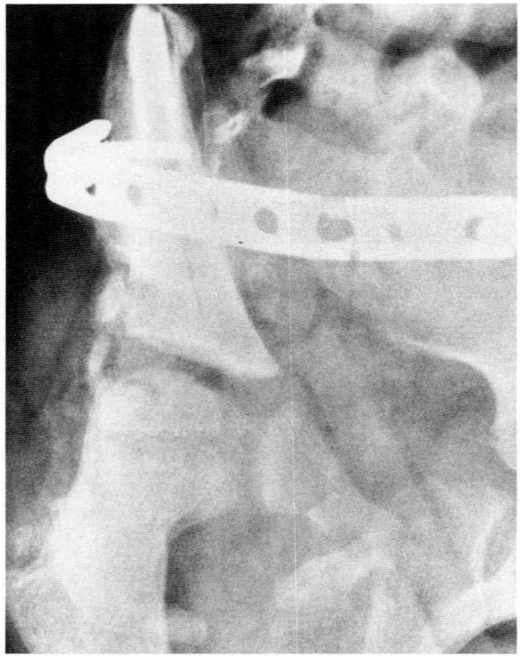

FIGURE 20-16. This 7-year-old boy was run over by a garbage truck. There was a significant degloving injury of the perineum that limited and delayed aspects of musculoskeletal care. The posterior disruptions eventually were stabilized with a plate. Ten weeks after the injury heterotopic bone is evident around the right hip.

Vertical Shear

With vertical shear the ring is broken in front and in back, and the free hemipelvis is shifted upward, inward, or outward. The free pelvic segment is displaced by spasm of the muscles whose origin is fixed to the floating piece (e.g., the psoas, adductors, gluteus maximus, lateral abdominal muscles). Leg length discrepancy results if upward displacement is sufficient.

Such fractures may be treated by skeletal traction using a pin through the distal femoral metaphysis. However, multiple system injury may preclude use of this method, because rigorous attempts at reduction may precipitate further retroperitoneal hemorrhage or nerve damage (traction or avulsion) and thus are contraindicated. Traction with 10 to 15 pounds, usually requiring a skeletal pin, may be necessary to reduce the fracture. After reduction is achieved, which is usually within a week, the position should be held. Countertraction should be maintained to prevent the child from inadvertently placing the injured leg in relative abduction. Open reduction is rarely indicated.

Bucket Handle Injury

With a bucket handle injury the pelvic ring is broken in front and back, and the floating pieces are rotated so the iliac crest is displaced medially and the ischial tuberosity laterally. This condition may be combined with some vertical shear. This type of injury, in effect, causes the reverse of an innominate osteotomy and thereby "uncovers" the femoral head. Again, this injury should be treated by skeletal traction or an external fixator whenever possible. It is important to reduce this deformity, as uncovering the femoral head, particularly in the young child up to 8 to 9 years of age, may cause relative or actual dysplasia of the acetabulum by the time growth is finished.

Lateral Compression

Lateral crushing injury folds the wing of the pelvis, hinged posteriorly on the sacroiliac joint or anteriorly at the pubis. However, the free edge of the fragment may be displaced centrally. When a child is run over, one ilium may be rotated externally at the sacroiliac joint and the other hemipelvis rotated internally.

Traction may be applied through the hip joint and proximal femur in an attempt to reduce it over time. Such reduction takes approximately 1 week and should be followed by maintenance of bed rest. Open reduction may be indicated, particularly in the small child in whom skeletal traction is not readily applicable. External fixation with a pelvic frame also may be used. Using the "lengthening" attachments, winging of a hemipelvis may be gradually reduced to a normal (or near-normal) anatomic position.

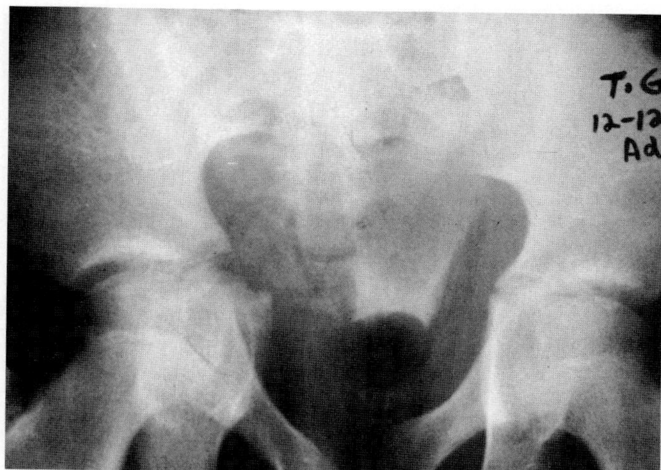

FIGURE 20-17. Fourteen-year-old girl with a central acetabular fracture through the still incompletely closed triradiate cartilage (as evident on the uninjured opposite side). The acetabular weight-bearing dome is intact with no central displacement of the femoral head. Because of other injuries this girl was treated nonoperatively with femoral traction and a good result. In retrospect, the osseous injury was not associated with significant articular cartilage injury, despite the apparent extent of osseous displacement.

ACETABULAR FRACTURES

Treatment of a pediatric patient with a fractured acetabulum is determined by the general condition, associated injuries and extent of skeletal maturation, particularly in the triradiate cartilage (14). Most authors have advised conservative treatment, especially in children. During and after closure of the triradiate cartilage the acetabular fracture patterns and treatment essentially are the same as in adults (Figs. 20-17 and 20-18) (10,13,30). The most important factor is the reestablishment of the superior dome and extraction of any loose fragments of bone, cartilage, or muscle that might be herniated into the defects, thereby reconstituting a normal relation between the femoral head and acetabulum. The future of the developing hip depends primarily on the condition of the weight-bearing portions of the acetabulum and femoral head, the potential for the development of ischemic necrosis in either the acetabulum or femoral head, an accurate femoral-acetabular relation, intrinsic stability of the joint, and age at time of injury.

Peripheral (Wall) Fractures

Peripheral acetabular fractures often are associated with dislocations of the hip, as they are in the adult. However, because of the structure of the child's acetabulum, particularly the pliable cartilaginous components such as the labral dislocations of the hip often occur without concomitant acetabular fracture or at least a radiologically evident (i.e., osseous) one. In the older child, posterior dislocation is more likely to displace a peripheral osseous acetabular fragment than is the less common anterior dislocation. The chance for displacement of an acetabular fragment also is influenced by the relative extent of ossification of the posterior and anterior walls. Any acetabular fracture that accompanies a hip dislocation should be reduced as accurately as possible, because it is an intracapsular injury in the child. Whether there are fragments within the joint is not always easy to determine, because portions of radiolucent cartilage may be displaced into the joint, particularly when there is separation of the fibrocartilaginous acetabular labrum away from the main hyaline cartilage. Any suggestion of limitation of motion or failure to attain complete, concentric reduction (widening of the radiolucent cartilage or joint space) should make one suspicious of this possibility. An arthrogram is often of benefit diagnostically. Depending on the age of the patient, the os acetabulum must be considered a source of roentgenographic "fracture." Large superior fragments should be viewed with caution and followed carefully through skeletal maturity in case they lead to subsequent acetabular dysplasia and hip subluxation. CT evaluation may be definitive.

Triradiate Injuries

Traumatic disruption of the acetabular triradiate physeal cartilage is an infrequent injury. Of the 84 pelvic fractures in children reviewed by Reed, only four had evidence of acetabular triradiate involvement (2). These injuries to the triradiate cartilage constitute physeal trauma comparable to fractures involving the physes of longitudinal bones

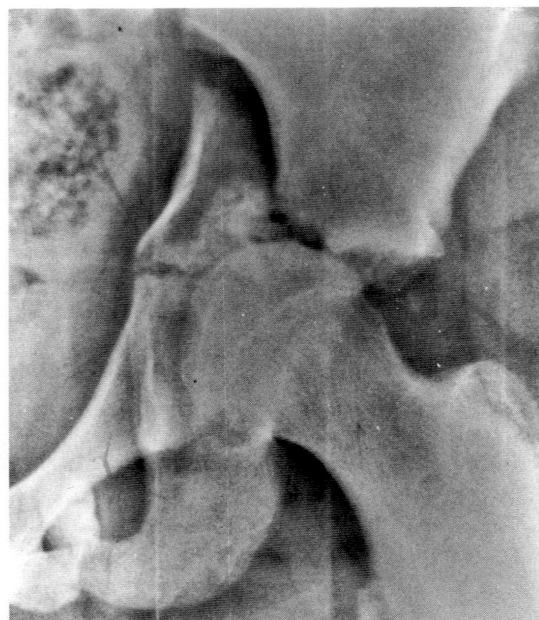

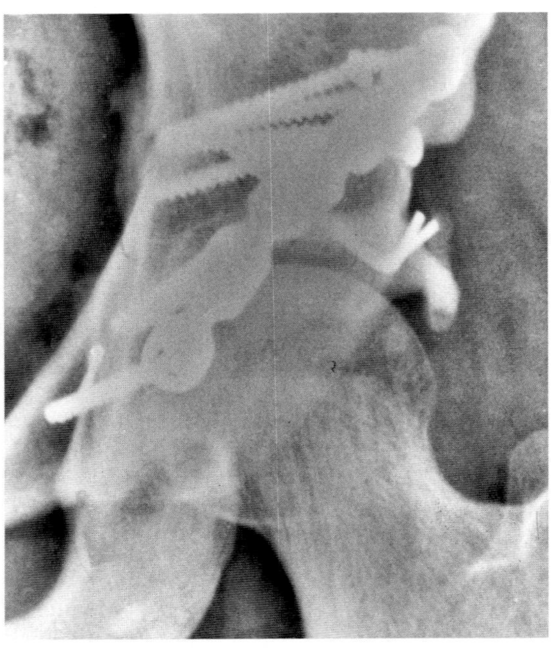

FIGURE 20-18. A: Central fracture of the acetabulum. The triradiate cartilage in this 12-year-old girl is still evident. This fracture is equivalent to a Type 2 growth mechanism injury, but because of patient age and impending closure of the physes of the triradiate cartilage, is more like an adult than a child's injury. **B:** Accordingly, the fracture was treated with open reduction and internal fixation.

(31–36). The potential for this injury should always be assessed whenever a single ramus fracture is noted. However, the bipolar anatomy of the triradiate cartilage and lack of ossified epiphyses until late adolescence may make classification of these injuries difficult. During adolescence the appearance of multiple secondary ossification centers additionally may make diagnosis confusing (Fig. 20-1).

If one of the pelvic bones (pubis or ischium) in a child is displaced and rotated at the symphysis pubis, then it must hinged elsewhere. In the skeletally immature patient, however, rather than injury to the entire hemipelvis, the forces may be summated at the triradiate cartilage, disrupting a portion (or all) of the triradiate end and the symphyseal end. Lateral compression forces in an adult may produce a hemipelvic disruption. In contrast, the child may sustain a quadrant disruption with rotatory disruption of the ischiopubic and triradiate units.

It is my experience that triradiate fracture is often overlooked and underdiagnosed in many children with seemingly solitary ramus fractures. If a ramus fracture is displaced, then there must be another injury that allows such hinging to occur. In the adult posterior (sacroiliac) disruption is likely. In the child there is a high probability of an unrecognized chondro-osseous separation at one or more arms of the triradiate cartilage. Such displacement, which may be subtle, is better detected by CT scans and reconstructions than routine radiography of the pelvis (Figs. 20-19 and 20-20).

These fractures are usually undisplaced and infrequently require open reduction. However, when a displaced Type 2

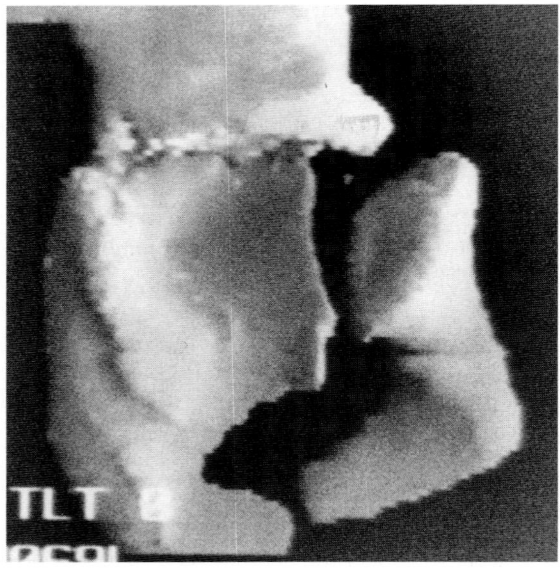

FIGURE 20-19. Pubic ramus fracture associated with triradiate cartilage injury at the "other end." Reconstruction of the computed tomographic scan shows outward rotation of the pubis at the triradiate cartilage and an additional displacement inferiorly at the junction of pubis and ischium. Also note the displacement of the ischium relative to the ilium at the posterior arm of the triradiate cartilage. These relatively subtle injuries require careful evaluation to detect and make informed decisions for management and prognosis.

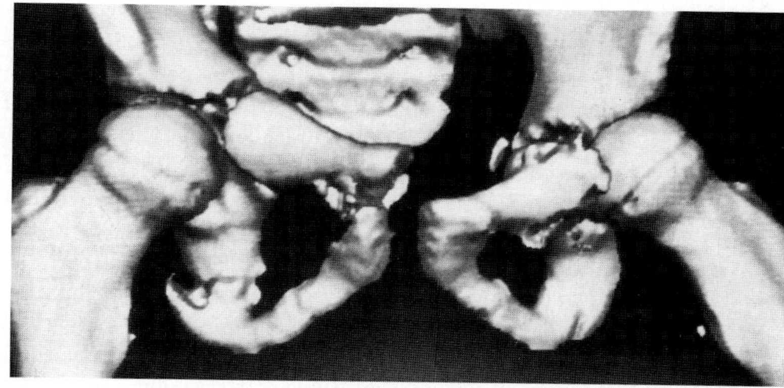

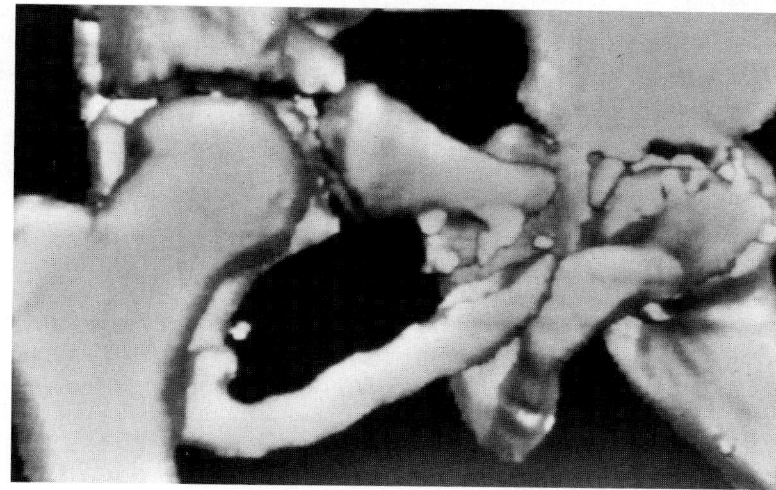

FIGURE 20-20. Computed tomographic reconstructions **(A,B)** of an ischiopubic fracture adjacent to the symphysis. There are "other end" fractures of the ischium next to the lesser trochanter and the pubis at the left triradiate cartilage. There is extensive bilateral injury.

growth mechanism is observed and CT scan shows joint disruption, open reduction may be indicated (Fig. 20-18).

The first pattern is a shearing-type injury owing to a blow to the ilium or the proximal end of the femur that causes a Type 1 or 2 injury at the interface of the two superior arms of the triradiate cartilage and the metaphyseal spongiosa of the ilium. A triangular medial metaphyseal fragment (Thurstan Holland sign) may be present. This fragment effectively splits the acetabulum into a superior (main weight-bearing) one third and an inferior (minimally weight-bearing) two thirds. The germinal zones contained within the bipolar physes would be unaffected by such a fracture mechanism, and so continued growth would be expected. Comparable disruption between the triradiate arms and the metaphysis of either the ischial or the pubic ramus is theoretically possible. Type 1 and 2 injuries appear to carry a favorable prognosis for continued (relatively) normal growth.

The second pattern is a displaced ramus fracture (more often involving the pubic ramus) in either the diaphyseal (analogous) segment or the metaphysis at the symphysis. The fulcrum of rotation becomes the inferior arm of the triradiate cartilage along with the anterior or posterior portion of the superior arm (contingent on whether the pubic or ischial ramus is involved). This rotational component at the physeal–metaphyseal interface of the triradiate cartilage is analogous to a displaced growth plate fracture in a long bone. Furthermore, there has to be subchondral separation from the contiguous articular cartilage. They are usually Type 1 or 2 growth mechanism injuries (Fig. 20-21 and 20-22).

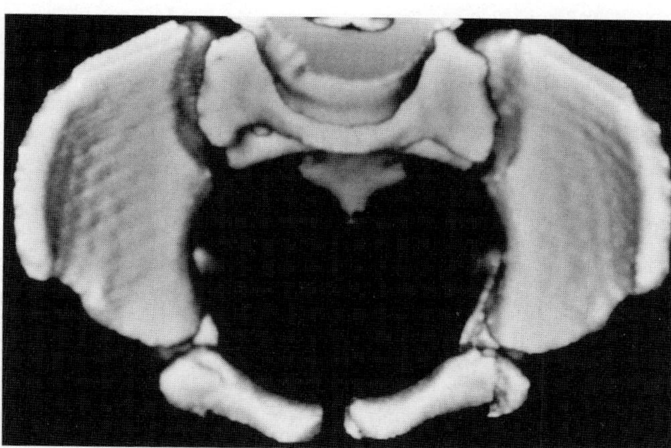

FIGURE 20-21. Bilateral Type 2 triradiate cartilage fractures.

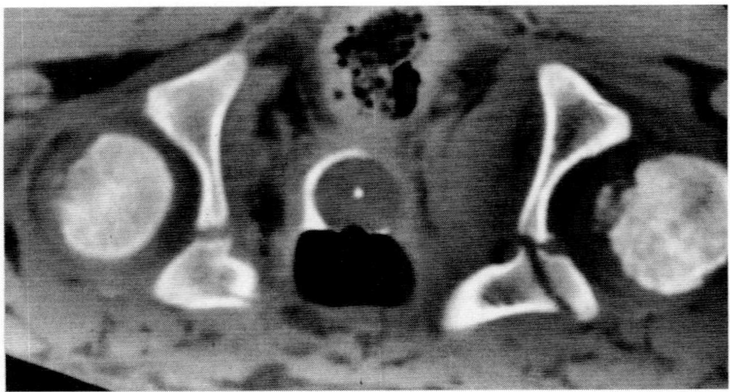

FIGURE 20-22. Computed tomographic (CT) scan of a bilateral pubic fractures. The CT scan revealed the extent of injury. One side had a greenstick fracture at the "other end" *(right)*, while the opposite side had a more obvious fracture extending into the left triradiate cartilage.

During the final normal stages of closure of the triradiate cartilage, severe trauma to the pelvis may result in a fracture across one or more of the regions of the arms of the triradiate cartilage (Fig. 20-23). This pattern, often occurring during adolescence, is analogous to the Tillaux fracture of the distal tibia, with the remodeling bone plate creating a region of temporary susceptibility to fracture until osseous remodeling across the physeal region is well under way. During this stage secondary (epiphyseal analogue) centers occur within the triradiate cartilage. These ossification regions should not be confused with a fracture or comminution in an adolescent being evaluated for acute pelvic trauma. Narrowing of the triradiate cartilage and displacement are difficult to detect roentgenographically, especially when other pelvic components are damaged.

The major subsequent problem is disparate growth of the acetabulum relative to the femoral head (31,32,36). The femoral head continues to grow, whereas the normal mechanism of concomitant hemispheric expansion of the acetabulum cannot occur responsively (Fig. 20-24). Growth may occur only at the periphery. Such growth at the periphery becomes increasingly subjected to pathologic pressure from the femoral head, causing eversional deformation, not unlike that seen in developmental hip disease. When the fracture occurs during adolescence, subsequent growth-related changes in acetabular morphology and congruency of the hip joint are unlikely. However, in young children, especially those who are <10 years old, acetabular growth abnormalities are a complication of this injury and may result in a shallow acetabulum similar to that seen in patients with developmental dysplasia of the hip.

The growth physes of the three pelvic bones extend continuously from the triradiate cartilage laterally into the discrete acetabular peripheral physis. Fusion of the triradiate cartilage may still leave the peripheral physis intact. Depending on the age of the child at the time of injury, this

A

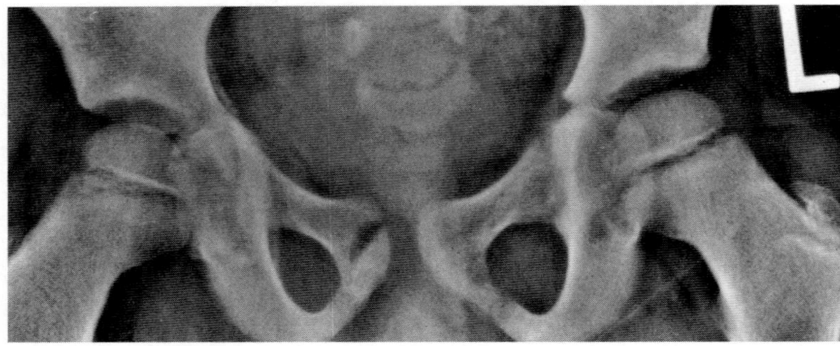

FIGURE 20-23. A: Pelvic fractures in an 11-year-old boy. This is evident on the patient's right side by the bone along the inner wall of the ilium and the obliteration of the triradiate compared to the opposite side. **B:** Computed tomographic scan showed the fracture involved both sides of the triradiate cartilage and, by definition, had to cross and displace this cartilage. **C:** Eight months later premature closure and bridging of the triradiate is evident. The patient's family refused resection of the osseous bridge.

B

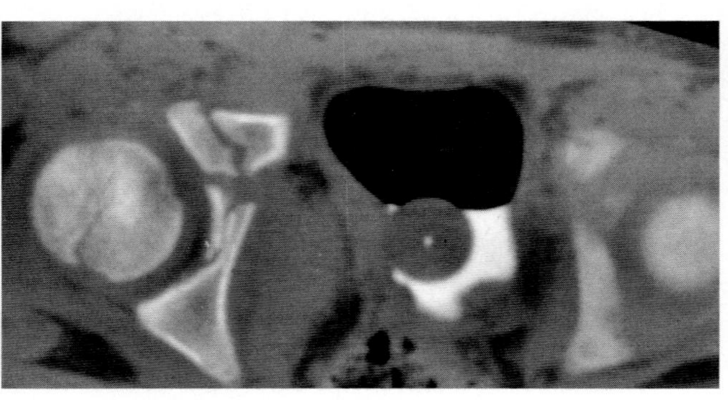

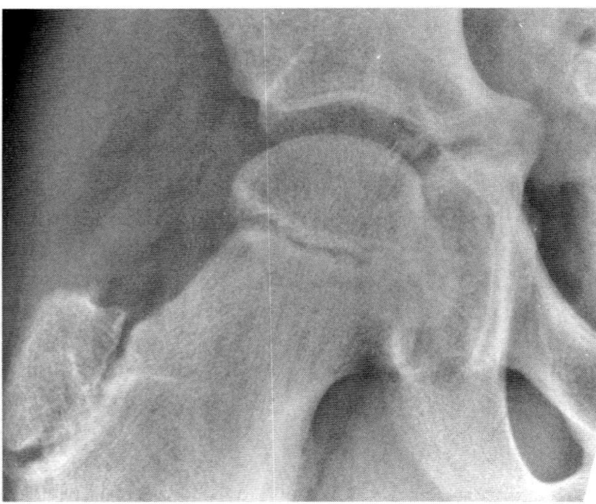

C

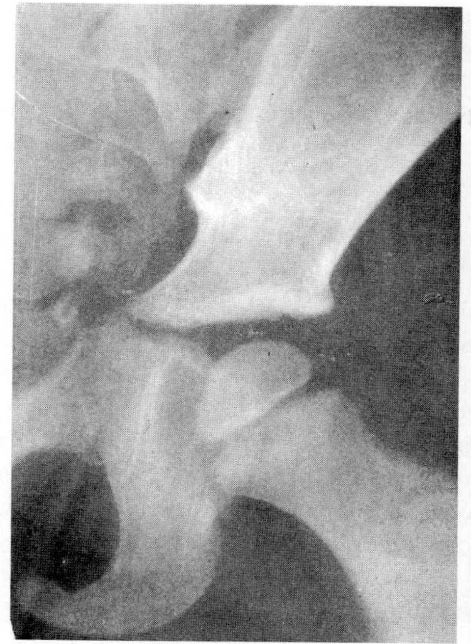
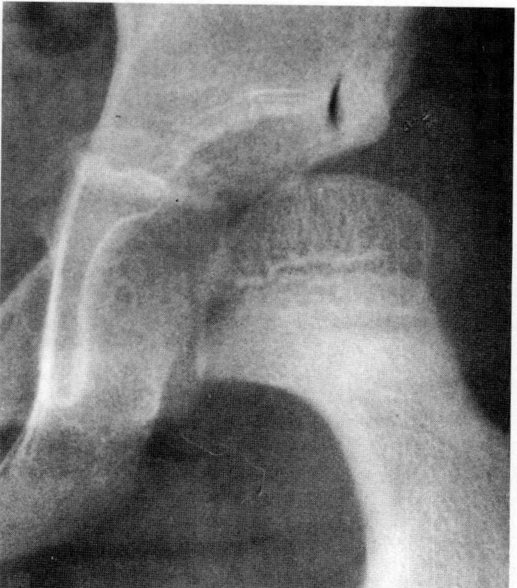
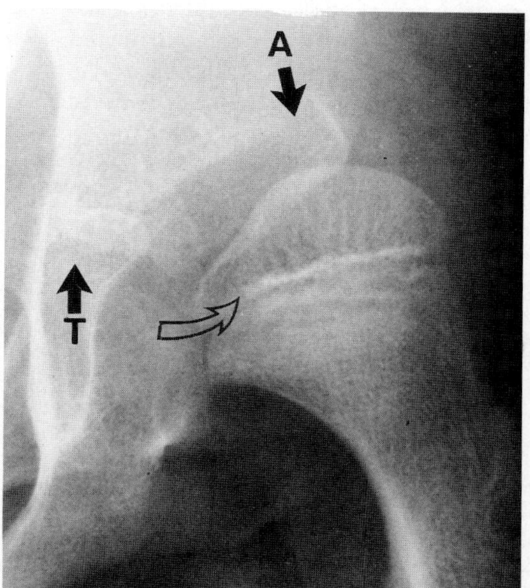

FIGURE 20-24. A: Three-year-old girl with multiple trauma after being hit by a car. The triradiate cartilage was injured, as evident by the medial shift of the pubic bone. **B:** This led to premature closure of the triradiate cartilage and a deformation of the acetabulum and femoral head. **C:** At 10 years of age she had closure of the triradiate cartilage *(T, arrow),* distortion of the superior acetabulum *(A, arrow),* and lateralization of the femur *(open arrow).* She subsequently underwent reconstructive surgery of the hip (shelf arthroplasty and varus osteotomy).

acetabular growth plate continues to grow, effectively enlarging the acetabulum laterally (i.e., circumferentially and posteriorly). The medial wall of the acetabulum becomes thicker and the acetabulum more shallow. Concomitantly, as the femoral head expands and is displaced laterally and superiorly (subluxates), it exerts increased pressure against the superior part of the acetabulum, impairing normal endochondral ossification and increasing the acetabular index, similar to the mechanism of developmental dysplasia of the hip.

Reconstructive surgery may be necessary in some of these children and must be individualized to the specific injury, concomitant pelvic deformation from other fractures, and the degree of anticipated growth. Shelf augmentation procedures offer a solution in many of these cases.

AVULSION FRACTURES

Avulsions are the most common type of pelvic chondro-osseous injury in the child, especially in the adolescent athlete (1,37–41). These regions may be avulsed prior to the appearance of secondary ossification (which frequently does not appear until late adolescence). In such absence of definitive radiologic diagnosis, the injury must be strongly suspected clinically, and treatment should be directed toward the presumptive injury. Several weeks later the diagnosis may be confirmed by the appearance of "metaphyseal" callus. Because of the thick periosteum and perichondrium, these fractures are not usually significantly displaced. Postinjury muscle function generally is not impaired by eventual healing in a mildly displaced position, even if a fibrous, rather than osseous, union results owing to the persistent tensile forces. However, significant displacement, which is much less common, may cause functional inefficiency of the attached muscles and may require open reduction or reconstruction for optimal muscle function. Complications are unusual, because these fractures ordinarily are associated with minor athletic stress, rather than major trauma.

When a musculotendinous unit is subjected to excess stress, whether an acute forceful, unbalanced overload or a less forceful but repetitive application, the contraction or contractions may be transmitted to the apophysis. This may result in a fracture at either the chondro-osseous interface or through a segment of the subchondral bone. The excessive, invariably repetitive demands of adolescent athletics make this age group especially susceptible to avulsion fractures.

Various studies suggest that iliac spine avulsions are the most common, whereas others list ischial injuries as being more frequent (38–41). Frequency is not as important as suspicion and recognition by the clinician. Rossi and Dragoni studied 203 avulsion fractures in 198 adolescent athletes. Five patients had multiple areas of involvement. The ischial tuberosity was involved in 109 cases, the anterior inferior iliac spine (AIIS) in 45 cases, the anterior-superior iliac spine (ASIS) in 39 cases, the superior corner of the pubic symphysis in seven cases, and the iliac crest in only three cases. The greatest number of cases involved soccer (74 patients) and gymnastics (55 patients).

The basic treatment protocol is to stop the evocative activity, prescribe rest (including bed rest), prescribe nonsteroidal antiinflammatory drugs, recommend appropriate positioning of the leg, and gradual resumption of activity. There should be protected weight bearing with crutches. Most avulsion fractures may be managed nonoperatively, with attention directed at minimizing tension in the musculotendinous insertion while the avulsion heals.

For competitive adolescent athletes conservative treatment of pelvic avulsion injuries may cause difficulties, despite good functional results. The disadvantages include a relatively long period of immobilization, use of crutches, risk of reinjury, alteration of functional length of involved muscles, disruption of normal training regimens, and the risk of missing a significant part of a sport season.

Acute injuries often have an obvious bone fragment. In contrast, the chronic pattern usually is associated with irregular changes in the metaphyseal equivalent bone, not unlike those seen in the gymnast's wrists (1). Confusion with neoplasia or osteomyelitis may be likely when there is irregular radiodensity and radiolucency and if the practitioner is not familiar with the injury patterns and radiographic appearances. If a biopsy is done, the callus may be misinterpreted as an osteosarcoma if there is not good communication between surgeon and pathologist. Such a mistake may lead to unnecessary and costly evaluation and inappropriate surgery.

Iliac Crest

Avulsion fracture of the iliac crest is a variation of "hip pointer," which is usually defined as an iliac crest contusion. Patients may sustain a direct blow to the crest, as from a football helmet (Fig. 20-25). Fractures of the anterior iliac apophysis may occur in adolescent runners. These are often stress fractures or may occur during sudden, severe contraction of the abdominal muscles associated with abrupt directional changes while running.

Symptoms may occur acutely or, at the other end of the spectrum, may persist for months following questionable injury. Some adolescent athletes have a posterior iliac crest apophysitis with pain localized at the posterior iliac crest. This condition may be duplicated by resistance to abduction with the hip flexed and the patient lying on the unaffected side.

To avoid the risk of further avulsion and more serious damage, crutches should be used for 5 to 7 days, followed by limited physical activity for approximately 4 weeks. Patients treated by rest and discontinuation of their usual athletic activity generally have complete relief of symptoms within 4 to 6 weeks and are able to resume training programs at that point.

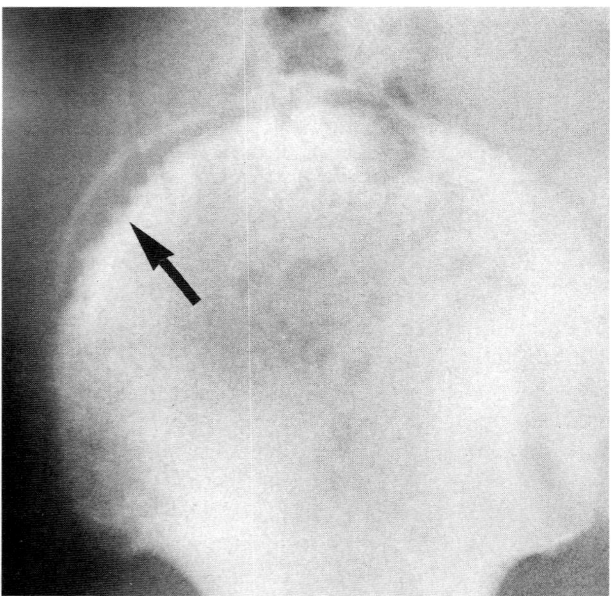

FIGURE 20-25. Avulsion injury of the iliac crest in a 16-year-old football player who was struck directly by a helmet. There is a distinct separation of the secondary ossification center in one section *(arrow)* relative to the rest of the crest.

More significant trauma may avulse significant portions of the iliac crest. The more violent the trauma, the greater is the risk of damage to growth potential, creating underdevelopment of the iliac wing (1,42). Growth disturbance of the entire ilium may be associated with premature fusion of the sacroiliac joint (1).

Physeal avulsion of a nonossified iliac crest may result in intestinal obstruction because of a lumbar hernia or entrapment of bowel segments (22,23). Damage to the iliac crest physis during early childhood may lead to growth discrepancy (Fig. 20-8). Olney and coworkers found that experimental splitting of the rabbit iliac apophysis significantly affected growth of the ilium (42). Altered iliac growth, development, and attainment of a normal shape and orientation might negatively affect the origin and vector efficiency of the adductor muscles, which could affect the biomechanics of the hip over time.

Iliac Spines

The ASIS serves as the attachment of the sartorius muscle and some of the tensor fascia lata, whereas the AIIS is the attachment for the rectus femoris muscle. The muscles arising from either spine cross two mobile joints, both of which are major hip flexors and may be under extreme force during vigorous athletic activity or an accident. Either iliac spine may be avulsed (43–48). The anterosuperior spine is probably injured more often than the anteroinferior spine (1). The classic presentation is an adolescent sprinter who feels a sudden, sharp pain in the groin on leaving the starting blocks. Less commonly repetitive stress of training may lead to insidious prodromal microfailure that can go on to complete avulsion (similar to the patterns of slipped capital femoral epiphysis and Osgood-Schlatter's injury).

Two mechanisms of injury have been proposed. The first is a forceful contraction of the sartorius and tensor fasciae

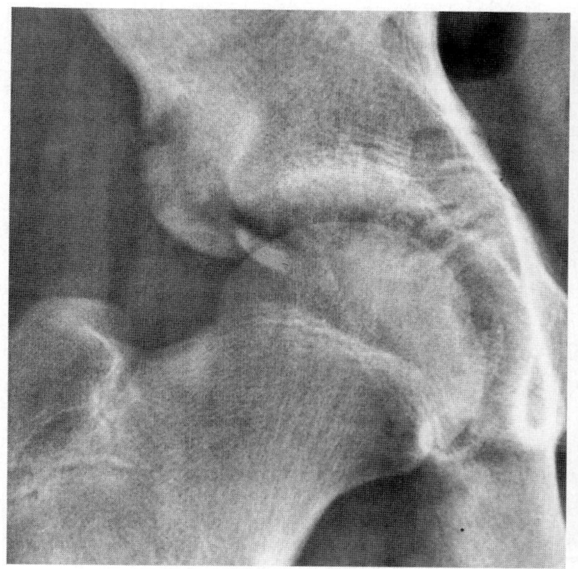
A

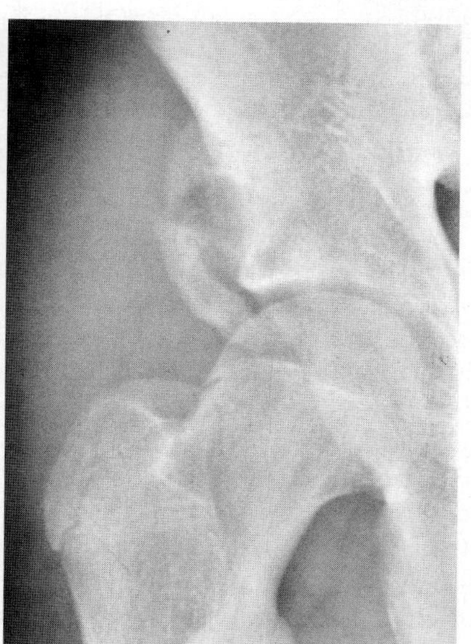
B

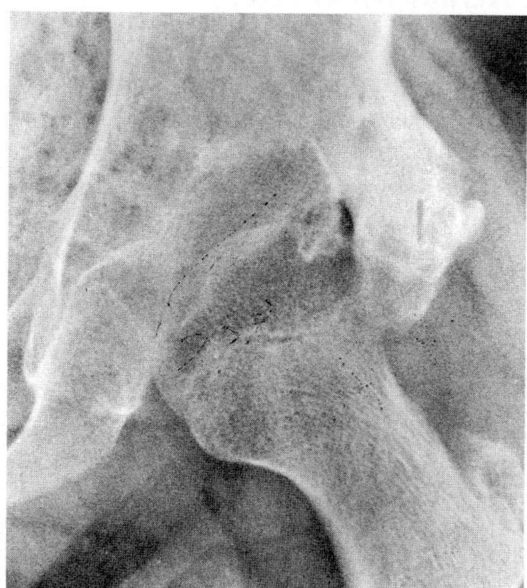
C

FIGURE 20-26. Avulsions of the anterior inferior iliac spine. **A:** Acute injury, with mild displacement. **B:** Appearance 3 months after a diagnosis of a "hip pointer." No x-ray studies were done initially. This film was obtained subsequently because of continuing complaints (groin pain). **C:** Appearance of extensive bone formation in an 11-year-old patient with multiple trauma and a head injury. **B,C:** The acute injury radiographs failed to discern the injury.

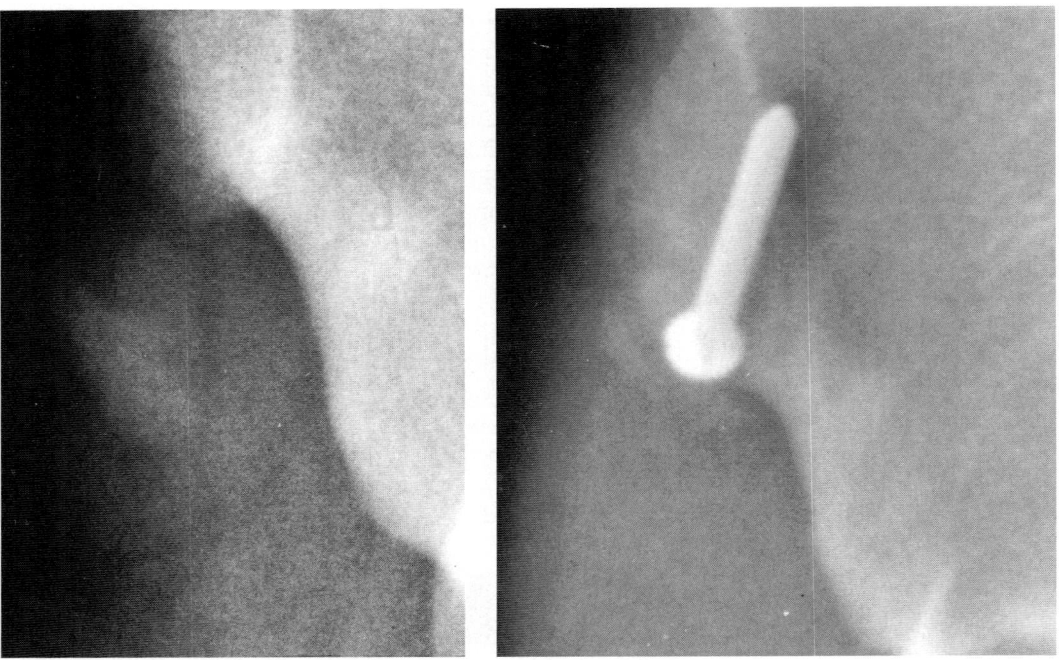

FIGURE 20-27. A: Acute avulsion of the anterior superior iliac spine. **B:** This was anatomically reduced and fixed internally.

lata muscles against a hyperextended trunk (e.g., while running, playing soccer), such as at the start of a race or while slipping. These areas also may be avulsed during a hip dislocation (46). The second is the sudden, repetitive move sprints. This injury pattern most frequently affects adolescent runners. Essentially the two joints are moving in opposite directions simultaneously.

Most patients complain of acute pain, which is usually severe enough to cause them to stop the activity. Pain is increased during active movement of the hip. A snap was felt by the patient in 45% of cases (48). Swelling and tenderness are often present.

Diagnosis may be difficult. In a young child the spine may be cartilaginous, and thus impossible to detect with routine radiography (Fig. 20-26). The adolescent usually has a fracture through the equivalent of metaphyseal bone, pulling off the cartilage and enough osseous tissue to be detected radiographically. Rarely, a secondary ossification center is evident in a cartilaginous disruption in the adolescent.

Usually these fractures do not separate significantly, although in rare instances they may be displaced several centimeters, especially when the trauma is repetitive. Winkler and coworkers described a displaced superior iliac spine that had led to formation of an extensively elongated osseous bar extending down from the superior spine owing to chronic, repetitive avulsion (49).

Treatment includes rest, minimal weight-bearing with the use of crutches, and discontinuation of athletic activities for 4 to 6 weeks. If a significant separation has occurred, open reduction may be indicated (Fig. 20-27). However, open reduction and internal fixation are rarely needed (1,50).

Exostosis formation of either the anterior-inferior iliac spine (AIIS) or anterior-superior iliac spine (ASIS) is caused by acute or chronic traction avulsion of the cartilaginous apophysis. The intervening gap is filled in with a combination of membranous and endochondral ossification. In the chronic situation the repetitive minimal avulsion/traction duplicates the same phenomenon as with limb lengthening through the growth plate (i.e., chondrodiastasis).

Ischial Tuberosity

Injury to the ischial tuberosity is a relatively frequent injury, especially in young athletes who experience acute or chronic abduction injuries of the leg (51–56). Irregularity of the apophysis of the ischial tuberosity has been termed Kremser's disease (1). The typical patient is a young adolescent athlete. Diagnosis often is difficult in these children. Ischial apophysiolysis often is diagnosed only after considerable time has elapsed since symptom onset. With formation of new bone, the diagnosis becomes obvious. In these delayed cases, commonly the precipitating injury is not considered significant by either the patient or the physician. This avulsed area may lead to nonunion, although not necessarily a symptomatic one (Fig. 20-28). Kujala and Orava presented an excellent review of the chondro-osseous maturation and injury patterns (51).

The mechanism of injury appears to be the action of the hip flexors on the pelvis, transmitted across the femoral head as a

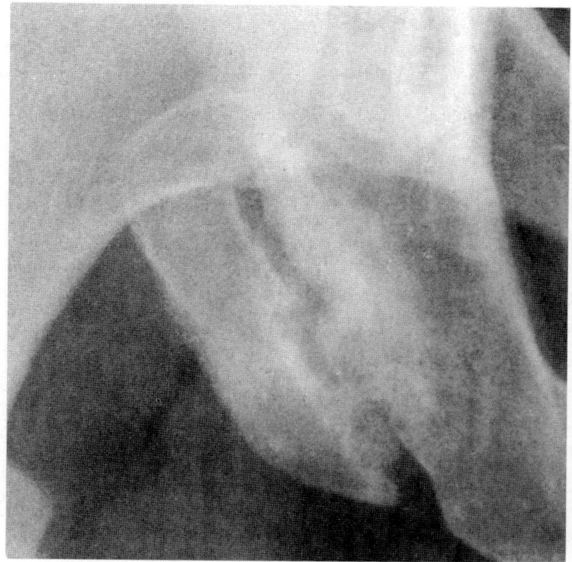
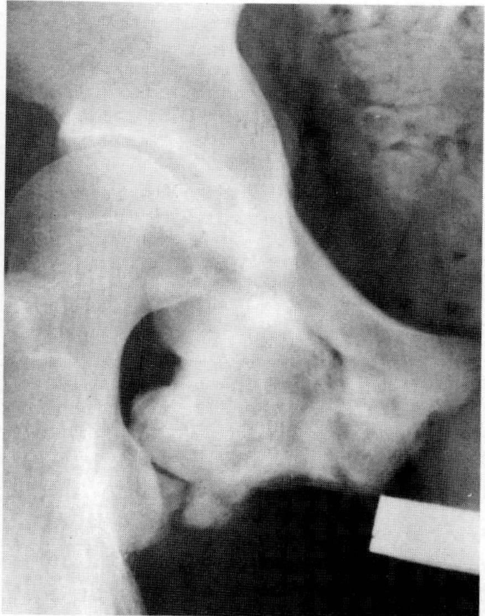

FIGURE 20-28. Ischial tuberosity avulsions that were not diagnosed acutely, but subsequently were evaluated because of pain during sports. **A:** Fourteen-year-old gymnast. **B:** Seventeen-year-old victim of motor vehicle-pedestrian accident 5 years earlier.

fulcrum, which tends to elevate the ischium. This elevation is counteracted by the hamstring muscle, which pulls downward and laterally, a force neutralized by the sacrosciatic ligaments. The degree of displacement of the ischial apophysis depends on the specific role of these ligaments. The most likely conditions for the injury are attained when a powerful muscle contraction takes place in the hamstrings with the pelvis fixed in flexion and the knee in extension. These conditions commonly occur with hurdling, gymnastics, and waterskiing, although many other sports are associated with the injury.

From an anatomic standpoint, an avulsion is likely to be partial (incomplete). The ischial tuberosity is roughly divisible into two portions, one for insertion of the hamstrings and the other for insertion of the adductor magnus. Thus the pattern of injury in a high hurdler could be different from that in a dancer doing a split.

Treatment may vary. Most patients with ischial apophysiolysis do well with rest and a protective program. Ideally, osseous union is demonstrable by roentgenography before strenuous exercises are again permitted. Failure to follow a protective program could result in avulsion fracture of the apophysis from a subsequent undisplaced injury. The possibility of contralateral involvement should always be kept in mind.

Avulsion fractures with significant separation ($\geq$1 cm) probably should be reduced anatomically by open reduction (Fig. 20-29). An attempt at closed reduction probably is

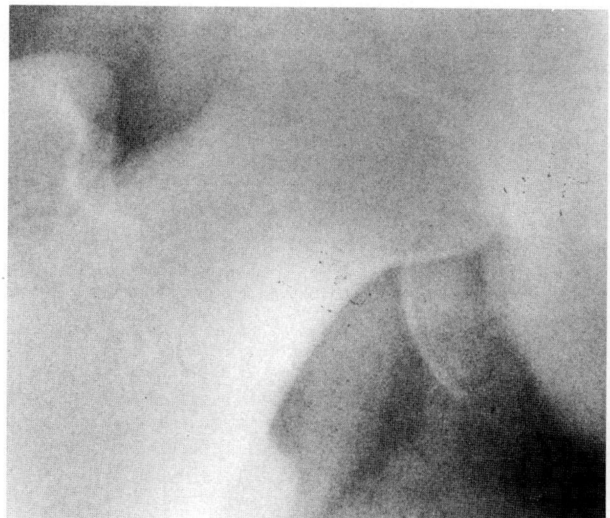
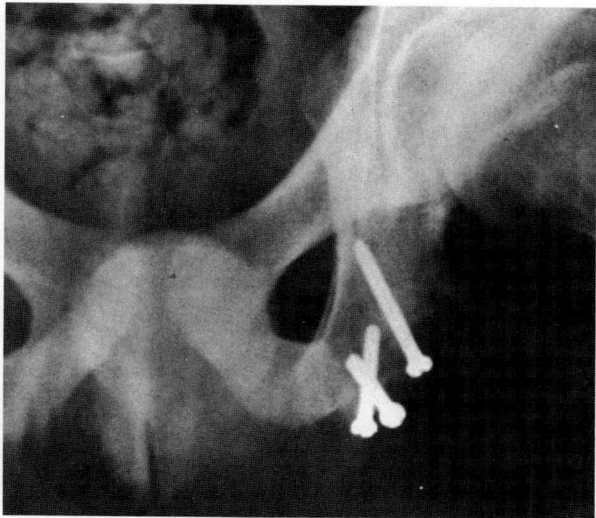

FIGURE 20-29. A: Acute avulsion of the ischial tuberosity in a 12-year-old gymnast. **B:** Appearance 3 years after open reduction and internal fixation in a similar case.

worthwhile and may be possible with direct pressure over the tuberosity. Open reduction of an avulsion fracture is a relatively straightforward procedure. Attachment may be made with cancellous screws (1,54).

The untreated avulsion fracture may unite spontaneously or may form a fibrous union with subsequent enlargement of the tuberosity. The symptoms include inability to sit comfortably on the enlarged, nonunited tuberosity and pain, with associated discomfort in the back or limb, especially while involved in excessive activity. The subsequent enlargement of the tuberosity may be irregular enough to suggest a tumor, and a diagnosis of osteogenic sarcoma or Ewing's sarcoma has been rendered in some cases. Sciatic-type pain is not a general feature of the older, chronic lesions; and if this symptom is encountered, one should rule out a coexistent herniated intervertebral disc before attributing neurologic symptomatology to this lesion.

Chronic injuries, when symptomatic, may be treated by excision of the ununited fragment and repair of the tendinous origin of the hamstrings or by fixation and bone graft.

Other Avulsion Injuries

The increased emphasis on competitive sports not only puts skeletally immature individuals at risk for the previously described avulsion injuries, it also may lead to unusual avulsions and stress fractures. As discussed in the section on anatomy, the pubic symphysis and ischiopubic synchondrosis are areas of progressive chondro-osseous growth and maturation. Repetitive use may cause strain and lead to chronic fatigue manifesting as pain (i.e., an incomplete or microscopic fracture of the evolving chondro-osseous interface) diagnosed as muscular avulsions (57). Stress fractures should be treated symptomatically, with the emphasis on decreasing or stopping the evocative activity.

Ischiopubic Osteochondrosis

The ischiopubic osteochondrosis region may be the site of stress fractures in young joggers and runners. Such fractures are nondisplaced. These injuries are more frequent in females, which may owe to differences in pelvic anatomy and running styles. The increased participation of young individuals in these sports leads to similar symptoms (groin/thigh pain) but with radiolucency/radiodensity or enlargement of the synchondrosis.

Treatment is symptomatic. Temporary cessation of the physical activity for 2 to 3 weeks usually alleviates the pain. Preactivity stretching may lessen muscle pull at the pelvic attachment.

Pubic Symphysis

In the adolescent the onset of midline pain at the symphysis may be due to a fatigue (tension) failure of the chondro-osseous origin of the gracilis muscle (58). Changes (radiographic) usually involve only one side of the symphysis. It is referred to by several names: osteitis pubis, pubic symphysitis, osteochondritis of the symphysis pubis, adductor injury, and gracilis syndrome.

Pain may be in the groin, perineum, or medial thigh and is usually gradually insidious in its onset. On examination there may be discrete tenderness at the symphysis. Radiographic proof is contingent on a cartilaginous avulsion (radiolucent) or a piece of subchondral bone along with a cartilage fragment. Fragment displacement is not significant. Reactive bone may form in the gap (similar to other apophyseal pelvic avulsions), sometimes leading to a small "exostosis." Chronic motion may also cause erosive irregularities in the bone margin, akin to gymnast's wrist. In Wiley's case the bone fragment was excised; histology was compatible with chronic avulsion failure (58).

REFERENCES

1. Ogden JA. *Skeletal injury in the child,* 3rd ed. New York: Springer-Verlag, 2000.
2. Reed MH. Pelvic fractures in children. *J Can Assoc Radiol* 1976;27:255–261.
3. Junkins EP, Nelson DS, Carroll KL, et al. A prospective evaluation of the clinical presentation of pediatric pelvic fractures. *J Trauma* 2001;51:64–68.
4. Silber JS, Flynn JM, Koffler KM, et al. Analysis of the cause, classification, and associated injuries of 166 consecutive pediatric pelvic fractures. *J Pediatr Orthop* 2001;21:446–450.
5. Torode I, Zieg D. Pelvic fractures in children. *J Pediatr Orthop* 1985;5:76–84.
6. Vazquez WD, Garcia VF. Pediatric pelvic fractures combined with an additional skeletal injury is an indicator of significant injury. *Surg Gynecol Obstet* 1993;177:468–472.
7. Quinby WC. Fractures of the pelvis and other associated injuries in children. *J Pediatr Surg* 1966;1:353–361.
8. Ismail N, Bellamare JF, Mollitt DL, et al. Deaths from pelvic fractures: children are different. *J Pediatr Surg* 1996;31:82–85.
9. Garvin KL, McCarthy RE, Barnes CL, et al. Pediatric pelvic fractures. *J Pediatr Orthop* 1990;10:577–582.
10. Silber JS, Flynn JM, Katz MA, et al. Role of computed tomography in the classification and management of pediatric pelvic fractures. *J Pediatr Orthop* 2001;21:148–151.
11. Magid D, Fisherman EK, Ney NR, et al. Acetabular and pelvic fractures in the pediatric patient: value of two- and three-dimensional imaging. *J Pediatr Orthop* 1992;12:621–625.
12. Potter HG, Montgomery KD, Pagdett DE, et al. Magnetic resonance imaging of the pelvis. *Clin Orthop* 1995;319:223–231.
13. Silber JS, Flynn JM. Changing patterns of pediatric pelvic fractures with skeletal maturation: implications for classification and management. *J Pediatr Orthop* 2002;22:22–26.
14. Biffl WL, Smith WR, Moore EE, et al. Evolution of a multidisciplinary clinical pathway for the management of unstable patients with pelvis fractures. *Am Surg* 2001;6:843–850.
15. Tile M. Pelvic fractures: operative versus nonoperative treatment. *Orthop Clin North Am* 1980;11:423–464.
16. Reichard SA, Helikson MA, Shorter N, et al. Pelvic fractures in children: review of 120 patients with a new look at general management. *J Pediatr Surg* 1980;15:727–734.

17. Lacheretz M, Herbaux B. Faut-il opérer les fractures instable du bassin chez l'enfant. *Chirurgie* 1988;114:510–515.
18. Barlow B, Rottenberg RW, Santulli TV. Angiographic diagnosis and treatment of bleeding by selective embolization following pelvic fracture in children. *J Pediatr Surg* 1975;10:939.
19. Canarelli JP, Collet LM, Ricard J, et al. Complications vasculaires des traumatismes pelviens chez l'enfant. *Chir Pediatr* 1988;28: 233–241.
20. McIntyre RC, Bensard DD, Moore EE, et al. Pelvic fracture geometry predicts risk of life-threatening hemorrhage in children. *J Trauma* 1993;35:423–429.
21. Bond SJ, Gotschall GS, Eichelberer MR. Predictors of abdominal injury in children with pelvic fracture. *J Trauma* 1991;31: 1169–1173.
22. Buchanan JR. Bowel entrapment by pelvic fracture fragments: a case report and review of the literature. *Clin Orthop* 1980;147: 164–166.
23. Nimityongskul P, Anderson LD, Powell RW. Small bowel incarceration associated with a central fracture dislocation of the hip in a child: case report. *Contemp Orthop* 1989;18:607–609.
24. Brereton RJ, Philip N, Buyukpamukcu N. Rupture of the urinary bladder in children: the importance of the double lesion. *Br J Urol* 1980;52:15–20.
25. Livne PM, Gonzalez ET Jr. Genitourinary trauma in children. *Urol Clin North Am* 1985;12:53–65.
26. Mark SD, Kesne TE, Vandemark RM, et al. Impotence following pelvic fracture urethral injury: incidence, aetiology and management. *Br J Urol* 1995;75:62–64.
27. Merchant WC III, Gibbons MD, Gonzales ET Jr. Trauma to the bladder neck, trigone and vagina in children. *J Urol* 1984;131: 747–750.
28. Reda EF, Lobowitz RL. Traumatic ureteropelvic disruption in the child. *Pediatr Radiol* 1986;16:164–167.
29. Heinrich SD, Sharps CH, Cardeaj A, et al. Open pelvic fracture with vaginal laceration and diaphragmatic rupture in a child. *J Orthop Trauma* 1988;2:257–261.
30. Heeg M, Fj H, Visserj D. Acetabular fractures in children and adolescents. *J Bone Joint Surg Br* 1989;71:418–421.
31. Bucholz RW, Ezaki M, Ogden JA. Injury to the acetabular triradiate physeal cartilage. *J Bone Joint Surg Am* 1982;64:600–609.
32. Delgado-Baeza E, Gil E, Serrada A, et al. Acetabular dysplasia associated with a lesion of iliopubic limb of the triradiate cartilage. *Clin Orthop* 1988;234:75–81.
33. Heeg M, Visser JD, Oostvogel HJM. Injuries of the acetabular triradiate cartilage and sacroiliac joint. *J Bone Joint Surg Br* 1988;70:34–37.
34. Pina-Medina A, Pardo-Montaner J. Triradiate cartilage fracture associated with a transepiphyseal separation of the femoral head. *J Orthop Trauma* 1996;10:575–585.
35. Scuderi G, Bronson MJ. Triradiate cartilage injury: report of two cases and review of the literature. *Clin Orthop* 1987;217: 179–189.
36. Trousdale RT, Ganz R. Post traumatic acetabular dysplasia. *Clin Orthop* 1994;305:124–132.
37. Duclover P, Fillipe G. Les avulsions apophysaires du bassin, chez l'enfant. *Chir Pediatr* 1988;29:91–92.
38. Hösli P, Vilaer L. Traumatische Apophysenlösungen in Berich des Beckens und des koxalen Femurendes. *Orthopäde* 1995;24: 429–435.
39. Metzmaker JN, Pappas AM. Avulsion fractures of the pelvis. *Am J Sports Med* 1985;13:349–358.
40. Rossi F, Dragoni S. Acute avulsion fractures of the pelvis in adolescent competitive athletes: prevalence, location and sports distribution of 203 cases collected. *Skeletal Radiol* 2001;30: 127–131.
41. Sundar M, Carty H. Avulsion fractures of the pelvis in children: a report of 32 fractures and their outcome. *Skeletal Radiol* 1994;23:85–90.
42. Olney BW, Schier FJ, Asher MA. Effects of splitting the iliac apophysis on subsequent growth of the ilium; a rabbit study. *J Pediatr Orthop* 1993;13:365–367.
43. Deeham DJ, Beattie TF, Knight D, et al. Avulsion fracture of the straight and reflected heads of rectus femoris. *Arch Emerg Med* 1992;9:310–313.
44. Khoury MB, Kirks DR, Martinez S, et al. Bilateral avulsion fractures of the anterior superior iliac spines in sprinters. *Skeletal Radiol* 1985;13:65–67.
45. Mader TJ. Avulsion of the rectus femoris tendon: an unusual type of pelvic fracture. *Pediatr Emerg Care* 1990;6:198–199.
46. Meyer NJ, Schwab JP, Orton D. Traumatic unilateral avulsion of the anterior superior and inferior iliac spines with anterior dislocation of the hip. *J Orthop Trauma* 2001;15:137–145.
47. Resniche JM, Carrmco CH, Edeiken J, et al. Avulsion fracture of the anterior inferior iliac spine and abundant reactive ossification in the soft tissue. *Skeletal Radiol* 1996;25:580–584.
48. Rosenberg N, Noirnan M, Edelson G. Avulsion fractures of the anterior superior iliac spine in adolescents. *J Orthop Trauma* 1996;10:440–443.
49. Winkler AR, Barnes JC, Ogden JA. Break dance hip: chronic avulsion of the anterior superior iliac spine. *Pediatr Radiol* 1987;7:501–502.
50. Rajasekhar C, Kumar KS, Bhamra MS. Avulsion fractures of the anterior inferior iliac spine: the case for surgical intervention. *Int Orthop* 2001;24:364–365.
51. Kujala UM, Orava S. Ischial apophysis injuries in athletes. *Sports Med* 1993;16:290–294.
52. Miller A, Stedman GH, Beisaw NE, et al. Sciatica caused by an avulsion fracture of the ischial tuberosity. *J Bone Joint Surg Am* 1987;69:143–145.
53. Pruner RA, Johnston CE. Avulsion fracture of the ischial tuberosity. *Orthopedics* 1998;13:335–357.
54. Wooton JR, Cross MJ, Holt KW. Avulsion of the ischial apophysis: the case for open reduction and internal fixation. *J Bone Joint Surg Br* 1990;72:625–627.
55. Veselko M, Smrkolj V. Avulsion of the anterior-superior iliac spine in athletes: case reports. *J Trauma* 1994;36:444–446.
56. Kozlowski K, Campbell JB, Azouz EM. Traumatised ischial apophysis. *Australas Radiol* 1989;33:140–143.
57. Schneider R, Kaye JJ, Gheiman B. Adductor avulsion injuries near the symphysis pubis. *Radiology* 1976;120:567–569.
58. Wiley JJ. Traumatic osteitis pubis: the gracilis syndrome. *Am J Sports Med* 1983;11:360–363.

21

COMPLICATIONS OF PELVIC TRAUMA

DAVID E. ASPRINIO
DAVID L. HELFET
MARVIN TILE

INTRODUCTION

Permanent morbidity and chronic pain are common following pelvic fractures. The early complications have been outlined and discussed elsewhere in this text. This chapter discusses the late sequelae of major pelvic ring disruption. The earlier editions of this book demonstrated that the majority of unsatisfactory results were directly related to the musculoskeletal system and neurologic injury (1). The late morbidity of pelvic fractures is now recognized by the general orthopedic community (2). As the quality of prehospital and in-hospital care improves, an increasing number of patients are surviving injuries to which they previously succumbed. Early fracture fixation allowing for mobilization, upright chest positioning, and improved pulmonary function account directly for a portion of this improvement. These same interventions which have resulted in improved survival also have decreased long-term morbidity (3,4). The early teachings of Tile and others, which demonstrated that early reduction and internal or external fixation improves late results by decreasing the incidence of pain, malunion, nonunion, leg length discrepancy, and gait abnormality have been validated by others. As enthusiasm for surgical stabilization of the pelvis has grown and an increasing number of patients have been treated operatively, the number of iatrogenic complications related to this complex surgery have increased. In some cases the morbidity of treatment remains greater than the morbidity of injury itself.

The successful treatment of the late sequelae of pelvic ring injuries requires a comprehensive history, thorough physical examination, and use of appropriate diagnostic modalities to correctly determine the exact etiology of presenting symptoms. Posterior pelvic pain is the common symptom of many posttraumatic sequelae. Patient with complaints of pain frequently have malunion of the pelvic ring. Pelvic malunion may be manifested as painful or painless pelvic obliquity, leg length discrepancy, or gait abnormality. Alternatively, pain may be the manifestation of nonunion leading to instability of the posterior sacroiliac complex. Late complaints of pain also may be neurologic in origin. In many cases, determining the specific cause of pain may be more difficult than actually treating the responsible lesion. Gastrointestinal and genitourinary tract injuries are causes of late morbidity in a smaller percentage of patients. The majority of new literature pertinent to this chapter and that has been published in the last 5 years pertains to urologic injury and its sequelae, treatment, and prevention. When present or suspected these problems generally require involvement of an appropriate subspecialist for both evaluation and treatment.

Unfortunately, many patients continue to heal with deformity or develop nonunion following a pelvic fracture. In some patients, preexisting medical conditions preclude optimal initial stabilization. In others, early treatment is not rendered owing to the presence of associated injuries, failure to appreciate the severity of injury, or lack of technical expertise. Patient noncompliance with treatment and follow-up also contributes to the incidence of nonunion or malunion despite appropriate initial treatment and follow-up. The number of surgeons with extensive experience treating late pelvic deformity remains limited. This experience is discussed at length, but it remains difficult and challenging for even the most experienced practitioners.

The earlier editions of this book clearly detailed the importance of neurologic injury as a cause of late morbidity. Postinjury neurologic deficits remain common causes of late pelvic fracture morbidity. There remains a tendency to underdiagnose or underreport these injuries, particularly those affecting the sacral nerve roots (5). Little progress has been made in the actual treatment of neurologic injuries that occur at the time of trauma; however, numerous authors have reported on the benefits of intraoperative neurologic monitoring and its potential to decrease the incidence of iatrogenic injury.

Late genitourinary tract complications remain common in male patients and have received increased attention in recent years. These complications, usually secondary to urethral injury, include stricture and impotence. Recent reports have confirmed the association between symphyseal injuries and/or inferior pubic ramus fractures and urethral injury. Some advances have been made in the prevention and treatment of late complications of genitourinary injury. Copeland and coworkers demonstrated that the incidence of female patients with genitourinary symptoms was greater than was previously suspected and that this incidence was related to the degree of initial and residual displacement of the pelvic ring (see Chapter 18). The incidence of genitourinary injury associated with childhood pelvic ring fractures also has been shown to be greater than that previously suspected. Early involvement and continued follow-up with a urologist are mandatory for optimal treatment of proven or suspected urologic injury. The reader is referred to the standard urologic literature and the references provided for further details on the late management of genitourinary injuries (6–12).

Late gastrointestinal complications are uncommon but they can also follow pelvic disruption. These complications have also received increased attention in recent years. Ryan described various hernias related to the type of pelvic fracture (13). Such hernias occur anteriorly through the disrupted rectus abdominus tendon or the posterior wall of the inguinal canal in association with lateral or vertical fractures. Chronic bowel obstruction—caused by entrapment of the bowel either by bone fragments or within the fracture itself—has been reported.

As in the most recent edition of this book, a primary focus of this chapter is those late sequelae of pelvic ring fractures that are either preventable or iatrogenic. The authors discuss the significance of and strategies for avoiding malreduction, malpositioned hardware, inadequate stabilization, and neurologic injury. The chapter also considers the incidence, prevention, and treatment of deep venous thromboembolism. Deep vein thrombosis (DVT) can result not only in pulmonary embolism, with its acute morbidity, but also in permanent postphlebitic syndrome and disability. The role for and risks of permanent or removable inferior vena caval filters also are considered.

MALUNION OR MALREDUCTION OF THE SACROILIAC JOINT

(See also Chapter 22.) Malunion resulting in leg length discrepancy of less than 1 cm, but with little additional functional or clinical significance, remains common following major disruption of the pelvis. A small number of patients are left with more significant malunion, resulting in leg length discrepancies of >1 cm. Malunion also may result in rotational deformities of the pelvis or fixed pelvic obliquity. Deformity of this degree can result in pain, gait abnormality, difficulty sitting, dyspareunia, difficult childbirth, and cosmetic complaints. The prevalence of severe deformity varies but has been estimated to be 5% of all major disruptions (14).

The primary effort should be directed at preventing such deformities by instituting the methods and principles outlined in previous chapters. A limited number of malunions are inevitable, and, on occasion, the orthopedic surgeon may be called on to manage such a case.

Significant advances were made in our ability to image the pelvis between the first and second editions of this book. These advances included improvement in the quality of two- and three-dimensional computed tomography (2DCT, 3DCT) and the development of magnetic resonance imaging (MRI). Advances have continued particularly with the development of computer software, which now allows for imaging and manipulation of images in multiple planes as well as the creation of 3D models. These ongoing developments have made it easier to diagnose and characterize the deformity and to develop a treatment plan.

Incidence

As indicated, most authors have stressed the frequent occurrence of late posterior pain in patients with malunion or sacroiliac joint malreduction. Holdsworth found that more than 50% of patients with a sacroiliac dislocation had continued pain and were unable to perform heavy work (15). Slatis and Huittinen found that, of 65 patients with unstable double vertical fractures, 32% had significant gait abnormalities and 17% severe pain (16). Tile and coworkers reported posterior pain to be a universal feature of all unsatisfactory results (14). The incidence of pain was clearly related to the type of fracture. Unstable shear fractures resulted in the greatest prevalence of posterior pain. Rubash and coworkers reported on seven cases of pelvic malunion and noted the frequency of posterior pain and pelvic obliquity (17). Henderson reviewed the results of nonoperative treatment of 26 patients with combined anterior and posterior pelvic injures. His review confirmed the direct relationship between the degree of displacement and long-term complications (18). Wright reported the results of surgery for 200 symptomatic malunions or nonunions (19). Almost all cases involved the pelvic ring posteriorly. Sacral nonunion or malunion was found to be most difficult to treat. Disuse osteoporosis and perineural scarring of the lumbosacral plexus were particularly problematic. Despite restoration of radiographically stable pelvic ring, pain persisted in 45% of the patients. McLaren retrospectively evaluated 43 patients at 5 to 9 years after injury (20). These patients were treated initially by a variety of methods and were divided into two groups based on degree of deformity. Of 26 patients with >1 cm of displacement in any plane, 70% complained of pain and 70% of functional disability. Only 12% of patients with <1 cm of deformity complained of pain, and only 18% of these patients had functional disabilities. Semba and coworkers also reported a significant correlation between pain and residual displacement of >1 cm (21).

It is extremely important to recognize that, despite malunion, many patients have no pain. This implies that the posterior pelvic weight-bearing complex has become stable. Malunion does not always result in pain, but pain is a frequent finding following malunion.

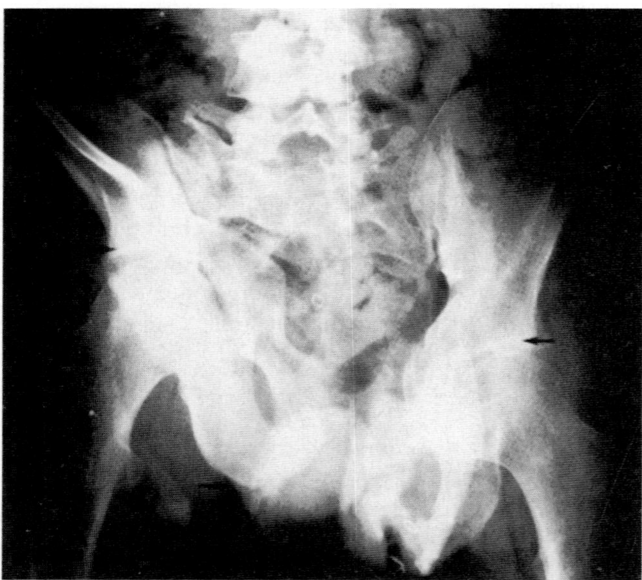

FIGURE 21-1. Anteroposterior radiograph of a pelvis demonstrates extreme malunion. This patient found it almost impossible to sit comfortably because of the marked elevation of the right ischial tuberosity *(black arrow).* The extreme upward rotation of the right hemipelvis resulted in the right hip joint being higher than the left *(black arrows),* and in leg length discrepancy.

Fracture Types

The frequency of malunion is clearly related to the fracture type. Malunions are most common following Type C (rotationally and vertically unstable) pelvic injuries. Most of the soft-tissue support of the hemipelvis, including the pelvic floor, is disrupted, allowing posterior and superior migration. Malunion is the inevitable result if displacement is not corrected by means of traction or by using one of the various forms of external or internal fixation or a combination of them (Fig. 21-1).

Type B lateral compression injuries, although vertically stable, also may result in malunion. The more severe lateral compression injury, despite an intact posterior tension band, may result in significant internal rotation deformity. The anterior bucket handle injury may result in impingement on the perineum and lead to symptoms, especially in women (Figs. 21-2 and 21-3). Given the oblique orientation of the pelvic ring, a severe internal rotation injury (i.e., bucket handle type injury) may result in significant leg length discrepancy.

Clinical Features of Malunion

Pain

Although pain is common, it is not inevitable in the presence of malunion. It is more common with some forms of malunion than others. In most cases posterior pain predominates and is generally *located* in the region of the sacroiliac joint. Pain owing to instability at the sacroiliac joint is more common following sacroiliac dislocation with nonanatomic reduction than with fractures through the sacrum and ilium.

Just as malunion does not automatically result in pain, not all pain can be attributed to malunion when both are present in the same patient. Other potential causes for pain must be excluded when both are present. Henderson discussed the difficulty that can be encountered in differentiating posterior pelvic pain from generalized low back pain in patients with a history of pelvic trauma (18). Isler suggested an injury to the L5-S1 facet to be the cause of pain in some posttraumatic states (22). Sacroiliac dislocation may lead to instability in the posterior weight-bearing arch with resulting chronic local pain. In addition to local pain, patients often have referred pain posteriorly as far as the ankle. The pain is usually worse with weight bearing and improves with rest.

Patients with significant pelvic obliquity secondary to malunion may complain of low back pain. This mechanical low back pain is worse with activity and improves with rest. Pain also may occur when the patient is sitting, especially if the malunion occurs in the area of the ischium or results in significant pelvic obliquity (Fig. 21-1).

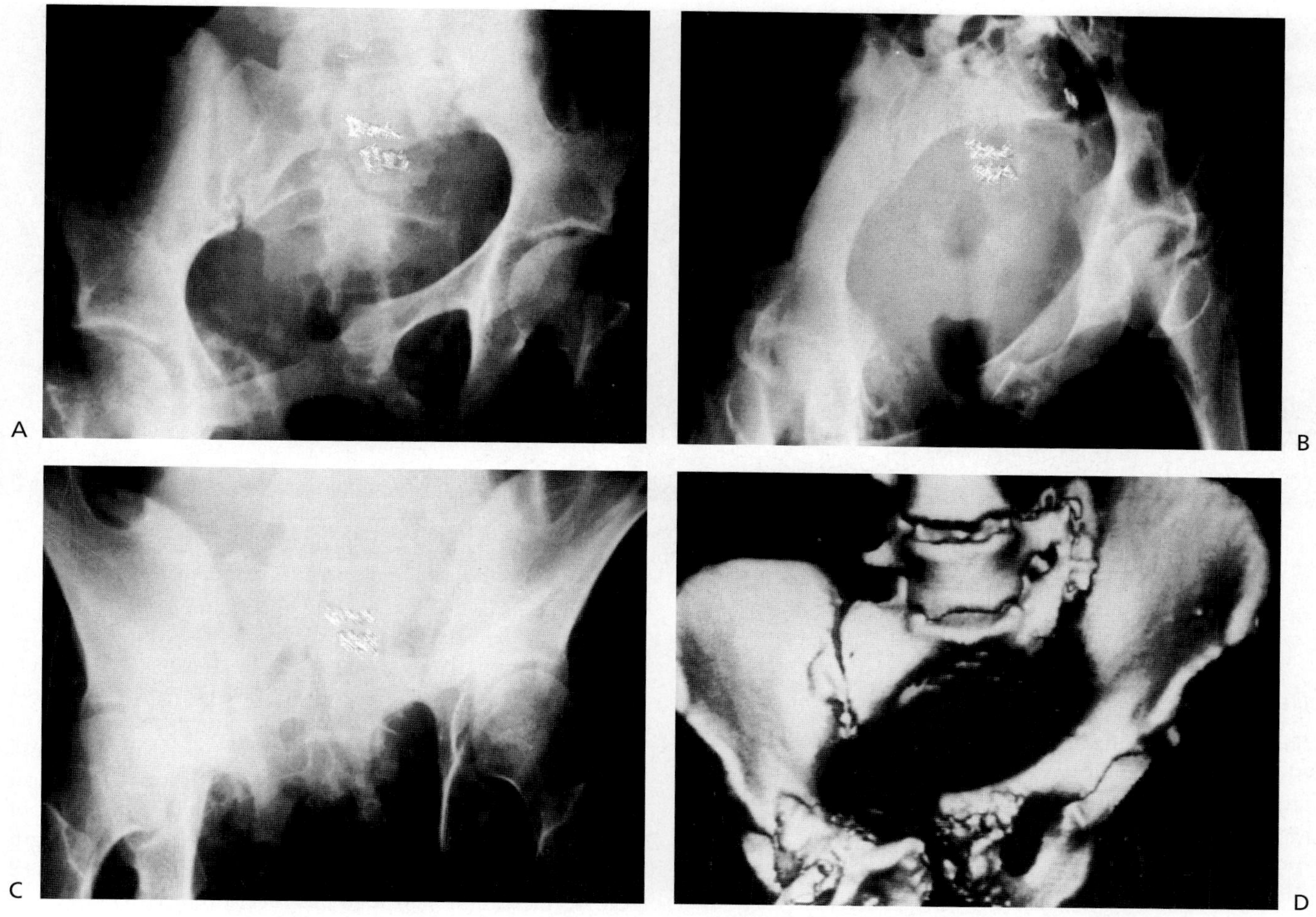

FIGURE 21-2. Anteroposterior pelvis **(A)**, inlet pelvis **(B)**, outlet pelvis **(C)**, and three-dimensional computed tomographic reconstruction **(D)** of a marked internal rotation deformity that impinged the urinary bladder.

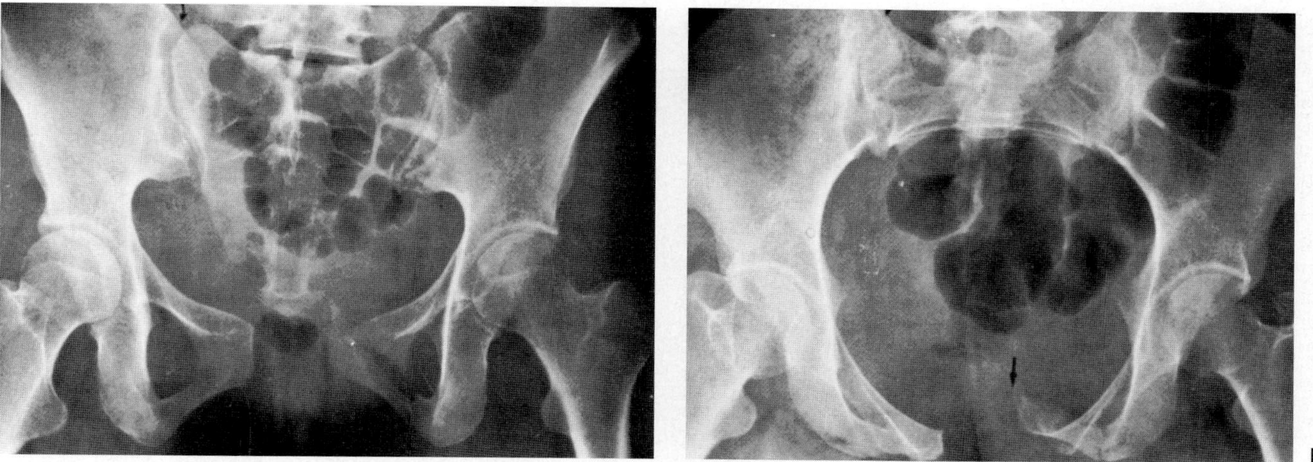

FIGURE 21-3. The anteroposterior **(A)** and inlet **(B)** radiographs demonstrate an unstable shear injury of the right hemipelvis in a 19-year-old woman. The pubic rami on the left side are rotated into the perineum *(black arrow)*. The unstable nature of the injury is shown by the sacroiliac subluxation *(curved arrow)*. (*Figure continues*)

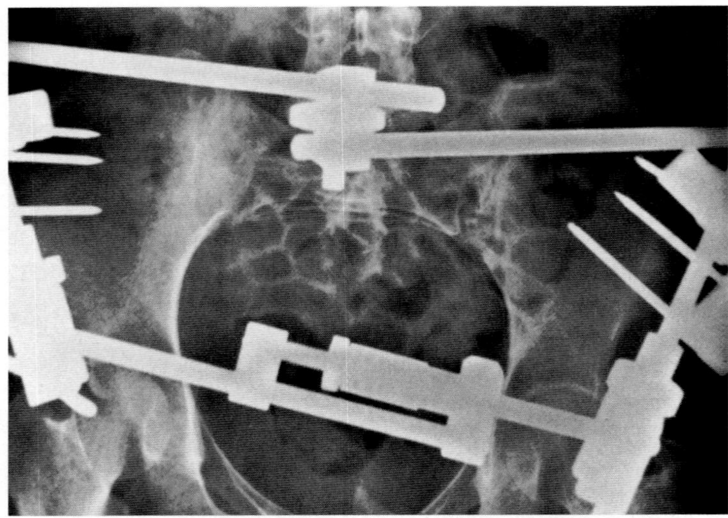

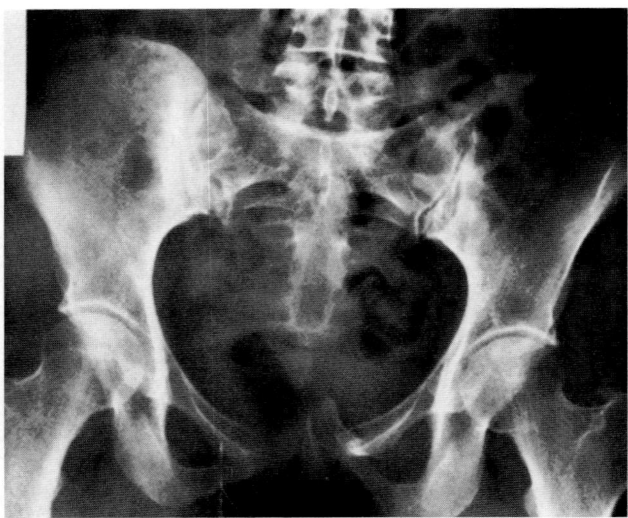

C D

FIGURE 21-3. ***(continued)*** The patient was treated with an external skeletal fixator **(C)**, no attempt was made to reduce the anterior fragment. **D:** The final result shows some sclerosis of the right sacroiliac joint and a bony mass protruding into the perineum. The patient continues to complain of right sacroiliac pain and anterior pain, including dyspareunia.

Deformity

Some patients complain of the bony deformity itself. On occasion, the rotated posterior superior spine appears as a large mass and is disturbing to the patient. Owing to its subcutaneous location, malunion of the sacrum, especially flexion deformities, may cause symptomatic deformities (Figs. 21-4 and 21-5).

Gait Abnormalities (Leg Length Discrepancy)

Malunion may occur in any plane. Isolated shortening in the coronal plane, as might be seen in a pure vertical shear injury, results in leg length discrepancy. Malunion following an injury associated with a rotational mechanism (i.e., lateral compression, anterior-posterior compression, or combined) may alter the position of the patient's foot, and therefore, the gait. In most cases rotation occurs on an oblique axis and also results in relative change in height of the acetabulum, causing an apparent secondary leg length discrepancy. In Tile's series, a leg length discrepancy of >2 cm occurred in nine of 248 patients (Table 21-1) (14).

Urinary Tract Symptoms

With severe internal rotation of the hemipelvis, the superior pubic ramus may impinge on the bladder. This may lead to

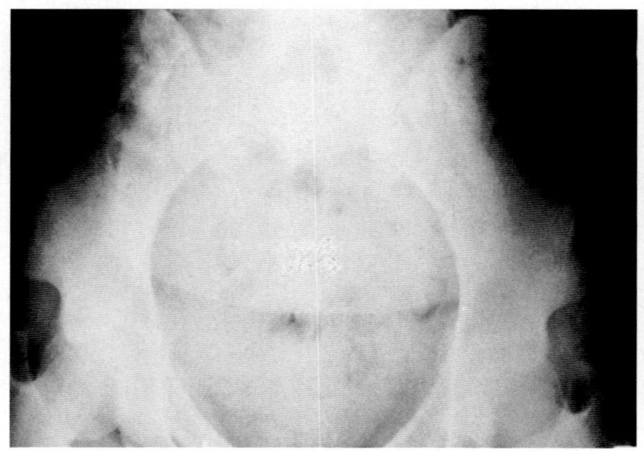

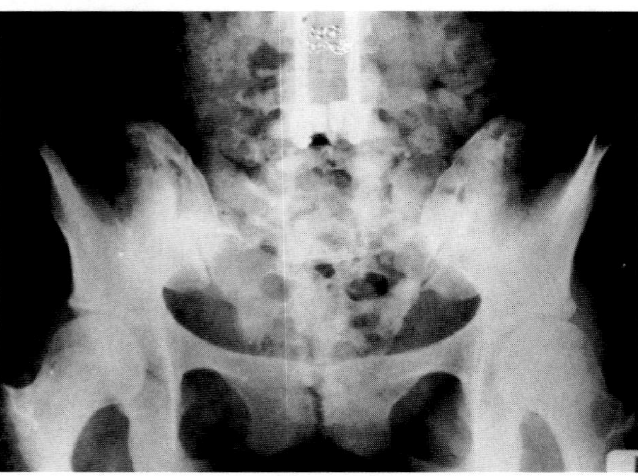

A B

FIGURE 21-4. (A–D) A 21-year-old who jumped three stories in a suicide attempt sustained multiple lumbar burst fractures and an H-type sacral fracture. Harrington distraction instrumentation resulted in flat back deformity, which exacerbated the flexed sacral pelvic deformity.

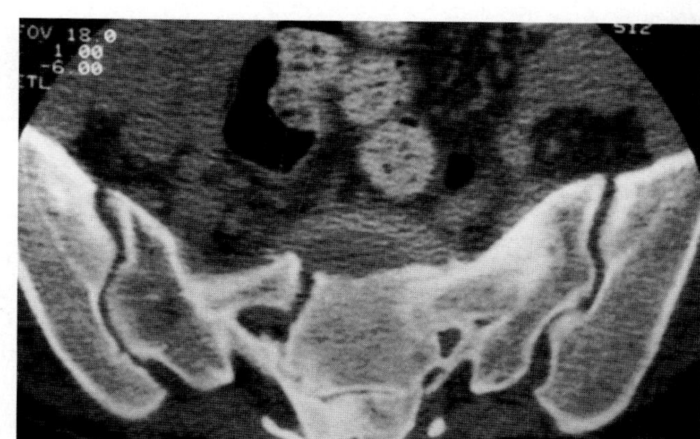

C

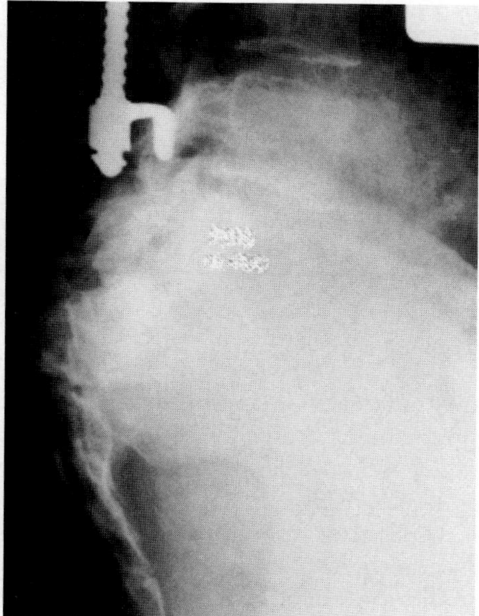

D

FIGURE 21-4. ***(continued)***

frequency of urination (Fig. 21-2). Cohen reported the case of a 43-year-old patient who presented 20 years after pelvic fracture with persistent dysuria. This was found to be secondary to a previously unsuspected penetrating bony spicule. Symptoms resolved following excision of the spicule (12). We recently encountered a similar patient who developed progressive dysuria beginning approximately 20 years following a pelvic ring fracture. Exploration revealed a bony spicule on which a calculus had formed.

Management

Prevention of clinically significant pelvic deformity should be the mainstay of treatment. When challenged by a patient with clinically significant complaints of pain, a gait abnormality, or a leg length discrepancy and an associated pelvic malunion, a careful and detailed assessment is mandatory. This includes a thorough history and physical examination. Extensive radiographic evaluation also is required. Initial

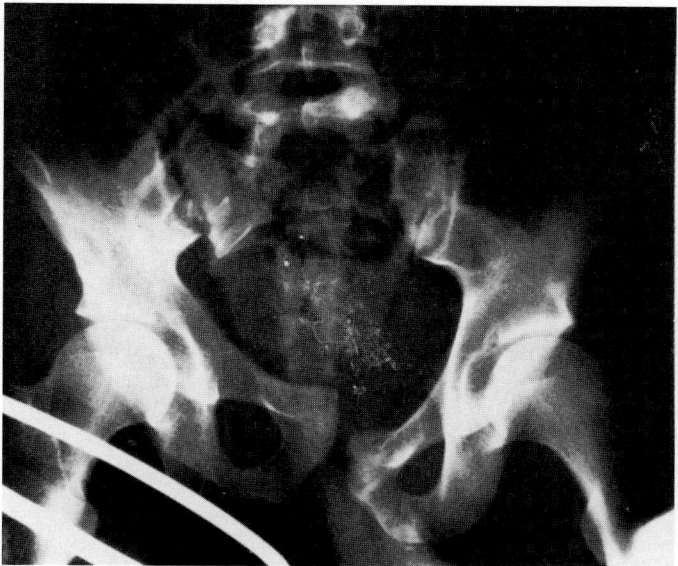

A

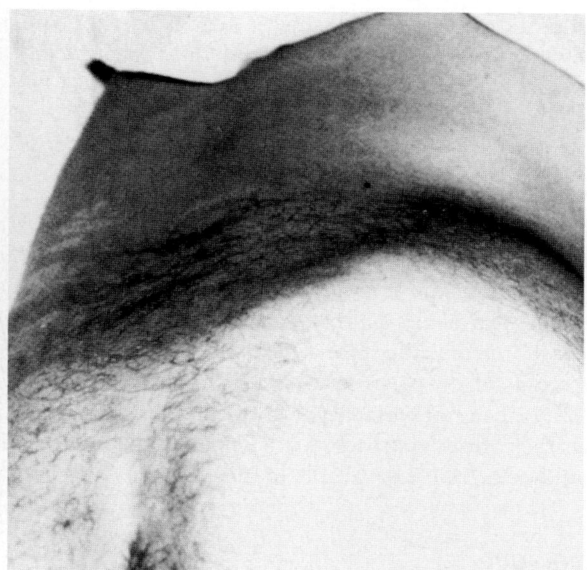

B

FIGURE 21-5. Major posterior displacement of the right hemipelvis **(A).** The malrotated, posteriorly displaced hemipelvis is seen clearly on the clinical photograph **(B).** The posterior superior iliac spine protrudes markedly on the right side.

TABLE 21-1. MAJOR FACTORS RESULTING IN UNSATISFACTORY RESULTS

Total number of patients	248
Sacroiliac pain	69
Nonunion	8
Malunion	22
Leg length discrepancy >0.2 cm	9
Permanent nerve damage	12
Impotence	7

assessment should include anteroposterior pelvis, pelvic inlet, and pelvic outlet radiographs. CT is most helpful in evaluating the posterior pelvic ring, including the sacroiliac joint (Fig. 21-6). 3DCT scan and software can be used to better evaluate the deformity and, in difficult cases, generate a model that can be used in preoperative templating. CT and MRI studies also can be used to assess the proximity and integrity of vital soft-tissue structures. These may be particularly helpful when planning surgery or when attempting to determine the cause of pain.

Many pelvic fracture patients have been emotionally and financially crippled by their injuries. Insurance issues, workers' compensation status, and ongoing litigation complicate patient assessment. It behooves the surgeon to carry out a careful evaluation and avoid embarking too quickly on surgical treatment. Careful consideration of the patient's personality and infirmity is essential. In Tile's experience, in many patients pain diminished over time and they were ultimately able to tolerate their symptoms without surgical intervention (14). This was especially true when the magnitude and potential risks of the surgical procedures were explained to them. The surgeon must realistically and honestly assess his or her experience and the chances of helping the patient and must then weigh the potential benefits against the risks.

Urinary Tract Symptoms

If the patient complains of urinary tract symptoms and x-ray examination reveals an internally rotated pubic symphysis or pubic rami, the surgeon must decide whether the most prudent treatment would be careful dissection of the bladder away from the rami with local ostectomy or an osteotomy of the pelvis to correct the entire deformity (Fig. 21-2). If the urinary tract symptoms are the only complaint, then the former approach is advisable. A urologic surgeon should be present or available in most cases.

Technique

Depending on the site of impingement a long paramedian or a transverse Pfannenstiel incision may be used. The extended Pfannenstiel incision or the inguinal portion of the ilioinguinal approach is necessary for more lateral impingement requiring exposure of the pelvic brim. The extraperitoneal Stoppa approach may be indicated in select cases. With a Foley catheter in place, the bladder can be dissected free from the pelvis. Using an osteotome, a large mass of bone may be removed easily, thereby freeing the bladder. This usually results in resolution of the patient's symptoms without need for further pelvic osteotomy.

Leg Length Discrepancy

If the patient's principal problem is a significant leg length discrepancy, then a variety of treatment options are available. The most appropriate treatment depends on the individual patient, the degree of discrepancy, the presence or absence of other complaints related to the pelvis (i.e., pain or neurologic dysfunction), patient age, comorbidities, and the anatomic lesion(s) resulting in the deformity. Minor discrepancy can be managed with a shoe lift in many cases. This is particularly true in older patients who would be at increased risk from a major surgical procedure. In children, leg length sometimes can be equalized by appropriately planned epiphysiodesis. Several approaches are possible for young adults with significant leg length discrepancy, but all have significant potential for surgical morbidity.

Limb Shortening

In a patient with a significant leg length discrepancy but no complaint of pelvic pain or deformity, the longer lower extremity can be shortened through the femur. Open techniques expose the patient to the risk of sepsis and other complications involving the normal lower extremity and may not be acceptable in all cases. These risks can be minimized by using the techniques of closed intramedullary shortening, as pioneered by Kuntscher (23) and modified by Winquist and coworkers (24). The extremity may be shortened with minimal morbidity using currently available techniques and instrumentation.

Limb Lengthening

Limb lengthening with bone grafting has been possible for many years but has been unreliable and not without complications. Distraction osteogenesis using techniques pioneered by Ilizarov has now become widely available. Distraction osteogenesis, although effective, remains a long and painful process with a high incidence of associated complications and should not be undertaken lightly, especially in adults.

Innominate Osteotomy

An innominate osteotomy is another possibility for a significant leg length discrepancy, especially one associated with

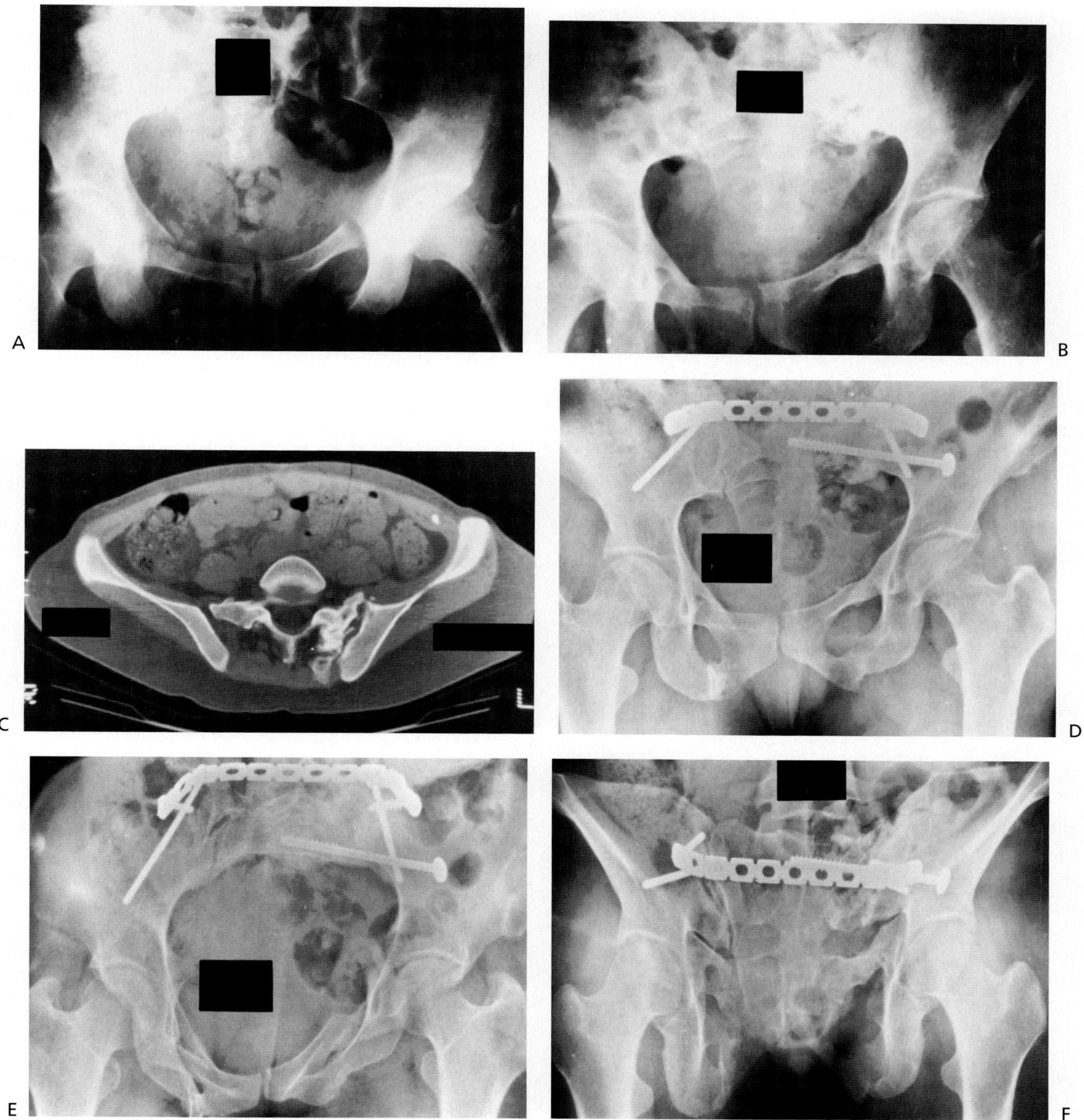

FIGURE 21-6. A,B: A 48-year-old woman continued to feel pain 18 months after a pelvic fracture. **C:** Computed tomography demonstrates sacroiliac malunion and/or nonunion. **D,E,F:** Open reduction and internal fixation and cancellous bone grafting relieved the pain.

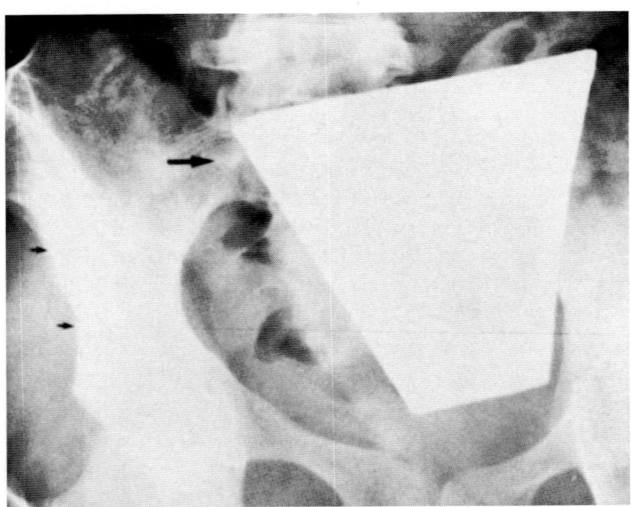

FIGURE 21-7. Anteroposterior radiograph of a 16-year-old girl who sustained a severe, unstable shear injury of the right hemipelvis at age 3 years. The sequelae—pelvic obliquity and leg length discrepancy—were corrected by a modified innominate osteotomy, using a rectangular bone graft rather than a triangular wedge. Leg length discrepancy of 2.5 cm was corrected by this mechanism, as noted on the radiograph. (Courtesy of Robert B. Salter.)

an internal rotation deformity of the pelvis (25). By externally rotating the distal fragment, the innominate osteotomy allows the internally rotated lower extremity to resume its normal position. Simultaneously, by opening the posterior aspect of the pelvic brim, 1.5 to 2.5 cm of leg length may be restored (Fig. 21-7).

Bilateral Innominate Osteotomy

Leg length discrepancy caused by fixed pelvic obliquity may be corrected by performing bilateral innominate osteotomies. An appropriate block of bone is removed from the lengthened hemipelvis and transferred to the shorter side, thus lengthening it. To reduce the load on the hip joint, the psoas tendon must be divided when lengthening the hemipelvis. The pelvic osteotomy may be stabilized with 4.5-mm screws or a well-contoured plate. This is a major procedure that should be reserved for adolescents or young adults.

Direct Osteotomy of Malunion Site

For patients with leg length discrepancy or pain rather than urinary complaints, a direct approach to the malunion site is possible. This particularly difficult procedure should be undertaken only after a thorough preoperative evaluation and only by very experienced pelvic surgeons. In their report, Rubash's group had an average operating time of 6 hours and an average blood loss of 1,200 mL (17).

Technical details vary with each case. Posterior malunion is generally approached directly. The fracture site should be recreated using power saws and osteotomes. Anterior malunion also requires a direct approach. The fracture site is recreated through malunion of the symphysis or inferior and superior pubic rami. Once the fracture has been recreated anteriorly and posteriorly, the femoral distractor and pelvic reduction clamps may be used to facilitate reduction of the malunion. Once reduced, stable anterior and posterior fixation is necessary. The type of fixation required varies with the lesion created. All of the methods of internal fixation previously discussed are potentially applicable. Standard principles of compression plating and lag screw fixation should be used posteriorly. The use of sacral bars posteriorly has fallen out of favor, owing to their inability to apply interfragmentary compression and the high incidence of fixation loss and migration. Anterior fixation generally involves plating the rami or symphysis. Intramedullary screw fixation also is possible. Occasionally, an external fixator is required. This surgery requires careful preoperative planning, including the surgical sequence. Staged anterior-posterior-anterior or posterior-anterior-posterior procedures may be necessary to osteotomize and mobilize the deformity prior to reduction and stabilization.

Reduction and stabilization of long-standing pelvic malunion may lead to iatrogenic lumbosacral nerve injury. It may be safer to perform staged procedures to minimize this risk. The first stage consists of "anterior and posterior" pelvic osteotomy and the placement of a distal femoral traction pin. After 10 to 14 days of traction with careful monitoring of the neurologic status of the limb, the pelvic wounds are reopened and the pelvis reduced and stabilized using the appropriate form of internal fixation. Intraoperative neurologic monitoring is recommended for one-stage corrections. Early technology involved monitoring of somatosensory evoked potentials (SSEPs). With the use of this technology there is a delay between an event and its being recorded. As the technology has evolved, monitoring of motor evoked potentials (MEPs) has become possible, allowing for instantaneous recording of an event.

The postoperative program depends on the degree of stability achieved. When stable plate and screw fixation is obtained anteriorly and posteriorly, the patient can be rapidly mobilized, bearing no weight on the involved extremity. If adequate stable fixation is not achieved, at least 6 weeks' bed rest is required before mobilization.

Sacroiliac Arthrodesis

Anatomic reduction of a long-standing malreduced sacroiliac joint cannot be obtained in many cases. Arthrodesis is generally the treatment of choice. Techniques for fusion are described in the following.

NONUNION

(See Chapter 22.) Nonunion following a pelvic ring disruption was once considered rare (26). In 1973, Pennal made the initial presentation of his series of pelvic nonunion to the annual convention of the Canadian Orthopaedic Association (27). This series of 42 patients with delayed union or nonunion of the pelvis, was subsequently published by Pennal and Massiah in 1980 (28). The patients included 39 men and three women whose average age was 25 years. The mechanism of injury was vertical shear in 17, lateral compression in 15, anteroposterior compression in seven, and miscellaneous causes in three.

Of the 42 patients, 24 were treated nonoperatively and 18 operatively. The principles of surgery involved stabilization of the nonunion and bone grafting. Of the 18 surgically treated patients, 15 achieved union and most were relieved of their symptoms.

The 24 patients who did not have surgery were treated with plaster casts and other forms of immobilization, for an average of 8.4 weeks. Of this group only 10 achieved union. Results were significantly worse in the nonoperative group. The authors concluded that posterior nonunion of the pelvic ring was significantly symptomatic and that operative treatment could usually relieve the symptoms. In a review of pelvic ring disruption in Southern Ontario and Toronto, Tile identified eight cases of nonunion (14). All results were classified as unsatisfactory because of continued pain, but only one patient required further surgical treatment.

Rubash and coworkers reviewed eight cases of pelvic nonunion, following either vertical shear or lateral compression fractures (17). Of the eight, six were treated originally by nonoperative means and two with external fixation. All of the patients had posterior pain and instability and all subsequently underwent open surgical procedures, with internal fixation and bone grafting. Union was achieved in all eight cases and resulted in symptomatic relief.

With the routine use of CT to seek the causes of pelvic pain, nonunion is more commonly recognized. Wright and coworkers presented 200 patients with pelvic nonunion or malunion, all of whom underwent surgery (19). For nonunion, the authors recommended bone grafting and stabilization of all "three columns" of the pelvis (anterior, middle, and posterior). The most problematic group of patients were elderly or osteopenic patients with sacral nonunion. For this group, the authors identified adjunctive screw and wire techniques to achieve stability.

Between 1984 and 1995 Matta and coworkers treated 37 patients with nonunion, malunion, and combined nonunion malunion of the pelvic ring. Thirty-two of 37 patients were satisfied with their eventual outcome (see Chapter 23).

The mainstay of treatment should be prevention. Pelvic nonunion continues to occur even when patients are treated by experienced and skilled surgeons; however, the incidence appears to be small. Cole and coworkers reported only one nonunion in 60 operatively treated pelvic fractures. Van den Bosch and coworkers reported one nonunion in 37 operatively treated patients.

Predisposing Factors

Type of Injury

The unstable vertical shear–type fracture with massive injury to the soft tissues, especially the sacrotuberous and sacrospinous ligaments, is the fracture type that most commonly predisposes to nonunion (Fig. 21-8). The fracture through the posterior weight-bearing portion of the pelvis renders its unstable. Soft tissues interposed in the sacroiliac joint or between the adjacent sacrum or ilium may prevent union. This has been clearly described in published pathology reports (29) and is commonly seen at surgery in the acute clinical case.

Lateral compression injury is the second most prevalent fracture type leading to nonunion. Nonunion that follows lateral compression injury is usually anterior, at the pubic rami, and is often relatively asymptomatic. The anteroposterior compression (open-book) fracture does not usually disturb the posterior tension band of the pelvis. The main weight-bearing forces continue to be transmitted through the sacroiliac joints into the femora. A wide disruption of the symphysis pubis, however, may result in rotational instability of the pelvis. Patients who have sustained such an injury may complain of anterior symphyseal pain. Two such patients were found in Tile's series (14).

Miscellaneous fractures of combined mechanisms may involve the acetabulum and pelvic ring and also may result in nonunion. It was once felt that acetabular fractures with so-called central dislocation always united. Nonunion of acetabular fracture does occur, as demonstrated by the patient shown in Fig. 21-9. Treatment of acetabular nonunion, alone or in combination with pelvic injury, is a particularly difficult problem. Patients commonly have severe symptoms secondary to the nonunion itself and to rapidly progressive posttraumatic osteoarthrosis of the hip. Postoperative results are rarely excellent, and primary or eventual arthrodesis or total hip arthroplasty is not uncommon.

Poor Immobilization

The chance of developing a nonunion also is related to the method of treatment. In the rare circumstance where nonoperative means are chosen to manage an unstable pelvic injury, immobilization must be prolonged. Even with prolonged immobilization, nonunion is possible. The average period of immobilization for patients who develop nonunion was 6 to 8 weeks in previously reported groups. This is clearly an inadequate period of immobilization for these difficult fractures. In young people, shear fractures through cancellous bone may exhibit delayed union in all areas of the body, including the pelvis. Conversion of the unstable cancellous fracture to a stable one, using interfragmentary compression, usually prevents delayed union or nonunion. If nonoperative treatment is attempted, bed rest must continue until union is complete. In Type C vertically and rotationally unstable injuries, this usually requires 12 to 16 weeks of immobilization.

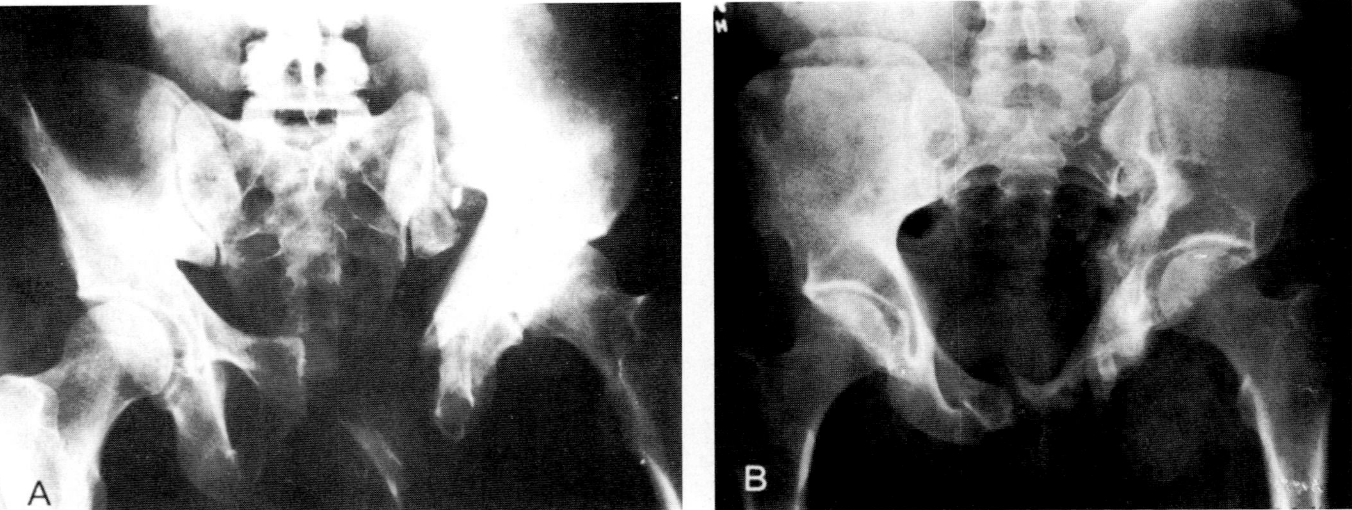

FIGURE 21-8. A: Anteroposterior radiograph demonstrates a completely unstable left hemipelvis following a mine-shaft accident. The superior and inferior pubic rami were surgically debrided through an open perineal wound. A complete lumbosacral nerve plexus injury, as well as many other lower extremity fractures, complicated this case. The pelvic fracture was neglected. **B:** The final anteroposterior radiograph indicates nonunion through the sacroiliac joint and symphysis pubis and persistent left hemipelvis instability and pain.

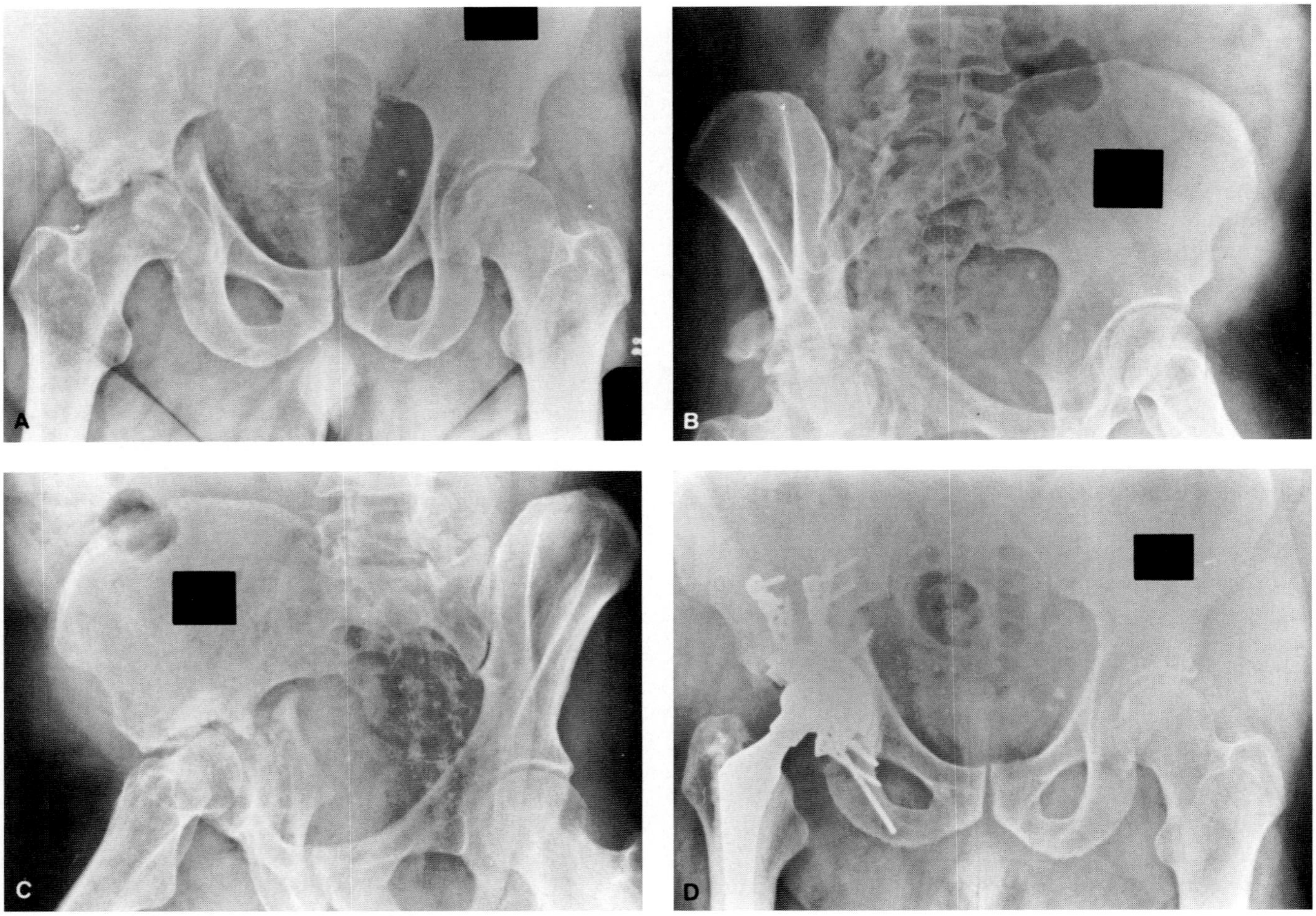

FIGURE 21-9. Two cases of acetabular nonunion. **A–C:** A 50-year-old man was treated for 8 weeks with traction, for an acetabular fracture and an associated fracture of the femoral head. **D:** After 11 months he had a markedly limited, painful range of motion. He responded well to open reduction and internal fixation and total hip replacement.

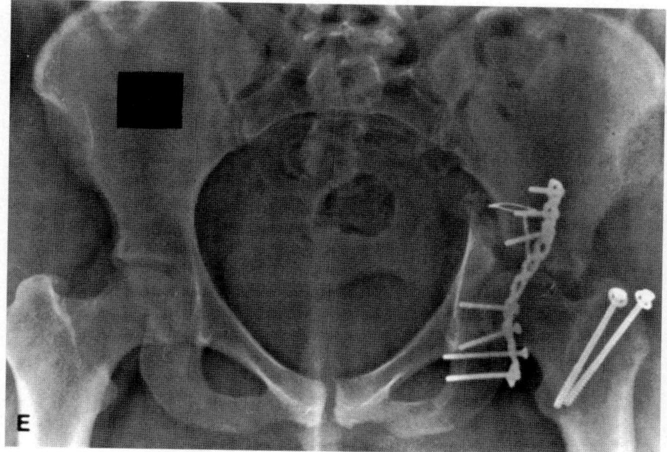

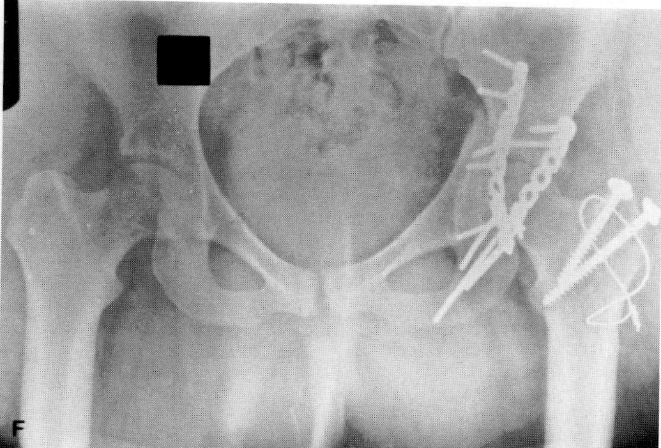

FIGURE 21-9. ***(continued)*** **E,F:** A 26-year-old, 320-lb woman was injured in a motor vehicle accident. She underwent Enders nailing of the left humerus and open reduction and internal fixation of the left acetabulum. She developed nonunion of the left humerus and left acetabulum. The acetabular nonunion followed early loss of fixation 1 week after open reduction and internal fixation and iliac crest cancellous bone grafting. The humerus did well, but the acetabulum requires ongoing treatment with nonsteroidal antiinflammatory drugs, owing to severe arthrosis.

Pathoanatomy

The common occurrence of soft-tissue interposition in cases of posterior pelvic ring disruption has been discussed elsewhere. This soft-tissue interposition at the fracture site prevents compression of the cancellous bone in the posterior aspect of the pelvis and may predispose to nonunion. With sacroiliac dislocation, interposed tissues may prevent anatomic reduction and predispose to continued pain.

Location

The location of the pelvic nonunion has a marked influence on the patient's symptoms. The integrity of the posterior sacroiliac complex is the key. Assuming the poster weight-bearing area is stable, nonunion occurring anteriorly may be completely asymptomatic. Pain is likely if nonunion develops through the sacrum or ilium—and almost certain if the sacroiliac joint is not anatomically reduced or unstable. Nonunion of the ischial tuberosity, although rare, is usually symptomatic (Fig. 21-10).

Clinical Features

Pain is the predominant feature of posterior nonunion, whereas anterior nonunion may be painless. Posterior pain is commonly located in the sacroiliac region and may be severe. It is associated with weight bearing and occurs most commonly after long walks or attempted running. This pain may preclude heavy work or athletic activity. The pain may be referred to the posterior aspect of the extremity and may extend distally as far as the ankle.

Instability

Instability may be a clinical symptom or a sign. Patients do not usually complain of clinical instability in the same sense as they do of knee instability. Objective instability often can be demonstrated by either clinical or radiologic examination. In more obvious cases of nonunion, instability of the hemipelvis may be demonstrated clinically by manipulating the pelvis. The so-called push–pull maneuvers often are helpful. Radiographs then may be used to confirm the diagnosis.

In more subtle cases, the diagnosis of instability cannot be made clinically. Radiographic means are necessary. An anterior-posterior radiograph taken with the patient standing on one foot and then on the other (the so-called "stork position") may reveal a clear shift in the pelvis superiorly and posteriorly, confirming the diagnosis. In other cases dynamic assessment under fluoroscopy is helpful.

Gait Abnormalities

A significant leg length discrepancy results in a noticeable limp. As in patients with malunion, Trendelenburg's sign, with an associated lurch, is common. Pelvic obliquity also may give rise to compensatory scoliosis and chronic low back pain.

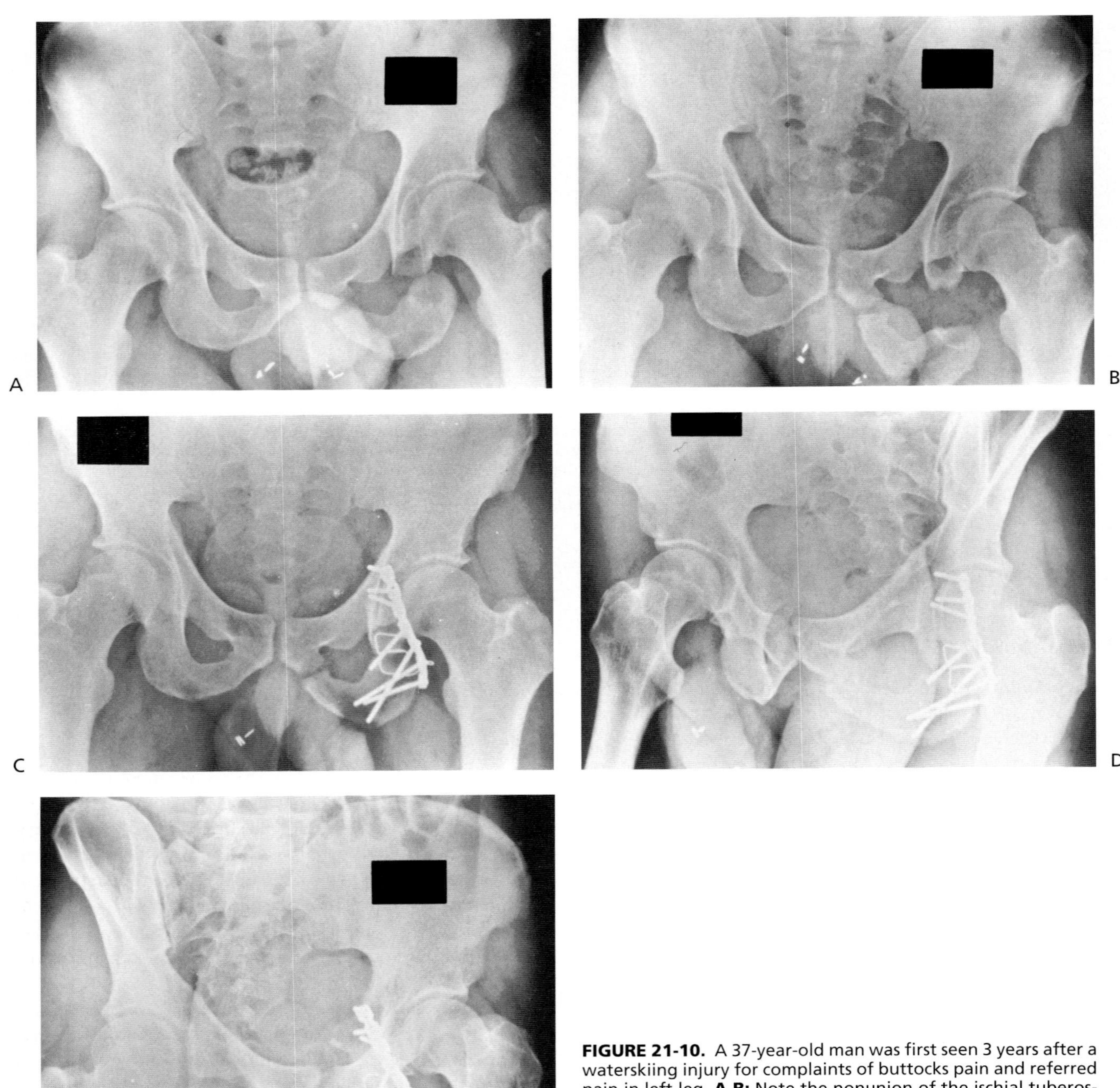

FIGURE 21-10. A 37-year-old man was first seen 3 years after a waterskiing injury for complaints of buttocks pain and referred pain in left leg. **A,B:** Note the nonunion of the ischial tuberosity fragment. **C,D,E:** He was treated with open reduction with internal fixation and iliac crest bone graft. Three months after surgery, he was free of pain.

Clinical Deformity

A significant deformity, occasionally seen in these patients, usually is related to marked pelvic obliquity.

Hernia

Disruption of the symphysis pubis usually is accompanied by avulsion of the rectus abdominis. This allows an anterior hernia to develop. Occasionally, the bladder is caught within the symphysis, leading to instability as well as urinary symptoms.

Clitoral Stimulation

An unusual case report involved a young woman who, following a pelvic injury, complained of constant clitoral stimulation on bearing weight (T. Porter, personal communication, 1983). The clitoris was constantly irritated by the displaced and unstable symphysis. Eventually, surgery was performed to disengage the clitoris and stabilize the symphysis.

Radiographic Appearance

Plain Radiographs

Nonunion can be hypertrophic or atrophic. In Fig. 21-11 both types are demonstrated in a single patient, a young logger who was struck by a tree and sustained an unstable pelvic disruption. In spite of appropriate nonoperative treatment, he developed both anterior and posterior nonunion. The superior public ramus and sacroiliac nonunion were hypertrophic, whereas the inferior pubic ramus nonunion was atrophic. This is clearly seen on the radiograph and was confirmed on the bone scan, which shows increased uptake at the superior ramus and sacroiliac joint and no uptake at the inferior ramus. Bone grafting resulted in union at all three sites and relieved the patient's symptoms.

Plain radiographs, including anteroposterior, pelvic inlet, and pelvic outlet views, are adequate for initial evaluation of either atrophic or hypertrophic nonunion. In many cases, additional studies are necessary to characterize the posterior lesion. Oblique radiographs may be very helpful and often clearly show the posterior nonunion site (Fig. 21-12).

Computed Tomography

The CT scan remains the diagnostic study of choice for evaluating the posterior pelvic ring. Most scanners currently in use allow for rapid scanning with fine cuts and in many cases allow for 3D reconstruction. The presence of a sacroiliac dislocation or nonunion of the sacrum and ilium is easily determined by this method. In most cases CT should be performed before surgery is recommended (Fig. 21-12B).

Technetium Bone Scan

The technetium polyphosphate bone scan may be helpful in determining the vascularity and activity of the nonunion. Hypertrophic or vascular nonunion appears "hot" and atrophic, poorly vascularized nonunion, "cold." This information may guide treatment decisions and help to determine when bone grafting is necessary.

Magnetic Resonance Imaging

CT is clearly the most helpful imaging technique for the diagnosis of nonunion; MRI may be helpful in the soft-tissue component of the injury.

Management

Assessment

Not all patients with delayed union or nonunion require surgery. In some cases, pain diminishes with time (Fig. 21-13). Careful assessment of the patient and injury must be made before recommending a major operative procedure. Important factors to assess include the patient's age, general medical condition, issues raising the possibility of secondary gain, and expectations. In appropriately selected patients, surgical stabilization of the pelvic ring has clearly been shown to improve symptoms.

Principles of Management

The principles of surgical treatment are stable fixation of the pelvic ring and bone grafting of the nonunion when necessary. Because most cases that require treatment involve both the anterior and posterior aspect of the pelvic ring, surgery usually needs to be directed to both the anterior and posterior lesion. The only exception is an open-book type fracture, which results in an unstable symphysis but no vertical disruption of the posterior ring.

Technique

Anterior

Symphysis Pubis. The symphysis is commonly approached through a Pfannenstiel incision (30,31). A Foley catheter should be inserted at the onset of surgery involving any anterior approach. The bladder should be carefully identified and dissected free of the symphysis. A pelvic reduction clamp attached to screws on either side of the symphysis pubis or a large reduction clamp placed in each obturator foramen can be used to reduce the pubic diastasis. Care must be taken to retract and protect the bladder while reduction is being carried out.

To stabilize the symphysis pubis, the same plating techniques previously recommended in the treatment of acute injuries are used. Bone graft placed across the symphysis pubis helps to ensure union.

Pubic Rami. If the patient has a nonunion of the superior ramus, a direct surgical approach should be performed. In the treatment of hypertrophic nonunion, raising osteoperiosteal flaps in the manner of Phemister, followed by application of a bone graft may suffice. An anterior stabilization of the superior pubic ramus nonunion with a compression plate and cancellous bone grafting is the treatment of choice (30,31).

Nonunions of the inferior ramus are often atrophic and usually occur in or near the ischial tuberosity, where they interfere with sitting (Fig. 21-10). The surgical approach

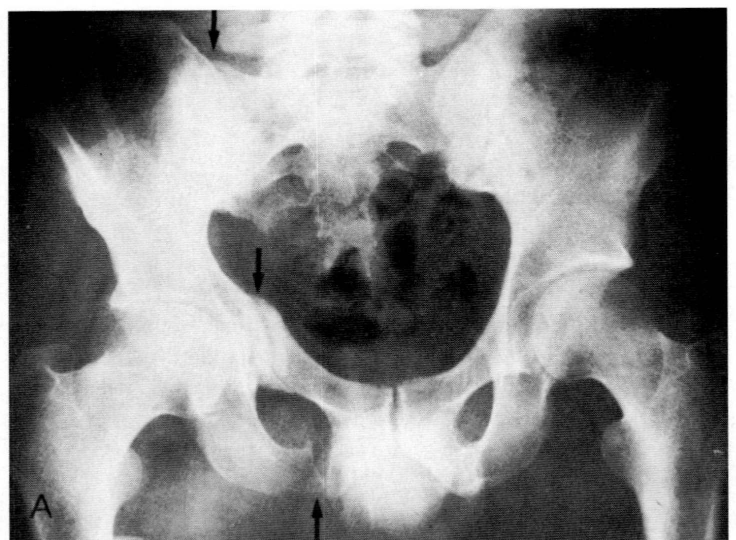

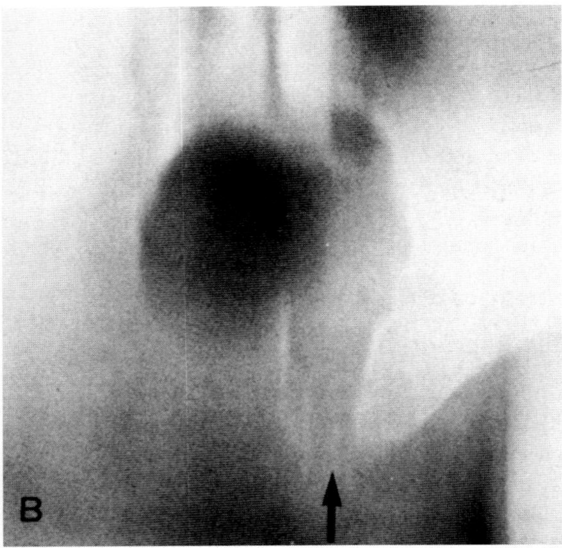

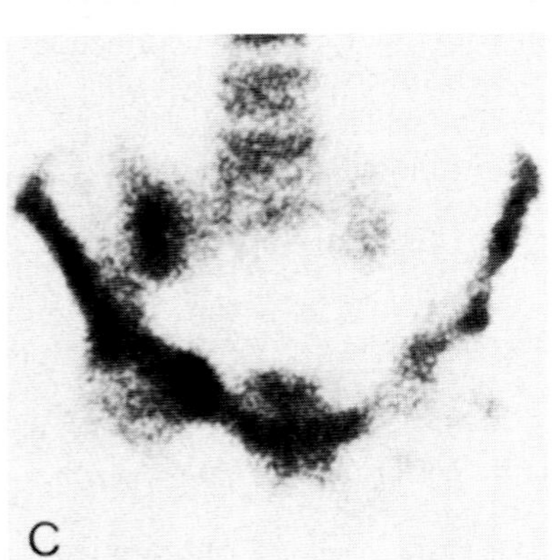

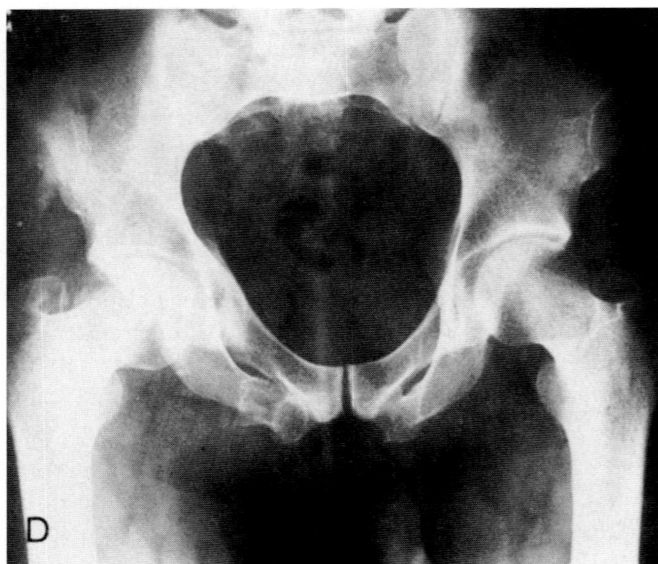

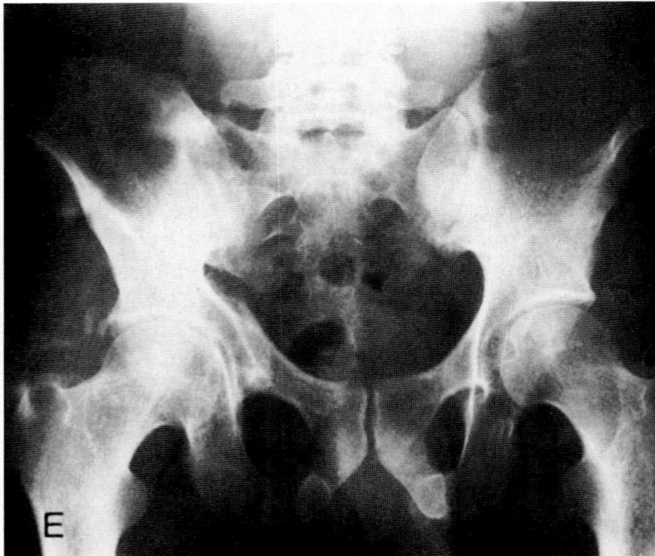

FIGURE 21-11. Anteroposterior radiographs demonstrate pelvic nonunion. **A:** The three arrows indicate three sites of nonunion: posteriorly through the sacroiliac joint and anteriorly through the superior and inferior pubic rami. The sacroiliac and superior pubic ramus nonunions are hypertrophic, whereas that through the inferior ramus is atrophic. **B,C:** The evidence on the tomogram and on the technetium polyphosphate bone scan indicate increased uptake at the sacroiliac joint and superior pubic ramus and no uptake at the inferior ramus. The patient complained of pain in the sacroiliac area as well as difficulty in sitting. After bone grafting in all three sites and stabilization with an external skeletal frame, the final anteroposterior **(D)** and inlet **(E)** radiographs, taken 18 months after that surgery, demonstrate bony healing of all three nonunions.

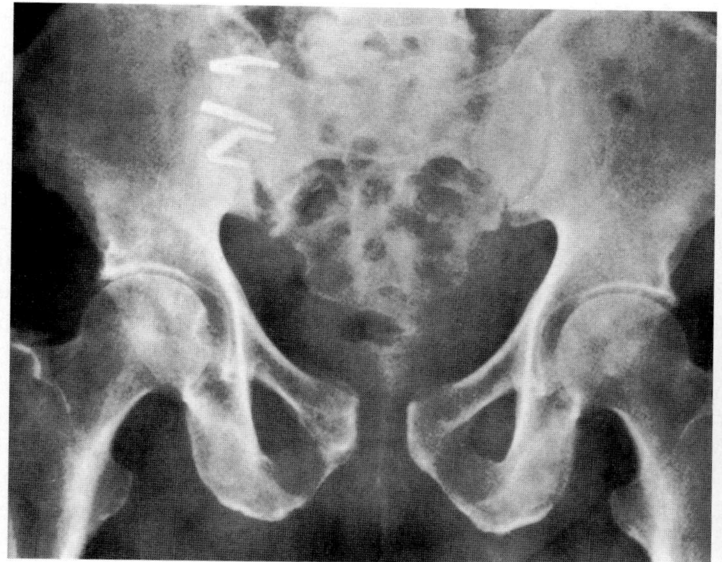

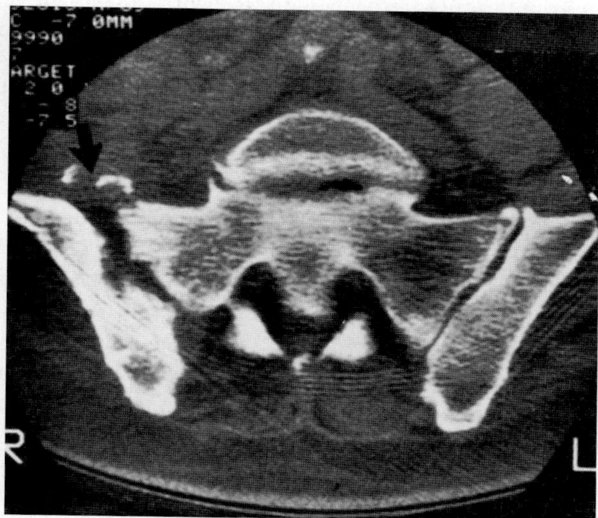

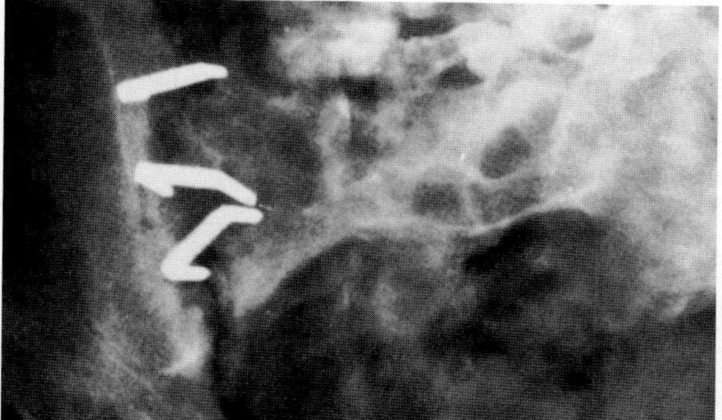

FIGURE 21-12. In the diagnosis of nonunion an anteroposterior radiograph may be very misleading. **A:** The surgeon looking at this view cannot be sure of the state of the right sacroiliac joint after surgery. **B,C:** Computed tomography and the oblique radiograph clearly demonstrate the nonunion.

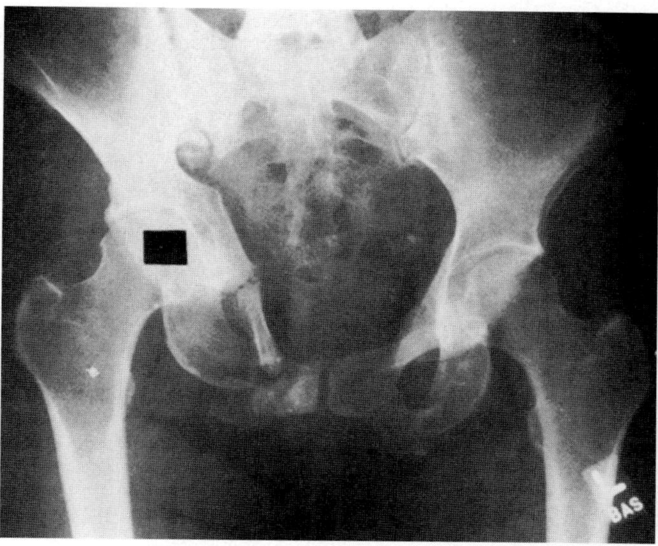

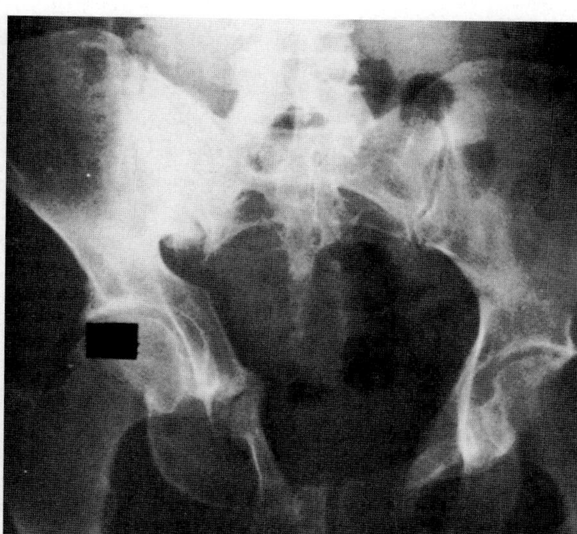

FIGURE 21-13. A: A patient first seen 18 months after an unstable right pelvic disruption who had nonunions of the right sacrum and of the superior and inferior pubic rami complained of significant pain and leg length discrepancy. When seen $3\frac{1}{2}$ years later she still had evidence of nonunion posteriorly and inferiorly, although the superior pubic ramus appeared to be uniting. **B:** At that time, her symptoms had lessened and her pain had become tolerable, with no surgical intervention.

depends on the precise location of the nonunion. In some cases, it may be approached directly with the patient in the lithotomy position. Osteoperiosteal flaps are raised and cancellous bone grafting performed. Internal fixation of the inferior ramus often is difficult to achieve. Long cancellous lag screws should be placed across the nonunion if this is technically possible. Evolving techniques for use of computer-assisted placement will likely prove helpful in the future. If the nonunion is more proximal, it may be exposed through a standard Kocher-Langenbeck approach. The posterior column of the acetabulum may be visualized distal to the ischial tuberosity. This approach allows open reduction with internal fixation using lag screws and plate fixation. An interfragmentary wire tension band can be used as an aid to reduction and to counteract the tensile forces of the hamstring musculature on the ischium.

Posterior

Restoration of posterior pelvic stability is the key to relieving the symptoms of pelvic nonunion. Occasionally, achieving stable fusion of the symphysis pubis anteriorly restores enough posterior stability to eliminate the pain. In most cases the posterior lesion should be approached directly. The sacroiliac joint may be approached either anteriorly or posteriorly (30,31). The posterior approach is favored because stable interfragmentary compression is easier to obtain.

Posterior Approach. A longitudinal incision is made just lateral to the posterior superior and posterior inferior spine. With sacroiliac joint lesions, all fibrous and cartilaginous tissues are then excised from the sacroiliac joint, and local cancellous graft bone is placed in the defect. Stabilization then can be obtained by any of the methods described. The most favored method involves using 6.5-, 7.0-, or 7.3-mm cannulated iliosacral screws placed across the joint. A lateral plate may be required to serve as a washer. Studies have shown purchase to be significantly improved when the sacral bodies are engaged. In addition, the posterior tension band plate, a 3.5- or 4.5-mm reconstruction plate, fixed and embedded in both posterior superior iliac spines with screws, may provide additional support. Where possible, anterior internal fixation should be used, rather than an anterior external fixator that cannot restore as much stability to the pelvis. Although no large series comparing anterior external fixation with open stabilization of the pelvic ring in the treatment of nonunions exist, recent articles have suggested internal stabilization to be superior to external fixation in treatment of acute injuries.

If the nonunion involves the sacrum, the site should be exposed, fibrous tissue removed, and bone graft applied. The same methods of internal fixation previously described should be used to obtain compression. Compression may not be possible when the sacral foramina are involved. If the nonunion is through the ilium, plate and screw fixation is used along with autogenous iliac crest bone graft.

Anterior Approach to the Sacroiliac Joint. Anterior exposure of the sacroiliac joint is not difficult. An incision is made just lateral to the iliac crest and the iliacus and psoas musculature

A

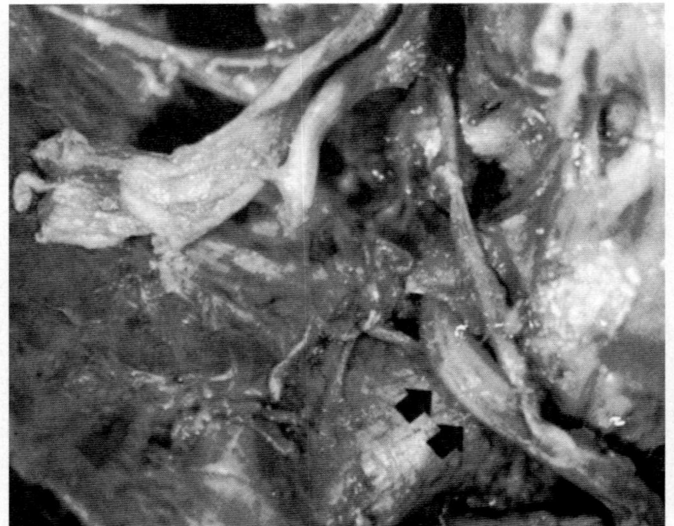

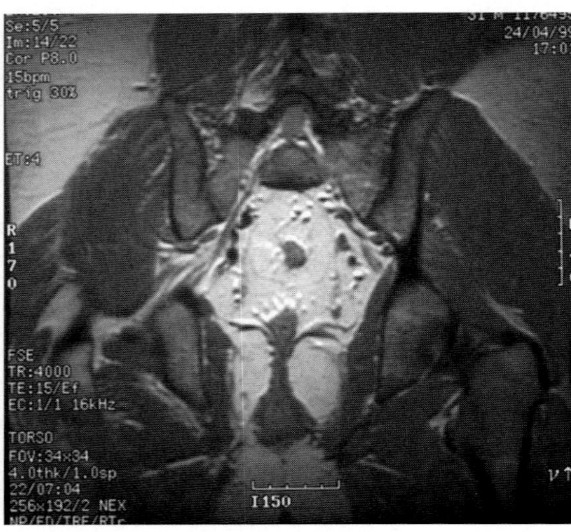

B

FIGURE 21-14. A: This anatomic dissection of the lumbosacral plexus shows the precarious position of the L5 nerve root as it crosses superiorly over the sacrum and sacroiliac joint. Fractures through the sacrum, which often extend up to the transverse process of L5, may sever this nerve or severely damage it by traction. The nerve also is at risk as it crosses the sacroiliac joint. **B:** Pelvic magnetic resonance imaging showing the nerve roots exiting the cauda equina, the injury is noted on the left side.

is stripped from the inner aspect of the iliac wing as far posteriorly as the sacroiliac joint. The L5 nerve root must be identified and protected as it tracks inferiorly over the sacral ala (Fig. 21-14). The joint may be opened, cleared of fibrous tissue, and bone grafted. Anterior plating, as described, may provide stable fixation, but it lacks the interfragmentary compression desired for fusion. The addition of a percutaneously placed cannulated iliosacral screw is recommended if feasible. This supplements the anterior plate and provides the necessary interfragmentary compression.

After Care

Weight bearing is forbidden, in order to allow bony union. This may require bed-to-chair transfers or crutch walking for 6 to 12 weeks, depending on the nonunion site, quality of the bone or fixation, and individual patient considerations. If radiographic union is progressing, a graduated program of mobilization may be commenced with progressive weight bearing after 6 to 12 weeks.

The complexity and magnitude of these procedures mandates that they be undertaken only by surgeons familiar with pelvic anatomy and advanced techniques of internal and external fixation.

Nerve Injury

Permanent nerve damage is a common cause of disability following pelvic disruption. The overall prevalence of *neurologic* injury in pelvic trauma, including those cases in which it is temporary, is believed to be between 10% and 15% (14,32). If one considers only unstable vertical shear fractures, the prevalence rises to 40% to 50% (33). The prevalence of nerve injury is clearly related to the site of the posterior lesion (5,34,35). Denis and colleagues classified sacral fractures based on direction, location, and level of fractures and reviewed 236 fractures (5). Zone I fractures occurred lateral to the sacral foramina and resulted in 5.9% rate of neurologic injury. Zone II injuries involved the foramina, and 28.4% of patients had neurologic injury. Zone III fractures occur medial to the sacral foramina and resulted in the highest percentage of neurologic injuries (56.7%). Of deficits associated with zone III fractures, 76% affected bowel, bladder, and/or sexual function.

The definitive work on this subject remains that of Huittinen and Slatis, who reviewed 85 patients with unstable pelvic fractures (33). Of that group, 31 (41%) were found to have a significant injury to the lumbosacral plexus. Of the 31, 22 demonstrated definite motor signs, whereas 26 had clinically significant sensory findings. The motor roots most often involved were L5 and S1. Surprisingly, eight of 31 cases had motor involvement of L4. Sensory involvement was most common in the sacral nerve roots, S2 to S5, but also in L5. These authors attempted to correlate the severity of nerve damage with the type of pelvic disruption. All patients had posterior disruption of the pelvic ring, but there appeared to be no clear distinction between nerve injuries that resulted from a sacral fracture and those that resulted in the setting of a sacroiliac dislocation. The authors also noted that the severity of the bone injury posteriorly did not correlate with the severity of injury to the neural elements. Clinically, the nerve injury usually was permanent.

As a result of this clinical study, Huittinen and Slatis carried out a careful cadaver dissection of 42 victims of high-energy trauma that fractured the pelvis. This dissection was complemented by radiographic and histologic examination. This meticulously done study added much to our understanding of the nerve injuries associated with pelvic disruption. The unstable pelvic disruptions in this group of patients who died from their injuries were extremely complex. The preponderance of bilateral unstable posterior injuries attests to the overall injury severity. The prevalence of genitourinary complications was 33%, also indicative of the high-energy nature of these injuries. Forty different injuries to the nerves were noted at various levels in 20 of 42 autopsies.

Traction injuries were found in 21 cases, disruption of the nerve in 15 cases, and compression injury in four cases. Virtually all areas of the lumbosacral plexus were involved, including the roots of the cauda equina in six cases, the obturator nerve in four, the lumbosacral trunk in 12, the superior gluteal nerve in 11, the anterior primary ramus of the L5 nerve root in two, and the anterior primary rami of S1 through S3 in five (see Chapter 2). The lumbosacral trunk and superior gluteal nerve commonly sustained traction injuries, whereas compression injuries were common to the anterior primary rami of the three sacral nerves and were owing to fractures through the sacrum. Most complete disruptions were encountered in the roots of the cauda equina, and they were often multiple. Surprisingly, all injuries to the obturator nerve were at the level of the sacroiliac joint, not at the obturator foramen. All injuries, including the traction injuries, were confirmed by histologic investigation. The traction injuries to the lumbosacral trunk and superior gluteal nerve were usually found in hemipelvis disruptions marked by external rotation and posterior and superior displacement. Comminution and impaction of the lateral mass caused compression of the sacral nerves. The authors also contrasted disruptions of the cauda equina, occurring distal to the intervertebral foramen, with extraforaminal disruptions seen in the cervical spine. The nerve roots in the lumbar spine exit in a longitudinal fashion; such that the nerve root avulsion occurs far distal to the intervertebral foramen and examination of the nerves following laminectomy often fails to reveal the site of trauma.

Harris and colleagues described four cases of lumbar nerve root avulsion complicating unstable fractures of the pelvis (36). Myelographic evidence of diverticula at the root level was found in all four cases. The authors suggested that the presence of a diverticulum in a lumbar myelogram did not imply avulsion of the nerve root because some recovery was observed in their patients. In addition, the neurologic deficit and clinical findings did not correspond to the location of the diverticulum. The authors suggested that the dural root sleeve may be ruptured without causing permanent damage to the nerve root. None of the patients was subjected to surgical exploration. Sidhu and Dhillon reported a similar case involving an 18-year-old motorcyclist who initially had flaccid paralysis of right leg following a right sacroiliac dislocation (37). Lumbar myelography revealed meningoceles at the L3-S2 nerve roots. Four months later, he had recovered completely except for residual footdrop. Barnett and Connolly added an additional case of an intradural avulsion of a nerve root with associated sacroiliac dislocation (38). These authors felt, in contrast to other investigators, that myelography clearly indicated a nerve root avulsion and therefore a contraindication to surgery. Schied and associates reported a prevalence of 50% for nerve injury in patients with sacral fractures, which led to fair to poor results in spite of adequate reduction and stabilization (39).

Diagnosis

Early and careful neurologic examination is mandatory for all patients. Helfet and colleagues demonstrated a significant increase in the incidence of nerve injury when patients were assessed by an independent examiner (40). Sensory examination of the perineum is a critical component of this assessment. Failure to complete this portion of the examination will overlook a large percentage of sacral nerve injuries. Permanent damage to the sacral nerves may cause late genitourinary dysfunction. Early urologic consultation and cystometry is recommended in any case where sacral nerve injury is suspected. Late attempts to evaluate sacral nerve function clinically often are complicated by complex psychosocial and medicolegal issues.

The motor strength of all lower extremity muscles should be carefully documented. Evaluation of the upper lumbar nerve roots, especially the fourth lumbar root, is particularly important. For example, a 15-year-old girl was struck by a motor vehicle while cycling. She sustained an open and markedly unstable pelvic ring disruption, which was treated with early open reduction and internal fixation. Although her fracture healed rapidly, the end result was compromised by the presence of a lacerated femoral nerve. The same patient also sustained an intimal tear of the femoral artery; however, her collateral circulation maintained the viability of the limb.

Electrodiagnostic studies are becoming more sophisticated and valuable. These studies, which traditionally were useful for diagnosis and prognosis, are now available as an intraoperative aid, to avoid iatrogenic injury (40–42). As a consequence of their ability to diagnose and prognosticate, perioperative studies may indirectly alter treatment decisions and may assist in the selection of an optimal rehabilitation regimen. Older modalities for assessing nerve conduction were of only limited use in assessing very high lesions. Improved techniques for testing cortical-evoked response now allow assessment of more proximal lesions.

Consultation with a neurosurgeon or neurologist with special interest in peripheral nerve injury may be helpful.

Management

Huittinen and Slatis demonstrated that the vast majority of injuries are either traction injuries or compression injuries (33). Repair of major peripheral nerves has been reported but remains only minimally successful. Intrapelvic nerve repair of the lumbosacral plexus historically has been a low-yield procedure, but advances in neurophysiology and repair may make such procedures more feasible in the future. Injuries to the femoral nerve have been treated successfully by direct nerve repair. If surgical repair of the femoral nerve is contemplated, myelography or MRI (Fig. 21-14B) is recommended to rule out spinal nerve avulsion, but this comes with the caveat that previous studies have suggested a large percentage of false-positive results. Attempted nerve repair should never by undertaken lightly, as some patients end up worse off because of an apparent increase in causalgic pain. If the injury is peripheral and nerve repair is attempted, it should be performed by a surgeon thoroughly versed in all aspects of nerve repair. Matejcik correlates the likelihood of successful treatment of peripheral nerve injury to the specific treatment rendered and to the delay to definitive treatment. Injuries treated with neurolysis resulted in the best outcome. Injuries that were possible to treat using direct suture technique fared better than those requiring nerve grafting.

The primary treatment of lumbosacral nerve injury must be directed toward reduction of the fracture. In some cases the damage done by compression or traction on the nerve at the time of injury may preclude any recovery. However, early reduction and stabilization prevents continued traction on the stretched nerve root and may decompress nerves entrapped at the fracture site. Some data suggest that decompression of entrapped sacral nerve roots, on either an acute or delayed basis, may ultimately improve prognosis (43).

Iatrogenic Complications

Enthusiasm for surgical stabilization of the pelvis has resulted in the development of new instrumentation and new techniques. Surgical approaches have been developed to address fractures in previously difficult to approach locations. Although these approaches are now familiar to a greater number of orthopedic surgeons, only a limited number have extensive experience. These approaches place neurologic and vascular structures at significant risk. The value of cadaveric dissection prior to undertaking surgery cannot be overestimated. Although changes in implant design, including such things as the development of pelvic reconstruction plates that allow for easier contouring may have made surgery easier, the basic principles of stable fixation using lag screws and compression plating must be remembered. Technological improvements in the quality of image intensifiers with better visualization and decreased radiation dosage has led to increased use of percutaneous and fixation techniques for the sacrum and sacroiliac joint. A limited window for safe passage of these screws is present (see Chapter 15). This has led to a variety of complications, including foraminal encroachment, injury to the cauda equina, and vascular injury (Figs. 21-15 and 21-16). Even in the hands of experienced surgeons, these techniques remain dangerous

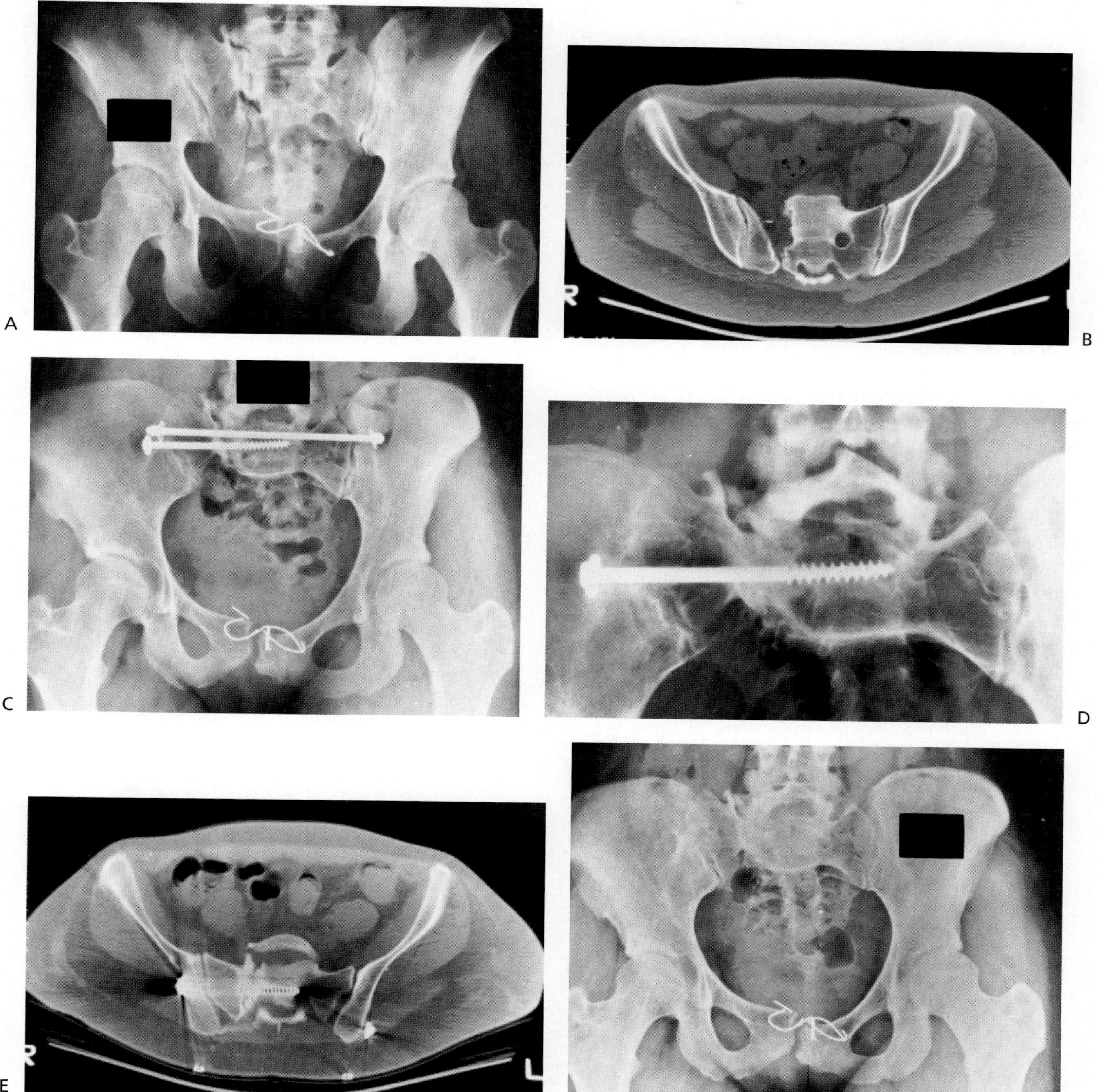

FIGURE 21-15. A,B: A 29-year-old patient underwent open reduction and internal fixation for painful sacral nonunion. Postoperatively, her low back pain resolved, but her radicular symptoms were exacerbated. **C,D,E:** Workup revealed a screw in the vertebral canal. **F:** After the screw was removed, the radiculopathy improved.

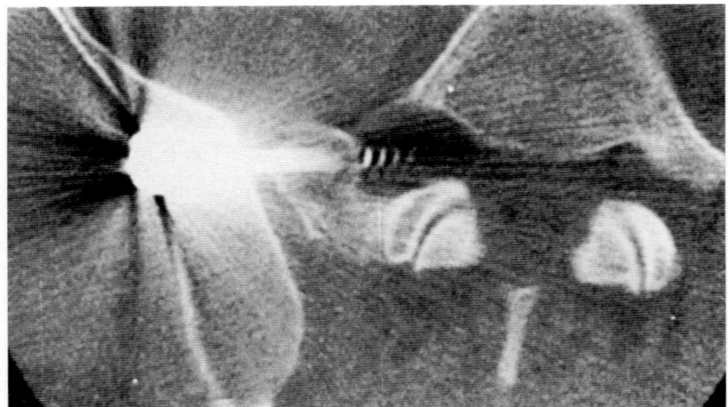

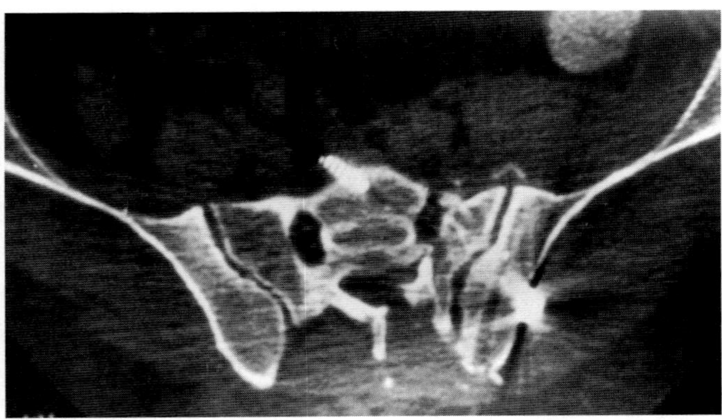

FIGURE 21-16. Computed tomography demonstrates possible complications of percutaneous screw placement: in the S1 intraforamen **(A)**, in the pelvis **(B)**, in the region of the iliac vessels.

and difficult. Computer-assisted placement using fluoroscopy or CT scan is an evolving technique that may ultimately decrease but will not eliminate the risk of complications. Anterior plating of the symphysis and pubic rami risks injury to the bladder, spermatic cord, round ligament, and neurovascular structures. Fixation may be difficult to obtain in this often osteoporotic region, and failure of fixation almost can be guaranteed if adequate posterior fixation is not obtained (Fig. 21-17). Anterior plating techniques for sacroiliac joint disruptions risk injury to the L5 nerve root as it courses over the sacral ala.

All surgical procedures about the pelvis carry a significant risk of soft-tissue complications and infection, particularly if performed following open fracture. There may be significant injury to the soft tissues; even with closed fractures. Initially the extent of subcutaneous degloving is often masked. Late reconstructive procedures following infection and soft-tissue loss are extremely challenging.

Aggressive perioperative nursing care is necessary to prevent progression of soft-tissue injury. Optimal care often includes the use of pressure relief mattresses designed to prevent decubiti. Patients remain at risk for soft-tissue breakdown postoperatively, particularly over the subcutaneous sacrum, especially when posterior surgical procedures have included placement of hardware. Recessing hardware and attention to closure of soft tissues and deep fascia can minimize these risks.

DEEP VEIN THROMBOSIS

DVT is recognized as a common sequela of pelvic and lower extremity trauma (44,45). The incidence of DVT proximal

FIGURE 21-17. A: A 35-year-old patient underwent open reduction and internal fixation of the symphysis for an open-book pelvic fracture-dislocation, for which two plates were used. In the early postoperative period he fell; therefore, the fixation failed. **B:** He developed a persistent sinus and eventually, this screw was extruded.

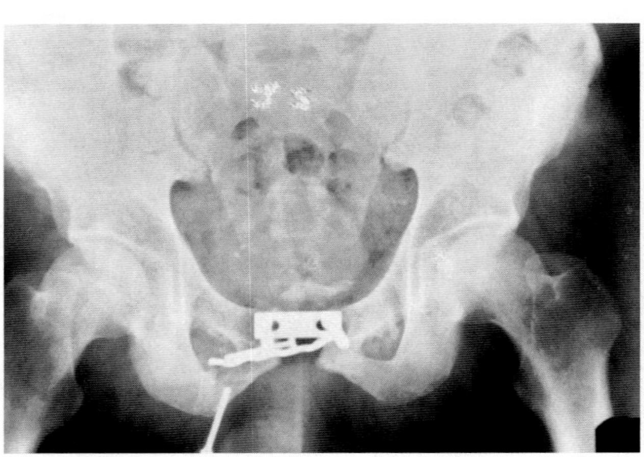

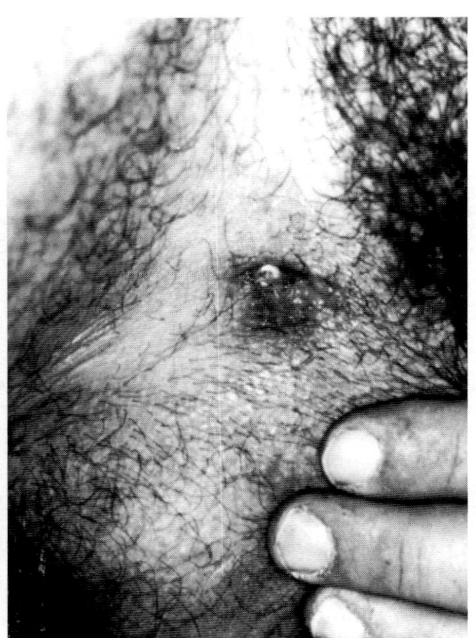

to the popliteal trifurcation is reported to be 40% to 60% following pelvic fractures (2). The acute complications of DVT, discussed elsewhere in the text, include—most importantly—a reported 4% to 22% rate of pulmonary embolism (PE) (46) and consequent mortality of 2% to 3%.

The natural history of DVT is multifactorial and unpredictable. The long-term sequelae are not well established. Postphlebitic syndrome may result in nonspecific complaints such as heaviness and pain. Objective findings, including edema and trophic changes or ulceration, have been reported to occur in two thirds of patients within 3 years of proximal thrombosis. Severity is highly variable. Thrombosis often begins at the time of injury as a consequence of intimal damage, hypercoagulable state, and local or systemic stasis. The prevalence of DVT associated with pelvic fracture trauma mandates prophylaxis whenever possible. Thrombosis may be prevented in a significant percentage of patients through early resuscitation, fracture reduction, and/or stabilization, patient mobilization, and pharmacologic or mechanical methods or prophylaxis. At least one study demonstrated that as many as 7% of trauma patients could not be treated by any of the available mechanical or pharmacologic modalities (47,48).

Once established, further progression of thrombosis can be halted pharmacologically, thus allowing a more rapid and complete recanalization. The optimal treatment modality for proven thrombi, and the appropriate duration of therapy has not been determined. Most authorities continue to recommend initial treatment with full heparin anticoagulation, although the use of therapeutic-dose low molecular weight heparin (LMWH) has gathered some recent support. After full anticoagulation with intravenous heparin and conversion to oral warfarin, treatment has historically been continued for 3 to 6 months, maintaining a prothrombin time of approximately 1½ to 2 times normal. Owing to variability in prothrombin time, most clinicians now recommend monitoring of INR and maintaining a range of 2 to 3.

A significant percentage of patients with pelvic fractures and proven DVT initially are not candidates for anticoagulation (44,46). This patient population includes those refractory to anticoagulation, those with ongoing hemorrhage or impending surgery, and those with an acute or chronic bleeding diathesis. The development of techniques for vena caval interruption has significantly improved the ability to prevent pulmonary emboli in a large number of patients with established DVT.

Early techniques for inferior vena caval interruption involved extraluminal ligation, plication, or stapling. In addition to requiring an extensive open surgical procedure, these techniques resulted in a high incidence of inferior vena caval thrombosis (49). Early intraluminal methods of caval interruption also resulted in a high incidence of inferior vena caval thrombosis (60% to 70%) (49). This incidence was substantially reduced with the development of new filter designs (49,50).

The previous edition of this book noted ongoing complications of filter placement in a significant number of patients (49,50). Device-related complications included migration (29%), tilt (7%), penetration of vessel wall (9%), device failure (2%), and insertion site thrombosis (22%). More recent reports using newer designs and techniques have suggested a much lower incidence of early complications. The risk of late complications such as inferior vena cava thrombosis and post-phlebitic syndrome with the use of new filter designs is not yet known. Early series of patients undergoing placement of inferior vena caval filters often included those with limited life expectancy secondary to malignancy or other disease. Older studies may not be applicable to a group of young trauma victims. Sekharan and coworkers recently reported 5-year follow-up results in 108 young trauma victims who had undergone prophylactic placement of filters. Although no major complications were reported, only 36 patients were available for follow-up and only 33 were seen (51). Langan and coworkers reported similar results. Removable inferior vena caval filters have been used in Europe for more than 15 years. Given concerns with the potential long-term morbidity of permanent filters they are a theoretically attractive alternative; however, only three reports are available in the literature. Because a greater number of removable filters are used in controlled trials it is expected that their risks, benefits, and indications will be better defined. Most practitioners still feel short-term anticoagulation is required to prevent acute thrombosis following inferior vena cava filter placement. The optimal duration of treatment is as yet undetermined, although most practitioners have adopted 3 months as a general guideline.

The prophylactic regimen chosen remains the choice of the individual clinician. Recent literature has suggested the clinician choose a treatment regimen based on the risk:benefit ratio and strength of data. Strength of data is a product of the methodology through which it was derived. Following an extensive literature review Geerts and coworkers (see Chapter 9) made four recommendations for the treatment of trauma patients:

1. Trauma patients with an identifiable risk factor for thromboembolism should receive prophylaxis if possible. If there is no contraindication the use of LMWH is recommended as soon as it is safe to do so. (This was a strong [Type 1A] recommendation based on the risk:benefit ratio and methodology through which efficacy of LMWH was shown to be effective.)

2. Initial use of mechanical prophylaxis was recommended in cases where use of LMWH would be delayed because of concerns with bleeding. This recommendation (Type 1C) was strong with respect to the potential risk:benefit ratio; however, the methodology through which supporting data had been gathered was deemed relatively weak.

3. A screening duplex ultrasound was recommended in

patients at high risk for thromboembolism who had received suboptimal prophylaxis. This was also a Type 1C recommendation for the reasons previously outlined.

4. Inferior vena caval filter insertion received a Type 1C+ recommendation when a proximal DVT was identified and anticoagulation was recommended. Again, the potential risk:benefit ratio was deemed high; however, the supporting evidence had been obtained from observational studies or extrapolated from studies on dissimilar groups of patients. Despite these flaws in methodology the evidence was deemed compelling, thus earning a C+ recommendation. The use of an IVC filter for prophylaxis was not recommended (Type 1C).

Antithrombotic therapy remains a rapidly evolving field. The preceding recommendations should serve only as guidelines. The interested reader is referred to Geerts' original article (see Chapter 9), but cautioned that guidelines are likely to change. New pharmacologic agents directed toward specific sites in the coagulation cascade remain under development and study. Optimal patient treatment will require ongoing attention to new developments and findings.

CONCLUSION

In the almost two decades that have passed since the first edition of this book was published, there has been a greater understanding of those factors that lead to late morbidity following pelvic ring fractures. Early and appropriate intervention has resulted in a decreased percentage of patients developing significant complications. New techniques, equipment, and greater familiarity with surgical approaches have improved our ability to treat the complications that inevitably occur. The primary goal of the clinician should remain the prevention of complications through the use of those modalities detailed in this text.

REFERENCES

1. Tile M. *Fractures of the pelvis and acetabulum.* Baltimore: Williams & Wilkins, 1984.
2. Poole GV, Ward EF, Griswold JA, et al. Complications of pelvic fractures from blunt trauma. *Am Surg* 1992;58:225.
3. Riemer BL, Butterfield SL, Diamond DL, et al. Acute mortality associated with injuries to the pelvic ring: the role of early patient mobilization and external fixation. *J Trauma* 1993;35:671.
4. Bone LB, Johnson KD, Weigelt J, et al. Early versus delayed stabilization of femoral fractures. *J Bone Joint Surg* 1989;71:336.
5. Denis F, Davis S, Comfort T. Sacral fractures: an important problem. *Clin Orthop* 1988;227:67.
6. Colapinto V. Trauma to the pelvis: urethral injury. *Clin Orthop* 1980;151:46.
7. Diekmann-Guiroy B, Young DH. Female urethral injury secondary to blunt pelvic trauma. *Ann Emerg Med* 1991;20:1376.
8. Schneider RE. Genitourinary trauma. *Emerg Med Clin North Am* 1993;11:137.
9. Ellison M, Timberlake GA, Kerstein MD. Impotence following pelvic fractures. *J Trauma* 1988;28:695.
10. Barach E, Martin G, Tomlanovich M, et al. Blunt pelvic trauma with urethral injury in the female: a case report and review of the literature. *J Emerg Med* 1984;2:101.
11. Perry MO, Husmann DA. Urethral injuries in female subjects following pelvic fractures. *J Urol* 1992;147:137.
12. Cohen ES, Scherz HC, Parsons CL. Voiding dysfunction secondary to penetrating bony fragment 20 years after pelvic fracture. *J Urol* 1989;141:606.
13. Ryan EA. Hernias related to pelvic fractures. *Surg Gynecol Obstet* 1971;133:440.
14. Tile M, et al. *Disruptions of the pelvic ring.* Presented to the Combined Meeting of English Speaking Orthopedic Surgeons. Cape Town, South Africa, March, 1982.
15. Holdsworth FW. Dislocations and fracture dislocations of the pelvis. *J Bone Joint Surg* 1948;30B:461.
16. Slatis P, Huittinen VM. Double vertical fractures of the pelvis. *Acta Chir Scand* 1972;138:799.
17. Rubash HE, Nelson DD, Mears DC. *Reconstructive surgery of the pelvis.* Presented to the American Academy of Orthopedic Surgeons. New Orleans, 1982.
18. Henderson RC. The long-term results of nonoperatively treated major pelvic disruptions. *J Orthop Trauma* 1989;3:41.
19. Wright MS, Mears DC, Gordon RG, et al. *Results of treatment of two hundred pelvic malunion/nonunions.* Presented at the American Association of Orthopedic Surgery Annual Meeting, 1993.
20. McLaren AC, Rorabeck CH, Halpenny J. Long-term pain and disability in relation to residual deformity after displaced pelvic ring fractures. *Can J Surg* 1990;33:492.
21. Semba RT, Yasukawa K, Gustilo RB. Critical analysis of results of 53 Malgaigne fractures of the pelvis. *J Trauma* 1983;23:535.
22. Isler B. Lumbosacral lesions associated with pelvic ring injuries. *J Orthop Trauma* 1990;4:1.
23. Kuntscher G (Rinne HHH, trans). *Practice of intramedullary nailing.* Springfield, IL: Charles C Thomas, 1967.
24. Winquist RA, Hansen ST Jr, Pearson RE. Closed intramedullary shortening of the femur. *Clin Orthop* 1978;136:54.
25. Salter RB. Innominate osteotomy in the treatment of dislocations and subluxation of the hip. *J Bone Joint Surg* 1961;43:518.
26. Dunn AW, Morris HD. Fracture and fracture dislocation of the pelvis. *J Bone Joint Surg* 1968;50A:1639.
27. Pennal GF. *Pelvic non-unions.* Presented at the Canadian Orthopaedic Association Annual Meeting. June 1973.
28. Pennal GF, Massiah KA. Nonunion and delayed union of fractures of the pelvis. *Clin Orthop* 1980;151:124.
29. Bucholz RW. The pathological anatomy of Malgaigne fracture-dislocations of the pelvis. *J Bone Joint Surg* 1981;63A:400.
30. Kellam JF, McMurtry RY, Paley D, et al. The unstable pelvic fracture. *Orthop Clin North Am* 1987;18:25.
31. Helfet DL. Internal fixation of pelvic fractures. *Techn Orthop* 1989;4:67.
32. Failinger MS, McGanity PLJ. Current concepts review: unstable fractures of the pelvic ring. *J Bone Joint Surg* 1992;74A:781.
33. Huittinen VM, Slatis P. Nerve injury in double vertical pelvic fractures. *Acta Chir Scand* 1971;138:571.
34. Majeed SA. Neurologic deficits in major pelvic injuries. *Clin Orthop* 1992;282:222.
35. Raf L. Double vertical fractures of the pelvis. *Acta Chir Scand* 1966;131:298.
36. Harris WR, Rathbun JB, Wortzman G, et al. Avulsion of lumbar roots complicating fracture of the pelvis. *J Bone Joint Surg* 1973;55A:1436.

37. Sidhu JS, Dhillon MK. Lumbosacral plexus avulsion with pelvic fractures. *Injury* 1991;22:156.
38. Barnett HG, Connolly ES. Lumbosacral nerve root avulsion: report of a case and review of the literature. *J Trauma* 1975;15: 532.
39. Schied DK, Kellam JF, Tile M. Open reduction and internal fixation of pelvic ring fractures. *J Orthop Trauma* 1991;5:226.
40. Helfet DL, Schmelling GJ, Mast JW. Somatosensory evoked potential monitoring in the surgical treatment of acute displaced acetabular fractures: results of a prospective study. *Orthop Trans* 1992;16:221.
41. Vrahas M, Gordon RG, Mears DC, et al. Intraoperative somatosensory evoked potential monitoring of pelvic and acetabular fractures. *J Orthop Trauma* 1992;6:50.
42. Helfet DL, et al. SSEP monitoring in pelvic fractures. *J Orthop Trauma* in press.
43. Rai SK, Far RF, Ghovanlou B. Neurologic deficits associated with sacral wing fractures. *Orthopedics* 1990;13:1363.
44. Kudsk KA, Fabian TC, Baum S, et al. Silent deep vein thrombosis in immobilized multiple trauma patients. *Am J Surg* 1989;158: 515.
45. Buerger PM, Peoples JB, Lemmon GW, et al. Risk of pulmonary emboli in patients with pelvic fractures. *Am Surg* 1993;59:505.
46. Rogers FB, Shackford SR, Wilson J, et al. Prophylactic vena cava filter insertion in severely injured trauma patients: indications and preliminary results. *J Trauma* 1993;35:637.
47. Shackford SR, Davis JW, Hollingsworth-Fridlund P, et al. Venous thromboembolism in major trauma. *Am J Surg* 1990;159:365.
48. Shackford SR, Moser KM. Deep vein thrombosis and pulmonary embolism in trauma patients. *J Int Care Med* 1988;3:87.
49. Ferris EJ, McCowan TC, Carver DK, et al. Percutaneous inferior vena caval filters: follow up of seven designs in 320 patients. *Radiology* 1993;188:851.
50. Crochet DP, Stora O, Ferry D, et al. Vena Tech-LGM filter: long term results of a prospective study. *Radiology* 1993;188:857.
51. Sekharan J, Dennis JW, Miranda FE, et al. Long term follow-up of prophylactic Greenfield filters in multisystem trauma patients. *J Trauma* 2001;51(6):1087–1090.

22

MALUNION AND NONUNION OF THE PELVIS: POSTTRAUMATIC DEFORMITY

MICHAEL D. STOVER
JOEL M. MATTA

INCIDENCE

The three-dimensional structure of the pelvis, composed of the two innominate bones and the sacrum, relies on a complex ligamentous network to provide stability. Rarely does an injury to a single area occur and injuries can involve ligamentous disruptions with associated dislocations or fractures with or without displacement. Most patients also present with associated injuries to other organ systems. An individual's associated injuries, the pattern of injury, and amount of displacement ultimately determine the initial treatment to the pelvic ring. Despite an increased understanding of pelvic injury, malunions and nonunions of the pelvic ring continue to occur. Malposition or instability of the pelvis following treatment may be secondary to fractures that heal with residual displacement, along with other areas that may not have achieved structural bone healing or ligamentous repair. This makes it difficult to separately discuss malunions and nonunions of the pelvic ring, because the two entities may commonly coexist in a single complex posttraumatic deformity. Regardless of the method of treatment, authors have estimated that as many as 5% of all fractures remain in an unsatisfactory position following injury (1).

ETIOLOGY

Malunion and nonunion of the pelvis can occur after any form of treatment, but most commonly is the result of nonoperative care (2–5). Residual deformity results when the degree of stability or displacement is misunderstood on initial or subsequent radiographic and clinical evaluation. Pelvic stability following injury depends on the mechanism of injury, type of injury (fracture or dislocation), and the amount of displacement. A stable injury pattern is commonly referred to as one that can withstand physiologic forces without further displacement (6). The difficulty with this description is defining the amount and duration of force that is physiologic, making determination of pelvic stability difficult at times. Therefore, how to evaluate for deformity and stability are the most important concepts physicians involved in the initial treatment of pelvic fractures need to comprehend.

External fixation may provide a degree of stability to the pelvis in the resuscitation of patients but this modality as the sole treatment in globally unstable pelvic fractures will likely result in deformity (6,7). Deformity also can result from operative treatment of fractures or dislocations if inadequate reduction and/or fixation is obtained at the time of surgery. What constitutes an acceptable and stable reduction is important to understand by the operating surgeon. This can be defined differently for various patient populations as the pattern of injury, bone material, and/or ability to cooperate with postoperative activity restrictions can affect fixation choices, or resulting outcome (8–10). A delay in definitive internal fixation owing to a patient's associated injuries or comorbidities can make reduction more difficult and require a greater understanding of surgical care (11). Patients with multiple traumatic injuries or preexisting medical problems are candidates for transfer to individuals and institutions well equipped to care for these fractures. Obtaining a near anatomic reduction with appropriate fixation of unstable fractures is the most reliable method to maintain fracture position until union and decrease the incidence of healing with residual displacement or instability (12). The development of less invasive methods for stabilization of pelvic ring injuries may decrease the acute morbidity associated with operative care in some settings (13), but these methods should not be used at the expense of an adequate reduction.

Prevention of deformity is the best treatment and inherent to any treatment modality is the need for radiographic monitoring of the fracture until union. Serial radiographic examination may reveal occult fracture or fixation instability early in the treatment course, making revisions in the treatment plan less difficult.

DEFORMITY

Specific deformities of the pelvis following injury can be complex, and may include translational and/or rotational displacement. Traditionally, a common point of reference to describe deformity for each hemipelvis is the posterior zone of injury (i.e., ilium, sacrum or SI joint), because this is the point around which most deformity occurs. Anatomic descriptions of translational deformity include caudad/cephalad, anterior/posterior (ventral/dorsal), and medial/lateral displacements. Rotational deformity also occurs around the posterior sacroiliac complex, resulting in flexion/extension, internal/external, and abduction/adduction malrotation. Specific views of the pelvis best depict remaining deformity after injury (Fig. 22-1). The appearance of the obturator foramen and specific anatomic features of the pelvis assist in the determination of deformity. Rotational displacements can be inferred from the anterior-posterior view, with internal rotation or external rotation resulting in the appearance of a obturator oblique or iliac oblique type view, whereas flexion and extension result in a more cephalad or caudad view of the pelvis, respectively.

Multiple translational and rotational displacements may be described within a single posttraumatic deformity, attempting to define the residual position of the hemipelvis following treatment. A typical deformity following an anterior-posterior compression mechanism includes cephalad-translation with external rotation and abduction of the hemipelvis. Lateral compression results in internal rotation with flexion and adduction of the hemipelvis. Dickson and Matta described a common deformity that can result after external fixation (14). Additional deformities can occur within the innominate bone. Often occurring in the rami, these deformities may be a source of morbidity in posttraumatic deformity and complicate subsequent treatment.

DEFINITION

Despite improved understanding of pelvic pathoanatomy (15), including the factors that contribute to instability following injury (16,17), and what may be necessary to regain this operatively (18,19), anatomic healing of the pelvis can be difficult to obtain. Therefore, many fractures heal with residual displacement. Commonly, initial radiographic fracture displacement of 1 cm cephalad and/or 15 to 20 degrees of rotation of the hemipelvis are thought to be acceptable. Less displacement may be tolerated with dislocations within the pelvic ring. These numbers represent estimates of what may be acceptable deformity at eventual union of the fracture. Greater displacements may represent malunion, because healing outside of these parameters has been associated with diminished clinical results (7,20–28), although this view is not universally held (29,30).

The diagnosis of nonunions may be difficult. Traditional radiographs may not reveal the nonunion, because it can be out of the radiographic plane or obscured by internal fixation. Some areas of the pelvis also may be slow to heal and take 6 to 12 months to unite. Areas of bridging bone may develop, but are insufficient to provide stability to the pelvic ring. Progression of fracture healing should be seen on serial radiographs, and the patient should show signs of clinical improvement with less pain or tenderness on examination. Continued pain, loss of fracture position, broken or altered position of internal fixation, no radiographic progression toward union or residual sacroiliac joint or pubic symphysis diastasis all provide clues of continued instability owing to nonunion or stability. Radiographs (anterior-posterior, obliques) centered on the area of interest, tomograms, and computed tomography (CT) scans may help to determine the extent of fracture union. Residual instability may be demonstrated with stress radiographs, including single-leg standing views (31).

SYMPTOMATOLOGY

Pain is the most common complaint following fractures of the pelvic ring. It is not limited to those fractures felt to be unstable at the time of injury (29), but is very prevalent after nonoperative treatment of the unstable fractures (20,32). Pain is also commonly reported following successful reconstruction (25,27). The etiology can be complex and related to adjacent tissue injury at the time of fracture. Lumbosacral articulations (33,34) and neurologic injury (35) are implicated as possible additional pain generators following pelvic trauma.

Deformity can be a source of pain and dysfunction following injury. Specific fractures of the anterior ring have been implicated, as having a propensity toward causing difficulties, and these so-called "tilt" fractures are com-

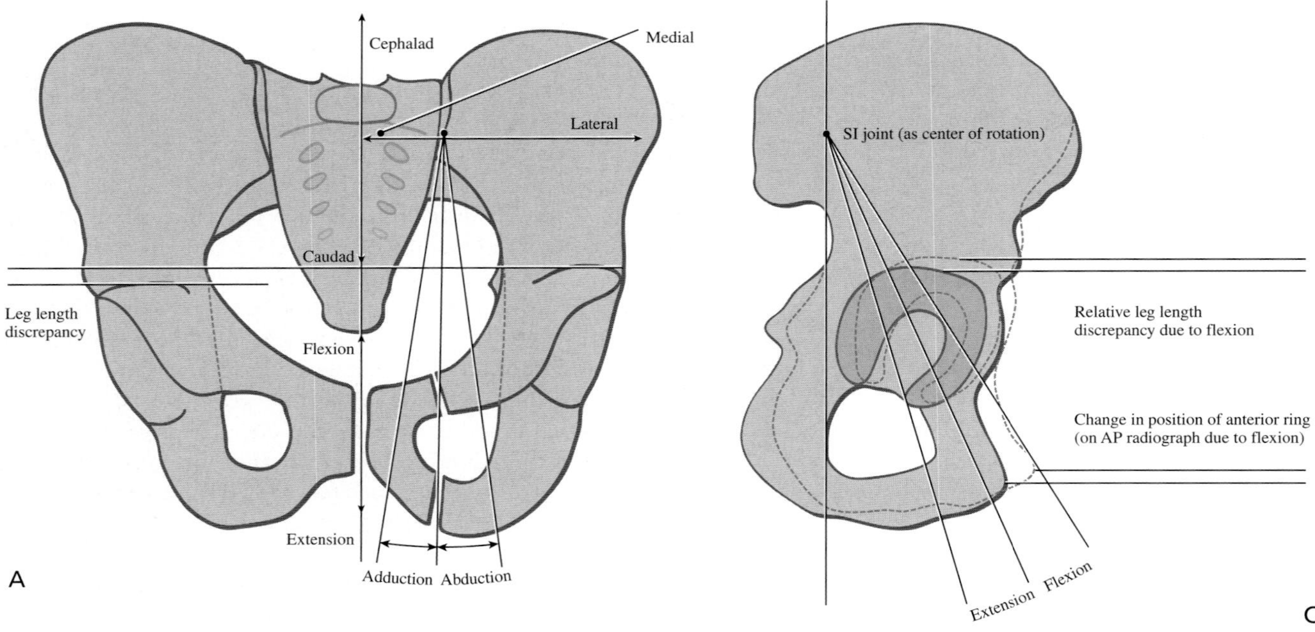

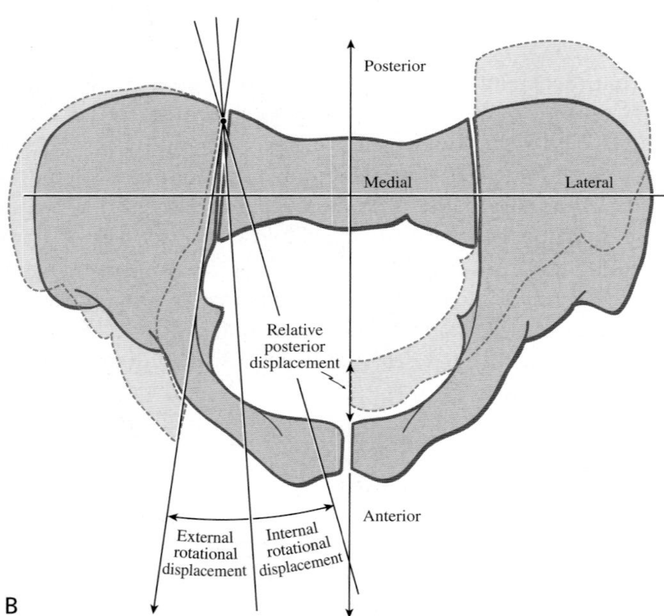

FIGURE 22-1. A: Most information regarding deformity can be obtained from the anterior-posterior (AP) pelvis. Leg length inequality (from cephalad displacement) is determined from line drawn perpendicular to the longitudinal axis of the body. Medial/lateral displacements and rotational displacements, especially abduction and adduction, also can be determined. Careful attention to the evaluation of the obturator foramen and specific anatomic features of the pelvis aid in determining rotational displacement. **B:** The caudad view frequently exhibits the greatest displacement. The view best depicts internal and external rotation of the hemipelvis, as well as medial/lateral displacements. The relative anterior or posterior displacements also are visible, but because of the physiologic tilt of the pelvis, true displacement in this direction should be determined from the computed tomography scan.**C:** Lateral view of the hemipelvis depicting flexion/extension deformity. This information is not readily available radiographically. The position of the anterior pelvic ring with respect to the posterior ring on the AP or cephalad views will help determine flexion extension rotation from these views. Cephalad/caudad displacement of the anterior ring may be apparent on the AP radiograph, resulting in the appearance of a more outlet or inlet view, respectively.

monly an indication for acute open reduction and internal fixation (ORIF) (Fig. 22-2). Residual displacement of anterior ring fractures can cause dyspareunia, urinary frequency, and chronic constipation in addition to pain. Although unlikely to cause biological difficulties with fertilization, pelvic injuries affect sexual function and may complicate subsequent delivery in the presence of deformity (36). Continued displacement or instability of posterior ring elements, especially sacral fractures, may result in persistent nerve root compression, irritation, and pain. Typical posterior and cephalad displacement of the pelvic ring results in a prominence along the posterior buttock or flank, making lying supine difficult or painful in some individuals. Residual cephalad and rotational displacement of

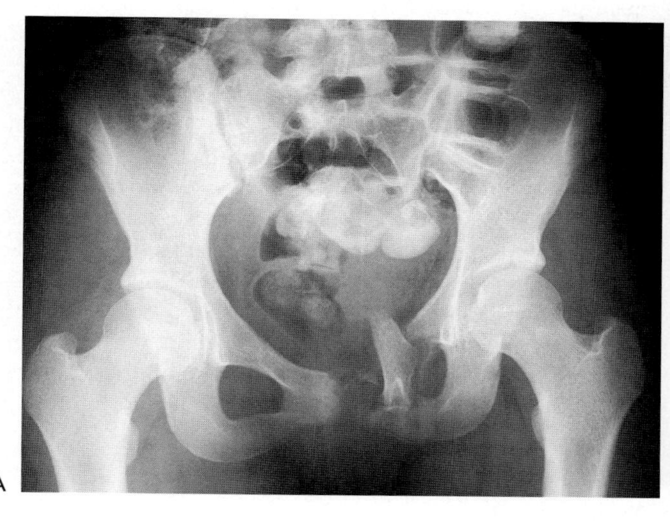
A

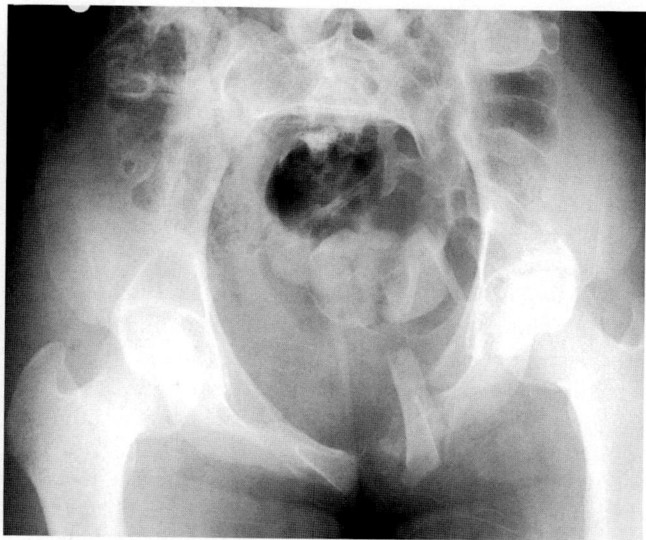
B

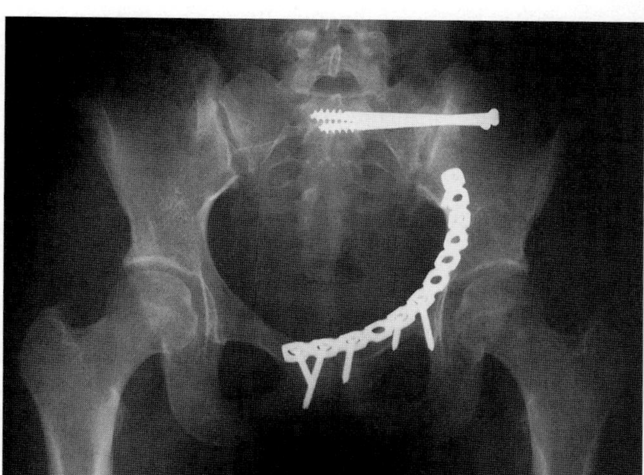
C

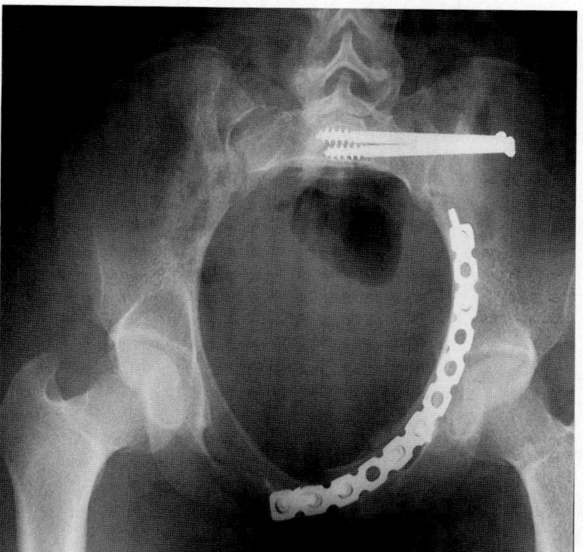
D

FIGURE 22-2. A,B: Two months following injury referred for residual displacement of L SI joint, fracture dislocation of pubic symphysis, "tilt fracture." Posterior-superior displacement of the pelvis through the SI joint, anterior deformity of the sacrum, and rotation of the pubis is apparent. **C,D:** One year following pelvic ring reconstruction and SI joint fusion performed through a single approach. Fusion obtained with acceptable alignment and clinical result.

the hemipelvis repositions the hip socket and ischial tuberosity, affecting limb length and rotation. These deformities may affect gait, sitting balance, and ultimately function, even in the absence of pain. Prolonged deformity may alter sitting or gait sufficiently to bring about compensatory motion with resulting pain and disability.

Hemipelvic instability, whether occult or obvious, also can be a source of pain. The patient may describe a sensation of limb shortening or pistoning during weight-bearing activities. Loading pain is characteristic, and occurs in the area of instability or nonunion.

PATIENT EVALUATION

History and Physical Examination

A detailed history of the injury mechanism, associated injuries, and initial treatment are necessary. Radiographs at the time of injury and during the subsequent treatment can help to define the pattern of injury, the progression of deformity, and possible areas of continued instability. If not adequately supplied by the individual or family, then obtaining the medical records from the treating hospital or physician may be necessary.

The patient's current symptoms should be documented. Pain should be quantified and the location, duration, and alleviating and exacerbating factors should be queried. Does the patient experience any numbness, paresthesias, or weakness in the lower extremities? Specific questions regarding bowel and bladder functions, or difficulties with sexual function should be asked. Finally, a description in the patient's terms of current functional difficulties should be obtained.

The patient's medical and surgical history should be detailed. The physiologic age of the patient impacts treatment decisions more than the chronological age. A full list of medications, as well as past and current narcotic needs, may give insight into the patient's requirements during the long-term or perioperative period.

Physical examination of the pelvis may reveal areas of tenderness. At times, gross instability of the pelvis can be demonstrated manually, during standing or gait. Obvious deformity can be visualized with asymmetry of skin folds, or prominence in the area of the greater trochanter or posterior pelvis. Less obvious deformities of the pelvis can be palpable along the posterior or anterior pelvic ring. Rectal and/or vaginal examinations reveal other deformities and diagnose impingement on the organs of the true pelvis.

Apparent leg lengths and hip rotation determine the effects of pelvic malposition on the lower limbs. Provocative maneuvers of the sacroiliac joint may implicate this region as a source of the patient's symptoms. A complete neurologic examination is needed to evaluate the effects of injury or treatment.

Radiographic Evaluation

Full radiographic evaluation of the pelvis is required. This includes anterior-posterior (AP), caudad, cephalad, and 45-degree oblique views of the pelvis to provide specifics of the areas injured and the resultant deformity. Overall pelvic deformity takes into consideration information from all of the views. The leg limb inequality is best determined on the AP view, and is quantified by determining the different positions of the superior articular surface of the acetabulum along a line parallel to the longitudinal axis of the body (spine, midposition of sacral promontory and body) (Fig. 22-1A). Evaluation of relative AP position is improved with the use of the caudad and cephalad views. Frequently, the caudad view demonstrates the greatest displacement. The oblique views provide additional information regarding fracture deformity within the innominate bone. A single-leg standing film may demonstrate the presence of persistent fracture or dislocation instability.

CT scans increase detail for each specific injury and can provide additional information on the status of fracture healing. CT is the best modality to quantify true posterior displacement. Internal/external rotational deformity also can be quantified using the CT scan at the level of the quadrilateral surface, and two-dimensional reconstructions in the coronal plane can reveal the amount of abduction or adduction of the hemipelvis. Three-dimensional reconstructions improve understanding of the true position of the pelvis in space, allowing visualization of the global deformity defined in part by each of the proceeding radiographic studies. The specific details provided by plain radiographs or computed tomography is lost with reconstruction, and this should not be the sole method of evaluation.

Along with determination of deformity, the amount of bone material and ability to obtain fixation and maintain the reduction following correction are important. Severe osteoporosis may be associated with age or disuse, and may be a relative contraindication to reconstruction.

Treatment

The evaluation of a patient following pelvic fracture treatment is to determine the symptoms, deformity, and existing disability. Distinguishing whether or not a given deformity is fixed or if continued instability exists, and whether or not these can be correlated with the patient's symptoms and physical and radiographic findings determines the ultimate treatment plan. This is more important than any set number for amount or degree of displacement in determining treatment. Indications for surgical treatment include pain, pelvic instability, and clinical problems related to pelvic deformity (sitting difficulties, limb shortening, and organ impingement) (2,4,5).

If it is determined that the patient would benefit from surgery based on history, physical examination, and radiographic evaluation, then the surgeon needs to determine if the individual is an appropriate candidate for surgical reconstruction. A full medical evaluation is needed and the patient should be able to comprehend and psychologically cope with an extensive surgery and rehabilitation. The patient's expectations of what can be accomplished with a surgery are important to understand. The patient should be given a detailed description of what the surgery involves, potential complications, and expected outcome.

The patient needs to understand that reconstruction is a prolonged surgery, requiring multiple incisions and is associated with an average blood loss of nearly 2,000 cc. Most patients require a blood transfusion during treatment. These surgeries are more difficult than primary pelvic reconstructions, and are associated with complications in 20% of patients, which can include bladder, nerve, or vascular injury during the procedure, with possible loss of reduction, persistent nonunion, or pain at follow-up (2). The after treatment requires limited weight bearing on the extremity for at least 3 months, with a gradual return to function over 6 to 12 months.

The patient can be informed that most benefit from the procedure, with improvements expected in sitting balance, limp, and cosmetic deformity. In the presence of demonstrable nonunion or instability, pain relief can be predictable, and an improvement in pain following reconstruction is common (2–5,37). Following this discussion, the patient should be left to make the final decision after understanding the realistic goals of surgery and accepting the risk of potential complications.

Once the decision has been made to proceed with surgery, certain elements should be in order. Expected blood loss should prompt the surgeon to bank autologous blood prior to surgery, and plan for blood salvage during the procedure. One may elect to use neurologic monitoring (38–41). Urologic or vascular colleagues should be made aware of your plans for surgery, and be available in case of emergency. A radiolucent table, fluoroscopic imaging, reduction instruments, and implants of various sizes should be available.

The surgeon then needs to develop a surgical strategy. Understanding the deformity and necessary surgical maneuvers required for reduction can be improved with the use of models created from CT data. The goal of surgical treatment is dependent on the findings of the patient evaluation and radiographic studies. The time since injury also influences technique. If instability or nonunion exists with little deformity, then the goal is to obtain stability of the pelvic ring with eventual bone union or joint stabilization, which may include fusion. The technique in the absence of deformity requires direct exposure, the possible application of bone graft, and fixation. With less delay since the time of injury or limited deformity, surgery may be done in one or two stages to approach the anterior and/or posterior ring (Fig. 22-2) (2,42).

In the presence of malunion or instability associated with significant deformity (Fig. 22-3), the goal is to obtain adequate correction of the deformity, along with stable reduction and fixation of the pelvic ring. This most commonly

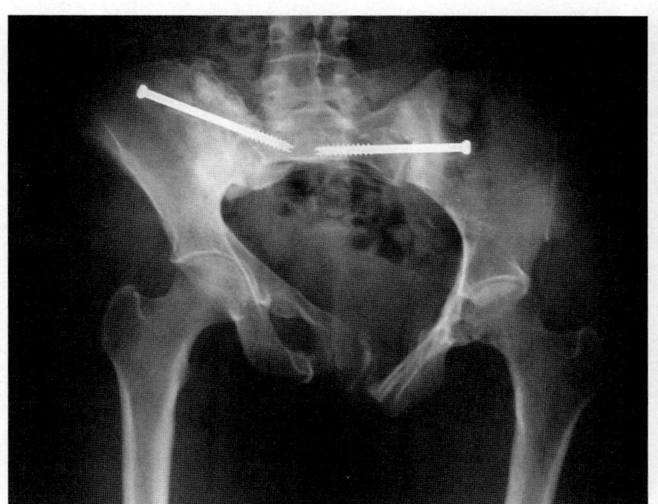
A

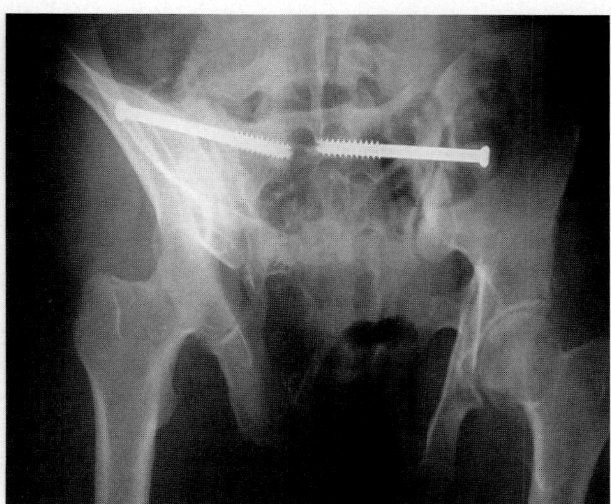
B

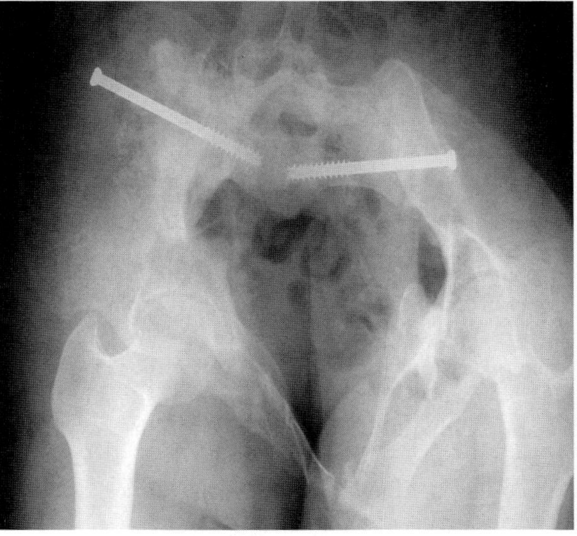
C

FIGURE 22-3. A–C: Complex posttraumatic deformity complicating initial fixation. Deformity is not limited to one side. Right hemipelvic internal rotation and adduction are accompanied by cephalad/posterior displacement. Left hemipelvis is abducted and extended. The deformity is complicated by multiple anterior ring fractures with resulting deformity. *(Figure continues)*

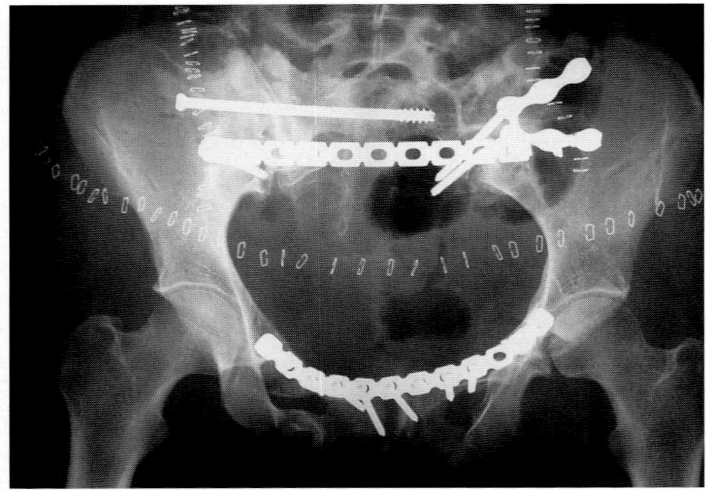

D

FIGURE 22-3. ***(continued)*** **D–F:** Reconstruction required four stages for correction of bilateral deformity. The surgery was successful, reestablishing gross pelvic morphology with minimal residual limb length discrepancy. The pelvis healed without complication and patient has had substantial improvement in the preoperative symptoms. (Courtesy of J. Matta.)

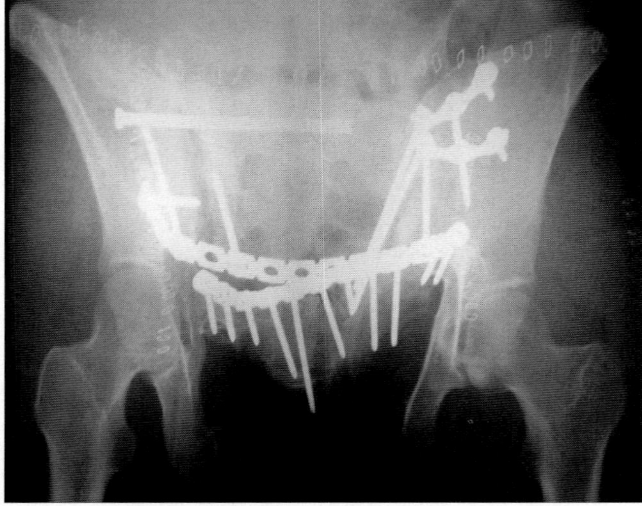

E

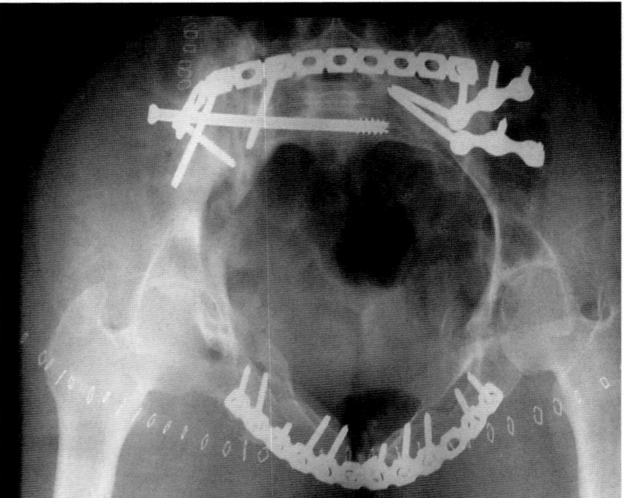

F

requires multiple stages in order to create an unstable environment in both the anterior and posterior ring to allow for correction of deformity in multiple planes. In order to accomplish this, extensive scar and callous resection, release of ligaments, and osteotomies are required (43). Anterior and posterior approaches to the pelvic ring are necessary to perform appropriate debridement and osteotomies. The approaches are best performed with the patient in the supine and prone positions in order to take full advantage of each approach. This necessitates multiple wound closures and repositioning of the patient during the procedure. The sequence of the approaches is anterior-posterior-anterior, or posterior-anterior-posterior (2,44). The sequence chosen should allow the majority of the reduction maneuver to be performed through the second approach after appropriate release of structures in the back and front of the pelvis. This decision depends on the type of initial injury, whether dislocations or fractures are present in the anterior or posterior ring, and the deformities that require correction. The posterior approach is typically used for the correction of translational deformity. Control and correction of rotational deformity can be difficult and require excessive force when working close to the axis of rotation in the posterior pelvis without the benefit of a lever arm. Therefore, anterior reduction maneuvers are best suited for correction of rotation and some translation, especially in the anterior posterior direction. Following reduction, stable internal fixation of the exposed portion of the pelvis should be obtained. The third or final approach then can be used to fine tune the reduction on the opposite side, and obtain fixation on this side of the pelvic ring. In addition to typical reduction maneuvers, novel methods for reduction have been developed in order to provide sufficient force to overcome the significant deforming forces created by scarring and healing in long-standing malunions (Fig. 22-4). The use of femoral distractors, external fixators, spinal pedicle screws, and unique screw clamp devices commonly are required. These unique methods typically require a stable environment

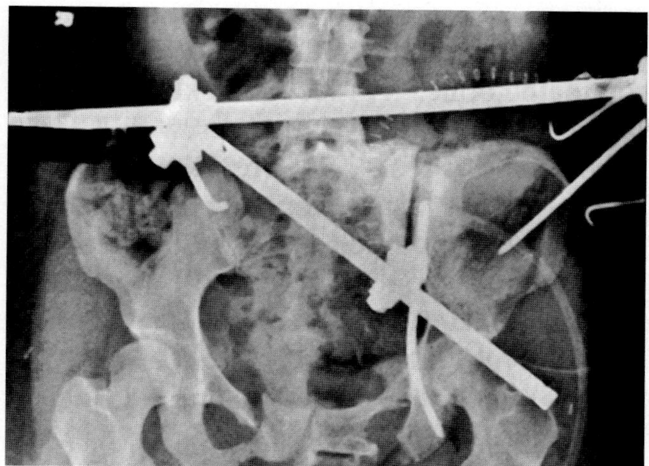

FIGURE 22-4. The novel use of the external fixator in the correction of deformity. (From: Fig. 2D from Ref. 2, with permission.)

(hemipelvis, spine) to work from in order to transmit force to and reduce the deformed hemipelvis. Deformity of both sides of the pelvis requires complex sequential release and reduction of each side of the pelvis. Without a normal hemipelvis to build to or use to generate the forces necessary for reduction, complete correction of deformity becomes much more difficult, and the goals of correction may be modified in this setting (2).

Following reduction, the choices for fixation usually are adapted from those used in treatment of acute pelvic injury. Due to the forces overcome to obtain reduction and the poor bone material that may be present from disuse or injury, larger implants, increased points of fixation, and supplementation of iliosacral screw fixation posteriorly may be necessary (Fig. 22-3).

CONCLUSION

Prevention of pelvic malunion and nonunion is the goal of pelvic injury treatment. Despite improved knowledge and education in the treatment of these injuries, significant residual deformity following treatment continues to occur. This may be a source of pain and disability to the patient. In the presence of nonunion or continued instability, the source of the problem may be clear. In the setting of fracture healing with residual deformity, the etiology may not be as obvious. Surgical reconstruction of these difficult problems remains an option for the well-informed patient. Functional improvements related to deformity can be expected and the majority of individuals experience improvement in their pain symptoms. Surgical reconstruction is very difficult and associated with a higher rate of complications than acute treatment. A substantial experience in the treatment of pelvic ring injuries is essential prior to attempting to treat this difficult problem.

REFERENCES

1. Tile M. *Fractures of the acetabulum and pelvis,* 2nd ed. Baltimore: Williams & Wilkins, 1995.
2. Matta JM, Dickson KD, Markovich GD. Surgical treatment of pelvic malunions and nonunions. *Clin Orthop* 1996;329: 199–206.
3. Mears DC. Management of pelvic pseudoarthroses and pelvic malunion. *Orthopade* 1996;25:441–448.
4. Pennal GF, Massiah KA. Nonunion and delayed union of fractures of the pelvis. *Clin Orthop* 1980;151(124):124–129.
5. Vanderschot P, Daenens K, Bros P. Surgical treatment of post-traumatic pelvic deformities. *Injury* 1998;29(1):19–22.
6. Tile M. Pelvic ring fractures: should they be fixed? *J Bone Joint Surg* 1988;70B(1):12.
7. Lindahl J, Hirvensalo E, Bostman O, et al. Failure of reduction with an external fixator in the management of injuries of the pelvic ring. *J Bone Joint Surg* 1999;81B(6):955–962.
8. Dujardin FH, Hossenbaccus M, Duparc F, et al. Long-term functional prognosis of posterior injuries in high-energy pelvic disruption. *J Orthop Trauma* 1998;12:145–150.
9. Keating JF, Werier J, Blachut P, et al. Early fixation of the vertically unstable pelvis: The role of iliosacral screw fixation of the posterior lesion. *J Orthop Trauma* 1999;13(2):107–113.
10. Routt ML Jr, Simionian PT, Mills WJ. Iliosacral screw fixation: Early complications of the percutaneous technique. *J Orthop Trauma* 1997;11(8):584–589.
11. Matta JM, Tornetta P 3rd. Internal fixation of unstable pelvic ring injuries. *Clin Orthop* 1996;329:129–140.
12. Matta JM, Saucedo T. Internal fixation of pelvic ring fractures. *Clin Orthop* 1989;242:83–97.
13. Routt ML Jr, Kregor PJ, Simionian PT, et al. Early results of percutaneous iliosacral screws placed with the patient in the supine position. *J Orthop Trauma* 1995;9:207–214.
14. Dickson KD, Matta JM. Pelvic deformity following external fixation. 1998, unpublished.
15. Bucholz R. The pathological anatomy of Malgaigne fracture-dislocations of the pelvis. *J Bone Joint Surg* 1981;63A:400–404.
16. Olson SA, Pollak AN. Assessment of pelvic ring stability after injury. *Clin Orthop* 1996;329:15–27.
17. Vrahas M, Hern TC, Diangelo D, et al. Ligamentous contributions to pelvic stability. *Orthopedics* 1995;18:271–274.
18. Leighton RK, Waddell JP, Bray TJ. Biomechanical testing of new and old fixation devices for vertical shear fractures of the pelvis. *J Orthop Trauma* 1991;5:313–317.
19. Simionian PT, Routt ML Jr. Biomechanics of pelvic fixation. *Orthop Clin North Am* 1997;28(3):351–367.
20. Henderson R. The long-term results of nonoperatively treated major pelvic disruptions. *J Orthop Trauma* 1989;3(1):41–47.
21. Kellam JF. The role of external fixators in pelvic disruptions. *Clin Orthop* 1989;241:66–82.
22. Korovessis P, Biakousis A, Stamatakis M, et al. Medium and long term results of open reduction and internal fixation for pelvic ring fractures. *Orthopedics* 2000;23(11):1165–1171.
23. Majeed SA. External fixation of the injured pelvis. *J Bone Joint Surg* 1990;72B:612–614.
24. McLaren AC, Rorabeck CH, Halpenny J. Long term pain and disability in relation to residual deformity after displaced pelvic ring fracture. *Can J Surg* 1990;33:492–494.
25. Pohlemann T, Gansslen A, Schellwald O, et al. Outcome after pelvic ring injuries. *Injury* 1996;27(Suppl):B31–B38.

26. Semba RT, Yasukawa K, Gustillo RB. Critical analysis of results of 53 Malgaigne fractures of the pelvis. *J Trauma* 1983;23: 535–537.
27. Tornetta P 3rd, Matta JM. Outcome of operatively treated unstable posterior pelvic ring disruptions. *Clin Orthop* 1996;329: 186–193.
28. Van den Bosch EW, Van der Kleyn R, Hogervorst M, et al. Functional outcome of internal fixation of pelvic ring fractures. *J Trauma* 1999;47(2):365–371.
29. Miranda MA, Reimer BL, Butterfield SL, et al. Pelvic ring injuries. A long term functional outcome study. *Clin Orthop* 1996;329:152–159.
30. Nepola JV, Trenhaile SW, Miranda MA, et al. Vertical shear injuries: Is there a relationship between residual displacement and functional outcome. *J Trauma* 1999;46(6):1024–1030.
31. Chamberlain WE. The symphysis pubis in roentgen examination of the sacroiliac joint. *Am J Roentgenol* 1930;24:621–625.
32. Holdsworth FW. Dislocations and fracture-dislocation of the pelvis. *J Bone Joint Surg* 1948;30B:461–466.
33. Isler B. Lumbosacral lesions associated with pelvic ring injuries. *J Orthop Trauma* 1990;4(1):1–6.
34. Oransky M, Gasparini G. Associated lumbosacral junction injuries (LSJIs) in pelvic fractures. *J Orthop Trauma* 1997;11(7):509–512.
35. Reilly MC, Zinar DM, Matta JM. Neurologic injuries in pelvic fractures. *Clin Orthop* 1996;329:28–36.
36. Copeland CE, Bosse MJ, McCarthy ML, et al. Effect of trauma and pelvic fracture on female genitourinary, sexual, and reproductive function. *J Orthop Trauma* 1997;11(2):73–81.
37. Blohm D, Madsen F, Jensen J. Fractures of the pelvis—a survey of "nonunion" and "malunion" surgical results. *Ugeskr Laeger* 2000;162:6413–6415.
38. Helfet DL, Hissa EA, Sergay S, et al. Somatosensory evoked potential monitoring in the surgical management of acute acetabular fractures. *J Orthop Trauma* 1991;5:161–166.
39. Moed B, Ahmad BK, Craig JG, et al. Intraoperative monitoring with stimulus-evoked electromyography during placement of iliosacral screws. *J Bone Joint Surg* 1998;80(A):537–546.
40. Vrahas M, Gordon RG, Mears DC, et al. Intraoperative somatosensory evoked potential monitoring of pelvic and acetabular fractures. *J Orthop Trauma* 1992;6:50–58.
41. Webb LX, Araujo W, Donofrio P, et al. Electromyography monitoring for percutaneous placement of iliosacral screw. *J Orthop Trauma* 2000;14(4):245–254.
42. Frigon VA, Dickson KD. Open reduction internal fixation of a pelvic malunion through an anterior approach. *J Orthop Trauma* 2001;15:519–524.
43. Gautier E, Rommens PM, Matta JM. Late reconstruction after pelvic ring injuries. *Injury* 1996;27(Suppl 2):B39–B46.
44. Letournel E. *Fractures of the acetabulum and pelvis.* Ninth AFOR Course and Workshop. Paris, 1993.

23

OUTCOMES AFTER PELVIC RING INJURIES IN ADULTS

HANS J. KREDER

INTRODUCTION

Health Outcomes and Health Measurement

The goals of treatment are to prevent injury, disease, and death; minimize disagreeable symptoms; and maximize function and well-being. Health outcomes must be defined and measured in a consistent and valid manner to compare the degree to which competing treatment strategies succeed in achieving these goals.

Traditionally, evaluation of the end result of treatment focused on radiologic outcomes or crude nonvalidated measures of pain and function that did not facilitate comparison of results from one report to the next. With the advent of validated measurement instruments, deficits in physical, social, and emotional function subsequent to injury and disease now can be consistently quantified (1).

A condition may impact on: (a) the function and integrity of a body part; (b) the performance of an individual; and (c) the involvement of an individual in a social context (2). Post and coworkers developed these concepts into an operational definition that is pertinent to the discussion of instruments for health measurement (Table 23-1) (3). They suggested that objective and subjective aspects should be considered within each of the three dimensions (body, individual, society). Objective measures focus on the performance of the body part, the individual alone, and the individual in a social context, whereas subjective measures seek to determine the individual's perception and reaction to this performance for each dimension. When taken together, the components of this matrix-dimensional structure represent the concept of well-being.

Objective determination of impairment at the body or organ level involves measures such as joint range of motion, muscle strength, and physical disfigurement. Subjectively, individuals might complain of pain, stiffness, or weakness owing to dysfunction at the organ level. Such organ dysfunction might disable that person from performing a particular task (e.g., reaching, running, or lifting). This disability is objectively measurable using questionnaires that ask about certain activities. The subjective consequences of the inability to perform a given activity may be quite varied. One individual may experience no sense of disability despite not being able to run, whereas this same physical difficulty might result in a perception of severe personal disability for another individual. Finally, a person may be unable to work, provide care, or otherwise participate in normal social activities because of a disability, with corresponding subjective consequences unique to that individual.

Health measurement instruments that sample broad aspects of mental and physical well-being are known as "generic" instruments. These instruments can be used to compare the health effects of different diseases (i.e., renal failure versus arthritis), but they may not address all of the concerns that individuals with a specific condition might have. "Disease-specific" measurement instruments are intended to evaluate specific problems experienced by individuals with a particular health condition. Disease-specific instruments generally exhibit better evaluative properties than generic tools, but they are less useful for comparing disparate health conditions. To get a more complete picture of well-being, a generic questionnaire can be supplemented with a disease-specific instrument.

TABLE 23-1. NOMENCLATURE FOR MEASURING HEALTH

	Body	Individual	Society
Objective characteristics	Impairment	Performance (disability)	Involvement (handicap)
Subjective aspects	Somatic sensations	Perceived health	Domain-specific life satisfaction

Levels of Evidence and Evidence-Based Practice

Scientific evidence to support medical and surgical intervention lies at the core of modern medicine. The "strength" (or "level") of evidence is a term meant to quantify the level of confidence that an observed result is indeed correct (4–6). Treatment recommendations can be graded by considering the strength of evidence in support of a particular management strategy. More recently, the concept of study quality has been extended to allow grading of studies concerning diagnosis, prognosis, and economic analysis (6). Evidence-based practice involves awareness, by the practicing clinician, of the strength of evidence in support of the treatment that he or she is recommending to a particular patient in the clinical setting (7).

The grade of recommendation that can be made regarding treatment options or the effect of potential prognostic factors with respect to pelvic ring injuries is grade C to D.

Functional Outcome Following Pelvic Ring Injuries

Overview

An assessment of functional outcome alone, without consideration of complications, provides an incomplete picture regarding outcome. The previous chapter covers some of the potential problems associated with pelvic ring injuries and their treatment. This information should be considered carefully when discussing treatment outcome and prognosis.

When describing the prognosis of pelvic injuries or comparing treatment options, few publications have used validated functional outcome tools to measure the end result. Moreover, those that have used such instruments often have applied them retrospectively, reporting results at a mean follow-up time within a wide range of follow-up assessment. Majeed noted that patient function improved over the first 18 months and then stabilized (8). In a prospective cohort of 366 patients with pelvic ring injuries evaluated at 6 weeks, 6 months, and annually thereafter (125 patients now at 2 years), we noted that scores in most functional domains plateau between 6 months and 1 year (Table 23-2).

Gruen and coworkers were among the first to use a validated assessment tool in describing the functional outcome after Type B and C pelvic ring injuries (9). They used the Sickness Impact Profile (SIP) (10) to describe 48 patients at a minimum of 1 year (mean 17.5 months) following Type B and C injuries. Disability as measured by the SIP was moderate for all patients in work and recreation. Although the results did not reach statistical significance, Type B1 fractures were associated with the greatest degree of disability, followed by Type C fractures, with B2 and B3 fractures demonstrating the lowest degree of disability in overall SIP scores and physical function, psychosocial function, sleep, work, home management, and recreation subscores. The same center also evaluated these 48 patients with the Oswestry back pain score (11), which is a validated measure of disability related to low back pain (12). The reported overall Oswestry score of 13.26 ± 15.41 (range 0 to 52.5) is consistent with minimal disability related to low back pain. The scores were worst for type C3 fractures (mean Oswestry score = 30.125 ± 15.8); however, the trend did not reach statistical significance. All reductions in this series of 48 patients were reportedly within 2 mm.

The Short Form (SF)36 (13,14) was first used by Oliver and coworkers to describe the outcome of 35 patients with Type B and C injuries at a mean follow-up of 2 years (range 16 to 28 months) (15). They noted a physical component score of 67.1 ± 26.3, which represents approximately 14% impairment compared with the U.S. normal population. There was no statistically significant difference between Type B and C injuries, although a separate analysis of B1 fractures was not reported. We have noted that Type B1 fractures are associated with functional results more in line with Type C fractures (Table 23-2). Therefore, their inclusion with Type B2 and B3 groups make it difficult to detect a difference between Types B and C in a small group of patients. Van den Bosch and coworkers noted significantly worse SF36 scores at 35.6 months (4 to 84 months) compared to the Dutch normal population for all but role emotional and mental health domains in 28 patients with unstable pelvic ring injuries treated operatively (16). The reported physical function score was 67.2 (standard deviation [SD] not given).

Cole and coworkers (17) evaluated 64 surgically treated Type C pelvic ring injuries with SF36 questionnaires at a mean follow-up of 36 months (range 5 to 74 months). They noted significant impairment in function with an overall mean physical function score of 61, mean role physical score of 47, and a mean bodily pain score of 61 (SDs not given). Patients with associated extremity injuries scored signifi-

TABLE 23-2. FUNCTION AFTER PELVIC FRACTURE

	Type B1	Type B2	Type C
N			
Completed 6 weeks	45	87	91
Completed 6 months	38	76	46
Completed 1 year	24	53	32
Completed 2 years	20	26	28
Gender			
Percent male	37 (82%)	40 (46%)	59 (65%)
Age			
Mean (years)	40.9	38.9	36.2
Mechanism			
Motorized vehicle	29 (64%)	64 (74%)	63 (69%)
Fall	8 (18%)	7 (8%)	9 (10%)
Sport, incl. bike	3 (7%)	6 (7%)	5 (6%)
Industry/other	5 (11%)	10 (11%)	14 (15%)
Associated Injuries			
Glasgow Coma Scale	14.7	13.3	13.6
Injury Severity Score	22.3	26.7	34.3
Spine	8 (18%)	18 (21%)	26 (29%)
Upper extremity	17 (38%)	25 (29%)	29 (32%)
Lower extremity	23 (51%)	32 (37%)	39 (43%)
Nerve Injury	4 (9%)	6 (7%)	11 (12%)
Vascular injury	2 (4%)	1 (1%)	3 (3%)
Bladder/urethral	4 (9%)	10 (11%)	20 (22%)
Open pelvic injury	1 (2%)	1 (1%)	8 (9%)
Function at 6 weeks			
SF36			
PCS_Z	−1.7	−2.8	−4.6
PF_Z	0.6	−1.3	−1.6
BP_Z	−2.0	−1.6	−4.1
MFA			
Overall	39.2	40.6	46.1
Lower extremity	56.2	56.4	63.8
Function at 6 months			
SF36			
PCS_Z	−2.1	−2.0	−2.4
PF_Z	−2.9	−2.0	−2.2
BP_Z	−1.3	−0.8	−0.9
MFA			
Overall	35.5	35.4	32.5
Lower extremity	48.3	44.8	41.8
Function at 1 year			
SF36			
PCS_Z	−2.5	−1.6	−2.7
PF_Z	−2.0	−1.0	−1.3
BP_Z	−1.3	−1.3	−2.6
MFA			
Overall	39.2	34.7	37.7
Lower extremity	54.4	43.1	49.1
Function at 2 years			
SF36			
PCS_Z	−2.6	−1.4	−2.3
PF_Z	−3.0	−1.6	−2.1
BP_Z	−1.6	−1.0	−1.3
MFA			
Overall	43.5	29.9	36.3
Lower extremity	52.3	39.0	39.6

cantly worse in almost all SF36 subscores than those without associated injuries. There was apparently no association between SF36 scores with ISS or the precise type of posterior pelvic ring injury.

Nepola and coworkers reported on 33 patients with Type C fractures and residual vertical posterior displacement of >2 mm (mean 18.1, range 2 to 52 mm) (18). Twenty-eight patients had been treated with anterior external fixation only, whereas five were treated nonoperatively. By analyzing the raw data presented in the publication, we found that the mean SF36 scores for physical function (70.3 ± 22.8), bodily pain (67.0 ± 23.8), and the physical component score (PCS) (42.2 ± 11.5) were all significantly below the normal population mean, but they were not statistically significantly lower than one SD below the normal population mean. There was no difference in SF36 scores with or without the presence of a sacral fracture in these patients.

Before validated instruments were widely used, Majeed developed a scoring system that evaluated pain, standing, sitting, sexual intercourse, and work performance (8,19). This instrument has not been validated to date. Lindahl used the Majeed score to evaluate 110 patients with unstable Type B and C pelvic injuries that had been treated with external fixation alone at a mean of 4.1 years (range 1 to 11 years) (20). The Majeed score was worst in Type C injuries (15% good and excellent), followed by Type B1 injuries (50% good and excellent). Type B2 injuries had the best outcome, with 74% good or excellent. Dujardin also noted that Type C fractures had the worst outcomes using the Majeed scoring system (21). At a mean follow-up of 4.58 years (18 months to 11.5 years), 27% of Type C fractures had a "poor" Majeed scores compared with 11% "poor" results in Type B1 fractures and no "poor" results in Type B2 fractures. Majeed scores were best for iliac wing fractures and SI fracture dislocations and worst for sacral fractures and pure SI dislocations. In Type B1 and C fractures, pure sacroiliac joint dislocations were associated with much worse Majeed scores compared to individuals with sacral fractures or fracture dislocations. The quality of reduction and presence of associated injuries may have contributed to the observed difference in scores between Tile types and the nature of the posterior injury for both of these studies. Type C fractures were associated with residual neurologic deficits in up to 40% of patients versus less than 10% in Type B fractures. Residual displacement was higher in the Type C fractures with posterior displacement >15 mm for the majority of Type C fractures in Lindahl's study (20). The evidence regarding a potential relationship between residual displacement and outcome is discussed on p. 414.

Instead of using ad hoc summary scores, other authors preferred detailed narrative descriptions to evaluate treatment outcome before the advent of validated instruments. Tornetta noted excellent results following open reduction and plating of the anterior pelvic ring in 29 patients with Type B fractures at a mean follow-up of 39 months (range 12 to 84 months) (22). Seventy-six percent had no limp, 96% had no pain or pain only with strenuous activity, and 83% returned to work (75% of these to their original jobs). There were no urologic or sexual problems identified. Despite plate breakage in four of 29 patients, this was not associated with deterioration in function and did not require reoperation. The same center evaluated operatively treated Type C fractures at a mean follow-up of 44 months (range 12 to 101 months) and noted that 63% ambulated without a limp or aides, 63% reported no pain or pain only with strenuous activity (23). Eighty-four percent overall returned to work, with 67% able to return to their usual work activity. Approximately 13% of the patients had sexual problems. Associated residual neurologic injury was noted in 35% of all patients.

Pain

Many authors have included an assessment of pain in their evaluation of patient outcome after pelvic ring injuries. Pohlemann and coworkers noted that only 34 of 58 patients (59%) were pain-free at a mean follow-up of 28 months (range 12 to 58 months) after surgical stabilization for unstable Type B and C injuries (24). Eighty-nine percent of the patients with Type B injuries were pain-free at follow-up, compared with only 30% of patients with Type C injuries.

It is generally accepted that pain is most severe after Type C injuries. Keating and coworkers noted that 85% of patients with Type C pelvic ring injuries had pain (11% severe and disabling) at a mean follow-up of 19 months (range 13 to 48 months) (25). Lindahl noted pain of moderate to severe nature in 47.5% of Type C injuries, compared with 37.5% open book injuries and 6.5% of lateral compression fractures. The Type C injuries had 40% neurologic deficits compared with 10% in Type B injuries. Associated lower extremity and lumbosacral injuries were associated with worse pain in Type C fractures at a mean follow-up of 36 month (range 5 to 74 months) (17). All patients treated by external fixation or without surgery for the anterior pelvic ring lesion complained of anterior pubic tenderness.

Few have commented regarding the location of pain after pelvic ring injury. Hakim found that Oswestry back pain scores were in the minimal disability range (13.26 overall, range from 0 to 52.5) at 1 year in B and C injuries fixed within 2 mm of anatomic (11). The scores were worst in Tile C3 fractures (mean 30.125, SD 15.8); however, the results were not statistically significant. Van den Bosch found that 61% of 37 patients with Type B and C pelvic injuries complained of pelvic pain while sitting; however, the location of pain was not precisely identified.

Return to Work and Recreation

Gruen and Hakim noted that at 1 year 76% of patients with Type B and C pelvic ring injuries who were employed prior to their injury had returned to work, with 14% requiring job modifications (9,11). Tornetta and coworkers noted a similarly high rate of return to work in patients with unstable pelvic ring injuries (22,23). Other authors have experienced less successful results with Type C injuries in terms of reintegration into the work force. Keating and coworkers noted that at a mean follow-up of 19 months (range 13 to 48), only 46% of Type C fractures had returned to their original work and 30% were on long-term disability (25). Cole and coworkers found that in Type C fractures evaluated at a mean of 36 months (range 5 to 74 months) only 41% of previous full-time workers were able to return to full-time work. Twenty-eight percent who had previously been employed full time were unemployed and 12% of previous full-time employees were employed part time (17).

There is little information available regarding impairment of recreational activities after pelvic ring injury; however, it is evident that significant restrictions in recreational activity are common. Keating and coworkers noted that only 31% of 37 patients with Type C pelvic ring injuries who were treated with iliosacral screws resumed their preinjury recreational activities at 19 months (range 13 to 48 months) (25). Thirty-one percent of patients had restricted their recreational activities and 38% were unable to perform any recreational activities.

Urologic Complaints

In a controlled study matching women with pelvic fractures to normal controls (extremity fractures without pelvic trauma) Copeland and coworkers noted urinary complaints in 21% of subjects versus 7% of controls (26). Within subjects, residual pelvic displacement ≥5 mm resulted in significantly more urinary problems than anatomically reduced pelvic injuries. Symptoms included prolonged or painful micturition and incontinence. Pohlemann and coworkers found that incontinence was more common with Type C injuries (presumably owing to sacral nerve injury), whereas problems with micturition were more commonly associated with Type B injuries (27). Residual displacement of the anterior pelvic ring is thought to be related to the development of painful or prolonged micturition; however, this has not been well studied. Nepola and coworkers reported a series of patients with residual posterior vertical displacement of the pelvic ring after Type C injury. They were unable to identify an association between sexual dysfunction or urologic problems and residual displacement (18).

Sexual Function

Type C injuries are associated with a higher risk of sexual problems than unstable Type B injuries (22,23,27). Pohlemann found erectile dysfunction in five of 40 men (12.5%) with unstable pelvic ring injuries (24). All of the men with erectile dysfunction had sustained Type C injuries. In a review of 64 Type C pelvic ring injuries, Cole and coworkers noted 19% dyspareunia in women, and 30% erectile impairment in men (17).

Corriere and coworkers noted normal erections in only 18 of 50 men (36%) with pelvic fractures and associated urethral disruptions (28). All men had undergone delayed one-stage urethroplasty. Routt and coworkers reported on 23 patients with urologic injuries treated at the same time as fixation of unstable Type B and C pelvic ring injuries (29). Three of the 18 men in this case series (16.7%) admitted to impotence at follow-up.

Copeland and coworkers noted that dyspareunia was more common with unstable pelvic fractures that had residual posterior pelvic displacement of ≥5 mm as compared with anatomically reduced injuries (43% versus 25%) (26).

Neurologic Outcomes

Nerve injury after Type C fractures is common, especially when the posterior lesion consists of a sacral fracture. Nerve dysfunction is not likely to recover fully when it occurs (23). Pohlemann and coworkers noted peroneal nerve dysfunction in 10 of 30 patients (33%) with Type C pelvic ring injuries treated with internal fixation (27). Another 12 patients (40%) reported variable sensory loss. After Type B injuries, nine of 28 patients (32%) experienced minor sensory deficits; however, there were no motor deficits in this group (27).

Keating and coworkers noted a 34% incidence of neurologic injury in Type C fractures; however, the incidence was 56% when only the Type C injuries with sacral fracture were considered (25). None of the nerve deficits recovered completely at a mean follow-up of 19 months (range 13 to 48 months). Tornetta and coworkers agreed that nerve injuries were more common after sacral fracture than pure sacroiliac joint dislocation (23). None of the nerve injuries in Type C fractures that they evaluated recovered fully despite anatomic reduction.

Range of Motion and Strength

Hakim and coworkers noted decreased lumbar spine range of motion, lift strength, stride length, and self-selected walking speed in patients with unstable Type B and Type C pelvic ring injuries compared with the normal population (11). Walking speed was most impaired with less difference from normal for stride length and lumbar mobility (9,11).

Factors Related to Outcome

Time to Fixation

Matta and Tornetta suggested that pelvic ring injuries should undergo definitive internal fixation before 21 days following injury based on their experience (30). They were able to achieve reduction to within 4 mm in 70% of patients with unstable pelvic ring injuries treated within 21 days versus 55% in those operated after 21 days; however, the difference was not statistically significant.

Worker's Safety Insurance Board/Litigation

Dujardin found that work-related injuries were associated with worse Majeed scores at mean follow-up of 4.6 years (range 18 months to 11.5 years) as compared with non–work-related injuries (21). Sixty-eight percent of those injured at work fell into the fair or poor range on the Majeed score compared with 45% fair and poor results for patients not injured at work ($p < 0.05$). Both groups of patients appeared to have a similar injury and demographic profile, although no formal statistical adjustment was made.

Open Pelvic Fractures

Brenneman noted a significant difference in SF36 physical function and role physical scores after open versus closed pelvic ring injuries, although the open fracture group contained more Type C fractures and more severe associated injuries, potentially accounting for these findings (31). Ferrera found that seven of 15 individuals with open pelvic ring injuries required assistance with activities of daily living. Six of the eight patients who remained independent had a stable pelvic ring injury that did not require surgical stabilization (32).

Residual Displacement

Few studies have examined the issue of patient function in relation to the quality of reduction in pelvic ring injuries using validated patient questionnaires. Keating and coworkers noted a trend toward worse SF36 scores, less likelihood to return to work, and less likelihood to resume normal leisure activities in patients with residual posterior displacement ranging from 1.4 cm to 2.3 cm versus those with anatomic reductions following Type C pelvic fractures treated with iliosacral screw fixation, but the numbers were too small to establish statistical significance ($p = 0.20$) (25). No details were given regarding the precise nature of the residual displacement.

Nepola and coworkers reviewed 33 patients at a mean of 7.2 years after Type C pelvic ring injuries, all with residual vertical posterior displacement of over 2 mm (range 2 to 52 mm) (18). Although the authors reported no overall association of vertical displacement and SF36 scores, a reanalysis of their data after stratifying by sacral involvement reveals that residual vertical displacement and bodily pain were significantly correlated (Spearman's rho $= -0.593$, $p = 0.025$) in patients where the posterior injury was a sacral fracture but not in patients without sacral fracture. Sacral fractures are associated with a higher likelihood of nerve injury, which may affect outcome.

Using his nonvalidated score, Majeed noted that patient function and anatomic result were correlated; however, he noted that a poor anatomic result could be associated with good or excellent function (8). Dujardin and coworkers noted improved Majeed scores in patients with Type B1 and C pelvic ring injuries that were left with <5 mm residual vertical and anterior-posterior displacement versus those with >5 mm displacement at a mean follow-up of 4.6 years (range 18 months to 11.5 years) (21). There was also a trend for better scores with less residual displacement in Type B2 pelvic ring injuries; however, the result was not statistically significant. The quality of the reduction seemed to be particularly important in pure SI joint dislocations, and least important in iliac wing fractures (21).

Lindahl and coworkers noted that in Type B1 and B2 injuries with residual rotation and vertical displacement at the pubic symphysis = 10 mm the pain and Majeed scores were worse than if displacement was <10 mm (20). They also noted that residual vertical displacement of ≥ 10 mm at the posterior ring in Type C fractures was associated with worse pain and Majeed scores compared with injuries that healed with <10 mm residual posterior vertical displacement.

Tornetta and Matta noted no difference in pain for Type C fractures reduced to within 4 mm versus those reduced to 4 to 10 mm (23).

Copeland and coworkers noted more urinary complaints in women with pelvic fractures displaced ≥ 5 mm versus anatomically reduced pelvic injuries (33% versus 14%) (26). Dyspareunia was also more common in patients with residual displacement (43% versus 25%). Initial displacement was related to an increased likelihood of requiring cesarean section (80% versus 15%) even after adjusting for previous cesarean section.

Operative Versus Nonoperative

The effects of the pelvic ring injury, associated neurologic injury, and residual displacement are difficult to disentangle. It may be that these factors are more important than the type of treatment in determining the final outcome. The more unstable the injury, the more difficult it is to control displacement using nonoperative means, leading many surgeons to recommend operative reduction and stable fixation for these injuries as a matter of routine. Lindahl noted that malunion was very common (64%) in patients with unstable Type B and C pelvic ring disruptions treated with external fixation with or without traction, however he removed the external fixation frame early at a mean of 6.4 weeks (range 6 to 11 weeks) (20).

Some have argued that fixation of even relatively stable pelvic ring injuries may speed patient recovery by improving mobility and reducing pain (Routt ML, personal communication, 1999); however, there is little direct evidence in the published literature regarding this issue. Prospective comparative studies are needed to evaluate the potentially beneficial effects of early stabilization, risks of surgery, and risks associated with traction and other conservative treatment methods.

Pohlemann and coworkers noted that there tended to be less residual posterior displacement with Type C pelvic ring injuries after fixing both the front and back (27). They noted that there seemed to be a correlation between good reduction and good clinical outcome, although no validated tools were used and no statistics were reported. Despite an excellent reduction, there was still a 20% rate of "fair" clinical results, suggesting that other factors were important in determining patient function besides the quality of reduction.

Cole and coworkers noted that pain in Type C pelvic ring injuries was worse at a mean follow-up of 36 months (range 5 to 74 months) when there were associated lumbosacral injuries or associated musculoskeletal injuries involving the lower extremities (17). The authors also noted that all patients who were treated either nonoperatively or with external fixation (versus internal fixation) for the anterior pelvic ring injury complained of anterior pubic tenderness.

In a review of 31 patients at a mean follow-up of 35.6 months, Van den Bosch and coworkers noted that posterior pelvic fixation was associated with better SF36 scores in patients with Type B and C pelvic ring injuries versus those with only anterior pubic ring fixation plus or minus external fixation (16). The amount of residual displacement was not quantified and precise type of posterior injury was not reported. The fact that six of 31 patients (19%) had leg length discrepancy >1 cm (three patients >2 cm) suggests that reduction was not anatomic in at least some of the patients.

CONCLUSION

A displaced pelvic ring injury results in significant long-term functional compromise and pain in most patients. Although a well-reduced pelvic ring injury is more likely to be associated with good functional outcome than a malunited fracture, even anatomically reduced injuries can be associated with severe residual pain, impairment, and disability. Functional outcome is worst for Type C injuries, followed by Type B1 injuries. Type B2 injuries generally have the best outcome.

Nerve injuries are most common when the posterior injury involves a displaced sacral fracture (Type C injuries). They are unlikely to resolve completely. Sexual dysfunction, prolonged and painful micturition, and incontinence are observed in a significant minority of patients with displaced pelvic ring injuries.

Prospective outcome studies are needed to better understand the relationship among outcome, type of injury, treatment, and residual displacement.

REFERENCES

1. Kreder HJ, Wright JG, McLeod R. Outcome studies in surgical research. *Surgery* 1997;121:223–225.
2. World Health Organization. *International Classification of Functioning, Disability and Health (ICF).* Geneva: World Health Organization, 2002.
3. Post MW, de Witte LP, Schrijvers AJ. Quality of life and the ICIDH: towards an integrated conceptual model for rehabilitation outcomes research. *Clin Rehab* 1999;13:5–15.
4. Cook DJ, Guyatt GH, Laupacis A, et al. Clinical recommendations using levels of evidence for antithrombotic agents. *Chest* 1995;108(Suppl):227S–230S.
5. Guyatt GH, Sackett DL, Sinclair JC, et al. Users' guides to the medical literature. IX. A method for grading health care recommendations. Evidence-Based Medicine Working Group. *JAMA* 1995;274:1800–1804.
6. Sackett DL, Strauss SE, Richardson WS, et al. *Evidence based medicine: how to practice and teach EBM,* 2nd ed. Toronto: Churchill Livingstone, 2000.
7. Kreder HJ. Evidence-based surgical practice: what is it and do we need it? *World J Surg* 1999;23:1232–1235.
8. Majeed SA. External fixation of the injured pelvis. The functional outcome. *J Bone Joint Surg Br* 1990;72:612–614.
9. Gruen GS, Leit ME, Gruen RJ, et al. Functional outcome of patients with unstable pelvic ring fractures stabilized with open reduction and internal fixation. *J Trauma* 1995;39:838–844.
10. Bergner M, Bobbitt RA, Carter WB, et al. The Sickness Impact Profile: development and final revision of a health status measure. *Med Care* 1981;19:787–805.
11. Hakim RM, Gruen GS, Delitto A. Outcomes of patients with pelvic-ring fractures managed by open reduction internal fixation. *Phys Ther* 1996;76:286–295.
12. Fairbank JC, Couper J, Davies JB, et al. The Oswestry low back pain disability questionnaire. *Physiotherapy* 1980;66:271–273.
13. Ware JE Jr, Sherbourne CD. The MOS 36-item short-form health survey (SF-36). I. Conceptual framework and item selection. *Med Care* 1992;30:473–483.
14. Ware JE Jr, Kosinski M, Bayliss MS, et al. Comparison of methods for the scoring and statistical analysis of SF-36 health profile and summary measures: summary of results from the Medical Outcomes Study. *Med Care* 1995;33(Suppl):AS264–AS279.
15. Oliver CW, Twaddle B, Agel J, et al. Outcome after pelvic ring fractures: evaluation using the medical outcomes short form SF-36. *Injury* 1996;27:635–641.
16. Van den Bosch EW, Van der KR, Hogervorst M, et al. Functional outcome of internal fixation for pelvic ring fractures. *J Trauma* 1999;47:365–371.
17. Cole JD, Blum DA, Ansel LJ. Outcome after fixation of unstable posterior pelvic ring injuries. *Clin Orthop* 1996;(329):160–179.
18. Nepola JV, Trenhaile SW, Miranda MA, et al. Vertical shear injuries: is there a relationship between residual displacement and functional outcome? *J Trauma* 1999;46:1024–1029.
19. Majeed SA. Grading the outcome of pelvic fractures. *J Bone Joint Surg Br* 1989;71:304–306.
20. Lindahl J, Hirvensalo E, Bostman O, et al. Failure of reduction with an external fixator in the management of injuries of the pelvic ring. Long-term evaluation of 110 patients. *J Bone Joint Surg Br* 1999;81:955–962.
21. Dujardin FH, Hossenbaccus M, Duparc F, et al. Long-term functional prognosis of posterior injuries in high-energy pelvic disruption. *J Orthop Trauma* 1998;12:145–150.
22. Tornetta P, Dickson K, Matta JM. Outcome of rotationally unstable pelvic ring injuries treated operatively. *Clin Orthop* 1996;(329):147–151.
23. Tornetta P, Matta JM. Outcome of operatively treated unstable

posterior pelvic ring disruptions. *Clin Orthop* 1996;(329): 186–193.
24. Pohlemann T, Gansslen A, Schellwald O, et al. Outcome after pelvic ring injuries. *Injury* 1996;27(Suppl):B31–B38.
25. Keating JF, Werier J, Blachut P, et al. Early fixation of the vertically unstable pelvis: the role of iliosacral screw fixation of the posterior lesion. *J Orthop Trauma* 1999;13:107–113.
26. Copeland CE, Bosse MJ, McCarthy ML, et al. Effect of trauma and pelvic fracture on female genitourinary, sexual, and reproductive function. *J Orthop Trauma* 1997;11:73–81.
27. Pohlemann T, Tscherne H, Baumgartel F, et al. [Pelvic fractures: epidemiology, therapy and long-term outcome. Overview of the multicenter study of the Pelvis Study Group]. *Unfallchirurg* 1996;99:160–167.
28. Corriere JN, Rudy DC, Benson GS. Voiding and erectile function after delayed one-stage repair of posterior urethral disruptions in 50 men with a fractured pelvis. *J Trauma* 1994;37: 587–589.
29. Routt ML, Simonian PT, Defalco AJ, et al. Internal fixation in pelvic fractures and primary repairs of associated genitourinary disruptions: a team approach. *J Trauma* 1996;40:784–790.
30. Matta JM, Tornetta P. Internal fixation of unstable pelvic ring injuries. *Clin Orthop* 1996;(329):129–140.
31. Brenneman FD, Katyal D, Boulanger BR, et al. Long-term outcomes in open pelvic fractures. *J Trauma* 1997;42:773–777.
32. Ferrera PC, Hill DA. Good outcomes of open pelvic fractures. *Injury* 1999;30:187–190.

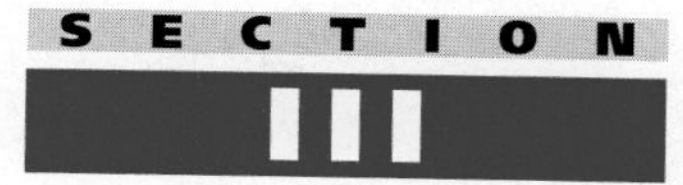

FRACTURES OF THE ACETABULUM

24

INTRODUCTION AND NATURAL HISTORY OF ACETABULAR FRACTURES

MARVIN TILE

INTRODUCTION

In the first edition of this book, I began the section on acetabular fractures with the statement, *"Fractures of the acetabulum remain an enigma to the orthopedic surgeon."* That statement is still true, although great strides have been made to the management of this fracture in the past decades. As we begin the new millennium, many questions about acetabular injuries remain unanswered, but the questions are different: Can we agree on what sorts of fractures are best treated operatively and what sorts nonoperatively (especially those fractures occurring in the older age group)? What is the role of total hip arthroplasty in management? Finally, many questions on the safest and most useful surgical approach, techniques of reduction, and avoidance of complications have been answered, but questions remain on the role of minimally invasive techniques. In spite of general acceptance of the principles in management of articular fractures—namely, *anatomic reduction, stable fixation, and early motion*—factors such as comminution and complications continue to result in about 20% of patients having less than perfect results. Acetabular fractures are relatively uncommon; therefore, the average orthopedic surgeon never gains wide experience with them, so the question of who should treat acetabular fractures is important. Clearly, this has become a subspecialty within orthopedic trauma; therefore, these fractures should only be operated on by surgeons with some specialized training. In the past decade, the literature has reached a greater consensus, but some problems remain, and few studies incorporating standard outcome measures are available.

The surgeon perusing the literature must learn to read between the lines. Only fractures of similar type and severity may be logically—and productively—compared; otherwise the results are meaningless. Comparison of a relatively undisplaced crack fracture of the acetabulum with a severely displaced centrally dislocated one is like comparing an apple to an orange (Fig. 24-1); yet the literature is full of such comparisons.

As readers will see in the ensuing paragraphs, a critical appraisal of the reports in the literature reveals a high degree of agreement between the authors; namely, that if displaced fractures involving the weight-bearing surface of the acetabulum are left unreduced, patients fare poorly, no matter what the treatment.

Therefore, if a fracture to this major weight-bearing joint is displaced, causing *incongruity or instability to the hip joint,* the ideal treatment is: (a) anatomic reduction to prevent secondary osteoarthritis; and (b) early motion to restore function to the joint. Joint congruity may be achieved and maintained by closed means, in which case the results usually are satisfactory. However, if incongruity between the femoral head remains after closed reduction, surgical intervention is the only logical alternative, but only when it is technically possible. This principle of fracture care is widely accepted; however, many factors can prevent the surgeon from achieving the desired goals. The age of the patient is important, especially as it relates to the state of the bone. Osteopenia may prevent stable fixation; the secondary consequence is loss of reduction. Extreme comminution and the complications associated with these difficult procedures can compromise the end result, even in the hands of experienced surgeons.

In summary, anatomic reduction and stable fixation are the mainstays of treatment for unstable, incongruous fractures of the acetabulum. Nonoperative care (meaning early ambulation and protective weight-bearing) gives good results for fractures that are stable and congruous. The role of skeletal traction should be limited to emergency care only; its role in definitive care should be very limited.

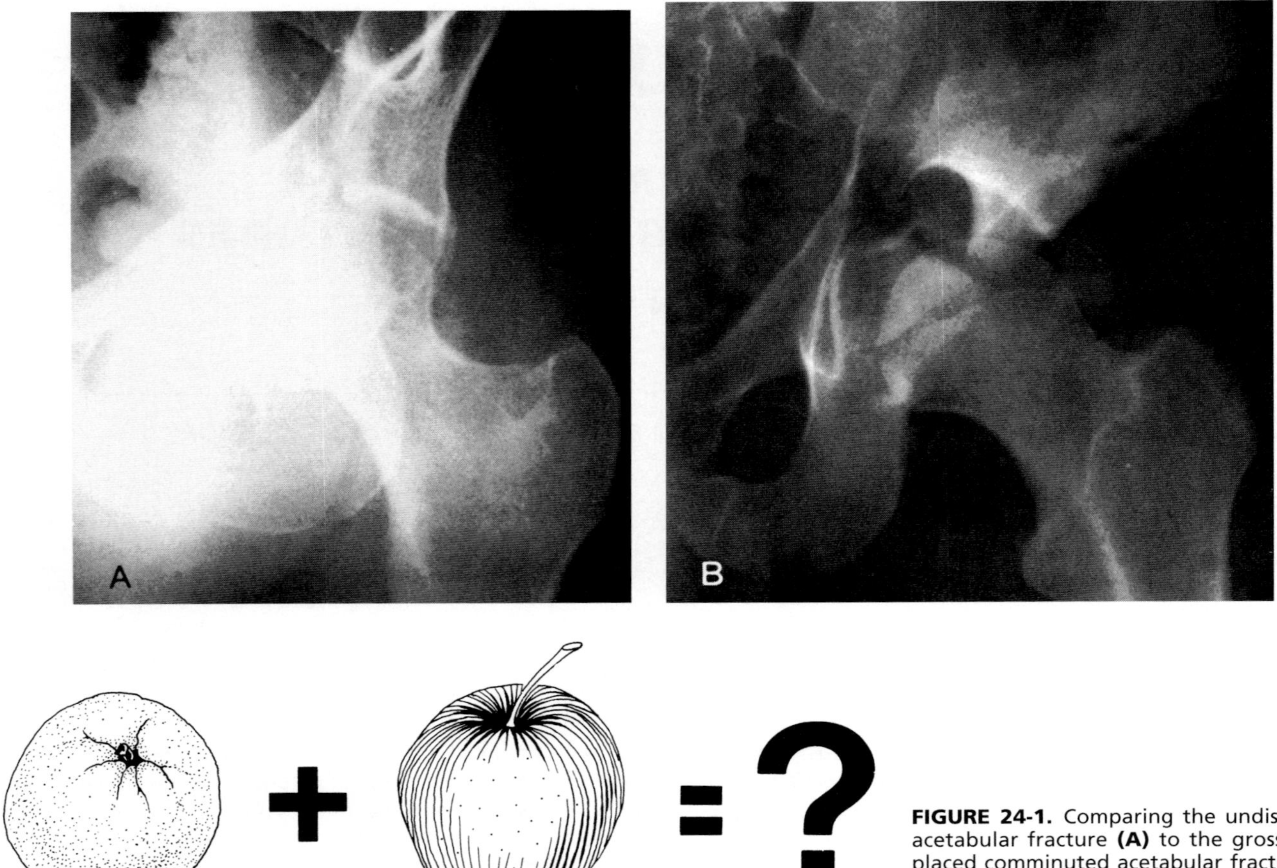

FIGURE 24-1. Comparing the undisplaced acetabular fracture **(A)** to the grossly displaced comminuted acetabular fracture associated with a pelvic ring disruption **(B)** is like comparing an orange to an apple **(C).**

Finally, there may be a role for early total hip arthroplasty in the older patient with extreme comminution, but only in cases where the hip is incongruous or unstable. If secondary congruity is present (e.g., both-column fracture in the same elderly population), then it is wise to treat the patient nonoperatively by early ambulation and progressive weight bearing, with the expectation of a satisfactory result. If not, then late total hip arthroplasty may be performed when necessary.

NATURAL HISTORY

The major authors on this subject, whether they recommend closed or open treatment, agree on this basic principle: Congruity between the femoral head and the acetabulum is essential for consistently good results. Anyone who assesses the overall results of this injury in the various published reports may be left with a confusing picture, because the proportion of significantly displaced fractures varies from article to article. It is not the overall results that are important, because they could reflect a large proportion of the "inconsequential fractures," those in which the superior or posterior acetabular wall is intact. The results of the significantly displaced fractures are more relevant. In any review of the important articles, only like fractures should be compared.

Early reports in the literature had so few cases as to be insignificant, but even so, trends were established (1–9). In 1961 Rowe and Lowell reported on 93 fractures in 90 patients who received their initial treatment at the Massachusetts General Hospital (10). This article has been frequently quoted by those who favor nonoperative treatment of acetabular fractures. A careful study of this paper, however, emphasizes the importance of relating the final result to the type of fracture. As expected, patients with linear crack fractures without displacement fared extremely well. On the other hand, patients with fractures of the posterior rim associated with a posterior dislocation required open reduction if instability of the hip persisted after closed reduction; otherwise, results were poor. All six of 17 patients treated by closed management had a poor result. Of the 11 patients who had a satisfactory result, eight were treated by open reduction and internal fixation; the stability of the remaining three fractures after reduction obviated surgery.

The results of the 26 cases in which the superior weight-bearing dome was involved were related directly to the degree of congruity between the femoral head and the dome that was achieved. If the dome was reduced to anatomic position, 13 of 15 patients had a satisfactory result, whereas without that reduction, 10 of 10 had a poor result. *

The largest group of patients (29) had a fracture of the medial wall and/or the anterior column. Twenty-six percent were older than 40 years, and all had an intact superior dome. When congruity could be restored by reduction and maintained by traction, 90% achieved a satisfactory clinical result, and 83% a satisfactory radiologic result. Therefore, a good result may be expected if congruity is restored between the femoral head and the dome. These authors concluded that the final result was related to: (a) restoration of perfect congruity between the femoral head and the dome fragment; (b) the amount of femoral head damage; and (c) the stability of the joint after reduction.

Lessons are to be learned by careful examination of this classic paper. First, high-energy injuries that result in hip instability (the posterior types) and/or disruption of the acetabular roof or dome, especially in younger persons, require anatomic reduction (usually open) for satisfactory long-term results. For older persons who sustain medial wall or anterior column disruption, satisfactory results may be obtained by traction that maintains relative congruity of the femoral head and the acetabulum. Many of the patients in this older age group were those with both-column fractures with secondary congruence, which are known to have a good prognosis with nonoperative care.

Larson, and the groups of Carnesale and Pennal came to similar conclusions (11–13). In Pennal's series of 103 patients (Table 24-1), 66 had residual displacement at the time of review and 72% had radiographically demonstrable degenerative changes. Of the 37 who had little displacement, only 30% had these changes.

In 1964, Judet and coworkers recommended open reduction and internal fixation for all displaced acetabular fractures (14). They proposed a classification of these fractures, based on the pattern of injury. Subsequently, in further reports and in their published text (15), they reported the results of the surgical treatment of 350 cases of acetabular fracture. Using strict criteria, 75.2% were rated *very good* (i.e., a normal or nearly normal hip), 8.3% good, and 16.5% poor. The satisfactory results varied with fracture type in their classification. More interesting was the close correlation between the clinical result and the quality of reduction achieved: Of the 74% of patients for whom anatomic reduction was achieved, 90% had a satisfactory clinical result. For the 26% of the fractures that were imperfectly reduced, the statistics

TABLE 24-1. RESULTS OF ALL TREATMENT METHODS

Displacement	Cases (No)	Degenerative Change (%)	Average Hip Rating
Residual pelvic displacement	66	72	14.5
No residual pelvic displacement	37	30	16.1

Source: Pennal GF, et al. Results of treatment of acetabular fractures. *Clin Orthop* 1980;151:115.

are these: The result was judged satisfactory for 55% when the head was centered under the acetabular dome; for 54.2% when there was loss of parallelism of the joint space; for 11% when protrusion was present; and for 9% when the attempt to reconstruct the acetabular dome failed. The combined operative complications accounted for 16% of the poor results.

Senegas and colleagues recommended closed reduction under general anesthesia for all displaced acetabular fractures (16). In 42 of 71 cases, congruity between the femoral head and the dome of the acetabulum was not achieved. In the 28 patients who were managed surgically through the lateral transtrochanteric approach, 85% had satisfactory results and only 15% unsatisfactory ones. Malreduction, avascular necrosis, and heterotopic calcification accounted for the poor results.

Ruggieri and associates discussed the results of follow-up on 188 surgically treated acetabular fractures in a cohort of 356 such injuries (17). Anatomic reduction resulted in good long-term results if complications were avoided. Early complications included avascular necrosis (four cases), sciatic nerve palsy (six cases), deep infection (three cases), heterotopic ossification (12 cases), and Sudeck's atrophy (12 cases). The investigators were able to follow 58 patients for 5 years. Their rate of "radiographic osteoarthritis" was 12%, 9% clinically significant. After 10 years, an additional 32 patients (16%) had radiographic osteoarthritis, of which 12.5% were clinically significant.

In 1986, Matta and coworkers did a retrospective radiographic analysis of 204 acetabular fractures. Sixty-four displaced fractures included in this analysis were also assessed clinically, and 43 of these were treated surgically. Average time of follow-up was 3.7 years (18). In this paper they introduced the concept that the percentage of intact dome could be used to determine whether to manage a fracture nonoperatively, an approach based on the biomechanics studies of Day and coworkers (19). If a 45-degree angle was maintained in the dome, nonoperative treatment could reasonably be considered, but if the angle was smaller than 30 degrees, operative treatment was indicated. Of the 21 displaced fractures treated in traction for an average of 7 weeks,

* In the report, only eight of ten case results were judged poor; however, the only two patients whose result was reported satisfactory had been treated with cup arthroplasty. This really represents failure of primary treatment.

TABLE 24-2. CLINICAL GRADE OF 64 FRACTURES TREATED BY OPEN AND CLOSED METHODS

Method of Treatment	Total	Grade			
		Poor	Fair	Good	Excellent
Closed	21	12	4	4	1
Open	43	15	11	17	0

Source: Matta JM, et al. Fractures of the acetabulum. *Clin Orthop* 1986;205:224.

TABLE 24-4. DISTRIBUTION OF CLINICAL GRADES WITHIN EACH RADIOGRAPHIC GRADE

Radiographic Grade	Clinical Grade			
	Poor	Fair	Good	Excellent
Excellent	0	0	2	0
Good	1	1	13	1
Fair	3	11	6	0
Poor	23	3	0	0

Source: Matta JM, et al. Fractures of the acetabulum. *Clin Orthop* 1986;205:234.

results for only five (24%) were good to excellent; for 16 (76%) results were fair to poor. Of 43 fractures treated surgically (all through posterior approaches and only three with an additional Smith-Petersen approach), 17 of 43 were good to excellent (40%), and 26 fair to poor (60%) (Table 24-2). There was good correlation between the clinical and radiographic results (Tables 24-3 through 24-5). The complications, other than inability to obtain anatomic reduction, included wound infection (9%), iatrogenic nerve injury (9%), pulmonary embolism (2%), and avascular necrosis (9%) in the operative group and 24% in the nonoperative group. The investigators concluded that closed treatment is satisfactory for displaced fractures only if the weight-bearing dome is intact. Anatomic reduction, in the absence of complications, significantly improves the prognosis. The radiographic results correlate closely with the clinical result, and open reduction and internal fixation is recommended for the majority of displaced acetabular fractures. Preferably, such techniques should be undertaken by surgeons with specific interests and training.

Matta and colleagues, in 1988 reported on his prospective study of 121 cases of displaced acetabular fractures (minimum displacement, 5 mm) in 118 patients (20). Most were young victims of motor vehicle trauma: 23 were treated in traction; 98 by open reduction and internal fixation—through a Kocher-Langenbeck approach in 55 cases, an extended iliofemoral approach in 19, and an ilioinguinal approach in 26. Seventy-four fractures were reviewed at a minimum of 26 months' follow-up. Closed treatment with traction resulted in six of nine (66%) good to excellent results. These were largely both-column fractures with secondary congruence. Open reduction and internal fixation resulted in 54 of 65 (83%) good to excellent results (Tables 24-6 and 24-7). Radiographic analysis indicated that displacement of 3 mm or more was unsatisfactory, <3 mm was satisfactory, and <1 mm was anatomic. Using these criteria, 91% of results were satisfactory and only 63% anatomic. Figures 24-2 and 24-3 are graphic examples of the learning curve: They demonstrate how, for any surgeon, the number of unsatisfactory cases declines with experience and the number of anatomic reductions increases.

In 1989, Goulet and Bray discussed operative treatment of complex (associated-type) fractures (21). Of a total of 116 cases 31 fell into these categories, including 13 with fractures of both columns, seven T types, and 11 others with an average of 21 months' follow-up. Their average age was 30 years, the injury severity score 15, and the interval from injury to surgery rather long—on average, 13.5 days. The authors recommend two approaches rather than a single extensile approach, the anterior approach being ilioinguinal, the posterior one Kocher-Langenbeck. A fracture table was not used. The patient was in a floppy lateral position, and an AO distraction was recommended. Again, the clinical results corresponded well to the anatomic radiographic results. Radiographically, anatomic reduction was achieved in 26 of 31 cases. Clinically, 24 results were good to excellent; seven, fair to poor. There was one instance of deep infection, one of avascular necrosis, and one of heterotopic ossification that required excision. Follow-up time is short in this series; but, again, findings point out the correlation

TABLE 24-3. CLINICAL AND RADIOGRAPHIC GRADE OF 64 ACETABULAR FRACTURES AT FOLLOW-UP

Grade	Poor (%)	Fair (%)	Good (%)	Excellent (%)
Radiographic	41	31	25	3
Clinical	42	23	33	2

Source: Matta JM, et al. Fractures of the acetabulum. *Clin Orthop* 1986;205:234.

TABLE 24-5. COMPARISON OF CLINICAL GRADE FOR FRACTURES REDUCED TO 3 MM DISPLACEMENT AND FRACTURES NOT REDUCED

Reduction	Total	Poor	Fair	Good	Excellent
Displacement ≤13 mm	11	0	1	10	0
Displacement >3 mm	53	27	14	11	1

Source: Matta JM, et al. Fractures of the acetabulum. *Clin Orthop* 1986;205:234.

TABLE 24-6. CLINICAL RESULTS IN 74 PATIENTS

	Closed Treatment (No)	Open Treatment (No)
Excellent	3	14
Good	3	40
Fair	-	10
Poor	3	1

Source: Matta JM, Merrit PO. Displaced acetabular fractures. *Clin Orthop* 1988;230:96.

TABLE 24-7. OVERALL RESULTS IN 74 PATIENTS

	Clinical (%)	Roentgenographic (%)
Excellent	22	45
Good	58	35
Fair	14	14
Poor	6	6

Source: Matta JM, Merrit PO. Displaced acetabular fractures. *Clin Orthop* 1988;230:96.

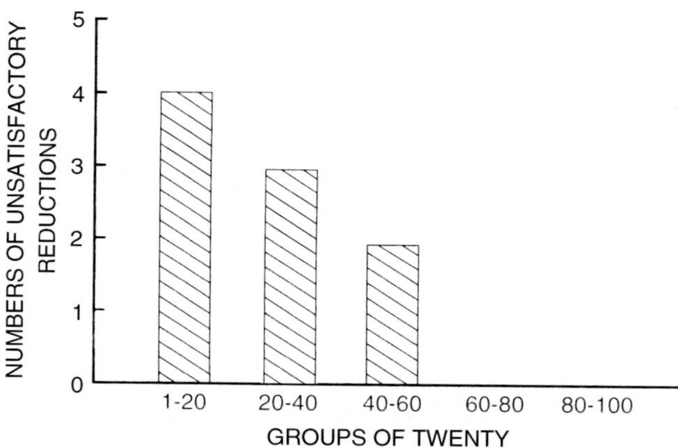

FIGURE 24-2. Number of unsatisfactory reductions per group of 20 for the first 100 surgical cases. (From: Matta IM, Merritt PO. Displaced acetabular fractures. *Clin Orthop* 1988;230:83, with permission.)

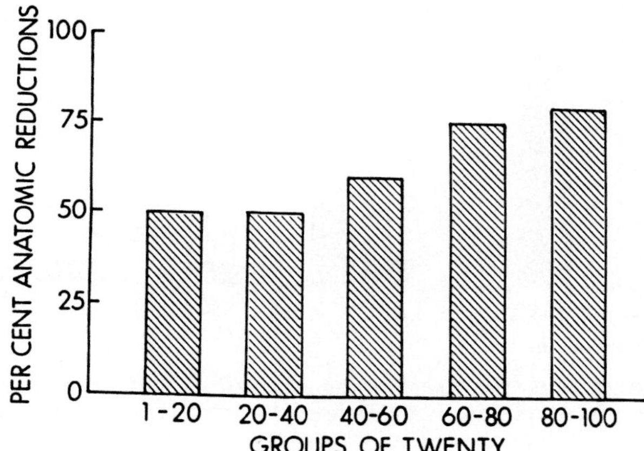

FIGURE 24-3. Percentage of anatomic reductions per group of 20 for first 100 surgical cases. (From: Matta IM, Merritt PO. Displaced acetabular fractures. *Clin Orthop* 1988;230:83, with permission.)

TABLE 24-8. CLINICAL AND ROENTGENOGRAPHIC RESULTS IN 58 PATIENTS

Result	Clinical (No) (%)	Roentgenographic (No) (%)
Excellent	18 (31)	22 (38)
Good	25 (43)	20 (34)
Fair	7 (12)	5 (9)
Poor	8 (14)	11 (19)

Source: Pantazopoulos T, Mousafiris C. Surgical treatment of central acetabular fractures. *Clin Orthop* 1989;246:61.

between anatomic reduction and clinical results of surgery, *if complications are avoided.* With the use of two separate incisions the complication rate was low.

Pantazopoulos and Mousafiris in 1989 reviewed 58 of a total of 65 available patients who had been treated with open reduction and internal fixation of their pelvic fractures, on average, $5\frac{1}{2}$ years earlier (22). Most of the fractures were of the associated complex variety, and those polytrauma victims were of a young age group. In virtually all cases, definitive treatment was delayed and the patient was treated in skeletal traction until surgery. According to Matta's classification of radiographic reduction, 38% of reductions were anatomic; 43%, satisfactory; and 19%, unsatisfactory. Table 24-8 shows that 74% of the patients had good to excellent results, and this correlated with the 72% satisfactory radiographic appearance. Again, the correlation between surgical reduction and clinical results was good (Table 24-9). Overall, 31% of the patients had radiographic evidence of osteoarthritis. Other complications included one infection, which resulted in a fused hip; two pulmonary emboli, which resolved; five sciatic nerve injuries, none of which resolved completely; six cases of heterotopic ossification that restricted motion more than 30%; and five cases of avascular necrosis.

In 1989 Ylinen and colleagues reviewed 74 patients with 75 fractures in a 7-year follow-up, but were able to recall only 43 for direct follow-up (23). Twelve of the patients had died (two from injuries resulting from a second episode of trauma). In general, this was also a polytrauma group, but the average age was much older: 37 years for the men (47 patients) and 52 years for the women (27 patients). Also in

TABLE 24-9. CORRELATION OF SURGICAL REDUCTION AND CLINICAL RESULTS

Surgical Reduction	Clinical Result				
	Total	Excellent	Good	Fair	Poor
Anatomic	22	12	6	3	1
Satisfactory	25	5	16	2	2
Unsatisfactory	11	1	3	2	5

Source: Pantazopoulos T, Mousafiris C. Surgical treatment of central acetabular fractures. *Clin Orthop* 1989;246:61.

this series were a large number of posterior wall fractures, which have not been discussed in any recent articles. It was interesting, however, in reviewing four posterior wall fractures treated conservatively and six treated operatively, that the mean hip score was the same. Two of the operatively treated patients developed avascular necrosis. If posterior wall fractures are eliminated, only 34 acetabular fractures remain for review–plus a large number of cases treated without operation. This series is difficult to summarize. Ten of the eleven single-column fractures were treated nonoperatively; results were good, except for one case of avascular necrosis and one of rheumatoid arthritis. The patients who had transverse or T fractures had much poorer results (16 were treated nonoperatively and three operatively). There was good correlation between the clinical and radiographic results. Of the both-column fractures, one was treated nonoperatively with an excellent result, and three were treated operatively; two of them developed osteoarthritis. There was one deep infection that resulted in a poor clinical outcome. The findings of this article are not statistically significant, but they are interesting, as, again, they indicate that the controversy between operative and nonoperative approaches to these difficult fractures has not been resolved.

Spencer reviewed 25 patients older than 65 years whose unilateral acetabular fracture was managed nonoperatively, in traction (24). Fourteen of the injuries were "low-energy" (owing to falls); the remaining 11 were caused by powerful forces. Seventeen patients showed no displacement on initial radiographs but later exhibited displacement. Seven patients (30%) had an unsatisfactory result, owing to a displaced posterior column, osteoporosis, delayed diagnoses, a too-brief period of traction, or early weight bearing. The findings from this series point out the special problems of managing this fracture in elders, whose osteoporotic bone becomes a major factor.

Heeg and coworkers reported a series of 54 acetabular fractures treated operatively (average follow-up, 9.6 years) (25). Fifty-two patients sustained high-energy injuries; their average age was 34 years. Anatomic reduction was achieved in 36 patients (67%), 31 of whom reported a good to excellent functional result (Table 24-10). At follow-up, 10 patients had undergone arthrodesis or total hip arthroplasty. Again, the correlation between quality of reduction and end result was clear, but seven poor results were related to heterotopic ossification and two to complications of surgery.

TABLE 24-10. RELATION OF FUNCTIONAL RESULTS TO CONGRUENCY AFTER REDUCTION

Result	Number	Congruent	Not Congruent
Excellent	26	25	1
Good	7	6	1
Fair	4	—	4
Poor	17	5	12

Source: Heeg M, Klasen HJ, Visser JD. Operative treatment for acetabular fractures. *J Bone Joint Surg* 1990;72B:384.

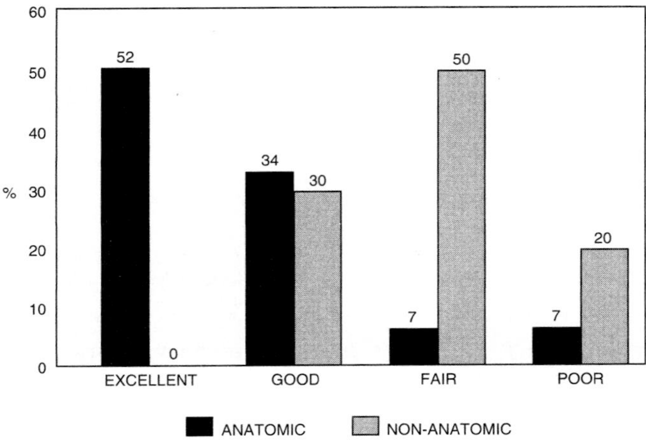

FIGURE 24-4. The results (acetabular fracture score) of anatomic and nonanatomic fracture reduction. (From: Kebaish A, Roy A, Rennie W. Displaced acetabular fractures: long-term follow up. *J Trauma* 1991;31:1539, with permission.)

Kebaish and colleagues reviewed 90 patients with displaced acetabular fractures who were followed for an average of 8 years. Fifty-four were treated operatively; 36, without operation (26). The correlation between anatomic reduction and good to excellent functional outcome was sustained: With anatomic reduction 86% excellent or good results and only 30% with residual displacement (Fig. 24-4). When open reduction was the method of treatment, the end result also correlated with the experience of the surgeon (Fig. 24-5), an observation made by our group as well (27). In general, the "operative group" of patients fared better than the "nonoperative group" (Fig. 24-6).

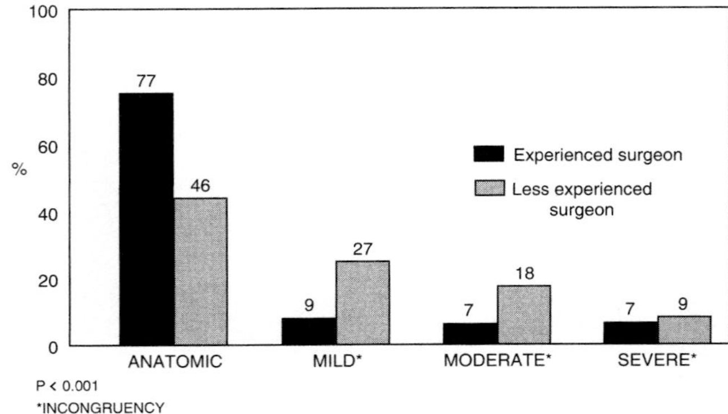

FIGURE 24-5. The quality of reduction achieved by experienced pelvic trauma surgeons and by less experienced ones. Mild incongruence is defined as up to 4 mm of fracture displacement; moderate, 4 to 10 mm; and severe, >10 mm. (From: Kebaish A, Roy A, Rennie W. Displaced acetabular fractures: long-term follow up. *J Trauma* 1991;31:1539, with permission.)

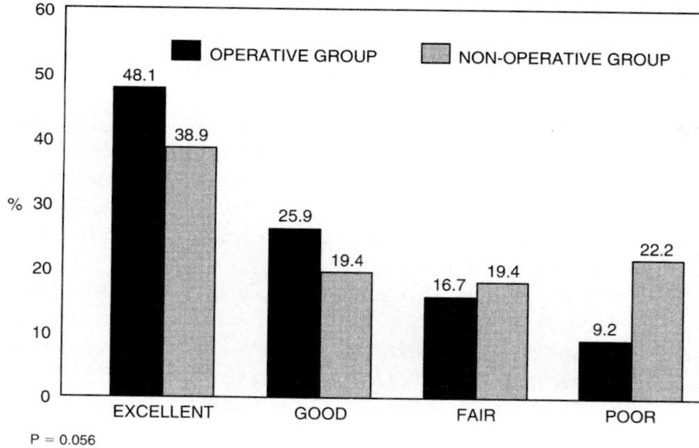

FIGURE 24-6. The results (acetabular fracture score) achieved in the operative group and in the nonoperative group. (From: Kebaish A, Roy A, Rennie W. Displaced acetabular fractures: long-term follow up. *J Trauma* 1991;31:1539, with permission.)

Letournel has reported on the largest series to date, and his work must be considered the gold standard at this time, as reported by David Helfet earlier.

Recent updated results from Letournel, Matta, and our group at Sunnybrook, as well as others, continue to show the close correlation between restoration of joint congruity and the excellence of the clinical outcome (15,20,27). The major complications continue to be heterotopic ossification and failure to achieve reduction or to maintain it in osteoporotic bone. Iatrogenic nerve damage is diminishing, owing to care at protecting the vulnerable nerves at surgery, and/or use of monitoring techniques in some centers (28).

SUMMARY OF THE NATURAL HISTORY

What may we deduce from studying the literature? A critical analysis reveals that the following major factors determine the outcome of an individual acetabular disruption (i.e., its natural history).

1. The degree of displacement of the fracture producing an unstable and incongruous hip joint.
2. The damage to the weight-bearing dome. This includes the degree of comminution, the presence of bone fragments in the joint, and the amount of damage to the articular cartilage of the femoral head.
3. The adequacy of the reduction. This includes restoration of joint stability in posterior fracture dislocations and the achievement of perfect congruity between the femoral head and the acetabulum.
4. The late complications of the fracture, some of which are inherent in the fracture itself and some in the treatment. Examples include avascular necrosis of the femoral head, heterotopic ossification, chondrolysis, metal in the joint, sepsis, and sciatic, femoral, or superior gluteal nerve palsy.

Thus, the natural history of displaced acetabular fractures is similar to that of other fractures involving a weight-bearing joint: If, the joint is stable and congruous following reduction, then a satisfactory result may be expected; if it is not, then early joint destruction ensues.

Logical management dictates a return to the basic principle for a lower extremity joint fracture: A displaced fracture requires anatomic reduction, stable fixation, and early motion for an optimal result, *if this is technically possible.* The last phrase has concerned surgeons, because it bridges the gap between ideal and existent. In this particular region, complicated anatomy makes surgical restoration difficult. Add to this the problems of comminution, the difficulties of fixation, and the general impact on an already seriously ill patient, and we have a situation many surgeons deem insurmountable.

Although it is true that the risks of surgery are considerable, we must not succumb to such surgical nihilism but must instead resort to basic principles in an attempt to repair this fracture. In the past decade, many problems with respect to this fracture have been resolved, but many still remain, and they require further clarification.

In select cases of older patients early total hip arthroplasty is an option. Nonoperative treatment is indicated if the hip is congruous and stable. This is also true in older patients with a both-column fracture who exhibit secondary congruity of the hip.

In the future, we must further refine the existing classifications of these fractures, to reflect the factors that affect the natural history, thus enhancing the management of the patient. Also, it is now clear that the results of operative treatment depend much on the skill of the surgeon; therefore, specialized referral centers, which now exist in many parts of the world, are essential. Surgeons who manage these difficult fractures must have knowledge of both fracture care and hip anatomy, and must have spent some time in specialized training in this area. However, surgeons working in these specialized areas must keep an open mind about surgical outcomes. Certainly, in the older age group of patients with osteoporosis and complex fracture patterns (e.g., T fracture and both-column fracture), there is still room for clinical studies to determine optimal outcomes. The role of early total hip arthroplasty requires further study.

REFERENCES

1. Armstrong JR. Traumatic dislocation of the hip joint, review of 101 dislocations. *J Bone Joint Surg* 1948;308:430.
2. Cauchoix J, Truchet P. Les articulaires de la hanche (col du femur excepte). *Rev Chir Orthop* 1951;37:266.
3. Cave EF, ed. *Fractures and other injuries.* Chicago: Year Book, 1958.
4. Knight RA, Smith H. Central fractures of the acetabulum. *J Bone Joint Surg* 1958;40A:1.
5. Stewart MJ, Milford LW. Fracture-dislocation of the hip, an end result study. *J Bone Joint Surg* 1954;36A:315.

6. Thompson VP, Epstein HA. Traumatic dislocation of the hip, a survey of 204 cases covering a period of twenty-one years. *J Bone Joint Surg* 1951;33A:746.
7. Urist MR. Fractures of the acetabulum, the nature of the traumatic lesion, treatment, and a 2 year end result. *Ann Surg* 1948;127:1150.
8. Urist MR. Fracture dislocation of the hip joint, the nature of the traumatic lesion, treatment, late complications and end result. *J Bone Joint Surg* 1948;30A:699.
9. Westerborn A. Central dislocation of the femoral head. *J Bone Joint Surg* 1954;36A:307.
10. Rowe CR, Lowell JD. Prognosis of fractures of the acetabulum. *J Bone Joint Surg* 1961;43A:30.
11. Larson CB. Fracture dislocations of the hip. *Clin Orthop* 1973;92:147.
12. Carnesale PG, Stewart MJ, Barnes SN. Acetabular disruption and central fracture-dislocation of the hip. *J Bone Joint Surg* 1975; 57A:1054.
13. Pennal GF, Davidson J, Garside H, et al. Results of treatment of acetabular fractures. *Clin Orthop* 1980;151:115.
14. Judet R, Judet J, Letournel E. Fractures of the acetabulum: classification and surgical approaches for open reduction. *J Bone Joint Surg* 1964;46A:1615.
15. Letournel E. Diagnosis and treatment of nonunions and malunions of acetabular fractures. *Orthop Clin North Am* 1990;21: 769.
16. Senegas J, Liourzou G, Yates M. Complex acetabular fractures, a transtrochanteric lateral surgical approach. *Clin Orthop* 1980; 151:107.
17. Ruggieri F, Zinghi GF, Montanari G. Fractures of the acetabulum. *Ital J Orthop Traumatol* 1987;13:27.
18. Matta JM, Mehne DK, Roffi R. Fractures of the acetabulum: early results of a prospective study. *Clin Orthop* 1986;205:241.
19. Day WH, Swanson AV, Freeman MAR. Contact pressures in the loaded human cadaver hip. *J Bone Joint Surg* 1975;578:303.
20. Matta JM, Merritt PO. Displaced acetabular fractures. *Clin Orthop* 1988;230:83.
21. Goulet JA, Bray TJ. Complex acetabular fractures. *Clin Orthop* 1989;240:9.
22. Pantazopoulos T, Mousafiris C. Surgical treatment of central acetabular fractures. *Clin Orthop* 1989;246:57.
23. Ylinen P, Santavirta S. Outcome of acetabular fractures: a 7-year follow up. *J Trauma* 1989;29:19.
24. Spencer RF. Acetabular fractures in older patients. *J Bone Joint Surg* 1989;718:774.
25. Heeg M, Klasen H, Visser JD. Operative treatment for acetabular fractures. *J Bone Joint Surg* 1990;728:383.
26. Kebaish A, Roy A, Rennie W. Displaced acetabular fractures: long-term follow up. *J Trauma* 1991;31:1539–1542.
27. Powell JN. *Acetabular fractures: a report from the University of Toronto.* Presented at The Orthopedic Trauma Association. Dallas, TX, 1988.
28. Tile M. Symposium. The management of acetabular fractures. Part 1. *Contemp Orthop* 1992;301.

25

DESCRIBING THE INJURY: CLASSIFICATION OF ACETABULAR FRACTURES

MARVIN TILE

INTRODUCTION

Acetabular fractures are so complex that no "perfect" classification has been constructed yet. Because the type of injury depends on the precise position of the femoral head at the moment of impact, the number of specific fracture types appears to be infinite. Any classification can serve two purposes: (a) It can help individual surgeons make a logical management decision for any given patient; and (b) It allows surgeons to compare similar groups of patients treated by different methods.

Treatment of a given fracture depends on "defining the injury," that is, the assessment of all the patient factors and fracture factors described in Chapter 26 that make up the "personality" of the injury.

Because there are many variables in acetabular fractures, and they are difficult to fit into any classification, attempting to do so is like attempting to fit a square plug into a round hole (Fig. 25-1). These variables, which make up the "personality of the fracture," must be considered in decision making, because the prognosis of an individual fracture pattern is dependent on them (Table 25-1). These variables include the anatomic types, the degree of the causative force (low versus high energy), the direction of displacement, the presence or absence of a dislocation, the number of fragments, the presence of marginal impaction, and damage to the articular surface of the femoral head and/or the acetabulum, among others. All these factors are important in decision making; *they define the injury.* This is clearly different than *classifying the injury,* because all of the present classifications are anatomically based, and do not factor in all these elements. For example, a T fracture may be undisplaced or displaced. If displaced, one column may be more displaced than the other, and may be associated with a wall fracture ± a dislocation. Also, the fracture may be caused by high energy, with severe comminution, or by low energy, in an older individual with poor bone. The prognosis of any given such T fracture will vary widely, even though the present anatomic classifications regard them all as a T (Fig. 25-2). The AO modification of the Judet-Letournel added modifiers to try and capture these variables, but these are not widely used because of their complexity. Therefore, at best, the present classifications, which are all anatomically based, can be used as a rough guide to compare cases between centers and as a guide to treatment. *Individualized decision making* is mandatory for all trauma patients.

Anatomic Classification

The most widely used classification is that of Judet and Letournel (1), anatomically based and in which all the fractures are divided into two major types, elementary and associated or complex, each with subgroups (Table 25-2). Their classification rendered the description of these fractures—previously identified as central dislocation of the hip—more precise, and led to a new understanding of these diffi-

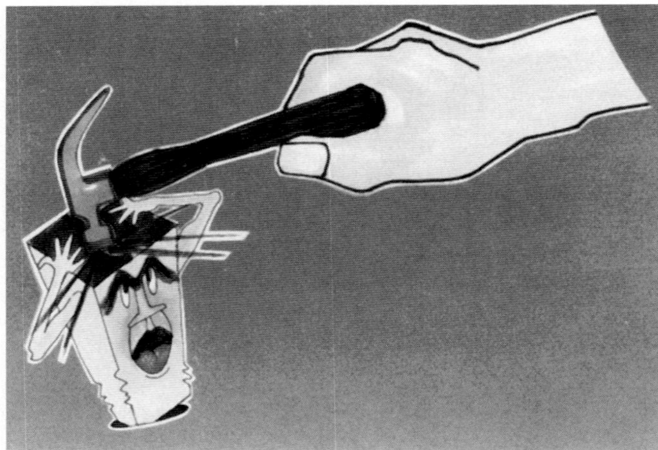

FIGURE 25-1. The use of the classification in individual decision making. A comprehensive classification is necessary for academic purposes such as prognosis and outcome studies. It is less important in individual decision making, because every trauma case is different. Thus, trying to force a square plug into a round hole is counterproductive.

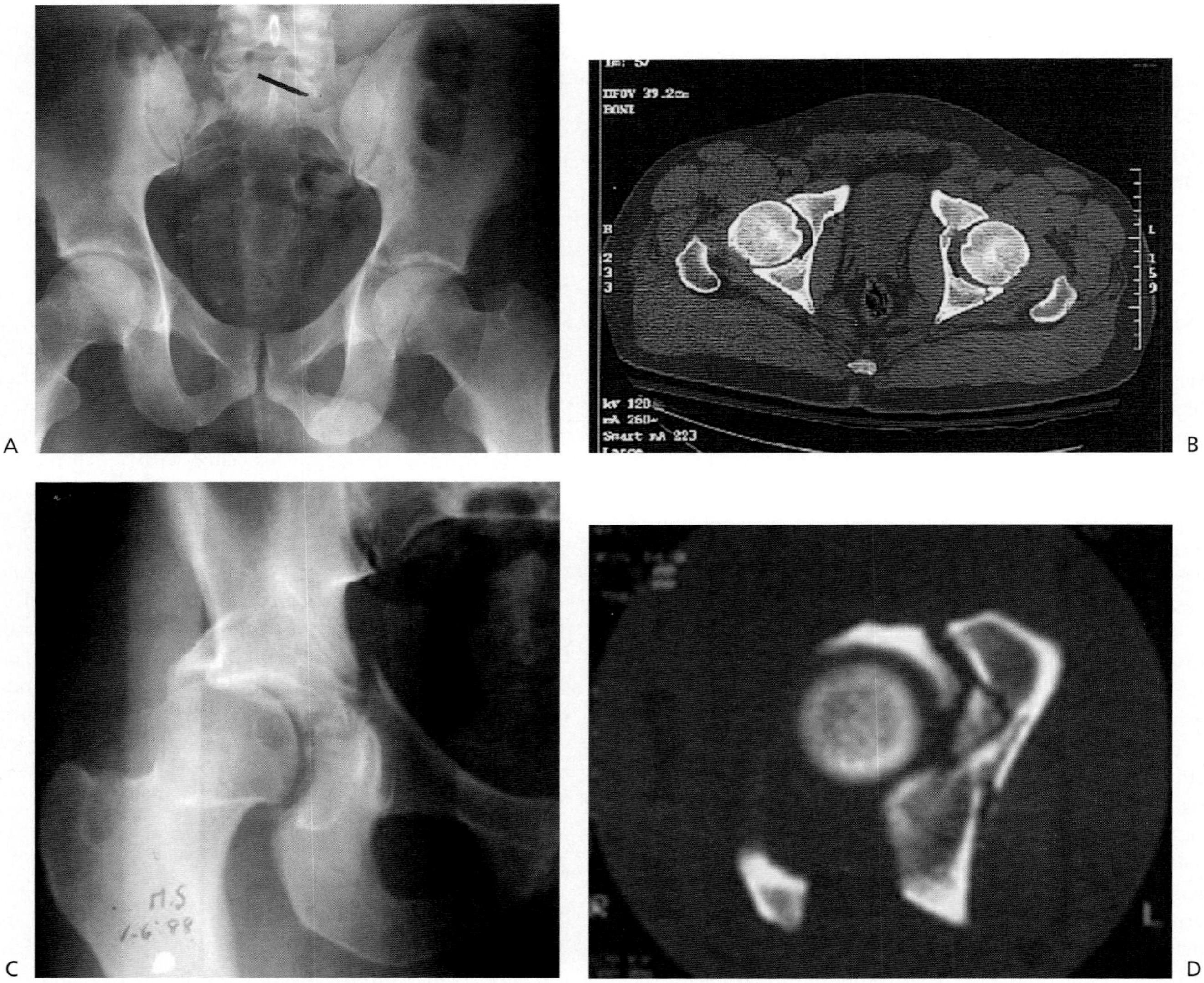

FIGURE 25-2. The prognosis of any given T type fracture varies widely, even though the present anatomic classifications regard them all as T fractures. For example, the anterior-posterior radiograph **(A)** and computed tomography **(B)** of a minimally displaced T fracture contrasted to a severely displaced fracture **(C)** and **(D).** It is obvious that the prognosis will be very different, but the classification is T fracture in both.

TABLE 25-1. VARIABLES AFFECTING THE PROGNOSIS OF THE ACETABULAR FRACTURES: "THE PERSONALITY OF THE INJURY"

Anatomic type
Degree of causative force (high vs low energy)
Degree and direction of displacement
Hip dislocation (y/n)
Degree of comminution
Articular damage to femoral head or acetabulum
Marginal articular impaction
Patient factors

cult fractures. Their contribution to this field cannot be underestimated. Understanding the anatomic types led to approaches and methods of surgically fixing these fractures, which at that time were largely treated with skeletal traction and long hospital stays; and, had poor results for displaced fractures. However, the classification does not address many of the factors discussed previously (Table 25-1) that affect the natural history, namely, the degree and direction of displacement, comminution, the integrity of superior weight-bearing surfaces, and the presence or absence of dislocation. Therefore, in the anatomic classification, any type may be simple (e.g., undisplaced) or very complex (i.e., comminuted and grossly displaced). For an investigator reviewing cases of any type (e.g., a transverse or T fracture), the lack of this information would be a major handicap. For example, a transverse fracture may be undisplaced or displaced. It may be comminuted and associated with a central or posterior dislocation of the femoral head, which are all important prognostic indicators. Perhaps future modifications will include these factors in each of the anatomic types.

AO Classification (Modification of Judet-Letournel)

For the purpose of case comparison, the ideal would be the development of a universal classification of all fractures that allows all surgeons to "speak the same language." In the past decade, the AO group (Table 25-3) has attempted to attain this elusive goal (1). By uniting such organizations as SICOT (Société International Chirurgie Orthopédique et de Traumatologie) and the Orthopaedic Trauma Association behind this classification, some agreement has been reached on extremity fractures, both diaphyseal and articular types. Helfet, working with committees of these organizations, including Letournel, achieved consensus on a classification for fractures of the acetabulum, which are extremely complex (D. Helfet, personal communication, 1993). It was difficult to fit all the variables into the alphanumeric code adopted by the group.

The general principles of the universal classification are admirable. Fractures are classified into three main types—A, B, and C—in increasing order of severity; the A group being the least severe, and C the most severe (Fig. 25-3) (2). Finer distinctions within these groups are possible, and, owing to the addition of subgroups, a complete classification has developed, one I shall describe later in this chapter.

However, the AO Comprehensive Classification is still mainly an adaptation of the anatomic classification of Judet-Letournel. In all other articular fractures, the progression from A to B to C goes from single articular fractures (A) to the "bag of bones" (C), as seen in the elbow or pilon fractures (Fig. 25-4). Because the anatomic classifications are similar, and do help with operative decision-making, I believe that retention of the anatomic classification is needed, with the addition of the AO (A to C), which will be of prognostic importance. The AO classification attempts this with the subtypes, the group using the Judet-Letournel should also adopt some type of scale of comminution for prognostic purposes.

Classification According to Direction of Displacement

In the previous edition of this text, our proposed classification incorporated all of Judet and Letournel's subtypes but placed them in a different format. The fractures were described anatomically, but *direction of displacement* was highlighted. This focus figured large in the decision-making process. For example, all the posterior-type fractures, whatever their type, share some characteristics. Fractures of the posterior wall, the posterior column, transverse, or T with posterior wall displacement, are usually caused by a blow to the flexed knee (e.g., dashboard injury); therefore, associated knee injuries are common (Fig. 25-5A). Posterior dislocation of the hip is common if an associated posterior wall fracture is present. Almost invariably this leaves the hip potentially unstable after closed reduction (Fig. 25-5B,C). Therefore, posterior fracture types usually require open reduction and internal fixation to restore hip stability (Fig. 25-5D–J). Finally, the addition of a posterior dislocation affects the prognosis significantly, because the prevalence of avascular necrosis and of sciatic nerve lesions is much increased.

The direction of the displacement is important for deciding what surgical approach is to be used. For example,

TABLE 25-2. JUDET-LETOURNEL CLASSIFICATION

Elementary fractures
Posterior wall
Posterior column
Anterior wall
Anterior column
Transverse
Associated fractures
T-shaped
Posterior wall plus posterior column
Posterior wall with transverse
Anterior column or wall with transverse
Anterior column or wall with posterior hemitransverse
Both columns

TABLE 25-3. COMPREHENSIVE CLASSIFICATION: FRACTURES OF THE ACETABULUM

Type A: *Partial articular* fractures, *one column* involved
- A1: Posterior wall fracture
- A2: Posterior column fracture
- A3: Anterior wall or anterior column fracture

Type B: *Partial articular* fractures (transverse or T-type fracture, *both columns* involved)
- B1: Transverse fracture
- B2: T-shaped fracture
- B3: Anterior column plus posterior hemitransverse fracture

Type C: *Complete articular* fracture (both-column fracture; floating acetabulum)
- C1: Both-column fracture, high variety
- C2: Both-column fracture, low variety
- C3: Both-column fracture involving the sacroiliac joint

transverse fractures may rotate anteriorly or posteriorly. T fractures may be displaced in only one column (anterior or posterior), while the other remains undisplaced. The correct surgical approach should be obvious to a surgeon who has all this information.

Summary of Comprehensive Classification

In this edition, we use the AO modification of the Judet-Letournel, and point out the similar nomenclature in the Judet-Letournel (Tables 25-2 and 25-3). Brandser and Marsh (3) have suggested a further modification, based on the same anatomic types, but divide them into wall, column, and transverse fractures. Their suggestion, which is aimed at radiologists, has merit; however, we will not adopt it because it does not appreciably change existing classifications; rather, it just rearranges the types.

The AO classification is based on the anatomic site, the segment, the type, group, and subgroup, and modifiers (4). An alphanumeric code is used for its suitability for computers. The acetabulum is anatomic location 62. The fractures may be divided into Type A (partial articular fractures), Type B (transverse or T fractures in which a portion of the articular surface of the acetabulum is still connected to the intact ilium, and, therefore, to the axial skeleton), and Type C, the both-column fracture, in which no portion of the acetabulum is connected to the intact ilium, nor, therefore, to the axial skeleton. In effect, Pattern C is a "floating acetabulum." This classification with subgroups is described in Table 25-2. Although, in order of severity, it attempts to follow the principles of the comprehensive long bone classi-

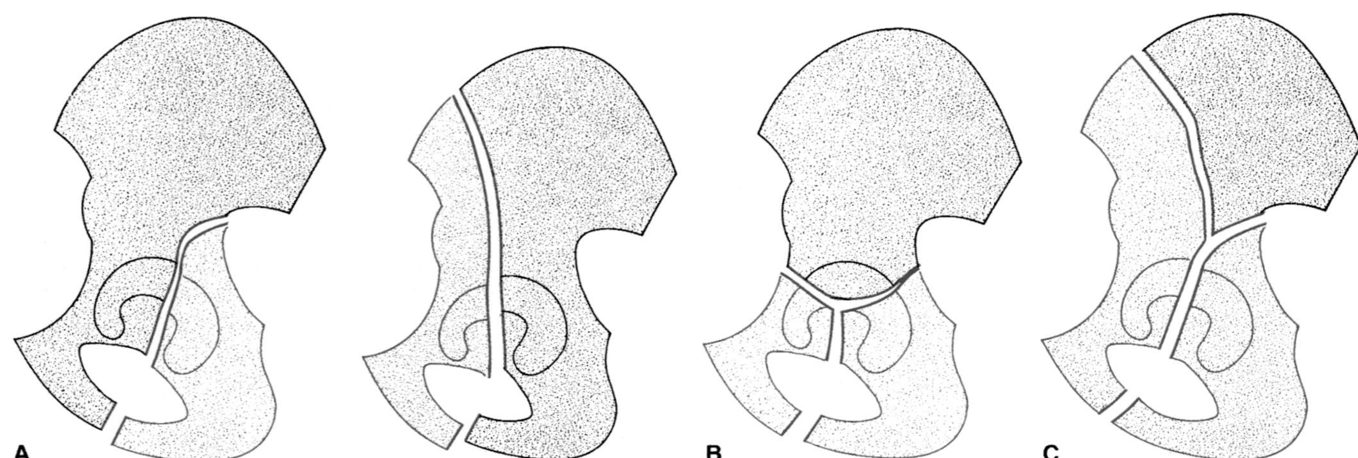

FIGURE 25-3. Universal classification of acetabular fractures. **A:** Type A: Fractures of one column or one wall, for example, A1-2, posterior column and anterior column. **B:** Type B1: Transverse or T-type fractures involving both columns but by definition always leaving a fragment of articular cartilage attached to the proximal ilium and, thus, to the axial skeleton, as in Fig. 25-2B. **C:** Type C: Both-column fracture of the acetabulum. By definition, no portion of the articular surface remains attached to the axial skeleton because fracture of both columns of the ilium is proximal to the joint.

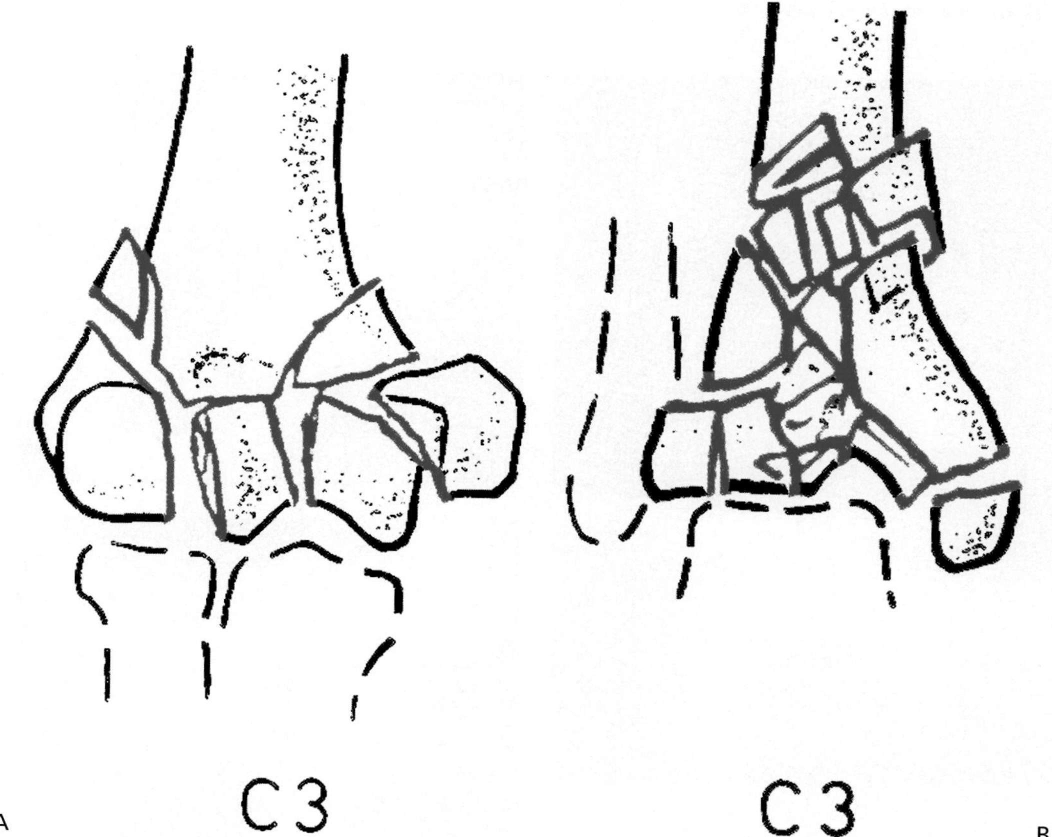

FIGURE 25-4. AO C types—severe comminution, "the bag of bones" as seen in the distal humerus **(A)** and the pilon **(B).**

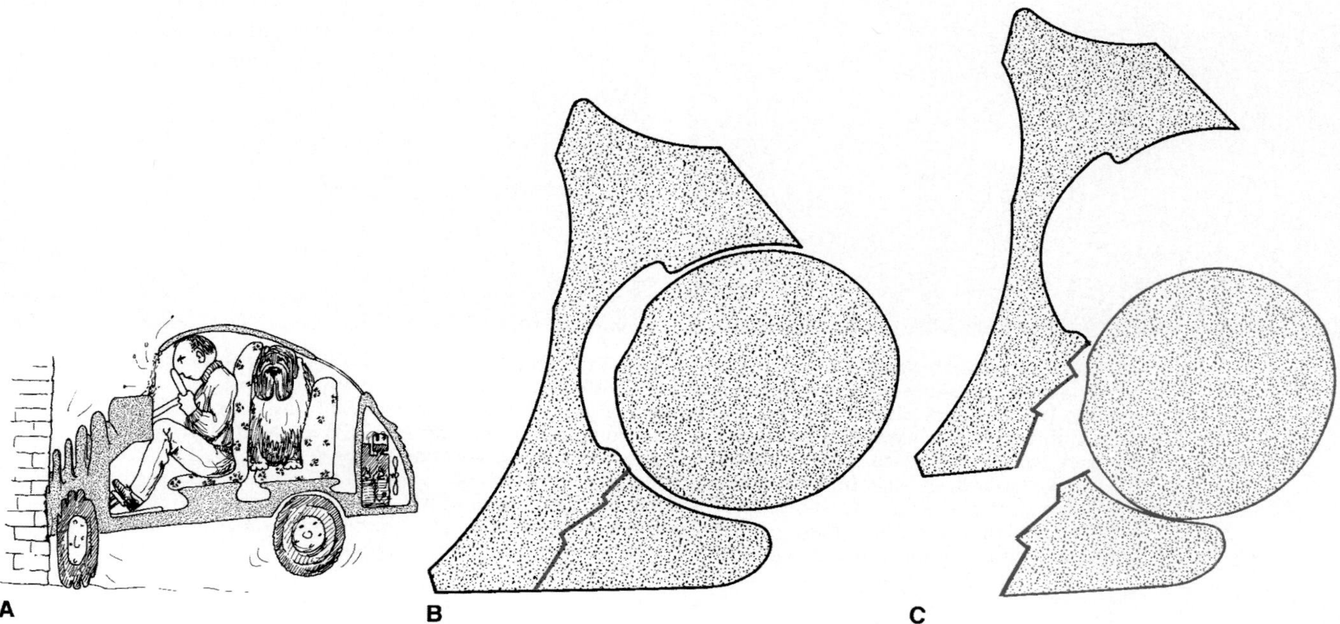

FIGURE 25-5. Posterior type fractures of the acetabulum. Posterior fractures of the acetabulum, including those of the posterior wall and the posterior column, with or without transverse or T configuration, are commonly caused by a blow to the flexed knee on the dashboard of a motor vehicle **(A).** Associated knee injuries, including patellar fractures and posterior subluxation of the knee as well as posterior dislocation of the hip, are common. Fractures of the posterior wall associated with posterior dislocation of the hip virtually always require open reduction and internal fixation because of potential instability of the hip **(C).** *(Figure continues)*

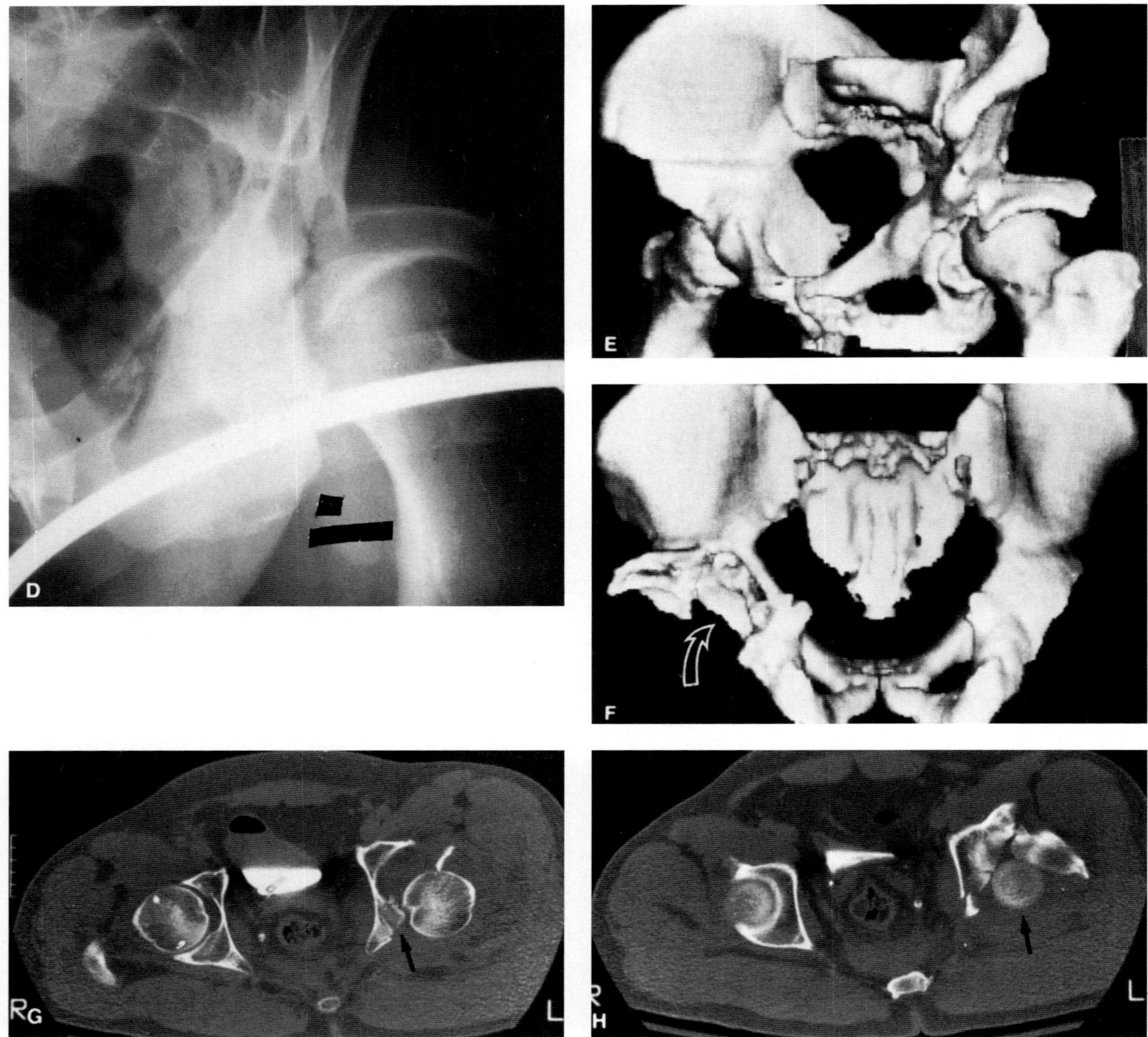

FIGURE 25-5. *(continued)* When the femoral head is relocated, the posterior wall stays unreduced, leaving the entire posterior aspect of the femoral head uncovered and the hip potentially unstable **(D).** Posterior dislocation of the hip with a large associated posterior wall fragment as seen on this obturator view. The three-dimensional computed tomography (3DCT) image shows the exact anatomy, the size of the fragment, and the posterior dislocation of the femoral head **(E).** The posterior 3DCT view **(F)** with the femoral head subtracted shows the entire anterior and posterior aspect of the hip uncovered. This instability of the femoral head is best seen on the axial CT **(G),** which also indicates marginal impaction and on a view **(H)** taken through the superior dome showing the dislocated position of the femoral head and the large fragment.

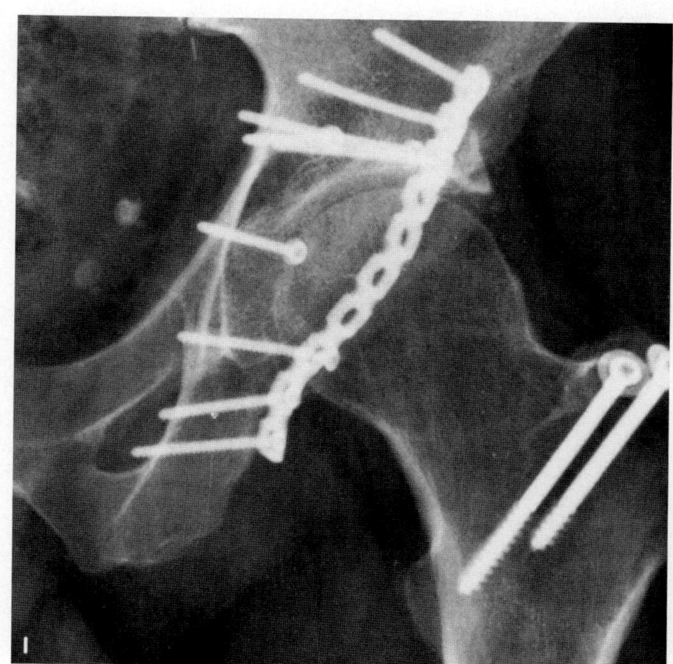

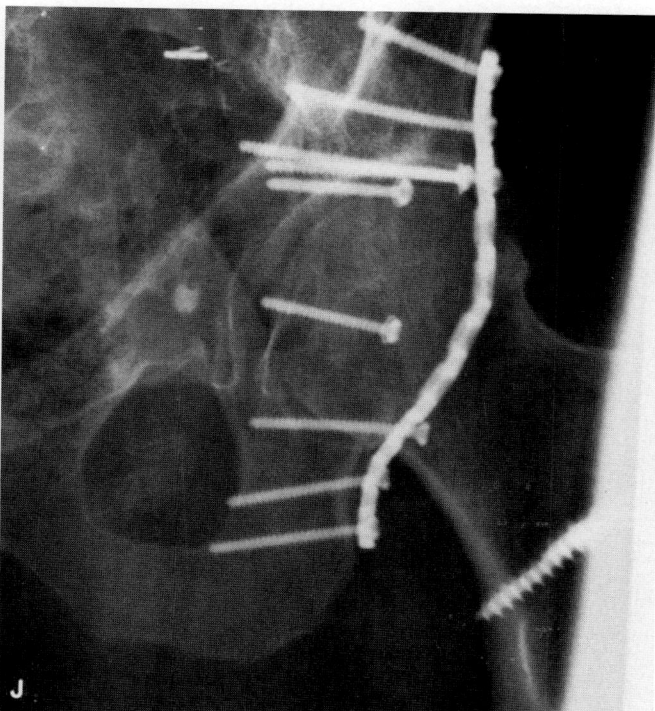

FIGURE 25-5. ***(continued)*** Open reduction and internal fixation of the posterior wall fragment were essential to restore stability to the joint. These were performed through a posterior Kocher-Langenbeck approach with removal of the greater trochanter to allow exposure of the superiorly placed fragment. Anatomic reduction with stable internal fixation using interfragmental lag screws and a posterior buttress plate is seen on the iliac oblique **(I)** and obturator oblique **(J)** views.

fication, it must make some compromises because of the complexity of these fractures. For example, a T fracture, although it is a B-type lesion, often is a much more severe injury than a C-type both-column fracture.

HOW TO USE THE CLASSIFICATION FOR INDIVIDUAL DECISION MAKING

Although a comprehensive classification is necessary for investigational purposes such as prognosis and outcome studies, it is less important in making decisions on individual cases. In trauma, every case is different; therefore, trying to force a square plug into a round hole is counterproductive (Fig. 25-1). The *surgeon must know the basic fracture types, but even more important, must be able to interpret the radiographs and draw the fracture lines on a dry skeleton (Fig. 25-6). Even experienced acetabular surgeons do this before every operation; consequently, it is absolutely essential that all surgeons adopt this preoperative practice.*

The acetabulum is much less of a mystery than is commonly believed. A study of its anatomy reveals that it is made up of two columns and two walls (Fig. 25-7). All of the anatomic fracture types are permutations and combinations of that pathoanatomy. Therefore, theoretically, the possibilities include fractures of the anterior, posterior, and/or both columns (Fig. 25-7A). If both columns are fractured together, then we arbitrarily call that a *transverse fracture.* If both columns are fractured (transverse) and also separate from each other, then we call that a T fracture. A portion of the acetabular articular surface is connected to a portion of intact ilium, and thus to the axial skeleton in both the transverse and T fracture (Type B).

Also, the acetabulum has an anterior and a posterior wall, and either may be fractured in association with an anterior or posterior dislocation (Fig. 25-7B). The femoral head also may be centrally dislocated through the quadrilateral plate. Fractures of the wall may be associated with many other fracture types.

The *both-column fracture* (1), arbitrarily so-named by Judet and Letournel, is really a variant of the T fracture in which the transverse break runs through the ilium above the acetabulum and thus disconnects all articular cartilage from the axial skeleton (the floating acetabulum) (Fig. 25-7C). In this type, the posterior column usually is separated and displaced, and may be associated with a posterior wall fracture.

Therefore, simply by applying thorough knowledge of anatomy, the surgeon can outline all of the possible fracture

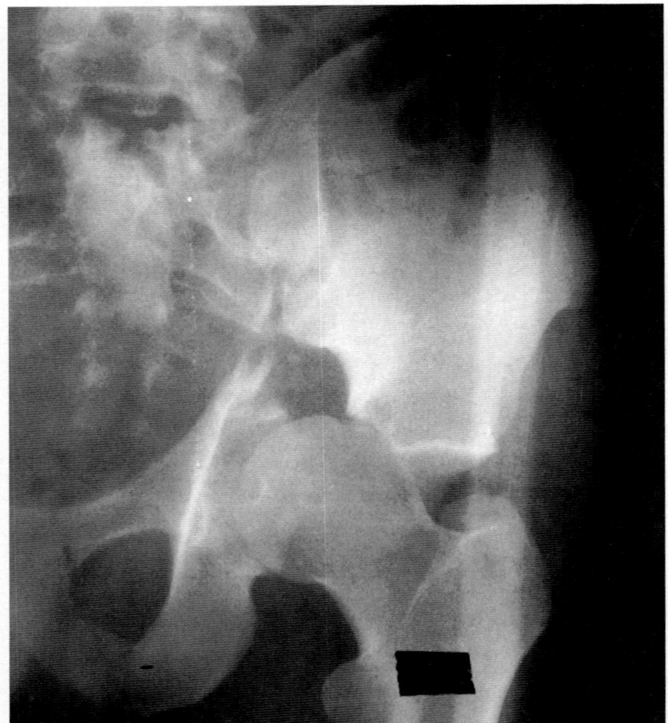

A

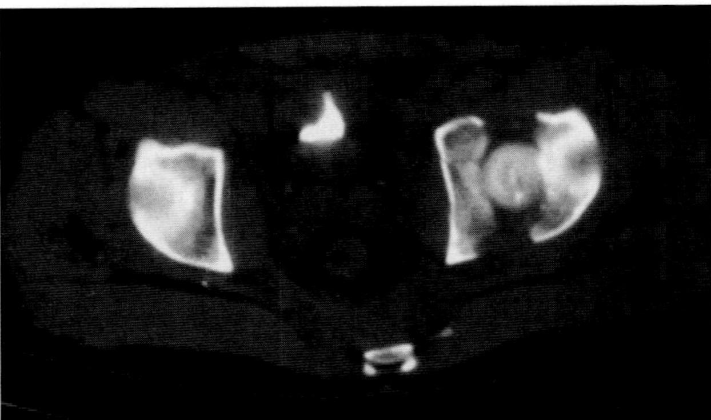

B

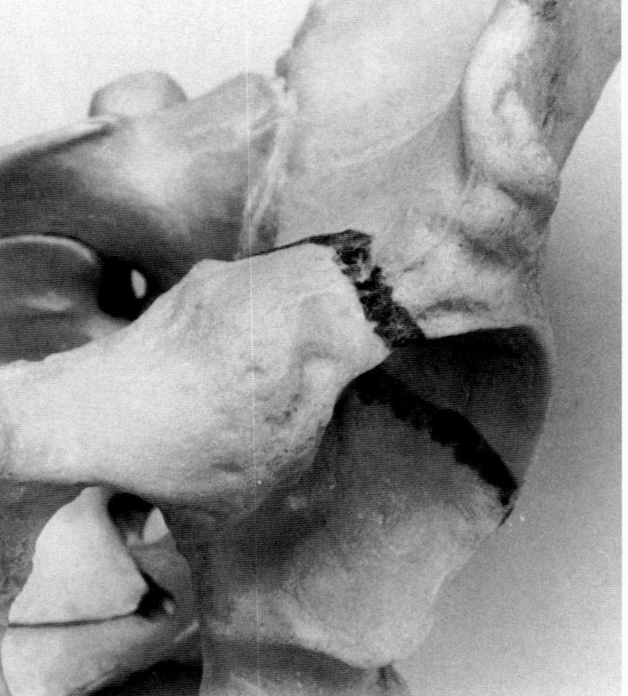

C

FIGURE 25-6. Radiographic interpretation and ability to draw fracture lines on a dry skeleton. The surgeon must know the basic fracture types but even more important must be able to interpret the radiographs and draw the fracture lines on a dry skeleton, in order to make decisions about the operative approach, method of fixation, and other technical points. Transverse fracture of the left acetabulum is noted on the anterior-posterior radiograph **(A)** and the classic appearance on the CT image **(B).** Before the surgery the surgeon should draw the fracture line or lines in their entirety on a dry skeleton **(C).**

types without having to memorize a complex classification. Furthermore, various landmarks on the radiographs can lead the surgeon to logical treatment decision making for each patient.

Other factors must be assessed carefully in order to define the personality of the fracture. The surgeon must define not only the type of fracture but also the factors that affect the prognosis; namely, (a) the degree of displacement; (b) the degree of comminution or impaction; (c) the exact position of the fracture, especially involvement of the acetabular dome; and (d) the presence of a dislocation—posterior, central, or (rarely) anterior (Table 25-1).

A logical management decision should follow further assessment of the limb, the patient, and the surgeon's own experience. Therefore, the treatment of the individual patient depends most on the assessment of each individual case by an experienced examiner.

COMPREHENSIVE CLASSIFICATION

Type A: Partial Articular Fractures

In Type A fracture patterns, only one portion of the acetabular articular surface is involved; the remainder of that surface remains intact. Thus, only one column and/or a corresponding wall is involved (i.e., the anterior column, anterior wall, or both; or the posterior column, posterior wall, or both). Dislocations, either anterior or posterior, associated with the corresponding appropriate wall or columns are relatively common with these Type A fractures, especially posterior dislocations.

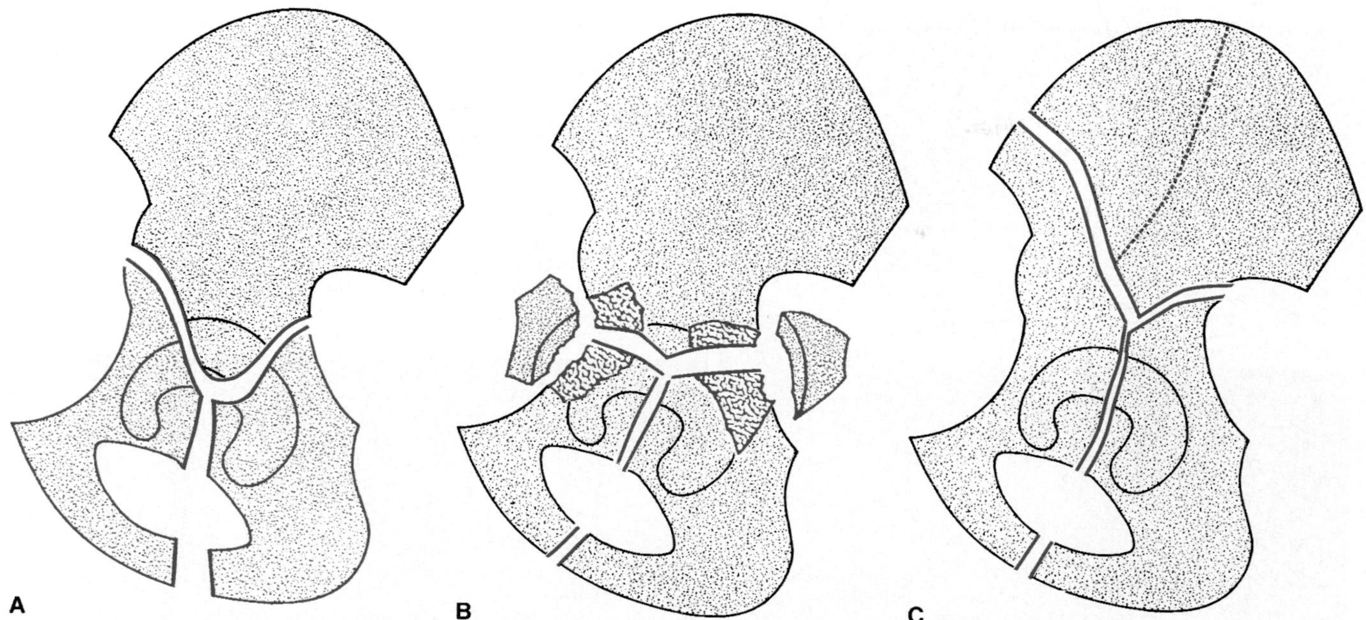

FIGURE 25-7. Anatomic fracture types of the acetabulum, permutations and combinations. The acetabulum is made up of two columns, anterior and posterior, and two walls, anterior and posterior. All of the fracture types other than the so-called both-column type are permutations and combinations of that anatomy. **A:** The anterior column may be fractured, the posterior column fractured, or both columns fractured together, which we call transverse. The T fracture is a transverse component with both columns separated from each other. **B:** The anterior wall may be fractured, a lesion often associated with anterior dislocation, or the posterior wall may be fractured, almost inevitably with posterior dislocation of the hip. These fractures may occur in isolation or in combination with anterior column and posterior column fractures as well as transverse and T fractures. **C:** The both-column fracture, by definition, divides the ilium proximal to the hip joint; therefore, no portion of the articular surface of the hip remains attached to the axial skeleton. In reality, this both-column fracture is a type of T fracture occurring proximal to the joint. All of these fracture types are theoretically possible from a study of the anatomy, and all occur with varying frequency in practice.

A1: Posterior Wall Fractures

We have seen that all posterior fracture types share common characteristics, the main one being a posterior wall fragment (Fig. 25-5). Other typical findings follow.

1. They are usually caused by a blow to the flexed knee (dashboard injury); therefore, associated knee injuries are common.
2. Posterior dislocation of the hip is common, and almost always present when the posterior wall is fractured.
3. The addition of a posterior dislocation greatly affects the prognosis, because the prevalence of avascular necrosis and sciatic nerve lesions is markedly increased.

The posterior wall fracture described here is isolated, and is usually associated with a dislocation. However, the posterior wall fracture, if associated with any other fracture type (e.g., a posterior column A2, transverse B1, B2 T fracture, or associated both-column C fracture), dictates the behavior of the pattern. Thus, the association of a posterior wall fracture with any anatomic fracture type is extremely important, because it signifies potential posterior instability of the hip following closed reduction. The presence of a posterior wall fracture usually directs the surgeon to open reduction and internal fixation of the fragment, unless the fragment is so small that the hip remains stable in all positions.

Posterior wall fractures always involve the posterior articular surface. The fragment may be single or multiple, large or small, high or low (Fig. 25-8). Impaction of the acetabular margin is not infrequent as the head dislocates (Fig. 25-5). If the fragment or fragments are large, reduction of the dislocation may not be followed by reduction of the fracture; therefore, the hip joint may remain unstable. Open reduction is mandatory to avoid repeat dislocation and instability. Excellent results should be achieved if the fragment is anatomically reduced and stabilized. On occasion, the fragment contains a large portion of the superior weight-bearing surface. Early accurate open anatomic reduction is essential to restore joint congruity and prevent early degenerative arthritis (Fig. 25-9).

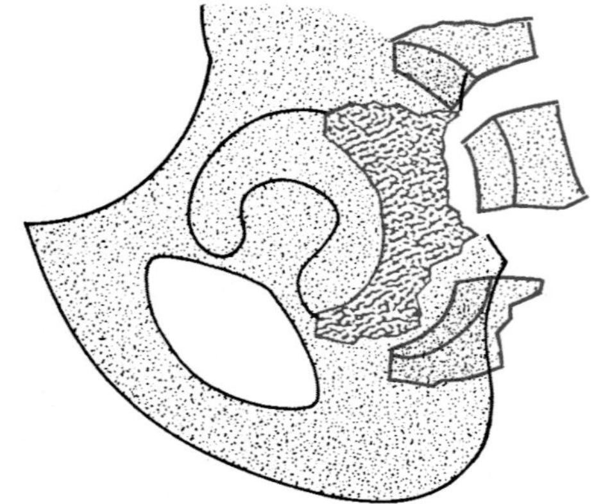

FIGURE 25-8. Subclassification of posterior wall fractures. Posterior wall fractures may be single or multiple, large or small, and involve superior, immediate posterior, or inferior portions of the wall. Impaction is frequent.

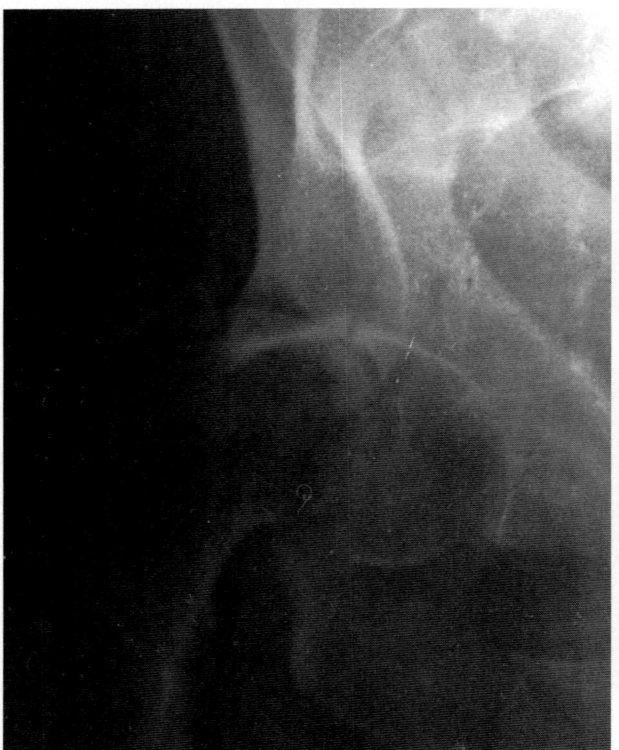

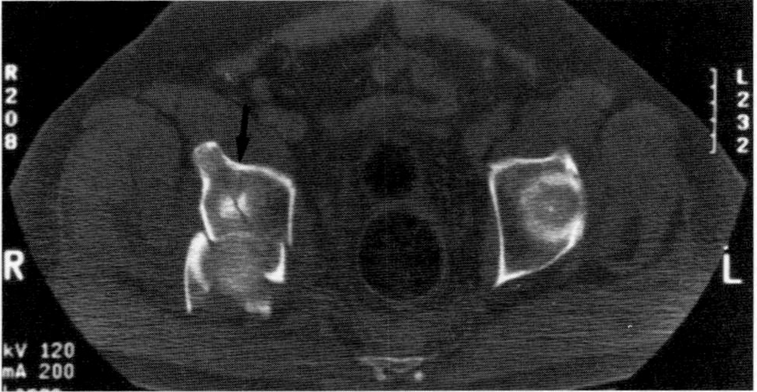

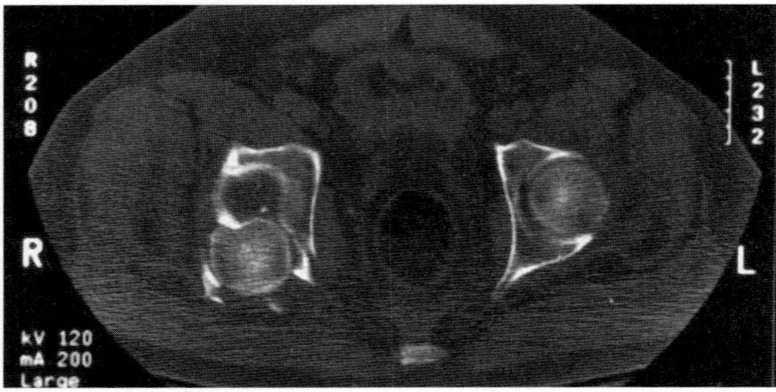

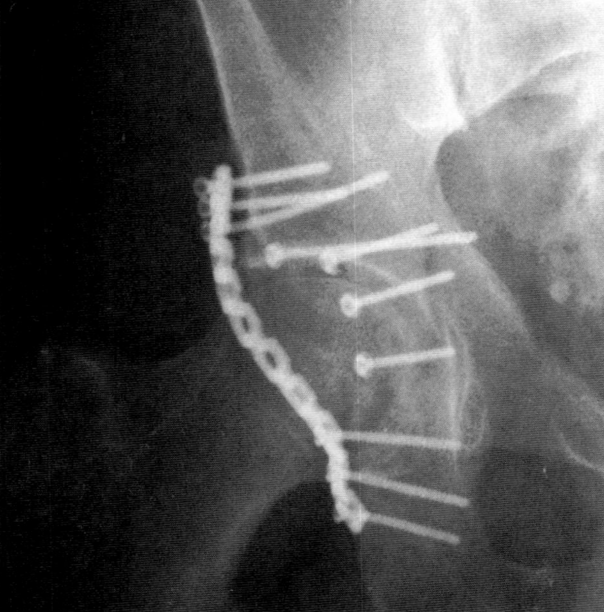

FIGURE 25-9. Posterior dislocation of the hip with an extremely large superiorly placed fragment, as noted on the anterior-posterior radiograph **(A),** and especially on computed tomography (CT) **(B)** taken directly through the roof of the acetabulum. The fragment extends through the roof and is associated with an undisplaced transverse component. The displaced head with a marginally impacted fragment is noted on the CT image **(C).** Anatomic fixation of the fragment with intrafragmental screws and a posterior buttress plate to prevent redisplacement of the transverse component is noted **(D).**

To account for all of these variables, groups and subgroups have been added to the universal classification of this fracture (Fig. 25-10).

A1-1: Pure Fracture-Dislocation (One Fragment)

Type A1-1 is a pure fracture-dislocation with one large fragment posteriorly. The fragment may be posterior 1, posterior-superior 2, or posterior-inferior 3 (Fig. 25-8). The posterior and posterior-inferior types may leave the hip unstable in flexion and internal rotation; the posterior-superior type is extremely unstable, even when the hip is extended. Very often, the hip cannot be kept in the reduced position, and this particular type requires emergency surgery.

A1-2: Pure Fracture Dislocation (Multiple Fragments)

In subgroup A1-2, the posterior wall is greatly fragmented, which makes operative repair difficult. The fragments also may be posterior 1, posterior-superior 2, or posterior-inferior 3. (Fig. 25-11).

A1-3: Pure Fracture Dislocation with Marginal Impaction

Type A1-3 has a very important prognostic indicator (Fig. 25-12A). The dislocating femoral head may drive one or more fragments of the posterior acetabular margin into the underlying cancellous bone. At surgery, these fragments are seen to lie at an angle of 90 degrees to the femoral head and the acetabular margin (Fig. 25-12B). Failure to recognize them at surgery may prevent anatomic reduction of the posterior wall. Also, these fragments may have lost their blood supply; consequently, they may collapse in the postoperative period, even if anatomic reduction was achieved originally. They also may be placed posteriorly 1, posterior-superiorly 2, or posterior-inferiorly 3. They are particularly important in the posterior-superior location, because they are in the main weight-bearing area of the acetabulum.

A2: Posterior Column Fractures

Partial Articular, One-Column

The posterior column extends from the greater sciatic notch through the acetabulum into the center of the inferior pubic ramus (Fig. 25-13). Isolated detachment of this column is rare, but it is important to recognize it. The unique features of this fracture can be seen on the accompanying radiographs (Fig. 25-14). The posterior column with the associated posteriorly dislocated hip is markedly displaced on both the obturator and iliac oblique radiographs, whereas the anterior column is intact. Reduction of the hip dislocation may restore congruity and stability to the joint; however, sophisticated radiographic studies, including tomography and computed tomography (CT), usually reveal a significant "step" in the joint; thus, I favor open reduction and stable fixation in most instances.

Several subgroups of A2 fractures are recognized in the universal classification.

A2-1: Ischium

The column fracture remains within the ischium (Fig. 25-13A). It is really an extended posterior wall fracture, because it extends around the posterior margin of the posterior column into the quadrilateral plate.

A2-2: Through the Obturator Ring

This typical posterior column fracture extends through the obturator ring (Fig. 25-13A,B) preserving the teardrop (4). Occasionally, this fracture extends to involve the teardrop (D. Helfet, personal communication, 1993).

A2-3: Posterior Column Lesion Associated with a Posterior Wall Fracture

Group A2-3 are posterior column fractures associated with a fracture of a portion of the posterior wall (Figs. 25-

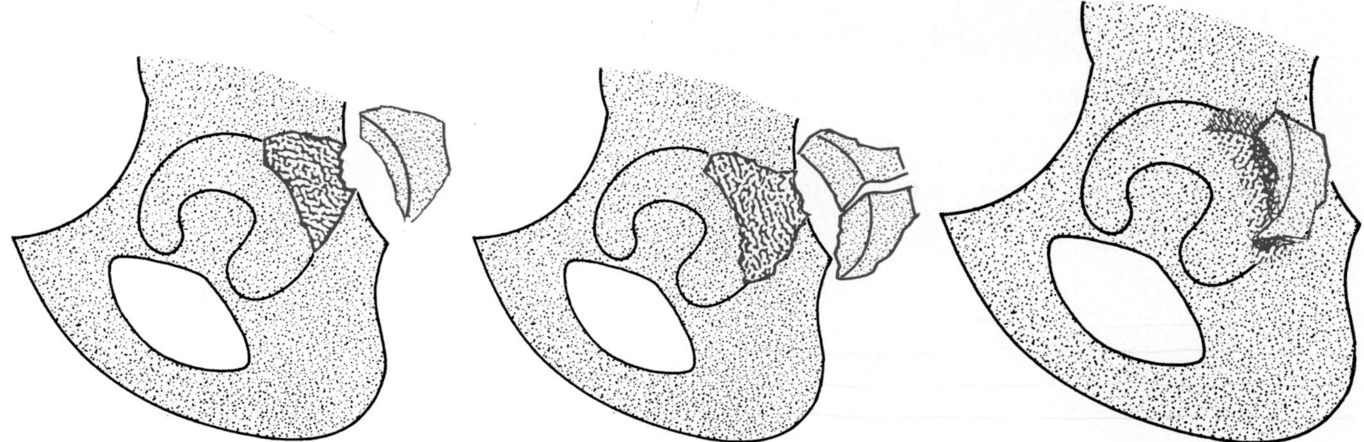

FIGURE 25-10. Subclassification of Type A1 posterior wall fractures. **A:** Type A1-1: a single fragment. **B:** Type A1-2: multiple fragments. **C:** Type A1-3: Posterior wall fragments associated with marginal impaction.

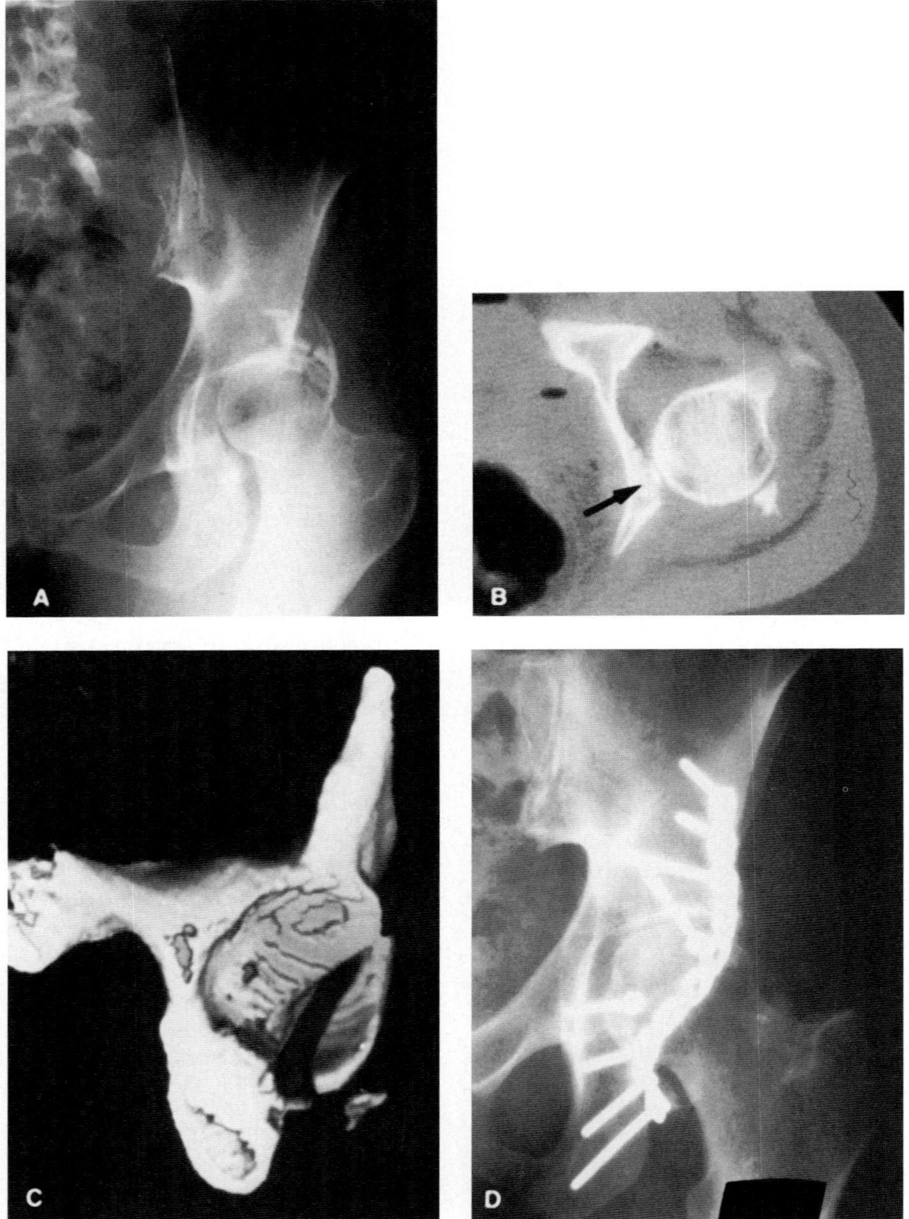

FIGURE 25-11. Fracture-dislocation with multiple fragments. **A:** Anterior-posterior view of the left hip showing a posterior dislocation and a large posterior fragment with a split. **B:** Axial computed tomography shows the dislocation and the usual marginally impacted fragment. **C:** The three-dimensional computed tomography image shows the large fragment with a split and another smaller fragment. **D:** Postoperative anterior-posterior radiograph shows the fixation with two interfragmental screws and a buttress plate.

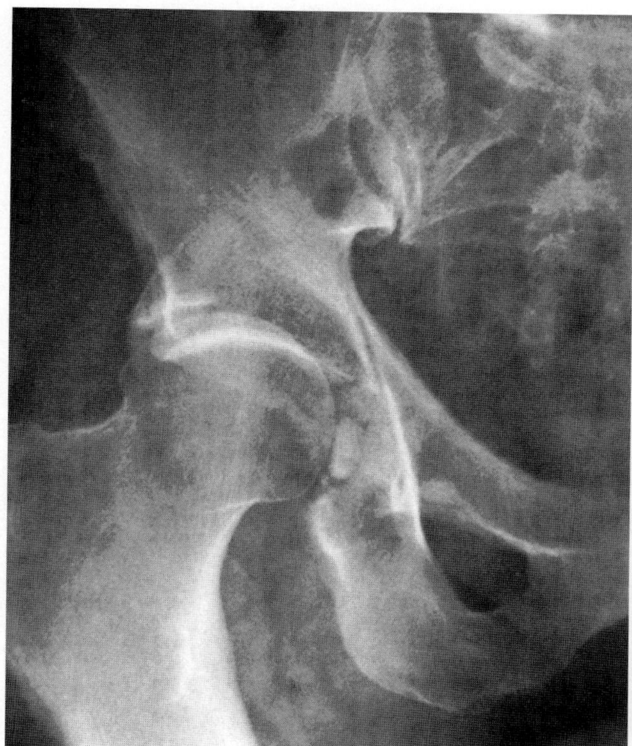

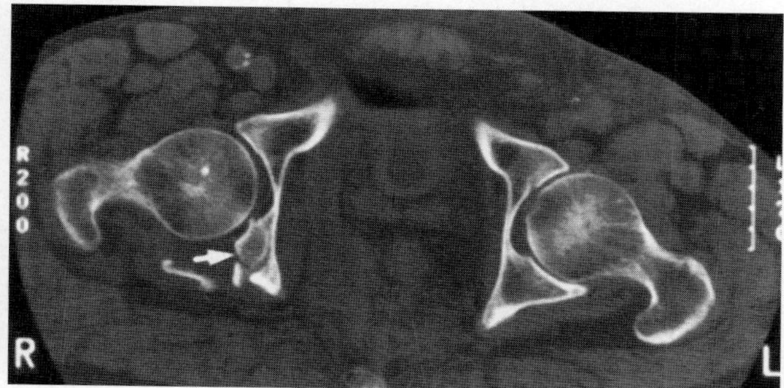

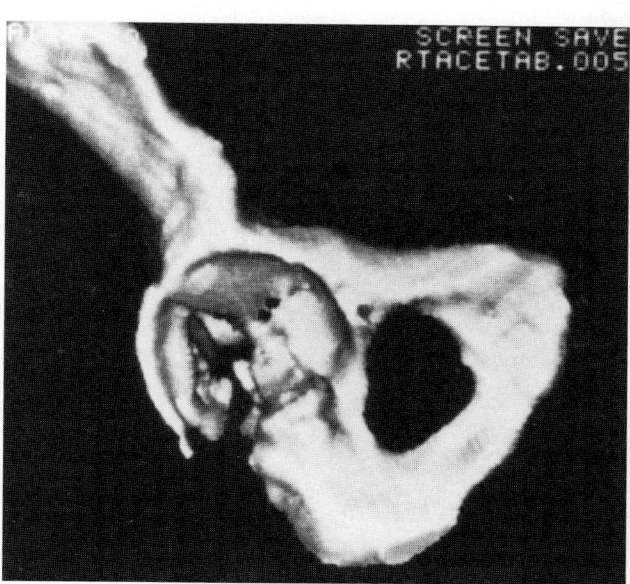

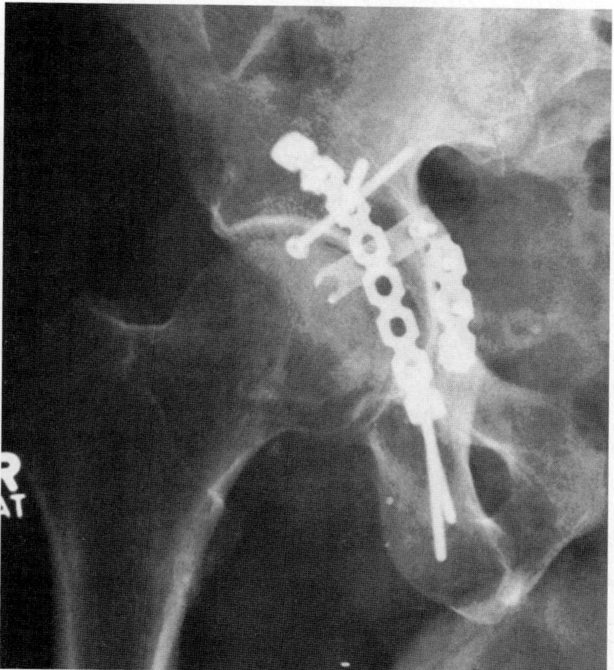

FIGURE 25-12. A: Anterior-posterior radiograph indicates a posterior fracture-dislocation of the hip with a large posterior wall fragment. **B:** Computed tomography shows a large impacted fragment *(arrow)* that is displaced. If it is not reduced and bone grafted, it will cause posterior incongruity of the joint. **C:** This is further identified on three-dimensional computed tomography. The dislocation was reduced and the fragments held by open reduction and internal fixation with intrafragmental screws, buttress plates, and a spring plate. **D:** The marginally impacted fragment was bone grafted to hold it in position.

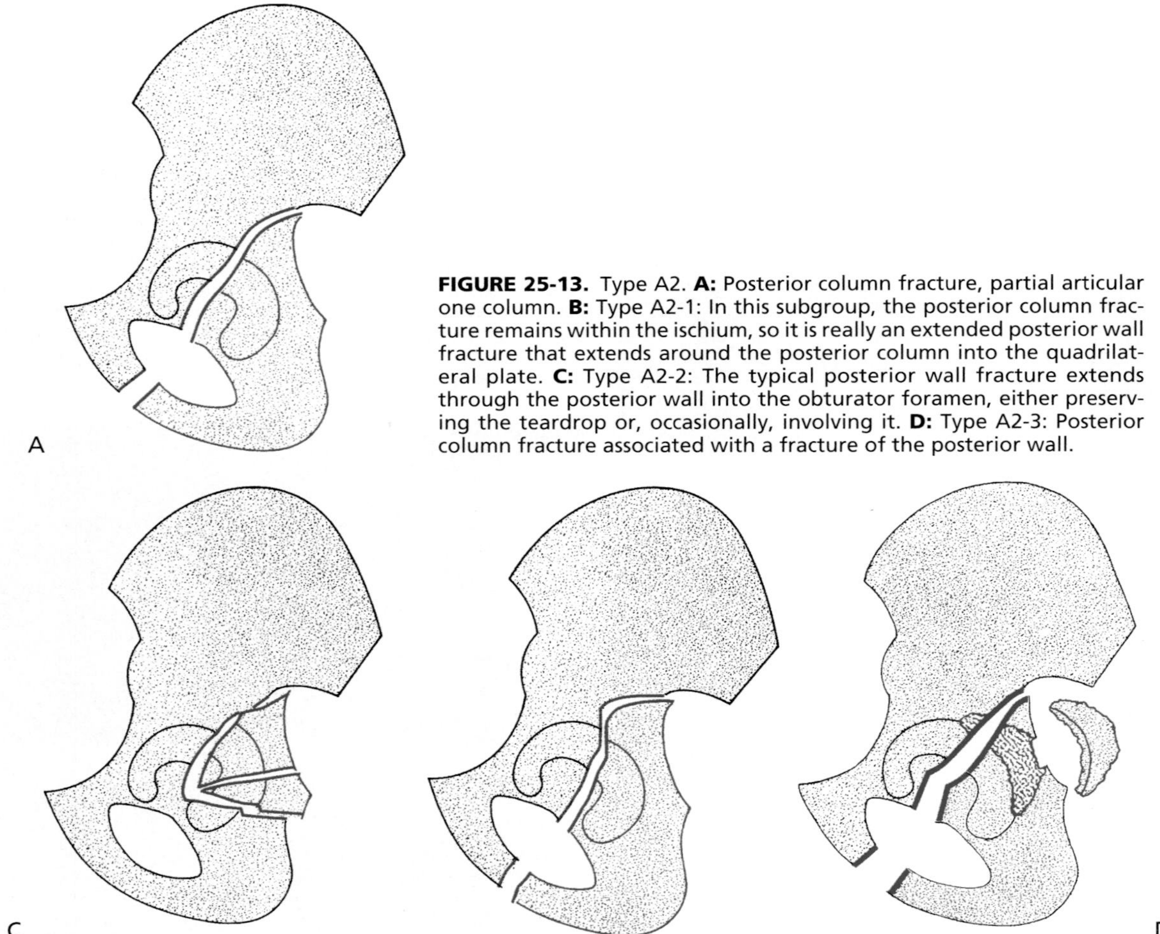

FIGURE 25-13. Type A2. **A:** Posterior column fracture, partial articular one column. **B:** Type A2-1: In this subgroup, the posterior column fracture remains within the ischium, so it is really an extended posterior wall fracture that extends around the posterior column into the quadrilateral plate. **C:** Type A2-2: The typical posterior wall fracture extends through the posterior wall into the obturator foramen, either preserving the teardrop or, occasionally, involving it. **D:** Type A2-3: Posterior column fracture associated with a fracture of the posterior wall.

13C and 25-15). The posterior wall fragment is important and must be characterized by its site—posterior, posterior-superior, or posterior-inferior—by the number of fragments and the presence or absence of marginally impacted fragments. Because the displaced posterior wall fracture usually renders the hip unstable, open anatomic reduction and internal fixation is required, as it is for most posterior types.

A3: Anterior Column and/or Wall, Partial Articular Fracture

Pure anterior fracture types always have been considered rare injuries—an insignificant percentage of all acetabular fractures (Fig. 25-16A). However, this is not really the case: Fractures of the superior pubic ramus (anterior column) often enter the hip joint with lateral compression types of pelvic ring disruption (Fig. 25-17). Thus, these injuries often are regarded as fractures of the pelvic ring rather than the acetabulum. Clearly, these injuries are caused by a blow to the greater trochanter when the leg is externally rotated.

In general, anterior fracture types rarely are associated with anterior hip dislocation, which is a relatively uncommon injury, as compared with posterior fracture types, which are almost always associated with posterior hip dislocation. Therefore, with anterior injury, complications are less frequent and the overall prognosis better than with other types.

Anterior partial articular fracture types are grouped as follows.

A3-1: Anterior Wall Fracture

Pure anterior wall fractures (Fig. 25-16B) are rare and are almost always associated with an anterior dislocation of the hip, caused by an abduction and external rotation force. The anterior wall fracture may produce one or multiple fragments, and some may be marginally impacted. The diagnosis is made by identifying the fracture of the anterior wall and confirming that there is no posterior injury. As in all wall fractures, the computed axial tomogram is invaluable for displaying the extent of the lesion.

A3-2, A3-3: Anterior Column Fractures, Partial Articular

The anterior column extends from the iliac crest to the

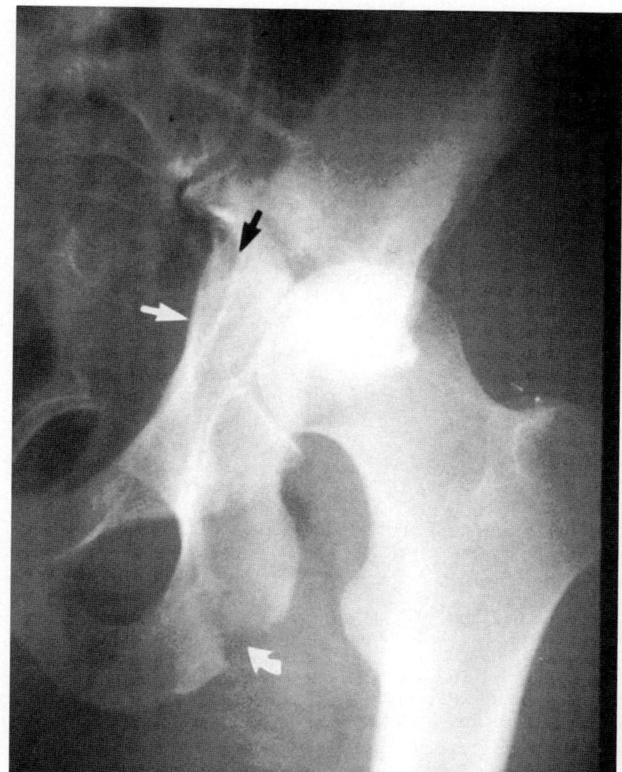

FIGURE 25-14. Type A2-3: Posterior column fracture associated with a posterior wall fracture. **A:** The unique features of this uncommon fracture are noted in the anterior-posterior radiograph. The *black arrow* indicates the iliopectineal line, which is intact, and the *white arrow,* the ilioischial line, which is displaced. The posteriorly dislocated hip joint has taken with it a posterior column fragment. The inferior margin of the posterior column fracture is through the ischial tuberosity and not in its more normal position through the obturator foramen *(curved arrow).* **B:** The unique features noted on the diagram depicting an axial view show the fracture entering the quadrilateral plate; thus, the posterior column is involved. **C:** The displaced posterior column is noted on computed tomography (CT), as is the intact anterior column. At the time of the CT the hip joint had been reduced. **D:** The features on three-dimensional computed tomography. It clearly indicates the posterior column fracture in the reduced position with the head subtracted.

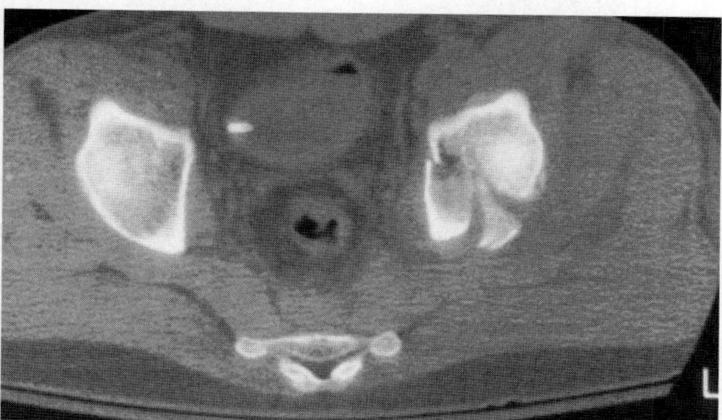

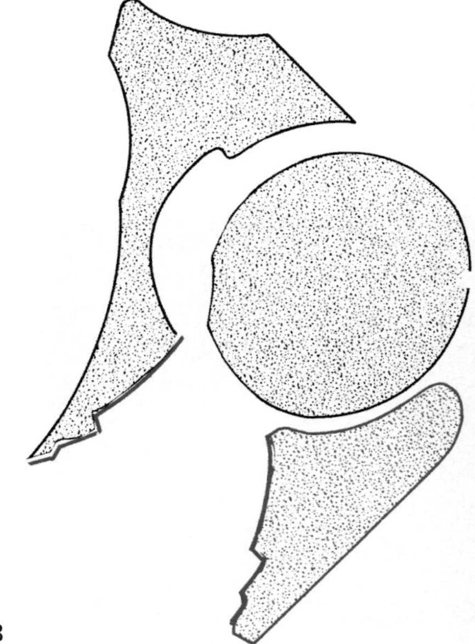

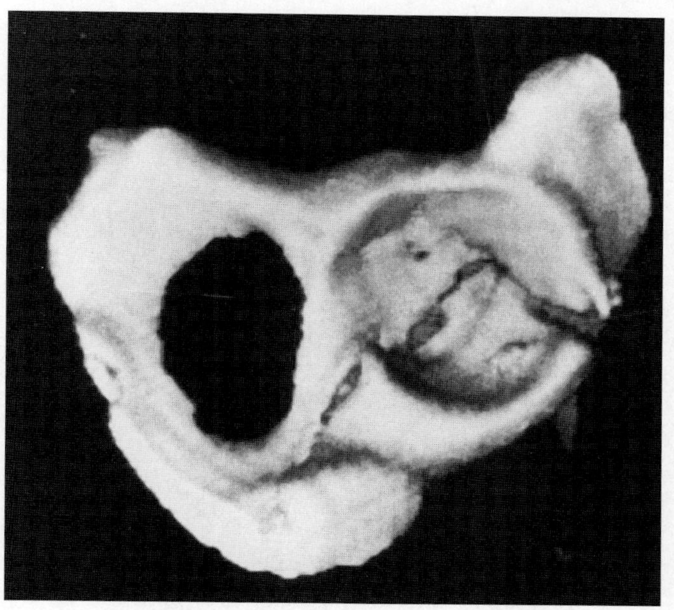

(*Figure continues*)

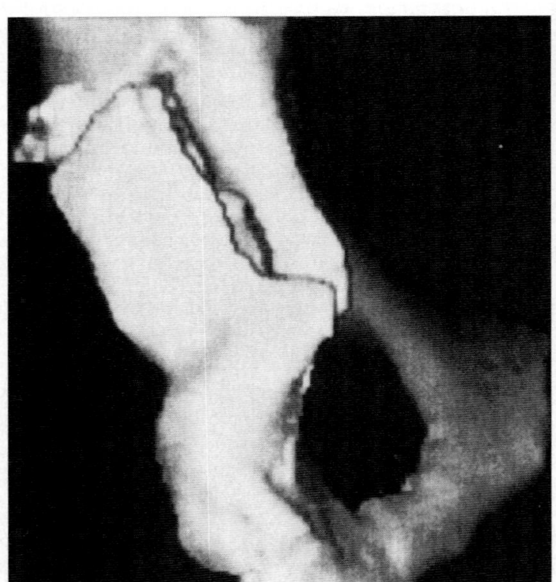
E

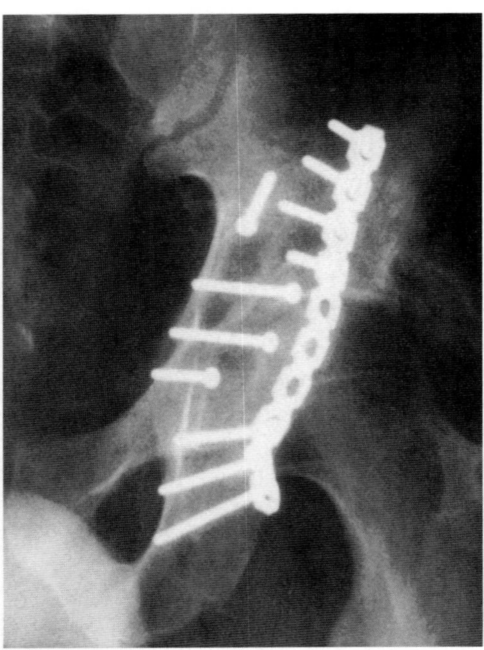
F

FIGURE 25-14. ***(continued)*** **E:** The direct posterior view shows the fracture of the posterior column. Because of incongruity, treatment consisted of open reduction and internal fixation using intrafragmental lag screws to fix the posterior column and a buttress plate to prevent redisplacement. **F:** Some heterotopic ossification has developed.

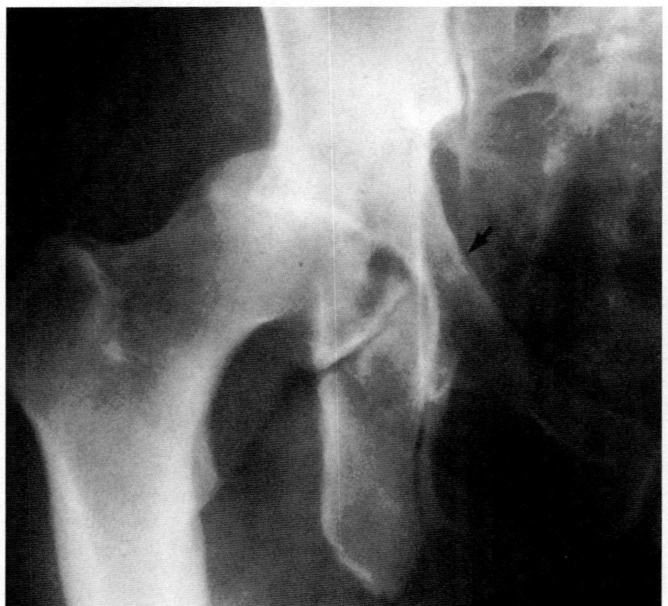
A

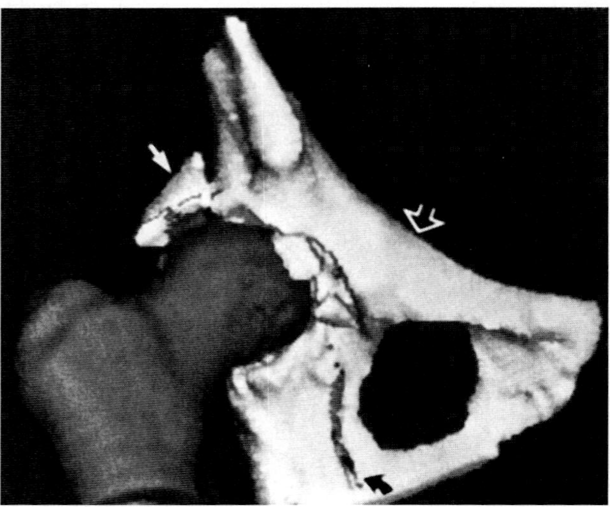
B

FIGURE 25-15. Posterior column fracture associated with a posterior wall fracture. Anterior-posterior radiograph **(A)** indicates a posterior dislocation of the right hip with a posterior column fracture associated with one of the posterior wall. The iliopectineal line is indicating the anterior column is intact *(black arrow),* but the ilioischial line is fractured at the ischial tuberosity as well as through the joint posteriorly. **B:** The three-dimensional computed tomography (3DCT) graphically illustrates the posterior wall fragment, the posteriorly dislocated hip, the posterior column fracture, and the intact iliopectineal line.

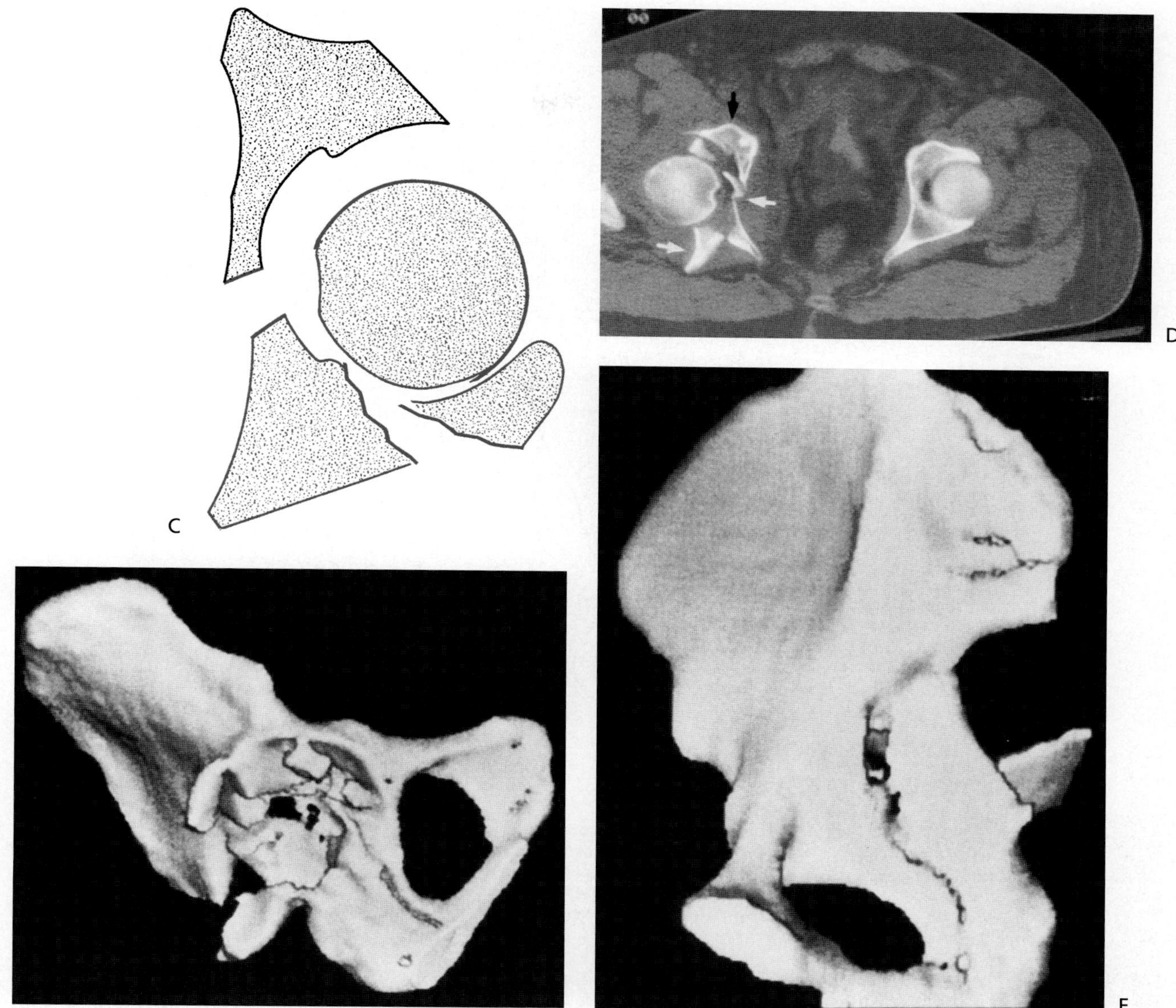

FIGURE 25-15. ***(continued)*** **C:** The classic axial CT features are noted in the drawing, which shows the posterior column fracture through the quadrilateral plate, the posterior wall fracture, and the dislocated femoral head. **D:** CT shows the intact anterior column *(black arrow)* and the markedly comminuted ischial column fracture and the associated posterior wall fracture. In this case, the posterior wall fracture is rotated 90 degrees to its normal position *(white arrow).* These features are also clearly seen on 3DCT, as viewed looking into the joint with the head subtracted **(E)** and from the quadrilateral plate medially **(F).**

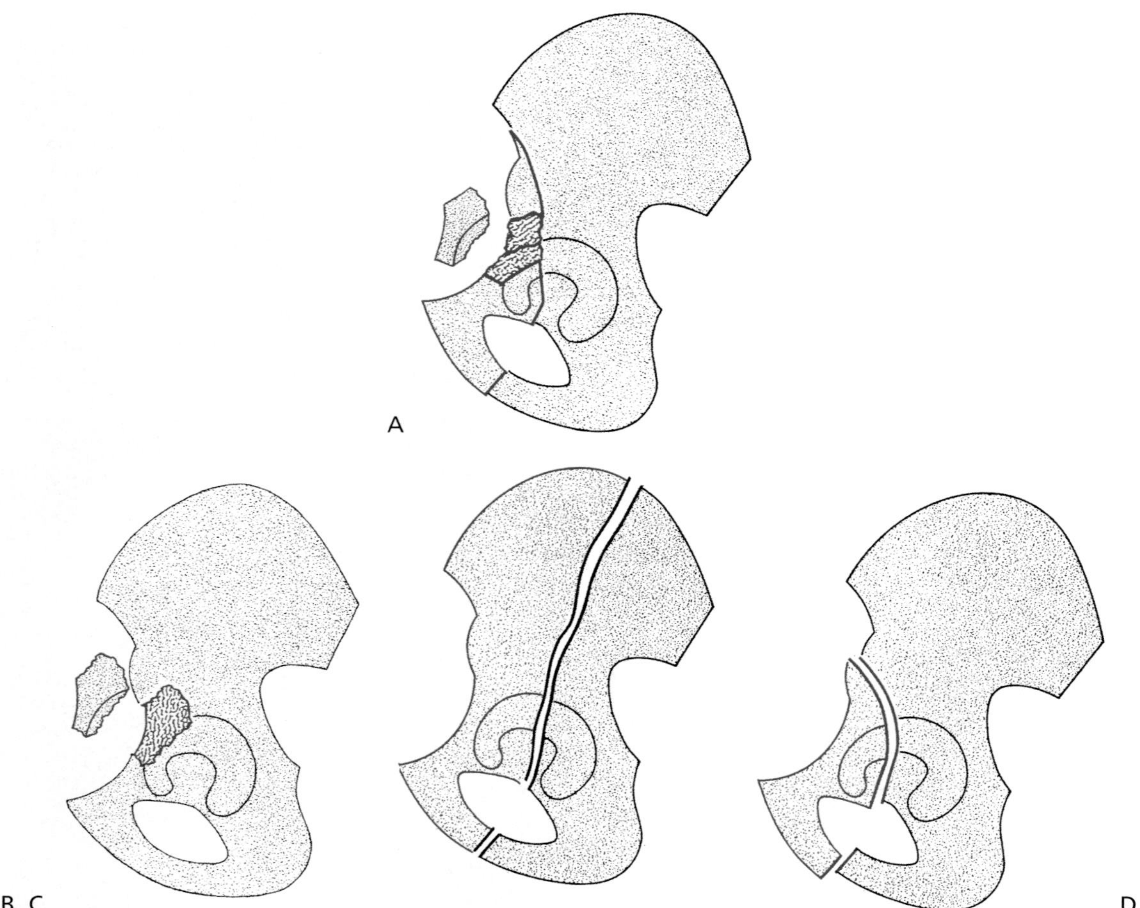

FIGURE 25-16. Type A-3: Anterior column fracture, partial articular, one column. **A:** The anterior partial articular types may involve the anterior column, or the anterior wall either separate or in combination. **B:** Type A3-1, the pure anterior wall fracture almost always is associated with an anterior dislocation of the hip (Fig. 25-13). The anterior column fracture may be high, reaching the iliac crest (Type C, A3-2) or low, reaching the anterior border of the ilium (Type D, A3-3).

anterior aspect of the acetabulum, and then to the superior pubic ramus and the symphysis pubis. Any portion of the anterior column can be fractured (Fig. 25-16C,D). Several types are recognized, a common one being fracture of the superior pubic ramus. Superiorly, the continuing force may separate the anterior column through any portion of its anatomy; that is, low (below the anteroinferior iliac spine, Type A3-3), intermediate (through the anterior part of the crest), or high (through the middle portion of the crest, Type A3-2). Anterior dislocation is uncommon.

The diagnosis is readily made when a fracture of the anterior column is associated with an *intact* posterior column. In general, the prognosis is favorable if the fracture is distal, because the important posterior-superior weight-bearing area of the acetabulum usually is preserved.

The low fracture types often separate a very small area of the acetabulum. This common injury often is overlooked as an acetabular injury and usually is considered a lateral compression-type pelvic ring disruption (Fig. 25-17). The superior ramus may be rotated slightly through the anterior tip of the acetabulum. The acetabulum is rarely sufficiently disturbed to require open reduction; therefore, the results usually are satisfactory. Occasionally, the superior ramus is markedly displaced at the symphysis; this is the tilt fracture of the pelvis. Only open reduction can derotate this fragment. Fixation with a threaded Steinmann pin usually is sufficient to stabilize the symphysis if the posterior pelvic ligaments are intact (Fig. 25-18).

The high fracture types disrupt the iliac crest somewhere above the anterior inferior iliac spine. Management depends on the degree of displacement; however, because the superior dome may be involved, open reduction often is indicated.

Anterior column fractures may be grouped as follows.

A3-2: Anterior Column (High Variety). The anterior fracture line reaches the iliac crest in Type A3-2 (Fig. 25-19).

A3-3: Anterior Column (Low Variety). The fracture line usually exits the anterior ilium below the crest in this type.

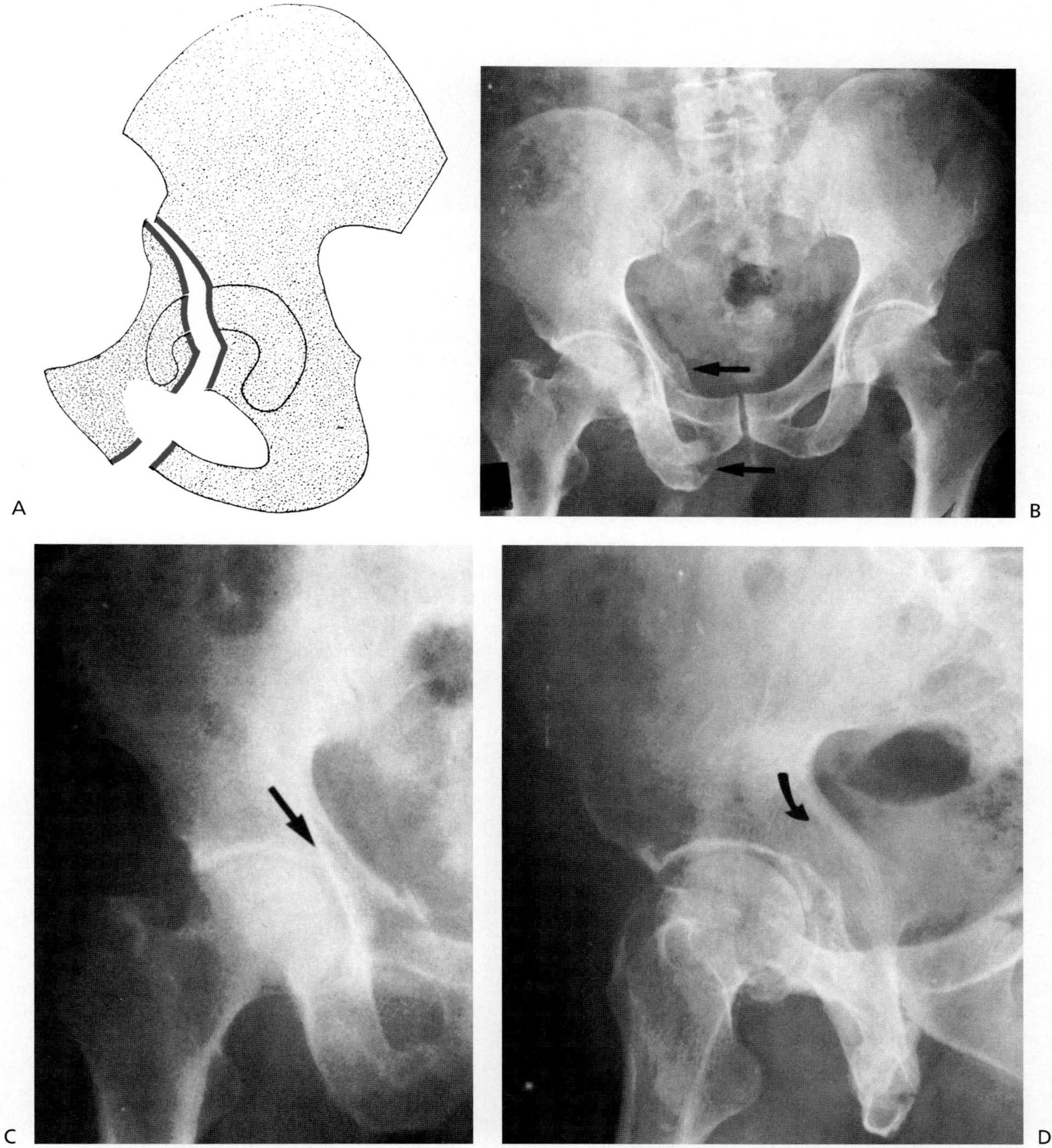

FIGURE 25-17. The diagram **(A)** demonstrates atypical anterior column fracture dividing the anterior column just under the anterior inferior iliac spine. The anterior-posterior radiographs of the pelvis **(B)** and acetabulum **(C)** clearly show the fracture through the anterior column with the intact posterior column clearly marked *(black arrow).* The iliac oblique view **(D)** demonstrates the intact posterior column. (*Figure continues*)

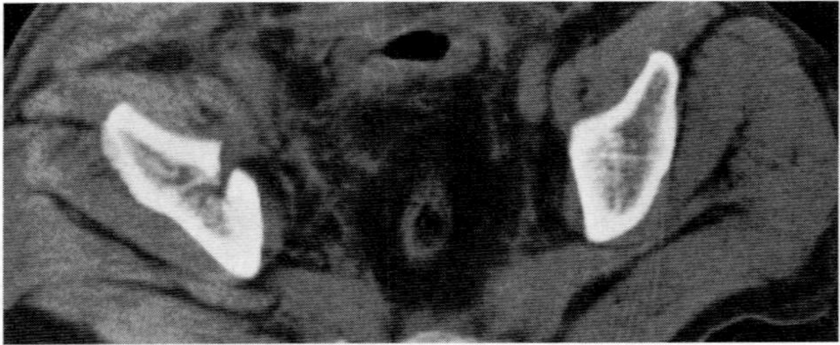

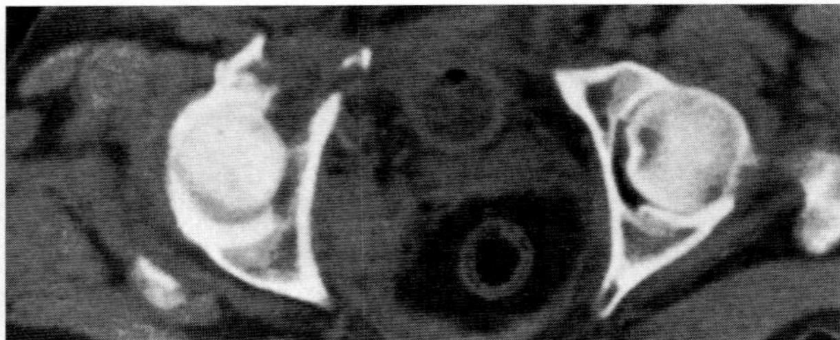

FIGURE 25-17. *(continued)* On computed tomography **(E,F)** the anterior column is split and comminuted and the posterior column is intact.

Also, as mentioned, the lateral compression pelvic fracture (B2) involving the superior ramus of the pelvis often enters the acetabulum, but very low (distal), and, therefore, usually does not require open reduction (Figs. 25-16D and 25-20).

Anterior column fractures may produce one fragment (designated by the suffix -a1), two fragments (-a2), or multiple fragments (-a3).

In the rare *associated anterior wall and anterior column fracture* (Fig. 25-21A–C), the posterior column remains intact. CT (Fig. 25-21D,E) clearly shows the anterior dislocation of the femoral head, as well as the intact posterior column. Another example (Fig. 25-21F–H) demonstrates this injury on three-dimensional CT (3DCT).

Type B: Transverse or T Type (Partial Articular) Fractures

B1: Transverse Fractures

Transverse fractures divide the hemipelvis into two parts through some portion of the acetabulum; therefore, both columns are divided. The line of division in the acetabulum is variable, but usually it runs through the superior rim of the acetabular fossa, and occasionally proximal or distal to this area (Fig. 25-22A). The fracture also exhibits varying degrees of obliquity, in both the vertical and horizontal plane (Fig. 25-22B).

Displacement may vary from minimal to complete central dislocation of the femoral head, which lies inside the

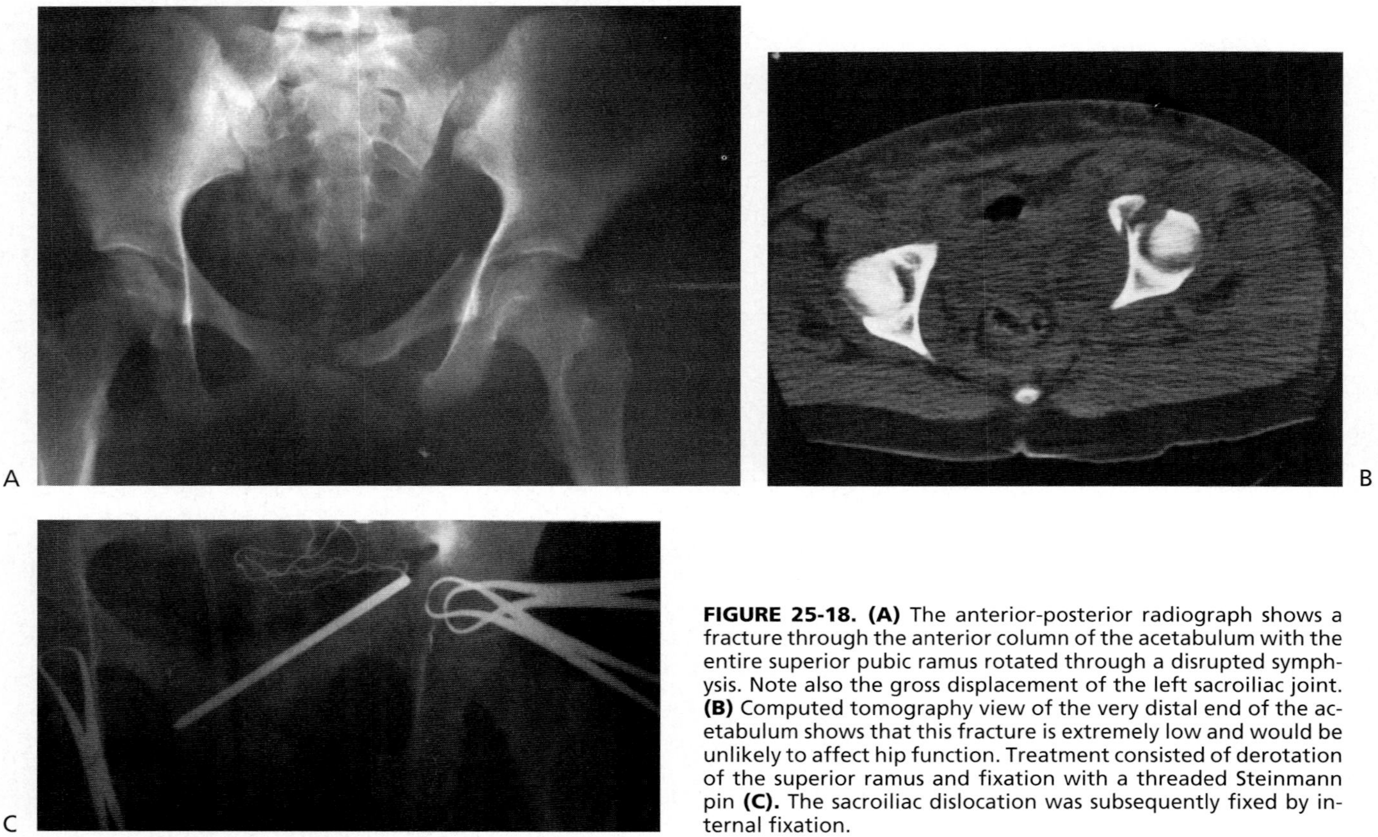

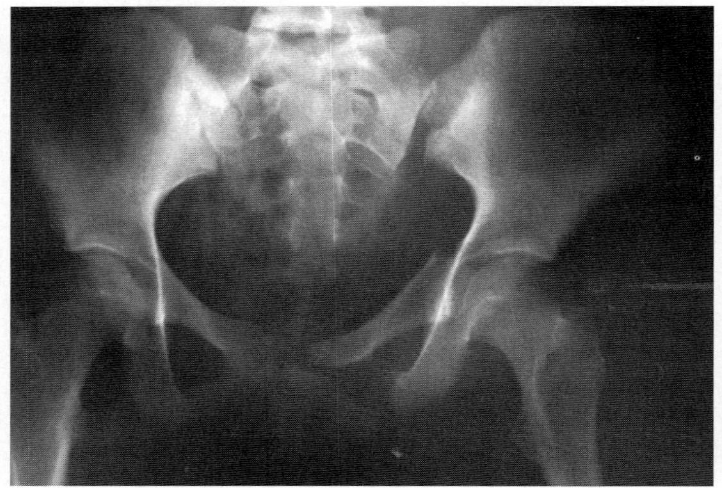

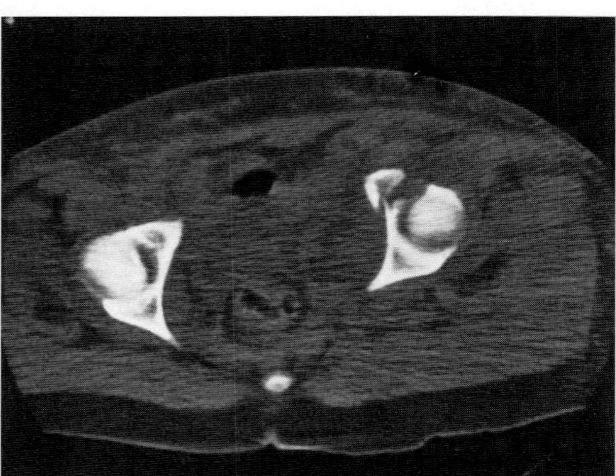

FIGURE 25-18. (A) The anterior-posterior radiograph shows a fracture through the anterior column of the acetabulum with the entire superior pubic ramus rotated through a disrupted symphysis. Note also the gross displacement of the left sacroiliac joint. **(B)** Computed tomography view of the very distal end of the acetabulum shows that this fracture is extremely low and would be unlikely to affect hip function. Treatment consisted of derotation of the superior ramus and fixation with a threaded Steinmann pin **(C)**. The sacroiliac dislocation was subsequently fixed by internal fixation.

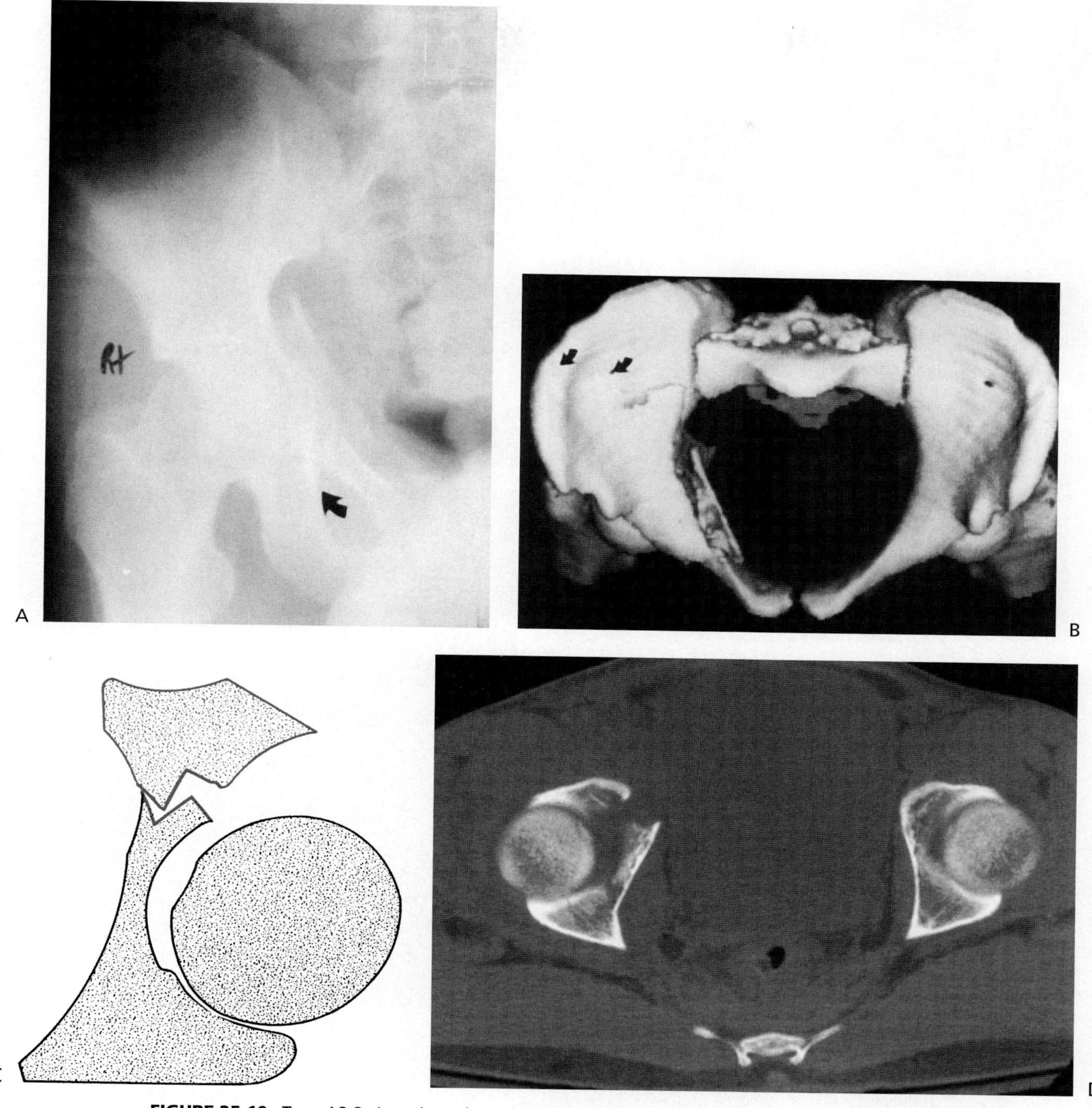

FIGURE 25-19. Type A3-2: Anterior column high variety lesion. **A:** Anterior-posterior radiograph shows a fracture through the anterior column with an intact posterior column, as noted on the ilioischial line *(black arrow).* **B:** The nature of this anterior fracture is better seen on three-dimensional computed tomography (3DCT). The anterior lesion is a greenstick fracture that reaches the iliac crest *(black arrows).* There also is a greenstick fracture of the quadrilateral plate, which does not reach the posterior column. The typical axial computed tomography (CT) appearance of this anterior column fracture is noted on the diagram **(C)** and the associated CT **(D).** The greenstick nature of this fracture of the quadrilateral plate is clearly seen on the CT **(D).**

(*Figure continues*)

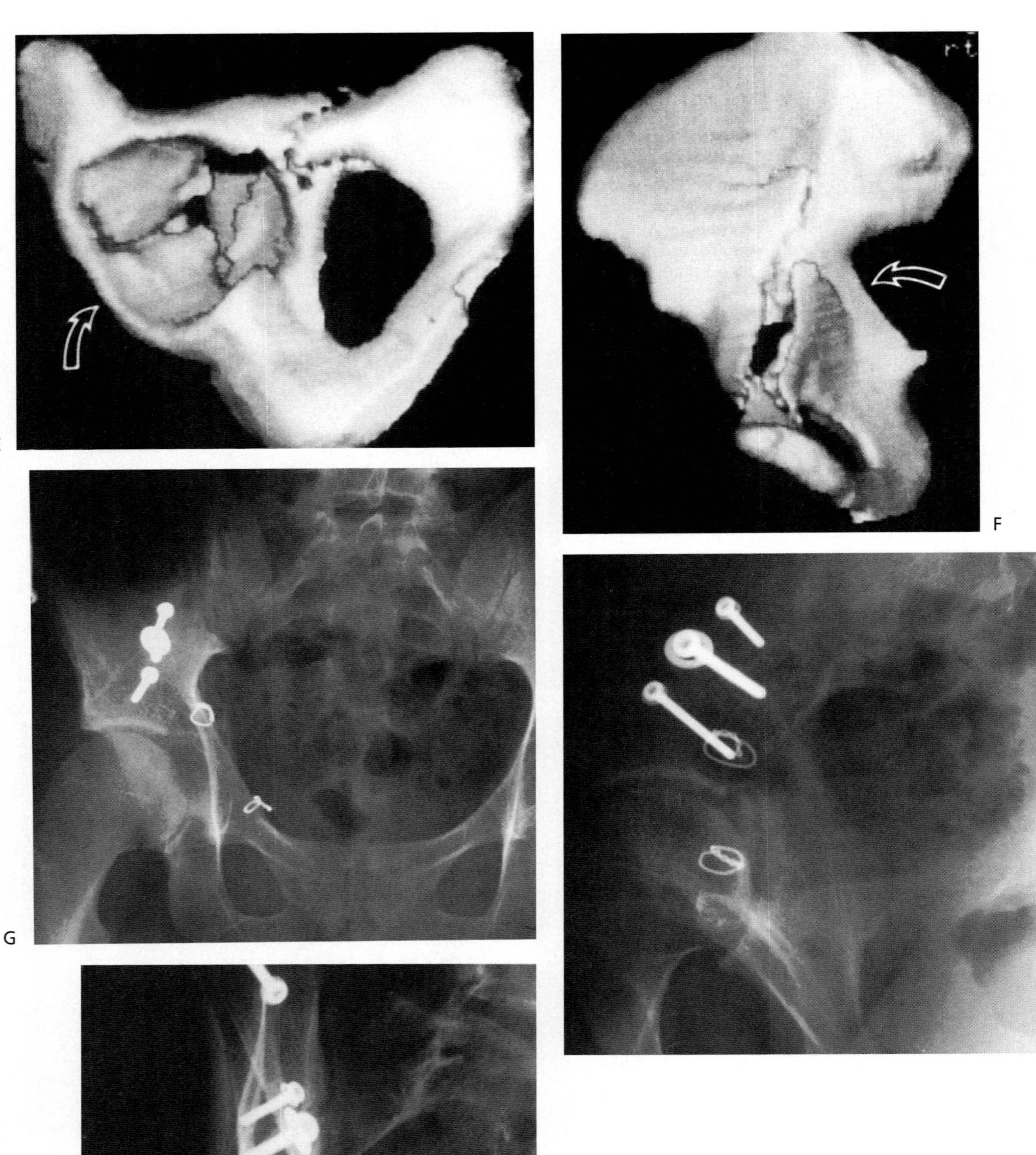

FIGURE 25-19. ***(continued)*** **E,F:** The 3DCT views show the intact posterior column, both seen into the acetabulum with the head subtracted **(E),** and looking at the medial aspect of the quadrilateral plate **(F)** *(white arrows).* **G–I:** Open reduction and internal fixation through an anterior approach resulted in anatomic reduction and fixation using lag screws and interosseous wires to hold the greenstick quadrilateral plate fracture in excellent position.

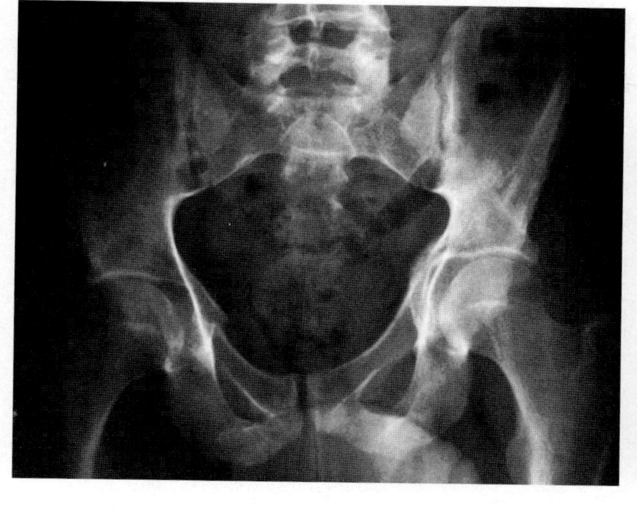
A

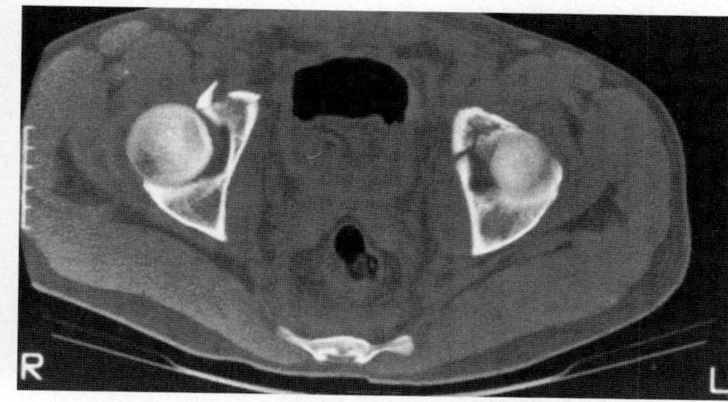

B

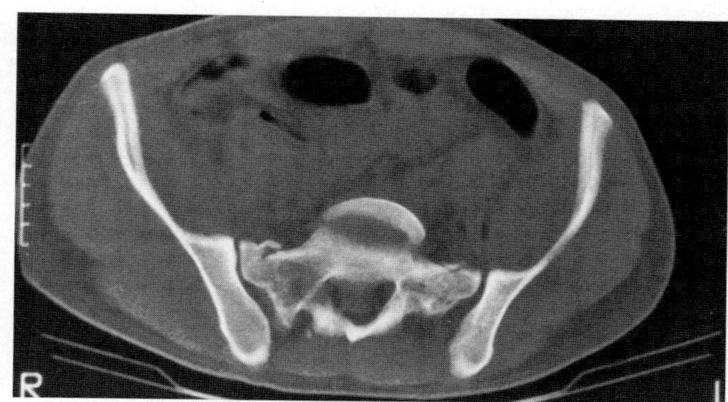

C

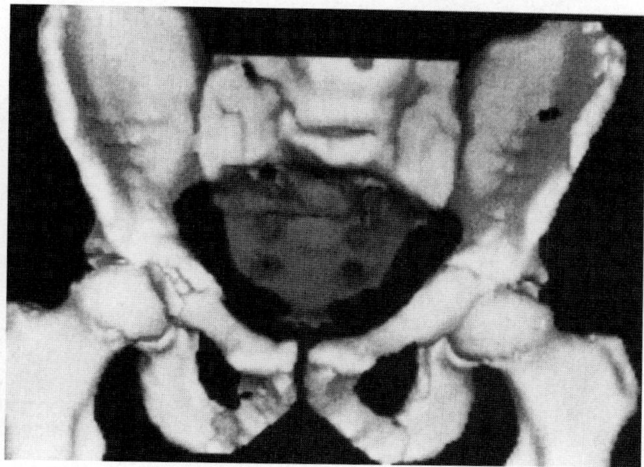
D

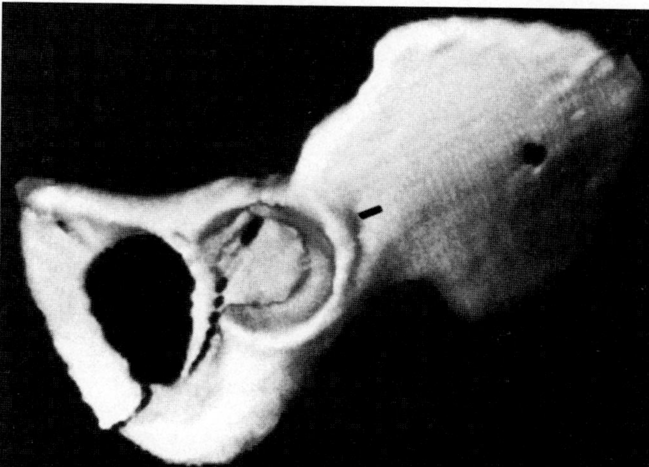
E

FIGURE 25-20. Type A3-3: Anterior column low variety. Anterior-posterior radiograph of a 24-year-old man struck from the side in a motor vehicle accident. **A:** The patient sustained bilateral fractures, which appeared to be lateral compression injuries to the pelvis (Type B-2). **B:** Computed tomography (CT) indicates that both superior ramus fractures have entered the hip joint, the left side through the roof with minimal displacement on the right farther distal. **C:** CT view through the sacroiliac joints show a compression fracture through the right sacrum with 1 cm overlap and very minimal compression through the left sacrum, confirming the picture of the injury. **D:** The three-dimensional computed tomography (3DCT) view shows the lesions through the sacrum bilaterally and the superior ramus fractures entering the hip joint. **E:** The 3DCT shows the location of the anterior column through the left hip with a marked resemblance to the drawing in Fig. 25-16D.

pelvis against the proximal fragment. Obviously, the amount of displacement and presence of central dislocation have great prognostic significance. Most commonly, the distal fragment moves inward, rotating around the symphysis pubis, but with complete central dislocation the proximal fragment may also rotate, usually through a disrupted sacroiliac joint (Fig. 25-23).

These fractures and the T types described in the following commonly are caused by high-energy shearing forces; consequently, although they look simple, they often have the worst prognosis of any acetabular fracture.

B1-1: Infratectal

This low transverse fracture may be managed nonoperatively; however, congruity is often sustained by the remaining medial wall (Fig. 25-24A).

B1-2: Juxtatectal

A B1-2 fracture shears through the junction of the acetabular fossa and the articular surface (Fig. 25-24B).

B1-3: Transtectal

A B1-3 fracture shears the articular surface through the major weight-bearing roof area; therefore, it has the worst prog-

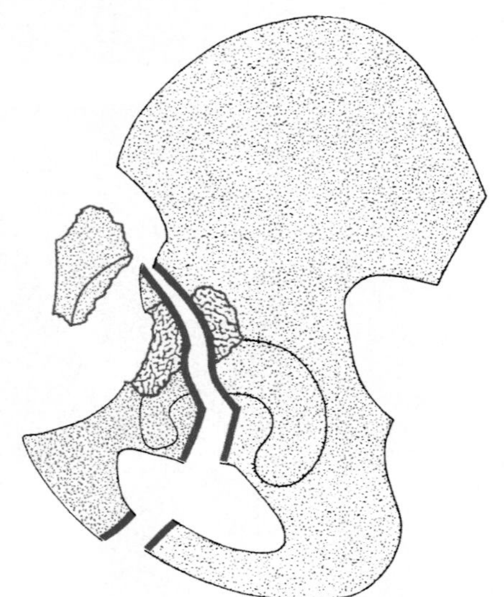

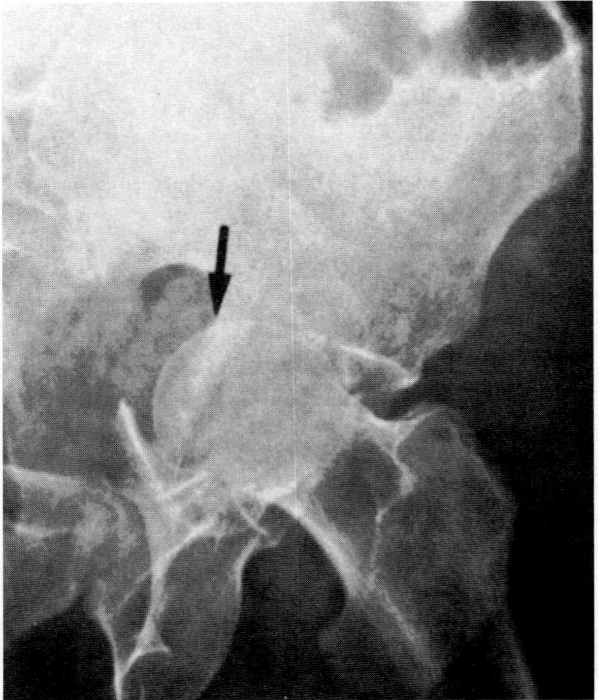

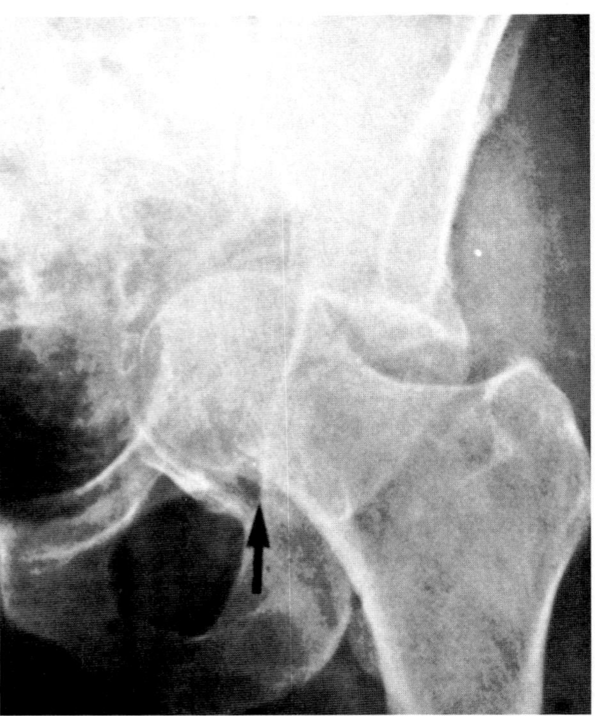

FIGURE 25-21. Associated anterior wall and anterior column fracture. **A:** Diagram demonstrates a typical anterior wall and anterior column fracture. The iliac oblique **(B)** and obturator oblique **(C)** radiographs clearly show the disruption of the anterior column and the anterior wall associated with an anterior dislocation of the hip. The posterior column outlined by the *black arrows* is intact.

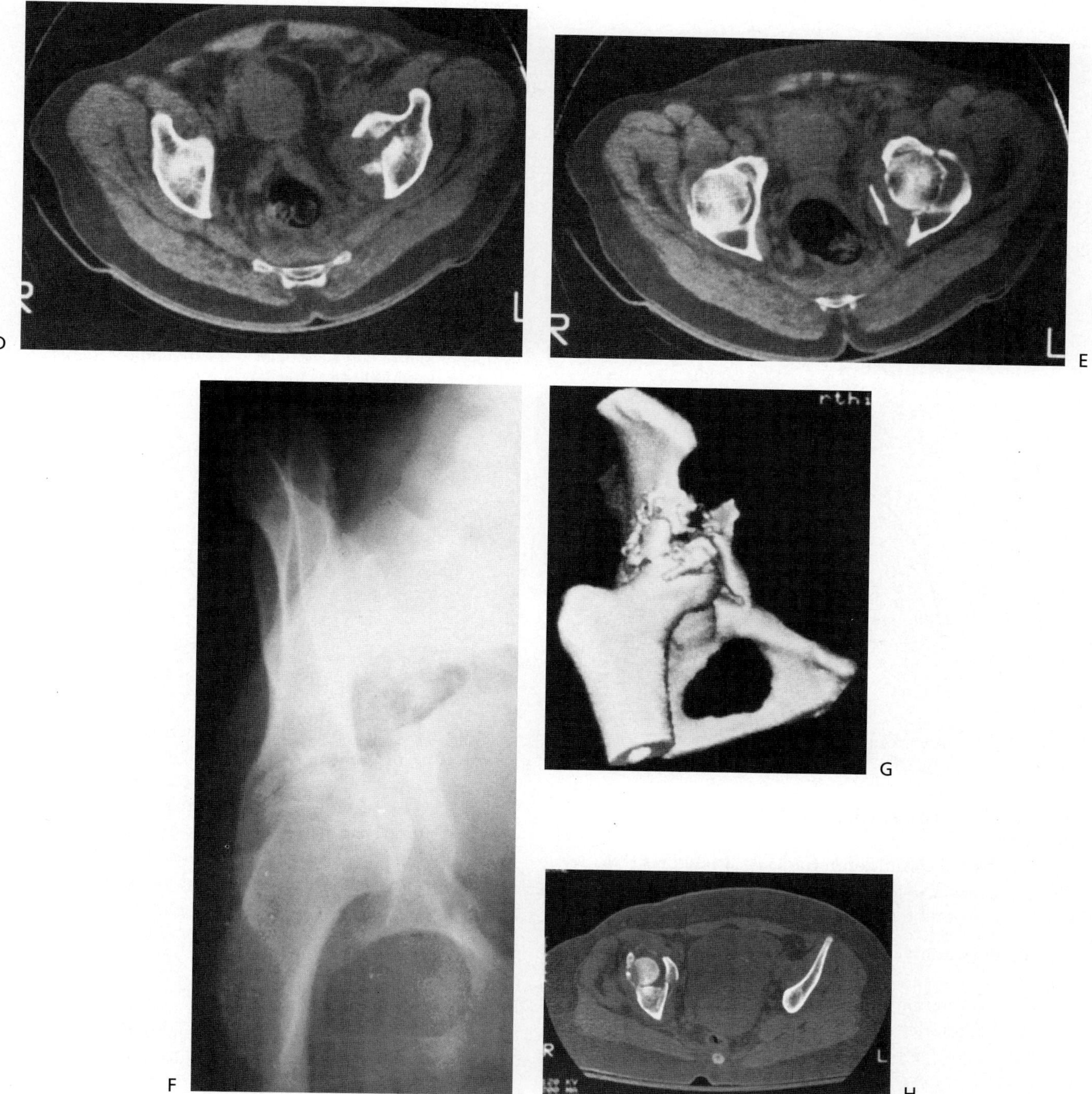

FIGURE 25-21. ***(continued)*** **D,E:** Computed tomography (CT) views taken through the dome and 1 cm distal to the dome of the left hip joint show an intact posterior column and a split comminuted anterior column with an anterior dislocation. **F:** Another example of an anterior column fracture associated with an anterior wall and anterior dislocation of the hip. The lesion is seen clearly on three-dimensional computed tomography **(G)** as marked fragmentation of the anterior wall and on axial CT **(H).**

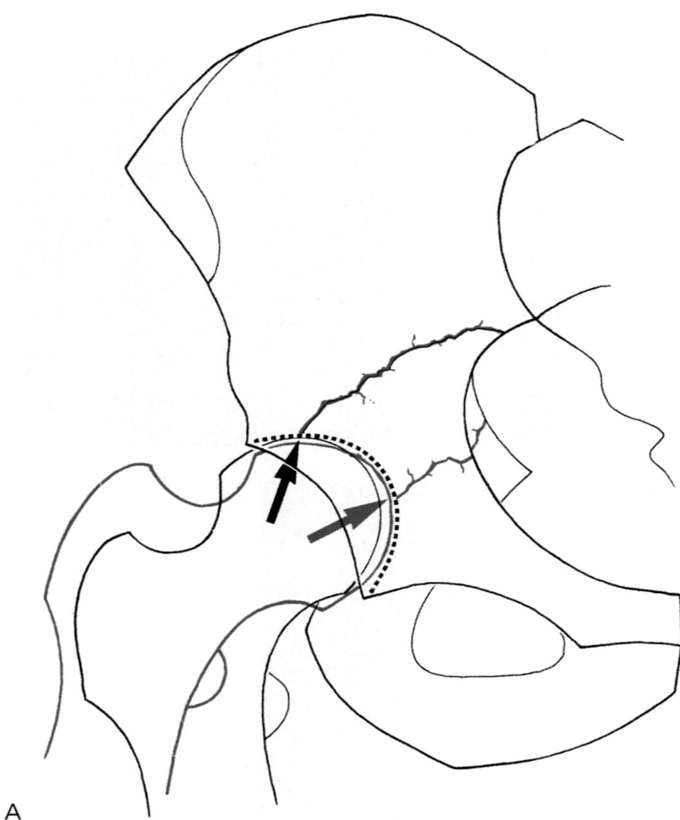

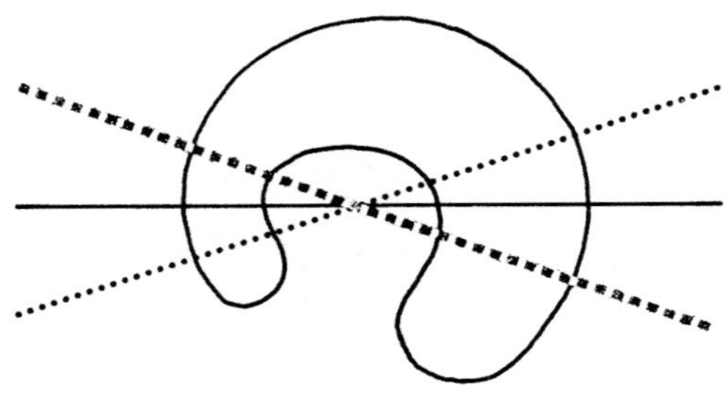

FIGURE 25-22. The line of division of the acetabulum in the transverse fracture is variable but usually occurs at the superior rim of the acetabular fossa though occasionally farther distal **(A).** Also, the fracture may exhibit varying degrees of obliquity in both the vertical and the horizontal plane **(B).**

nosis of the three groups—the transverse as well as the T group (Fig. 25-24C).

Associated Transverse (B1) and Acetabular Wall Fractures

In the universal classification for Type B fractures (Fig. 25-25), the presence of the modifier "a" designates the presence of a posterior wall fragment, as follows.

(a1): Pure transverse fracture; no posterior wall involvement

(a2): + Posterior wall, single fragment

(a3): + Posterior wall, multifragmentary

(a4): + Posterior wall, multifragmentary with marginal impaction

The association of a transverse fracture with a posterior wall fracture is common (about 20% of all cases). Also, it is usually associated with extremely high energy, and usually with posterior dislocation of the hip. The prognosis for this type must be guarded for these reasons.

The major component may be the posterior wall, and only an "insignificant" transverse crack might be noted on the radiographs. The physician must beware, especially in young patients; however, this transverse component may displace secondarily if it is not fixed at the time of open reduction and internal fixation of the posterior wall (Fig. 25-26).

The degree of difficulty is much increased when both the transverse component and posterior wall are grossly displaced. It is essential that the sinister nature of this injury be recognized by accurate diagnosis of the posterior wall fragment. Common complications—sciatic nerve palsy and avascular necrosis—are caused by the *posterior injury.* Careful radiographic study separates this group from pure transverse fractures. Computed axial tomograms are especially useful for identifying posterior lesions (Fig. 25-25).

B2: T Fracture, Partial Articular

In addition to the transverse component of the fracture (Fig. 25-27), T fractures split the acetabulum vertically (Fig. 25-27A). The transverse limb may be oriented in any plane or through any part of the acetabulum, usually at the superior part of the acetabular fossa, as in pure transverse fractures (Fig. 25-23). The vertical limb usually splits the central portion of the acetabulum and the inferior pubic ramus, which distinguishes this injury from the pure transverse type. Other possibilities for the vertical fracture are seen in Fig. 25-27B and include a more anterior or posterior limb; occasionally, such a lesion does not split the obturator foramen at all. As for the pure transverse fracture, the degree of femoral head displacement is variable, but central dislocation is more common because this is generally a more high-energy injury.

(Text continues on page 459)

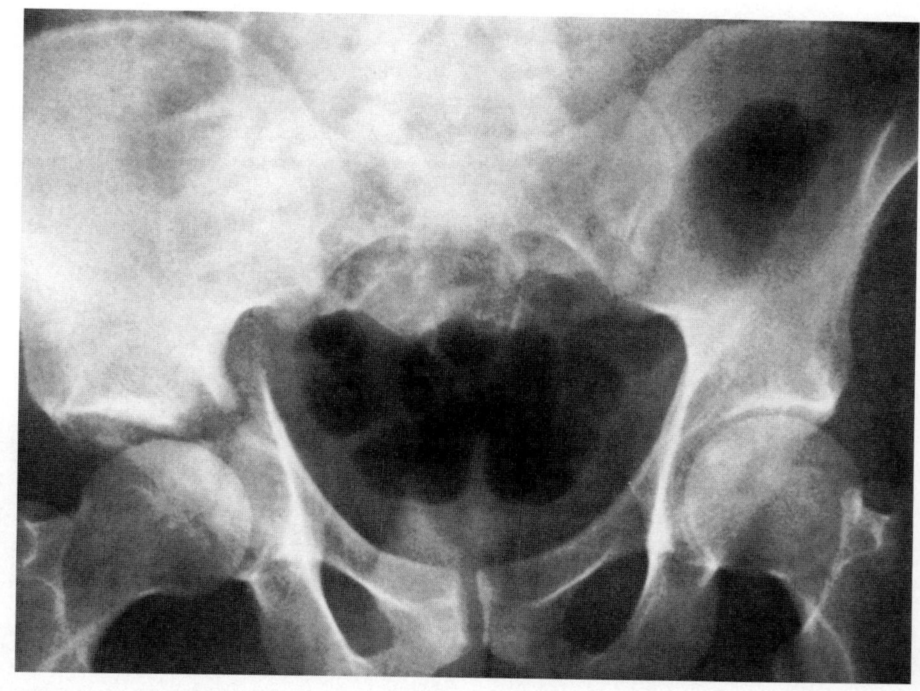
A

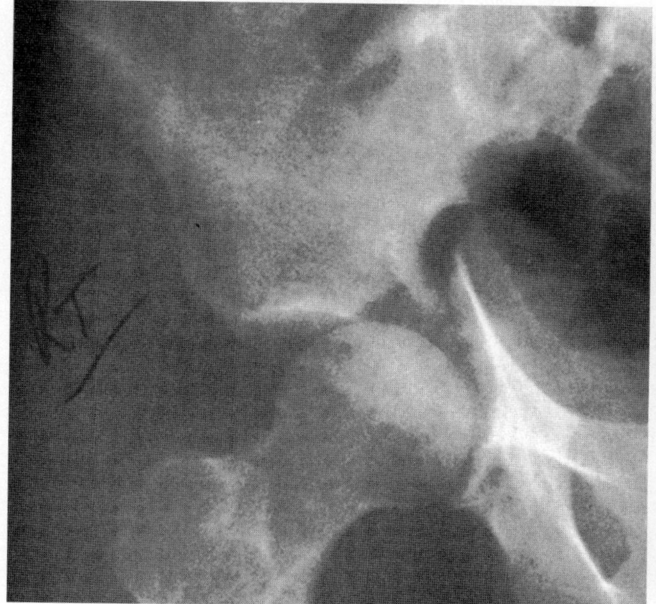
B

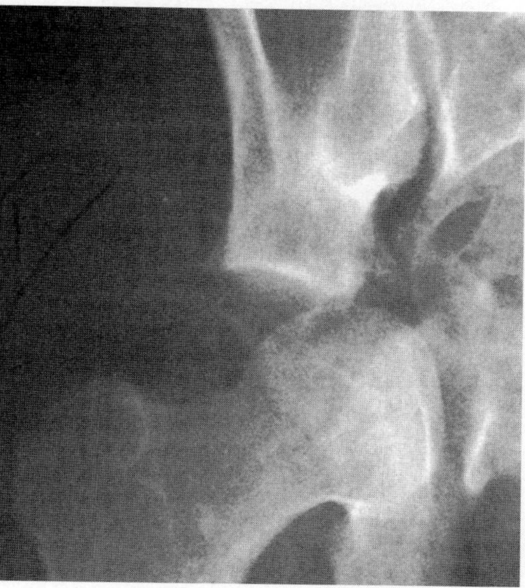
C

FIGURE 25-23. Transverse fracture. The anterior-posterior radiograph **(A),** iliac oblique **(B),** and obturator oblique views **(C)** show a typical transverse fracture in a 29-year-old man who was involved in a motor vehicle accident. (*Figure continues*)

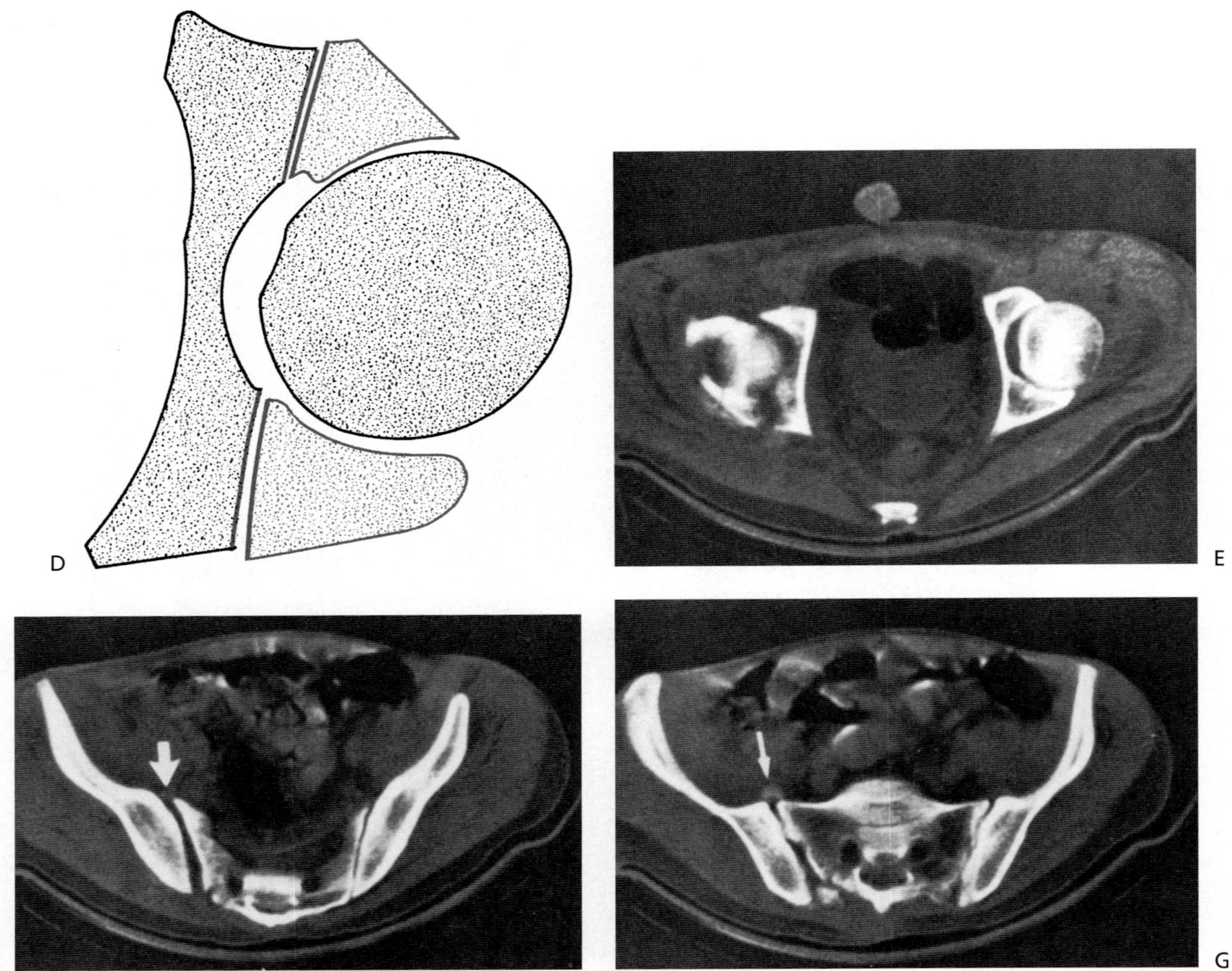

FIGURE 25-23. ***(continued)*** **D:** Diagram shows the direction of the transverse fracture in the acetabulum, as does CT **(E).** The rotation in this transverse fracture is not only through the distal fragment but also through the proximal fragment with rotation through the sacroiliac joint, as noted on CT **(F,G).** At 4 weeks a small amount of anterior callus was noted *(white arrow).*

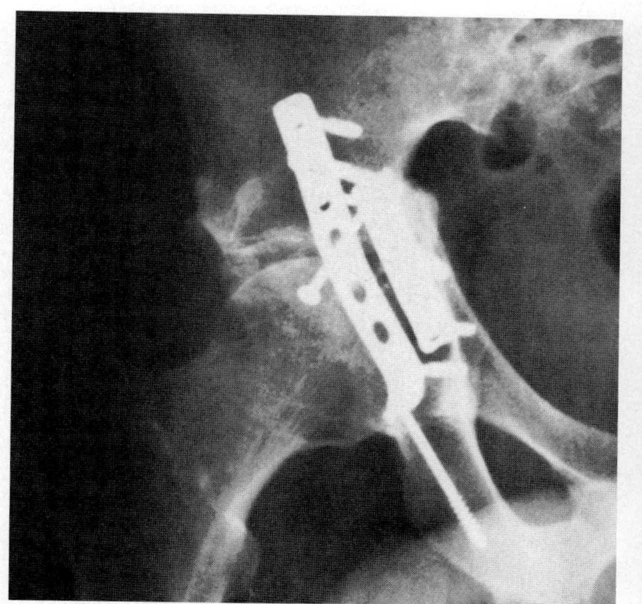

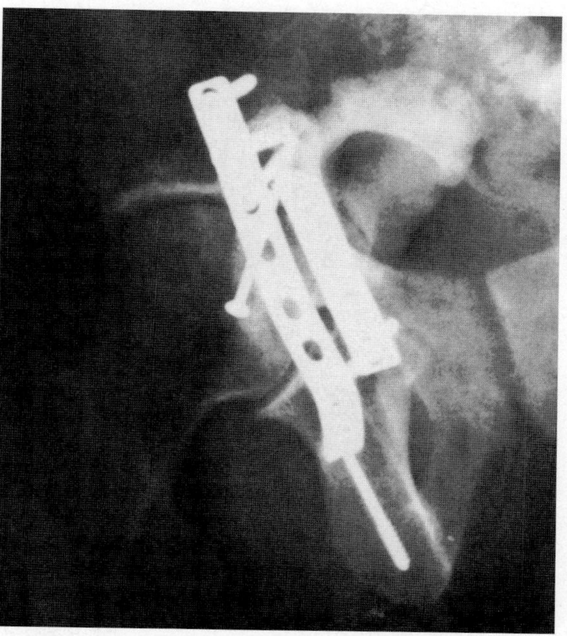

FIGURE 25-23. ***(continued)*** Four weeks after the injury the fracture was approached posteriorly and fixed with two plates **(H,I),** which improved the congruity of the joint.

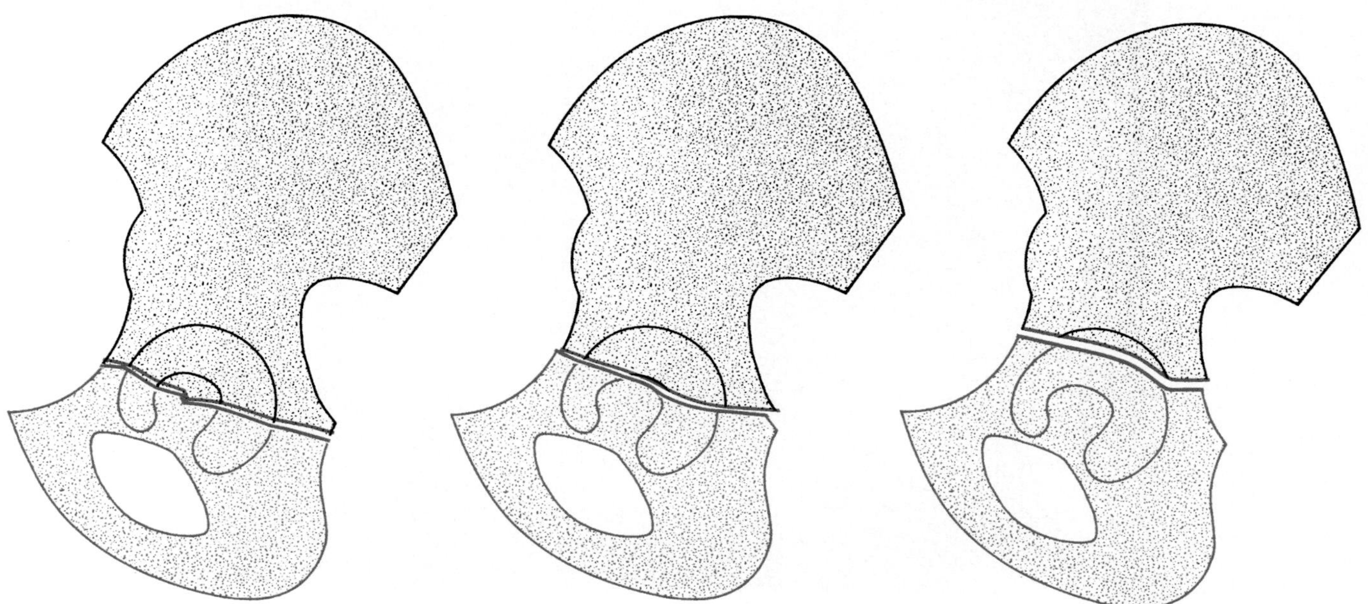

FIGURE 25-24. Subclassification of transverse fractures. The transverse fractures may be subclassified as infratectal (B1-1, A), juxtatectal (B1-2, B), and transtectal (B1-3, C). Type B1-3 shears through the articular surface and has the worst prognosis.

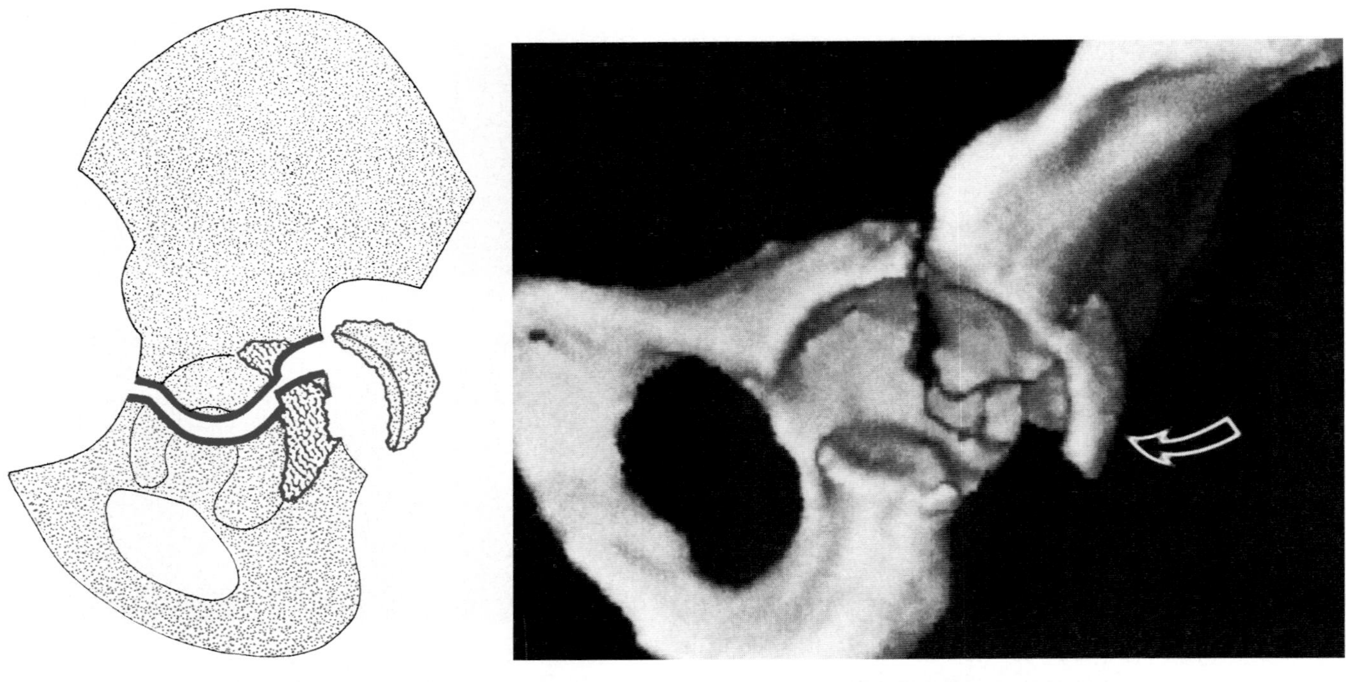

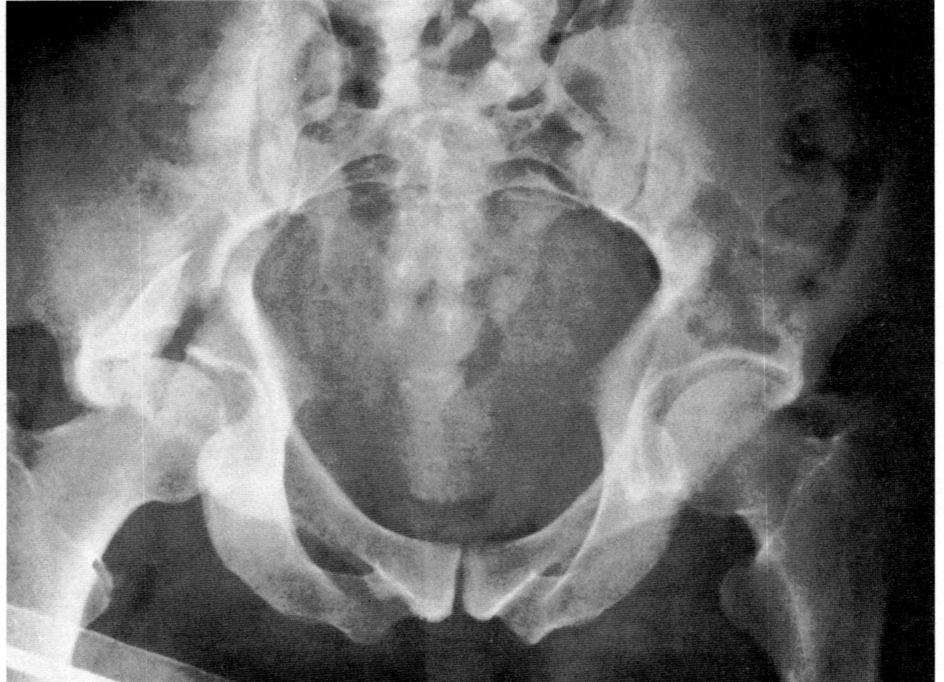

FIGURE 25-25. Associated transverse (B1) lesion with posterior acetabular wall fracture. The posterior wall fracture may be associated with a transverse fracture of the acetabulum, as shown in the diagram **(A1)** and in the three-dimensional computed tomography image **(A2).** Note the obliquity of the transverse fracture and the large posterior wall fragment. A typical example is seen in the anterior-posterior **(B),** iliac oblique **(C),** and obturator oblique **(D)** radiographs of this 46-year-old physician injured when his single-engine plane crashed into a tree **(F,G).**

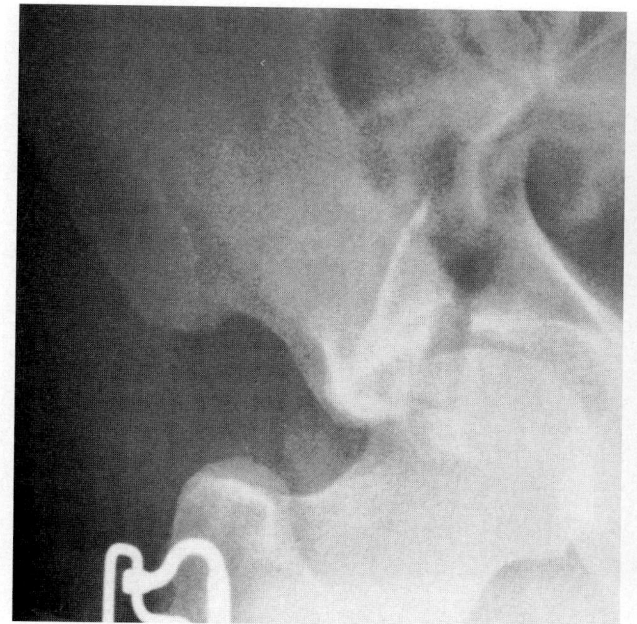

C

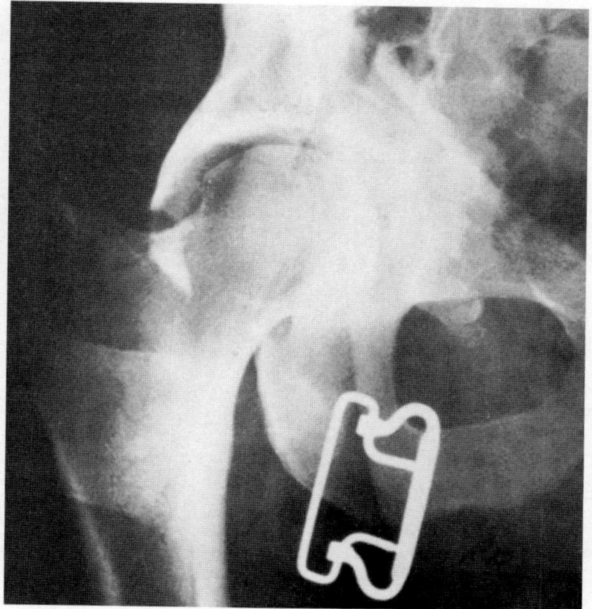

D

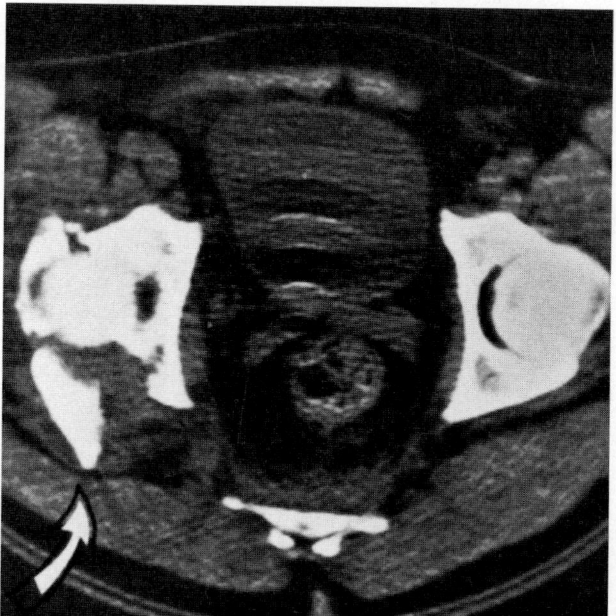

E

FIGURE 25-25. ***(continued)*** **E:** Computed tomography shows gross displacement of the large posterior wall fragment through which the posterior dislocation of the hip had occurred. A view of the cockpit and position of the engine **(F,G)** clearly demonstrates the mechanism of injury–a so-called dashboard injury.

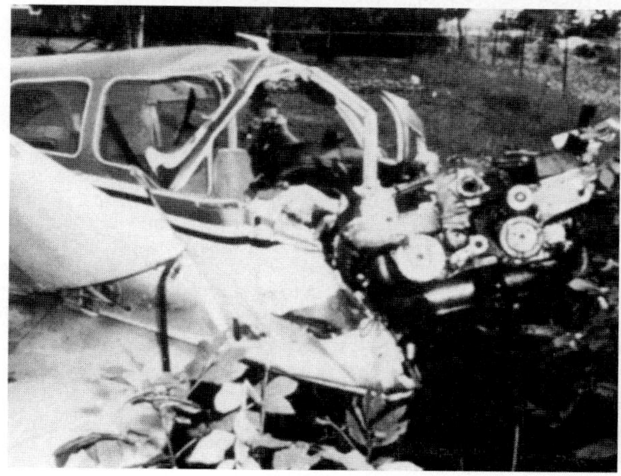

F

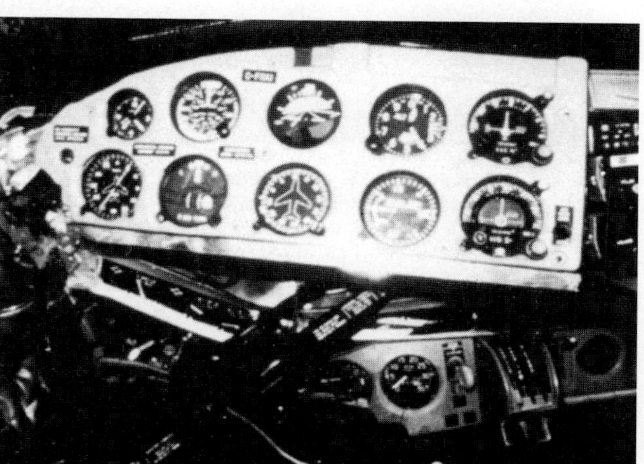

G

(*Figure continues*)

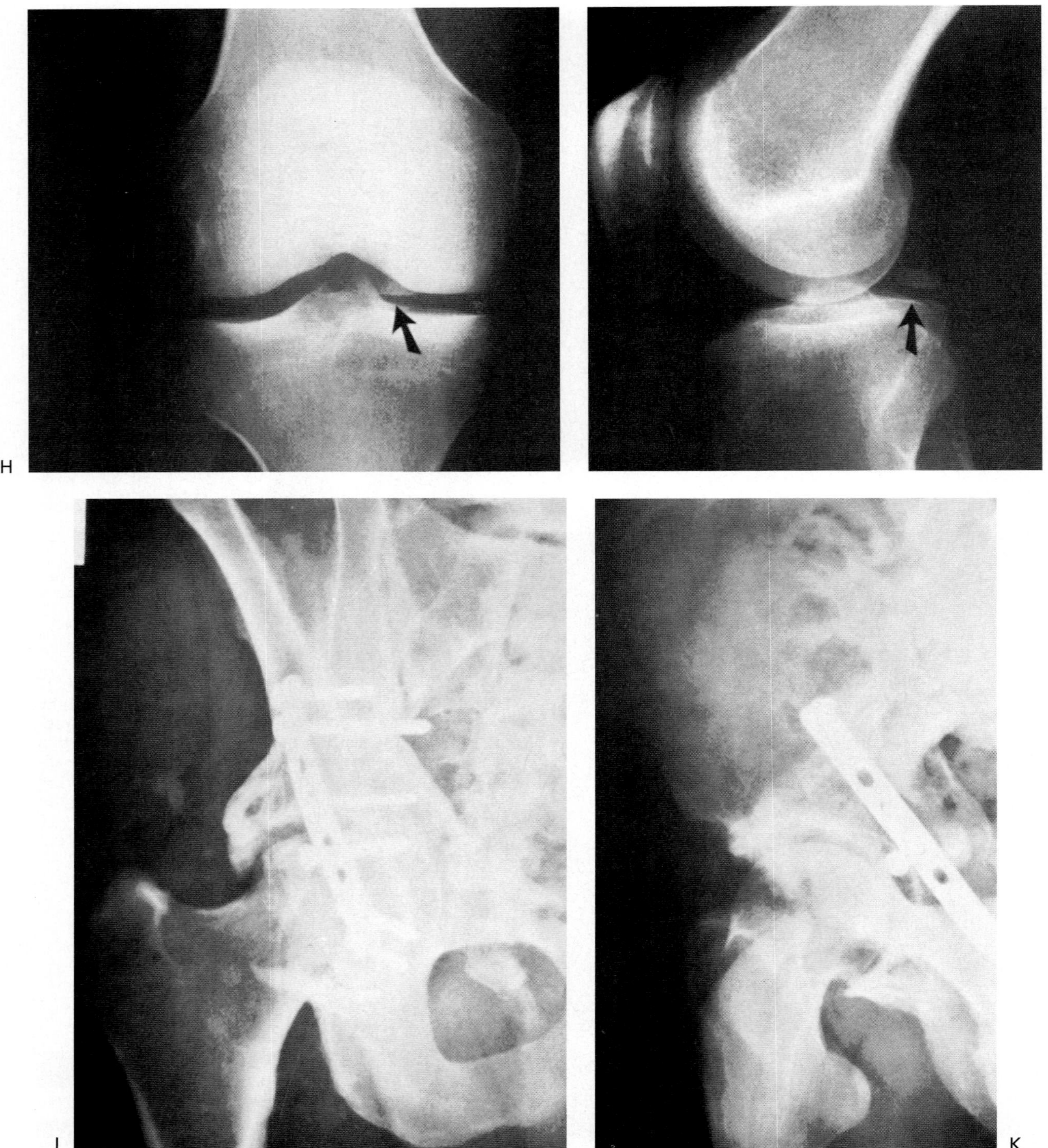

FIGURE 25-25. ***(continued)*** **H,I:** The patient sustained bilateral posterior subluxation of the knees; on the left side, with avulsion of the tibial end of the posterior cruciate ligament *(black arrow).* The fracture was fixed through a posterior approach. **J,K:** The 3-year follow-up radiographs indicate good congruity with slight heterotopic ossification posteriorly that did not affect the range of motion.

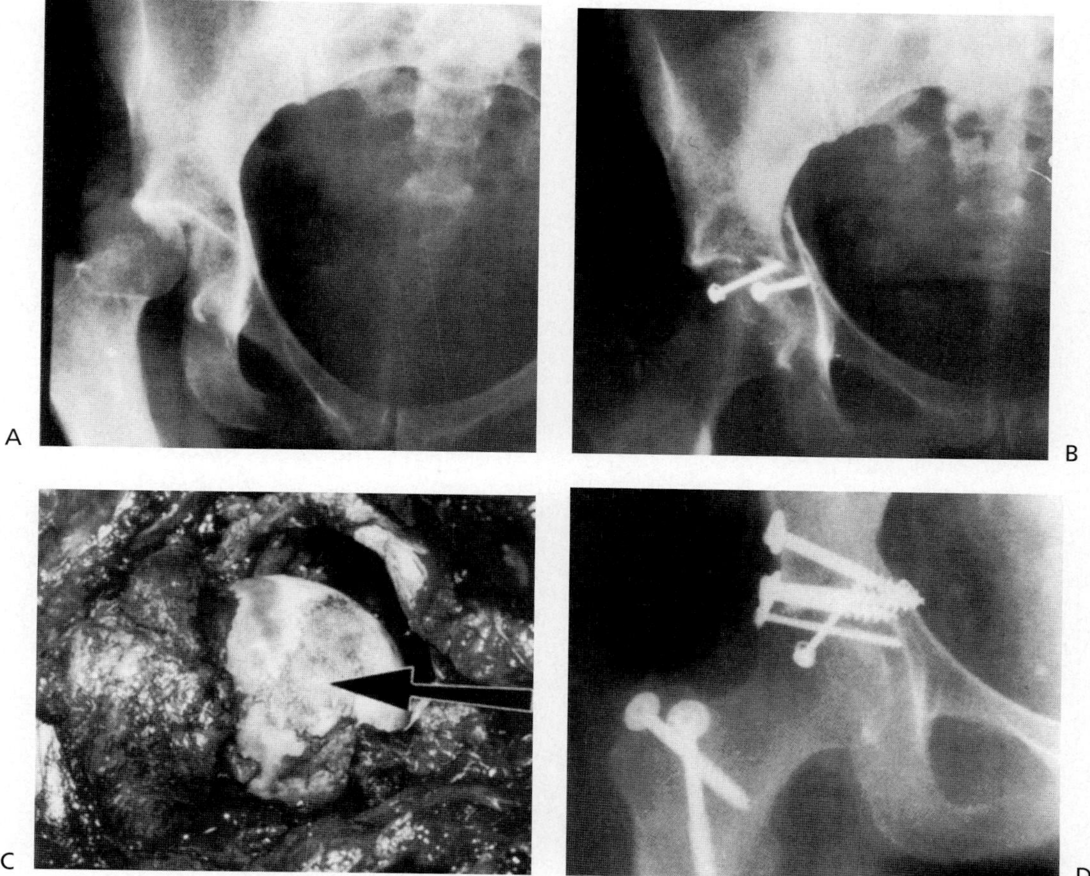

FIGURE 25-26. Pressure necrosis of articular cartilage. **A:** Anterior-posterior radiograph of the right hip of a 48-year-old woman with a posterior fracture-dislocation. **B:** The postoperative radiographs at 6 weeks shows the fixation of the posterior wall fracture. The previously undisplaced transverse fracture of the acetabulum displaced some time during the 6 weeks. **C:** Intraoperative photograph shows the large zone of pressure necrosis of the articular cartilage on the femoral head *(arrow)*. **D:** Postoperative radiograph shows the transverse fracture of the acetabulum fixed with four interfragmental screws. The reduction is anatomic. In spite of the large zone of pressure necrosis, the patient had an excellent result 9 years later. (From: Schatzker I, Tile M. *The rationale of operative fracture care.* Heidelberg: Springer-Verlag, 1987, with permission.)

Recognition of the T component has great surgical significance. Anatomic open reduction of a *pure transverse fracture,* through either a posterior or anterior approach, perfectly reduces both columns; however, if the columns are split by the vertical limb of the T, open reduction of either the anterior or posterior column does not reduce the other column (Fig. 25-27C). In these circumstances, anatomic restoration of the acetabulum can be obtained only by a direct approach to both columns.

A careful study of the radiographs should lead to the diagnosis. As noted in the following example, on the AP view of the pelvis (Fig. 25-28A), the posterior column is widely displaced, the anterior minimally so. The vertical limb is most often identified by the fracture of the inferior pubic ramus (Fig. 25-28B, *white arrow*). CT is particularly accurate for identifying the vertical split (Fig. 25-28C, D, *black arrow*).

In all recent reports, the T fracture had the worst prognosis of any type. The success rate for anatomic reduction, even in the most expert centers, was no higher than 60%; also, damage to the head and articular surfaces is extensive and complications are common. T fractures have been further classified by the level of the transverse component and the location of the stem component. The modifier *a allows classification of T fractures associated with posterior wall fractures, as for transverse fracture. Thus, T fractures may be classified as follows (Fig. 25-29A–C).

B2-1: Infratectal

1. Stem component, posterior
2. Stem component, through obturator foramen
3. Stem component, anterior

B2-2: Juxtatectal

1. Stem component, posterior
2. Stem component, through obturator foramen
3. Stem component, anterior

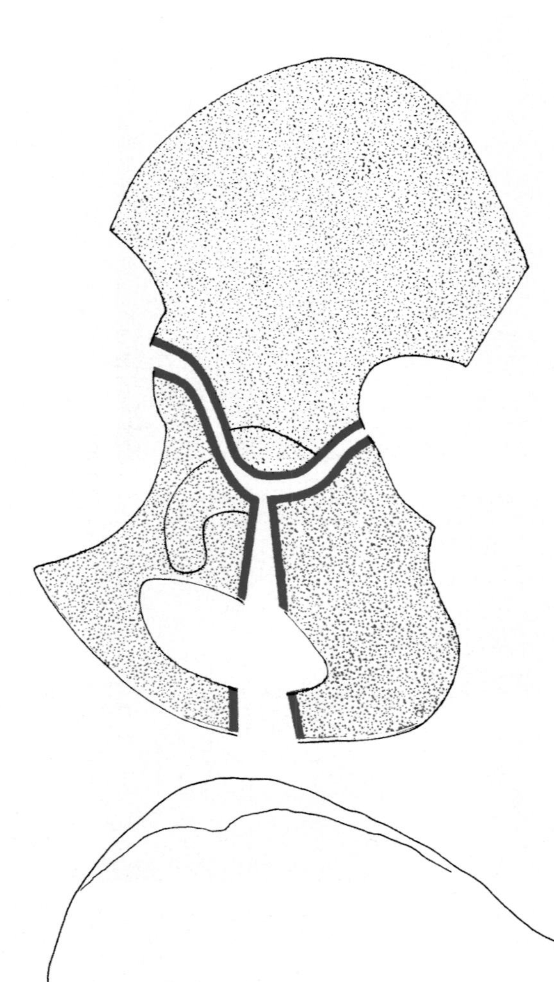

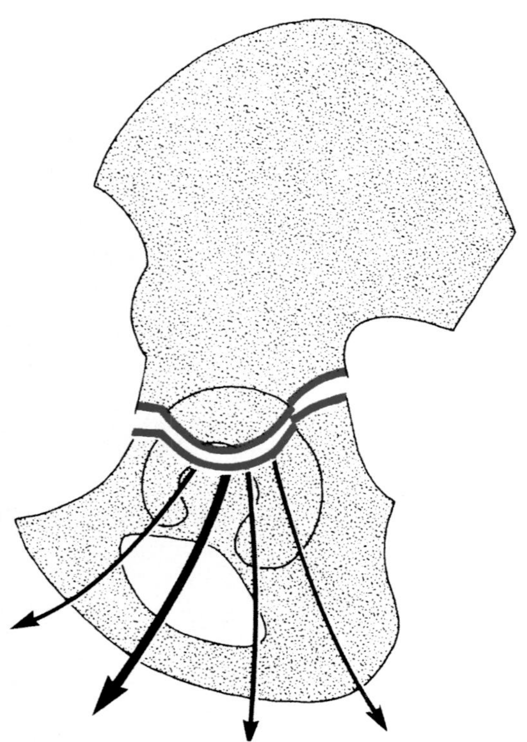

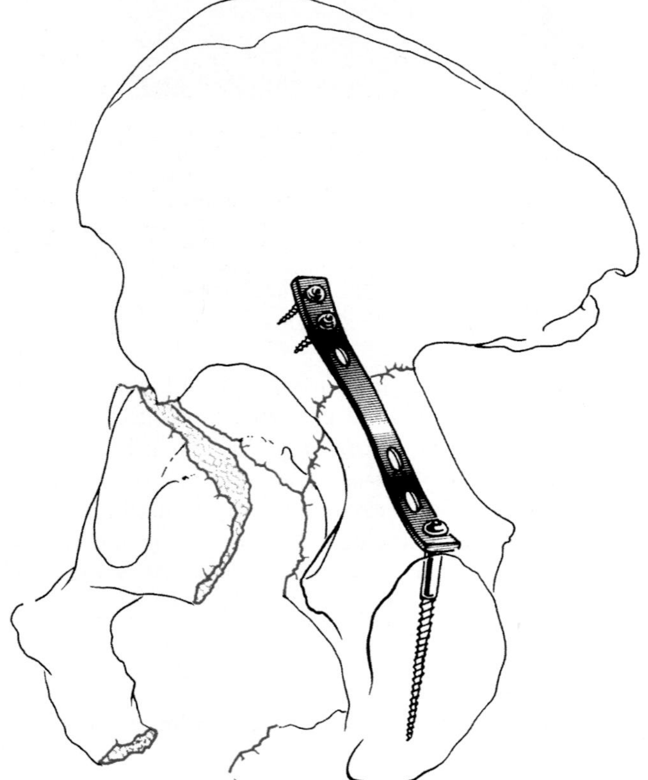

FIGURE 25-27. A: Type B2: T-shaped fracture. Diagram of a typical T-shaped fracture with the distal limb dividing the obturator foramen. The transverse limb of this fracture may be oriented in any plane or through any portion of the acetabulum, as previously discussed for transverse fractures. The vertical limb usually splits the central portion of the acetabulum **(A),** but other possibilities for the vertical limb are noted in **(B),** where the limb exits anteriorly or posteriorly and involves the obturator foramen not at all. Recognition of the T component is important surgically because fixation of one column does not necessarily reduce the opposite column, as one would expect in a pure transverse fracture **(C).**

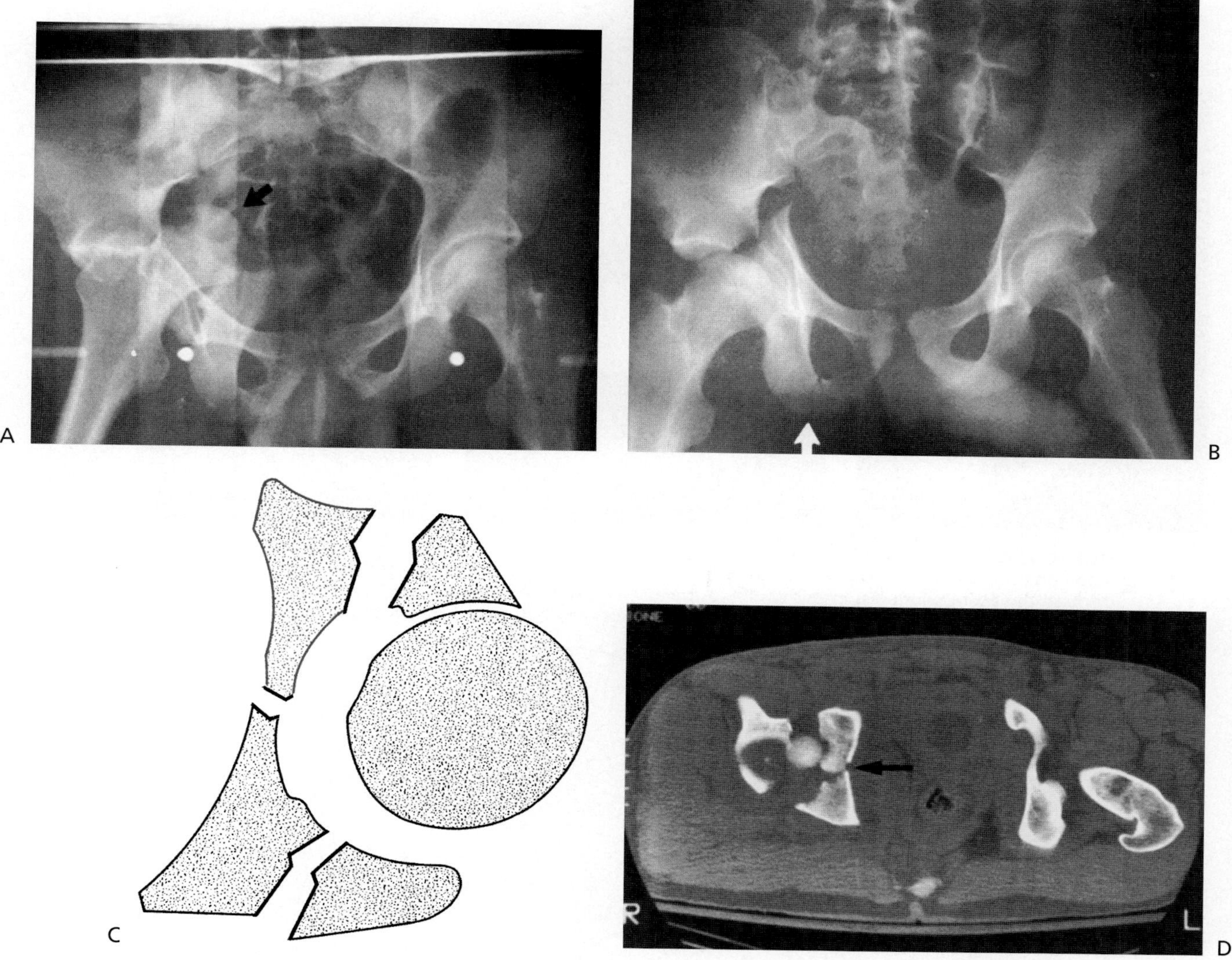

FIGURE 25-28. T-shaped fracture. Anterior-posterior radiograph shows central protrusion of the femoral head into the pelvis. **A:** Closed reduction was required to pull the head out of the pelvis to prevent cartilage necrosis because open reduction was to be delayed, in this case because of other injuries. **B:** The postreduction radiograph shows the head out of the pelvis, but with persistent incongruity. The transverse fracture is noted through the roof of the acetabulum, the T shape of this injury was determined by the fracture of the inferior pubic ramus *(white arrow).* The diagram **(C)** shows the pathognomonic features on axial computed tomography (CT), with the division of the quadrilateral plate dividing the two columns, as well as the transverse fracture in the anterior-posterior direction. **D:** In this case, the axial CT mirrors the drawing. The two columns are divided *(black arrow).*

(*Figure continues*)

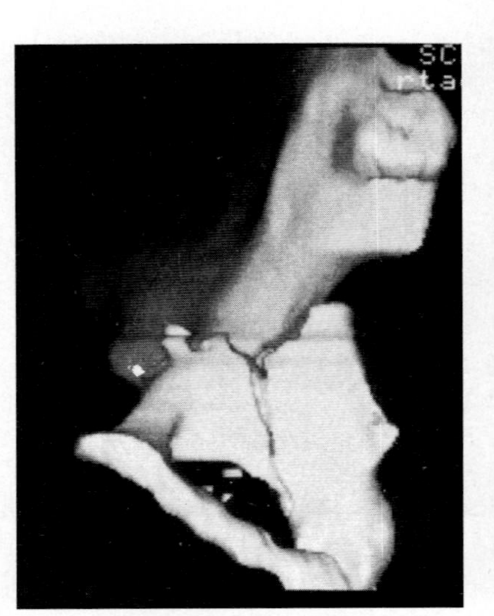

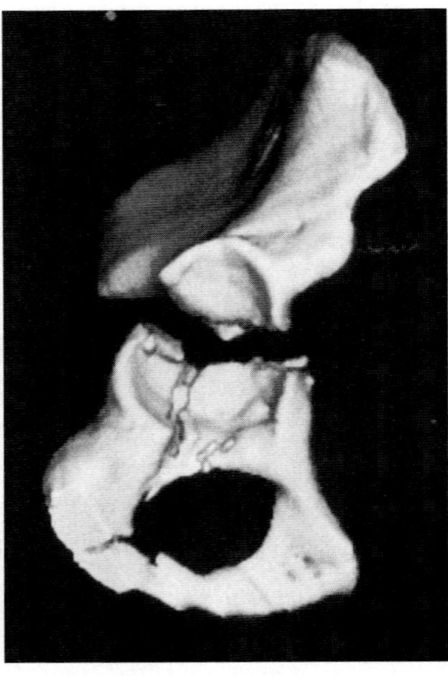

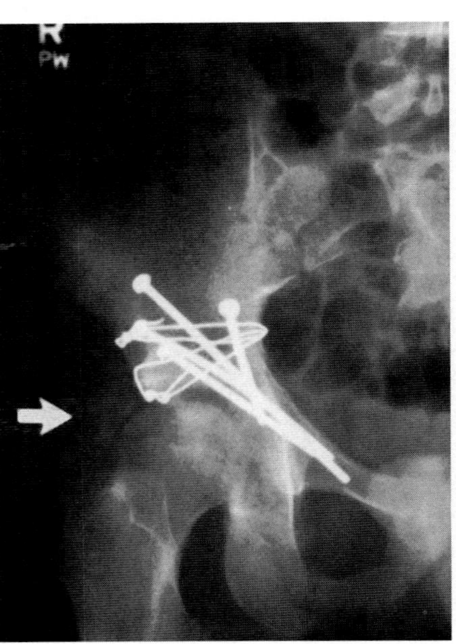

E,F G

FIGURE 25-28. ***(continued)*** The three-dimensional computed tomography really shows the T shape on both the medial view of the quadrilateral plate after closed reduction **(E)** and the view through the acetabulum **(F).** In this case, the fracture was reduced surgically and held with cerclage wires and lag screws. **G:** The *white arrow* indicated early heterotopic ossification.

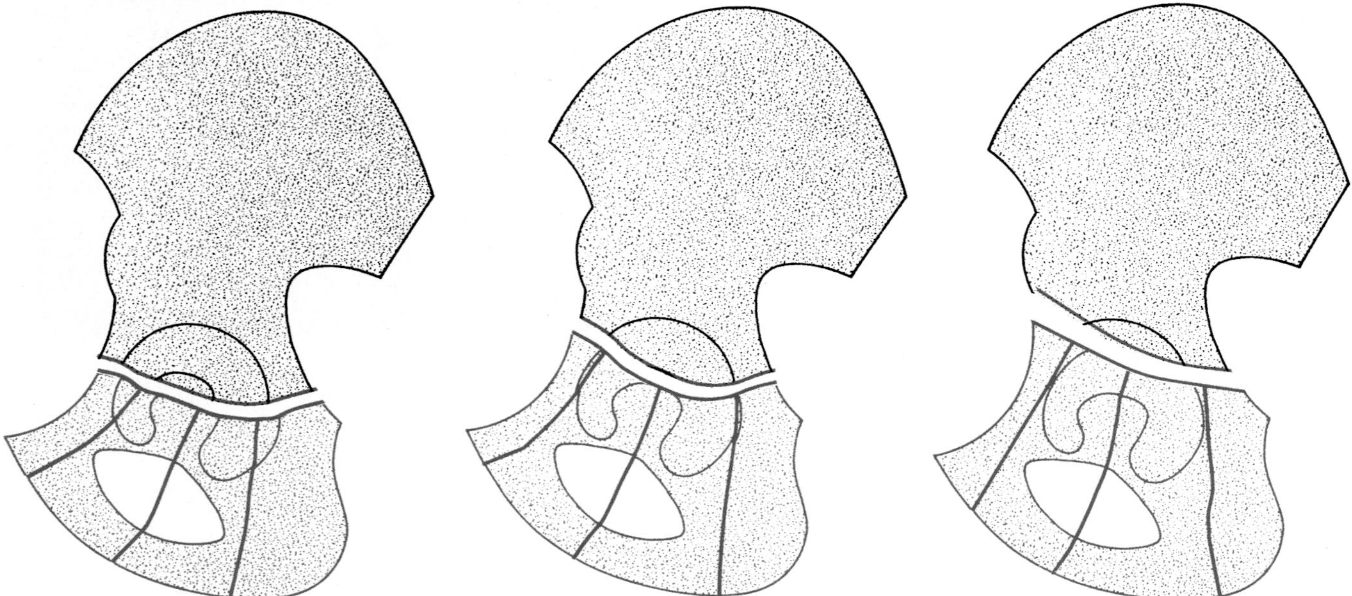

A, B C

FIGURE 25-29. Type B2: T-shaped fracture subclassification. The T-shaped fractures have been further classified by the level of the transverse component and the location of the stem. Also the modifier *a allows classification of the T fractures associated with posterior wall fractures, as noted in the transverse fractures previously described. Therefore, the T fractures may be classified as follows.

A. Type B2-1: Infratectal transverse
   1: Stem posterior
   2: Stem through obturator foramen
   3: Stem anterior
B. Type B2-2: Juxtatectal
   1: Stem posterior
   2: Stem through obturator foramen
   3: Stem anterior
C. Type B2-3: Transtectal
   1: Stem posterior
   2: Stem through obturator foramen
   3: Stem anterior

B2-3: Transtectal

1. Stem component, posterior
2. Stem component, through obturator foramen
3. Stem component, anterior

These progress generally in order of severity; thus, the designation has prognostic significance.

T Type Associated with Posterior Wall Injury. The very important T types associated with a posterior wall injury are designated by the modifier "a," like the B1 transverse types (Fig. 25-30). Therefore, the following is suggested.

(a1): No posterior wall fracture
(a2): + Posterior wall, single fragment
(a3): + Posterior wall, multifragmentary
(a4): + Posterior wall, multifragmentary with marginal impaction

The T fracture (B2) (Fig. 25-30) with a posterior wall fragment, usually with a posterior dislocation, in general, has a poorer prognosis; consequently, the use of these modifiers becomes extremely important in separating "apples from oranges."

B3: Anterior Column with Posterior Hemitransverse Lesion

This not uncommon fracture type (Fig. 25-31), really a variant of the T fracture, is best seen on CT or 3DCT. In this group, an anterior column fracture associated with a posterior hemitransverse fracture (Fig. 25-32), the femoral head is anteriorly dislocated or subluxed, lesions best seen on the obturator oblique view (Fig. 25-32A,B) or on CT (Fig. 25-32D–F). Note that the posterior column on the iliac oblique view (Fig. 25-32C) is fractured but not displaced.

Although this fracture is relatively uncommon, its recognition is surgically important. An unwary examiner could fail to recognize the major anterior thrust of the injury, demonstrated on the obturator oblique view, and would approach it posteriorly. Anatomic reconstruction and stable fixation of the posterior column will not restore the more major displacement of the anterior column, or even the anterior subluxation of the femoral head (Fig. 25-33). In this example, the anterior column with the femoral head has remained unreduced, resulting in rapid destruction of the hip.

This group has also been subgrouped according to the level of the anterior wall, with the modifier **a to designate the degree of comminution (Fig. 25-31).

B3-1: Anterior wall
B3-2: Anterior column (high variety)
B3-3: Anterior column (low variety)

The modifier *a is used as follows.

(a1): Anterior column in one fragment
(a2): Anterior column in two fragments
(a3): Anterior column in more than two fragments

Variants of the T Fracture

As mentioned, not all fractures can be put neatly into a slot. Variants do occur, and that is why individual decision making becomes extremely important. The fracture illustrated by Fig. 25-34 is a Type T fracture with marked posterior displacement and minimal displacement of the anterior column. One can hope to achieve a good result only by careful consideration of all aspects of the fracture.

Type C: Both-Column Fracture, Complete Articular

This fracture divides both columns above the level of the acetabulum, through the ilium in the coronal plane, with a T extension into the joint (Fig. 25-35). It is really a variant of the T fracture but is sufficiently different to merit a separate name. The transverse component divides the ilium above the acetabulum in the coronal plane, whereas the T fracture fractures the posterior column through the joint. One could regard this as "the floating acetabulum;" however, the articular surface is no longer connected to the axial skeleton, so it is classified as a complete articular fracture. Central dislocation of the head is common because this injury usually is caused by powerful forces. Comminution of the ilium and acetabulum likewise is frequent. Injuries to the acetabular wall also must be sought, because they affect the prognosis.

The major radiographic features (Fig. 25-36) include a centrally dislocated femoral head, a fracture into the ilium, and the characteristic *spur* sign. This sign, best seen on the obturator view, represents the transverse limb of the iliac fracture as it passes above the acetabulum (Fig. 25-36C,D). The fracture line is in the coronal plane.

Although this fracture may look terrible at first glance (Fig. 25-36), much of the distortion on the plain radiograph may be through the ilium above the joint. Even though in the universal classification, this type has been labeled Type C (the most severe), in fact most Type B fractures may have more severe consequences and a poorer prognosis. However, the complexity of acetabular fracture types is such that some compromises had to be made in formulating the universal classification.

The appearance on CT, especially 3DCT, is characteristic (Fig. 25-37), showing the articular fracture oriented in the coronal plane. These fractures also may exhibit comminution, especially of the acetabular roof. A separate rotated triangular roof fragment of articular cartilage certainly heralds a much poorer prognosis, especially if the fragment has been devitalized during surgery.

The *both-column fracture* (Type C) also is amenable to nonoperative care in some cases because the anterior and posterior columns may line up around the femoral head, allowing *secondary congruence* (Fig. 25-36). Many groups and subgroups have been identified because of the complexity of this fracture pattern and its relative frequency. Also,

(Text continues on page 470)

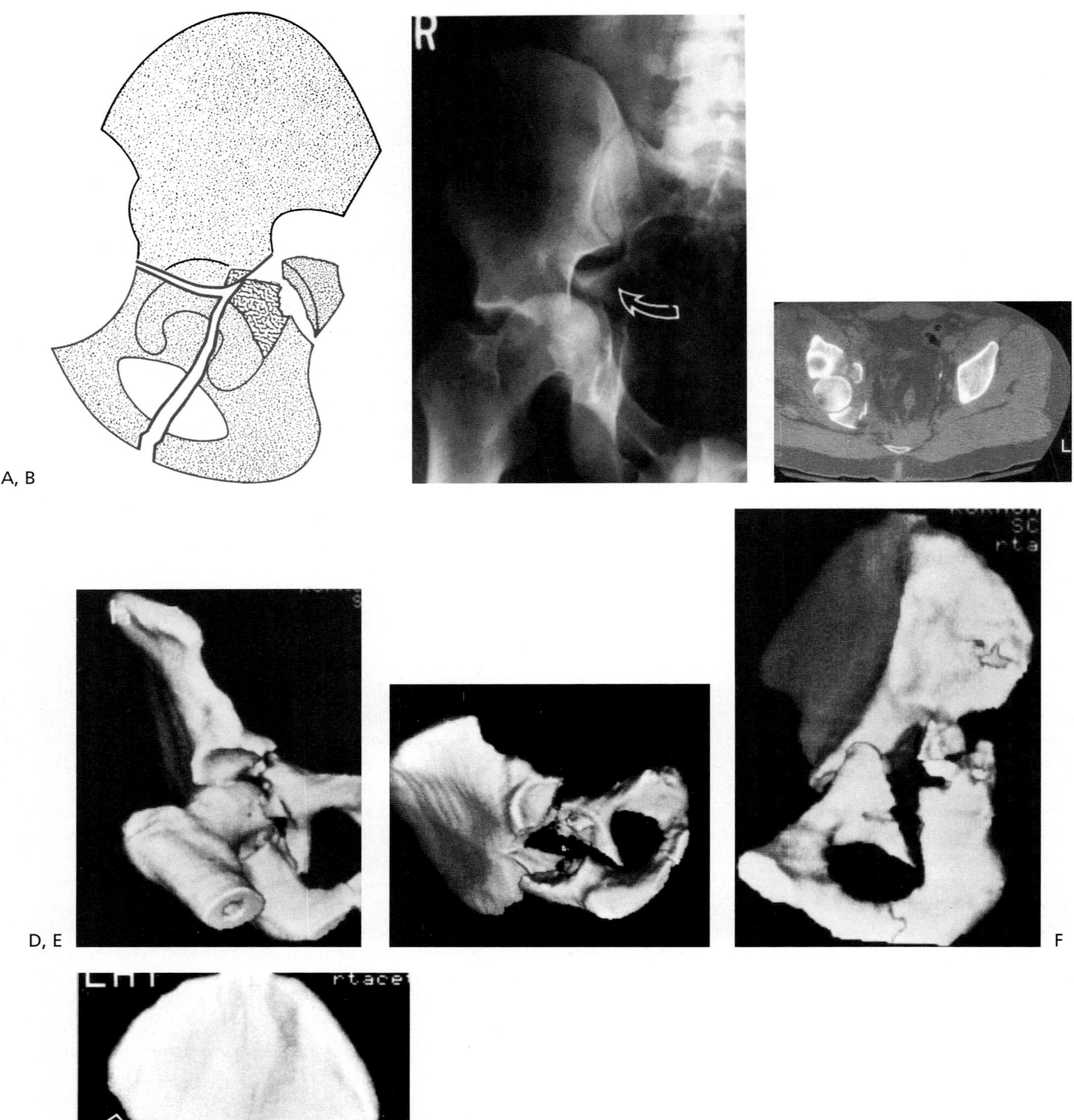

G

FIGURE 25-30. A: T-shaped fracture with posterior wall fragment. The diagram **(A)** shows a typical transtectal T-shaped fracture with a large posterior wall fragment. The anterior-posterior radiograph **(B)** shows a typical case with a posterior dislocation and a large posterior wall fragment rotated 180 degrees *(white arrow).* **C:** Computed tomography shows the posterior dislocation and the nature of the T fracture. The exact pathoanatomy is best seen on three-dimensional computed tomography. **D:** The femoral head is noted to be dislocated. **E:** The T fracture is seen through the obturator foramen more clearly with the head subtracted. The T fracture is viewed **(F)** from the medial quadrilateral surface and **(G)** the rotated posterior wall fragment, the articular surface pointing away from the joint *(white arrow).*

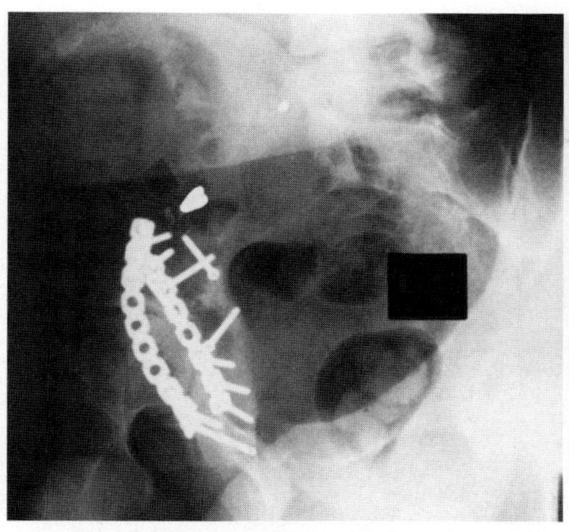

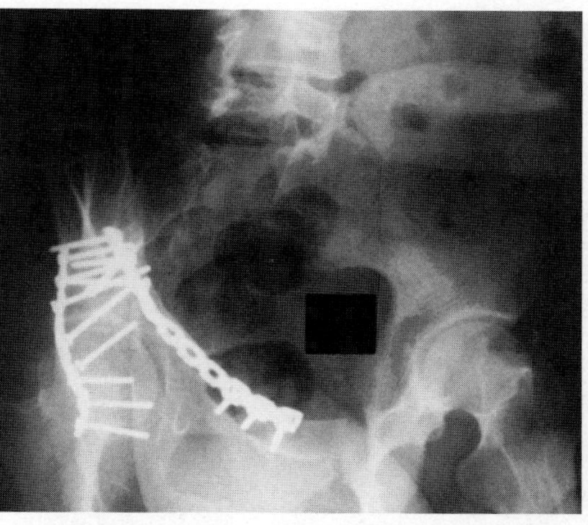

FIGURE 25-30. ***(continued)*** The postoperative radiographs, including the iliac oblique view **(H)** and the obturator oblique view **(I),** show anatomic reduction, fixation of the posterior wall fragment with two lag screws, and fixation of the columns with lag screws and buttress plates. This T fracture was approached through an individual anterior ilioinguinal and posterior Kocher-Langenbeck approach.

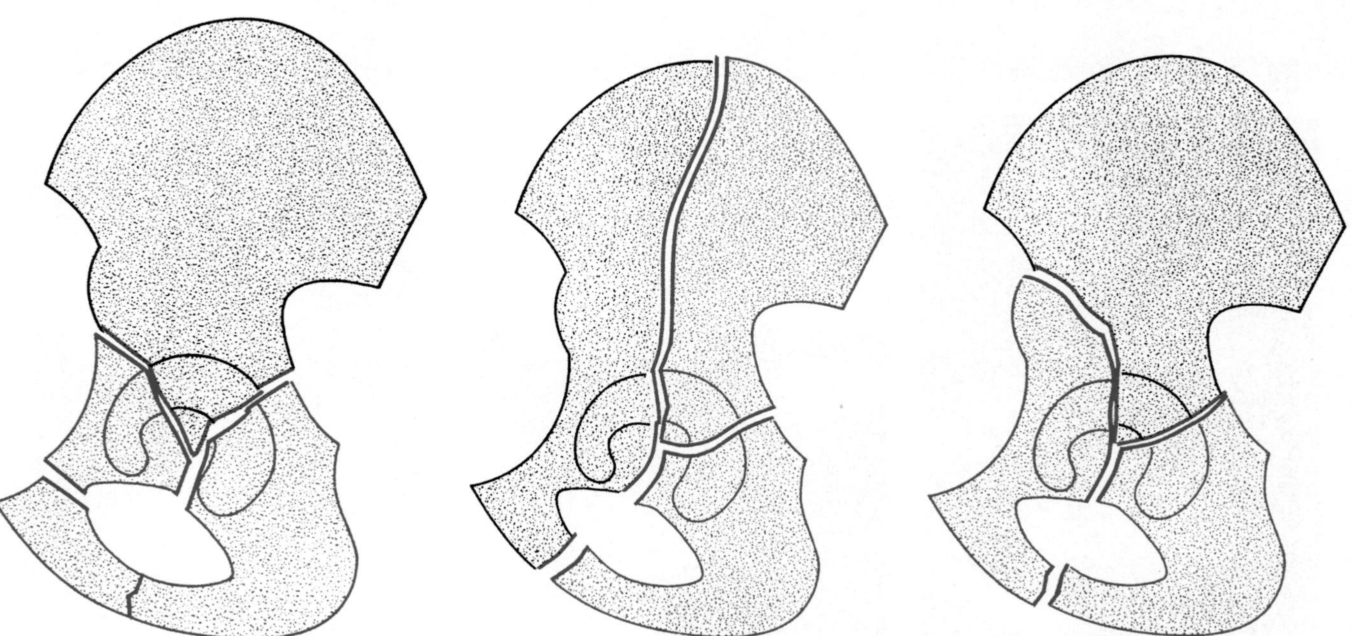

FIGURE 25-31. Type B: Anterior column with posterior hemitransverse fracture. This variant of the T fracture is best seen on computed tomography or three-dimensional computed tomography. The displacement of the head is anterior; the posterior fracture is undisplaced. This is extremely important in surgical decision making. The three subtypes are related to the anterior fracture: **(A)** Type B3-1: Anterior wall fracture with posterior hemitransverse lesion; **(B)** Type B3-2: Anterior column, high variety with posterior hemitransverse lesion; and **(C)** Type B3-3: Anterior column, low variety.

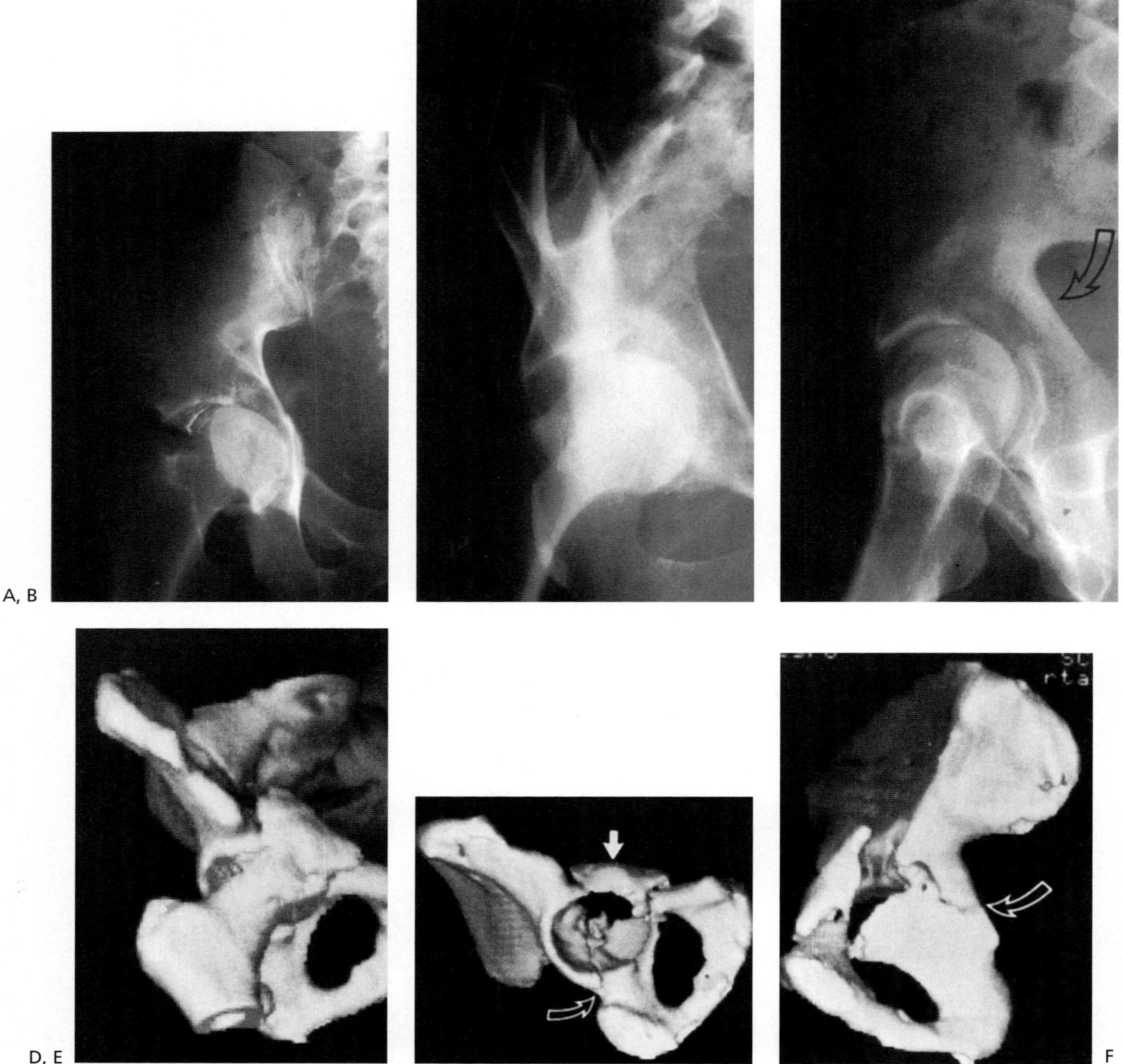

FIGURE 25-32. Typical example of Type B3, anterior plus posterior hemitransverse fractures. **A:** Anterior-posterior radiograph shows a fracture through the acetabulum with marked incongruity. The direction of displacement of the head is much more clearly delineated in the obturator oblique view **(B),** which shows anterior displacement of the head on the anterior column. The head is being impinged on by the corner of the acetabular fracture. The iliac oblique view **(C)** shows the intact posterior column *(black arrow).* The pathoanatomy is best seen on the three-dimensional computed tomography. **D:** With the femoral head in place, anterior subluxation is noted. **E:** With the head subtracted, displacement of the anterior column *(solid white arrow)* and the undisplaced nature of the posterior hemitransverse *(arrow)* are clearly noted. **F:** This is further clarified in the quadrilateral plate view.

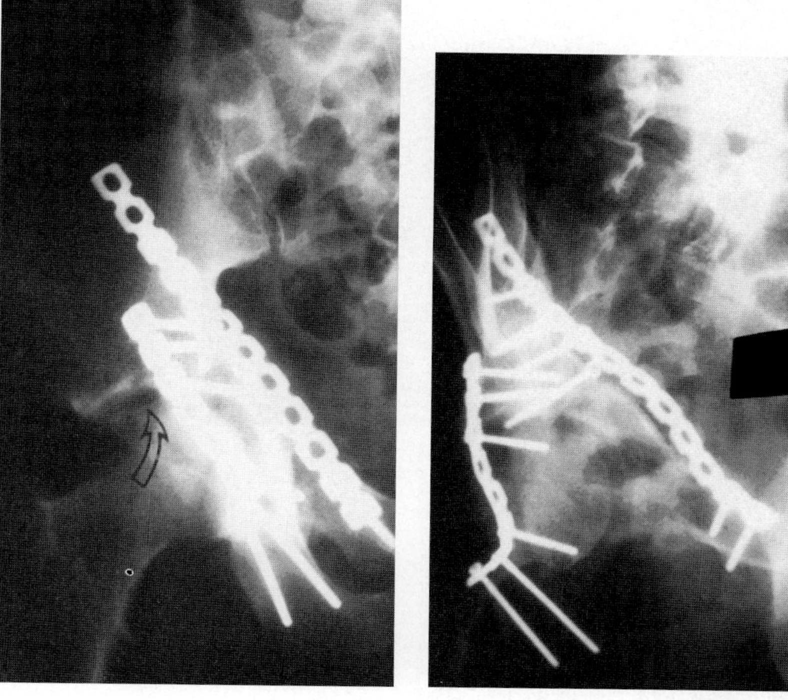

G,H

FIGURE 25-32. ***(continued)*** Open reduction and internal fixation through two simultaneous approaches allowed anatomic reduction, as noted in the anterior-posterior view **(G)** and the obturator oblique view **(H)**. Note the notching of the femoral head *(black arrow)*, which will adversely affect the long-term outcome.

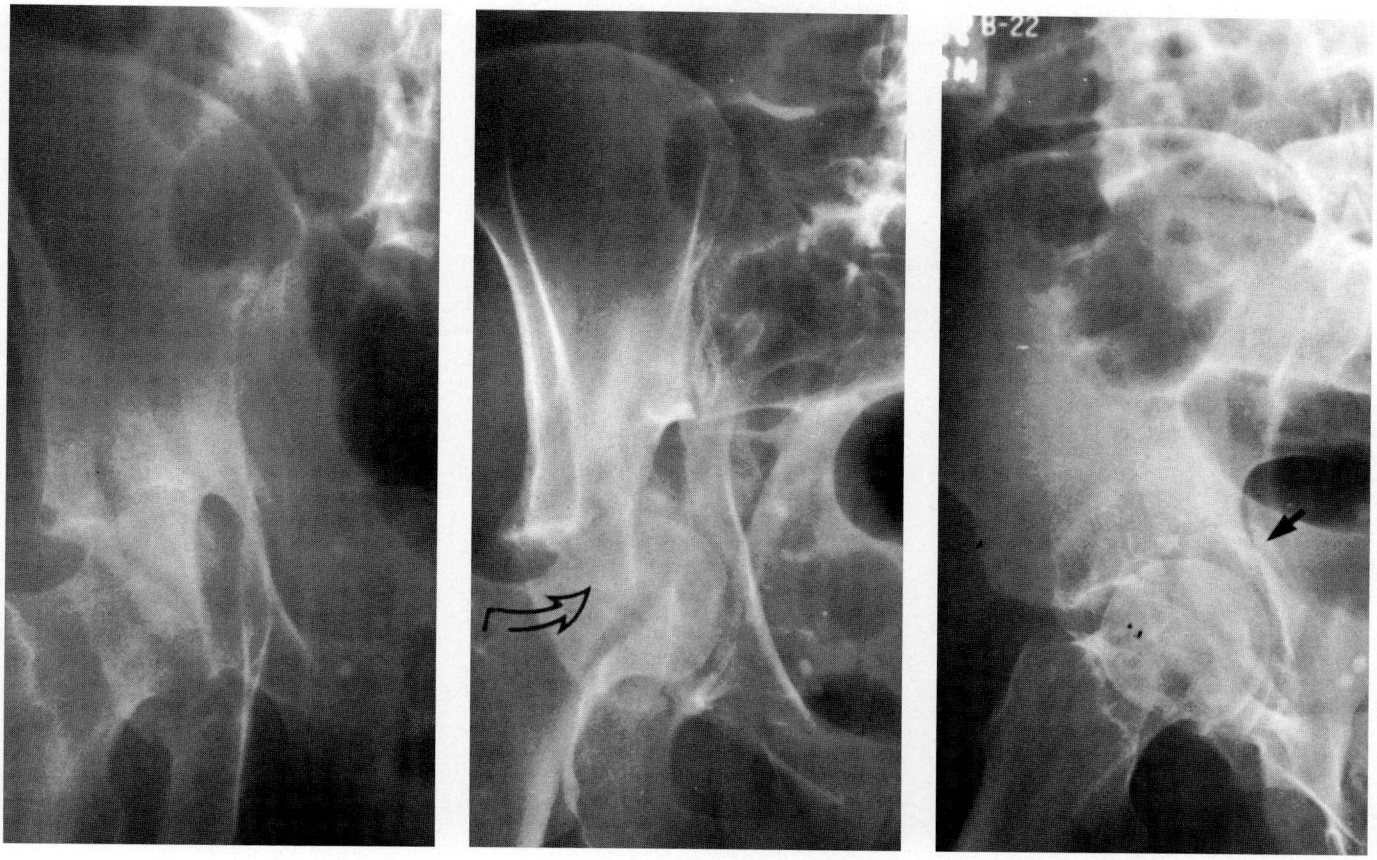

A, B

C

FIGURE 25-33. Importance of correct decision making in the anterior with posterior hemitransverse fracture. The anterior-posterior radiograph **(A)**, obturator oblique view **(B)**, and iliac oblique view **(C)** clearly demonstrate the marked anterior displacement of the femoral head associated with a virtually undisplaced posterior column *(black arrows)*. (*Figure continues*)

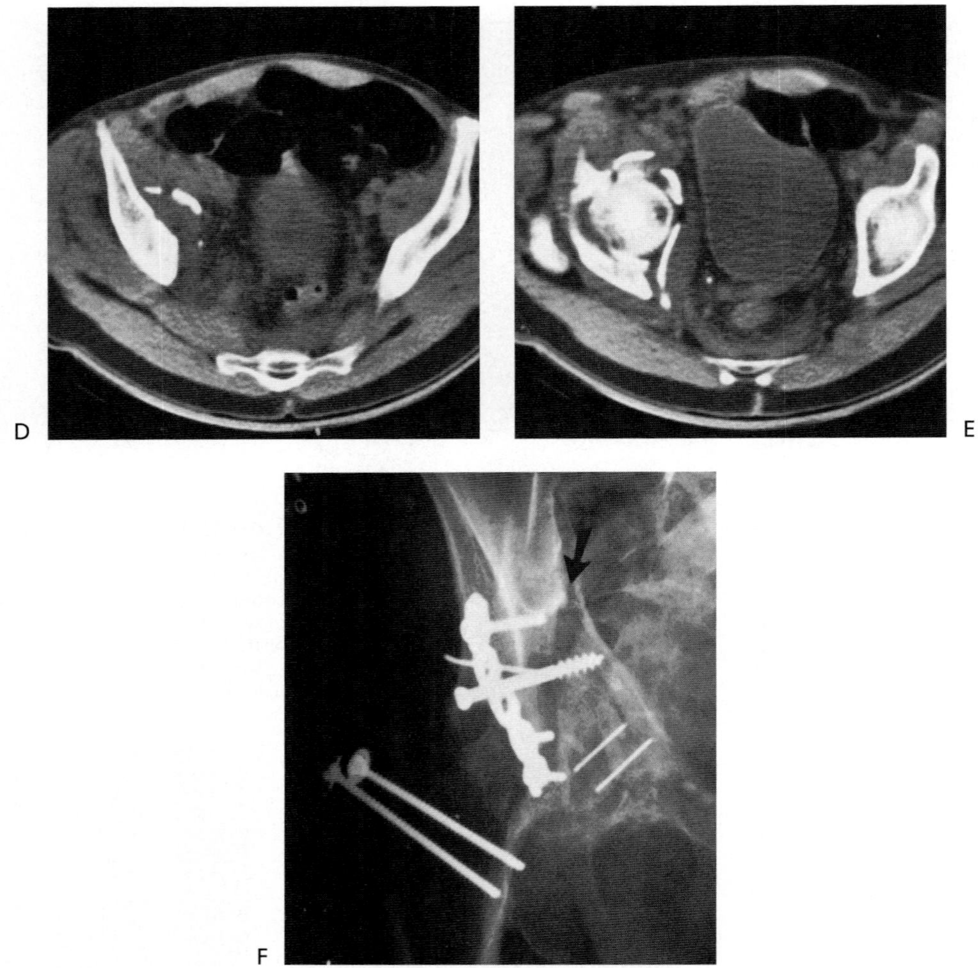

FIGURE 25-33. ***(continued)*** The computed tomography (CT) **(D)** shows anterior displacement, and the anterior displacement of the femoral head also is best seen on CT **(E).** The fracture was reduced through a transtrochanteric triradiate approach. The anterior subluxation of the head and the anterior column fragment were not reduced *(black arrow),* resulting in rapid dissolution of the joint **(F).**

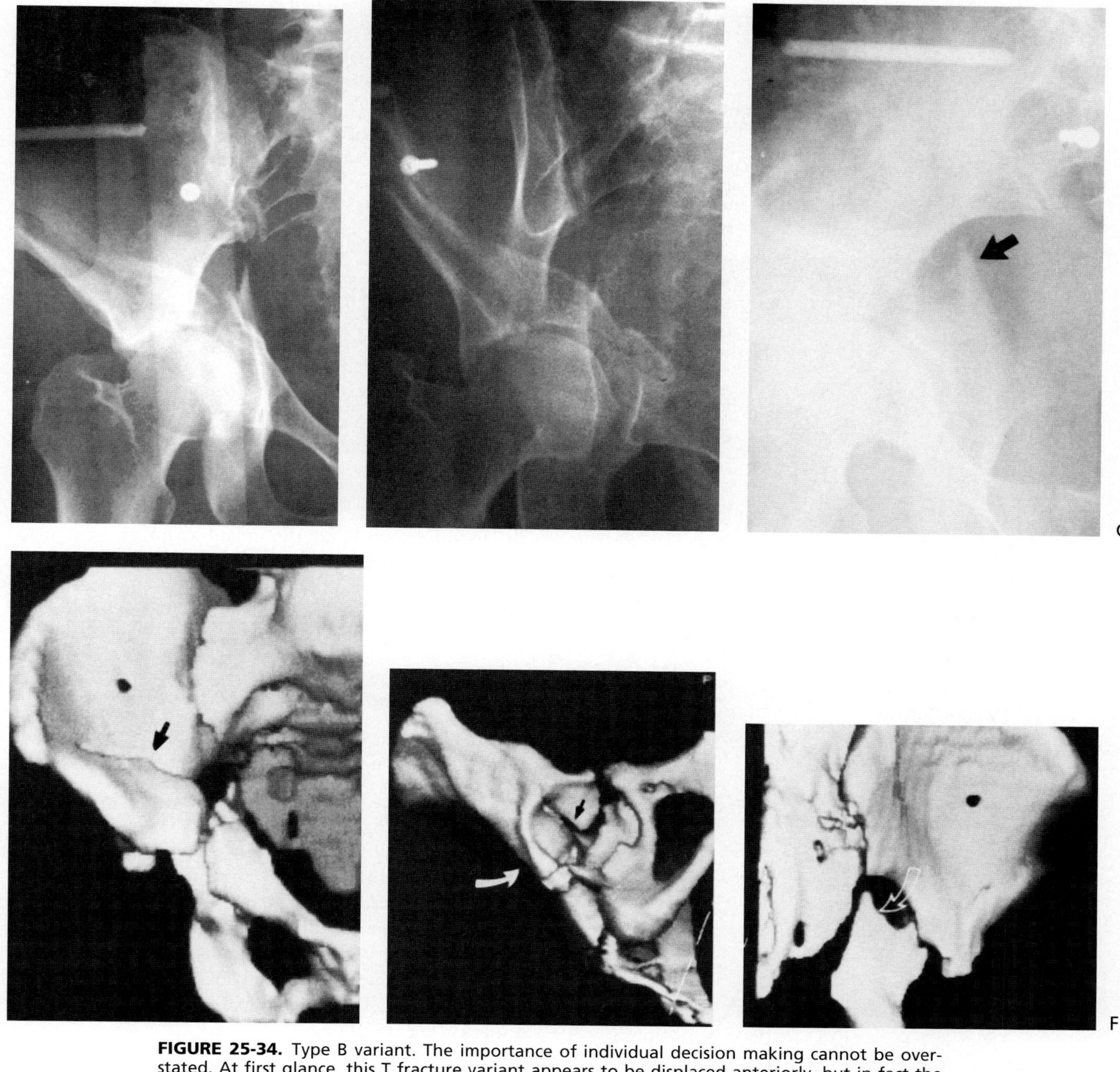

FIGURE 25-34. Type B variant. The importance of individual decision making cannot be overstated. At first glance, this T fracture variant appears to be displaced anteriorly, but in fact the posterior column is markedly displaced. This can be seen on the anterior-posterior **(A),** obturator oblique **(B),** and iliac oblique **(C)** *(black arrow)* views. The anterior column is split coronally, like a Type C fracture, as noted on the three-dimensional computed tomography (3DCT) **(D,E),** very much like a both-column Type C lesion *(white arrow).* A portion of the posterior wall is attached to the axial skeleton, making this a true T type fracture *(white arrow).* The marked displacement of the posterior column is noted in **(F).** *(Figure continues)*

FIGURE 25-34. *(continued)* G: The 3DCT is more helpful in determining the pathoanatomy than the axial view computed tomography. Open reduction and internal fixation through a triradiate approach resulted in anatomic reduction **(H).**

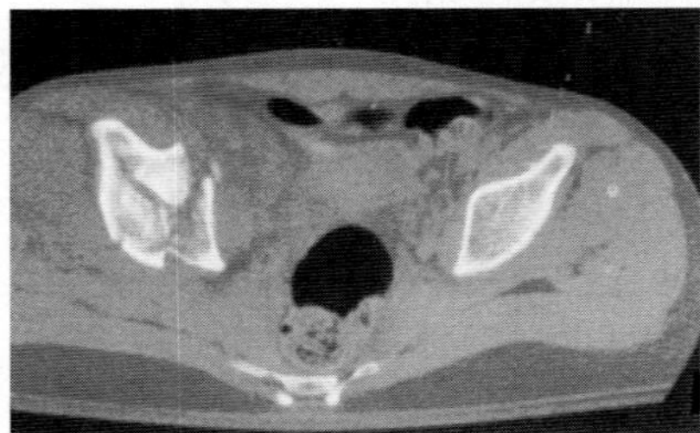
G

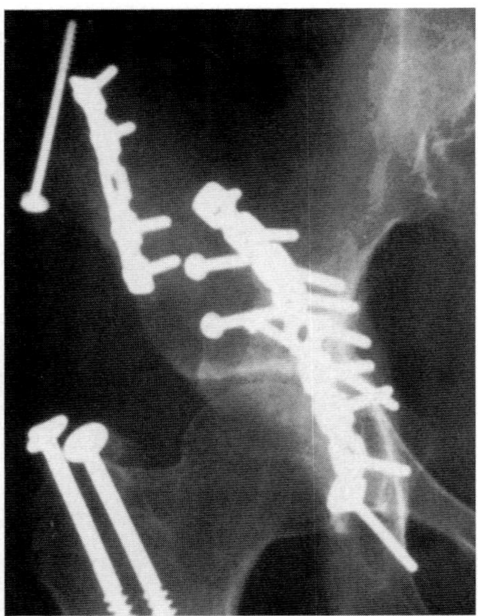
H

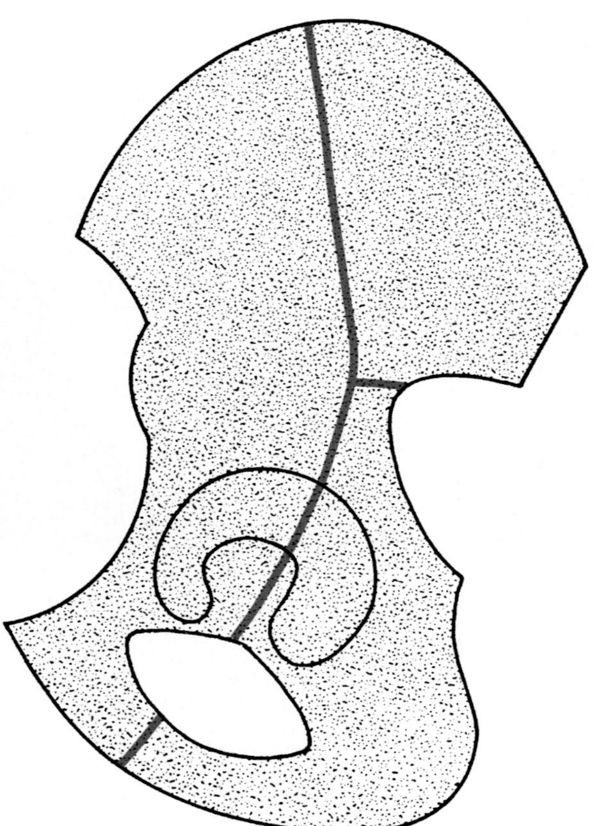

FIGURE 25-35. Type C: Both-column complete articular fracture in which all segments of the acetabular articular surface are separated from the axial skeleton. The fracture is truly a floating acetabulum and can be considered a T variant, the T segment in the ilium proximal to the joint and the vertical limb usually crossing the obturator foramen.

the modifiers allow for the introduction of other major prognostic factors, especially associated posterior wall fractures with posterior dislocation of the hip.

The major groups are characterized by level of the fracture in the ilium.

C1: Both-Column Fracture, High Variety

In this group the iliac fracture exits through the iliac crest. The subgroups are as follows (Fig. 25-38).

C1-1: Each column is a single fragment, that is a typical configuration (Fig. 25-38A).

C1-2: The posterior column is a single fragment, the anterior column two or more fragments (see Fig. 25-38B).

C1-3: A posterior wall fragment is present as well as the posterior column. Modifiers are used to describe the number of fragments of the anterior column (a1, a2, a3) and the number of fragments and complexity of the posterior wall (b1, b2, b3, b4). These modifiers are also used in C2 and C3 varieties (Fig. 25-38C).

C2: Both-Column Fracture, Low Variety

In the C2 group, the anterior column exits below the iliac crest, usually just proximal or distal to the anterior inferior spine. The same subgroups are used as in C1, and are as follows.

C2-1: Each column, single fragment (Fig. 25-39A).

C2-2: Posterior column, single fragment. The anterior column has at least two fragments (Fig. 25-39B).

C2-3: The posterior column has an associated posterior wall fragment. The same modifiers are used as described (Fig. 25-39C).

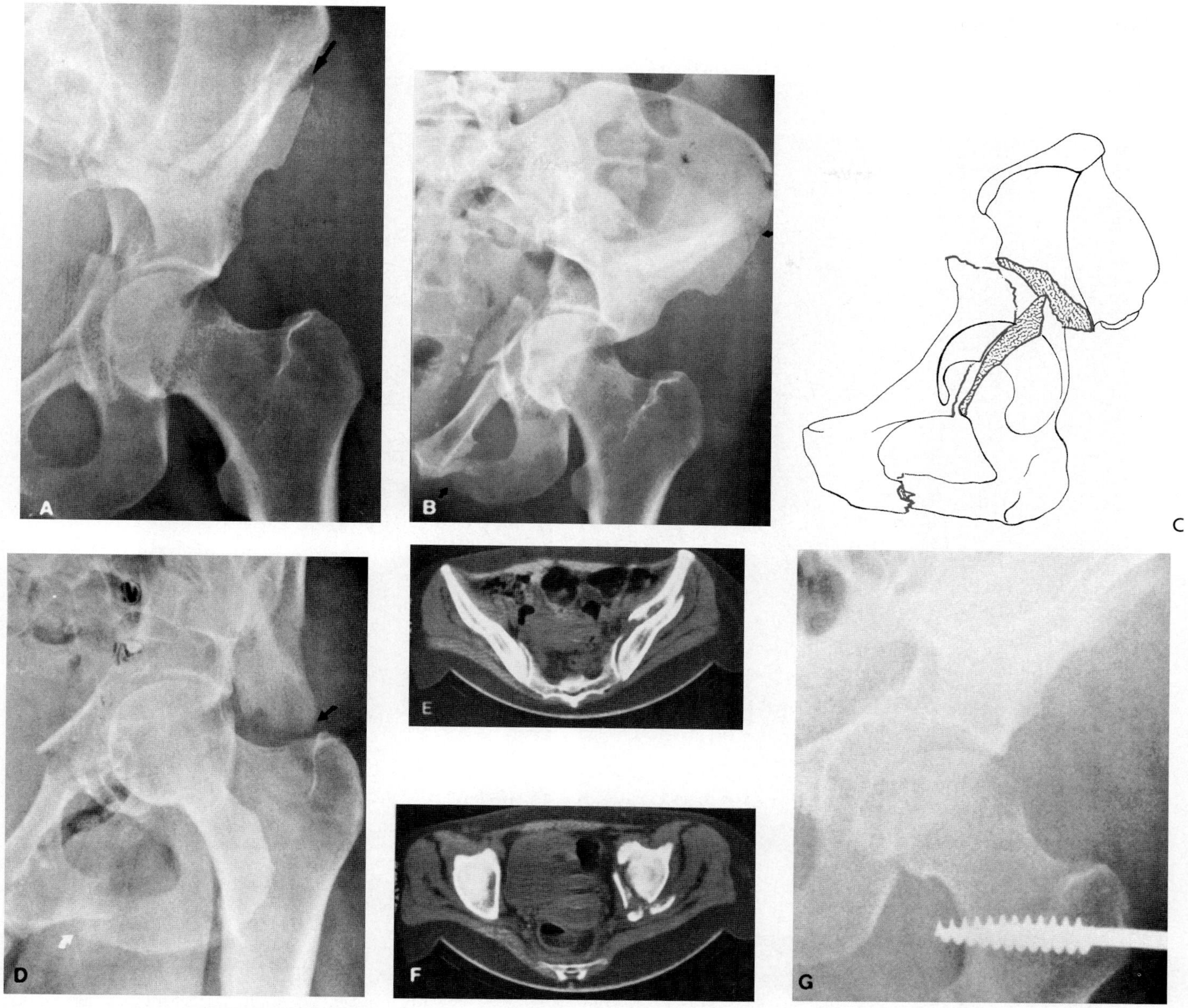

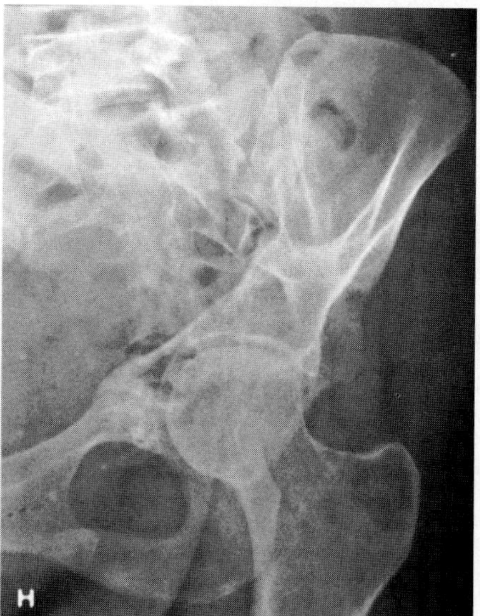

FIGURE 25-36. Radiographic appearance of a Type C both-column fracture. The anterior-posterior radiograph **(A)** shows the typical appearance of a both-column fracture where the fracture of the anterior column exits through the iliac crest above the anterior superior spine *(black arrow).* The unusual appearance on the anterior-posterior view is owing to the anterior, column fracture superior to the hip joint in the ilium. The entire joint is displaced medially and has the appearance of congruity. This is further noted on the iliac oblique view **(B).** The pathognomonic feature of this injury, the so-called spur sign, is best seen on the obturator oblique view, as seen in the drawing **(C)** and the radiograph **(D).** On this drawing and radiograph it is noted that the entire hip joint is separated from the axial skeleton by a fracture through the ilium above the joint. The tip of the spur *(black arrow)* is the extraarticular fragment of the remaining ilium, the entire joint being displaced medially and internally rotated. Typically, also, the posterior column fracture splits the distal fragment, in this case through the obturator foramen *(white arrow).* The coronal nature of the iliac fracture is seen clearly on the computed tomography (CT) **(E)** and the comminution on the CT **(F).** In this case trochanteric traction was applied through an "unrecommended" pin **(G).** Healing occurred, and 17 years after the injury the patient has an excellent result, 92 on the Harris hip rating **(H).**

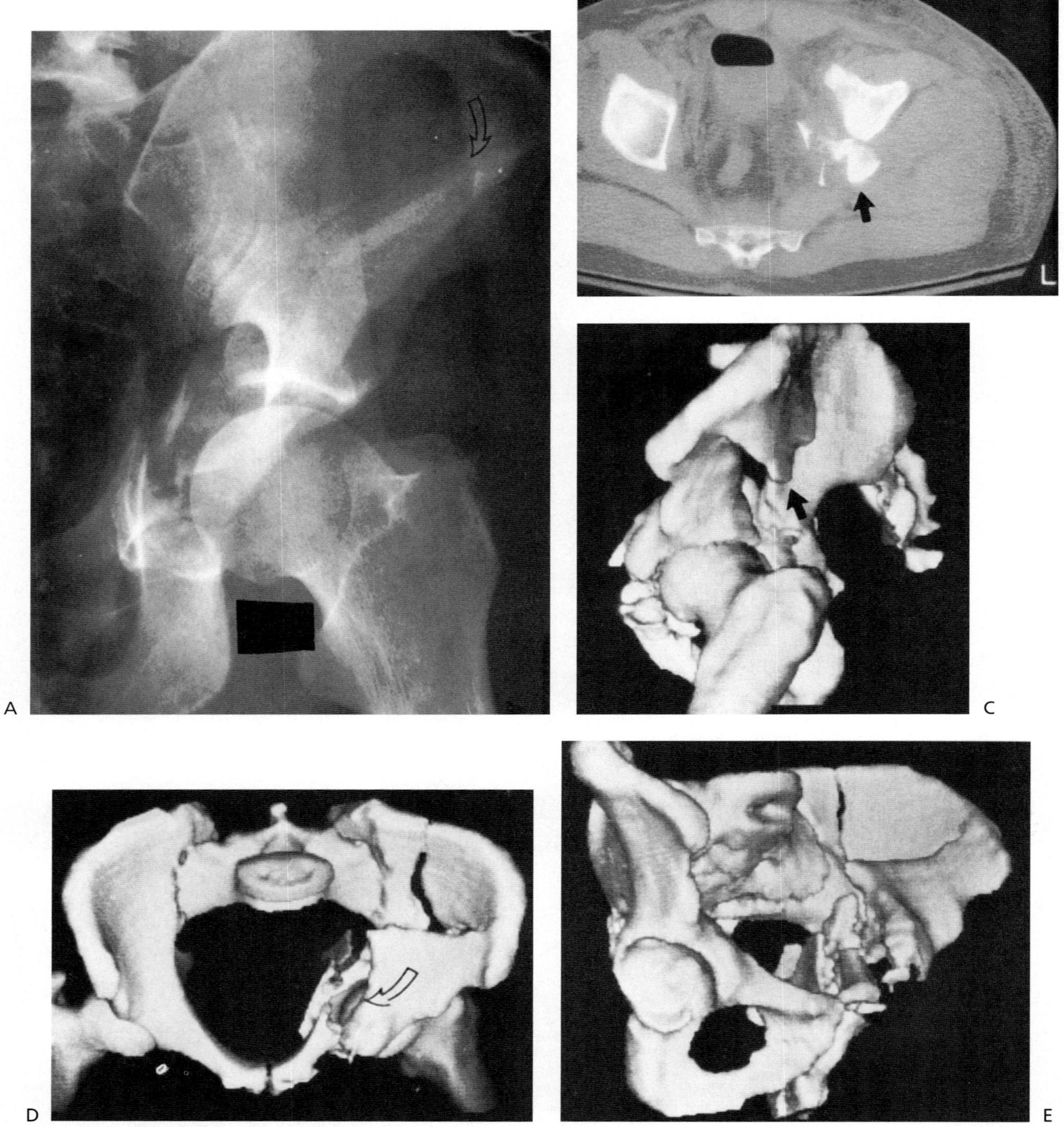

FIGURE 25-37. Characteristic both-column fracture radiographs, including three-dimensional computed tomography (3DCT). **(A)** The anterior-posterior radiograph shows the typical appearance of a both-column fracture. The anterior column fracture extends to the iliac crest and separates off a V-shaped portion *(black arrow).* **(B)** The axial computed tomography view through the area of the dome shows the coronal split as well as the spur sign, indicating the extraarticular portion of the iliac fracture *(black arrow).* This corresponds to the spur sign on 3DCT **(C)** *(black arrow).* Note in this view that the entire hip joint has been medially displaced and internally rotated, leaving behind the ilium, which makes up the so-called spur. The characteristic 3DCT **(D)** shows the flap of anterior column, the split V section extending almost to the posterior spine, and the coronal split along the pelvic brim with the femoral head peeking through *(black arrow).* This pathoanatomy is seen again in **(E).**

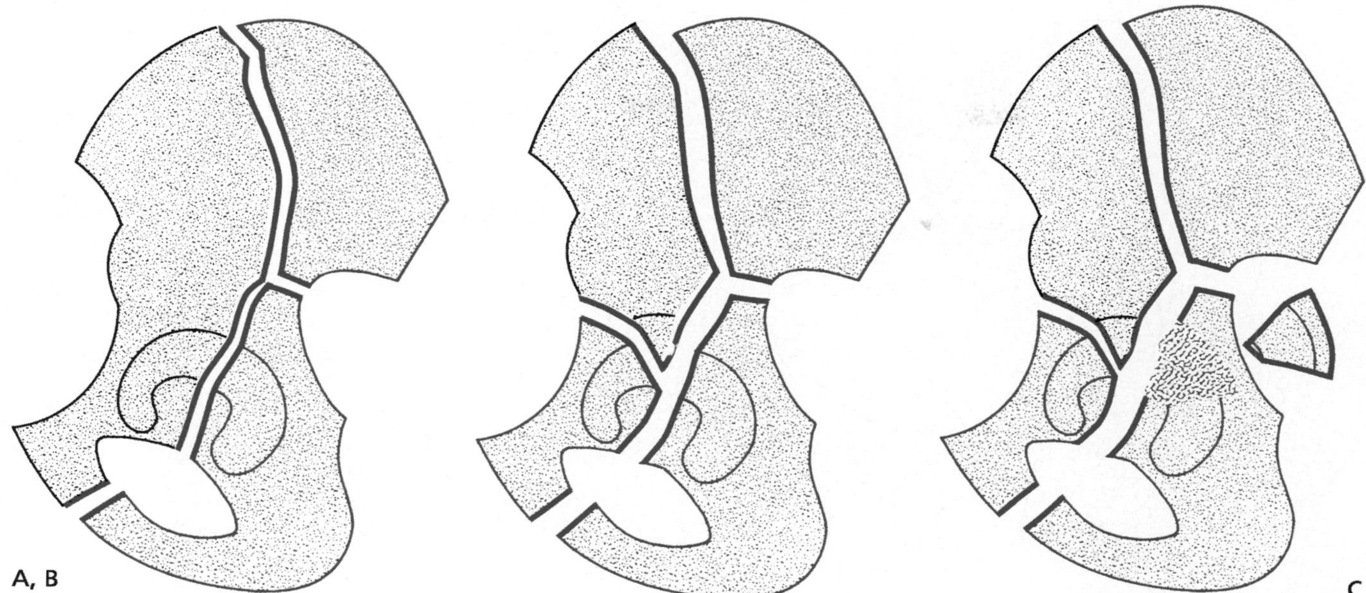

FIGURE 25-38. Type C both-column fracture, high variety. In this group the fracture line of the anterior column reaches the iliac crest. Subtypes include **(A)** C1-1, each column a single fragment; **(B)** C-2, the posterior column a single fragment, the anterior column two or more; and **(C)** C1-3 a posterior wall fragment associated with a fracture of the posterior column, with one or more fragments in the anterior column. This type has the added problem of potential instability of the hip should the posterior wall fracture not be anatomically reduced and fixed.

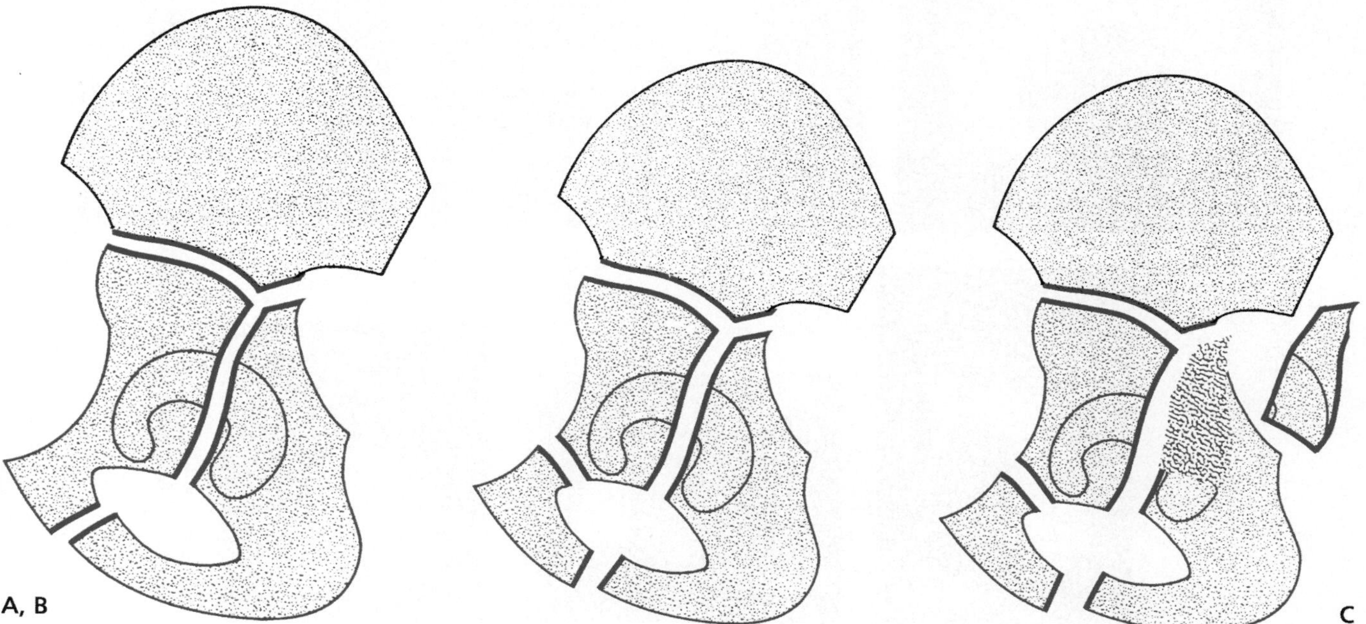

FIGURE 25-39. Type C2 both-column fracture, low variety. In this group the anterior column fracture exits below the iliac crest, usually proximal or distal to the anterior inferior spine. The subgroups are the same ones used in C1. **A:** C2-1, each column a single fragment. **B:** C2-2, the posterior column a single fragment, the anterior column two or more. **C:** C2-3, the posterior column has an associated posterior wall fragment.

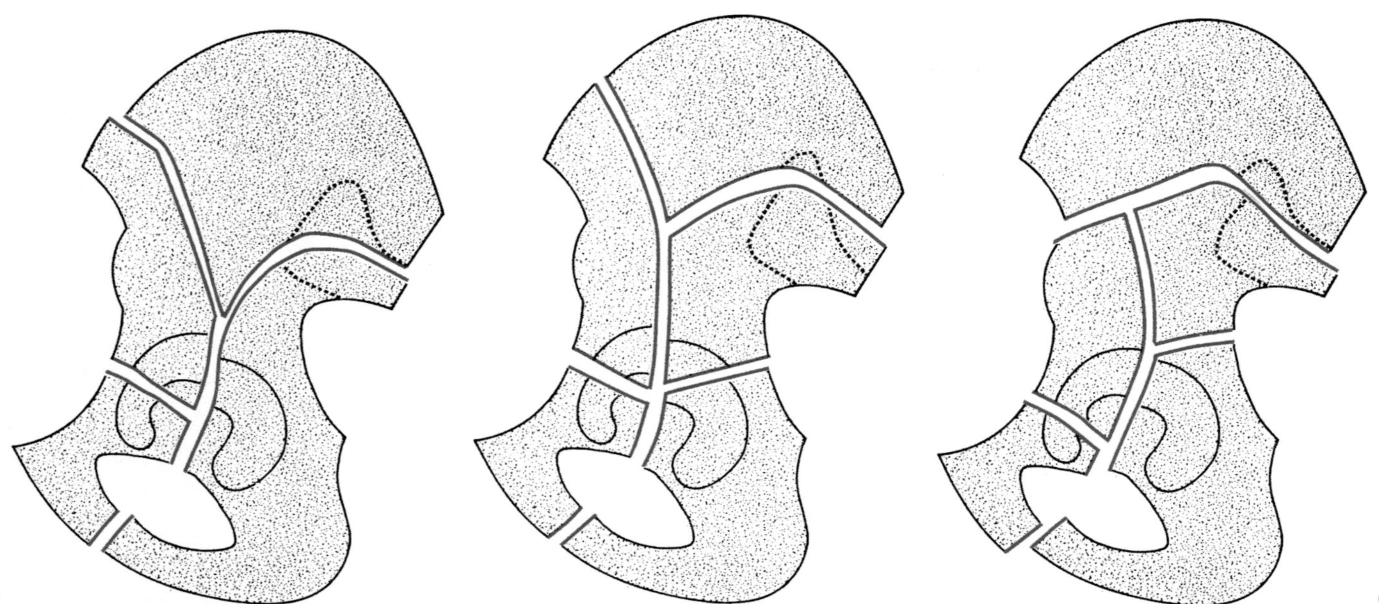

FIGURE 25-40. Type C3 both-column involving the sacroiliac joint. In this group the iliac fracture line enters the sacroiliac joint. **A:** Type C3-1, the posterior column is a single fracture entering the joint; the anterior column fracture may be of any variety previously described. **B:** Type C3-2, the posterior column entering the joint is multifragmental, the anterior column high. **C:** Type C3-3, the posterior column entering the joint is multifragmental, the anterior column low.

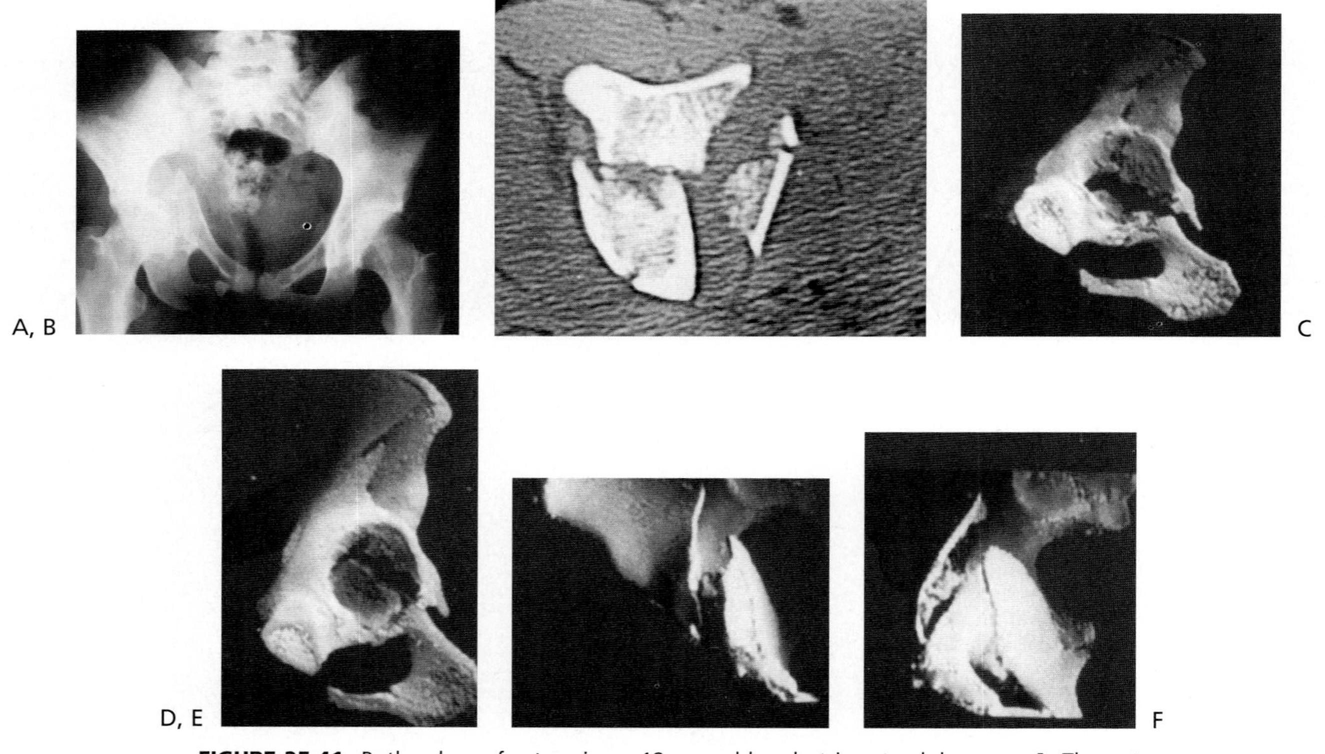

FIGURE 25-41. Both-column fracture in an 18-year-old pedestrian struck by a car. **A:** The anterior-posterior radiograph shows the medially displaced head and the fracture through the anterior column of the ilium above the fracture. **B:** The coronal nature of this fracture is noted on the computed tomography (CT). The three-dimensional computed tomography (3DCT) **(C)** shows the extent of the anterior column displacement and, on **(D),** the extension of the fracture posteriorly. The 3DCT looking medially at the pelvic brim **(E)** shows the coronal split along the brim, best seen in **(F).** It clearly shows a greenstick fracture of the posterior column. Because of incongruity in the dome in the roof fragment, open reduction and internal fixation through an anterior approach was undertaken and resulted in anatomic reduction.

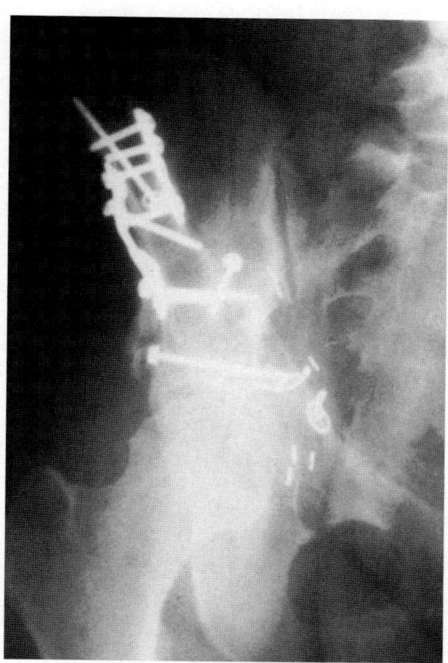

FIGURE 25-41. ***(continued)*** **G:** The result after 5 years is excellent.

C3: Both-Column Fracture Involving the Sacroiliac Joint

In this group the iliac fracture line enters the sacroiliac joint. Several subgroups have been identified.

C3-1

The posterior column is a single fragment (Fig. 25-40A). Modifiers follow.

(a1): High anterior column lesion
(a2): Low anterior column lesion
(a3): High, multiple fragments
(a4): Low, multiple fragments

C3-2

The posterior column is in multiple fragments. The anterior column fracture is high (Fig. 25-40B).

C3-3

The posterior column is in multiple fragments. The anterior column fracture is low (Fig. 25-40C).

Many modifiers are possible, as described, which identify cases with significant prognostic indicators, namely posterior wall fractures, with or without comminution and/or marginal impaction and anterior column comminution (Fig. 25-41).

The both-column Type C fracture remains an enigma, because it is still unclear which method of treatment yields the best overall outcome.

REFERENCES

1. Judet R, Judet J, Letournel E. Fractures of the acetabulum. Classification and surgical approaches for open reduction. *J Bone Joint Surg* 1964;46A:1615.
2. Muller ME, Nazarian S, Koch P, et al. *The comprehensive classification of fractures of long bones.* Berlin: Springer-Verlag, 1990.
3. Brandser E, Marsh JL. Acetabular fractures: easier classification with a systematic approach. *AJR Am J Roentgenol* 1998;171(5): 1217–1228. Review.
4. Muller ME, Allgower M, Schneider R, et al. *AO manual on internal fixation,* 3rd ed. Heidelberg: Springer-Verlag, 1990.

26

DEFINING THE INJURY: ASSESSMENT OF ACETABULAR FRACTURES

MARVIN TILE
JOEL RUBENSTEIN
DOUGLAS MINTZ

INTRODUCTION

Precise diagnosis of fractures is crucial because the anatomic relationships of the acetabulum are so complex and the choice of surgical approach so important. A careful clinical assessment outlines the patient's general status and the forces that produced the injury, but only a complete radiographic examination can reveal the exact nature of the fracture. Together, these patient factors and fracture factors "define the injury personality" and lead to logical decision making; first, as to the type of treatment, and second, by surgical approach if necessary.

CLINICAL ASSESSMENT

History

As always, the patient's general medical profile and posttrauma status are important, as the surgical decision often depends on these variables. The age of the patient, the condition of the bone (whether osteopenic or not), and the general medical, cardiac, and respiratory status figure prominently in decision making. The patient may be able to outline the mechanism of injury, which should give the surgeon some insight into the fracture. Different fracture patterns are produced when force is directed at the greater trochanter and when it is directed through the knee joint, the latter the so-called dashboard injury. With the dashboard injury, associated lesions in the knee are common.

Physical Examination

Careful general assessment is mandatory. As with pelvic ring disruption, hemorrhage may be profuse, and major associated injuries are common. Examination of the limb may reveal posterior subluxation of the knee, a fractured patella, or a sciatic nerve lesion. Because nerve injury is relatively common, careful neurologic assessment must be made and recorded before any treatment, closed or open, is undertaken.

Local examination is helpful in determining the mechanism of injury. Inspection may reveal bruising at the greater trochanter or knee. The position of the limb suggests a dislocation: internal rotation, a posterior dislocation; external rotation, an anterior dislocation. Manipulation of the hip may reveal the degree of instability.

RADIOGRAPHIC ASSESSMENT

An accurate anatomic diagnosis, essential for decision making and especially for surgical planning, can be arrived at by conducting an extensive radiographic assessment. The plain radiographs, including the oblique views advocated by Judet and Letournel, when combined with the newer techniques of cross-sectional imaging with computed tomography (CT) and magnetic resonance imaging (MRI) provide an accurate description of the fracture pattern and the surrounding soft tissues.

Pelvic Views

Because many acetabular fractures are associated with either pelvic ring disruption or an ipsilateral sacroiliac injury, the three standard pelvic views—anteroposterior, inlet, and outlet—may be helpful.

Acetabular Views

In addition to the standard anteroposterior radiograph of the hip, we recommend the two oblique views recommended by Judet, Judet, and Letournel (1). Careful study of these three views, the anteroposterior, the iliac oblique, and the obturator oblique, in most cases enable the surgeon to render an accurate anatomic diagnosis. When studying these views, the surgeon should have a dried pelvis at hand; otherwise, the various lines and columns may be confusing. The introduction of three-dimensional computed tomography (3DCT) has not diminished our need to obtain the three radiographic views; it has, in fact, made it more important, because a study of the same three views seen in a 3D format enhances understanding of the fracture pattern.

Anteroposterior View

All of the six major landmarks may be seen on the anteroposterior view (Fig. 26-1): the ilio-pectineal line, the pelvic brim, or border of the anterior column; the ilioischial line, the border of the posterior column; the roof, the teardrop, or medial wall of the acetabulum; the anterior border of the acetabular wall; and the posterior border of the acetabular wall.

The teardrop is a complicated anatomic structure, representing a confluence of lines that are projected from different coronal planes. The base of the teardrop is the upper border of the obturator fossa, the lateral border is the midportion of the acetabular (cotyloid) fossa, the medial border is formed by the outer wall of the obturator canal merging posteriorly with the outline of the quadrilateral surface of the ilium.

Obturator Oblique Views (Fig. 26-2)

The obturator oblique view is obtained by elevating the affected hip 45 degrees from the horizontal by means of a wedge and directing the beam through the hip joint. Raising the injured hip positions the hemipelvis in internal rotation, allowing us to see the entire obturator foramen. In

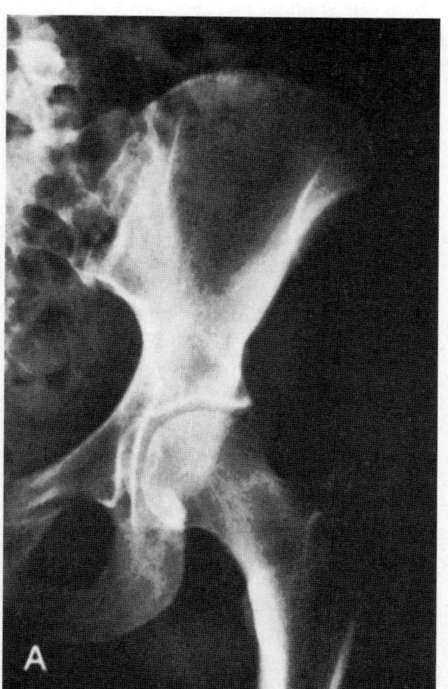

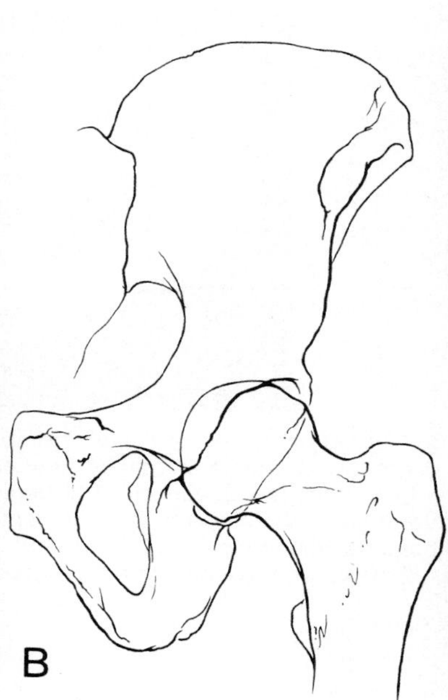

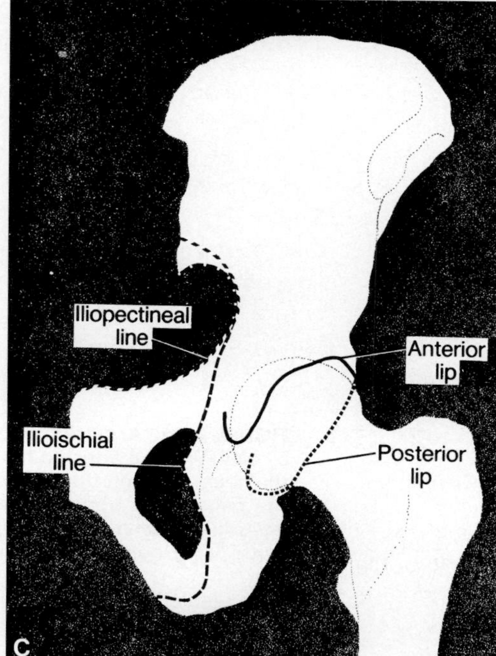

FIGURE 26-1. A: Anteroposterior radiograph of the left hemipelvis. **B:** Diagram demonstrates the anatomic landmarks visible on the anteroposterior radiograph. **C:** Diagram outlines the major landmarks. (The same lines are used in Figs. 26-2D and 26-3D.)

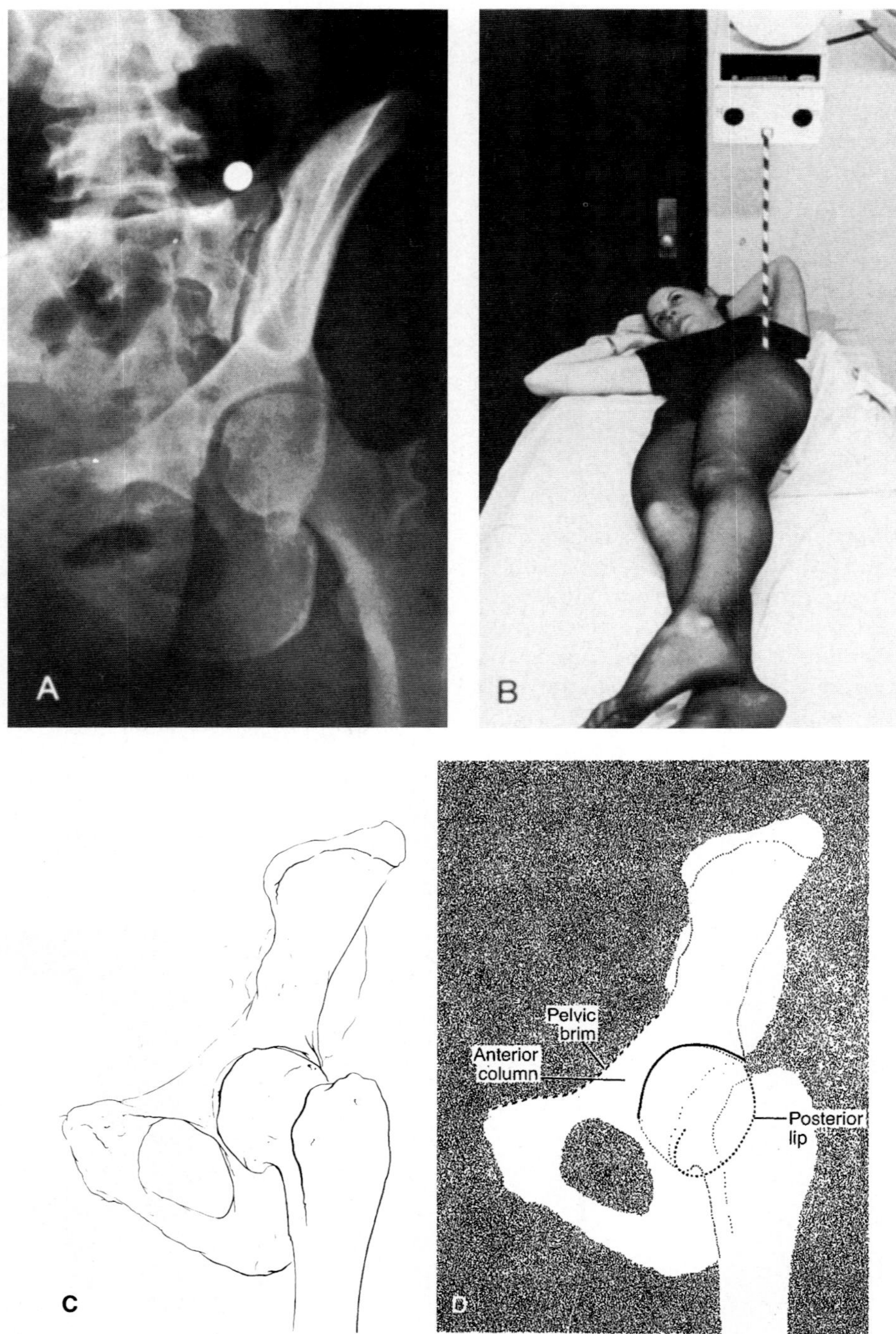

FIGURE 26-2. A: Obturator oblique radiographic view of the left hemipelvis. **B:** This view is taken by elevating the affected hip 45 degrees from the horizontal by means of a wedge and directing the beam through the hip joint with a 15-degree upward tilt. This demonstrates the anatomy of the pelvis on the obturator oblique view. **C:** Diagram. **D:** This demonstrates the important anatomic landmarks by various lines, as explained in Fig. 26-1C. In this view, note particularly the pelvic brim, indicating the border of the anterior column and the posterior lip of the acetabulum.

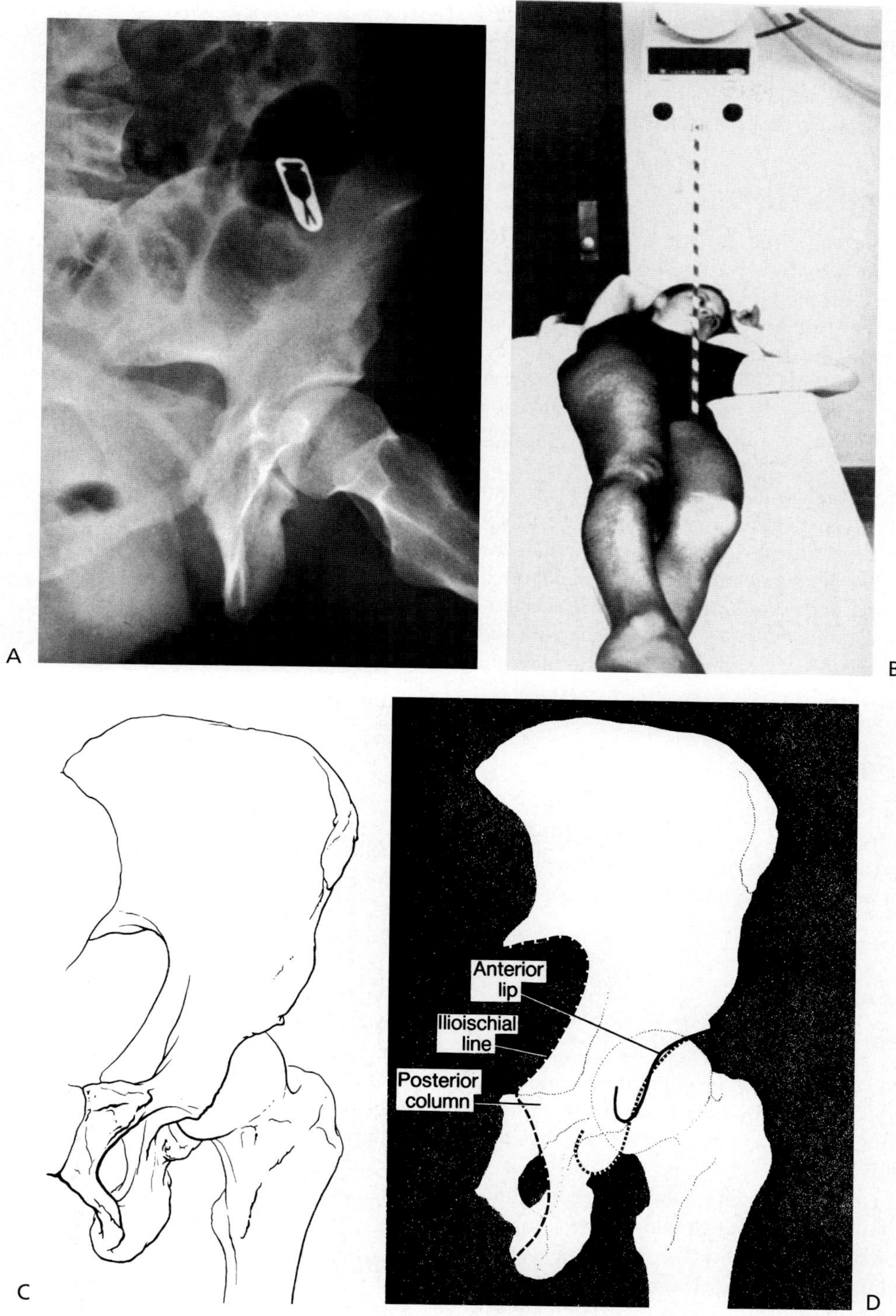

FIGURE 26-3. A: Iliac oblique radiographic view of the left hemipelvis. This view is taken by rotating the patient into 45 degrees of external rotation by elevating the uninjured side on a wedge **(B). C:** Diagram demonstrating the anatomic landmarks of the left hemipelvis on the iliac oblique view, further clarified **(D)** by the various lines, as explained in Fig. 26-1C. This view best demonstrates the posterior column of the acetabulum, outlined by the ilioischial line, iliac crest, and anterior lip of the acetabulum.

addition to the obturator foramen, this view outlines the anterior column and the posterior lip of the acetabulum, and the iliac wing is seen perpendicular to its broad surface, allowing us to see the so-called spur sign, which indicates a both column fracture above the true acetabulum.

Iliac Oblique View (Fig. 26-3)

For the iliac oblique view, the patient is rolled into 45 degrees of external rotation by elevating the uninjured side. The beam is centered on the hip joint, just below the anterior-superior spine and midway between the spine and the midline. On this view, the entire iliac wing is seen but the obturator foramen disappears. This view clearly outlines the posterior column, including the ischial spine, the anterior border of the acetabulum, and the full expanse of the iliac wing.

On occasion, an acutely injured patient has a great deal of pain when attempts are made to rotate the pelvis. In such cases it may be easier to tilt the x-ray tube (rather than the patient) 45 degrees in both directions. The view obtained shows an exaggerated but accurate picture of the acetabulum. Although an accurate diagnosis can be made with the views already described, more sophisticated techniques are helpful.

Tomography (Fig. 26-4)

Plain tomograms have become less important since the advent of CT; however, they may be very helpful if CT is not available. Especially useful is the ability to see small fragments in the joint and impacted fractures at the acetabular margin.

Computed Tomography

Plain Computed Tomography

CT has revolutionized diagnostic imaging of musculoskeletal diseases, and this is especially true of acetabular trauma, because a 3D picture of the fracture is vital for diagnosis and treatment of such injuries.

Conventional axial CT imaging consists of contiguous or overlapping thin sections through the area of injury to provide optimal image quality in the shortest time. At our institution, 3-mm contiguous sections are obtained through the fracture plus 5-mm sections through the remainder of the pelvis using a bone algorithm for edge definition. One important advantage of CT is that the examination can be completed without moving or turning the patient, which is not possible with the conventional radiographic views (2).

Crucial to interpretation of the axial CT images is an understanding of the normal cross-sectional anatomy of the acetabulum, as described in several previous reports (3–5).

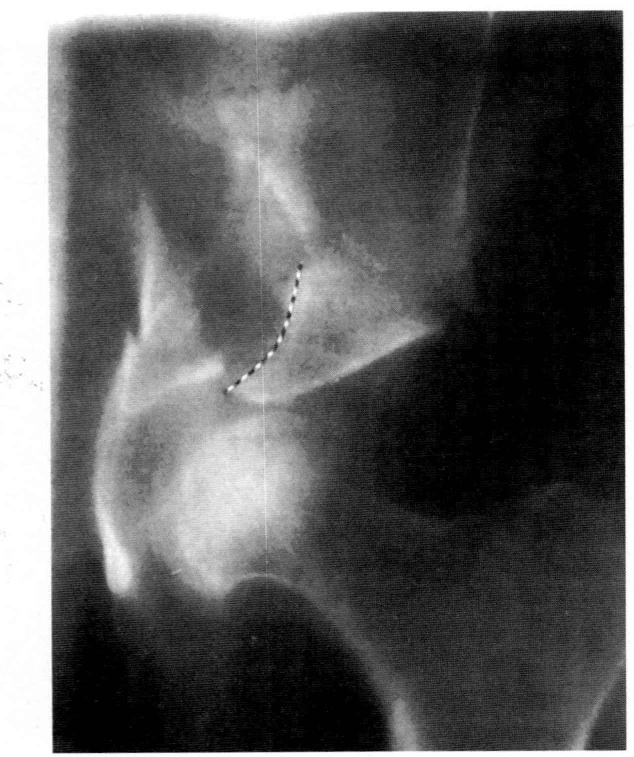

FIGURE 26-4. Tomogram shows a dome fragment rotated 90 degrees. This fragment remained unreduced in spite of attempted closed reduction and traction.

Excellent anatomic correlation has been obtained by sectioning a cadaver pelvis into axial slices that correspond to the CT sections (Fig. 26-5).

Routine axial images have proven more sensitive than plain films for demonstrating the location and extent of acetabular wall fractures (Fig. 26-6), the degree of comminution and impaction of the weightbearing acetabular dome (Fig. 26-7), intraarticular fragments (Fig. 26-8), injury to the femoral head (Fig. 26-9), pelvic hematoma (Fig. 26-10), and sacroiliac joint integrity (6–8). Although dislocations of the hip are usually apparent on plain films, CT may also occasionally demonstrate a dislocation that is not apparent on routine radiographs (Fig. 26-11).

Multiplanar Reconstruction

Multiplanar reconstructions (MPR) are capable of producing multiple sequential coronal and sagittal images of varying thickness. One protocol uses consecutive 4-mm-thick axial slices at 3-mm intervals through the area of interest, requiring 2 to 10 minutes for reconstructions (9). Newer software provides instantaneous reconstruction. Although MPR still requires mental integration to establish an overall impression of the fracture, the series of images does add perspectives that are not available with axial sections alone.

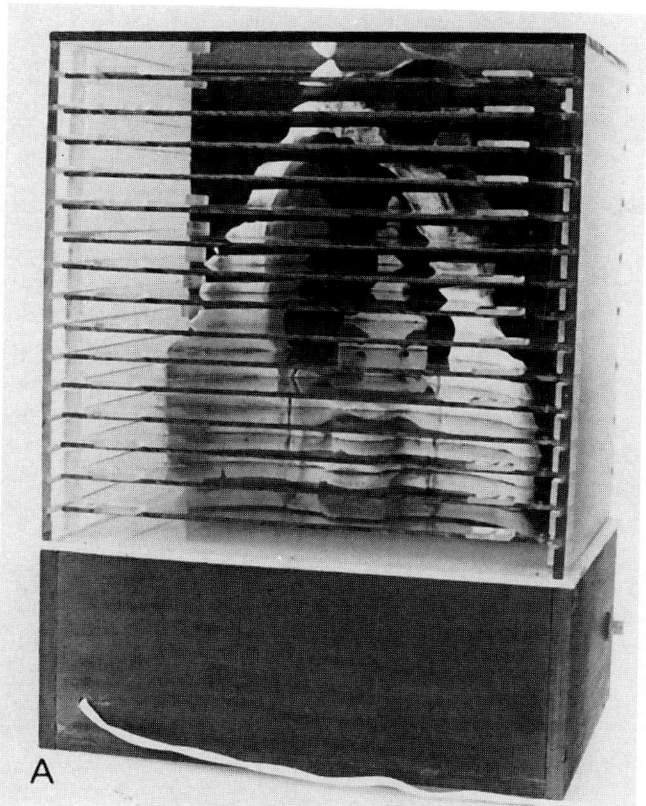

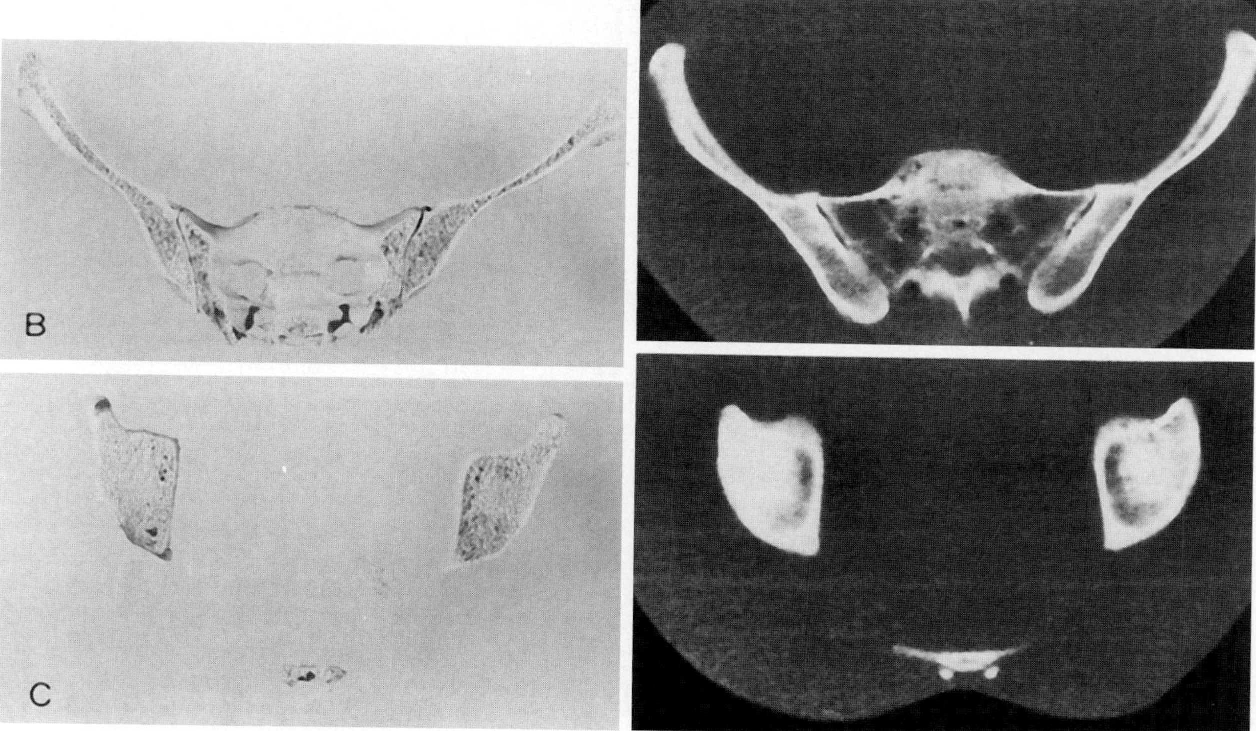

FIGURE 26-5. A: A pelvis was embedded in clear acrylic and then sliced, as shown. This allows the surgeon and the radiologist to compare the various anatomic slices with the computed tomography (CT) image at the same level, and also to see where that particular slice fits into the pelvis as a whole. This facilitates interpretation of CT images of acetabular fractures. Sequential slices through the pelvis on the left are compared to the CT scan at that level on the right. **B:** The segment through the sacroiliac joints.

(*Figure continues*)

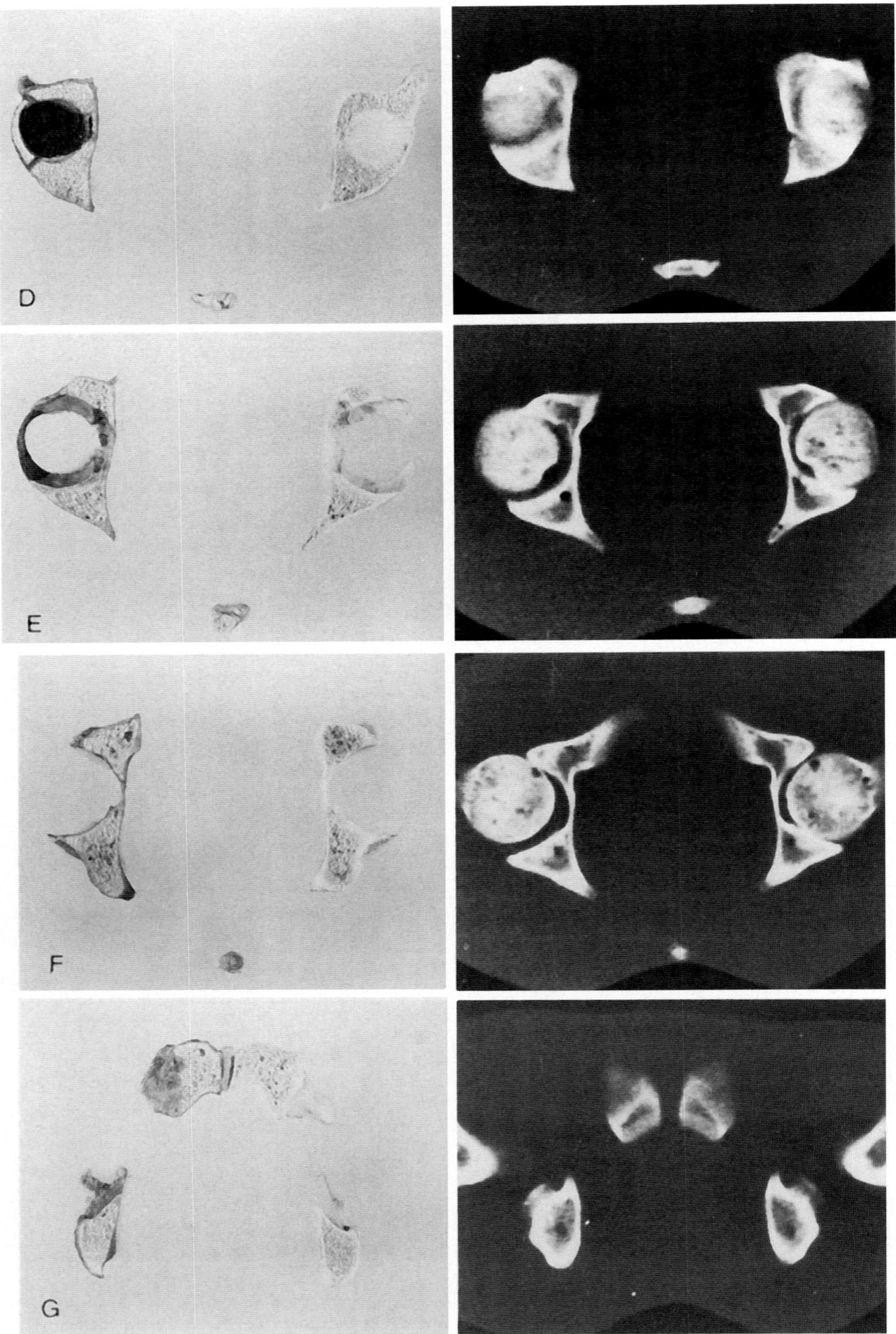

FIGURE 26-5. ***(continued)*** **C:** These slices are just cephalad to the dome of the acetabulum, whereas in **(D)** the slice has gone through the dome of the acetabulum. In this view **(D),** the articular cartilage of the dome is clearly outlined, as is the anterior column, the posterior column, and the medial wall of the acetabulum. **E:** A bone slice 1 cm from the dome. **F:** A slice through the central portion of the acetabulum. **G:** The pelvis beyond the acetabulum, through the symphysis pubis.

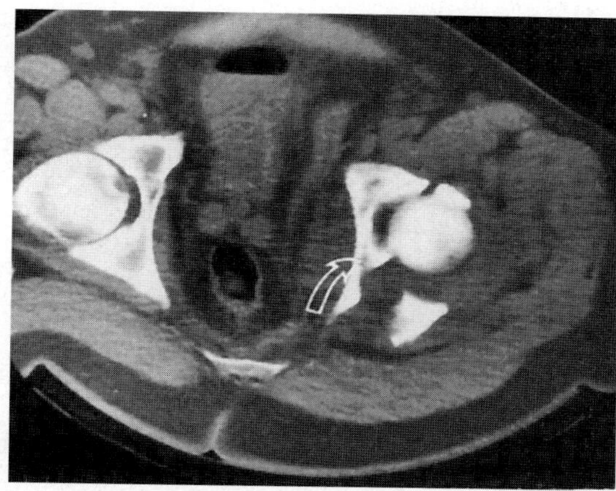

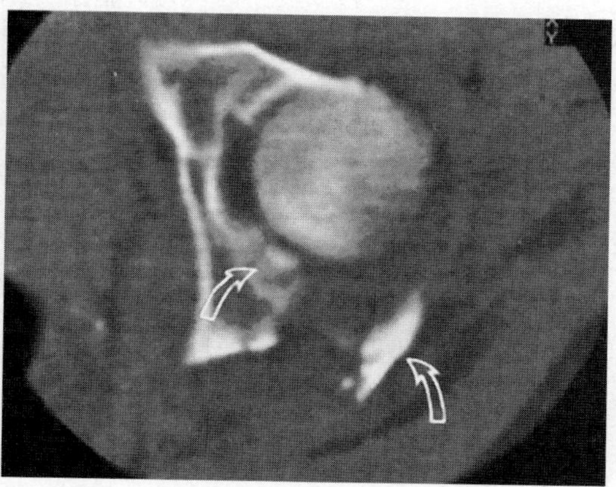

FIGURE 26-6. A: Computed tomography (CT) demonstrates a transverse fracture of the acetabulum; both the anterior column fracture and the large posterior wall fracture are clearly seen. The arrow points to a comminuted rotated bony fragment. **B:** CT through the central portion of the acetabulum. Note the large displaced posterior wall fracture on the lower right. The other arrow on the left points to an impacted fracture of the articular surface. These depressed articular fractures are best seen with CT.

Three-Dimensional Computed Tomography

Sophisticated software has made 3DCT a more valuable visual tool for defining acetabular fractures. Of particular advantage is the ability to subtract unwanted structures, such as the femur, in order to demonstrate the exact fracture pattern (Fig. 26-12A) and to view the 3DCT image from any perspective (Fig. 26-13). This is particularly true for complex displaced fractures, which are difficult to describe verbally, and for which mental reconstruction of the axial sections into a 3D configuration is a time-consuming effort (Fig. 26-14). Thus, 3DCT is obviously important for deciding which fractures require operative intervention, and especially in preoperative planning for those injuries (10,11). The technology in this area is improving rapidly. A 3DCT image still is not as accurate as plain CT for examining precise anatomic details such as marginal impaction and bone in the joint. For this precise detail, sagittal and coronal reconstructions may be very helpful (3) and aid in decision making (Fig. 26-15).

Should surgery be the chosen treatment option, 3DCT is invaluable in planning the operative approach. The ability of surgeons to examine the fracture with "virtual reality" from all directions enables them to choose the correct operative approach, so valuable in preventing complications.

RADIOGRAPHIC INTERPRETATION

Proper interpretation of all radiographic data is essential for logical decision making. On plain radiographs, it is necessary to examine all the lines described on all the views—anteroposterior, obturator oblique, and iliac oblique. If

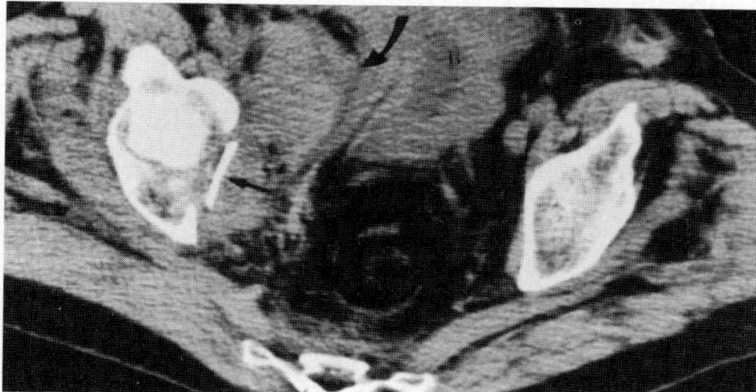

FIGURE 26-7. Axial computed tomography view through the dome segment shows centrally displaced medial cortex *(straight arrow)* with otherwise intact weight-bearing surface. Note hematoma *(curved arrow)* displacing the urinary bladder *(B).*

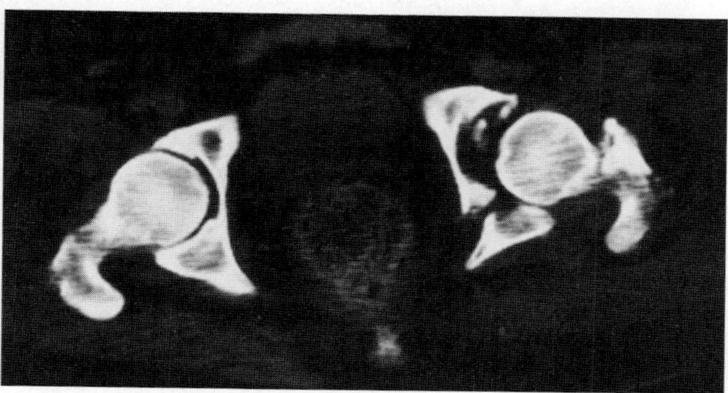

FIGURE 26-8. Intraarticular fragments that were not apparent on plain films, associated with posterior wall fracture and joint space widening.

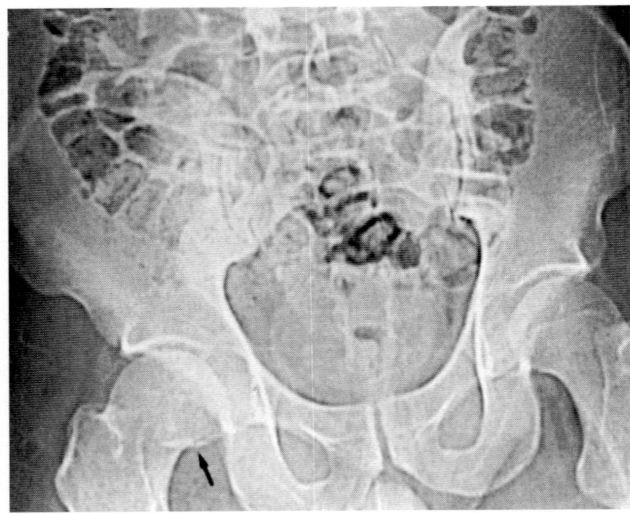

A

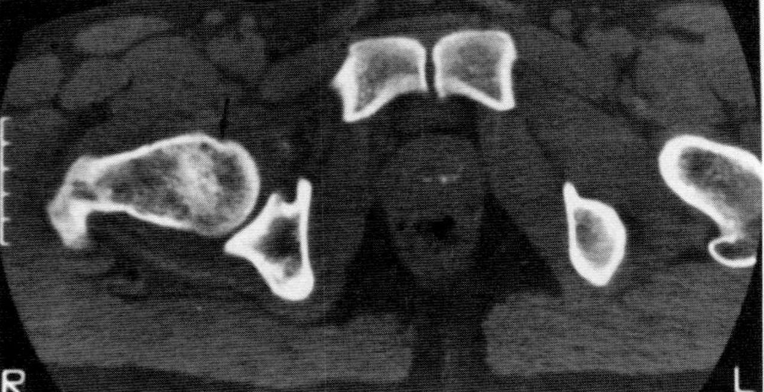

B

C

FIGURE 26-9. A: Postreduction film of right hip following posterior dislocation. Slight irregularity of inferior margin of right femoral head. **B:** Computed tomography (CT) shows large osteochondral fracture of right femoral head, which was not appreciated on plain film. **C:** Impacted fracture of the anterior surface of the femoral head *(arrow)* following posterior dislocation.

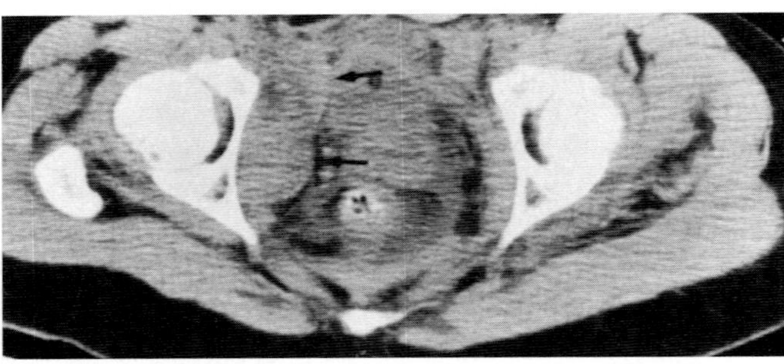

FIGURE 26-10. Large pelvic hematoma along medial wall of right acetabulum *(arrows).*

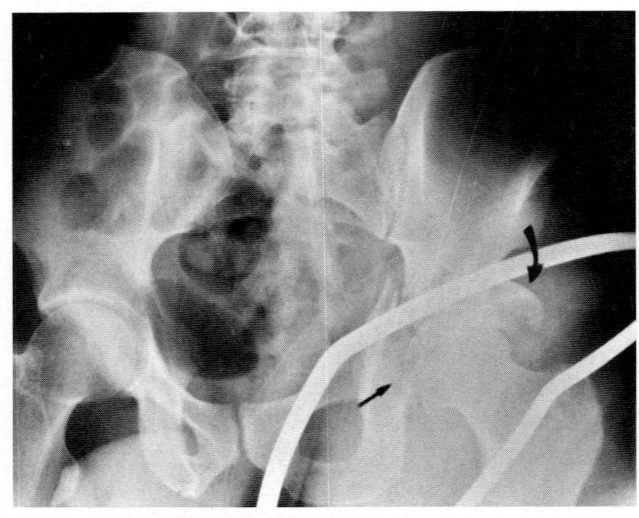

A

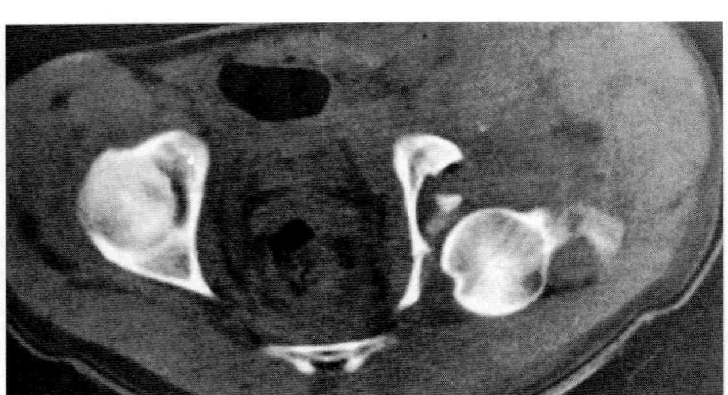

B

FIGURE 26-11. A: Radiograph of a fracture of the left acetabulum with intraarticular bony fragments *(straight arrow)* and displaced posterior wall fragment *(curved arrow).* The femoral head appears concentric within the acetabulum. **B:** Computed tomography (CT) shows posterior dislocation that was not appreciated on plain film and confirms the presence of intraarticular fragments that prevented reduction. The posterior wall is not visualized, owing to displacement shown on plain film.

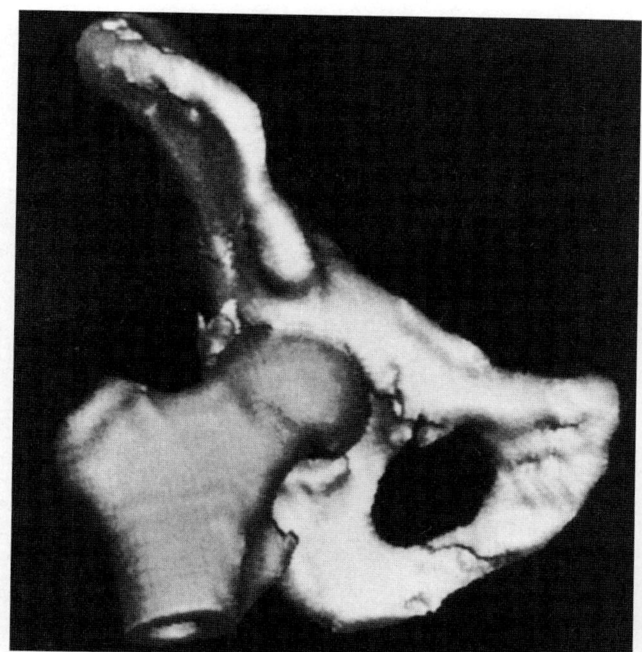
A

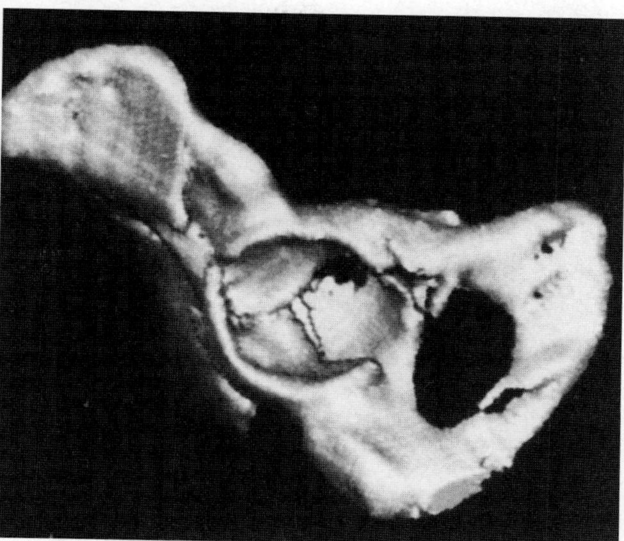
B

FIGURE 26-12. A: A 3DCT view of right hip with femur in place. **B:** Right femur has been edited from the 3D image, revealing a T fracture of the acetabulum.

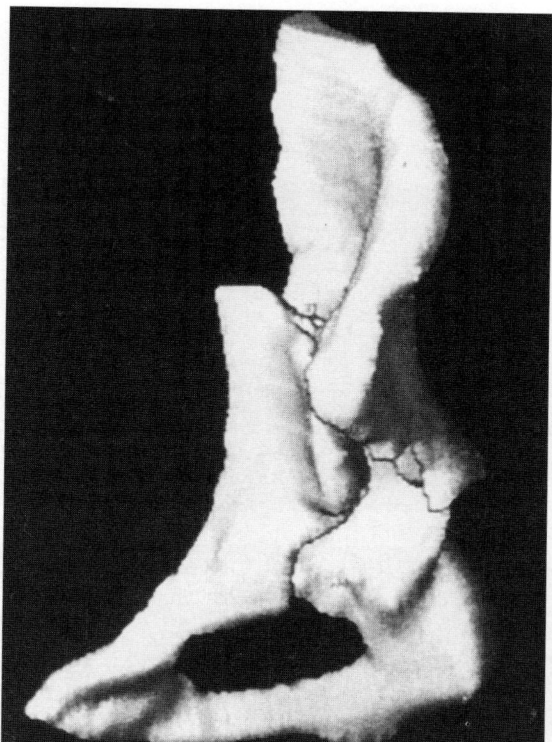
A

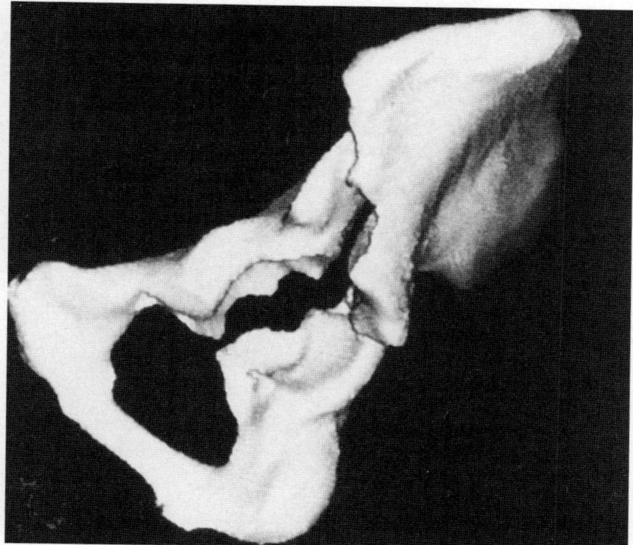
B

FIGURE 26-13. Three-dimensional computed tomography images of the left acetabulum define a T fracture from the anterior **(A)**, left anterior oblique **(B)**, and medial surface **(C)** of the hemipelvis.

(*Figure continues*)

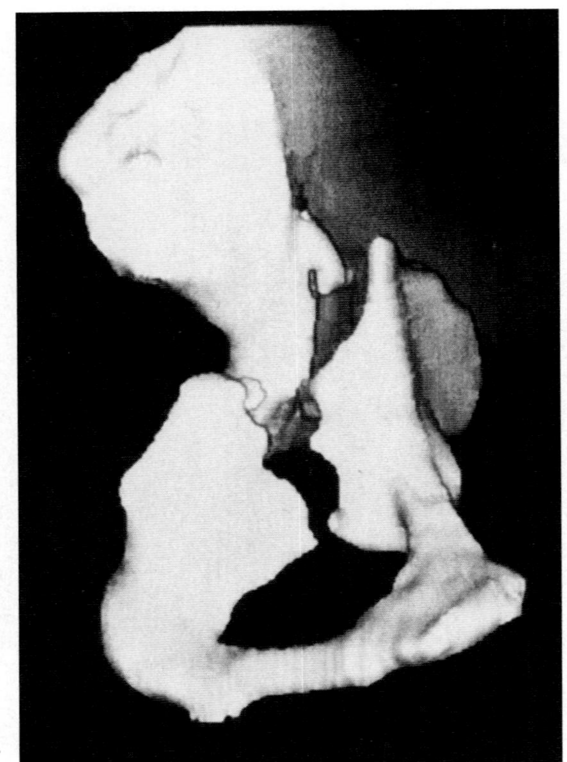

C

FIGURE 26-13. ***(continued)***

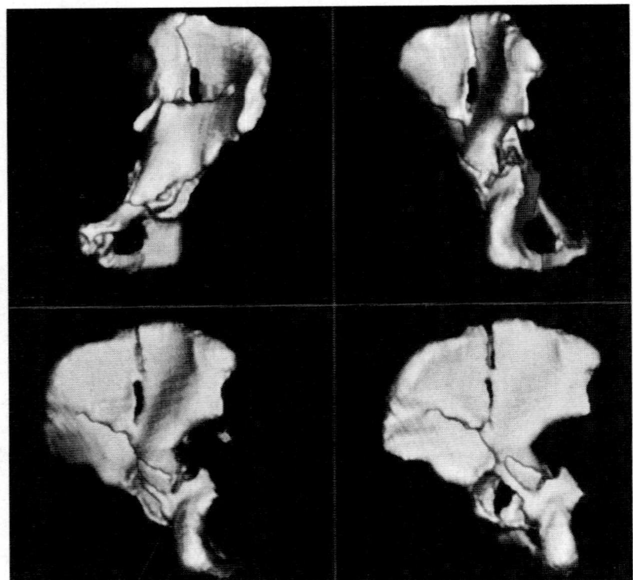

FIGURE 26-14. Composite three-dimensional computed tomography images of a complex both-column fracture of the right acetabulum and iliac wing viewed from different projections.

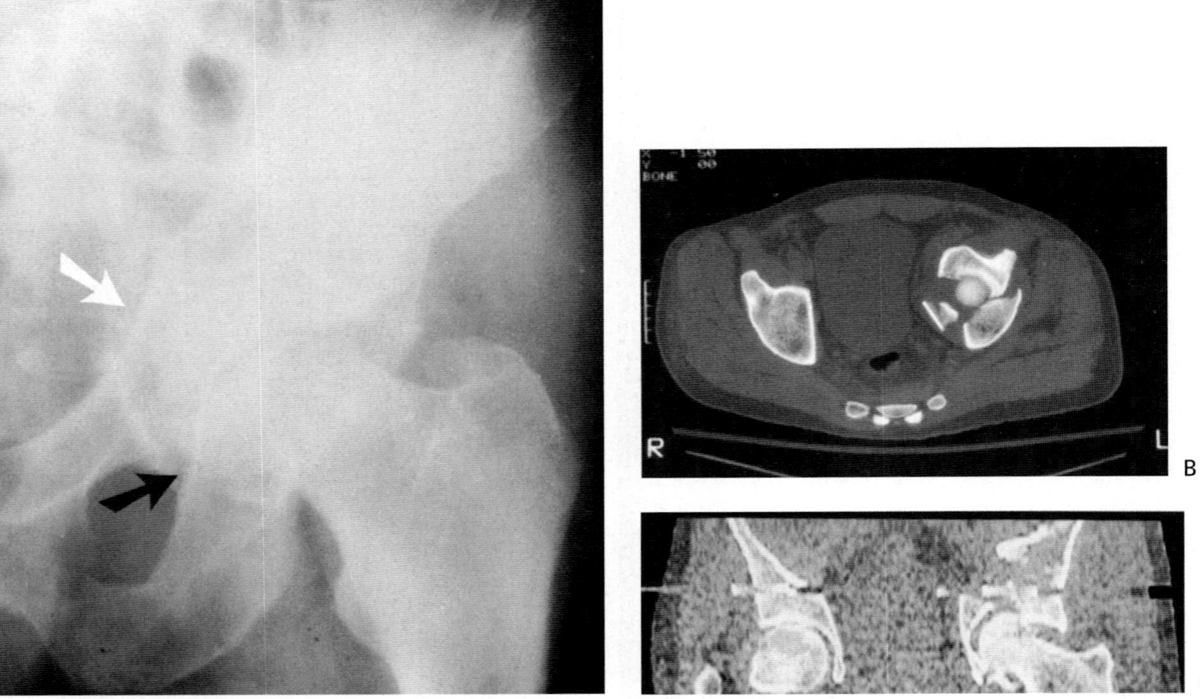

FIGURE 26-15. A: Anteroposterior view of a complex anterior column-type injury. Note the ilioischial line *(black arrow)* is intact, whereas the iliopectineal line and the femoral head are grossly displaced medially *(white arrow).* The head displacement can be seen clearly on computed tomography **(B)** and on sagittal reconstruction **(C).**

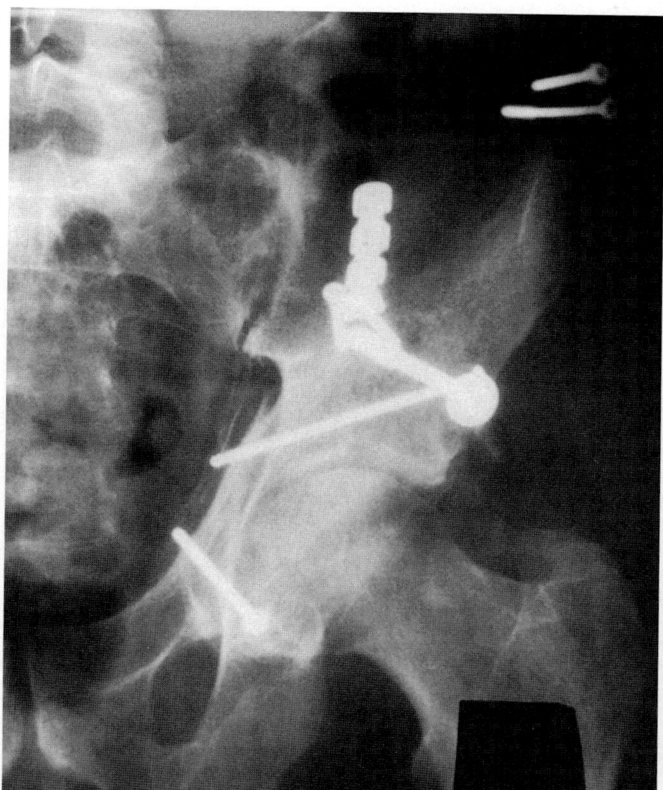

D

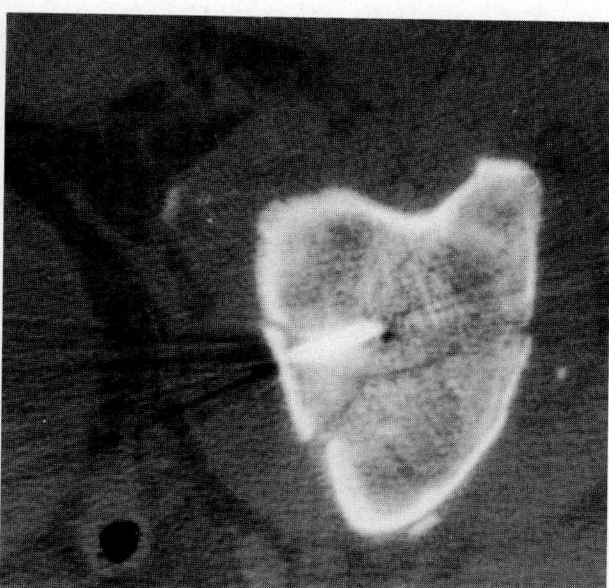

E

FIGURE 26-15. ***(continued)*** The postoperative radiograph **(D)** shows marked improvement in the position; however, perfect anatomic reduction could not be obtained because the surgery was performed more than 21 days after the injury occurred. Computed tomography (CT) image through the dome of the acetabulum shows almost anatomic reduction **(E).** Postoperative evaluation of the reduction, even with metal in place, is both possible and desirable. Modern software can eliminate the scatter from the metal. Postoperative CT is also valuable to detect metal in the joint.

only one line, the iliopectineal (anterior column) (Fig. 26-15A) or the ilioischial (posterior column) (Fig. 26-16A), is interrupted, then a single-column fracture is suspected (Type A). If both lines are interrupted but a portion of the articular surface remains attached to the ilium, a transverse (Type B) is indicated (Fig. 26-17). Separation of the two columns in the transverse types (Type B), indicating a T-type fracture (B2, B3), is detected by examining the area of the obturator ring. If an inferior ramus fracture is seen, then further extension into the joint must be present, since a single fracture cannot occur in a ring structure. Thus, if a fracture is present in the inferior pubic ramus, the second fracture must go through the acetabulum (Fig. 26-18).

On CT, interpretation is further enhanced. Single-column fractures are seen as splits in the coronal plane (Fig. 26-15), side to side, whereas transverse fractures are seen as sagittal splits (front to back, anterior to posterior) (Fig. 26-17). T types show a transverse fracture but also a break into the quadrilateral plate, signifying division of the two columns from each other (Fig. 26-18).

The both-column fracture (Type C, floating acetabulum) is really a T-type with the transverse limb of the T above the joint, in the ilium in the coronal plane. Confusion arises because we forget that the ilium above the acetabulum lies at 90 degrees to the distal portion. Therefore, the spur sign, described by Judet and coworkers (1), seen on the internal rotation or obturator oblique view is pathognomonic (Fig. 26-19). As well, the fracture through the ilium separates all articular cartilage of the acetabulum from the axial skeleton; thus, the term floating acetabulum. The examiner looks for the fracture line above the joint in the ilium, to the iliac crest (Type C1), the anterior border of the ilium (Type C2), or into the sacroiliac joint on all three views. The diagnosis on CT is most easily made by confirming that no piece or fragment of the acetabulum connects to the ilium in sequential axial images. Also, the spur sign can be seen on CT. The 3DCT appearance of this type is also typical.

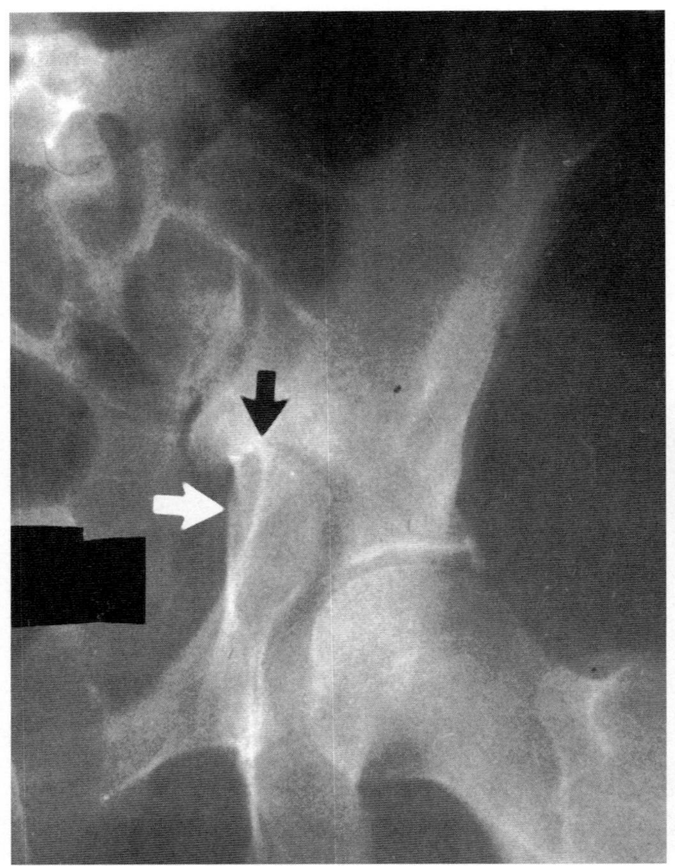
A

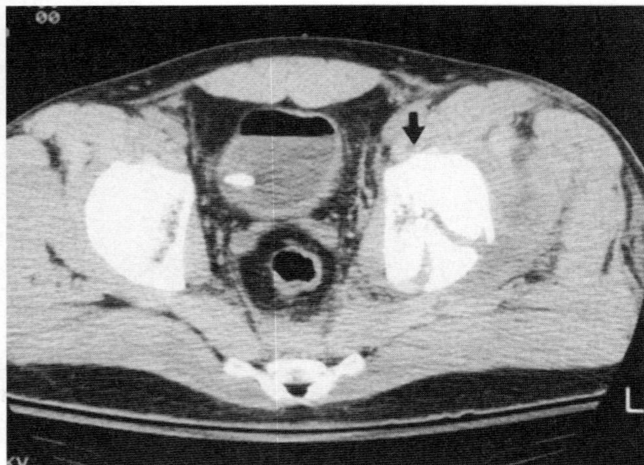
B

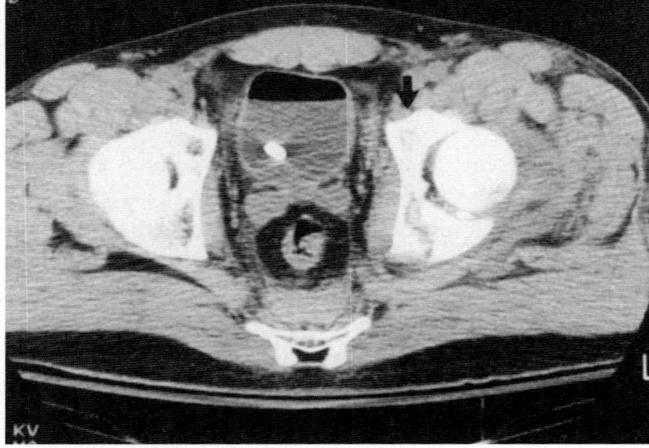
C

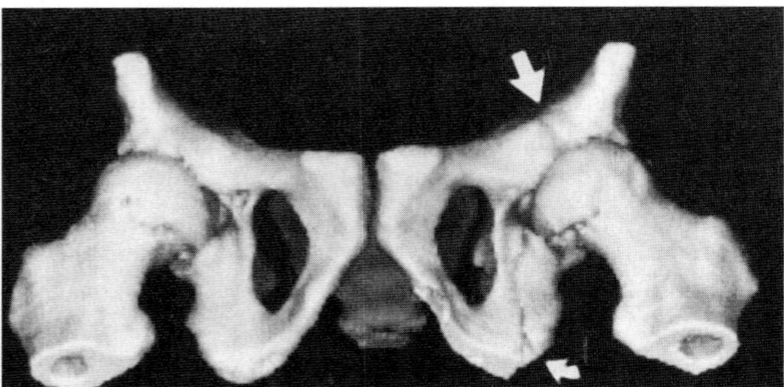
D

FIGURE 26-16. A: Anteroposterior radiograph indicates displacement of the posterior column *(white arrow)* with an intact anterior column *(black arrow).* This is confirmed on the axial computed tomography **(B,C);** the *black arrow* indicates the intact anterior column, the posterior column posterior wall fracture is noted. **D:** The 3DCT shows the intact anterior column *(straight white arrow)* and the fracture through the posterior column ischial tuberosity *(curved white arrow).*

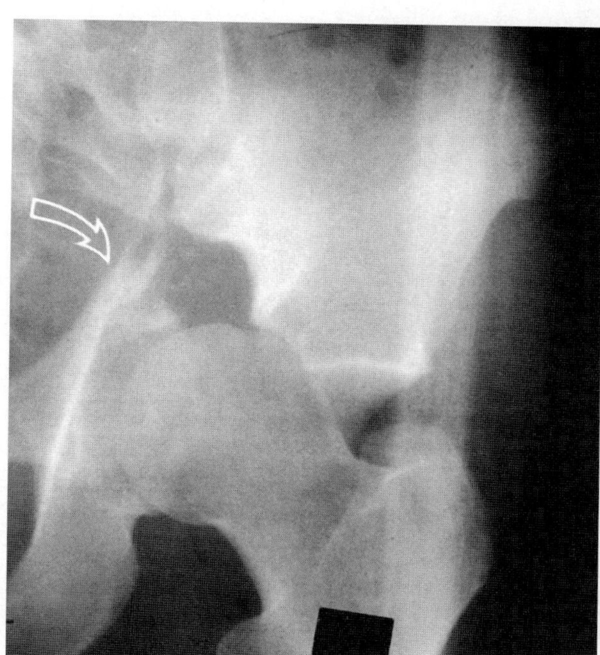

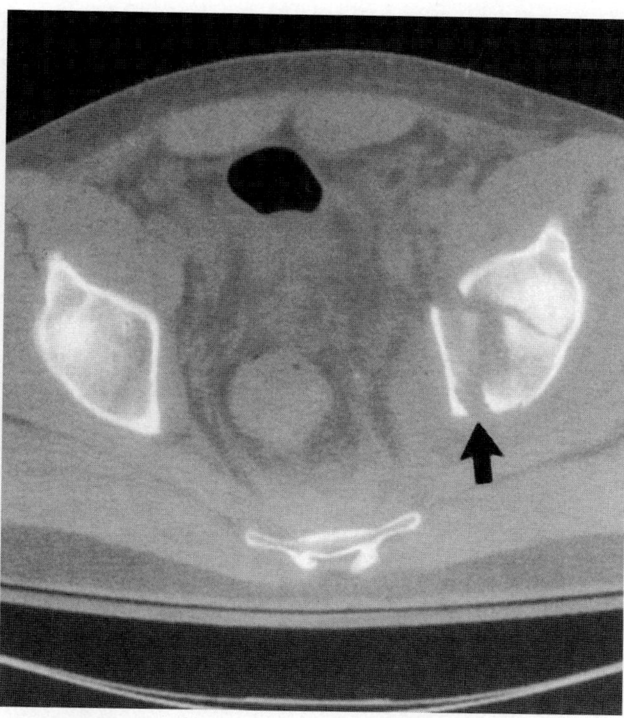

FIGURE 26-17. Transverse fracture. **A:** Note that both the anterior column *(iliopectineal line, white arrow)* and the posterior column *(ilioischial line, white arrow)* are displaced, indicating the transverse nature of this injury. **B:** Computed tomography shows anterior-to-posterior split, a feature of the transverse fracture. There is also a crack that laterally divides the columns, but no major crack in the quadrilateral plate.

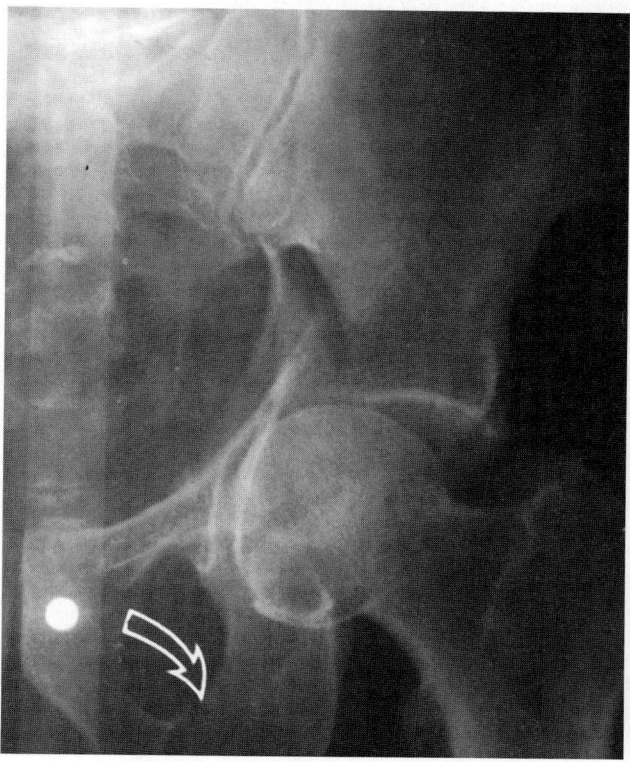

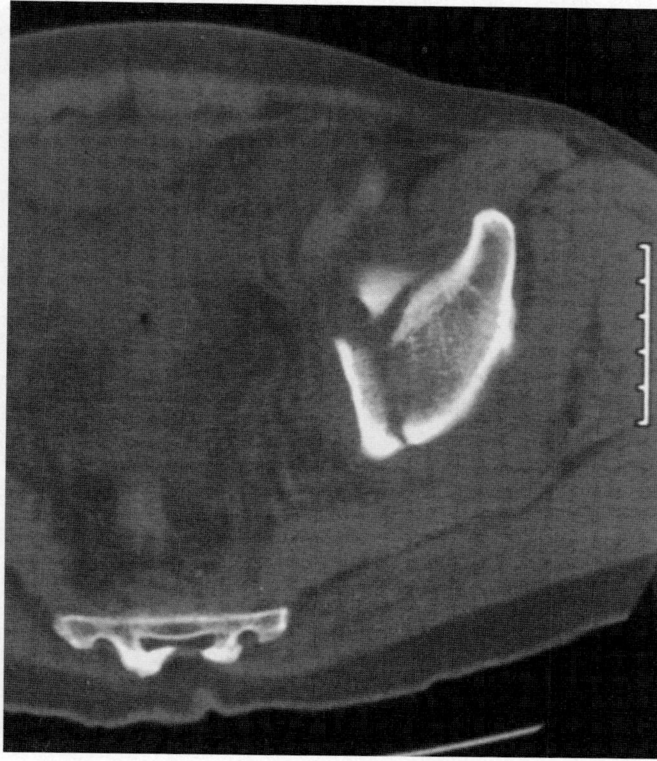

FIGURE 26-18. A: Anteroposterior radiograph demonstrates a T fracture. Note that both columns are fractured, leaving behind a fragment of articular surface. The head is in a position of medial subluxation. A split in the two columns is seen by the pathognomonic fracture through the inferior pubic ramus *(white arrow).* This is much more clearly visible on computed tomography **(B),** showing the nature of the T fracture.

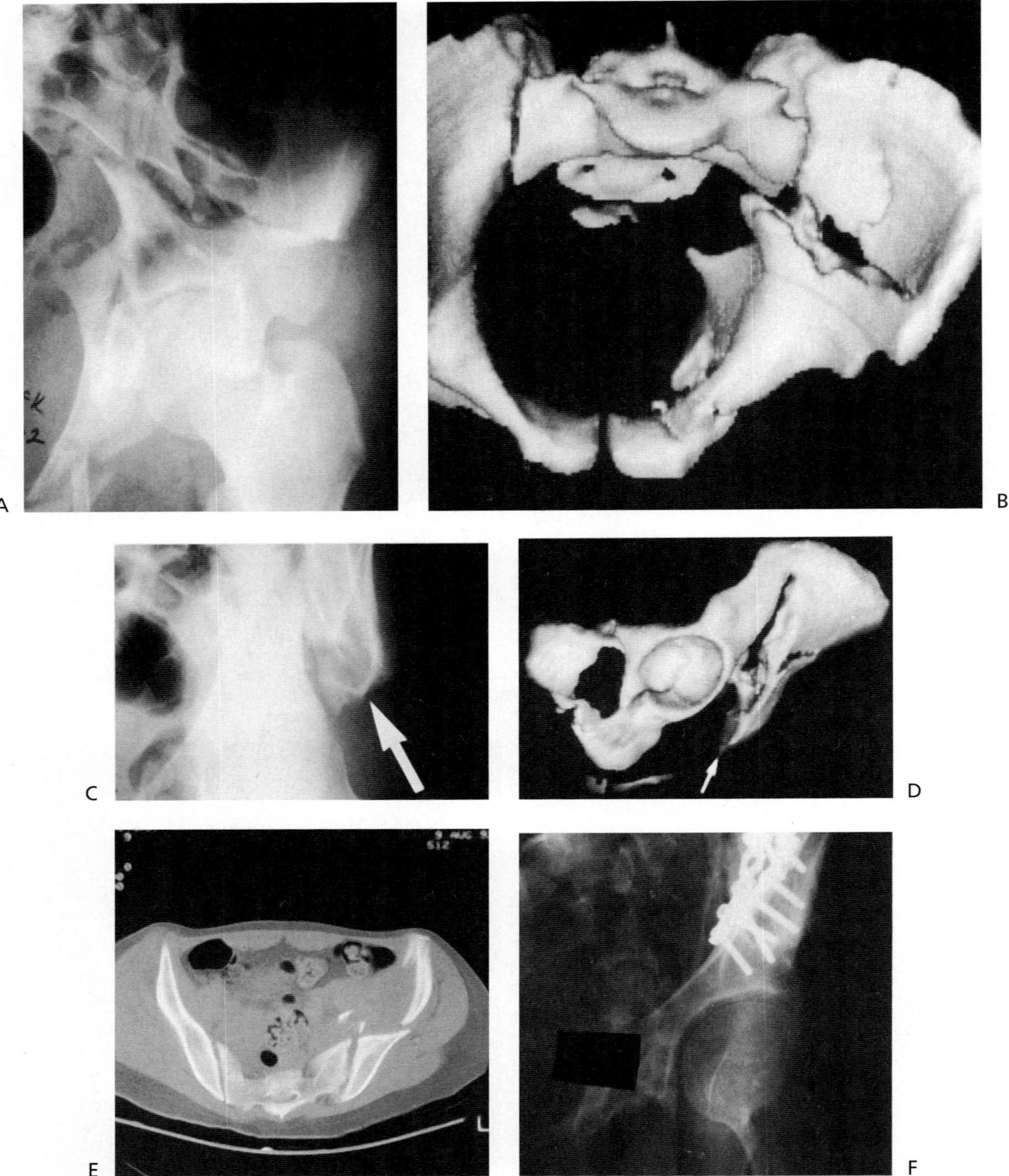

FIGURE 26-19. Radiographic features of the both-column Type C fracture. **A:** Inlet radiograph of the left hip clearly shows the fracture through the ilium superior to the joint, thus separating the articular surface of the hip joint from the axial skeleton. **B:** The comparable 3DCT view. **C:** The pathognomonic spur sign *(white arrow)* is created by the remaining nonarticular portion of the ilium. **D:** A 3DCT view provides a more realistic picture of the extraarticular spur sign and the entire articular surface of the hip joint in internal rotation. Note the good congruity of the joint, in spite of a fracture through the posterior column. **E:** Axial computed tomography shows the anterior opening of the sacroiliac joint and the split through the iliac wing. **F:** Because of the rotational deformity, the fracture of the ilium was fixed through an anterior approach.

POSTOPERATIVE ASSESSMENT

CT and 3DCT are invaluable tools for postoperative radiographic assessment. Modern techniques can eliminate metal scatter allowing good visualization of the accuracy of fracture reduction (Fig. 26-20A) and, even more important, of the location of the fixation devices. CT is invaluable for determining whether screws have entered the hip joint through the articular surface, and it should be performed whenever there is a question about that possibility (Fig. 26-20B).

In CT scans obtained after the placement of orthopaedic hardware, there is beam-hardening artifact created by the metal, such that plates and screws cause "streaks," which obscure regional anatomy. These streaks can be reduced by using higher imaging techniques (140 kVP and 300 + mAS). In our experience, axial (rather than helical) scanning, using the standard reconstruction algorithm (not the bone or detail algorithm) has been helpful in reducing artifact. With additional software modifications, artifact will be further diminished.

Imaging can also be performed to look for complications, including those directly related to the surgery such as suboptimal fracture reduction or inadvertent placement of instrumentation into the joint or adjacent neurovascular structures (Figure 26-21). Complications may also be related to the injury, including avascular necrosis, heterotopic bone formation, posttraumatic chondrolysis, and postoperative infection.

MAGNETIC RESONANCE IMAGING

MRI, modified by parameter adjustment to increase signal and diminish the artifactual frequency shifts (12) that occur in the presence of instrumentation, may be used to detect early osteonecrosis of the femoral head and sciatic nerve entrapment by heterotopic ossification and/or instrumentation (Figure 26-22).

MRI also can be used to define bony anatomy, but in general is not essential in determining the precise fracture type. It does, however, have the added benefit of being able to image articular cartilage and provide better definition of the soft tissues of the pelvis. Since small bony fragments can be difficult to detect on MR images, especially in inexperienced hands, CT remains the commonly used cross-sectional imaging modality. MR does add the benefit of being able to screen for occult deep pelvic venous thrombi while also imaging the fracture. At our institution, all preoperative acetabular fractures undergo CT scan, limited MRI, and MR venography of the pelvis.

MRI is a technique that takes advantage of the nuclear spins of protons, usually hydrogen, in our bodies. It does so by aligning the protons to an external magnetic field and applying radiofrequency (RF) pulses to bring them to a higher energy state. Once the "disturbing" RF pulse is turned off, the protons return to their initial energy state and release energy, which generates a voltage in a receiver coil. This is converted to digital data, which is then manipulated by a mathematical progression into a digital image. MRI provides superior soft-tissue contrast to any available imaging technique.

Some general principles are: (a) a higher field strength magnet (1.5 Tesla [T]) can provide a better anatomic image than a low-field strength magnet (0.3 T); (b) surface coils should be applied to the area of interest (e.g., hip) in order to obtain the best possible image; (c) instrumentation is not a contraindication to MRI, but special parameters must be used to decrease artifact from the instrumentation.

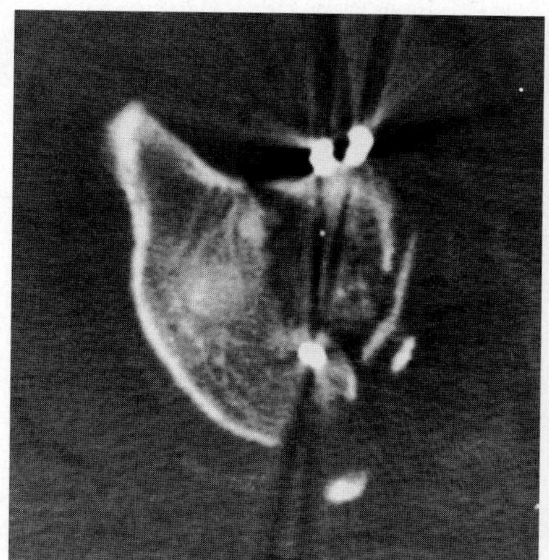
A

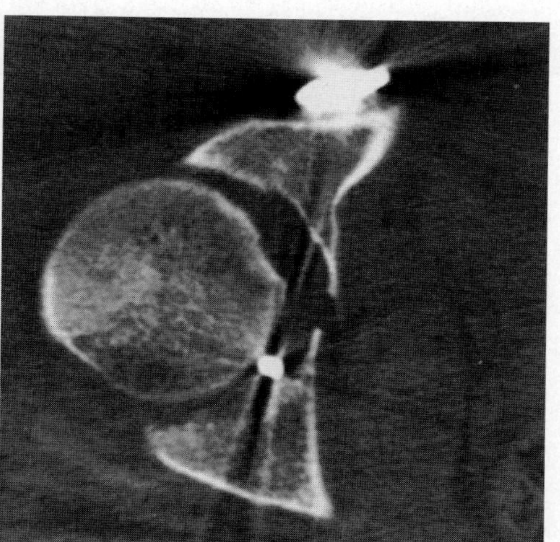
B

FIGURE 26-20. A: Postoperative computed tomography axial cut through the dome of the acetabulum shows slight metal scatter, but the fracture lines are clearly seen and the adequacy of the reduction can be assessed. **B:** The long posterior column lag screw is clearly within the joint and in this case was removed early in the postoperative period.

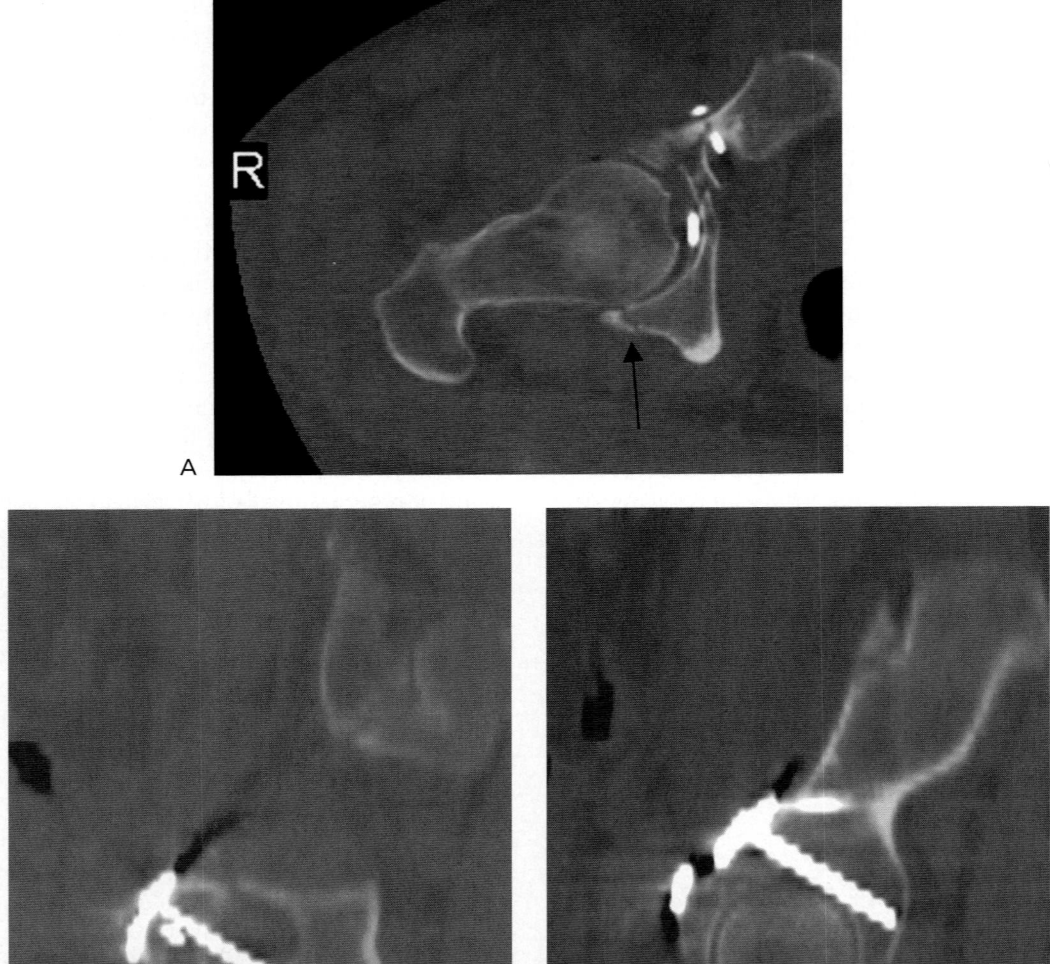

FIGURE 26-21. Computed tomography examination with instrumentation. **A:** Axial postoperative CT scan demonstrating a screw in the cotyloid fossa. Note the small posterior wall fracture *(arrow).* **B:** Reformatted sagittal screw image demonstrating the screw through the cotyloid fossa. **C:** Sagittal CT reformation showing another screw positioned near, but not extending into, the joint. Despite mild artifact, the screws are well demonstrated.

There are some contraindications to MRI, including patients with pacemakers and nerve MR stimulators, patients with recent (<6 weeks) arterial stent or venous filter placement, and patients with cerebral aneurysm clips. Relative contraindications include pregnancy, tremors, and metallic foreign objects in places where potential movement can cause damage (e.g., to the eye). If one is unsure about MR safety, there are available references to consult (13). Some external fixators have metallic joints that are relatively ferromagnetic and should not go into the magnet, and these may be tested with a hand-held magnet prior to entry into the large imaging bore magnet. The imaging magnet is extremely strong (about 25,000 times the earth's magnetic field) and can potentially fix a limb to the MR unit.

The utility of MR imaging in the assessment of acetabular fractures lies in its superior soft-tissue contrast, excellent anatomic detail, and multiplanar capabilities. MRI can distinguish cortical from cancellous bone, and articular cartilage from the fibrocartilaginous labrum. Injury causes characteristic abnormalities in both bone and soft tissue, yielding high signal on the fluid-sensitive sequences. Fat suppression techniques "rescale" the contrast range, making

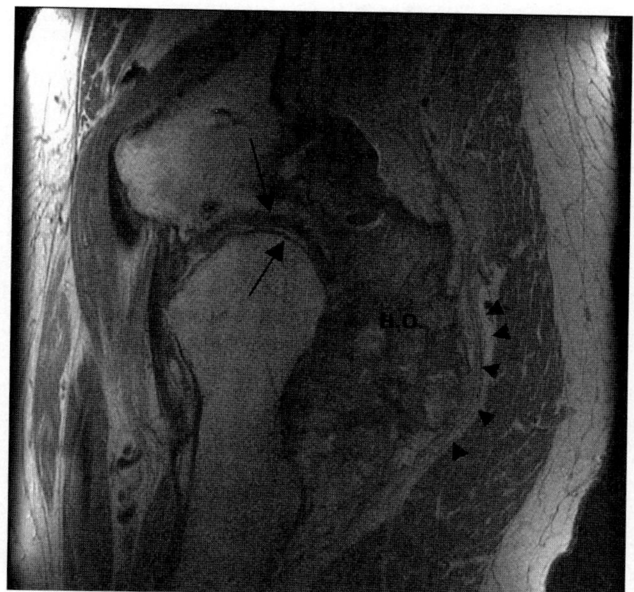

FIGURE 26-22. Heterotopic ossification displacing sciatic nerve. Sagittal MR image of the hip after repair of an acetabular fracture. Note the posterior displacement of the sciatic nerve *(arrowheads)* by heterotopic ossification (HO). Despite the presence of instrumentation, one can also see the full thickness cartilage loss over the femoral head and partial cartilage loss over the acetabulum *(arrows).*

fluid (including that found in fracture) and bone marrow changes more conspicuous (14). Fat suppression is thus an essential component of the trauma MR protocol. High-resolution techniques also allow for assessment of articular cartilage injuries of the femoral head and injury to the sciatic nerve (Figure 26-23). Owing to its superior contrast range, MR is more sensitive than CT in detecting occult femoral head injury or early ischemic change (15). Following acetabular fracture in the older patient with preexisting osteoarthrosis, MRI can be helpful in determining whether total hip arthroplasty is more prudent than reduction without joint replacement. Postoperatively, MRI can detect for delayed osteonecrosis and/or early arthrosis, even in the setting of operative fixation.

IMAGING OF COMPLICATIONS AND ASSOCIATED INJURIES

Nerve Injuries

In the preoperative setting, MR can be used to find the cause of a nerve palsy, including encasement by hematoma or displacement by bony fragment. Higher resolution techniques are able to visualize the individual nerve fascicles. Primary traction injury without a distinct change in nerve architec-

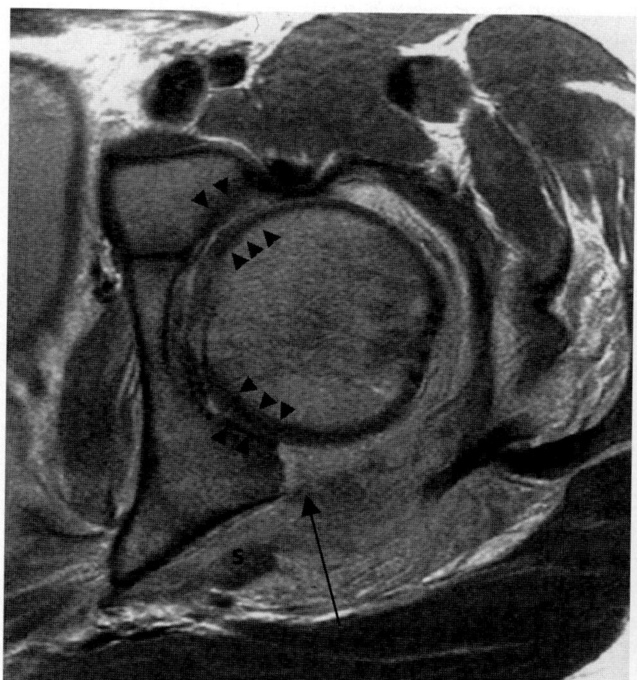

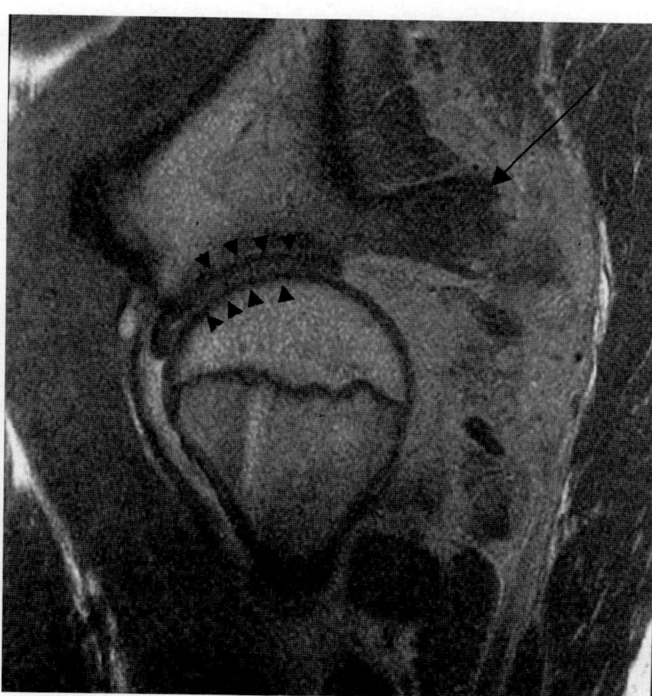

FIGURE 26-23. Preoperative MR examination. **A:** Axial MR image of the left hip in a skeletally immature individual after posterior hip dislocation with posterior wall fracture *(arrow).* There is hematoma adjacent to the sciatic nerve(s). Note the auricular cartilage over the femoral head and acetabulum *(arrowheads).* **B:** Sagittal imaging showing the displaced fragment *(arrow).*

ture may not be evident on MRI. The findings on MR do not predict a neurologic deficit, but can predict changes from baseline SSEP during operative reduction of acetabular fractures (16). Obliteration of the perineural fat plane is an important clue in detecting potential nerve injury. Defining nerve transsection preoperatively, however, is difficult, particularly if the nerve is encased in muscular or pelvic hematoma.

Vascular Injuries

Arterial injury is identified clinically as loss of blood pressure or drop in hemoglobin/hematocrit. The role of imaging can be both diagnostic and therapeutic. Conventional contrast arteriography can identify an actively bleeding artery or vein that can be embolized immediately following diagnosis. Unless continuous monitoring is available, MR arteriography is not recommended on unstable patients.

Venous Thrombosis

The incidence of DVT/PE after acetabular/pelvic trauma is reported to be between 14% and 61% (17–24), with a pulmonary embolus rate of about 2% (18,25,26). Thrombosis can occur in any of the pelvic and lower extremity veins. Detecting thrombi in pelvic veins can be problematic in that ultrasound is limited in large patients owing to inability to compress the veins. In trauma patients with an associated bowel ileus, there is artifactual loss of the ultrasound beam (27). Conventional contrast venography via dorsal foot vein cannulation cannot depict the internal iliac veins, and has limited visualization of the common iliac veins owing to rapid dilution of contrast by unpacified venous branches. CT angiography may also detect occult pelvic thrombi (28,29). If a patient has a contrast-enhanced CT or other conventional angiography, care must be taken to avoid contrast doses in excess of 300 cc in a 24-hour period, in order to prevent renal damage.

At The Hospital for Special Surgery, we use MR venography the day before surgery to screen for pelvic clots (Figure 26-24). If there is a thrombus, the patient has a vena-caval filter placed. MR venography has the benefit of being able to evaluate for pelvic clots noninvasively, and is added to the standard MR evaluation of the pelvis to define occult bony or soft tissue injury. We use 2D time-of-flight technique (TOF) with parameters. We scrutinize each of the axial source images, and do further evaluation of suspicious areas, including single regional cine examination (with peripheral gating to the cardiac cycle), in order to disclose transient diastolic backflow phenomena that may stimulate a thrombus (30). Additional acquisitions in the same area with more excitational pulses improve signal and better define the anatomy, allowing one to observe small inflowing vessels that cause turbulence and may stimulate a thrombus. In the instrumented patient, contrast-enhanced MR venography using 3D data sets allow for background subtraction techniques similar to conventional digital subtraction angiography, and are less subject to flow artifacts (23). With minimal pulse sequence parameter modification, the vessels may be well seen despite extensive stainless steel instrumentation. All MR venographic techniques share distinct advantages over conventional contrast angiography, which require direct arterial catheterization with its attendant risks, and the use of contrast agents that are potentially allergenic and nephrotoxic. Gadolinium agents have not been shown to be nephrotoxic, are freely removed during dialysis in renal compromise, and have a lower risk of contrast allergy (31). In the ideal setting, preoperative MR venography could be followed by placement of removable vena caval filters, when available, which can be used perioperatively in patients with thrombi, thus obviating the need for permanent vena caval filters and their associated complications (32).

A
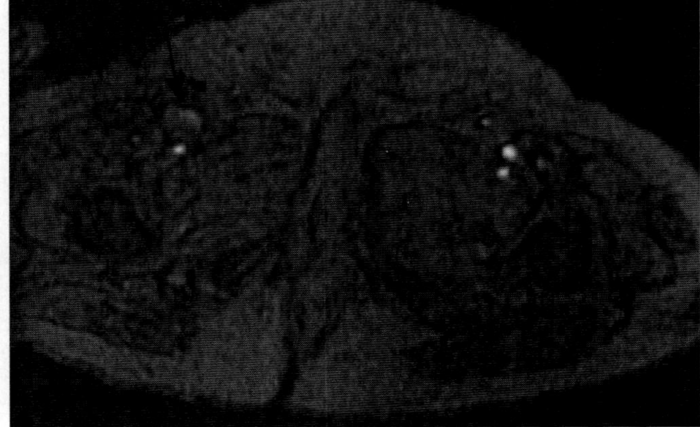

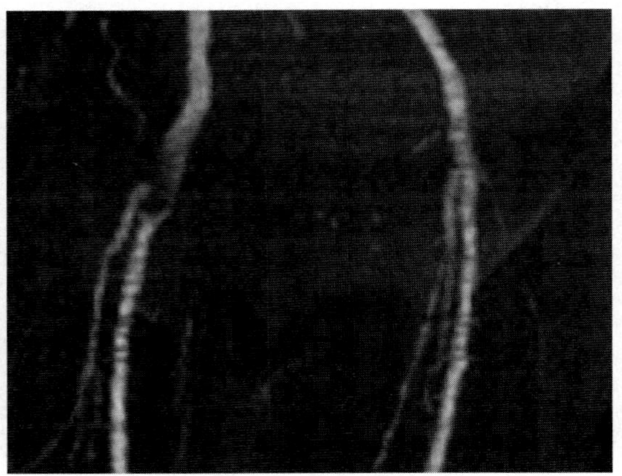
B

FIGURE 26-24. Magnetic resonance venography. **A:** Two-dimensional time of flight imaging demonstrates a filling defect in a dilated right common femoral vein *(arrow)*. **B:** The reconstructed venogram shows this filling defect on the right *(arrow)*.

CONCLUSION

Proper imaging of acetabular fractures allows for preoperative planning. Attention to detail both in obtaining the images and in interpreting them is important. As always, radiographic interpretation is most important. The cross-sectional imaging modalities of CT and MRI add information.

For CT, bony detail and multiplanar reformations can improve the understanding of a particular fracture and add information about intraarticular bodies and injuries to the femoral head. For MRI, soft-tissue abnormalities are evaluated, especially nerve injuries and deep vein thromboses. Cartilage injury and subtle femoral head injury that likely affect prognosis also can be identified.

Postoperative evaluation with radiograph, CT, and MRI is useful confirm adequate reduction and to diagnose and help treat the complications of acetabular fractures, as well as to serve as a baseline for heterotopic bone and fracture healing.

REFERENCES

1. Judet R, Judet J, Letournel E. Fractures of the acetabulum: classification and surgical approaches for open reduction. *J Bone Joint Surg* 1964;46A:1615.
2. Blumberg ML. Computed tomography and acetabular trauma. *Comput Tomogr* 1980;4:47.
3. Rubenstein J, Kellam J, McGonigal D. Cross-sectional anatomy of the adult bony acetabulum. *J Can Assoc Radiol* 1982;33:137.
4. Harley JD, Mack LA, Winquist RA. CT of acetabular fractures: comparison with conventional radiography. *AJR Am J Roentgenol* 1982;138:413.
5. Saks BJ. Normal acetabular anatomy for acetabular fracture assessment: CT and plain film correlation. *Radiology* 1986;159:139.
6. Sauser DD, Billimoria PE, Rouse GA, et al. CT evaluation of hip trauma. *AJR Am J Roentgenol* 1980;135:269.
7. Rubenstein J, Kellam J, McGonigal D. Acetabular fracture assessment with computerized tomography. *J Can Assoc Radiol* 1982;33:139.
8. Mack LA, Harley JD, Winquist RA. CT of acetabular fractures: analysis of fracture patterns. *AJR* 1982;138:407.
9. Fishman EK, Magid D, Mandelbaum, BR, et al. Multiplanar (MPR) imaging of the hip. *Radiographics* 1986;6:7.
10. Burk DL Jr. Three-dimensional computed tomography of acetabular fractures. *Radiology* 1985;155:183.
11. Scott WW Jr, Fishman EK, Magid D. Acetabular fractures: optimal imaging. *Radiology* 1987;165:537.
12. White LM, et al., Complications of total hip arthroplasty: MR imaging-initial experience. *Radiology* 2000;215(1):254–262.
13. Shellock FG. *Pocket guide to MR procedures and metallic objects: update 1999.* Philadelphia: Lippincott Williams & Wilkins, 1999.
14. Mirowitz SA, et al. MR imaging of bone marrow lesions: relative conspicuousness on T1-weighted, fat-suppressed T2-weighted, and STIR images. *AJR Am J Roentgenol* 1994;162(1):215–221.
15. Lang P, et al. Imaging of the hip joint. Computed tomography versus magnetic resonance imaging. *Clin Orthop Rel Res* 1992; 274:135–153.
16. Potter HG, et al., MR imaging of acetabular fractures: value in detecting femoral head injury, intraarticular fragments, and sciatic nerve injury. *AJR Am J Roentgenol* 1994;163(4):881–886.
17. White RH, et al. Deep-vein thrombosis after fracture of the pelvis: assessment with serial duplex-ultrasound screening. *J Bone Joint Surg Am* 1990;72(4):495–500.
18. Hammers LW, et al. Doppler color flow imaging surveillance of deep vein thrombosis in high-risk trauma patients. *J Ultra Med* 1996;15(1):19–24.
19. Geerts WH, et al. A prospective study of venous thromboembolism after major trauma. *N Engl J Med* 1994;331(24): 1601–1606.
20. Evans AJ, et al. 1992 ARRS Executive Council Award. Detection of deep venous thrombosis: prospective comparison of MR imaging with contrast venography. *AJR Am J Roentgenol* 1993;161(1): 131–139.
21. Carpenter JP, et al. Magnetic resonance venography for the detection of deep venous thrombosis: comparison with contrast venography and duplex Doppler ultrasonography. *J Vasc Surg* 1993;18(5):734–741.
22. Potter HG, et al. Magnetic resonance imaging of the pelvis. New orthopaedic applications. *Clin Orthop Rel Res* 1995;319: 223–231.
23. Montgomery KD, Potter HG, Helfet DL. Magnetic resonance venography to evaluate the deep venous system of the pelvis in patients who have an acetabular fracture. *J Bone Joint Surg Am* 1995;77(11):1639–1649.
24. Gruen GS, McClain EJ, Gruen RJ. The diagnosis of deep vein thrombosis in the multiply injured patient with pelvic ring or acetabular fractures. *Orthopedics* 1995;18(3):253–257.
25. O'Malley KF, Ross SE. Pulmonary embolism in major trauma patients. *J Trauma Injury Infect Crit Care* 1990;30(6):748–750.
26. Webb LX, et al., Greenfield filter prophylaxis of pulmonary embolism in patients undergoing surgery for acetabular fracture. *J Orthop Trauma* 1992;6(2):139–145.
27. Kremkau FW, Taylor KJ. Artifacts in ultrasound imaging. *J Ultra Med* 1986;5(4):227–237.
28. Loud PA, et al. Deep venous thrombosis with suspected pulmonary embolism: detection with combined CT venography and pulmonary angiography. *Radiology* 2001;219(2):498–502.
29. Shah AA, et al. Assessment of deep venous thrombosis using routine pelvic CT. *AJR Am J Roentgenol* 1999;173(3):659–663.
30. Catalano C, et al. Role of MR venography in the evaluation of deep venous thrombosis. *Acta Radiol* 1997;38(5):907–912.
31. Prince MR, Arnoldus C, Frisoli JK. Nephrotoxicity of high-dose gadolinium compared with iodinated contrast. *J Magn Reson Imag* 1996;6(1):162–166.
32. Bovyn G, et al. The Tempofilter: a multicenter study of a new temporary caval filter implantable for up to six weeks. *Ann Vasc Surg* 1997;11(5):520–528.

27

DECISION MAKING: NONOPERATIVE AND OPERATIVE INDICATIONS FOR ACETABULAR FRACTURES

MARVIN TILE
STEVEN A. OLSON

INTRODUCTION

The management of any fracture begins with logical decision making, which in turn requires careful clinical and radiographic assessment of the injury. Assessment of the "personality" of the injury also includes a careful appraisal of the patient, the limb, the fracture-dislocation, and, finally, the health care team (Fig. 27-1).

Logically, displaced fractures of the acetabulum should be managed like other intraarticular fractures of the lower extremity—*by anatomic reduction and stable internal fixation, followed by early motion.* If congruity cannot be obtained by closed means, open methods are indicated. Even if congruity can be obtained by closed means, some experimental evidence indicates that intraarticular fractures are better managed by anatomic open reduction and stable fixation (1,2). If the weight-bearing roof, especially the posterior aspect, is violated, open reduction may be the treatment of choice, even if closed reduction seems to restore stability.

All decision making, however, must take into account the *risk:benefit equation.* Open reduction and internal fixation of acetabular fractures is fraught with complications, even in expert hands. Therefore, the benefits gained must always be measured against the risks involved in the surgery.

Factors beyond the purely anatomic morphologic aspects of the fracture become important. Thus, in decision making, *patient factors* are clearly as important as *fracture factors.* Also important is the expertise of the health care team or the proximity of the patient to expert care.

More recently, total hip arthroplasty for select fractures has been advocated (3). The role of total hip arthroplasty in the primary and secondary treatment of these fractures is discussed in Chapters 43 and 44.

Therefore, the *treatment options* for the acute acetabular fracture available to the surgeon include:

Nonoperative Care
- Traction
- Early mobilization, limited and progressive weight bearing

Operative Care
- Open reduction, internal fixation
- Primary total hip arthroplasty

The role of all these treatment modalities should become clear after a careful assessment of the patient and the injury, as well as the experience and expertise of the surgeon and the health care team. What may be ideal treatment in an ideal setting, may be less than optimal and even dangerous in another; therefore, careful surgical judgment remains the pillar of logical decision making.

THE HEALTH CARE TEAM
THE PATIENT
THE LIMB
The Fracture
MORPHOLOGY
LOCATION
DISPLACEMENT
FORCES
COMMINUTION
SOFT TISSUES

FIGURE 27-1. The "personality" of an injury is determined by a careful appraisal of the patient, the limb, the fracture or dislocation, and the expertise of the health care team.

FACTORS IN DECISION MAKING

Patient Factors

Patient factors are as important as morphology in decision making for acetabular fractures. The personality of the patient includes factors such as age, general medical or posttrauma status, associated injuries, and future expectations. If the patient is young and has good bone and a definitive operative indication, internal fixation and stabilization should be the ideal treatment. Unfortunately, some of these patients have such severe associated injuries that acetabular reconstruction cannot be undertaken for several weeks.

If the patient is elderly, has poor bone that is unlikely to hold a screw, has comminution, and is in a questionable medical state, open reduction would be folly, and the results of nonoperative treatment often are surprisingly good in this age group (Fig. 27-2). This is especially true in patients with *a both-column fracture with secondary congruence.* In many cases in the older age group, the patient can be managed by early mobilization, with progressive weight bearing. If necessary, late total hip arthroplasty is preferable to an early surgical misadventure.

Obviously, many patients' injuries fall between these two extremes. Surgical stabilization is suitable for most if a strong indication exists, but sound surgical judgment must be exercised in all cases.

Also, current surgical wisdom demands early fracture stabilization for polytrauma patients, to allow them to assume the upright position for proper ventilation. In general, I agree with this principle; although it is more difficult to apply to the acetabulum than to any other fracture. If the acetabular fracture is relatively simple, such as a posterior column or posterior wall fracture, fracture stabilization may be achieved with relatively little risk to the patient. More complex types of fractures require much longer operating time and more blood; therefore, an injudicious open reduction in such a case may have the opposite effect; that is, it could jeopardize the patient's life.

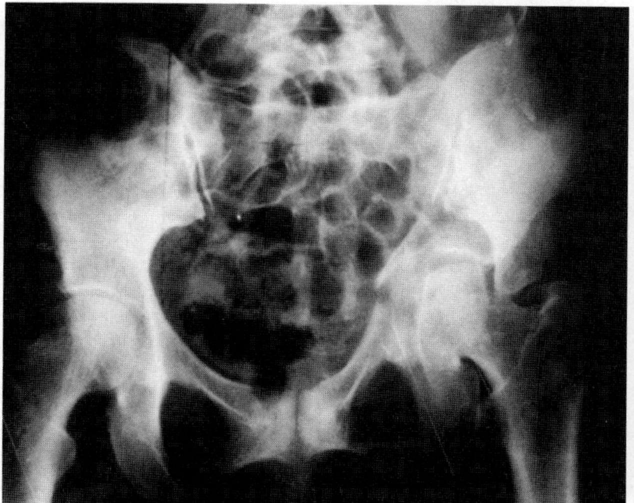

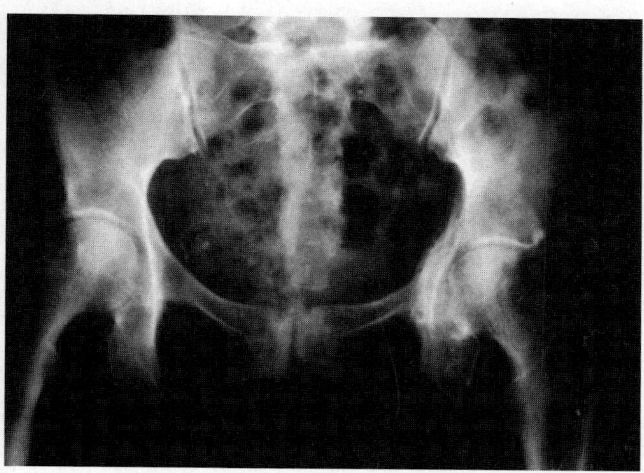

FIGURE 27-2. A: Anteroposterior radiograph of a severely comminuted both-column fracture in a elderly woman. **B:** Treatment in traction allowed reduction of the fracture and resulted in an excellent clinical and radiographic result.

No broad generalization will help the surgeon manage any particular patient. All the factors must be considered if one is to make an intelligent judgment.

Fracture Factors

To make treatment decisions, and after assessment of the patient, the surgeon must answer the following questions regarding the fracture:

- Is the hip stable or unstable?
- Is the femoral head congruous with the acetabulum?
- What is the degree of comminution?
- Is there a femoral head fracture?
- Is the fracture fixable, by me, by anyone?

If no adverse patient factors exist, then open reduction and internal fixation are indicated for instability or incongruity of the hip.

Instability of the Hip

Posterior

Because the stability of the hip joint, more than that of any other joint, depends on its bony architecture, a dislocation of the hip associated with a large posterior wall fragment may result in instability of that hip even after reduction of the dislocation (Fig. 27-3). Posterior dislocations associated with posterior wall fractures are notorious in this regard and, therefore, should be surgically stabilized. Also, following reduction, small fragments of bone may be retained in the joint, causing incongruity of the bony surfaces and other mechanical difficulties. As well as instability, posterior dislocations often produce impacted articular fragments, causing incongruity of the articular surfaces.

Only if the posterior fragments are small and the hip joint is stable through a full range of motion can nonoperative treatment be considered, as may be the case in a pure posterior dislocation of the hip. Thus, a posterior wall injury associated with a posterior dislocation of the hip is almost an absolute indication for surgery.

Anterior

Although less common, anterior wall fractures that result from anterior dislocation of the hip can also produce anterior instability of the hip (Fig. 27-4). These fractures also require stabilization to prevent anterior recurrent dislocation.

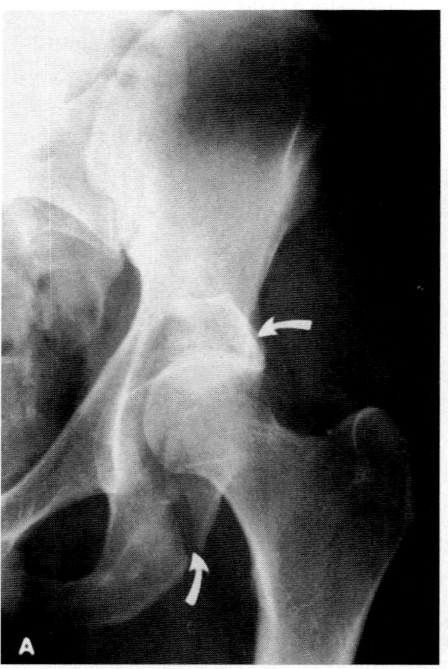

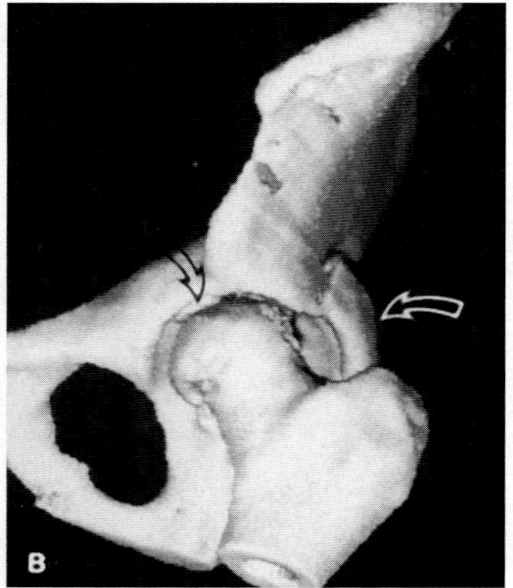

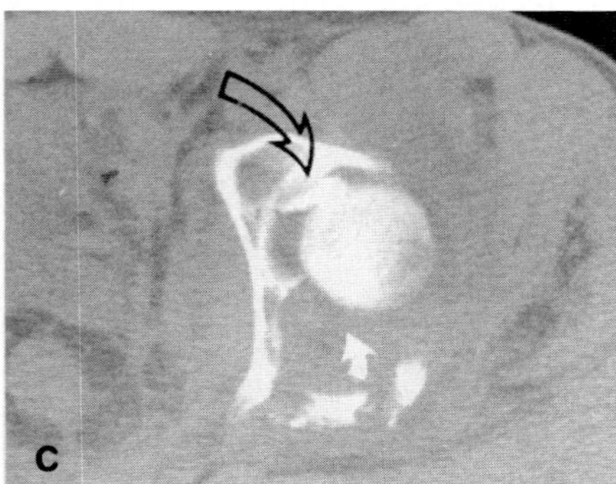

FIGURE 27-3. Posterior instability of the hip is an almost absolute indication for surgical stabilization. **A:** The anteroposterior radiograph of the left hip shows a posterior dislocation with a large posterior wall fragment and an extension through the posterior column *(white arrows)*. **B:** The three-dimensional computed tomography version of the same view shows the posterior subluxation, the large superior posterior fragment *(white arrow)* and also a free fragment of bone within the hip joint *(black arrow)*. **C:** This corresponds on the axial computed tomography to the interposed fragment of bone from the posterior column *(black arrow)*. Note also the complete absence of any bone to stabilize the femoral head *(white arrow)*.

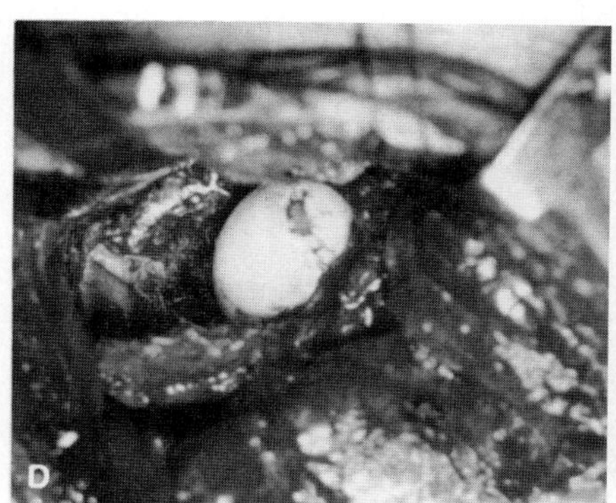

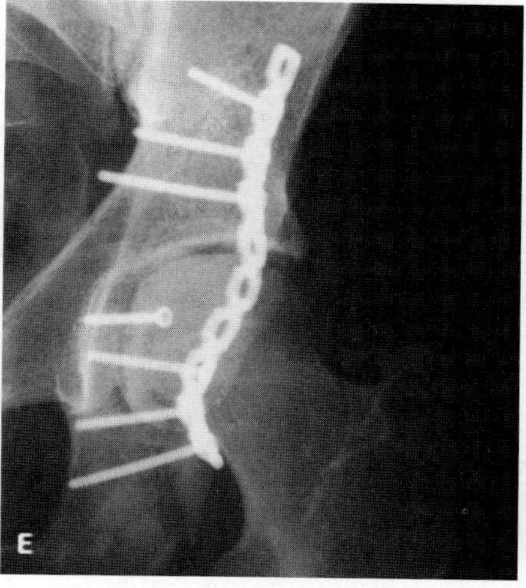

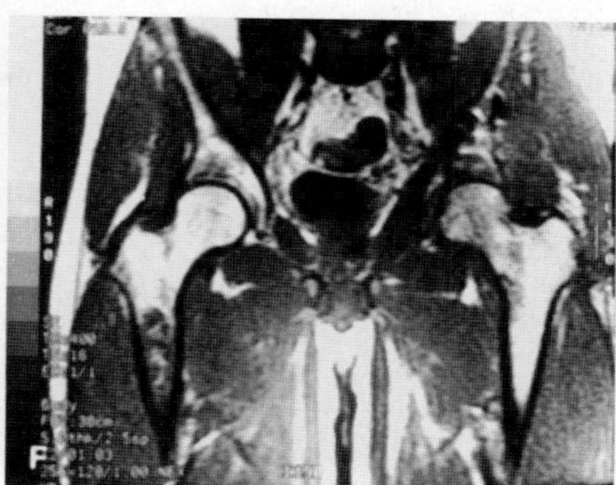

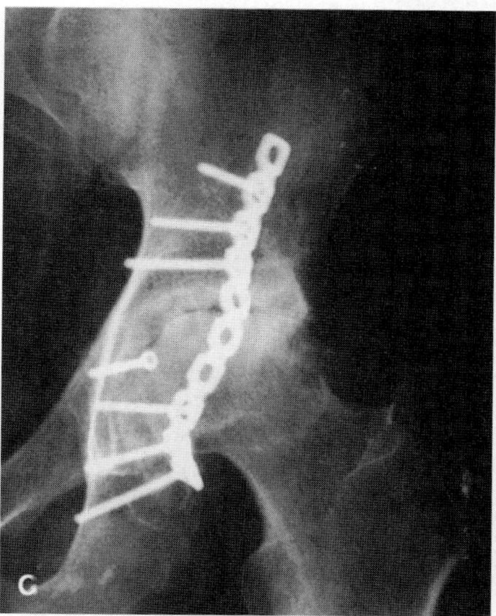

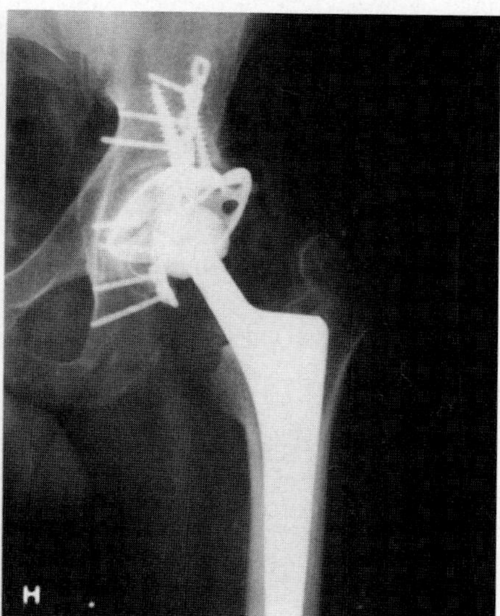

FIGURE 27-3. ***(continued)*** **D:** On the clinical photograph at the time of surgery an osteochondral lesion is noted on the femoral head as well as the marginally impacted fragment. **E:** The fracture was reduced anatomically and fixed with an interfragmental screw and a buttress plate. Unfortunately, in this case, the complication of avascular necrosis ensued. **F:** This was first diagnosed on the magnetic resonance image before collapse of the femoral head. **G:** This is noted in the anteroposterior radiograph. **H:** A hybrid total hip arthroplasty was performed.

Central/Medial

Also, the femoral head may be centrally unstable if a large fragment of the quadrilateral plate is fractured. This may occur even after open reduction and internal fixation, when the columns are restored but the quadrilateral plate is not. Failure to recognize this leads to an incongruous hip and a poor result. Although this is difficult to accomplish, the quadrilateral plate must be held in its anatomic position by spring plates, cerclage wires, or other means as necessary (Fig. 27-5).

Incongruity

Congruous is derived from the Latin *congruus* (to fit). Therefore, incongruity as applied to the hip joint means any alteration or inconsistency in the relationship between the femoral head and acetabulum. In general, the curve of the femoral head fits exactly into the dome of the acetabulum on all three radiographic views. Any distortion represents incongruity, but some types are more clinically important than others. The hip joint does not tolerate subluxation well

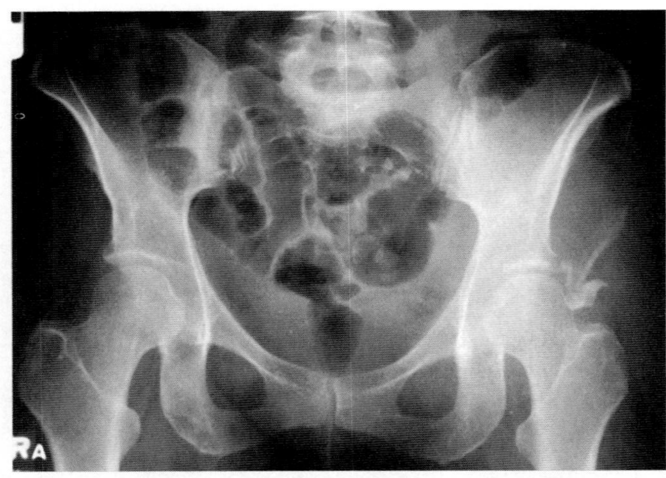

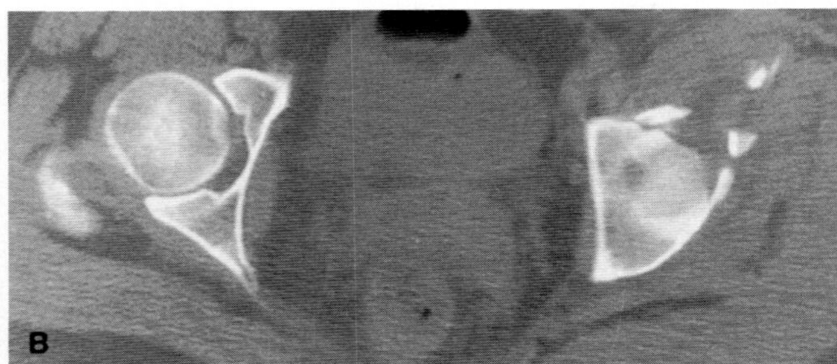

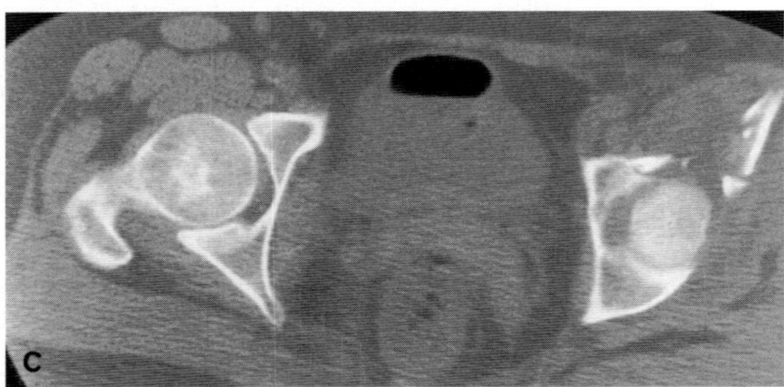

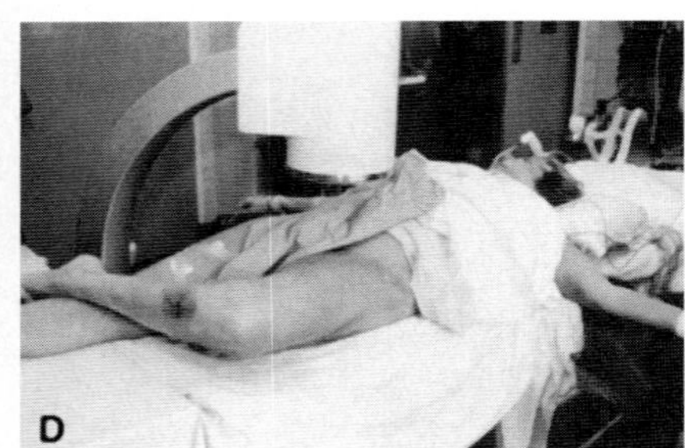

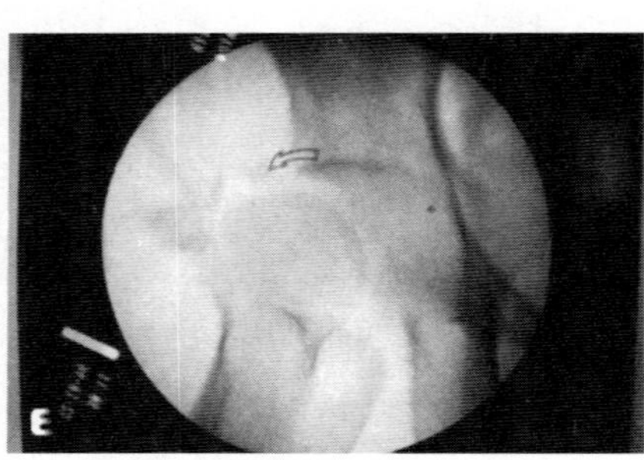

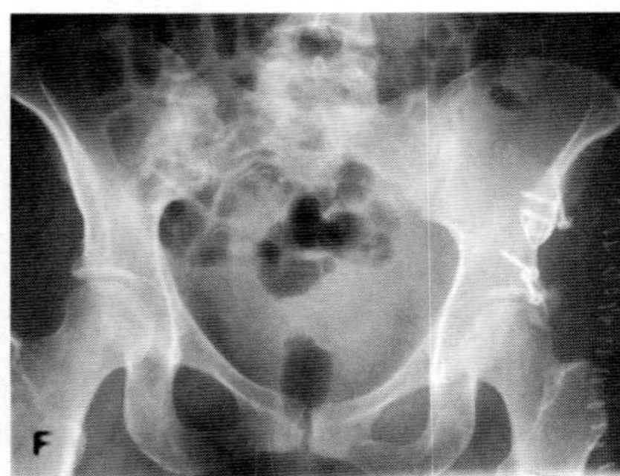

FIGURE 27-4. Anterior instability of the hip. A woman sustained an anterior dislocation of the left hip in a motor vehicle accident. The hip was reduced at the scene. **A:** When the patient was referred, the anteroposterior radiograph showed a reduced joint with a fracture of the anterior inferior iliac spine. **B,C:** The axial computed tomography images demonstrated the fracture pattern of the anterior wall. **D:** To determine hip instability and if open reduction and internal fixation were required, the patient was anesthetized and the leg was externally rotated. **E,F:** Under image intensification the hip joint subluxed anteriorly, thus, anterior hip instability was demonstrated and open reduction and internal fixation were required.

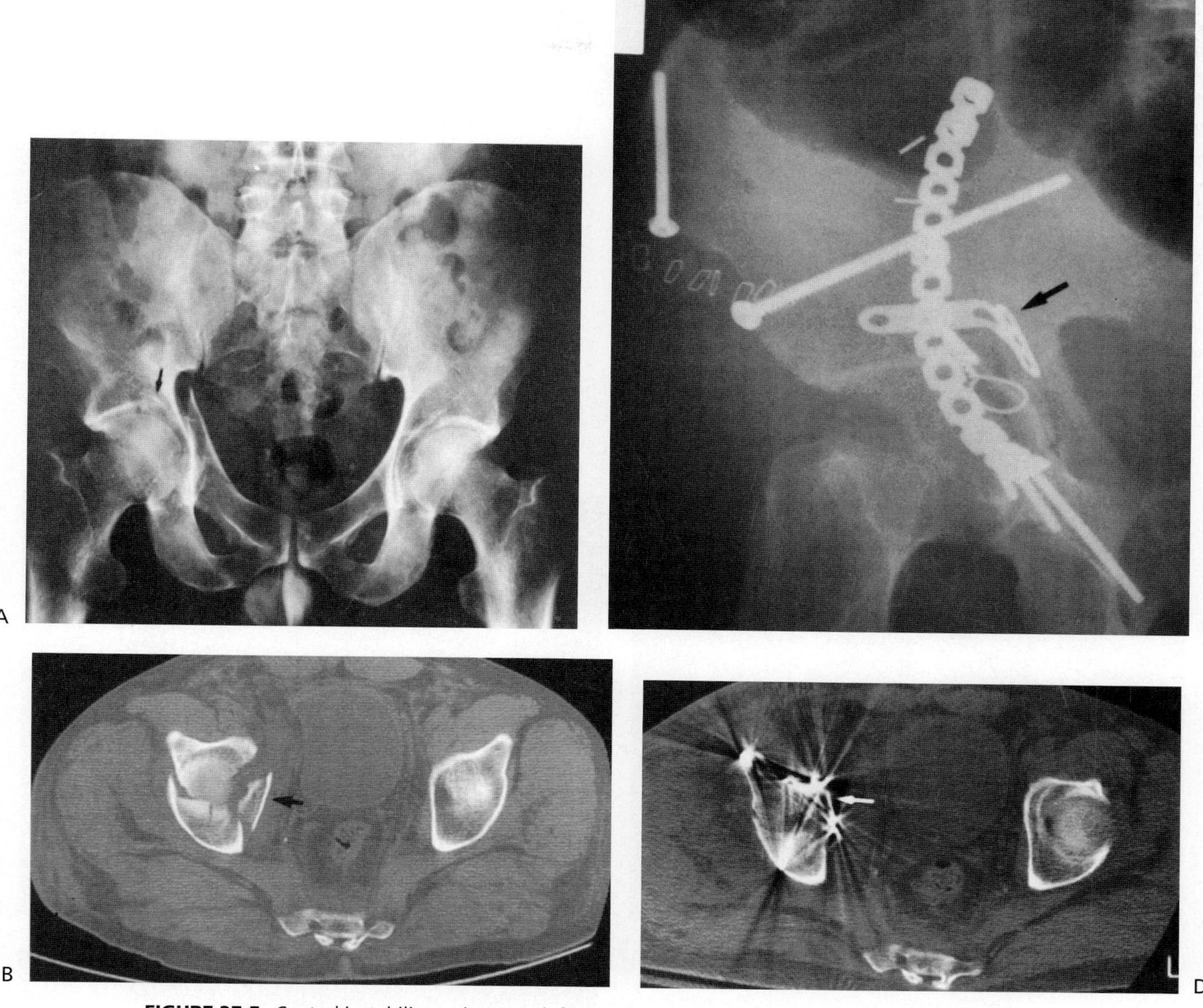

FIGURE 27-5. Central instability owing to a defect in the quadrilateral plate. **A:** Anteroposterior radiograph shows an impacted portion of the anterior area of the roof of the acetabulum, producing incongruity. **B:** Central subluxation is noted and appreciated only on the axial computed tomography (CT) view through the dome. Note the large fragment of quadrilateral plate displaced medially. This fragment is large enough to allow subluxation of the head if it is not surgically fixed *(black arrow).* **C:** Open reduction and internal fixation produced a congruous hip. The central quadrilateral plate fragment was held with a so-called spring plate *(black arrow),* as noted on the radiograph. **D:** Postoperative CT clearly shows the position of the spring plate holding the quadrilateral plate fragment in the anatomic position and the anatomic reduction through the superior dome cut on this CT view.

in any plane (Fig. 27-6). Loss of joint parallelism is less important than distortion of the acetabular joint surface produced by a transverse or T-type fracture through the roof of the acetabulum (Fig. 27-7). Also, displacement (especially) of the anterior column, may be distal, so that displacement of the column may not produce incongruity. This is much less likely with displacement of the posterior column or posterior wall. If the radiographic assessment of the hip joint reveals incongruity, then closed methods will fail and early osteoarthritis will ensue.

Gross incongruity between the femoral head and the acetabulum is obvious (Fig. 27-8), but more subtle cases are difficult to interpret (Fig. 27-9) and depend on the plane of the incongruity (i.e., coronal or sagittal, anterior or posterior, high or low) as well as the actual amount of displacement. Attempts have been made to measure incongruity from the plain radiographs. Matta has recommended the use of roof arc measurements (Fig. 27-10) (4). If the measurement is greater than 45 degrees, then the transverse component is usually low and the joint remains congruous; however, roof arc measurements are not helpful in the both-column fracture (Type C).

Three-dimensional computed tomography (3DCT) may be better for the evaluation of the acetabular weight-bearing surface (Fig. 27-8). By subtracting the femoral head, the area of dome involvement can be clearly seen. Also in T-type fractures, one column may be congruous or undisplaced, as noted on plane radiographs and on CT, whereas the other is incongruous. In those cases, the surgeon may choose internal fixation for the incongruous column only.

Any fracture pattern can exhibit incongruity, but those involving the roof of the acetabulum are more likely to do so, especially shearing-type transverse and T-type fractures

(Text continues on page 507)

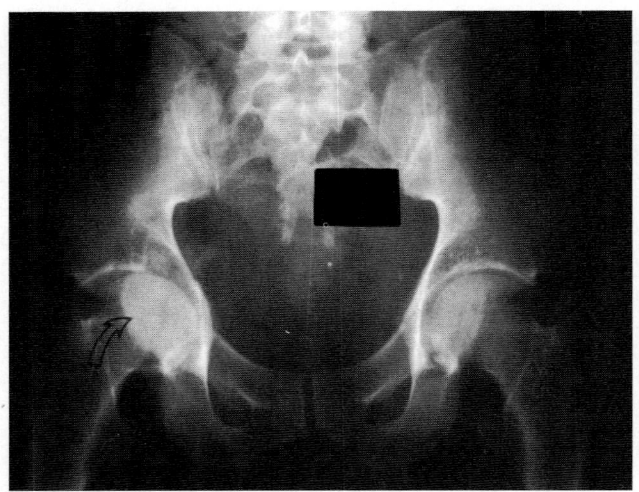
A

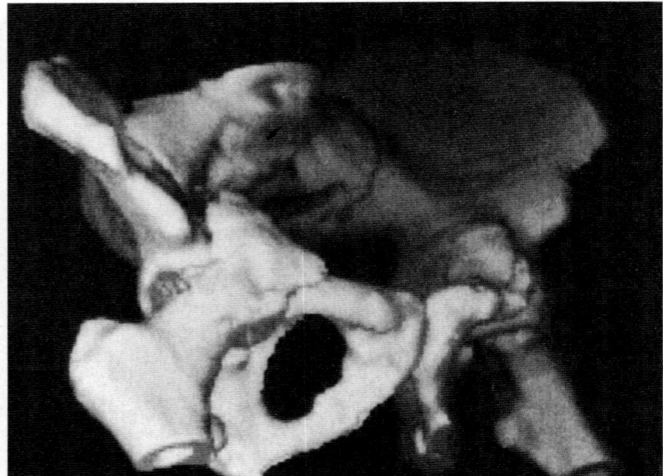
B

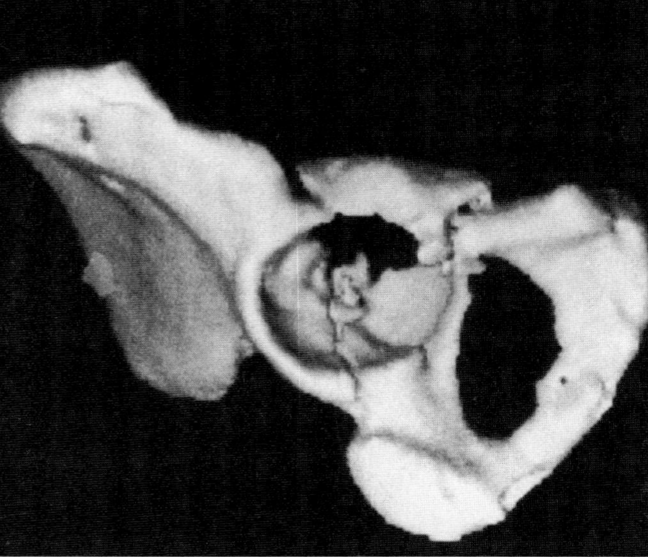
C

FIGURE 27-6. Incongruity. Subluxation of the femoral head in any plane is not tolerated by the joint. **A:** Anteroposterior radiograph indicates central subluxation of the head and lack of parallelism causing incongruity between the head and the acetabulum. **B,C:** In this instance, the migration of the head is anterior as well as central, as noted in the three-dimensional computed tomography, showing a classic anterior plus posterior hemitransverse fracture pattern (Type B3).

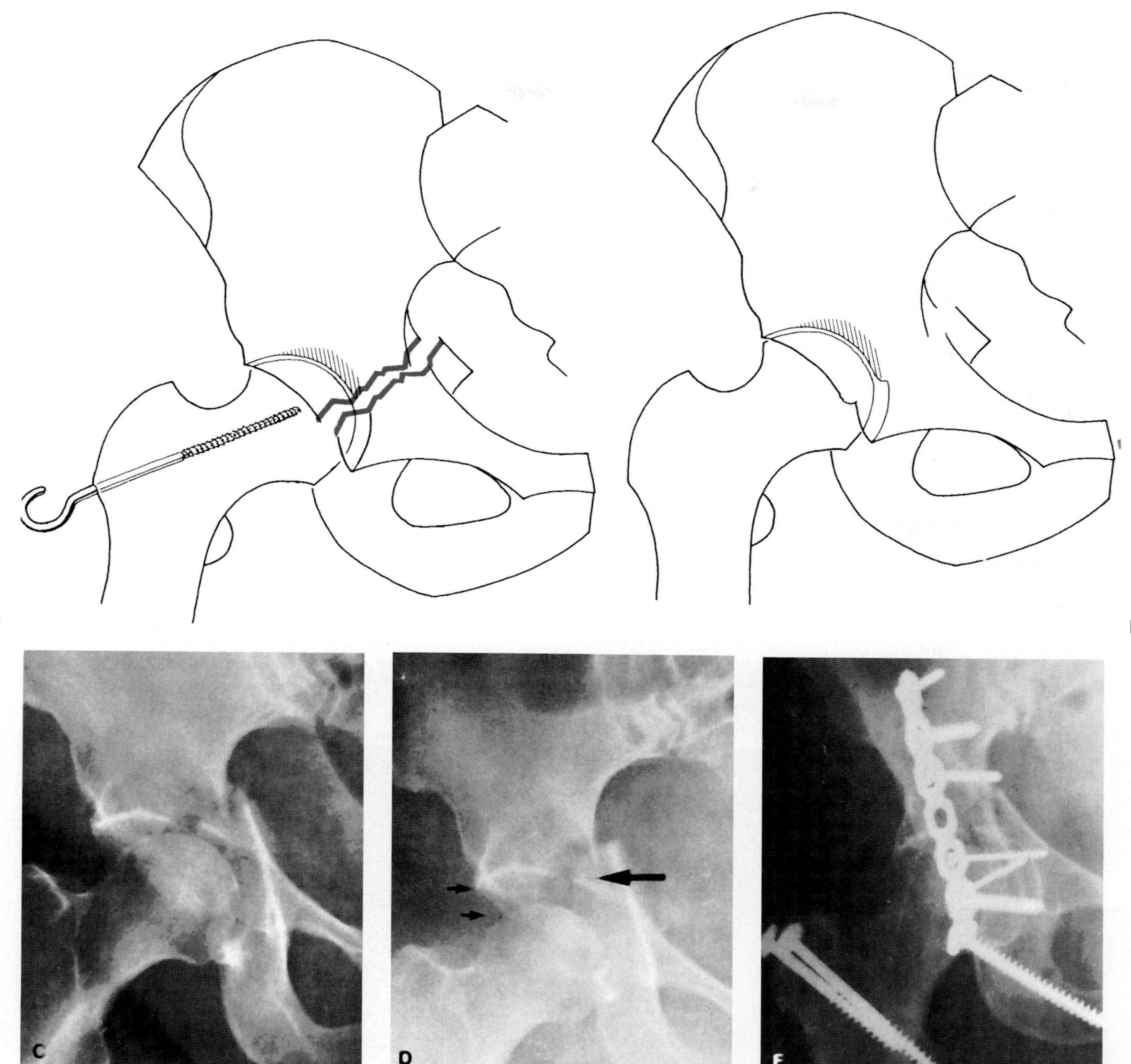

FIGURE 27-7. Incongruity produced by transverse fractures through the acetabular dome. **A,B:** If the fracture of the acetabulum is distal through the dome, the femoral head remains congruous to the acetabulum and nonoperative care will produce a good result as noted in the drawing. **C:** Contrast this to the high fracture of the acetabulum noted on the anteroposterior radiograph. **D:** Traction applied to that injury noted in the radiograph failed to reduce the medial wall *(black arrow).* (*Figure continues*)

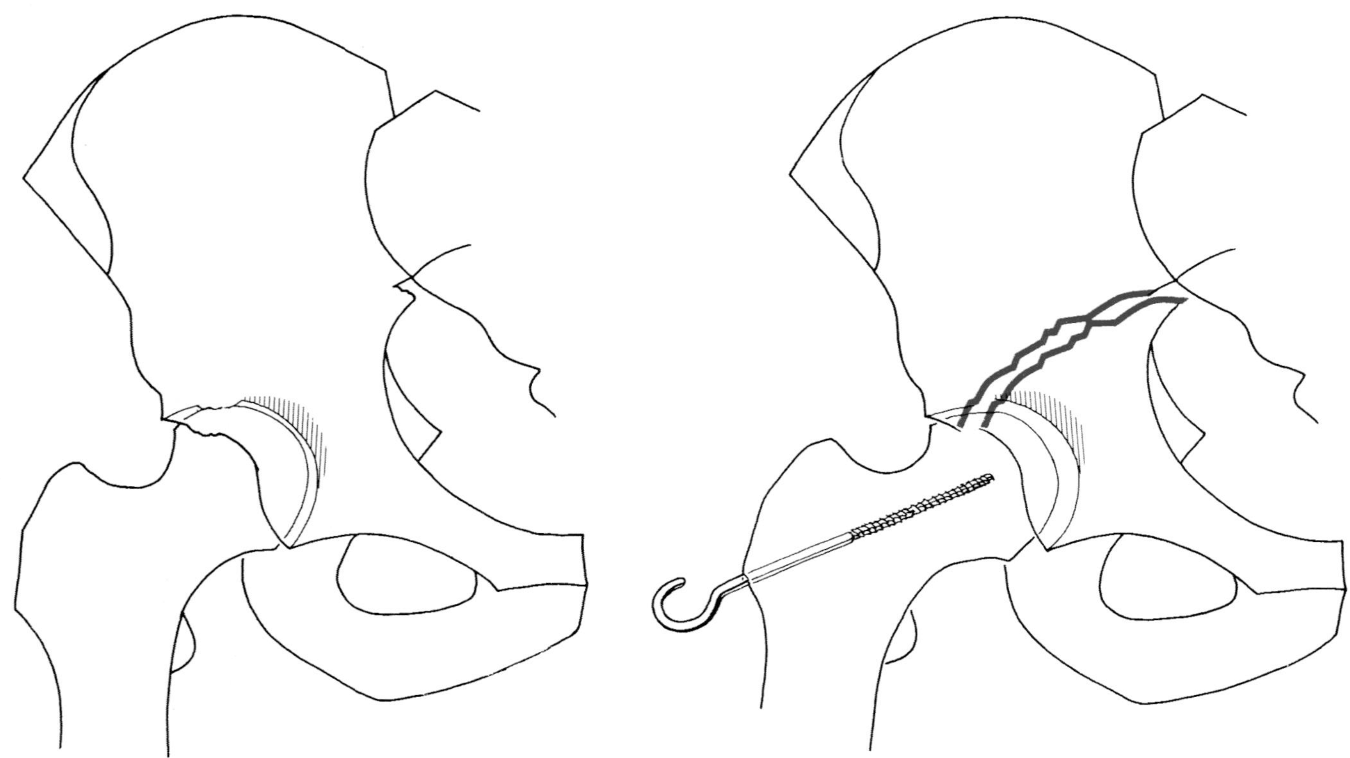

FIGURE 27-7. ***(continued)*** **F,G:** Even if the femoral head were left in that position for a long time, it would return to the original position of the medial wall and produce incongruity of the joint and early osteoarthritis, as depicted in the drawings. **E:** Therefore, a good clinical and radiographic result can be obtained only by anatomic open reduction and internal fixation.

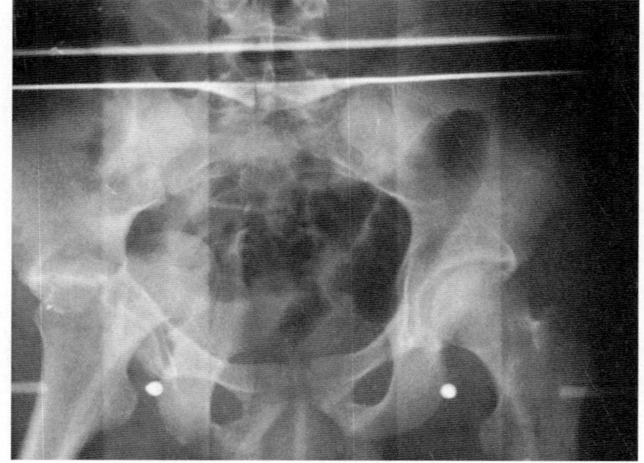

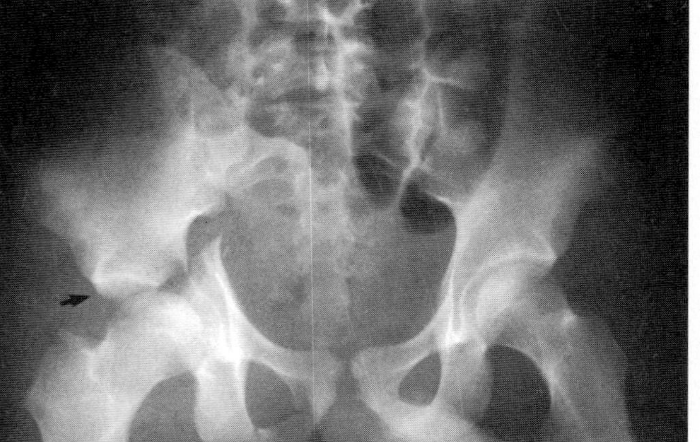

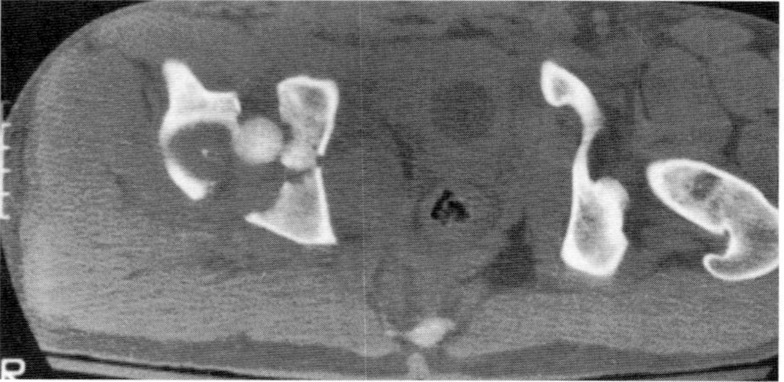

FIGURE 27-8. Gross incongruity between the femoral head and the acetabulum. **A:** Anteroposterior radiograph shows complete central protrusion of the femoral head within the pelvis. **B:** On the night of admission, the patient was given a general anesthetic so that the femoral head could be reduced, to prevent articular cartilage pressure necrosis. Congruity was not restored in this T-type fracture. **C:** Axial computed tomography shows the central dislocation of the head, the impingement on the lateral aspect of the head by the lateral fragment, and the classic nature of this T injury.

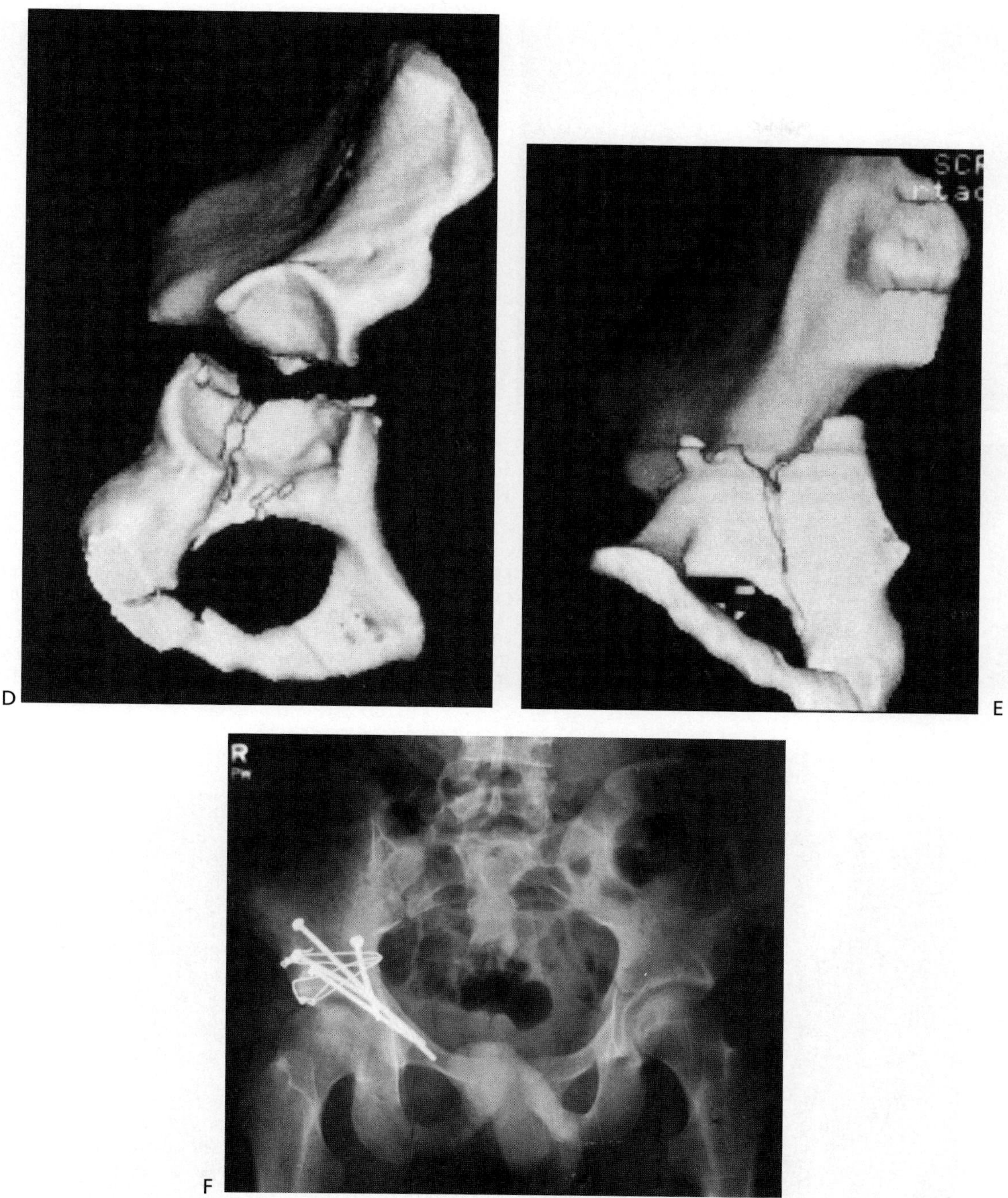

FIGURE 27-8. ***(continued)*** **D,E:** A three-dimensional computed tomography image shows the classic appearance of a T fracture with a grossly unstable transverse component. **F:** Open reduction and internal fixation using cerclage wires and lag screws achieved anatomic reduction.

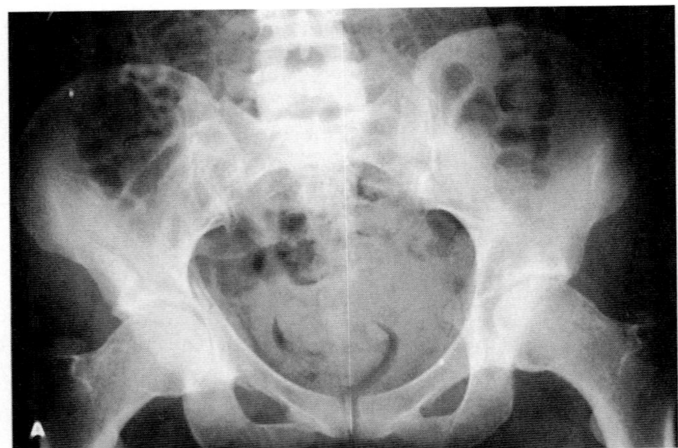

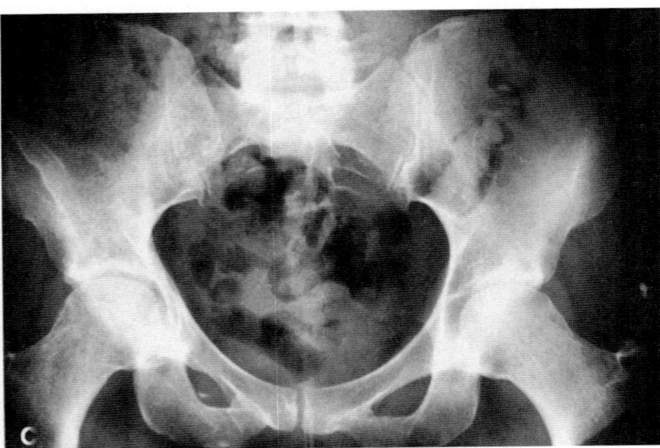

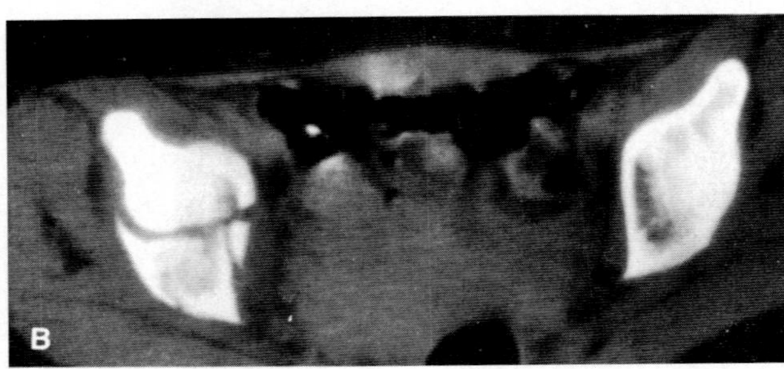

FIGURE 27-9. How much incongruity? **A:** Anteroposterior radiograph of a both-column fracture in a young woman injured while skiing. **B:** Axial computed tomography through the dome shows the coronal split and minimal incongruity. **C:** Treatment consisted of traction without operative intervention. The result at 9 years is excellent congruity of the hip. The patient is functioning normally.

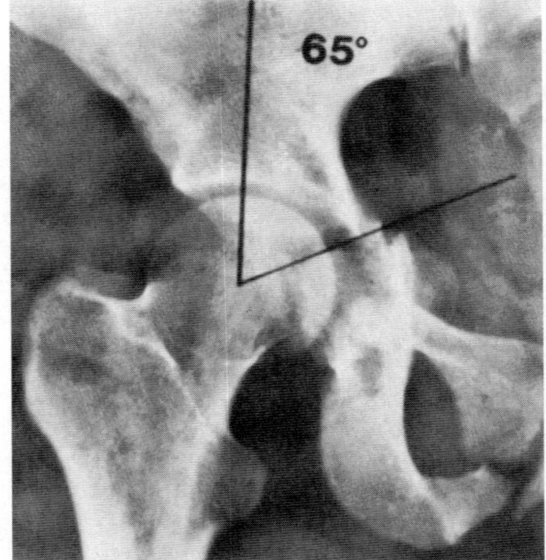

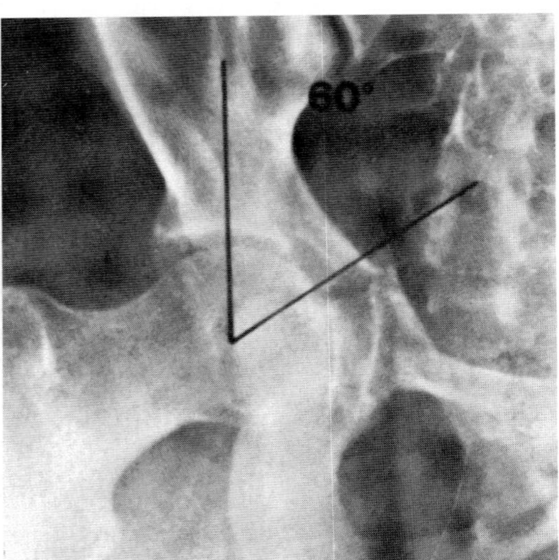

FIGURE 27-10. The anterior-posterior view **(A),** the obturator oblique view **(B),** and the iliac oblique view **(C)** of a T-shaped fracture show congruence of the femoral head out of traction and adequate roof arc measurements. Closed treatment is indicated. (From: Matta J. Operative indications and choice of surgical approach for fractures of the acetabulum. *Tech Orthop* 1986;1:18, with permission.)

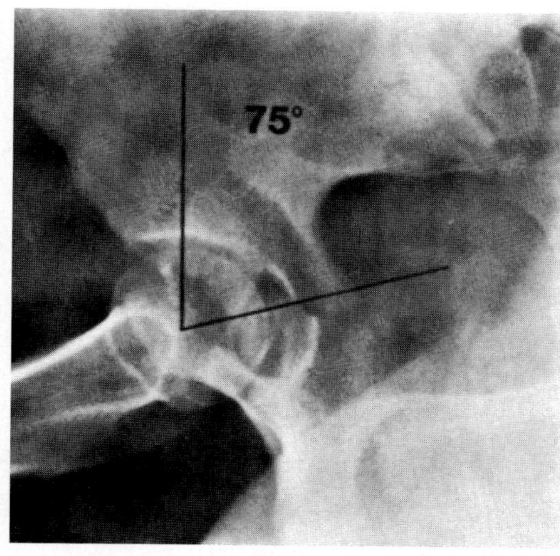

FIGURE 27-10. *(continued)*

and those fractures in which a triangular fragment of dome is separated.

The concept of congruity as it pertains to both-column fractures (Type C) is particularly difficult. Such fractures may appear grossly displaced through the ilium, whereas the joint, although medially displaced, may appear congruous (Fig. 27-11).

For purposes of decision making, the position of the posterior column in this pattern becomes extremely important.

For this fracture, Letournel has introduced the concept of secondary congruence (5). In this pattern, the split in the acetabulum is in the coronal plane. The two columns, anterior and posterior, of the acetabular articular surface surround the femoral head (Fig. 27-12), much as the twin towers of the prize-winning Toronto City Hall surround the circular Council Chamber (Fig. 27-12C). The two fragments of the acetabulum are separated from each other by a gap of varying size (3 to 4 mm), but both remain congruent to the femoral head (Fig. 27-11B). This may allow good function of the joint and a good long-term prognosis. It is paradoxic that nonoperative management may achieve good results in the most complex type of acetabular fracture, namely the both-column fracture (6).

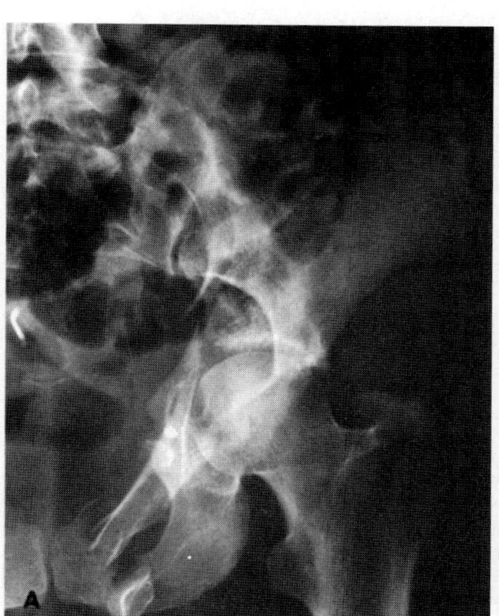

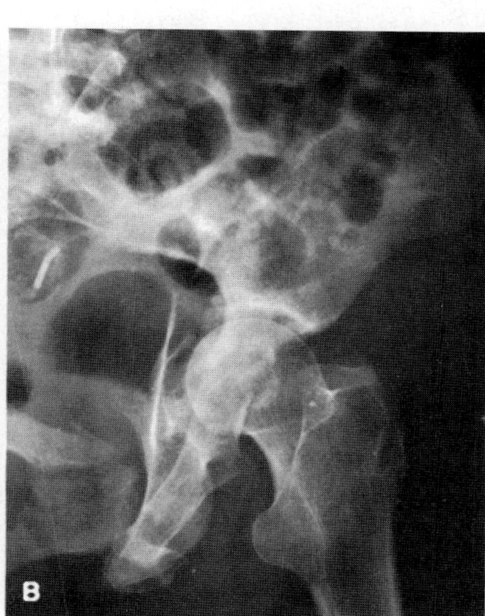

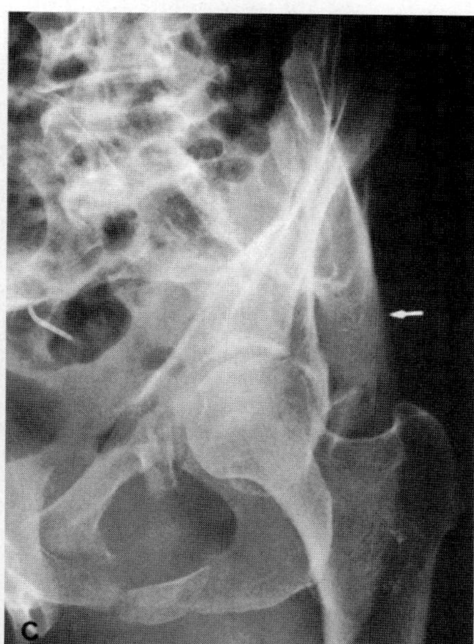

FIGURE 27-11. Both-column fracture secondary congruence. Anteroposterior **(A)**, iliac oblique **(B)**, and obturator oblique **(C)** radiographs of a typical both-column fracture of the left acetabulum. Note the spur on the obturator oblique radiograph **(C)** *(white arrow)*. *(Figure continues)*

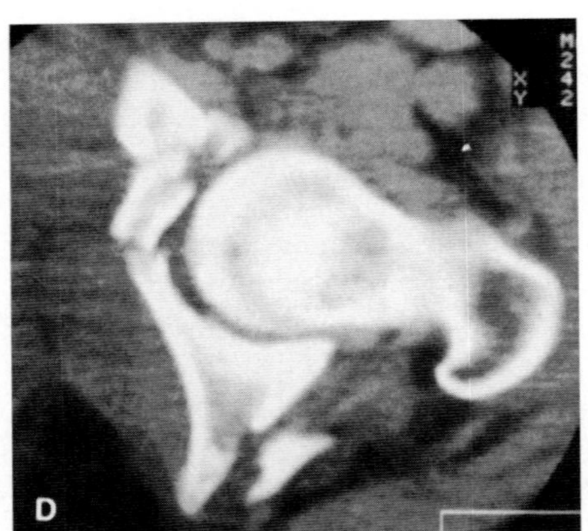

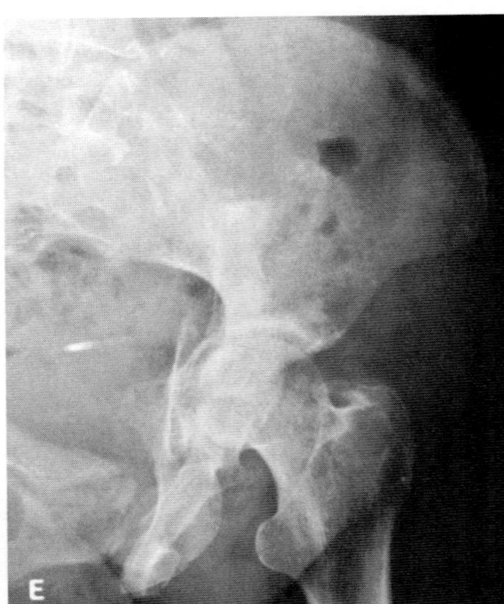

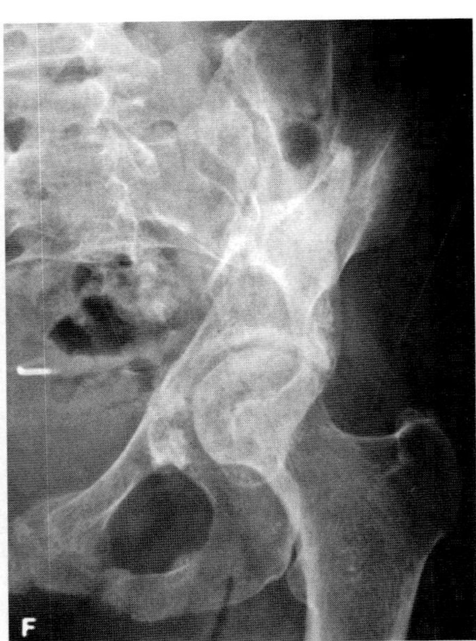

FIGURE 27-11. ***(continued)*** **D:** The axial computed tomography shows the femoral head well covered by the anterior and posterior column. The patient was treated with skeletal traction after closed reduction with the excellent congruity of the joint on the iliac oblique **(E)** and the obturator **(F)** view. The patient had an excellent clinical result 14 years after the injury.

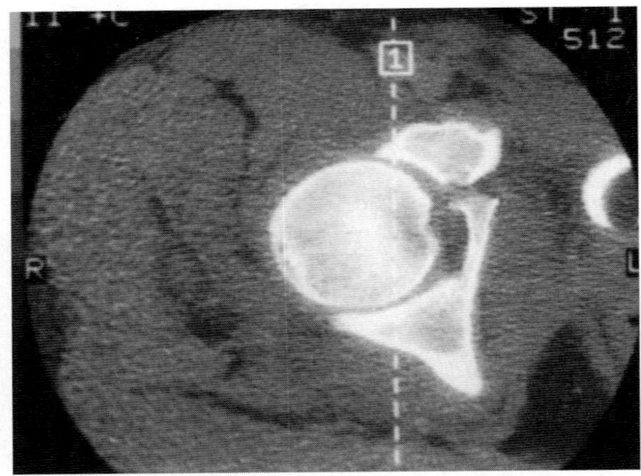

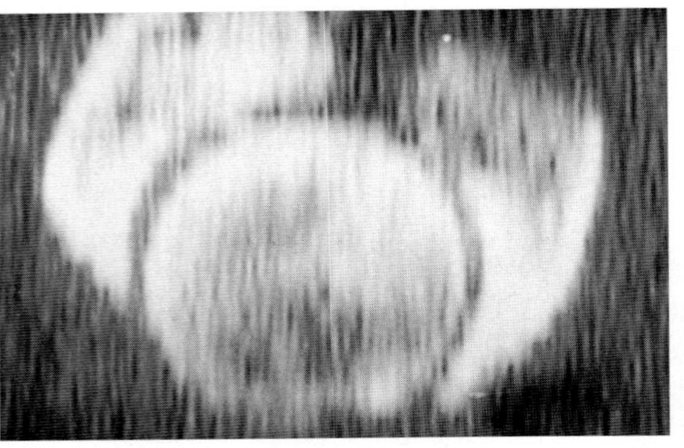

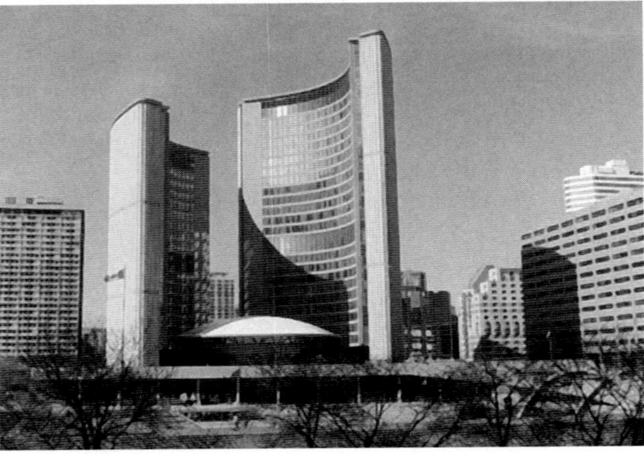

FIGURE 27-12. Secondary congruence. The two columns anterior and posterior to the acetabular articular surface surround the femoral head, even though they may be separated by a gap. This is best seen on the axial computed tomography **(A)** and the sagittal, reconstruction **(B).** The way the two columns embrace the femoral head bears an uncanny resemblance to Toronto's City Hall, whose twin towers surround the round council chamber **(C).**

Other Fracture Factors

Other important factors include the degree of comminution of the acetabular articular surface, the damage to the femoral head associated injuries in the limb, and finally the operability of the fracture by the attending surgeon or a pelvic surgical specialist. If any doubt exists, an opinion of such a specialist should be sought early, because undue delay will compromise the outcome.

NONOPERATIVE CARE

Indications

Historical Perspective

Over the past 50 years, various authors have reported characteristics of acetabular fractures that have resulted in posttraumatic arthritis of the hip (Table 27-1). The classification system of Judet and Letournel, now the most common descriptive classification of acetabular fractures used, was not available prior to 1964 (7). However, there is still value in some of these early reports. A review of work very early in the 20th century reveals that acetabular fractures that require traction to maintain concentric reduction of the femoral head and acetabulum resulted in a successful clinical outcome with nonoperative treatment in a minority of cases (13% to 30% satisfactory results) (8–10). In 1948, Urist noted that the integrity of the acetabular cartilage along the posterior rim of the acetabulum is a critical factor in the end result (11). He reported that in matched cases of posterior fracture dislocations of the hip treated conservatively and by open reduction, good function and little or no disability were shown when the joint surfaces were restored as perfectly as possible. However, he noted that this could only be accomplished on a consistent basis by open reduction and internal fixation.

In the 1950s, Knight and Smith, and Pennal noted that the primary objective of operative treatment of acetabular fractures was to restore the "weight-bearing vault" of the acetabulum (12,13). In 1961, Rowe and Lowell reported on a retrospective series of acetabular fractures, and identified those factors affecting clinical outcome (14). They noted the following risk factors: (a) disruption of the superior acetabulum or "weight-bearing dome;" (b) the loss of the normal relationship between the femoral head and the superior acetabulum (incongruence); (c) early or late posterior instability of the hip joint; and (d) severe impaction injuries of the femoral head.

In the early 1980s, following the observations of Rowe and Lowell, Matta developed the concept of roof arc measurements (15). These measurements, made on the anterior-posterior (AP) pelvis, iliac oblique, and obturator oblique views of the involved acetabulum afford an estimate of the area of the superior acetabular surface that remains intact following a displaced acetabular fracture (Fig. 27-13). Based on retrospective and prospective clinical series, Matta proposed criteria for indications for nonoperative treatment of displaced acetabular fractures (15). A similar assessment of the superior acetabulum can also be performed using computed tomography (CT) (16). The use of CT results in evaluation of the CT subchondral arc (Fig. 27-13). The subchondral arc results from the ring of subchondral bone seen in the CT cut through the superior acetabulum.

TABLE 27-1. NONOPERATIVE MANAGEMENT:

Fracture factors:
Hip stable and congruous
Guidelines to be correlated to patient factors
- Type A: Undisplaced fractures
- Type B: Minimally displaced fractures, (low anterior column, low transverse)
- Type C: Fractures with secondary congruence (both-column)

Patient factors:
Severe osteopenia, severe systemic illness making operative intervention high risk.

Criteria for Nonoperative Care

The authors proposed the following criteria for nonoperative treatment:

- The superior acetabulum is intact, as judged by the CT subchondral arc in the superior 10 mm of the acetabulum.
- The femoral head maintains a congruent relationship with the superior acetabulum on the AP, iliac oblique, and obturator oblique x-rays, with all three x-rays taken out of traction.
- There is no evidence of posterior instability of the hip (16).

Using these criteria, Olson and Matta reviewed a series of 23 patients treated nonoperatively (16). Eleven of these patients met all three criteria for nonoperative treatment. Nine of these 11 patients went on to have a good or excellent clinical result. Twelve patients did not meet the criteria for nonoperative treatment. Five of these 12 patients went on to have a good to excellent clinical result. Patients had greater than 1-year follow-up in this investigation (Fig. 27-14).

Dynamic Stress Views

More recently, Tornetta has modified the criteria as reported by Olson and Matta by including a dynamic stress view (17). Tornetta recommended taking the patient being

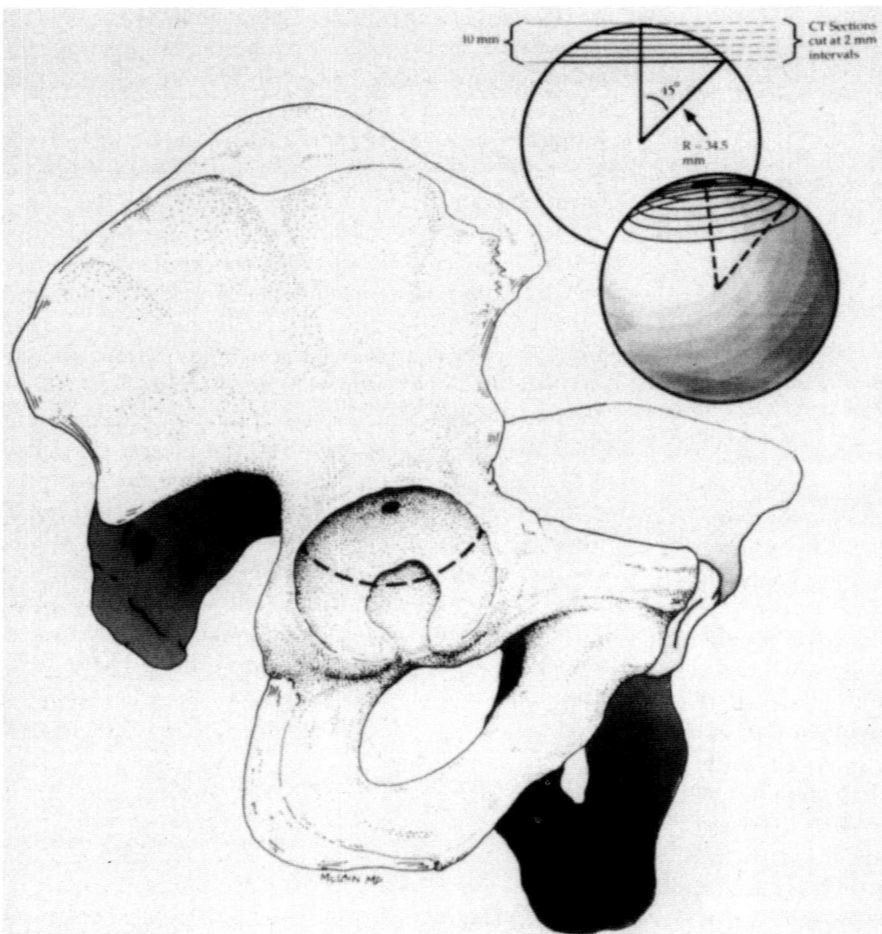

FIGURE 27-13. Illustration of the concept of computed tomography subchondral arc. The line shown in the acetabulum represents the level on the computed tomography (CT) image at 10 mm inferior to the vertex of the acetabulum. The circle along the subchondral bone at 10 mm inferior to the vertex is equivalent to a fracture line for which all three roof arc measurements are 45 degrees. Evaluation of the superior 10 mm of the acetabulum should be equivalent of a roof arc of >45 degrees in almost all cases. The inset diagram illustrates evaluation of the superior acetabulum by CT to 10 mm inferior to the vertex in 2-mm intervals. (From: Olson SA, Matta JM. The computerized tomography subchondral arc: a new method of assessing acetabular continuity after fracture (a preliminary report). *J Orthop Trauma* 1993;7:402–413, with permission.)

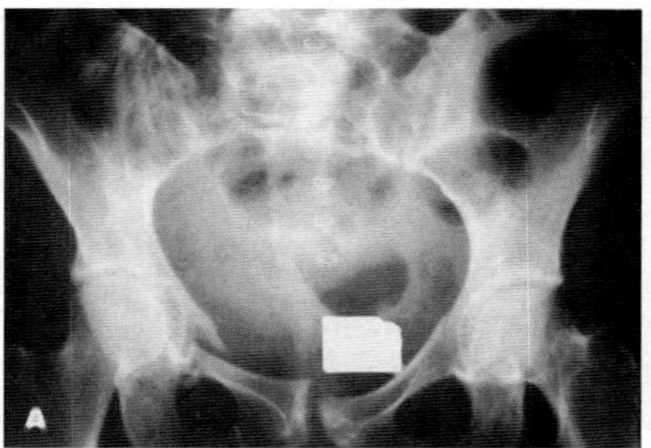

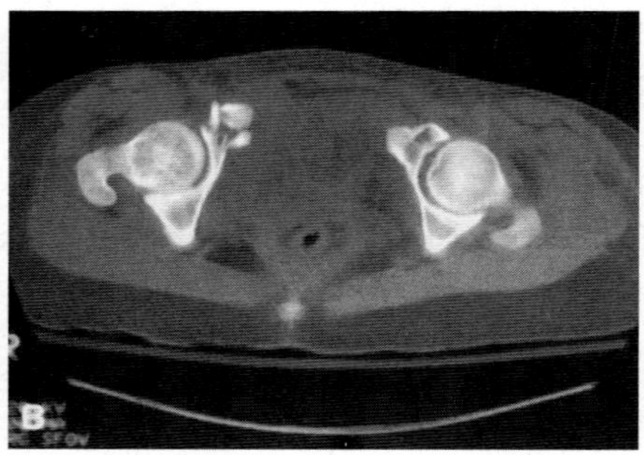

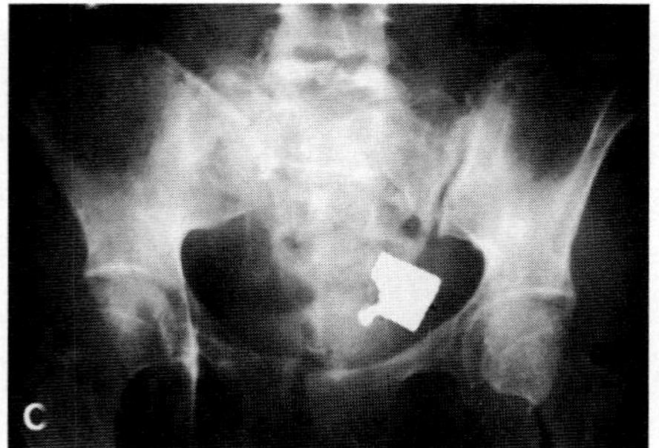

FIGURE 27-14. Distal anterior column fracture that is treated nonoperatively. **A:** Anterior posterior radiograph of a 27-year-old woman injured in a motor vehicle accident demonstrates bilateral anterior column injuries with greater displacement on the right, and minimal displacement on the left. In both instances, the anterior column is very distal and meets all three criteria for nonoperative treatment as outlined by Olson and Matta. **B:** Note that a distal computed tomography axial cut demonstrates the beginning of articular involvement on the right. This is well below the superior 10 mm of the acetabulum. **C:** Nonoperative care consisted of bed rest with no skeletal traction until the patient was comfortable. Excellent healing occurred with no evidence of hip incongruity and a good functional clinical result.

considered for nonoperative treatment to the operating room to undergo an evaluation under anesthesia consisting of range of motion of the hip with intraoperative fluoroscopy. If any evidence of subluxation or incongruence of the hip was noted with range of motion, then the patient was considered a candidate for operative treatment. If, however, the patient maintained a congruent relationship between the femoral head and the superior acetabulum, the patient was treated nonoperatively. With this protocol, 38 patients met all three of Olson and Matta's criteria and also were found to be congruent at the time of dynamic stress view. Out of 38 patients, 35 were found to have a good to excellent clinical result at an average of 2 years follow-up (17).

Secondary Congruence

The aforementioned criteria for nonoperative treatment are useful for fractures where a portion of the superior acetabulum is maintained in continuity with the posterior iliac wing. However, these indications do not apply to both-column acetabular fractures (18). The associated both-column acetabular fracture is unique because all of the articular segments of the acetabulum are disrupted from the intact posterior iliac wing. Typically these are complex, high-energy fractures with severe comminution that often require operative management. However, occasionally, this fracture pattern can occur in such a way that large fragments of the articular surface are displaced in a rotational manner that leads to a medialized hip center but maintains a relatively congruent relationship between the articular surfaces and femoral head (18). This condition is clinically known as *secondary congruence* (Fig. 27-12). In the event of secondary congruence, nonoperative treatment may be contemplated if there is a congruent relationship or parallelism between the subchondral bone of the acetabulum and femoral head on the AP, iliac oblique, and obturator oblique views of the acetabulum taken out of traction. The CT evaluation also may be helpful to determine congruence in this matter (Fig. 27-11). Management is similar to that for the other fracture patterns if nonoperative treatment is elected. The patient may undergo early constant passive motion (CPM) mobilization for maintenance of range of motion and articular healing. Ten to 30 lbs weight-bearing is instituted for the first 8 weeks. Weight-bearing then can be increased after that point. Typically there is some loss of rotation of the hip with this type of management (18).

As with any nonoperative management of articular fractures, serial x-rays are important to ensure that no late subluxation of the femoral head, or late loss of position of acetabular fragments are noted that would potentially compromise the result. Trochanteric traction is rarely, if ever, useful and is absolutely contraindicated if there is any consideration of operative management during the patient's course.

Other Indications

Other potential indications for nonoperative treatment of acetabular fractures include: (a) the nondisplaced acetabular fracture; (b) patients who have severe osteopenia such that benefit of open reduction and internal fixation may be lost because of the quality of the bone; (c) the patient with severe systemic illness or systemic compromise such that operative treatment is a greater risk than nonoperative treatment and the development of posttraumatic arthritis (16,19).

Methods of Nonoperative Care

Role of Skeletal Traction

Historically, skeletal traction was the only treatment option; however, today it has only a limited role in the definitive management of a displaced acetabular fracture. It is unnecessary in undisplaced or minimally displaced fractures that are stable and congruous. Open reduction and internal fixation should be the treatment of choice in displaced fractures, if traction is required to maintain the reduction. In most cases, adequate reduction cannot be obtained, making open reduction and internal fixation the desired treatment option (Fig. 27-7). Therefore, skeletal traction should be used in the acute situation, if surgery is delayed, to keep the femoral head away from the acetabulum (Fig. 27-8), and in the rare case of a patient who, usually polytraumatized, who is too sick to undergo a major operative procedure. Pressure necrosis of the articular cartilage may develop quickly, as noted in Fig. 27-15. Also, skeletal traction may be the only option if a surgeon or pelvic team is not accessible and referral is impossible.

Trochanteric traction is never indicated in the management of the acute fracture, because sepsis may occur at the pin site, making operative intervention risky; therefore, temporary skeletal traction should be supracondylar (Fig. 27-16).

Early Ambulation, Limited and Progressive Weight Bearing

Nonoperative management in this patient population consists of mobilization with protected weight bearing on the involved hip. Typically this involves minimal, 10- to 30-lb touchdown weight-bearing on the involved extremity. Occasionally, patients have bilateral injuries that would contraindicate immediate weight bearing on the opposite limb. In this case, patients are transferred in a bed to chair manner to mobilize. Active range of motion with CPM can begin early to facilitate maintenance of range of motion as well as articular healing (8). Weight bearing is subsequently allowed at 8 weeks postinjury.

As with any nonoperative management of articular fractures, the surgeon must be certain of the stability of the fracture. If there is any doubt, examination under anesthesia and image intensification (dynamic stress views) will dispel

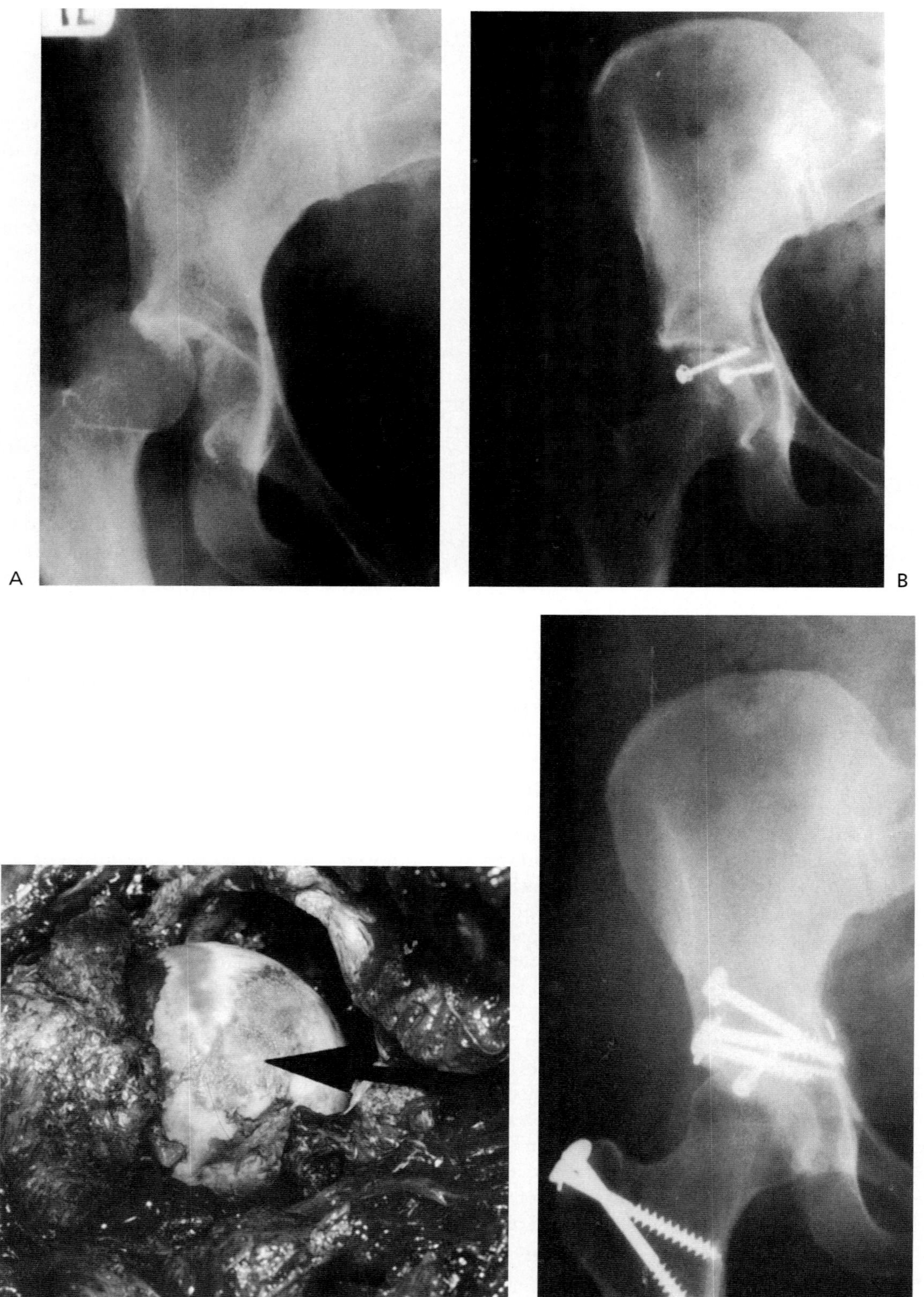

FIGURE 27-15. A: Anteroposterior radiograph shows a posterior dislocation of the hip. The transverse fracture associated with it was relatively undisplaced. **B:** The posterior wall fracture was fixed with two screws, the transverse component was not buttressed. After 6 weeks, the transverse fracture had flipped medially, causing incongruity of the joint. **C:** At reoperation, the femoral head exhibited a large area of pressure necrosis *(black arrow).* The posterior fracture was stabilized with lag screws, which restored anatomic congruity to the joint. **D:** In spite of the area of pressure necrosis, the patient remains asymptomatic 6 years after the injury. (From: Schatzker I, Tile M. *The rationale of operative fracture care.* Heidelberg: Springer-Verlag, 1987, with permission.)

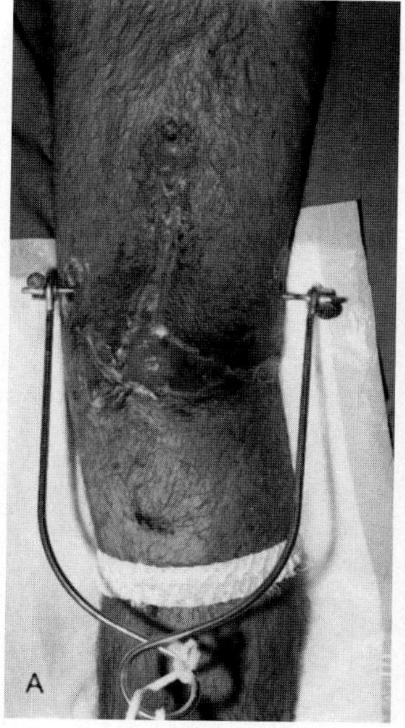

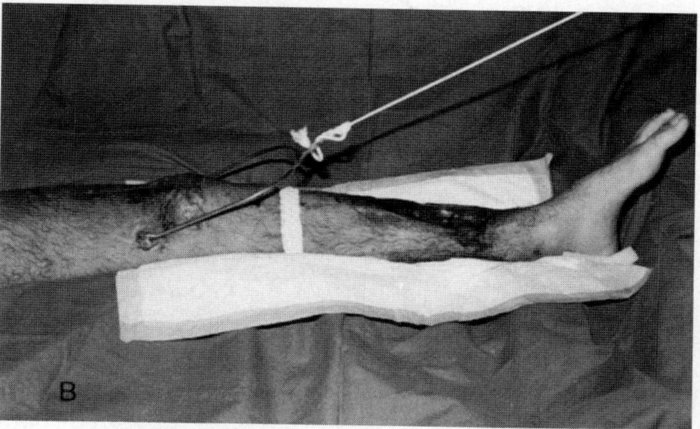

FIGURE 27-16. A: Photographs indicating the position of the supracondylar traction pin in the femur. **B:** This pin must be placed posteriorly enough so as not to enter the suprapatellar pouch, where it would interfere with flexion of the knee joint. This particular patient had an open fracture of his tibia, a quadriceps tendon rupture, and a fracture of the acetabulum. In this case, traction has been used temporarily before definitive open reduction and internal fixation of the acetabular fracture.

these doubts, as noted earlier in this chapter in the study of Tornetta (17).

Also, serial x-rays are important to ensure that no late subluxation of the femoral head or late loss of position of acetabular fragments is noted that would potentially compromise the result.

Comments on Specific Fracture Types

Undisplaced or Minimally Displaced Fractures

Fractures that exhibit only a linear crack and those with less than 3 mm of displacement may be managed nonoperatively. Great care must be taken, because some of these fractures, even those caused by minimal trauma, may displace. If there is any concern, dynamic stress views should be undertaken.

Distal (Low) Anterior Column Fractures

Low anterior column fractures most commonly are associated with pelvic disruption. This fracture usually involves the most distal and anterior portion of the acetabular dome; thus, the relationship between the femoral head and the dome is rarely significantly disturbed (Fig. 27-14).

Distal Transverse Fractures

Distal (low) transverse fractures are below the top of the acetabular fossa (an infratectal lesion). In this particular injury, the main portion of the acetabular dome is intact; therefore, closed reduction often produces a congruous joint (Fig. 27-7A). Also, in the displaced type, congruity can be achieved by closed reduction, but it usually cannot be maintained by traction (Fig. 27-7B).

Since the medial portion of the dome is intact to the level of the acetabular fossa, the femoral head is prevented from "redisplacing." The stable type of transverse fracture (Type B) must be contrasted with the transverse fracture that runs superiorly through the dome (transtectal, Type 1B) (Fig. 27-7C,D). In that particular unstable fracture, a congruous relationship between the femoral head and the acetabulum is difficult to maintain. The femoral head always has a tendency to displace medially with the medial wall of the acetabulum. With traction, the femoral head may be pulled laterally under the dome, so that the hip appears congruous (Fig. 27-7E), but if the medial wall of the acetabulum remains medially displaced the femoral head is redisplaced when the traction is released, resulting in rapid destruction of the joint (Fig. 27-7G). Therefore, for high transverse (transtectal) fractures (Type 1B) in which the medial fragment remains displaced, open reduction is required to maintain joint congruity (Fig. 27-7E).

The criteria of Olson and Matta are important (16).

1. The superior acetabulum is intact, as judged by the CT subchondral arc in the superior 10 mm of the acetabulum.

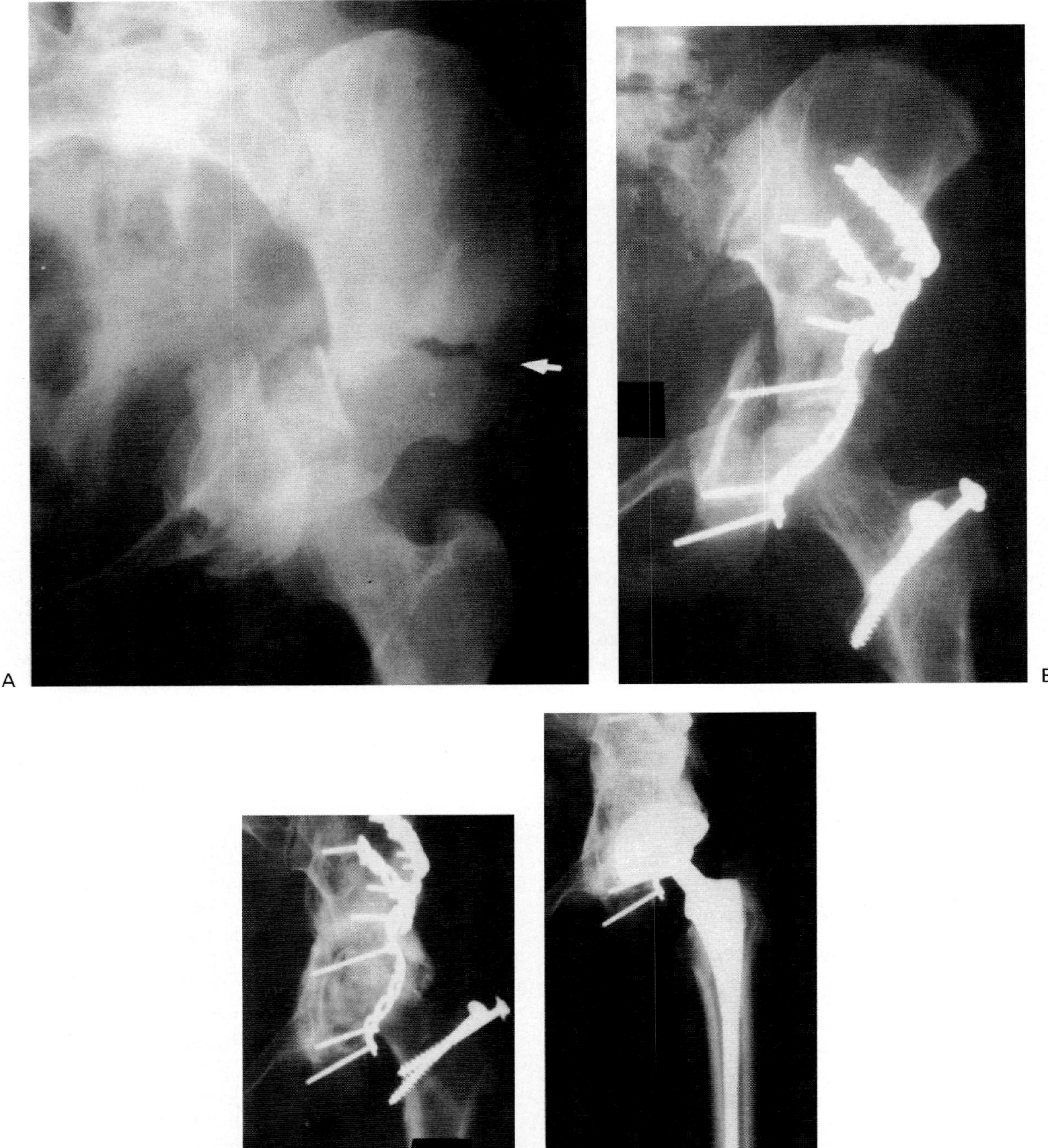

FIGURE 27-17. A: Both-column fracture with marked incongruity, as noted on the anteroposterior radiograph. Open reduction and internal fixation was performed, but not until 25 days after injury. **B:** Congruous reduction was not confirmed by the anteroposterior radiograph. **C,D:** Within a year dissolution of the joint occurred, requiring total hip arthroplasty.

2. The femoral head maintains a congruent relationship with the superior acetabulum on the AP, iliac oblique, and obturator oblique x-rays, with all three x-rays taken out of traction.
3. There is no evidence of posterior instability of the hip.

Both-Column Fractures

The both-column fracture (Type C) is unique, because the displacement is in the coronal plane, introducing the concept of secondary congruence.

The both-column fracture (Type C) occasionally can be managed by closed means. This fracture appears extremely

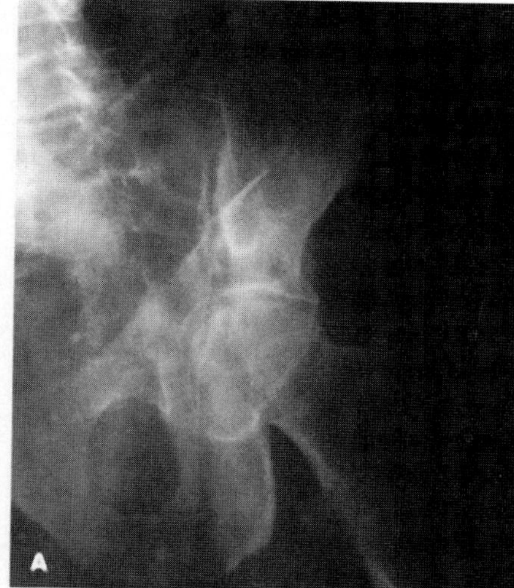

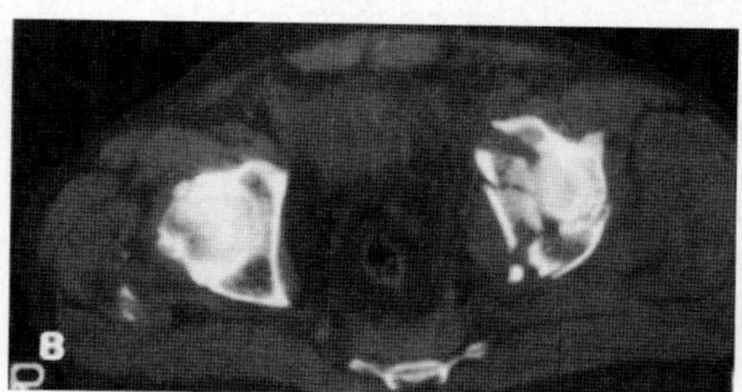

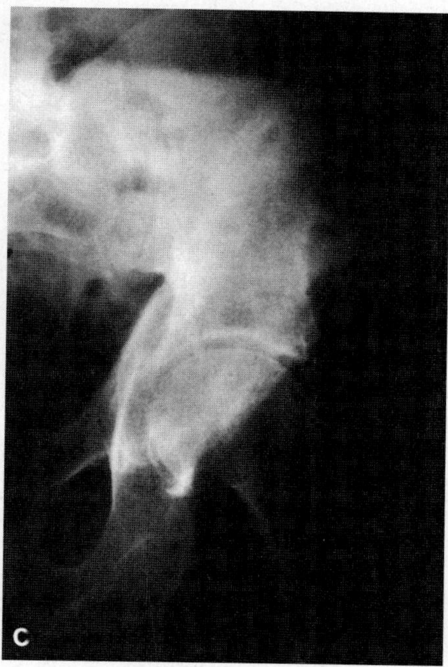

FIGURE 27-18. Both-column fracture in an elderly patient. **A:** The obturator oblique view indicates a both-column fracture of the left acetabulum with good congruity. **B:** The marked comminution in this fracture is best noted on the axial computed tomography. Treatment was traction for 8 weeks, resulting in excellent congruity between the femoral head and the acetabulum and an excellent clinical result 5 years after the injury. **C:** Considering the osteopenic bone and the severe comminution, it is likely that operative intervention would not have led to this excellent result.

complex on radiographs, but the complexity is caused by the major displacement of the extraarticular fracture of the ilium with complete medial displacement of the hip joint (Figs. 27-2 and 27-11).

In some of these fractures, secondary congruity may be maintained between the femoral head and the acetabulum with closed methods (Figs. 27-11 and 27-12), as has already been described. The definitive study of this fracture has yet to be done to determine if nonoperative or operative care produces the more desirable long-term outcome. Surgery for the fracture is challenging and, for less experienced operators, fraught with complications, and anatomic reduction is difficult to achieve. This fracture should be treated operatively by only experts working in an ideal environment; otherwise, it is certain that nonoperative care will produce a better outcome (Fig. 27-17).

If the hip is congruous on all three views, nonoperative care will suffice, especially in older patients (Fig. 27-18), but if there is gross distortion of the roof or posterior column, surgery is indicated (Fig. 27-19) (6).

OPERATIVE CARE

Operative management is indicated for an unstable and/or incongruous hip joint, no matter what the anatomic subgroup of the fracture. The final decision whether or not to operate, depends on other factors, especially *patient* factors.

There are clear indications for open reduction and internal fixation of displaced acetabular fractures (19). They can be summarized as follows: (a) >5 mm displacement of fractures involving the superior acetabulum (within the superior 10 mm of the CT subchondral arc); (b) loss of congruence (subluxation) of the femoral head with the acetabulum on any of the three plain radiographic views; (c) posterior wall fracture with associated demonstrated hip instability; and (d) an incarcerated osteochondral fragment with a nonconcentric reduction of the femoral head. Although there is uniform agreement about these criteria for open reduction, there continues to be controversy regarding some indications for operative intervention. These relative indications for open reduction also may be considered as relative indications for closed reduction (19). These include: (a) displacement of 2 to 4 mm in the superior acetabulum; (b) gross displacement of the remaining portions of the acetabulum such that a significant deformity would result; (c) >5 mm of marginal impaction, typically of the posterior wall; (d) 50% or more involvement of the posterior wall with a "stable" hip; (e) the polytrauma patient with an acetabular fracture that needs to be mobilized; and (f) the acetabular fracture associated with an intralateral femoral neck fracture or femoral head fracture that requires open reduction. Nonoperative treatment of these latter diagnoses is nearly as controversial as the operative treatment. Treatment of fractures with each of these injury characteristics needs consideration on a case-by-case basis, considering the fracture pattern, the

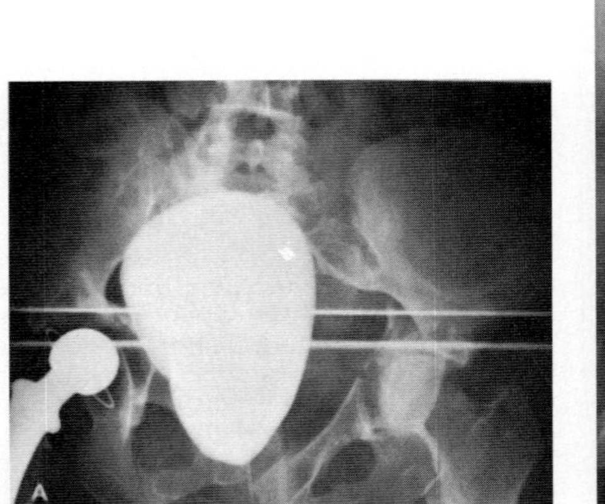
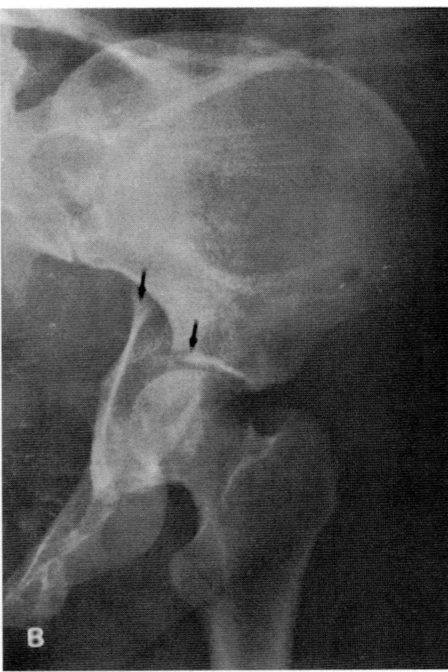
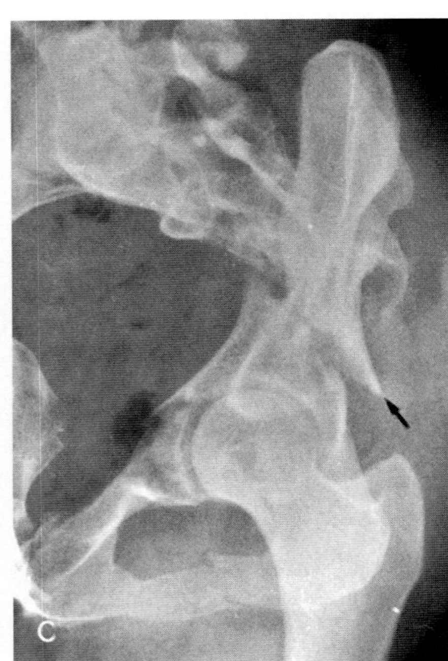
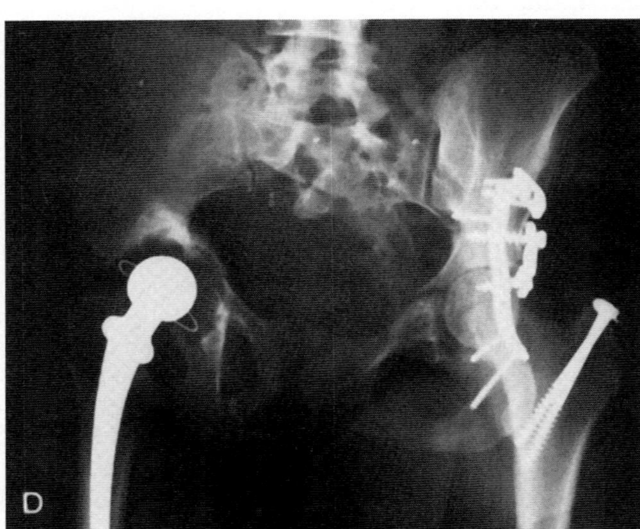
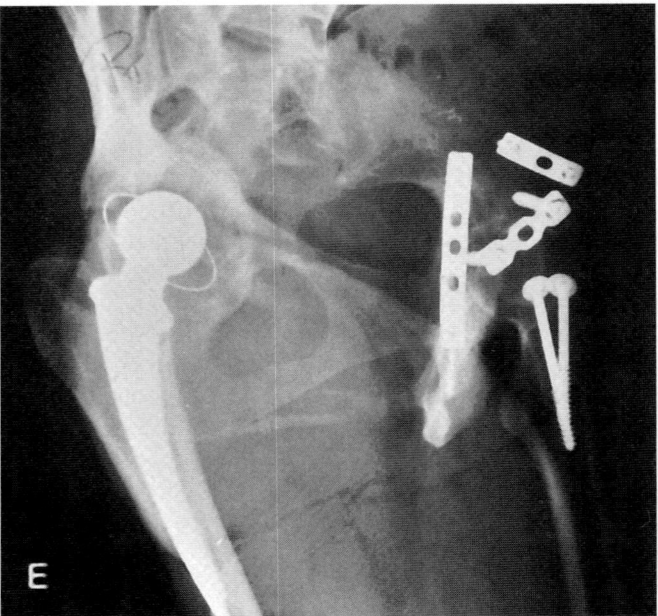

FIGURE 27-19. A: Cystogram shows a both-column fracture of the left acetabulum. Note the large retropelvic hematoma on the left side. A previous fracture of this young woman's right acetabulum was treated nonoperatively, and within 2 years she required total hip arthroplasty. **B:** The iliac oblique radiograph shows displacement of the posterior column *(medial black arrow)*. A component of the fracture enters the dome of the acetabulum and another, through the iliac crest anteriorly. **C:** The exact nature of this injury is best seen on the obturator oblique view, demonstrating the classic spur sign of the both-column fracture. **D,E:** Because this fracture entered the weight-bearing portion of the joint, internal fixation through a transtrochanteric approach was performed, as shown in the obturator oblique and the iliac oblique radiograph.

TABLE 27-2. OPERATIVE INDICATIONS: FRACTURE FACTORS

Hip unstable and/or incongruous
Guidelines to be correlated to patient factors
- A. *Instability:* Hip dislocation associated with,
  1. Posterior wall or column displacement
  2. Anterior wall or column displacement
- B. *Incongruity:*
  1. Fractures through the roof or dome
     - (a) Displaced dome fragment
     - (b) Transverse or T types (transtectal)
     - (c) Both-column types with incongruity (displaced posterior column)
  2. Retained bone fragments
  3. Displaced fractures of femoral head
  4. Soft tissue interposition

patient's systemic condition, as well as the expectations of the individual patient.

The biomechanical aspects of operative versus nonoperative treatment of acetabular fractures can be found in Chapter 5.

Indications (Table 27-2)

Those fractures that exhibit instability and/or incongruity are as follows:

Hip Instability

Fractures of the Acetabular Wall

Posterior Wall Types. All fractures of the posterior wall that are large enough to allow instability of the hip joint—no matter if isolated or associated with a posterior column or transverse fracture—require open reduction and internal fixation (Fig. 27-3). Such instability is virtually an absolute indication for surgery. If uncertainty exists about the stability of the hip joint, then it should be examined with the patient under general anesthesia. Surgery is mandatory if the femoral head dislocates posteriorly in any position of the joint. Failure to proceed will lead to dire consequences, such as redislocation of the femoral head (Fig. 27-20).

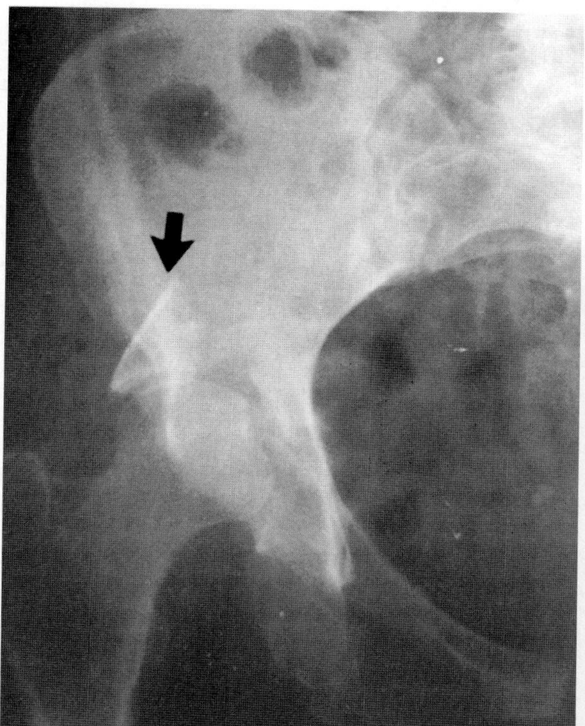
A

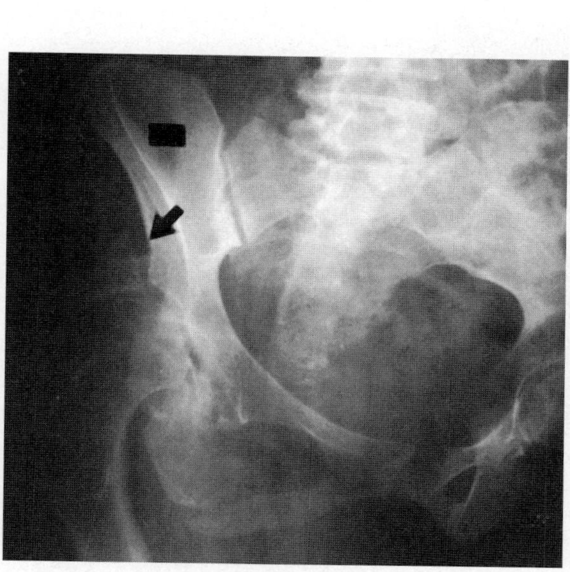
B

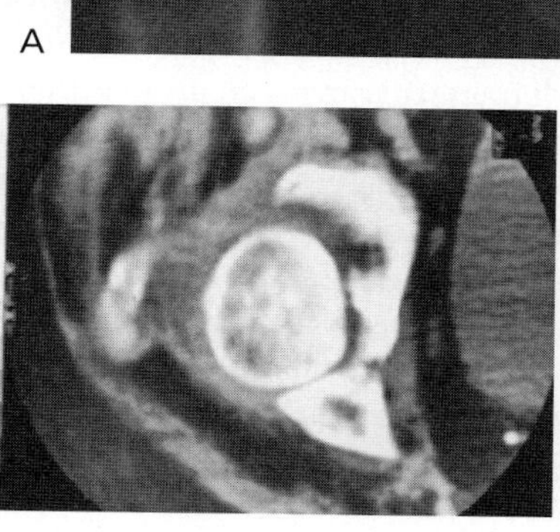
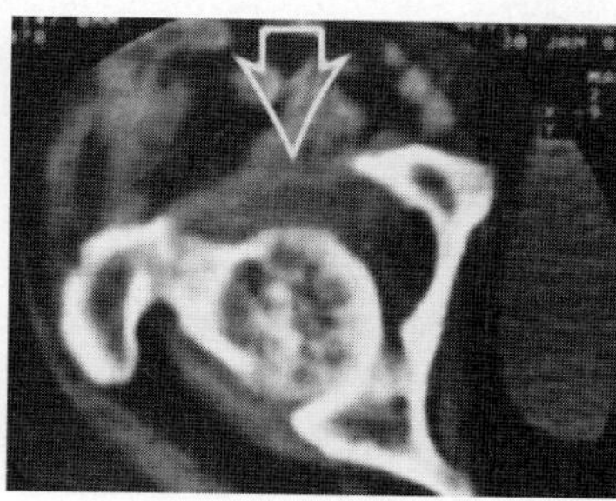
C,D

FIGURE 27-20. Displaced acetabular dome. **A,B:** Anteroposterior radiograph of the right hip and obturator oblique view show an unreduced acetabular fracture with a large superior posterior fragment from the dome *(black arrow).* **C,D:** The computed tomography cuts show marked subluxation of the femoral head that progressed early to degenerative arthritis and necessitated total hip arthroplasty within 1 year of trauma. This fracture required open reduction and internal fixation for hip stabilization and restoration of congruity.

Anterior Wall Fractures. Although less common, anterior wall or anterior column fractures may result in anterior dislocation of the hip and anterior instability (Fig. 27-4).

Incongruity

Fractures Through the Superior Weight-Bearing Dome or Roof (Transtectal)

Displacement of the acetabular dome may occur with any of the fracture types in our classification, depending on the level of the fracture. Thus, posterior, anterior, and transverse fractures all may involve the superior weight-bearing surface to some degree. Some subtypes are more likely than others to displace the dome. These subtypes may be summarized as follows.

Displaced Acetabular Dome (Roof) Fragment. All fracture types may involve the superior dome, often a triangular fragment of it. This superior triangular fragment often is rotated and rarely reduces anatomically in traction (Fig. 27-21). If it remains displaced, it must be anatomically reduced by open reduction and stabilized by internal fixation; otherwise, early degeneration of the joint can be expected. Such wall fractures rarely occur in isolation; usually they are part of a more complex fracture type, such as a transverse or T (Type B) or a both-column (Type C) lesion. Careful planning is required to achieve the goals of surgery.

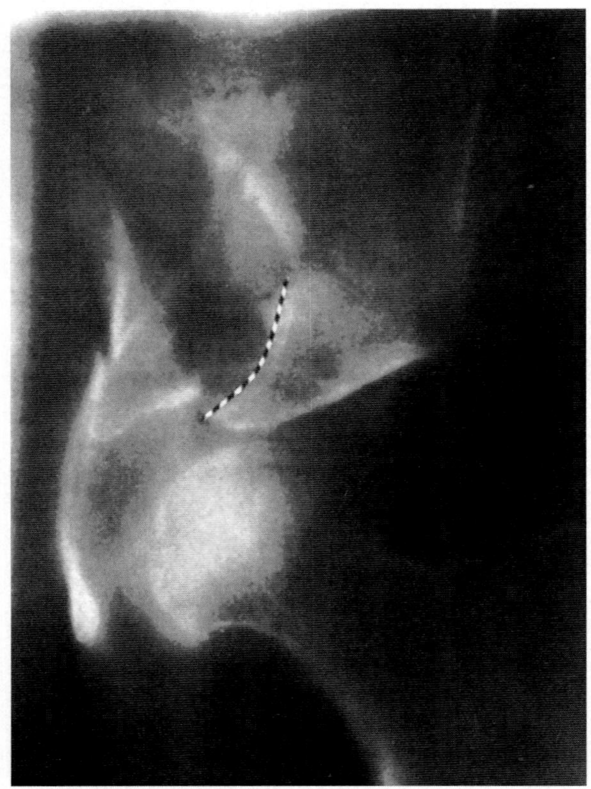

FIGURE 27-21. Displaced acetabular dome. Tomogram shows the dome fragment rotated 90 degrees. This fragment remained unreduced, in spite of an attempted closed reduction and traction.

Transverse Types (Type B). The new comprehensive classification describes transverse types in great detail (see Chapter 25). For our present purpose, they can all be divided into low fractures (infratectal, Type B2-1), which do not violate the dome, and high fractures (transtectal, Type B2-3), which do. As in all classifications, there are fractures in the gray zone (transtectal, Type B2-2). If the transverse component of the fracture is at or below the level of the superior border of the acetabular fossa, the hip may show no incongruity. If the dynamic stress views show good stability of the hip, a good result can be expected with nonoperative care (Fig. 27-22). Therefore, open reduction is indicated if the transverse limb of the fracture is high and traverses the dome, no matter whether it is a pure transverse type, T type, or anterior type (Fig. 27-23). Failure to do so usually results in early degenerative arthritis of the hip (Fig. 27-24).

Both-Column Fractures (Type C)

Type C fractures are most confusing to inexperienced surgeons and require further explanation. The main component of such fractures runs above the acetabulum through the ilium in the coronal plane. If the dome is not fractured, or, if fractured, it is not displaced, and if secondary congruity is achieved by the fragments lining up around the femoral head, this injury may be treated nonoperatively with satisfactory results, especially in older patients. The radiographic appearance shows malunion of the ilium, but, functionally, the hip will be satisfactory.

In younger patients with displacement of the columns, open reduction is indicated if there is a fracture component crossing the dome, or the uncommon presence of a posterior wall component with hip instability (Fig. 27-25). Surgical management of these difficult fractures only should be performed by surgeons with experience in pelvic and acetabular trauma.

Retained Bone Fragments

Retained bone fragments in the joint that are large enough to cause incongruity or to prevent reduction of a dislocation are an absolute indication for open reduction and removal of the fragments. Such fragments are often incarcerated during the reduction of a dislocation, thus preventing anatomic reduction of the hip (Fig. 27-26A). They are easily recognized on CT and should be surgically removed to prevent incongruity, mechanical derangement, and eventual destruction of the joint. These fragments should not be confused with avulsion fractures at either end of the ligamentum teres. These fragments are small, lie in the fovea, and do not cause incongruity, and, thus, do not require removal (Fig. 27-26B).

(Text continues on page 525)

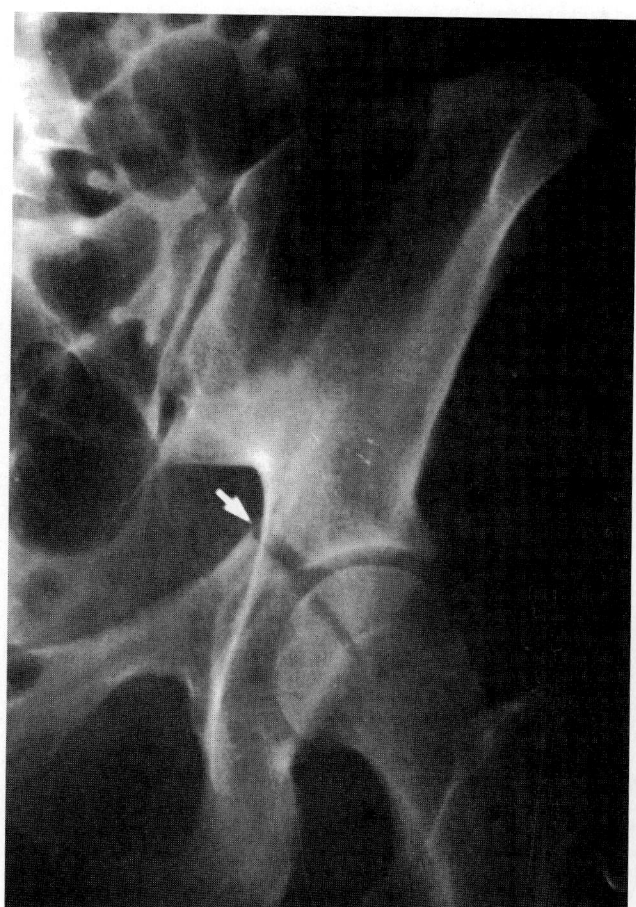

A

FIGURE 27-22. Skeletal traction for a transverse fracture. **A:** Anterior-posterior radiograph shows a transverse fracture of the left acetabulum with anterior gap and rotation confirmed on the axial computed tomography **(B)** and the three-dimensional computed tomography **(C, D).**

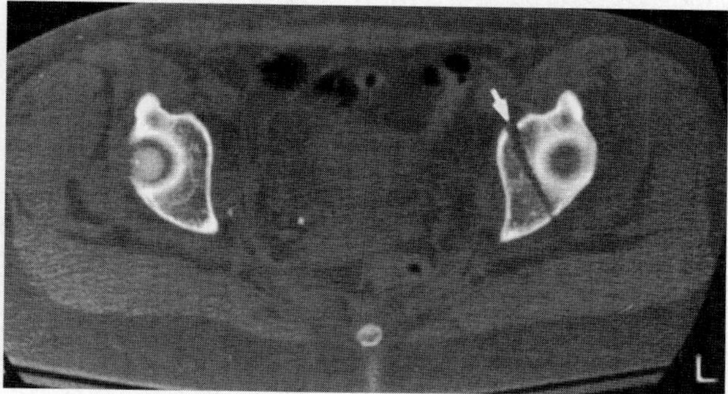

B

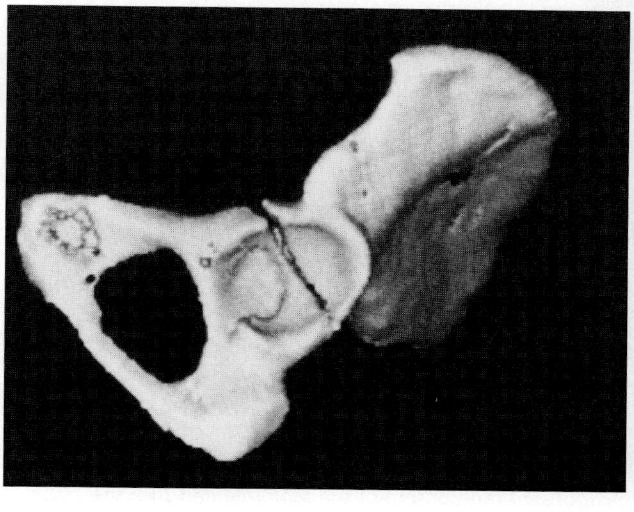

C

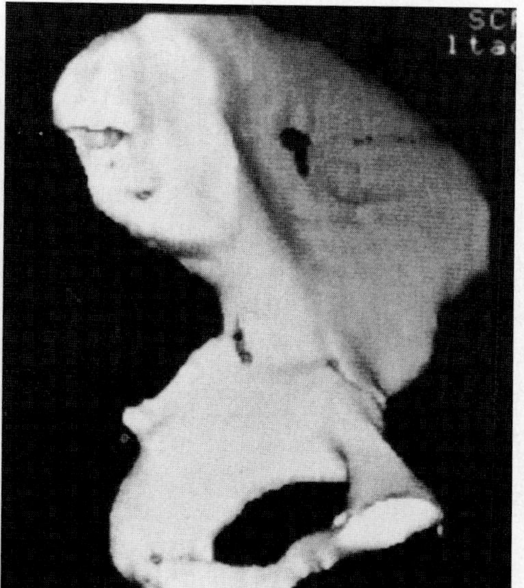

D

(*Figure continues*)

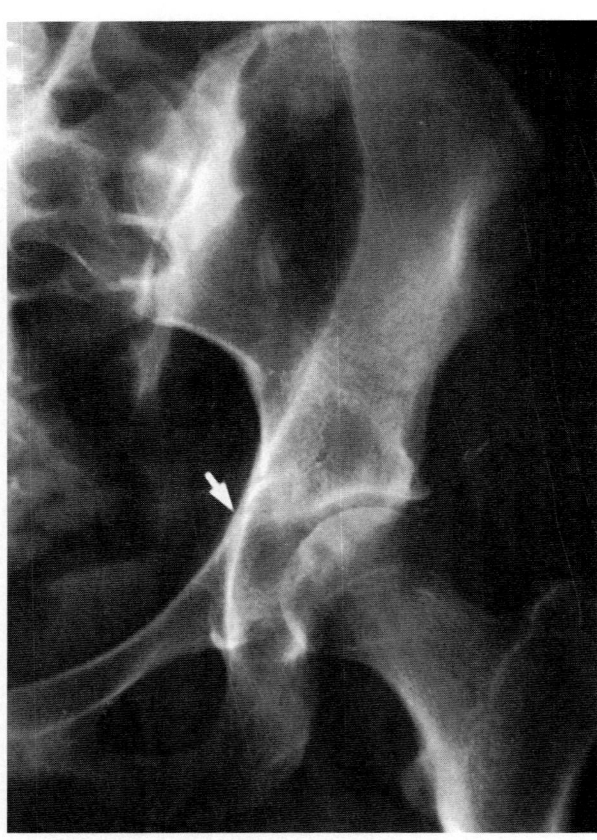

FIGURE 27-22. ***(continued)*** Skeletal traction was applied, which reduced the rotatory deformity, resulting in healing in the anatomic position **(E)** and an excellent clinical result in this 22-year-old woman.

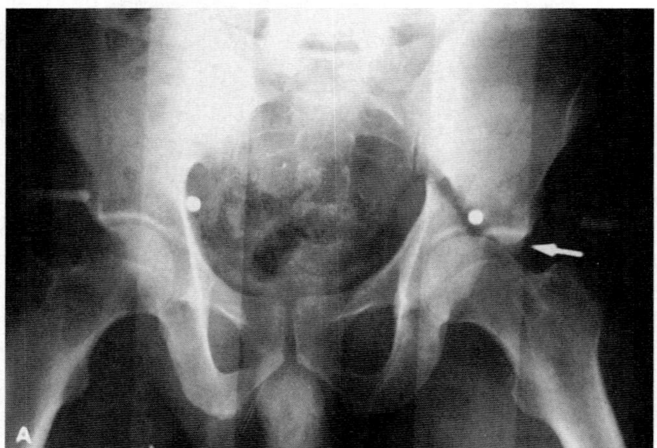

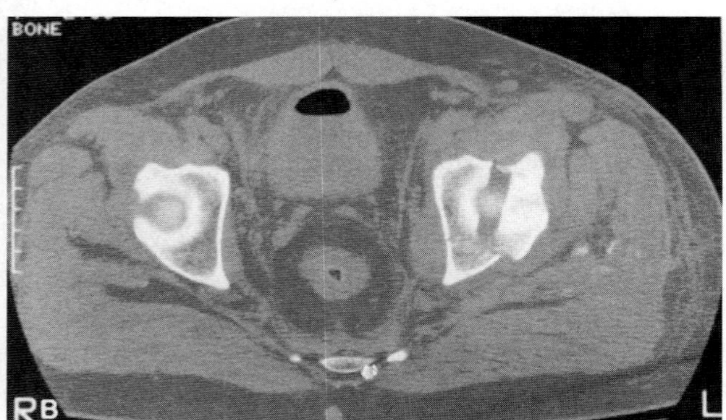

FIGURE 27-23. A: An anterior-posterior pelvis radiograph of a patient with a displaced transtectal transverse fracture of the left hip. The femoral head has translated with the ischial-pubic segment of the acetabulum. This results in an incongruent relationship of the femoral head with the residual intact superior acetabulum. **B:** A computed tomography image taken at the level of the roof of the acetabulum shows the displacement of the transverse fracture. The fracture line is in the sagittal plane consistent with a transverse fracture pattern.

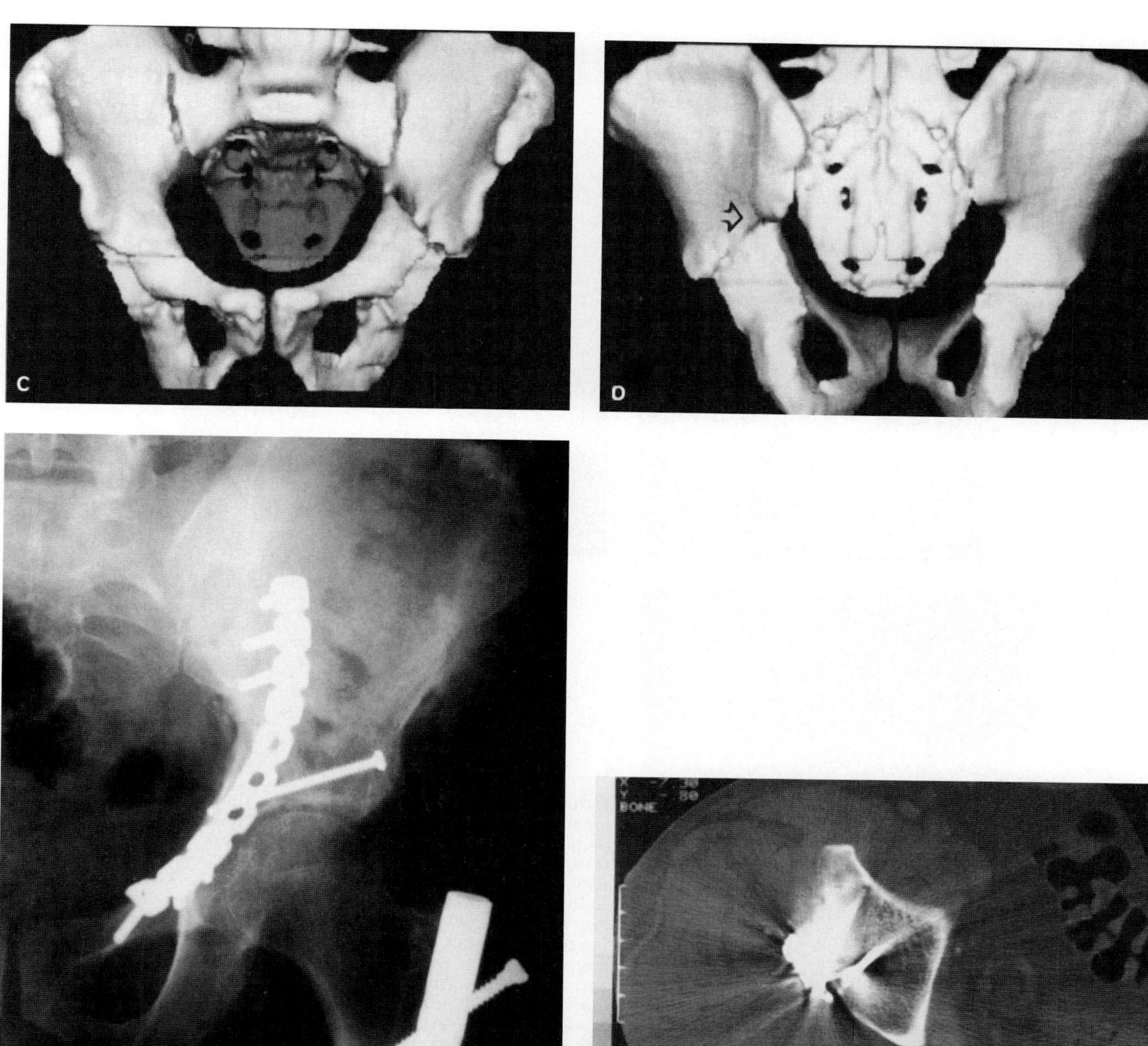

FIGURE 27-23. ***(continued)*** **C:** A three-dimensional (3D) reconstruction of the acetabulum with the subtraction of the femur demonstrates the displacement of the anterior component of the fracture. **D:** A 3D reconstruction of the acetabulum with the subtraction of the femur demonstrates the displacement of the posterior component of the fracture. **E:** Postoperative anterior-posterior pelvis radiograph shows restoration of the articular surface. Because the displacement was more extensive anteriorly an ilioinguinal approach was selected for this case. **F:** A postoperative computed tomography image demonstrates reduction of the fracture.

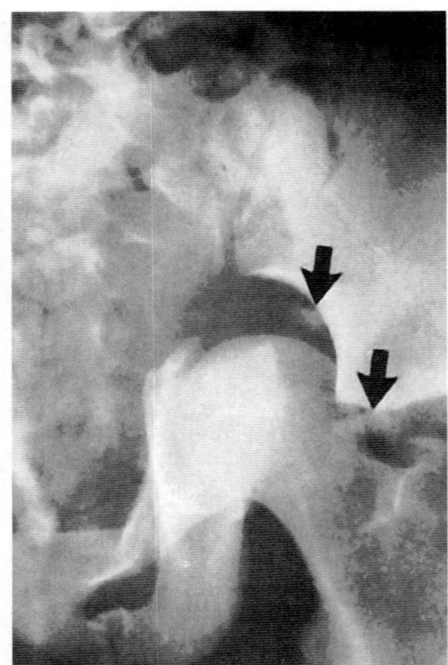

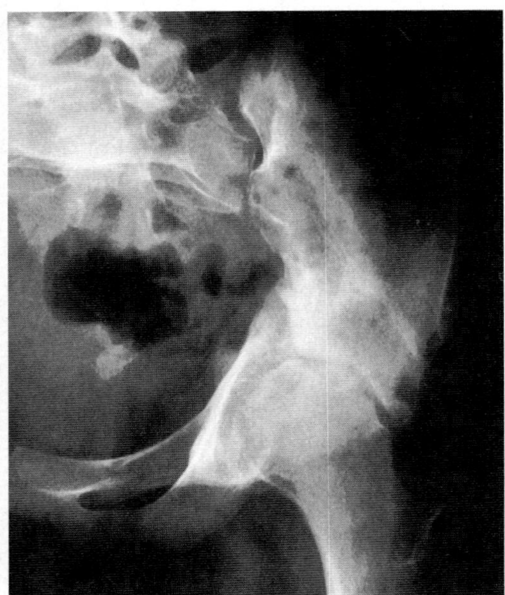

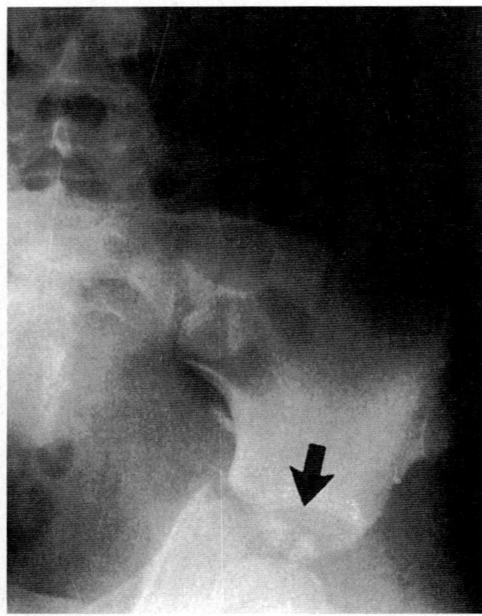

FIGURE 27-24. A transverse fracture with incongruity following attempted closed reduction. **A:** Anteroposterior radiograph of the left hip of a 17-year-old girl demonstrates a transverse fracture of the left acetabulum through the dome with central dislocation of the hip. The two *black arrows* point to loose bone fragments. **B:** Following closed reduction, the two fragments have been retained within the joint. In spite of traction, reduction is inadequate because of the bone fragments in the joint and incongruity between the femoral head and acetabulum. Definitive treatment consisted of traction maintained until the fracture healed. **C:** The result at 18 months. Note the severe narrowing and erosions on the superior weight-bearing margin of the femoral head. The patient's clinical result was poor. She had a 60-degree flexion deformity and continuous pain and required arthrodesis.

FIGURE 27-25. Both-column fracture. Open reduction and internal fixation was accomplished via a triradiate approach. **A:** Anteroposterior radiograph indicates a both-column fracture of the left acetabulum. The classic appearance is noted in the three-dimensional computed tomography (3DCT) **(B),** indicating the large anterior column fracture exiting the iliac crest above the acetabulum in the coronal plane. A further split in the anterior column is noted well posterior in the classic Y pattern of this fracture. This is better seen on the 3DCT **(C),** which also shows the spur sign posteriorly and the 3DCT **(D),** showing the disruption from the inside of the pelvis (i.e., to the quadrilateral plate). Open reduction and internal fixation were performed through an triradiate approach.

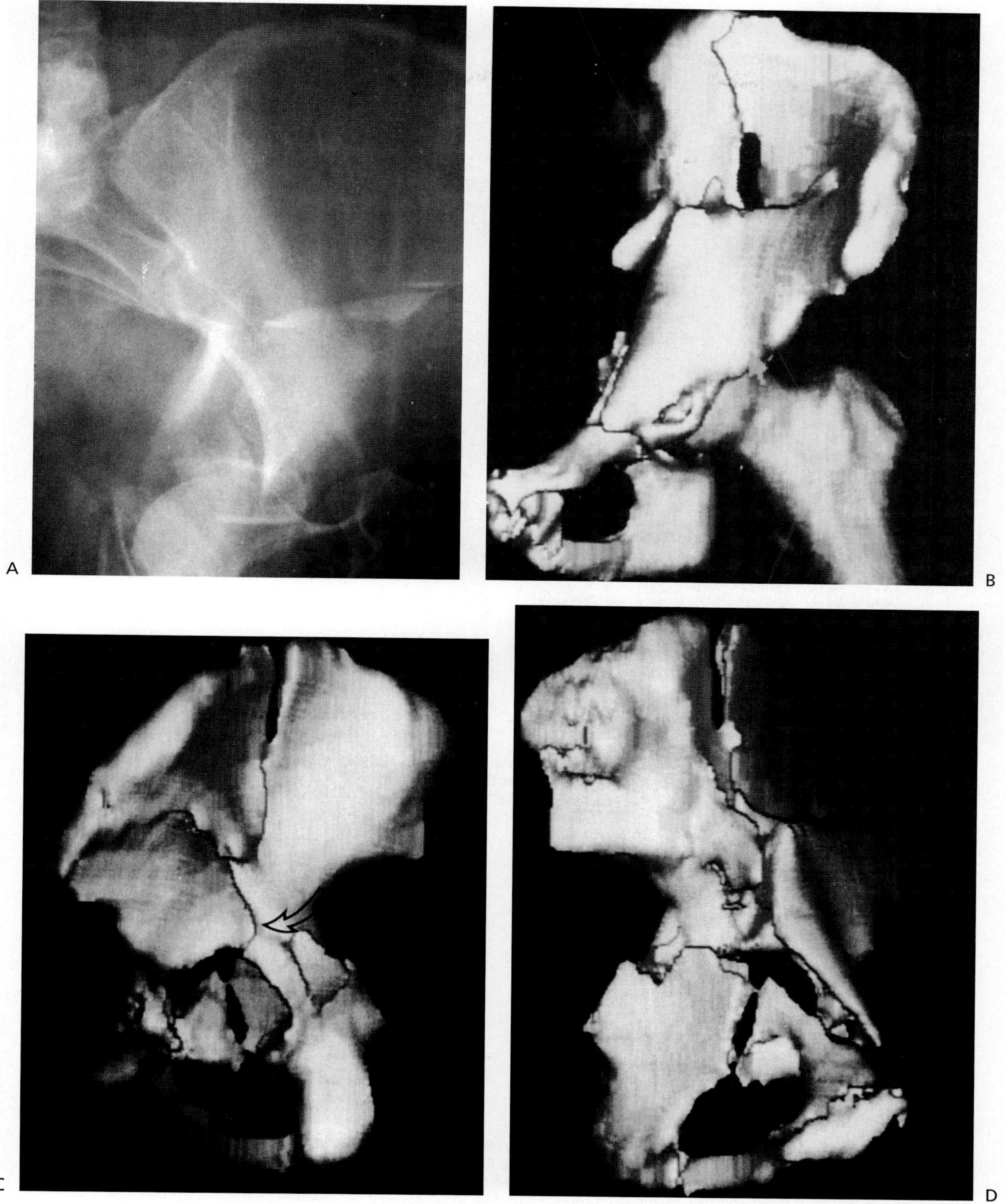

(Figure continues)

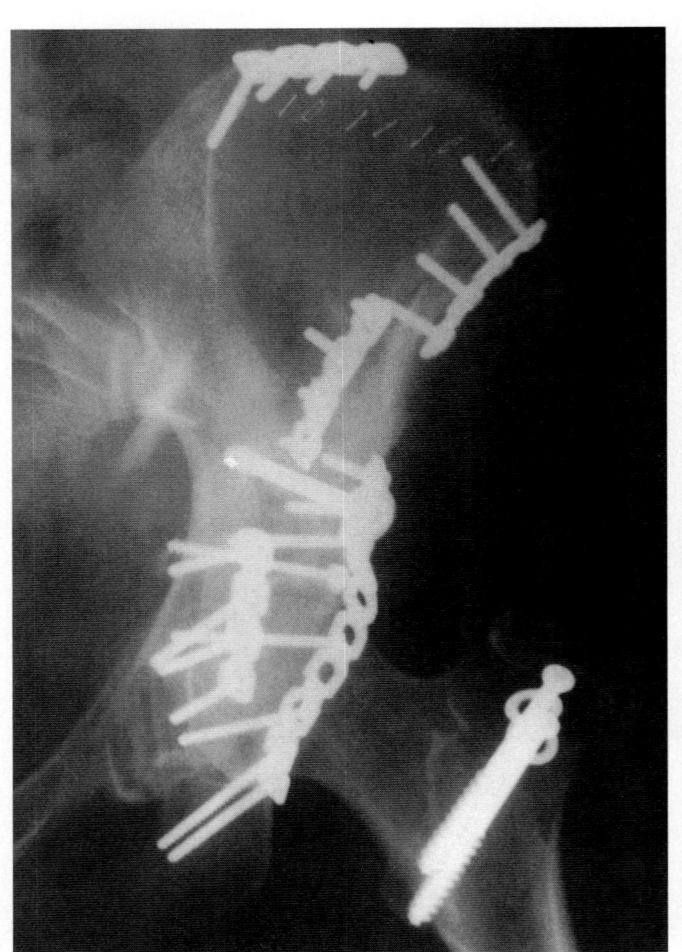
E

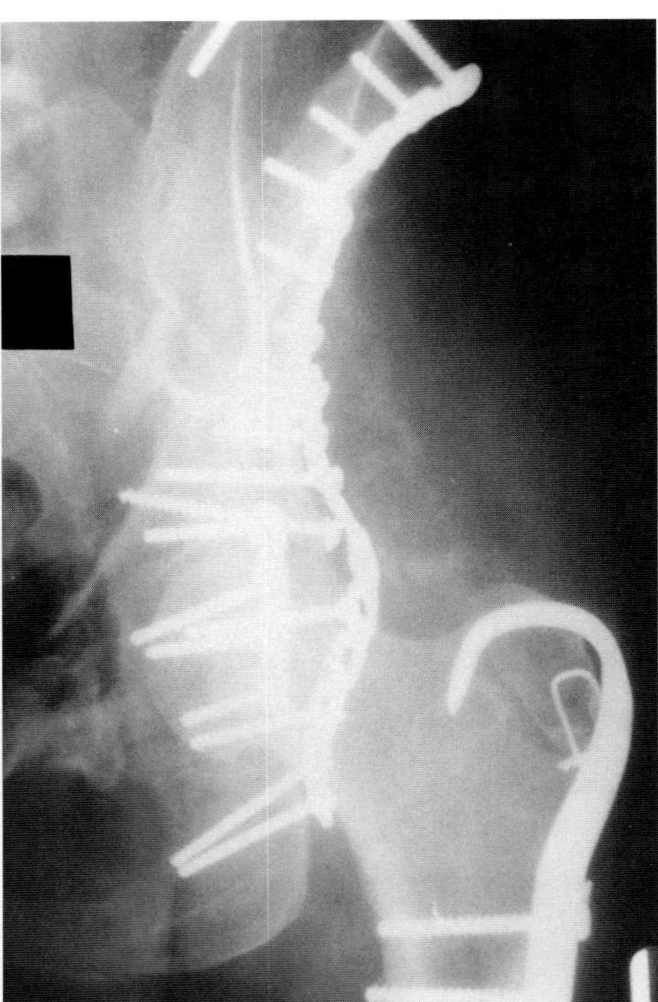
F

FIGURE 27-25. ***(continued)*** The postoperative radiograph **(E)** shows an excellent reduction, and the followup radiograph **(F)** shows slight heterotopic ossification and the unusual complication of nonunion of the trochanter, requiring secondary fixation.

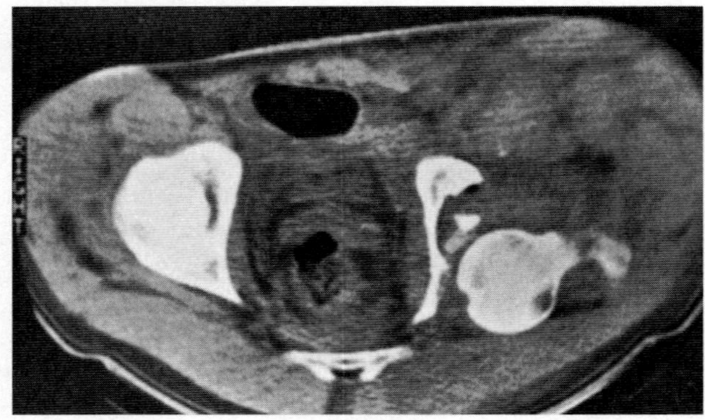
A

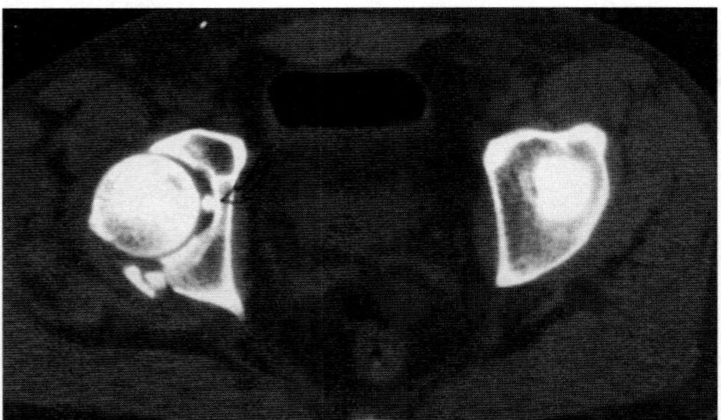
B

FIGURE 27-26. A: Computed tomography (CT) demonstrates a transverse fracture of the acetabulum; both the anterior column fracture and the large posterior wall fracture are clearly seen. The arrow points to a comminuted rotated bone fragment. **B:** CT shows an avulsed fragment from the femoral head and the ligamentum teres. Note that this fragment lies within the fovea and does not cause incongruity of the joint. Note also, in this particular case, marginal impaction of the posterior column fragment, which required open reduction and internal fixation.

Fractures of the Femoral Head

Displaced fractures of the femoral head usually require anatomic open reduction and internal fixation (Fig. 27-27). Occasionally, closed manipulation and maintenance of internal rotation lead to an excellent result.

Interposition of Bone or Soft Tissue

Large bone fragments prevent congruous reduction and require operative removal (Fig. 27-26A). Also, on reduction of a posterior dislocation, the capsule may be drawn into the joint, preventing anatomic reduction. Again, open reduction is required to restore congruity.

Other Factors That Favor Operative Intervention

In the Limb

Many factors in the limb influence the management decision.

Sciatic Nerve Lesion. Exploration of the nerve and the fracture is mandatory if sciatic nerve palsy develops during reduction or while the patient is in traction. Less clear-cut is the approach to management of a nerve lesion that occurs at the moment of injury. In most cases, the patient has posterior dislocation of the hip; therefore, surgery may already be indicated for the fracture. If so, the nerve should be explored at that time. The patient may be observed and the fracture treated by closed means in the absence of a dislocation and a specific musculoskeletal indication for open reduction. Recovery ensues in most cases; if not, late exploration by an expert in nerve repair may be indicated.

Associated Fracture of the Femur. Fractures of the ipsilateral femur are commonly associated with acetabular fractures (Fig. 27-28). Other methods must be used because effective traction to the hip is not possible in the presence of an unstable femoral fracture. Operative stabilization of the femoral fracture is mandatory in the presence of a displaced acetabular fracture (20). Open reduction and internal fixation of the acetabulum also is usually indicated because traction on the femur is undesirable following internal fixation, especially intramedullary nailing. This combined injury to the acetabulum and the femur is difficult to manage, requiring careful planning to obtain an optimal result (Fig. 27-28).

Ipsilateral Knee Disruption. Injuries to the knee, such as patellar fractures and posterior ligamentous disruptions, are common because many acetabular fractures occur when the flexed knee is driven into the dashboard of a car. Traction wires through a tibial or femoral condyle should not be used if knee surgery is necessary. A tibial wire exerts traction through an already unstable knee, and a femoral wire may limit motion and retard knee rehabilitation. Preferably, the acetabular fracture should be stabilized to allow early rehabilitation of the entire limb and no traction used.

Indications for Emergency Open Reduction and Internal Fixation

Irreducible Dislocation

If, even with general anesthesia and muscle paralysis, the femoral head cannot be reduced, early open reduction is mandatory (Table 27-3). The usual causes are: (a) large fragments of bone within the hip; or (b) soft-tissue interposition. The capsule or acetabular labrum may be caught in the joint, or the head may be "buttonholed" through the capsule.

Unstable Hip Following Reduction

Rarely the wall fragment is so large (Fig. 27-3) that the femoral head cannot be contained within the acetabulum, even with the limb in traction—in abduction, extension, and external rotation for a posterior dislocation, and in internal rotation, flexion, and adduction for an anterior lesion. In these circumstances, the surgeon should be prepared to carry on immediately with open reduction and internal fixation, or, alternatively, to refer the patient to a center that can deal with the situation urgently.

Increasing Neurologic Deficit

An increasing sciatic nerve deficit before closed reduction is an indication for urgent closed reduction; an increasing sciatic nerve deficit following closed reduction is an indication for urgent open reduction. Monitoring equipment should be used in this circumstance if it is available.

Associated Vascular Injury

Again, this is a rare indication that usually involves the anterior column of the acetabulum, penetrating the femoral artery.

Open Fractures

Open fractures of the acetabulum are rare, but when one is present, the principles of management for open fractures must prevail, including cleansing, debridement, and stabilization. Obviously, internal fixation in this circumstance should be done only under ideal conditions; thus, skeletal traction and secondary open reduction and inter-

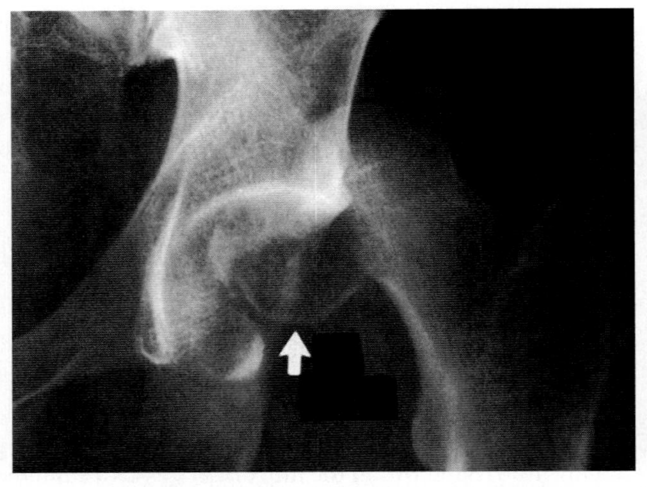

A

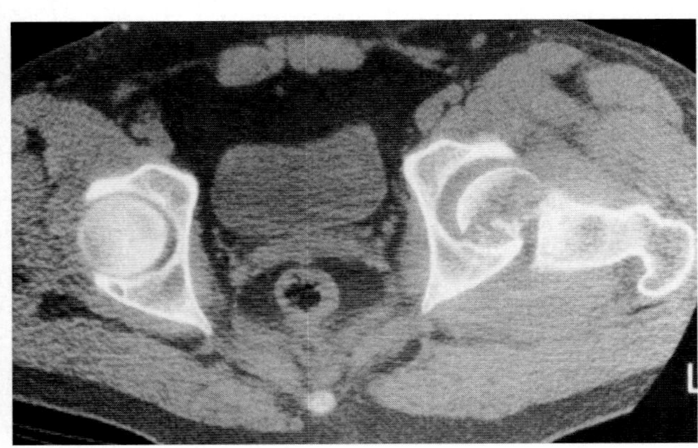

B

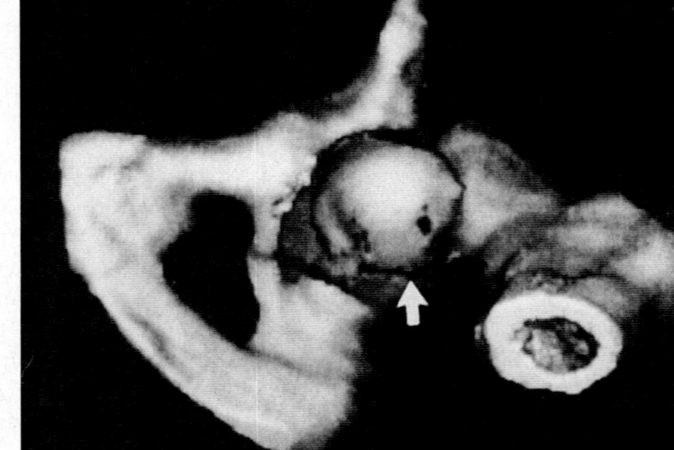

C

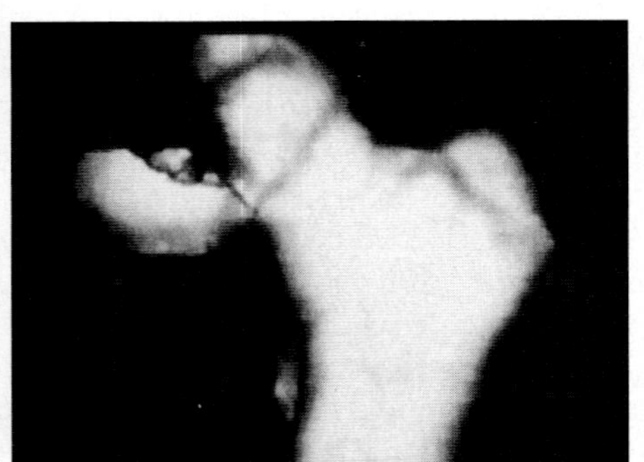

D

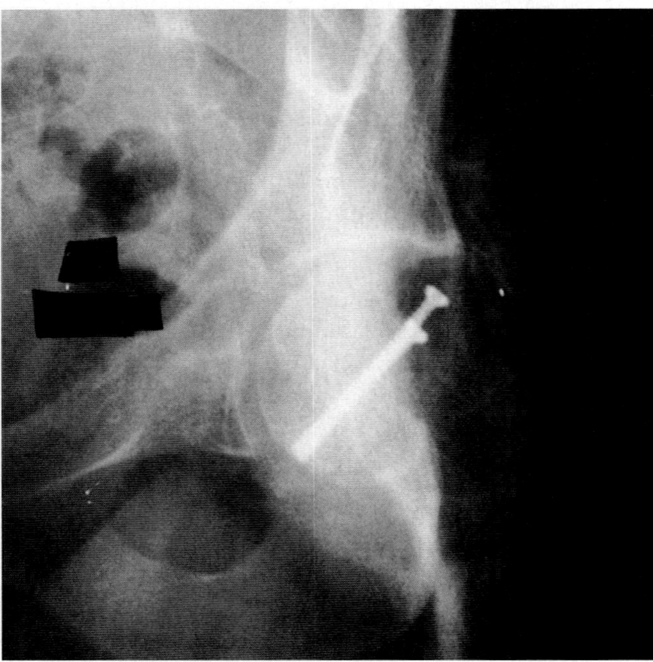

E

FIGURE 27-27. Fracture of the femoral head. **A:** Anteroposterior radiograph of the left hip, showing a posterior dislocation and a large fragment from the inferior portion of the femoral head remaining in the joint. This fracture is more clearly delineated on the axial computed tomography **(B)** and the three-dimensional computed tomography **(C,D).** Open reduction and internal fixation was performed through an anterior approach. Fixation of the fragment was held in a retrograde fashion by two screws. The anterior approach allowed the vascularity of the blood supply through the ligamentum teres artery to be preserved **(E).**

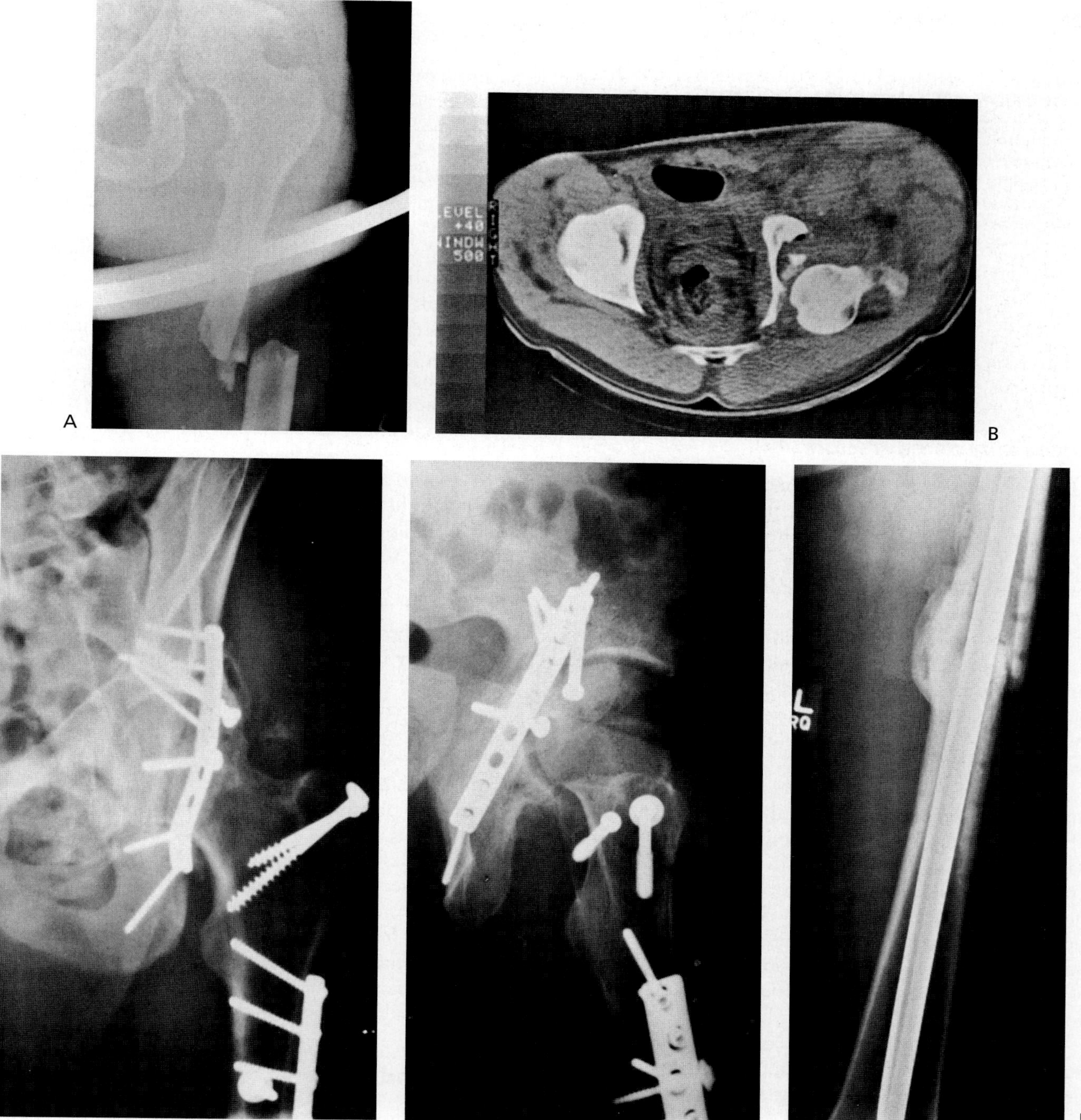

FIGURE 27-28. Anteroposterior radiograph shows a transverse fracture of the left acetabulum with a posterior wall fragment associated with a comminuted fracture of the shaft of the femur **(A).** This injury also included severe involvement of the left sciatic nerve. The severe nature of the injury is best seen on computed tomography, showing the posterior dislocation and the retained bone fragment **(B).** Because of the sciatic nerve lesion, the femoral and acetabular fractures were internally stabilized on the night of admission, the femur with a plate and interfragmental screws and the acetabulum through a transtrochanteric approach, using interfragmental screws for the posterior fragment and a neutralization 3.5-mm dynamic compression plate, as shown on the obturator oblique **(C)** and iliac oblique **(D)** radiographic views. Also, because we had planned to use the transtrochanteric approach to the hip, an intermedullary nail would have been technically difficult and undesirable. This patient had excellent restoration of congruity of his hip with an excellent clinical result. However, his femur failed to unite. Following a fracture through the plate at the site of the nonunion, an intermedullary nail was inserted **(E);** eventually this resulted in sound union. The peroneal division of the sciatic nerve never recovered. In this situation, primary stable plating of the femur allowed full control of the femoral head without concern that the femoral fracture would become displaced again.

TABLE 27-3. INDICATIONS FOR EMERGENCY OPEN REDUCTION AND INTERNAL FIXATION

1. Irreducible dislocation
2. Unstable hip following reduction
3. Increasing neurological deficit
4. Associated vascular injury
5. Open fractures

nal fixation may be the preferred option, depending on circumstances.

Operability of the Fracture

Having decided that the reduction is incongruous or that hidden instability is still present, as evidenced by a displaced posterior wall fracture, the surgeon must decide whether the fracture is operable or inoperable. This is often a difficult question, because it depends on the experience of the surgeon as ones experience grows, the number of cases that are truly inoperable falls. However, given a experienced surgeon, there are both patient factors and fracture factors that will lead to alternative treatment such as total hip arthroplasty, or nonoperative management of the fracture, with late total hip arthroplasty, if necessary.

Inoperable Injury or Poor Surgical Candidate

If the patient has any contraindication to surgery, it is far safer to continue with nonoperative treatment. The contraindications have been described; they include soft bone and a comminuted fracture in an elderly patient and, in a younger patient, such severe comminution that surgery would be hazardous. Finally, occasionally a patient's general state is so precarious that the major open reduction required to fix an acetabulum would jeopardize life.

Under these circumstances, closed treatment with supracondylar skeletal traction should be continued. If at any time a younger patient's general status improves, surgery can be carried out then. Traction should be continued for 8 to 12 weeks. At that time, the patient should be carefully assessed. Surprisingly, the patient may have little pain and a reasonably functional hip joint; if so, rehabilitation should proceed quickly (Fig. 27-2). At such time as the patient's symptoms warrant, if ever; a late reconstruction procedure should be performed (usually total hip arthroplasty; Fig. 27-29). With a concomitant fracture of the femoral head, early total hip arthroplasty may be the treatment of choice.

The younger the patient, the more the surgeon should be inclined toward restoration of the hip joint; for in older patients total hip arthroplasty is an option. If total hip arthroplasty is chosen, many precautions are in order, because early loosening of the socket is common (21). This is described further in Chapters 43 and 44.

Operable Fracture

If a complete assessment indicates that the fracture is operable (i.e., the surgeon feels he or she can achieve the goals of anatomic reduction and stable internal fixation), then that operative procedure should be carried out as soon as the patient's general status allows and the operating team can be assembled. The operability of any fracture depends on many factors, including the anatomic features, the degree of comminution, the general state of the patient, and the condition of the bone. Therefore the surgeon needs to ask two questions. *Can I fix the fracture? Can the fracture be fixed at all?*

These are two separate questions that must be answered quickly. If the decision is made in favor of surgery but available surgeons are not sufficiently experienced, early referral is essential, because delay increases the hazards of surgery and adversely affects the end result. As one's experience increases in this field, the number of cases that are truly inoperable becomes fewer (Fig. 27-30).

If surgery restores congruity to the joint, the results are improved, but if surgery fails to achieve stability and congruity, the results will not be improved and the patient will have been exposed to the added risks of surgery, which are formidable. The surgery is demanding and requires more than adequate human and material resources. A truism worth remembering is this: *The learning curve is hard on patients* (Fig. 27-31).

Alan Apley has observed, "The 'average surgeon' is average." I have paraphrased this to say that, in acetabular surgery, the superior surgeon has not only more experience, but lots of help, human and material help. No surgeon should attempt to fix these fractures operatively without such help and without first attending manual skill courses, including cadaver dissections.

Contraindications

The indications for surgery described here are valid only in ideal conditions. Many factors can make the conditions less than ideal, in which case the surgical risks are too great. These contraindications to surgery may reside in the patient, fracture, or surgical team.

Contraindications in the Patient

As described in the introduction of this chapter, patient factors may be as important as fracture factors in decision making. The fracture "personality" includes such considerations as the age and general medical or posttrauma status of the patient. Surgical stabilization may be indicated by the fracture pattern, but strong contraindications, such as osteoporotic bone or severe associated injuries, would dissuade even the most operatively minded surgeon. Traction methods may result in good outcomes, in some instances; however, for many reasons this is almost never used today. In these cases, a primary total hip arthroplasty remains an option.

Contraindications in the Fracture

Clear indications have been outlined, but these depend on the ability of the surgeon to achieve the stated goal of anatomic reduction and stable fixation. Rarely, a fracture may be so comminuted that it defies even the most expert and experienced surgeon. In those circumstances, where the fracture is deemed inoperable, it is far better to resort to nonoperative methods than to place an already traumatized patient at further risk. I might add that the number of inoperable cases one sees depends on the perception of the surgeon. Any surgeon's ability to see through the maze on the radiographs and CT images increases with experience, and the number of inoperable cases becomes few indeed.

Contraindications In the Surgical Team

Open reduction and internal fixation of this injury may be hazardous and should not be attempted by surgeons not experienced in this field. If the patient is injured in an area where expert help is not available, nonoperative methods should prevail. If a strong indication for operative treatment exists, the patient should be referred to a center whose surgeons are capable of managing this type of injury.

ROLE OF TOTAL HIP ARTHROPLASTY

The role of primary total hip arthroplasty is evolving rapidly, and is discussed fully in Chapter 43. Suffice it to say that, as in other fractures of joints, especially the elbow and shoulder, total hip arthroplasty should not be used for fractures that are best treated by open reduction and internal fixation. However, in older patients with poor bone or excessive comminution with a probable poor result, total

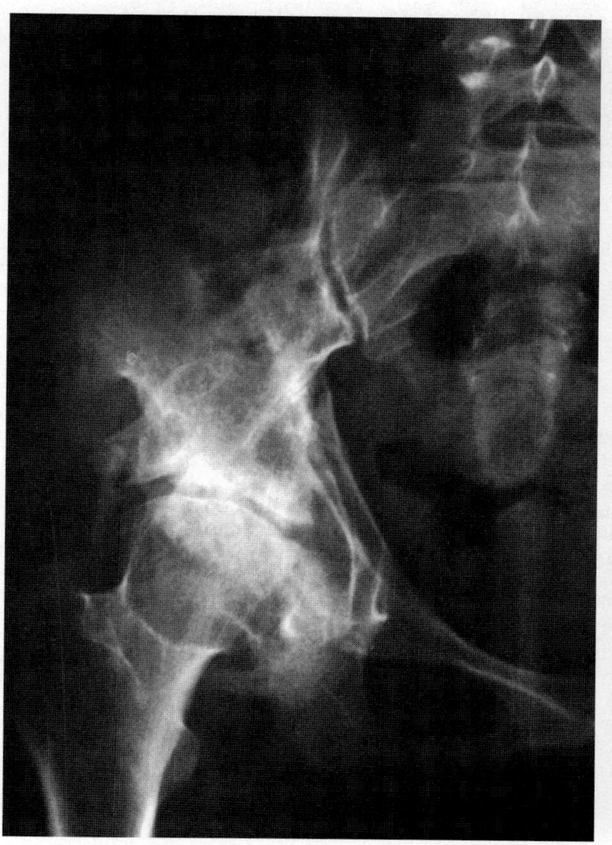

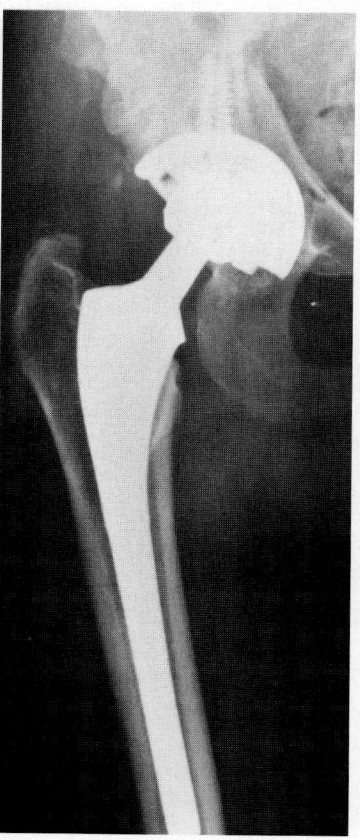

A B

FIGURE 27-29. A: Anteroposterior radiograph of a young woman who sustained a both-column fracture of the acetabulum at age 16 years. **B:** Sixteen years later symptoms of osteoarthritis became severe enough to warrant an uncemented total hip arthroplasty.

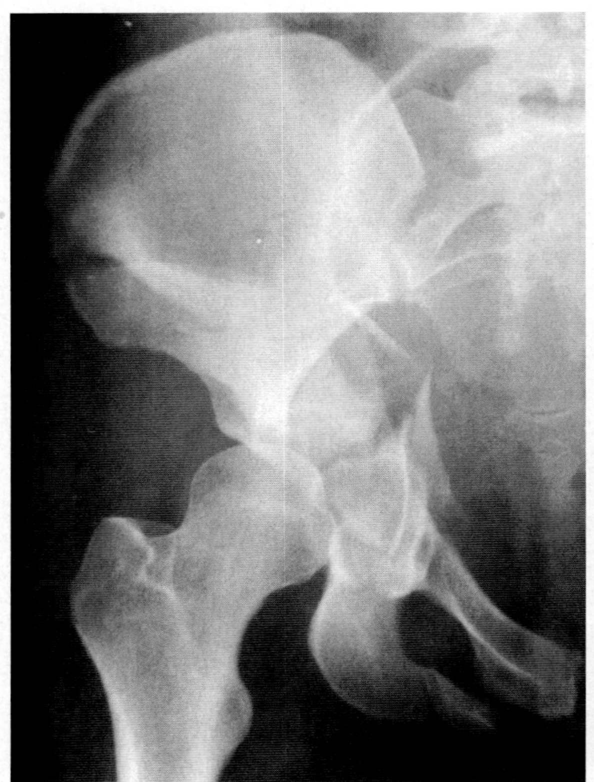
A

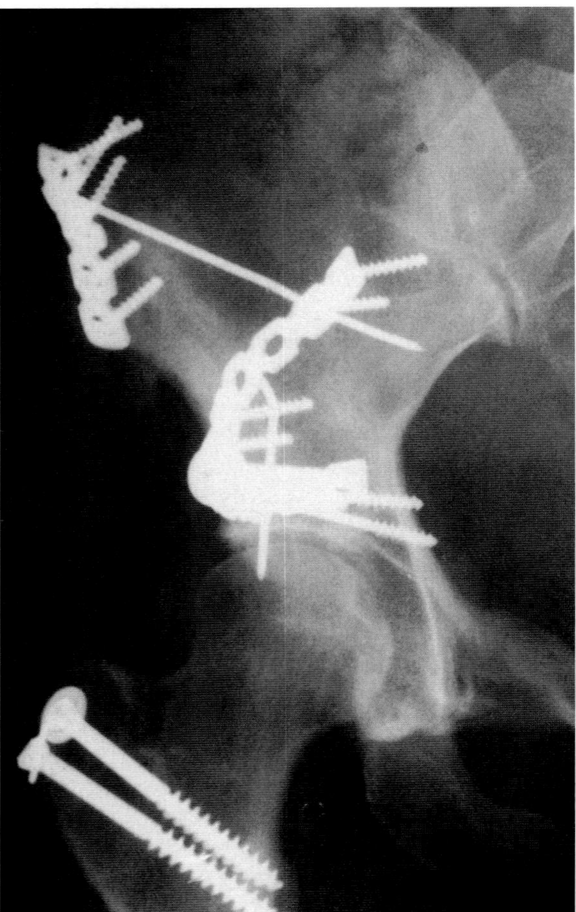
C

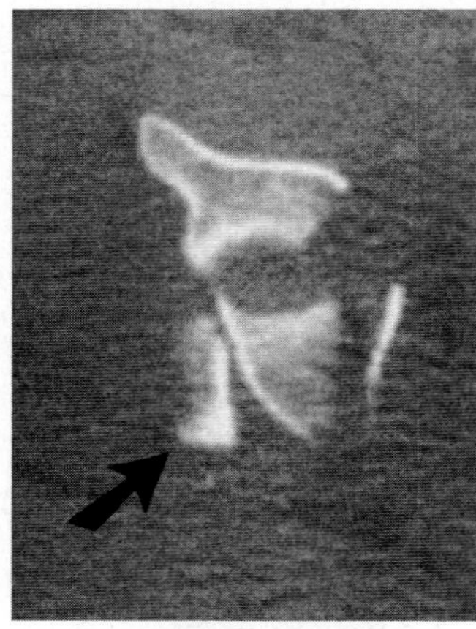
B

FIGURE 27-30. A: Anteroposterior radiograph of a young woman who sustained a both-column fracture in a motor vehicle accident. Note the marked comminution and the confusing picture. The question to be answered is, Is this fracture operable? The answer of course, is, yes, but to be successful, it requires careful scrutiny of the radiographs and, at operative intervention, an experienced surgeon. **B:** Computed tomography shows the coronal split and the spur sign. **C:** The postoperative radiograph shows a healed fracture with an anatomic reduction, 5 years following the injury. She remained well for 14 years, then developed severe osteoarthritis within 1 year requiring uncemented total hip arthroplasty with an excellent result.

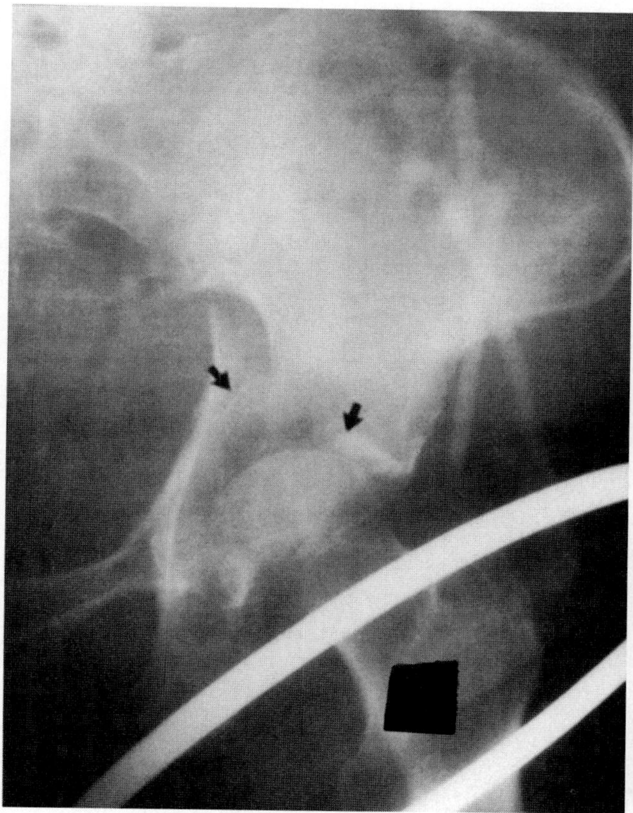
A

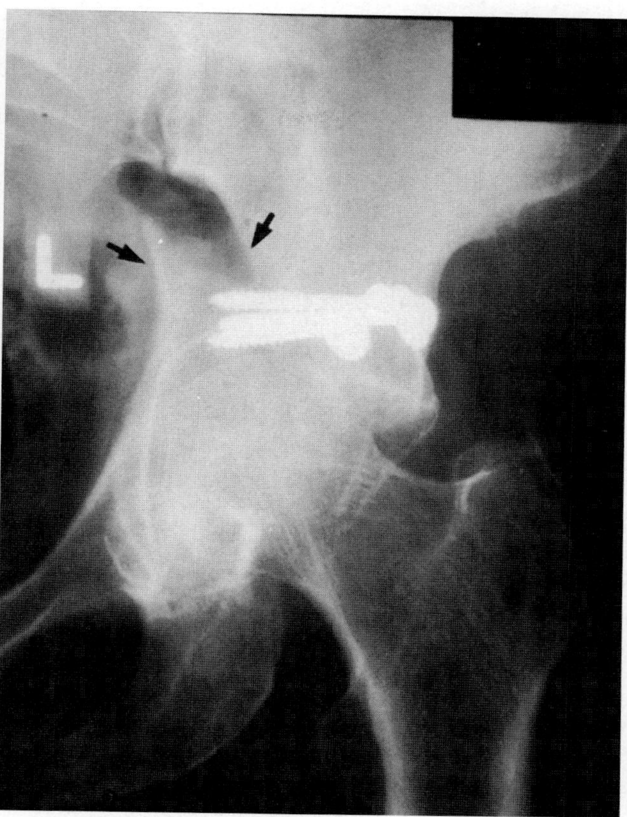

B

FIGURE 27-31. Anteroposterior radiograph shows a transverse fracture associated with a displaced posterior wall fragment **(A).** An attempted open reduction and internal fixation is seen in **(B).** The transverse fracture was not reduced and remains in the displaced position with the femoral head centrally dislocated. Early total hip arthroplasty was required. This case illustrates how the learning curve can be hard on patients.

hip arthroplasty should be considered. Techniques of fixing the acetabular component, the major technical challenge, are improving. Look at Chapters 43 and 44 for details.

REFERENCES

1. Mitchell N, Shepard N. The resurfacing of adult rabbit articular cartilage by multiple perforations through the subchondral bone. *J Bone Joint Surg* 1976;58A:230.
2. Salter RB, Simmonds DF, Malcolm BW, et al. The biological effect of continuous passive motion on the healing of full thickness defects in articular cartilage—an experimental investigation in the rabbit. *J Bone Joint Surg* 1980;62A:1232.
3. Mears DC, Velyvis JH. Acute total hip arthroplasty for selected displaced acetabular fractures. Two to twelve year results. *J Bone Joint Surg* 2002;84A:1–9.
4. Matta J. Operative indications and choice of surgical approach for fractures of the acetabulum. *Tech Orthop* 1986;1:18.
5. Letournel E. Acetabular fractures: classification and management. *Clin Orthop* 1980;151:81.
6. Halliwell S, Borkhoff C, Owen PJ, et al. *The associated both-column fracture: long term functional outcome of conservative versus surgical management.* Presented at the Canadian Orthopaedic Association Meeting. St. John's, Newfoundland, July 1999.
7. Judet R, Judet J, Letournel E. Fractures of the acetabulum: classification and surgical approach for open reduction. *J Bone Joint Surg* 1964;46A:1615–1645.
8. MacGuire CJ. Fractures of the acetabulum. *Ann Surg* 1926; 83:718.
9. Palmer DW. Central dislocation of the hip. *Am J Surg* 1921; 35:118.
10. Peet MM. Fracture of the acetabulum with intrapelvic displacement of the femoral head. *Ann Surg* 1919;70:296.
11. Urist MR. Fracture-dislocation of the hip joint: the nature of the traumatic lesion, treatment, late complications, and end results. *J Bone Joint Surg* 1948;30A:699–727, quote taken from page 725.
12. Knight RA, Smith H. Central fractures of the acetabulum. *J Bone Joint Surg* 1958;40A(1):1
13. Pennal GF. Central disloc ı of the hip. *J Bone Joint Surg* 1958; 40A:1435.
14. Rowe CR, Lowell JD. Prognosis of fractures of the acetabulum. *J Bone Joint Surg* 1961;43A:30.
15. Matta JM, Mehne DK, Roffi R. Fractures of the acetabulum: early results of a prospective study. *Clin Orthop Rel Res* 1986; 205:241.
16. Olson SA, Matta J. The computerized subchondral arc: a new

method of assessing acetabular articular congruity after fracture: a preliminary report. *J Orthop Trauma* 1993;7:402–413.

17. Tornetta P 3rd. Nonoperative management of acetabular fractures. The use of dynamic stress views. *J Bone Joint Surg Br* 1999;81(1):67–70.
18. Letournel E, Judet R. *Fractures of the acetabulum,* 2nd ed. New York: Springer-Verlag, 1993.
19. Olson SA, Matta JM. *Skeletal trauma, Vol. 1* 2nd ed. Philadelphia: Saunders, 1997.
20. Joyce JJ, Kellam JF, Tile M. The floating hip displaced acetabular fracture with an ipsilateral femoral shaft fracture. *J Bone Joint Surg Orthop Trans* 1988;12:708.
21. Romness DW, Lewallen DG. Total hip arthroplasty after fracture of the acetabulum. *J Bone Joint Surg* 1990;72B:761.

28

SURGICAL TECHNIQUES FOR ACETABULAR FRACTURES

DAVID L. HELFET
MARTIN BECK
EMANUEL GAUTIER
THOMAS J. ELLIS
REINHOLD GANZ
CRAIG S. BARTLETT
KLAUS A. SIEBENROCK

INTRODUCTION

Timing

Fractures of the acetabulum often pose so many diagnostic and technical problems that routine open reduction and internal fixation cannot be recommended as an emergency procedure. The exceptions, listed in Fig. 28-1, include dislocations that cannot be reduced by closed means and unstable posterior dislocations that cannot be held in the reduced position because of the marked deficiency of the posterior wall. Progressive or a sciatic nerve palsy that develops after reduction of the dislocation also should be considered a surgical emergency. Rare indications include open fractures of the acetabulum and those that involve significant vascular injuries. Surgery should be performed immediately in all these situations.

We believe it is advisable to wait 3 to 5 days in all other circumstances, to allow the patient's general status to stabilize. During this period, careful radiologic and computed tomographic (CT) assessment of the fracture can be carried out, to inform careful planning of the operative procedure. A difficult procedure then can be done on an elective basis with a more experienced operating team.

We should point out, again, that dislocations are surgical emergencies that should be reduced as soon as possible after the injury. Operative procedures may be delayed, but not reduction of displaced fractures or dislocations.

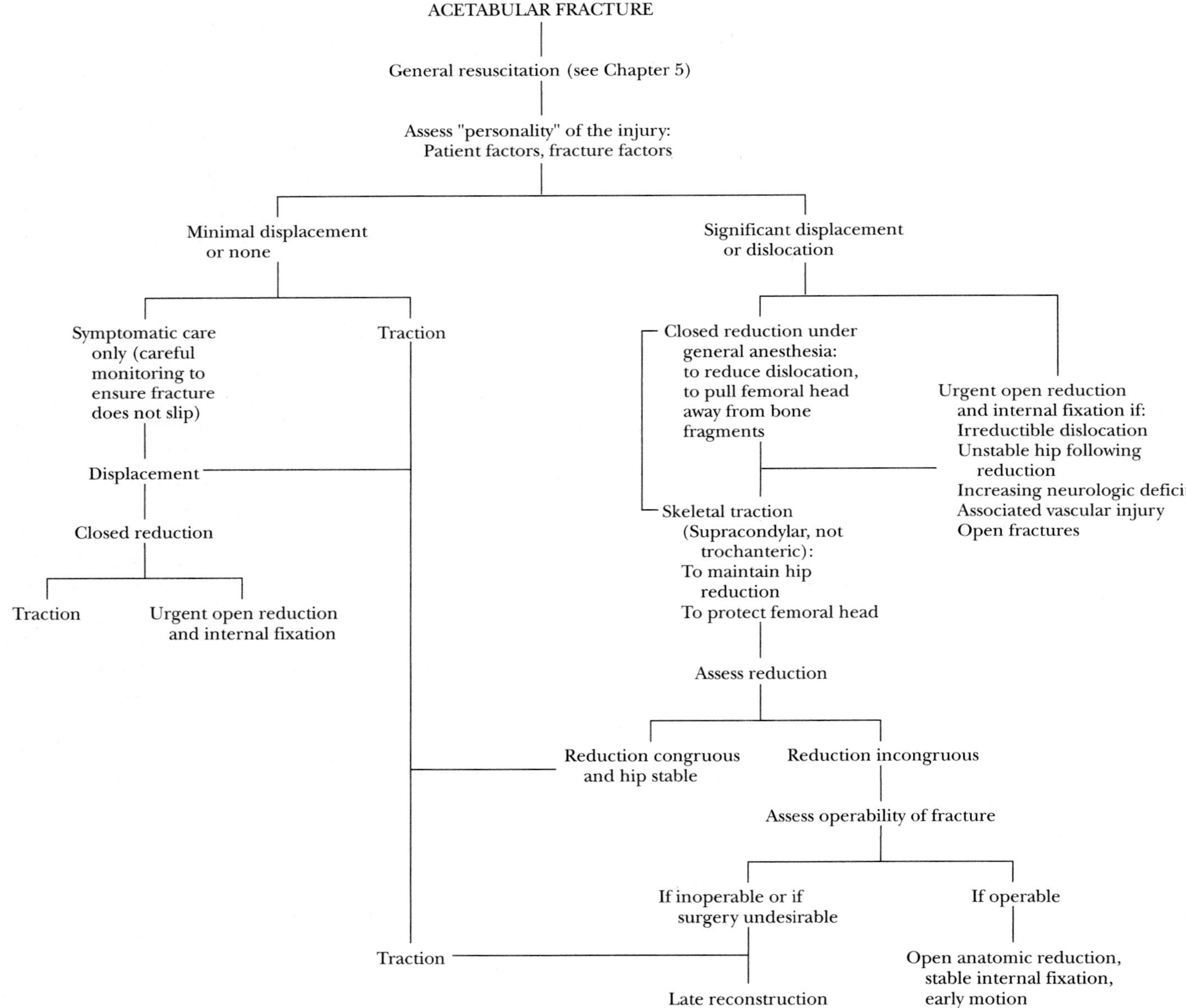

FIGURE 28-1. Management algorithm showing application of indications to the individual patient.

Antibiotics

Prophylactic antibiotics are used in all cases because of the magnitude of the operative procedure. The preferred drug is a cephalosporin given i.v. immediately preoperatively and for at least 48 hours thereafter; it is safe to discontinue coverage at that point if no complications have arisen.

Blood

Although bleeding should not be profuse, the possibility of major hemorrhage is real; therefore, 4 to 6 units of blood should be available for the operation. In centers so equipped, intraoperative cell saver blood replacement is being used successfully in order to mitigate the dependency on banked blood.

SURGICAL IMPORTANCE OF RECENT ADVANCES IN THE KNOWLEDGE OF THE BLOOD SUPPLY TO THE HIP AND ACETABULUM

Blood Supply to the Femoral Head

The intraosseous terminations of the medial femoral circumflex artery (MFCA), the lateral femoral circumflex artery (LCFA), the artery of the round ligament, and the intraosseous vessels are discussed extensively in the literature (1–7). There is general agreement that the deep branch of the MFCA is the most important contributor to the blood supply of the femoral head. It provides blood to two thirds to four fifths of the weight-bearing part of the femoral head (4–6,8,9). Branches of the LCFA supply the anterior joint capsule and femoral neck (6,10). The artery of the round ligament usually originates from the obturator artery, although occasionally it arises as a branch of the MFCA (6,11,12). Although some authors believe the artery of the round ligament is a major supplier of blood to the femoral head (1,6), its contribution in adults is most likely restricted to the perifoveal area (8,9,11–13). In addition, the intraosseous branches of the first perforating artery and the intraosseous vascular system supply the proximal part of the shaft and the neck of the femur. They anastomose with vessels within the femoral head, particularly in the caudal part of the head (4,6,8), but their primary contribution is limited to the femoral neck (5).

With respect to surgical implications, the extracapsular course of the medial femoral circumflex artery was delineated in a recent cadaveric injection study (14). After its origin from the deep femoral artery and the division of the ascending and superficial branches, the deep branch of the MFCA runs between the iliopsoas and the pectineus muscle in a dorsal direction. It then courses proximal to the lesser trochanter at the base of the femoral neck along the inferior border of the obturator externus muscle. The vessel runs anterior and cranial to the quadratus femoris muscle toward the intertrochanteric crest. The vessel emerges between the quadratus femoris and obturator externus muscle adjacent to their insertion into the proximal femur. At this point, one to two branches are given off to the greater trochanter. The main vessel, with a diameter of about 3 mm, runs along the intertrochanteric crest and crosses the tendon of the obturator externus posteriorly and the tendon of inferior gemellus, internal obturator, and superior gemellus anteriorly. It obliquely perforates the capsule (Fig. 28-2) just cranial to the insertion of the tendon of the superior gemellus and caudal to the tendon of the piriformis, where it ramifies into two to four subsynovial terminal branches (superior retinacular arteries) (Fig. 28-3). Twenty percent of the hips also have two vessels dorsoinferiorly (inferior retinacular arteries) (14), and the superior retinacular arteries may be slightly thinner in these cases. No vessels were found on the posterior aspect of the femoral neck. An important anastomosis exists between the medial femoral circumflex artery and a branch of the inferior gluteal artery. This branch of the inferior gluteal artery (IGA) runs along the inferior border of the piriformis, crosses posterior to the triceps coxae, and meets the deep branch of the medial femoral circumflex artery in the interval between quadratus femoris and obturator externus muscles. Its size correlates inversely to the size of the deep branch.

Surgical Implications

By understanding the anatomy of the MFCA, the surgeon can dislocate the hip via a Kocher-Langenbeck or Gibson approach with a trochanteric osteotomy without the risk of avascular necrosis (AVN)(15). The preservation of the blood supply to the femoral head during surgical dislocation of the hip was confirmed by continuous Laser Doppler flowmetry measurement (16). The same study revealed that tension on the retinacular arteries by tight suture of the joint capsule may obstruct the perfusion to the femoral head (16). The knowledge of the course of the MFCA with respect to the tendons of the external rotators and the distance to the intertrochanteric crest (Fig. 28-4) is a prerequisite to perform this type of surgery. Dislocation of the hip allows for evaluation and treatment of articular pathologies and also for anatomic reduction of the articular surface in acetabular fractures (17). The deep branch of the MFCA is protected by the obturator externus muscle (Fig. 28-5), which prevents the femoral head from displacing more than 11 cm (14). As long as the obturator externus is intact, the MFCA is not stretched during hip dislocation. If the obturator externus is torn, presumably the deep branch of the MFCA also is damaged and the femoral head is at risk for developing AVN.

Published descriptions of posterior surgical approaches do not give sufficient details to guide the surgeon in reconstructive surgery (18–20) and even propose the ligation of

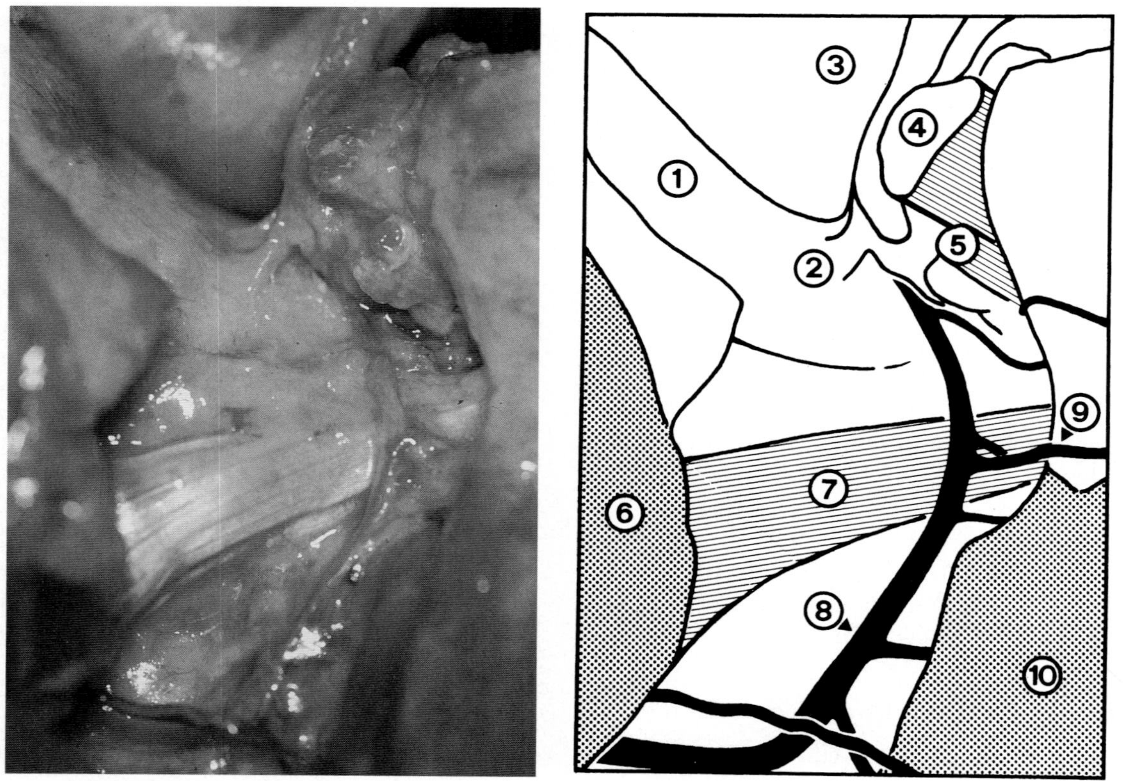

FIGURE 28-2. A: Photograph showing the deep branch of the medial femoral circumflex artery crossing the obturator tendon posteriorly and perforating the joint capsule at the level of the superior gemellus. **B:** Diagram showing the femoral neck *(1)*, the reflexion of the joint capsule *(2)*, anterior joint capsule *(3)*, cut piriformis tendon *(4)*, cut tendons of the triceps coxae *(5)*, muscle body of the triceps coxae *(6)*, obturator externus tendon *(7)*, deep branch of the medial femoral circumflex artery *(8)*, trochanteric branch *(9)*, and quadratus femoris muscle *(10)*.

the MFCA during exposure (21). Usually, section of the short external rotators close to their trochanteric insertion is recommended. However, this is close to the course of the deep branch of the MFCA. In addition, inclusion of the tendon of the obturator externus in the tenotomy risks iatrogenic damage to the deep branch of the MFCA. Therefore, we recommend dividing the external rotators about 1.5 cm medial to their trochanteric insertions while sparing the tendon of the obturator externus.

The branch of the inferior gluteal artery along the piriformis tendon is an important anastomosis to the deep branch of the MCFA. Preservation of this anastomosis may be advantageous in certain situations. For example, when the MFCA has to be sacrificed during radical tumor resection or is damaged in a combined proximal femur and acetabular fracture, preservation of this anastomosis will maintain femoral head perfusion (14).

Finally the metaphyseal vessels contribute as little to the epiphyseal blood supply in the adult (KA Siebenrock, unpublished data). This has been shown by Sevitt (5) and was proven using Laser Doppler flowmetry before and after osteotomy of the femoral neck. This knowledge opens new possibilities for femoral neck osteotomies in the adult, which would avoid some of the disadvantages of intertrochanteric osteotomies such as excessive limb shortening and chronic discomfort with blade-plates *in situ*.

Blood Supply to the Acetabulum

Information of the blood supply to the acetabulum is rare, with only few detailed descriptions (Fig. 28-6) (22–25). The blood supply to the external side is provided through the superior gluteal artery (SGA), IGA, the obturator artery (OA), and the MFCA. The fourth lumbar, iliolumbar artery, and obturator artery contribute to the intrapelvic blood supply. There also is an abundant intraosseous anastomotic network (23,26).

The main nutrient artery of the ilium measures about 1 mm in diameter and is the principal branch of the iliolumbar artery, which usually originates from the posterior trunk of the internal iliac artery (27,28), but also may originate from the obturator artery (29). It is the major source for the vascularization of the supraacetabular bone (14). Laser Doppler flowmetry of the acetabulum during periacetabular osteotomy showed a drop of about 40% of the original blood flow after selective coagulation of the nutrient artery

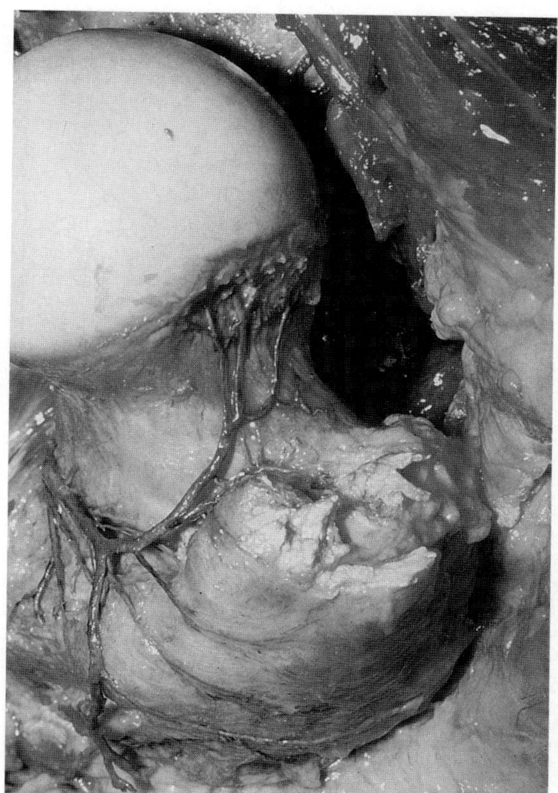

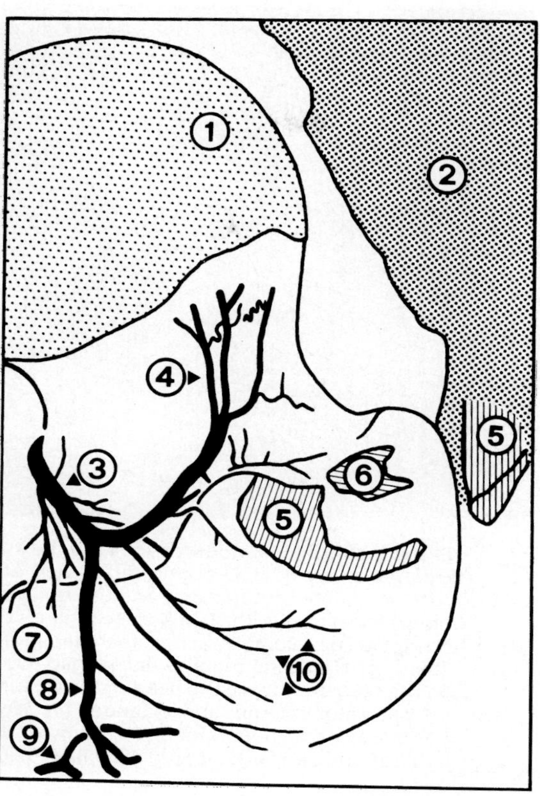

FIGURE 28-3. A: Photograph showing the perforation of the terminal branches into bone *(right hip, posterosuperior view).* The terminal subsynovial branches are located on the posterosuperior aspect of the neck of the femur and penetrate bone 2 to 4 mm lateral to the bone–cartilage junction. **B:** Diagram showing the head of the femur *(1),* gluteus medius *(2),* deep branch of the medial femoral circumflex artery (MFCA) *(3),* terminal subsynovial branches of the MFCA *(4),* insertion and tendon of the gluteus medius *(5),* insertion and tendon of piriformis *(6),* lesser trochanter with nutrient vessels *(7),* trochanteric branch *(8),* branch of the first perforating artery *(9),* and trochanteric branches *(10).* (From: Gautier E, Ganz K, Krugel N, et al. Anatomy of the medial femoral circumflex artery and its surgical implications. *J Bone Joint Surg* 2000;82-B:679–683, with permission.)

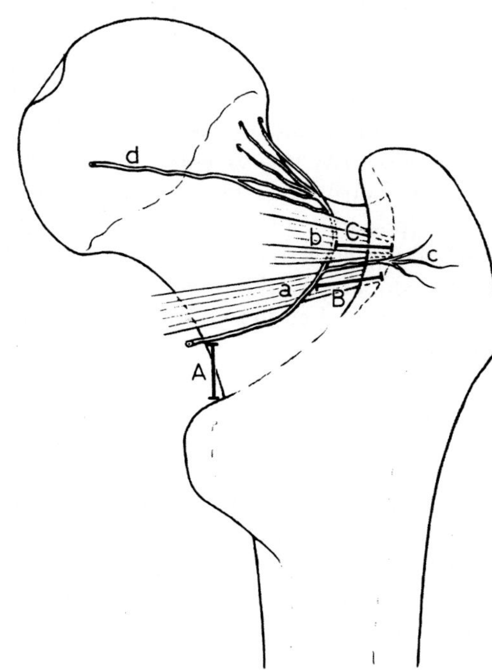

FIGURE 28-4. Diagram showing the course of the deep branch of the medial femoral circumflex artery (MFCA) with respect to the tendons of the: *(a)* the obturator internus; *(b)* obturator externus; *(c)* trochanteric branch; and *(d)* anastomosis to the inferior gluteal artery along inferior rim of the piriformis. Distances of the deep branch of the MFCA to the trochanteric crest at level of the lesser trochanter (A = 18.2 mm), insertion of the obturator externus tendon (B = 8.8 mm), and insertion of the obturator internus (C = 12.4 mm).

A

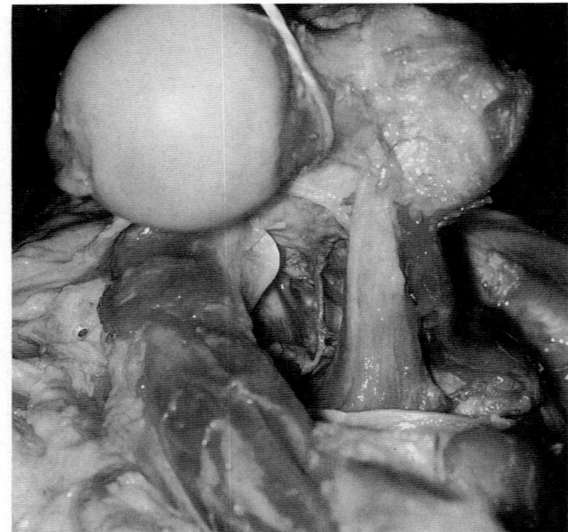

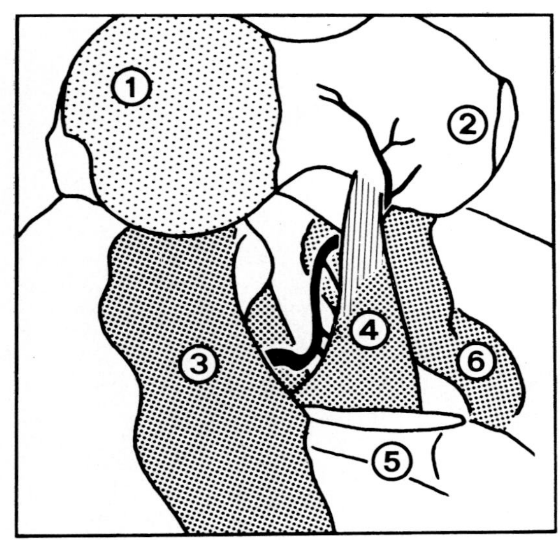

B

FIGURE 28-5. **A:** Photograph showing the integrity of the deep branch of the medial femoral circumflex artery (MFCA) during dislocation of the head of the femur *(right hip, superior view).* After complete capsulectomy and tenotomy of all external rotators, except for the tendon of the obturator externus, the head of the femur is dislocated with external rotation of the femur. There is no stretch or compression of the deep branch of the MFCA during dislocation and the normal course of the vessel remains unchanged. Obturator externus and its tendon protect the vessel. **B:** The diagram shows: the head of the femur *(1),* tip of the greater trochanter *(2),* rectus femoris *(3),* obturator externus and its tendon *(4),* acetabulum *(5),* and quadratus femoris *(6).* (From: Gautier E, Ganz K, Krugel N, et al. Anatomy of the medial femoral circumflex artery and its surgical implications. *J Bone Joint Surg* 2000;82-B:679–683, with permission.)

(30). The nutrient artery usually enters the innominate bone anterior to the iliosacral joint and lateral to the pelvic brim. However, in two of four hips it entered the bone medial to the pelvic brim, in one it originated from the obturator artery (29). The iliolumbar artery also gives a superior ramus to the anterior superior iliac spine and an inferior ramus to the anterior inferior iliac spine and to the iliopectineal eminence, where it anastomoses with a small branch of the deep branch of the SGA.

The principal blood supply to the external pelvis is provided by the SGA (23,29,31). The main stem of this vessel divides into a superficial branch to the gluteus maximus and a deep branch. The deep branch ramifies further into four rami; the superior ramus skirts the cranial border of the gluteus minimus and the inferior ramus traverses horizontally between the gluteus minimus and medius with the superior gluteal nerve to the tensor fasciae latae (27,28). These two vessels mainly supply the gluteus minimus and medius. The blood supply to the acetabulum is provided by the supraacetabular ramus and the acetabular ramus. The supraacetabular ramus courses well protected within the muscular body of the gluteus minimus and anastomoses with the acetabular ramus on the roof of the acetabulum (Fig. 28-7). It most commonly originates from the inferior ramus, but also can arise from the superior ramus or directly from the deep branch (29). The acetabular ramus originates from the deep branch and courses along the inferior border of the gluteus minimus to the posterior-superior acetabulum. After its anastomosis with the supraacetabular ramus at the midportion of the acetabular roof it continues to the interspinous crest, where it anastomoses with the ascending branch of the LCFA and with the iliolumbar artery.

The obturator artery contributes both to the intrapelvic and extrapelvic vascularization. It gives small branches to the quadrilateral plate during its intrapelvic course. After its emergence from the obturator canal it anastomoses with the IGA and occasionally with the deep branch of the MFCA anteriorly (13,14,29). The acetabular ramus enters the joint via the acetabular notch deep to the transverse ligament and supplies the round ligament and the floor of the fossa acetabuli. Anterior-inferiorly, two branches of the deep branch of the MFCA contribute to the vascularity of the acetabulum. One supplies the anterior-inferior joint capsule. The other runs along the lateral border of the pectineus muscle and supplies the anterior-inferior acetabulum. It continues to the iliopectineal eminence and anastomoses with the inferior ramus of the iliolumbar artery.

Anastomotic Network

Substantial communications between the intraosseous and periosteal vascular systems have been described (23,26). Periosteal anastomoses are found around the acetabulum and more peripherally at the edges of the iliac bone. The systems of the superior gluteal artery, the fourth lumbar and iliolumbar artery, and the superficial and deep iliac circum-

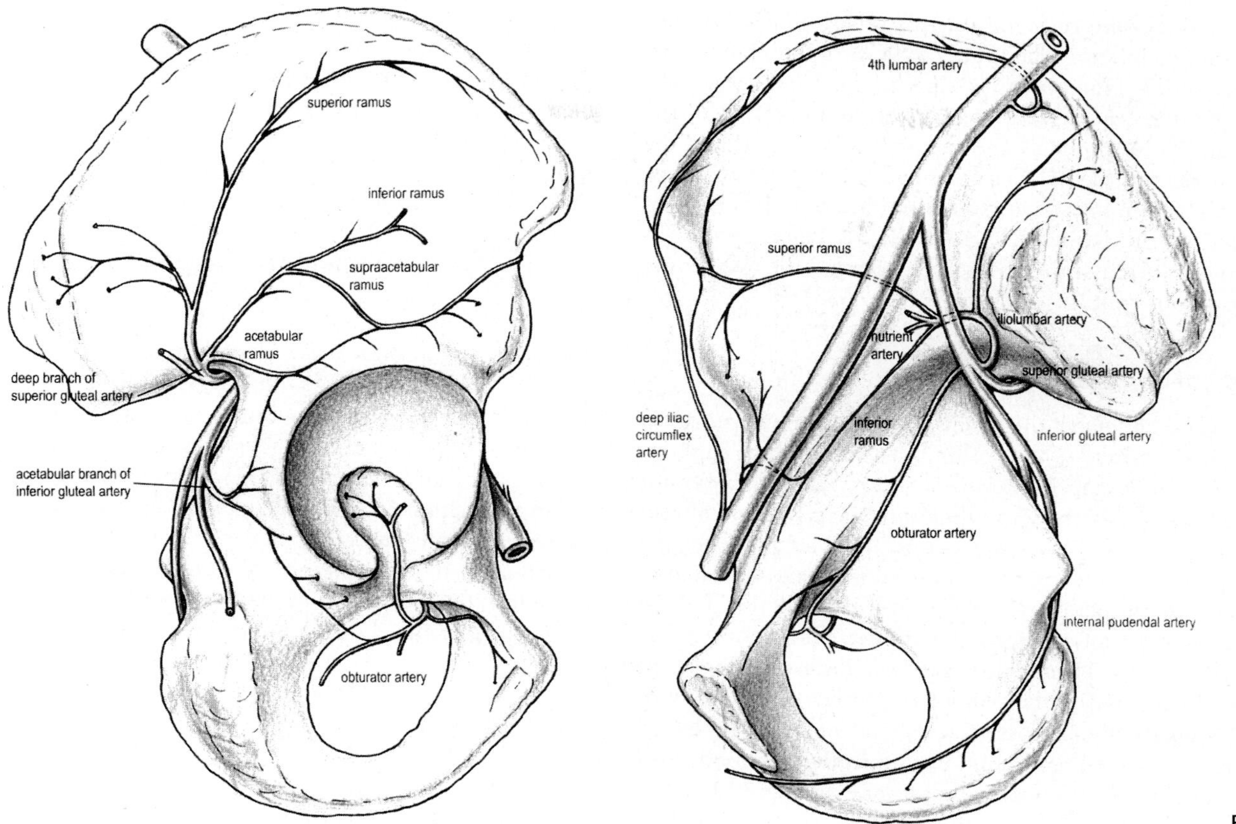

FIGURE 28-6. A: Diagram of the blood supply to the external side of acetabulum of a right hip. For reason of simplicity the medial femoral circumflex artery and its branches to the anterior-inferior acetabulum are omitted. **B:** Intrapelvic blood supply. The schematic drawing includes the blood vessels important to the acetabular blood supply; visceral arteries are omitted. In hips, where the nutrient artery enters medial to the pelvic brim, the inferior ramus of the iliolumbar artery originates directly from the obturator artery.

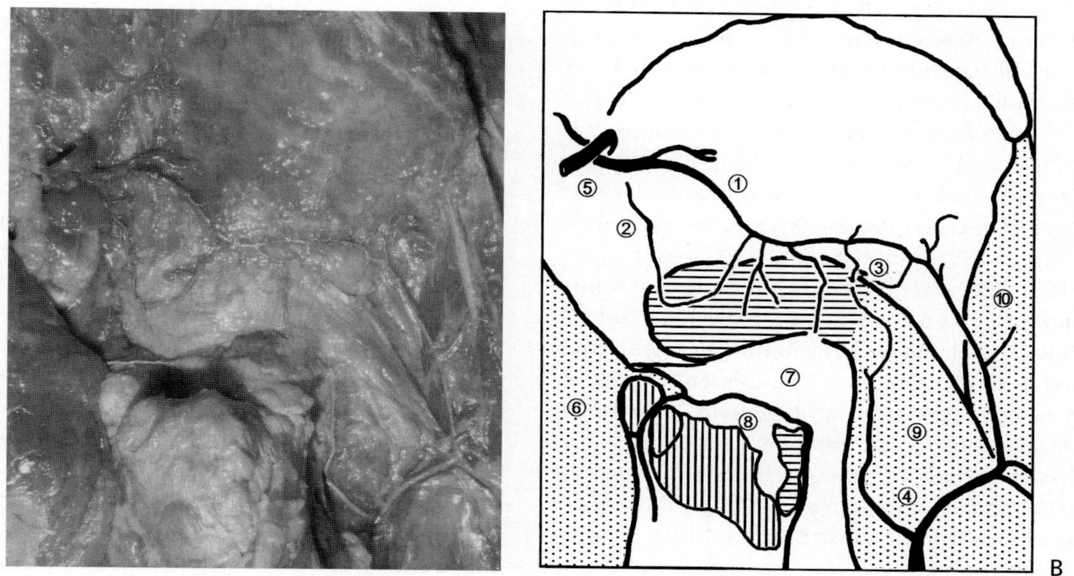

FIGURE 28-7. A: Anterior-lateral view of a right hip. The superior gluteal artery with the supraacetabular and acetabular ramus supplies the roof of the acetabulum. After their anastomosis they continue to the anterior inferior iliac spine and anastomose with the ascending branch of the lateral femoral circumflex artery (LFCA). **B:** The diagram shows: supraacetabular *(1)* and acetabular *(2)* ramus of the superior gluteal artery (SGA), anterior inferior iliac spine *(3)*, ascending branch of the LFCA *(4)*, sciatic notch with deep branch of the SGA *(5)* to the gluteus maximus, detached gluteus medius *(6)*, joint capsule *(7)*, greater trochanter *(8)*, rectus femoris muscle with reflected tendon *(9)*, and tensor fasciae latae *(10)*.

flex arteries converge at the anterior superior iliac spine. At the anterior inferior iliac spine the SGA, iliolumbar artery, and ascending branch of the LCFA anastomose. Periacetabular anastomoses exist between the obturator and IGA, the IGA and SGA, the SGA and the iliolumbar artery, and the iliolumbar and the MFCA. Irregularly, an extrapelvic anastomosis is found between the obturator artery and the deep branch of the MFCA (13,14,20), and between the intrapelvic portion of the obturator artery and the SGA at the interspinous crest (29,32).

Surgical Implications

The blood supply to the supraacetabular bone depends on the nutrient artery of the iliolumbar artery and the supraacetabular and acetabular ramus of the SGA. In a fracture or osteotomy of this area extending into the posterior column or sciatic buttress, the intraosseous blood supply from the iliolumbar artery is interrupted and the remaining vascularity relies on the periosteal blood supply through the SGA. In these cases or after an approach with detachment of the iliac muscle from the inside of the pelvis, additional stripping of the abductors should be avoided to prevent disturbances of the blood supply. The supraacetabular ramus is protected within the gluteus minimus during limited subperiosteal dissection of the supraacetabular bone surface (29). This allows for safe tunneling of the abductors to place a reduction clamp from the interspinous crest to the sciatic notch, if a substantial portion of the gluteus minimus muscle is left undisturbed near the hip joint.

Certain anatomic vascular variations can result in excessive intraoperative bleeding. The entry point of the nutrient artery of the ilium usually is lateral of the pelvic brim (33) and can be coagulated during the approach. However, if it enters the iliac bone medial to pelvic brim, as was the case in 50% of our specimens, quite often the nutrient ramus cannot be visualized and coagulated. In addition, a supraacetabular osteotomy always interrupts the nutrient artery and bleeding from its intraosseous course may be difficult to control.

The fragments in posterior wall fractures depend on the vascular supply from small branches of the IGA and the acetabular branch of the SGA. Visualization and protection of these vessels is difficult but may be important to preserve the viability of these posterior wall fragments. The role of the LFCA for the supraacetabular blood supply is poorly known, although there is an anastomosis with the supraacetabular and acetabular ramus of the SGA (Fig. 28-6). These anastomoses may contribute substantially to the remaining vascularity of superior and posterior wall fragments. However, often the only remaining blood supply for acetabular wall fragments is via the joint capsule. Although the exact blood supply to the joint capsule is not known, vessels from the SGA, IGA, LFCA, and MFCA contribute to the vascularization of the joint capsule. Capsulotomy or extensions of the ruptured joint capsule should be avoided if possible because the capsule may be the only remaining blood supply to the fragments in acetabular wall fractures. This also is true for spherical osteotomies close to the joint (34,35), where the only other source may be the acetabular ramus of the obturator artery. The Bernese periacetabular osteotomy (36,37) and osteotomies more distant to the joint should leave the OA, SGA, and IGA intact (29), providing sufficient perfusion of the acetabular fragment.

ANESTHESIA

Expert and experienced anesthesia is essential. General, regional, or combinations thereof are the types of anesthesia advocated, and depend on many factors, including the institution, patient factors, length of the procedure, and the need for intraoperative nerve monitoring. Obviously, regional is most preferable, not only intraoperatively, but also for postoperative pain management, but requires dedicated and involved anesthesiologists as part of the team.

NERVE MONITORING

Intraoperative monitoring of the nerves of the lower extremity has become standard practice in many centers to prevent nerve injury. Measurements of both sensory and motor evoked potentials are required and are being used successfully for this purpose.

SPECIFIC CONSIDERATIONS

Position and Use of the Traction Table

The position of the patient—prone, supine, or lateral—depends on the surgeon's operative approach. Universal use of a traction table is still a controversial recommendation. If a traction table is used because it is the surgeon's preference, then it is incumbent on that surgeon to choose a versatile one, that is, one that allows manipulating the limb in almost any position and still permits fluoroscopy. The Tasserit ("Judet"-type) table, especially designed for this purpose, was designed and deemed invaluable by Letournel and others as an intraoperative tool (38,39). Unfortunately, the Tasserit table is no longer commercially available! The assistance of an unscrubbed surgeon or a technician trained in its use was essential, to enable manipulation of the limb during the operation.

We rarely use a traction table for several reasons. First, we do not have a Tasserit table. Second, a fracture table with a central post may hinder unbridled fluoroscopic views intraoperatively. Third, the perineal post or fracture table may cause specific complications (e.g., pudendal nerve palsy). Fourth, the fracture table may limit full motion of the extremity (e.g., hip flexion with the ilioinguinal approach). Fifth, and most important, it is possible to achieve similar traction and limb positioning without the fracture table. Traction can be applied directly to the femoral head by various means, such as a sharp hook placed around the greater trochanter or a corkscrew driven into the femoral neck. Or even more elegantly, the femoral distractor can be applied intraoperatively to the pelvis and femur via Schantz screws and traction and limb positioning "dialed in." Therefore, we prefer to place the patient on a totally radiolucent table, which can rotate (Jackson, OSI in type) and drape the affected extremity "free," which allows full and unrestricted manipulation of the hip joint during surgery. Until the issue has been studied more rigorously, surgeon's preference dictates whether or not a traction table is used, but either way the patient must be intraoperative x-ray "visible."

SPECIFIC SURGICAL APPROACHES AND TECHNIQUES

Introduction

Prior to the classic work by Judet and coworkers (40,41) and Letournel (42–44), there was little understanding of the complex pathoanatomy and proper surgical management of acetabular fractures. However, following the introduction of their classification scheme and novel surgical approaches, the last three decades have seen improvements in surgical approaches, techniques of reduction, and implants, leading to more consistently good results (40–50). Unfortunately, the management of these difficult fractures remains a challenging problem.

The care of the patient with a pelvic injury begins with prompt resuscitation performed by a trained multidisciplinary trauma team and accurate assessment and stabilization of any life-threatening injuries. Once the patient has been stabilized, definitive treatment should only be undertaken by a surgeon experienced in handling such fractures.

A patient's functional outcome following an acetabular fracture is dependent on several factors—some controllable, but others injury-related and inevitable. Of the surgical factors, the most important is obtaining an anatomic reduction of the articular surface and fixation stable enough to allow early range of motion while avoiding both acute and late complications. The achievement of these goals can be a demanding and frustrating task, which cannot be achieved without the following resources (51): (a) An experienced surgeon who uses atraumatic techniques, including the preservation of the blood supply to the femoral head and articular fragments without causing undue additional trauma; (b) a knowledgeable nursing team able to produce readily the proper and necessary reduction and fixation devices, including the specialized pelvic reduction clamps, instruments, and implants; (c) an accomplished anesthetist able to paralyze the patient and able to respond to any eventuality; (d) ± a neurophysiologist to provide nerve monitoring; and (e) a fluoroscopy table and the ability to obtain intraoperative fluoroscopic or plain x-ray views of the pelvis and hip joint. A thorough understanding of the complex anatomy of the pelvis is necessary prior to surgical treatment because surgical outcomes greatly depend on an accurate diagnosis and an appropriately chosen and well-executed approach.

Indications for Surgery

(See also Chapter 27.) Because malreduction or subluxation of the hip joint can lead to abnormal loading of the articular cartilage with subsequent joint arthrosis (43,44,47,49, 50,52–56), acetabular fractures should be treated with the same principles granted to other intraarticular fractures. Therefore, the primary goal in their management is to perform an accurate reduction of the articular surface in order to obtain a congruent hip joint and therefore restore normal joint mechanics. To this end, the decision to perform surgery is based on many factors including the patient, the "personality" of the fracture, and the capabilities of the surgical team. However, the patient's medical condition (associated injuries, comorbidities, etc.), physiologic age, and functional needs are also key determinants of the treatment algorithm.

With respect to the injury pattern itself, indications for operative fixation include displacement of the articular surface, joint incongruity, unacceptable roof arc measurements, incarceration of an intraarticular fragment within the hip joint, and any subluxation of the femoral head (50,54,57–60). Although most authors now agree that anatomic reduction of the weight-bearing surface and concentric reduction of the hip are essential for long-term satisfactory results (38–40,44,49,50,57,61–75), the degree of hip joint incongruity that can be tolerated still is not known.

Helfet and Schmeling (65) observed that an articular step off of >2 mm or a gap of >3 mm was associated with a fourfold increase in joint space narrowing at early follow-up. This was confirmed in a prospective study by Matta (47), who achieved an anatomic reduction in 71% of 262 acetabular fractures, with 83% of these patients having good or excellent outcomes at an average follow-up of 6 years. Of the 29% with an imperfectly reduced acetabulum, good or excellent results were obtained in 68% of cases if the defect measured 2 to 3 mm, and only 50% if >3 mm. The most clearly predictive initial factor was damage to the femoral head. Malkani and coworkers (67) and Hak and coworkers (63) have used cadaver models to further support 2 mm or less as the appropriate prerequisite for an acceptable reduction.

The location of the fracture also is important. Matta and coauthors have shown that an intact 45-degree roof arc and a congruent hip joint are mandatory in order to achieve a satisfactory result (47,54,58,59). Other authors have noted that fractures involving generally >40% of the posterior wall will result in instability, whereas those affecting <20% of the wall are stable (50,76,77). Building on this knowledge, Olson (60) developed strict criteria for consideration of nonoperative treatment: (a) the articular surface must be intact in the superior 10 mm of the joint on computed tomography (CT); (b) without traction, the femoral head must remain congruent with the superior acetabulum on the anterior-posterior (AP) and 45-degree oblique views; and (c) a minimum of 50% of the posterior wall articular surface must be intact.

Such objective criteria cannot be considered absolute, as Tornetta (78) has demonstrated that although satisfying the preceding guidelines, some fractures still require stabilization because of dynamic instability. This particular entity can be identified be performing dynamic stress views while the patient is sedated or anesthetized. Finally, Olson and coworkers (71) have found that small defects in the posterior wall produce major changes in the articular contact area that may predispose to late posttraumatic degenerative changes even in the presence of clinical stability. Another controversy regards displaced both-column fractures that demonstrate secondary congruence, which some have argued may not routinely require operative reduction and stabilization, especially in the older patient (44,50,64,68,78). However, a recent biomechanical cadaver study has shown that abnormal increases in stress concentration still occur in the dome of the acetabulum adjacent to the fracture line in such cases (79).

Timing of Surgery

Fractures of the acetabulum often pose many diagnostic and technical problems. Therefore, acute open reduction and internal fixation rarely are indicated. Exceptions to this include dislocations that cannot be reduced by closed means, an incarcerated intraarticular fragment following closed reduction, and unstable posterior dislocations that cannot be held in the reduced position because of the marked deficiency of the posterior wall. The former should be considered a surgical emergency and a reduction of the dislocation performed as soon as possible after the injury. Progressive or sciatic nerve palsy that develops after reduction of the dislocation also should be considered a surgical emergency. Rare indications for emergent surgical intervention include an open fracture of the acetabulum and an anterior column fracture associated with a femoral artery lesion (51). In all other circumstances, the timing of surgery is more dependent on stabilization of associated visceral, skeletal, and soft-tissue injuries, the completion of all imaging studies necessary for careful preoperative planning, and the availability of an experienced surgeon. A difficult procedure then can be performed on an elective basis with a more experienced operating team, usually between the second and fifth day after the time of injury.

Although deferral of operative treatment for up to 2 weeks usually provides only a minor compromise to the ease of surgical reduction, delays of over a week should be avoided if possible. One study has noted an average time to surgery of 11 days for fractures with an acceptable reduction (80), whereas another demonstrated a correlation with poorer results when surgical stabilization was undertaken after 7 days (81). Beyond 2 weeks, an anatomic reduction becomes progressively harder to obtain because of the increasingly difficult task of meticulously taking down varying amounts of callus, organizing hematoma and granulation tissue (38,39,42,44,49,50,62,68,73,75,82–87). Letournel himself found that his rate of anatomic reduction dropped from 75% to 62% of cases in this group of patients (44).

Preoperative Planning

Because patients with acetabular fractures often present with associated visceral injuries and skeletal injuries to such structures as the pelvis, femur, and ipsilateral knee, the preoperative evaluation needs to begin with a thorough physical examination and appropriate trauma work-up. Accurate assessment of the patient's neurologic status also is mandatory because the incidence of preoperative, posttraumatic sciatic nerve compromise following acetabular fractures has ranged from 12% to 38% (44,49,57,59,88–92).

Another important part of the preoperative work-up includes both prophylaxis and surveillance for deep vein thrombosis (DVT), which has been reported to occur in as many as 35% to 60% of patients with pelvic fractures (93–96). Patients with acetabular fractures awaiting transfer to another institution for their definitive care are at especially high risk for DVT and require prophylaxis. Letournel (44) reported a 3% incidence of clinically evident DVT with four fatal and eight minor pulmonary emboli in a series of 569 patients, in spite of the majority receiving anticoagulant prophylaxis. In a prospective study, Geerts and coworkers (93) demonstrated a 60% incidence of DVT in patients with primary lower extremity orthopedic injuries and Kudsk and coworkers (94) demonstrated a 60% incidence of silent DVT by venography in patients with multiple trauma immobilized 10 days or more. Montgomery and coworkers (97) used magnetic resonance (MR) venography to evaluate 45 consecutive patients with a displaced acetabular fracture, noting 24 asymptomatic thrombi in the thigh and pelvis of 15 patients (33%). During the preoperative period, we prefer subcutaneous heparin combined with an intermittent pneumatic compression device, and magnetic resonance venography (MRV) to rule out a DVT (95,97,98). Although most studies have found MRV to be highly specific and sensitive (95,97–100), some have questioned its value (101,102). If a significant clot is diagnosed, most patients undergo placement of a vena caval filter and are treated with i.v. heparin prior to surgery.

A thorough understanding of the complex pathoanatomy involved is extremely important prior to attempting operative fixation. An accurate diagnosis of the basic fracture pattern can be accomplished with three basic roentgenograms described by Judet and coworkers (40): An AP view of the pelvis, an iliac oblique view of the acetabulum, and an obturator oblique view of the acetabulum. This initial roentgenographic survey, with accurate delineation of all fracture lines, provides vital information that dictates the treatment plan. If surgery is indicated, this information also helps the surgeon select the optimal surgical approach.

The addition of conventional CT scans with thin slice (1 to 3 mm) axial cuts allows for better appreciation of the extent of injury. Although CT provides little additional information regarding simple column fractures, it is particularly helpful in evaluating the integrity of the dome, posterior lip, sacrum, sacroiliac joint, and femoral head; and delineating the rotation of the columns and presence of intraarticular bony fragments (60,103,104). Although obtaining both the plain films and a CT scan may seem redundant, intraoperative decision-making and technique depends on a clear understanding of the former. These are superior for evaluating hip joint congruency and can be compared with intraoperative and postoperative images. Advances in imaging software technology have led to the development of three-dimensional computed tomography (3DCT), which can help provide a better understanding of the spatial relationship of the fracture pattern relative to the pelvis as a whole. Although its role is not yet altogether defined, it can be useful when viewed real time on a monitor, which allows visualization of the fracture from various projections. 3DCT scans can be used in conjunction with plain roentgenograms, including Judet views, and axial CT scans for teaching, to facilitate preoperative planning, and especially in late cases such as acetabular nonunions and malunions.

It is often helpful to transfer the fracture lines from these radiographic studies to a model pelvis. Such a 3D perspective can assist the surgeon in the selection of the optimal surgical approach, reduction technique, and method of fixation for the major fracture fragments. These decisions are made with the expectation that the entire procedure can be performed through a single operative incision.

Selection of the Optimal Surgical Approach

The surgeon must use a surgical exposure that will afford the best opportunity to restore joint congruency by anatomic reduction and stabilization of the articular surface, while resulting in the least morbidity. To this end, Mayo (48) has identified five major factors that affect this decision: (a) the fracture pattern; (b) the local soft-tissue conditions; (c) the presence of associated major systemic injuries; (d) the age and projected functional status of the patient; and (e) the interval from injury to surgery. Under most circumstances, the first of these—the fracture pattern—is the major determinant. Therefore, it is important to accurately classify the fracture using either the Letournel-Judet (42–45) (Table 28-1) or Comprehensive Classification (105) system (Table 28-2) (45). Importantly, any additional injuries to the pelvic ring also must be considered. Finally, it should be appreciated that the selection of the proper surgical exposure also is driven by the experience of the operating surgeon to a large extent.

When open treatment is indicated, the majority of acetabular fractures can be treated with a single more lim-

TABLE 28-1. GUIDELINES FOR CHOICE OF APPROACH TO ACETABULAR FRACTURES (LETOURNEL-JUDET)

Type of Fracture	Approach
Anterior	
CEPHALAD TO ILIOPECTINEAL Eminence	Iliofemoral
Complex patterns requiring exposure to the symphysis and quadrilateral plate	Ilioinguinal
Posterior wall or posterior column	Posterior Kocher-Langenbeck
Transverse, with posterior wall involvement	Posterior Kocher-Langenbeck, transtrochanteric; sequential or combined anterior and posterior approach
Transverse, no posterior wall	Approach depends on the level, obliquity, and displacement of the fracture; anterior and posterior combined/extensile
T type	Approach depends on pattern: may be posterior, anterior, extensile, or some combination
Both-column	Ilioinguinal, modified Ilioinguinal, extended iliofemoral, triradiate, transtrochanteric, or combined

TABLE 28-2. CHOICE OF APPROACH TO ACETABULAR FRACTURES (AO: COMPREHENSIVE CLASSIFICATION)

Type of Fracture	Approach
Type A: Partial articular, involving only one of the two columns	
A1 (POSTERIOR WALL FRACTURE)	Kocher-Langenbeck—lateral decubitus
A2 (Posterior column)	Kocher-Langenbeck
A3 (Anterior column or wall)	Ilioinguinal
Type B: Partial articular, involving a transverse component	
B1 (pure transverse)	Approach depends on the level and obliquity of the transverse component, direction of rotation, and the column with the major displacement. For most fractures, a Kocher-Langenbeck (prone) will be successful. For transtectal pure transverse (B1-2) and difficult associated transverse and posterior wall fractures (B1-3), an extensile approach may be preferred.
B2 (T-shaped)	If the major displacement is posterior, particularly in the infratectal or juxtatectal type, and there is an associated posterior wall fracture, then the Kocher Langenbeck should be utilized. When the major displacement or rotation is primarily anterior, then the ilioinguinal should be employed. The patient should be prepped for both exposures, in case a supplemental approach is required. For fractures, which are transtectal, comminuted, displaced, or of late presentation, an extensile approach may be required.
B3 (Anterior column and posterior hemitransverse)	Ilioinguinal
Type C: Fractures (complete articular: both-columns)	
C1 (High variety, extending to the iliac crest)	Ilioinguinal, unless there is complex involvement of the posterior column and/or wall, which will necessitate an extensile approach
C2 (Low variety, extending to the anterior border of the ilium)	Same as C1
C3 (Extension into the sacroiliac joint)	C3 Extended iliofemoral

ited anterior or posterior surgical approach (43,44,48,57, 65,72,106,107). Using the technique of indirect reduction with a single nonextensile approach in 84 complex acetabular fractures involving two columns, Helfet and Schmeling (65,108) reported a success rate of 91%, a deep infection rate of 0%, and an incidence of significant heterotopic ossification of 2%. Therefore, if an adequate preoperative evaluation of the patient and fracture pattern has been performed, then it is rare that a second surgical approach will be required. This is important because extensile exposures involve greater patient morbidity compared to single anterior or posterior approaches, including increased operative time, blood loss, infection, nerve injury abductor weakness, joint stiffness, and heterotopic ossification (39,44,48,49,54, 57,62,68,74,75,82,109–112).

However, for more complex fracture patterns involving both acetabular columns and those delayed past 2 to 3 weeks, an extensile or combined anterior and posterior surgical exposure may be necessary for visualization and reduction (39,42,44,49,50,62,67,68,72–75,82–84,87,107). An extensile approach also might be considered in lieu of the ilioinguinal should there be a nearby suprapubic catheter or colostomy, which presents a greater risk for infection (39). Although the extended iliofemoral approach (42–44) is presently the preferred extensile exposure for the surgical stabilization of acetabular fractures, other extensile approaches have been described. Senegas and coworkers (113) reported a transtrochanteric approach, which is a modification of the Ollier approach and allows limited exposure of the anterior column above the supraacetabular region. Another transtrochanteric approach that has been used in the past is a modification of the Gibson approach, which involves a straight lateral incision (21,74,114). Finally, Reinert and coworkers (115) described a T-shaped modification of the extended iliofemoral approach. Mears and Rubash (116,117) popularized the triradiate approach.

These later approaches require osteotomy of the greater trochanter, which carries the additional risk of nonunion and also has been associated with an increased risk of heterotopic ossification (109,111).

Perhaps blunt trauma to the gluteal muscle mass and peritrochanteric region is the most troubling finding when planning a posterior or extended approach. Contusions and abrasions over this region may herald the presence of the "Morel-Lavalle" lesion. The area is usually fluctuant secondary to a large hematoma and fat necrosis developing under the degloved skin and subcutaneous tissues. Despite their closed nature, these are associated with high rates of secondary bacterial contamination and must be addressed with surgical decompression, debridement, and drainage prior to definitive fracture care (118). Another relative contraindication for a posterior or extensile approach is the presence of a closed-head injury, which has the potential in and of itself to lead to massive heterotopic ossification (118–121). In these cases, the ilioinguinal approach has been recommended if the fracture pattern permits (121).

Fracture Patterns Affecting Primarily One Column

Fracture patterns that strictly involve only the posterior elements, such as the posterior wall (Type A1), posterior column (Type A2), and comminuted posterior variants are best exposed through the Kocher-Langenbeck approach. Prone or lateral positioning is at the discretion of the surgeon.

In contrast, fracture patterns that involve primarily the anterior aspect of the acetabulum, such as the anterior column (Type A3), anterior wall (Type A3), and anterior column with a posterior hemitransverse component (Type B3) are best suited for the anterior ilioinguinal approach. Anterior column variants, which exit in the vicinity of the iliopectineal eminence, are termed "low," as opposed to fractures with a large iliac fragment, which are described as "high" (122). In certain cases, such as with some of the "high" variants, a more limited exposure, such as the standard iliofemoral (Smith-Petersen) approach might suffice (51).

The choice of the proper approach for more complex fracture patterns may not be as straightforward.

Transverse Fracture Patterns

In the case of the pure transverse (Type B1) and the T-type (Type B2) fractures, the choice of the optimal approach depends on the column with the greatest involvement, direction of rotation and displacement, height of the fracture relative to the femoral head, obliquity of the transverse fracture, presence of impaction, and status of the acetabular walls. The degree of displacement and extent of wall involvement is best seen on CT (Figs. 28-8 and 28-9).

If the anterior column has the greatest displacement after preoperative assessment, then the ilioinguinal is the approach of choice. However, more commonly the posterior column demonstrates the major displacement and rotation. In these cases, particularly with an infratectal or juxtatectal fracture, the Kocher-Langenbeck approach should be used. The presence of an associated posterior wall fracture also mandates a posterior or extensile approach. Among the most difficult fractures are the high transverse (transtectal) and T-type fracture patterns with involvement of the weight-bearing dome. These variants often require an extensile approach or a combined anterior and posterior expo-

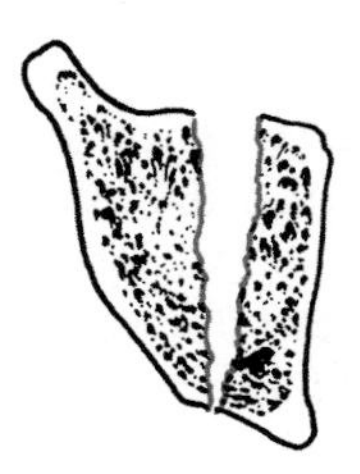

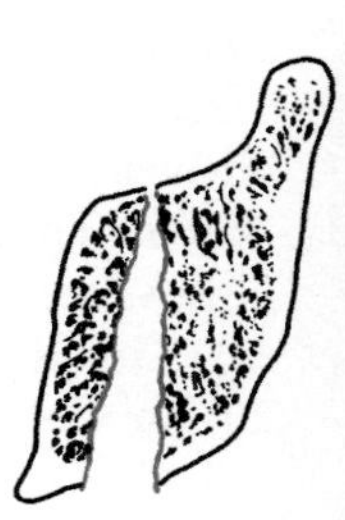

A

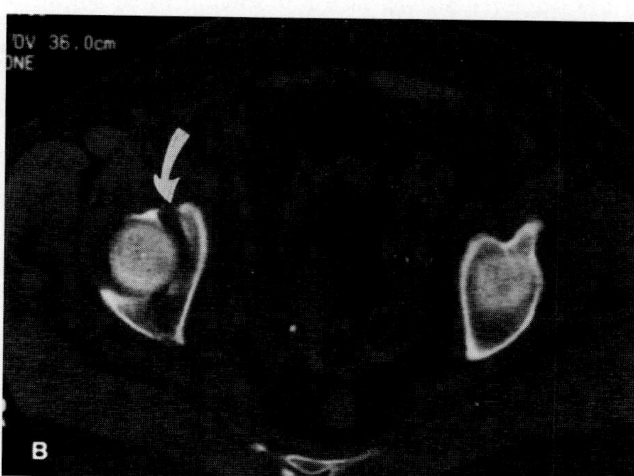

FIGURE 28-8. For transverse fractures of the acetabulum the choice of anterior or posterior approach depends on many factors, including the rotation of the transverse fracture. **A:** Here, the rotation is anterior (i.e., an anterior gap is noted on computed tomography, as depicted in the drawing **(A)** and the CT **(B)**). The approach should be anterior, whereas if the rotation is posterior and is associated with any major fragments of the posterior wall, the approach should be posterior (Kocher-Langenbeck).

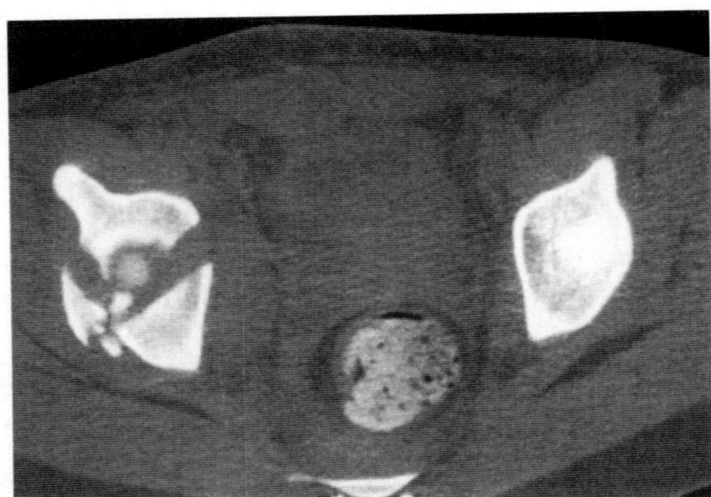

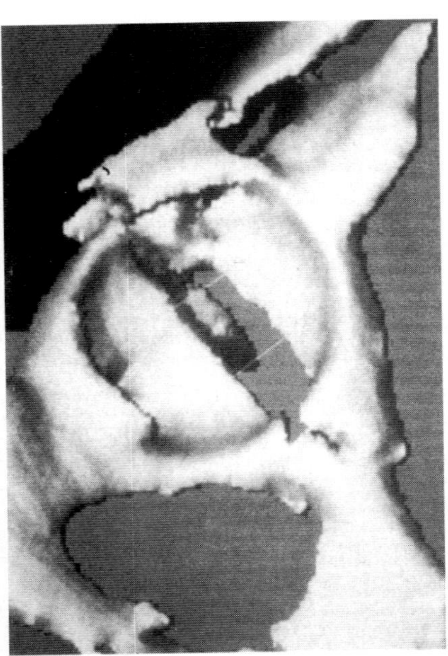

FIGURE 28-9. Computed tomography of both column fracture. **A:** Axial view revealing significant dome comminution. **B:** Three-dimensional reconstruction facilitating perception of fracture configuration. (From: Wiss D, ed. *Master techniques in orthopaedic surgery.* Philadelphia: Lippincott-Raven, 1998, with permission.)

sure in order to gain adequate access to the roof of the acetabulum to facilitate anatomic restoration of the articular surface.

Matta has provided some guidelines when determining whether the fracture should be approached from either a Kocher-Langenbeck or an extensile approach (123). He noted that in his experience, 80% of transverse plus posterior wall fracture patterns were amenable to the former but that the presence of two of the following three conditions mitigated more for an extensile approach: (a) transtectal transverse fractures, because the anterior displacement in these cases may be difficult to control from the posterior aspect of the pelvis, and precise reduction of the roof is imperative; (b) associated symphysis disruption and/or contralateral pubic rami fractures as the "hinge reduction" mechanism for the ischiopubic segment is lost; and (c) the presence of an extended posterior wall pattern, where posterior visualization gives no indication of the quality of the reduction of the transverse component of the fracture. (In such cases the surgeon must look to other areas, such as the articular surface or anterior column cortex.)

Clearly, the novice pelvic surgeon should not attempt a single nonextensile approach for complex transverse and T-type fracture patterns. In cases where the surgeon is uncertain regarding his abilities to reduce such fractures through a single approach but wishes to proceed in such fashion, the patient should be prepped and draped in the floppy lateral position (72,106–108). This will permit the use of a combined anterior and posterior approach, if necessary. If a combined approach is planned or should the anterior column reduction be found to be impossible through a Kocher-Langenbeck approach, the posterior column can be reduced and stabilized from the lateral decubitus position. Following this, the patient is turned to the semisupine position to permit anterior column reduction and fixation via the ilioinguinal approach. The disadvantage of using combined approaches in the floppy lateral position is that visualization of the fracture pattern from either approach is suboptimal. An alternative strategy is to extend an anterior limb from the midportion of the Kocher-Langenbeck incision to the anterior-superior iliac spine, effectively converting the approach to the extensile triradiate approach.

Finally, a simple alternative for difficult fractures, such as those with a split into the superior weight-bearing surface of the joint, is to perform a supplemental greater trochanteric osteotomy. This may facilitate the exposure without resorting to a combined or extensile approach. Removal of the greater trochanter will improve visualization of the posterior column and the superior and posterior aspects of the acetabulum, allow palpation of the anterior column, and lessen the traction on the superior gluteal vessels and nerve (17,51,82,124). For T-type or transverse fractures with posterior and superior wall involvement, this technique also allows palpation and visualization of the anterior portion of the fracture.

Both-Column Fractures

Associated both-column (Type C) fractures are the most impressive for their involvement and displacement of both the anterior and posterior columns, and their complete dissociation from the intact ilium and axial skeleton. In most cases, particularly when the posterior column is a single fragment that can be reduced anteriorly from within the pelvis, an ilioinguinal approach is in order. However, Matta has warned that a clear distinction must be drawn between reduction of both-column fractures and reduction of T-shaped fractures through the ilioinguinal approach, as the latter can be very difficult (125). This is because with both-column fractures, the joint capsule and acetabular labrum often remain firmly attached to both the anterior and posterior column fragments, allowing their reduction from within the pelvis by hinging them on their capsular attachments. In a T-shaped fracture, the posterior column is typically torn away from its capsular attachments and therefore cannot be easily hinged back into place.

Although the ilioinguinal is frequently the approach of choice, both-column fractures require excellent surgical access to the entire ilium, often necessitating an extensile approach such as the extended iliofemoral approach or triradiate, or combined anterior and posterior approaches. These alternatives are generally preferred when patients are taken to the operating room late or when there are complex fracture patterns that extend into the sacroiliac joint (Type C3), involve the weight-bearing dome, have fragmentation of the posterior column, or are associated with a posterior wall fragment large enough to require surgical stabilization.

Because extensile exposures are associated with the highest incidence of heterotopic ossification and postoperative morbidity (44,57,109,112,117,126,127), some surgeons have promoted the use of a simultaneous or sequential anterior and posterior approach to treat complex fracture patterns that involve displacement of both anterior and posterior structures (72,83,85,107,128).

Operating Room Preparation

General, regional, or combinations thereof are the types of anesthesia advocated, and depend on many factors, including the institution, patient factors, length of the procedure, and need for intraoperative nerve monitoring. Obviously, regional is most preferable (not only intraoperatively but also for postoperative pain management) but requires dedicated and involved anesthesiologists as part of the team. The addition of epidural catheterization also is beneficial because of reduced inhalation anesthetic requirement (48), reduced blood loss, and improved postoperative pain relief. Because of the magnitude of the operative procedure, prophylactic antibiotics are used in all cases. The preferred drug is a cephalosporin given i.v. immediately before surgery. A Foley catheter is placed in the patient's bladder and vascular access is obtained with two large-bore i.v. catheters. Patients with advanced age or significant medical conditions may require placement of an additional arterial or central line. Although bleeding should not be profuse, the possibility of major hemorrhage is real; therefore, 4 to 6 units of blood should be available during the operative procedure. We also routinely use an intraoperative cell saver to minimize patient exposure to homologous blood. This permits recycling of about 20% to 30% of the effective blood loss (118).

The patient is placed on a radiolucent operating table that allows intraoperative traction and fluoroscopy. The selection of the type of table to be used is controversial and based on the preference of the surgeon. The position of the patient is dictated by the surgeon's planned exposure: prone, supine, or lateral. All bony prominences are well padded and the patient supported on a bean bag.

With posterior and extensile approaches the sciatic nerve is in danger and constant vigilance and protection of the nerve is mandatory. Protection is afforded by the maintenance of knee flexion and hip extension throughout the procedure, because this position lessens tension on the sciatic nerve (44,129). When available, intraoperative sciatic nerve monitoring using both somatosensory evoked potentials (SSEPs) (73,90,91,130) and electromyography (EMG) (88,131) also have been shown to afford a degree of protective surveillance. Likely because of its ability to provide "real-time" information, the latter has been shown to be more sensitive and specific than the former (88,131). However, no EMG signal is produced in the absence of nerve irritation. In contrast, the advantage of SSEP is that a monitored signal represents intact nerve function. Recently, some have questioned the value of these modalities with two retrospective studies by experienced pelvic surgeons yielding results similar to those reported in monitored patients (132,133) and a high rate of false-negative readings when using SSEPs (132). Although controversial, these techniques should be considered especially in patients at risk for developing an iatrogenic sciatic nerve injury; that is, those already demonstrating preoperative nerve compromise and those with a fracture pattern that includes a posterior column or wall fracture. When used, we prepare the entire extremity free and insert sterile subdermal electrodes. The sensory electrodes are inserted adjacent to the common peroneal and posterior tibial nerves and the motor adjacent to the tibialis anterior, peroneus longus, and abductor hallicus.

SPECIFIC APPROACHES

Posterior Kocher-Langenbeck Approach

History

In 1958, Judet and Lagrange (41) combined the benefits of the Kocher (1907) and Langenbeck (1874) approaches to the hip to gain better access to the posterior column of the

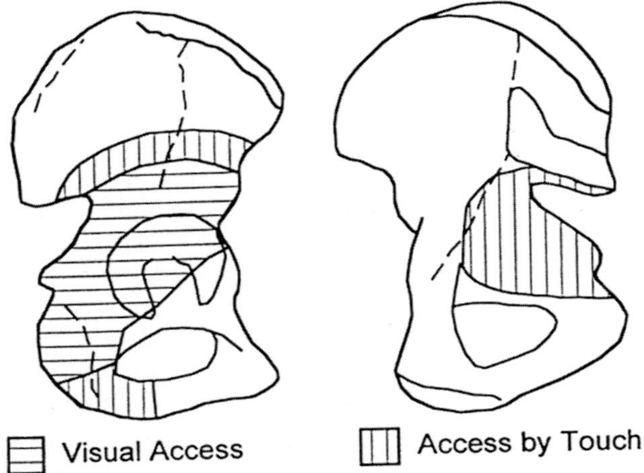

FIGURE 28-10. Access to the pelvis via the Kocher-Langenbeck approach. (From: Bartlett, CS, Helfet DL. The use of a single limited posterior approach and reduction techniques. *Semin Arthroplasty* 12:146. Philadelphia: WB Saunders, with permission.)

acetabulum through the greater and lesser sciatic notches (Fig. 28-10).

Indications

The posterior approach is recommended for isolated posterior wall fractures and isolated fractures of the posterior column. In experienced hands and with proper preoperative planning, it may also be used for transverse or T-type fractures of the infratectal or juxtatectal variety, especially those with associated posterior wall involvement.

Access

This approach (Fig. 28-10) provides direct access to the retroacetabular surface of the innominate bone (posterior column) from the ischium to the greater sciatic notch, including visualization of the entire posterior wall of the acetabulum.

Indirect access to the quadrilateral surface is possible by palpation through the greater and lesser sciatic notches, allowing assessment after the reduction of fractures involving the quadrilateral plate and pelvic brim (anterior column). The greater sciatic notch also provides a window for the placement of specially designed clamps to manipulate and reduce these fractures.

Position

The patient is positioned either in the lateral decubitus position or prone on pillows or bolsters. The distinction between these two different positions is dependent on the fracture pattern or "personality." The former simplifies intraoperative management, particularly for the anesthesia team, and is used primarily for posterior wall (Type A1) and simple posterior column (Type A2) fractures. In this position, the weight of the leg often hinders the reduction of transverse (Type B1) fractures, thus mitigating in favor of prone positioning. The hip is extended slightly and the knee flexed 90 degrees throughout the procedure to minimize the incidence of iatrogenic sciatic nerve injury (Fig. 28-11).

Advantages

This approach is well-known to most surgeons who perform hip reconstruction surgery or unipolar or total hip arthro-

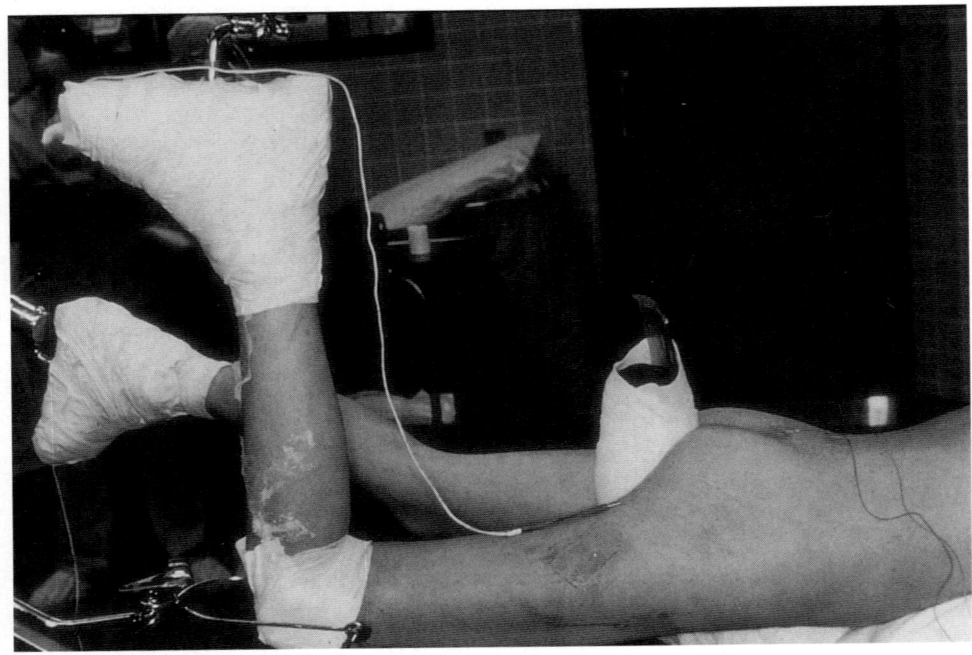

FIGURE 28-11. Patient prone on Judet fracture table with hip extended, knee flexed, and distal femoral skeletal traction in place. (From: Sledge CB, ed. *Master techniques in orthopaedic surgery: the hip.* Philadelphia: Lippincott-Raven, 1998, with permission.)

plasty. Muscle dissection is minimal, as is blood loss, and exposure is adequate for both the posterior column and posterior wall.

Disadvantages and Dangers

Superior Gluteal Neurovascular Bundle

One major limitation of the Kocher-Langenbeck approach is that the superior gluteal neurovascular bundle limits access to the superior iliac wing and is at risk during exposure of the greater sciatic notch and sciatic buttress. Therefore, the exposure is limited, especially if the transverse limb extends into the area of the greater sciatic notch (51). Injury to the bundle can result from severe displacement of the sciatic notch because of a high transverse fractures with marked medial rotation, or from an iatrogenic insult during surgery (48,134,135). Letournel (44) reported an incidence of 3.5% in his series. The neurovascular bundle is at greatest risk during exposure of the greater sciatic notch and must be protected from undue traction or damage by carefully placed retractors. Furthermore, the surgical team must use extreme caution when applying traction to the gluteus medius in order to better visualize the lateral wall of the ilium because this act may tear the artery, with disastrous consequences, or stretch the nerve, causing permanent paralysis of the hip abductors.

Vascular injury can occur either during the exposure or fracture reduction (44,48,134). Control of bleeding is crucial in this situation. Initially, packing of the area may provide hemostasis. Failing this, ligation of the bleeding vessel must be performed. The surgeon must avoid haphazardly placed vascular clips because the proximity of the superior gluteal nerve places it at risk of accidental ligation with disastrous results for the patient. Should a bleeding superior gluteal vessel retract into the pelvis in the midst of a posterior approach, an osteotomy of the sciatic notch can be performed to identify and control the bleeding vessel.

Sciatic Nerve

When this approach is used, the sciatic nerve is always in danger and therefore must be protected at all times (Fig. 28-12). To this end, the knee joint must be flexed and the hip extended throughout the procedure, and the nerve protected by the short external rotator muscles by way of a tagged suture in the conjoint tendon. The first assistant must maintain a constant watch, to ensure that any retraction of the nerve is gentle. Special retractors inserted into the greater or lesser sciatic notch with a small hook may be useful, but constant vigilance is still required. Although controversial, we also routinely perform intraoperative sciatic nerve monitoring using SSEPs and spontaneous EMGs. The neurotechnologist can detect sciatic nerve compromise through intraoperative monitoring of EMG activity (immediately) or via significant unilateral changes in amplitude and latency of the SSEPs. If nerve compromise is detected,

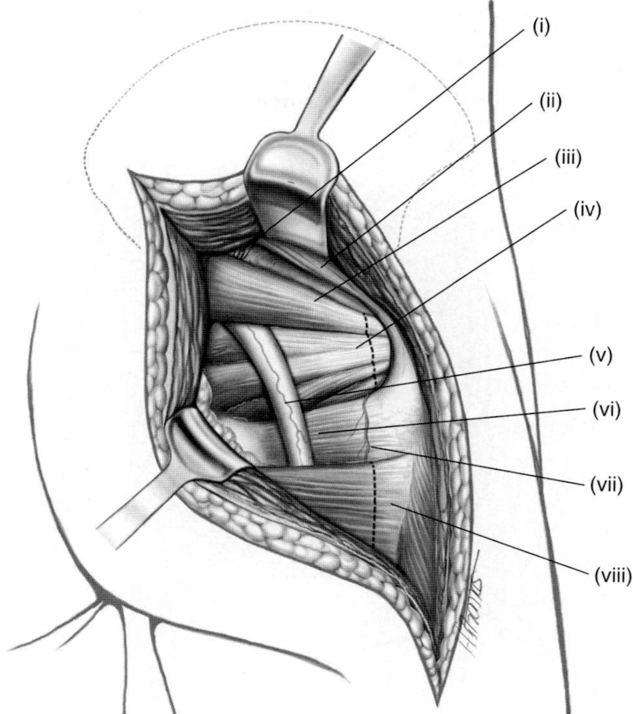

FIGURE 28-12. Posterior exposure of the sciatic nerve, tagging and incision of the piriformis and external rotators, right side. **(i)** Superior gluteal neurovascular bundle; **(ii)** gluteus medius; **(iii)** piriformis; **(iv)** external rotators: superior and inferior gemelli and obturator Internus; **(v)** sciatic nerve; **(vi)** quadratus femoris; **(vii)** medial femoral circumflex artery; **(viii)** tendonous femoral insertion of gluteus maximus. (From: Sledge CB, ed. *Master techniques in orthopaedic surgery: the hip.* Philadelphia: Lippincott-Raven, 1998, with permission.)

then the surgical team must promptly respond by releasing traction and removing any retractors that have placed against the nerve until the EMG activity ceases or the potentials return to baseline.

Pudendal Nerve

The pudendal nerve is at risk as it exits the pelvis through the greater sciatic notch and reenters through the lesser sciatic notch. It can be injured through vigorous dissection or poorly placed retractors around the ischial spine. It also can be injured through excessive traction on a fracture table at the level of the perineal post.

Medial femoral circumflex artery.

The medial femoral circumflex artery is at risk during exposure of the posterior column. Its branches are buried in the muscle of the quadratus femoris (Fig. 28-13) and can be injured if the quadratus femoris muscle is released at its insertion on the femur. The vessel emerges between the quadratus femoris muscle and obdurator extensus adjacent to the femor where it is at maximal risk.

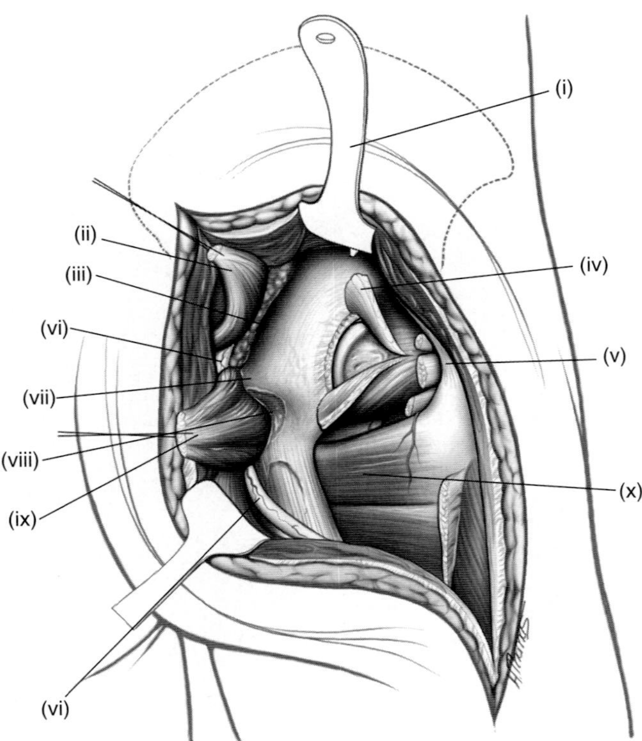

FIGURE 28-13. Completed exposure of the posterior column and wall and hip joint through the Kocher-Langenbeck approach, right side. **(i)** Hohmann retractor under the gluteus medius; **(ii)** piriformis; **(iii)** greater sciatic notch; **(iv)** posterior hip capsulectomy; **(v)** gluteus medius; **(vi)** sciatic nerve; **(vii)** ischial spine; **(viii)** lesser sciatic notch; **(ix)** obturator internus and gemelli; **(x)** quadratus femoris. (From: Sledge CB, ed. *Master techniques in orthopaedic surgery: the hip.* Philadelphia: Lippincott-Raven, 1998, with permission.)

Heterotopic Ossification

This complication occurs after all approaches to the outer aspect of the ilium with rates ranging from 18% to 90% (44,56,57,109,111,136). It is frequently noted along the gluteus minimus and the debridement of any necrotic muscle in this location may decrease the risk of its occurrence (137).

Hip Abductor Weakness

Posterior approaches had been associated with a significant loss of hip abductor strength, possibly because of careless dissection of the gluteus maximus muscle and damage to branches of the superior gluteal nerve. Dickinson and coworkers (138) noted that posterior approaches were associated with a 50% or greater loss of hip abductor strength at an average 21-month follow-up, with less than half of the patients demonstrating a normal gait, and seven of 22 having a residual Trendelenburg gait. On the other hand, Borrelli and colleagues (139), although still observing that poor functional outcome was associated with muscle weakness, noted that normal muscle strength could be regained in some patients and that most demonstrated only minor changes in gait at follow-up.

Surgical Technique

Prior to the surgical incision, all bony landmarks are outlined with a sterile marking pen, including the posterior-superior iliac spine, greater trochanter, and shaft of the femur. The incision for the Kocher-Langenbeck approach is then centered over the posterior half of the greater trochanter. It begins 5 cm distal to the posterior superior iliac spine, curves over the tip of the greater trochanter, and travels along the lateral aspect of the femoral shaft for approximately 8 cm, ending just distal to the insertion of the gluteus maximus tendon (Fig. 28-14).

The iliotibial band then is incised up to the greater trochanter until the fascia overlying the gluteus maximus muscle is encountered. This fascia then is incised and the underlying muscle gently split in line with its fibers by blunt dissection, with two fingers aiming toward the posterior-superior iliac spine (Fig. 28-15). If the gluteus maximus muscle is divided too far medially, the inferior gluteal neurovascular bundle may be compromised. Therefore, in order to not denervate a significant portion of hip abductor muscle, the muscle should not be split proximal to the first neurovascular pedicle. Next, the trochanteric bursa is incised and the gluteus maximus tendon partially released (if desired) at the level of its insertion into the femur to decrease tension. Occasionally, the detachment of a portion

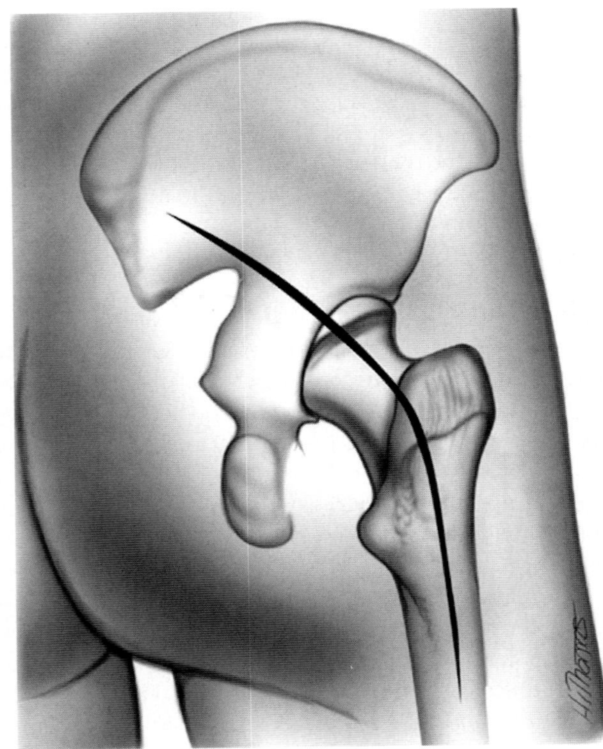

FIGURE 28-14. Surgical incision for the Kocher-Langenbeck approach, *right side.* (From: Sledge CB, ed. *Master techniques in orthopaedic surgery: the hip.* Philadelphia: Lippincott-Raven, 1998, with permission.)

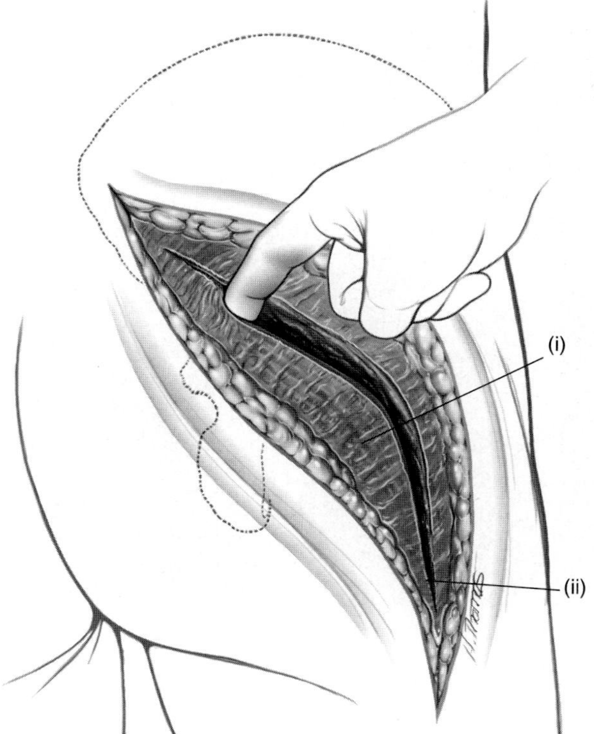

FIGURE 28-15. Finger splitting of the gluteus maximus proximal to the greater trochanter–this separates the upper one-third (blood supply: superior gluteal artery) from the lower two-thirds (blood supply: inferior gluteal artery), right side. **(i)** Fibers of gluteus maximus; **(ii)** iliotibial band. (From: Sledge CB, ed. *Master techniques in orthopaedic surgery: the hip.* Philadelphia: Lippincott-Raven, 1998, with permission.)

of the medius off the greater trochanter also improves visualization (M. Tile, personal communication, 2002).

At this point, it is imperative to identify and isolate the sciatic nerve, which can be consistently located along the medial aspect of the quadratus femoris muscle (Fig. 28-12). Fractures of the posterior wall or column of the acetabulum may have significant associated soft-tissue injuries, such as avulsion of the tendon of the piriformis muscle that can distort normal anatomy and place the sciatic nerve at risk for an iatrogenic injury. Once the sciatic nerve has been identified, it should be followed to its pelvic exit at the greater sciatic notch. After identifying the sciatic nerve, the short external rotators are visualized and placed on stretch by gentle internal rotation of the hip.

Exposure of the posterior column of the acetabulum is performed in a stepwise manner from the greater sciatic notch to the ischial tuberosity, avoiding injury to the sciatic nerve. The piriformis and the conjoined tendons of the obturator internus and gemelli (superior and inferior) muscles should each be isolated, tagged, released, and reflected from their femoral insertions (Fig. 28-13). It is at this junction of the procedure that an understanding of the architecture of the medial femoral circumflex artery is crucial. As the course of its ascending branch is constant in this area (14), the critical blood supply to the femoral head can be preserved by protecting the quadratus femoris muscle and releasing the external rotators 1.5 cm from their insertions (Fig. 28-13).

Once the piriformis muscle has been released, it is retracted back toward the sciatic notch to gain exposure of the superior aspect of the posterior column of the acetabulum. Additional exposure of this area is provided by a Hohmann retractor inserted into the ilium under the tendon of the gluteus medius muscle. However, caution also should be taken to identify and protect the superior gluteal neurovascular bundle as it exits the greater sciatic notch in the region of the sciatic buttress. Excess traction on the bundle from too vigorous a dissection, excessive retraction on the hip abductors, or poorly placed retractors in this area may tear the artery or stretch the nerve, leading to disastrous consequences (Fig. 28-13).

Retraction of the conjoined tendons of the obturator internus and gemelli allows elevation of the obturator internus muscle by blunt dissection exposing its bursa and the posterior column of the acetabulum (Fig. 28-13). After release of the bursa, the obturator internus muscle is then followed into the lesser sciatic notch where a blunt curved Hohmann or sciatic nerve retractor is carefully inserted. The dissection around the area of the ischial spine must be meticulous because the pudendal neurovascular bundle is at risk as it exits the pelvis through the greater sciatic notch and reenters through the lesser sciatic notch. Retraction of the conjoined obturator internus tendon gives access to the lesser sciatic notch and affords a measure of protection to the sciatic nerve and pudendal neurovascular structures, which cross over (posterior to) the tendon.

In contrast, although retraction of the piriformis tendon provides access to the greater sciatic notch, it does not provide protection for the sciatic nerve, which exits the notch deep (anterior) to the tendon. Although careful placement of blunt Hohmann retractors in the lesser and greater sciatic notches provides a clear exposure of the entire retroacetabular surface, the assistant must be vigilant regarding the sciatic nerve. This requires the maintenance of minimal and only intermittent tension, while balancing the protective soft-tissue layer of the tendon of the obturator internus between his retractor and the nerve.

For complex fracture patterns, dissection should be performed to allow placement of a finger through the greater sciatic notch in order to palpate the medial fracture line along the quadrilateral surface. This may require release of the sacrospinous ligament or osteotomy of the ischial spine (Fig. 28-16). If further exposure of the posterior-inferior aspect of the acetabulum is required, then the quadratus femoris muscle can be released from its pelvic origin along the ischium but not from its femoral insertion where the medial femoral circumflex artery is at risk. The bursa of the hamstrings overlying the ischial tuberosity can be cleared with an elevator to expose the tendonous origin of the hamstring muscles. In rare instances, when access to the superior

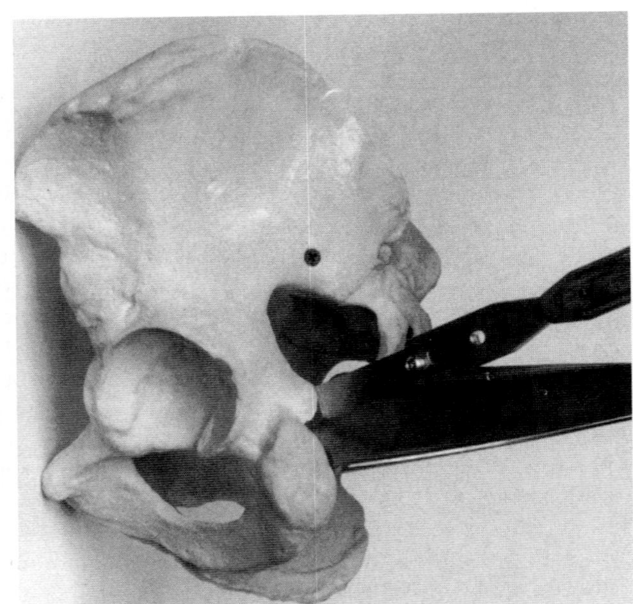

A

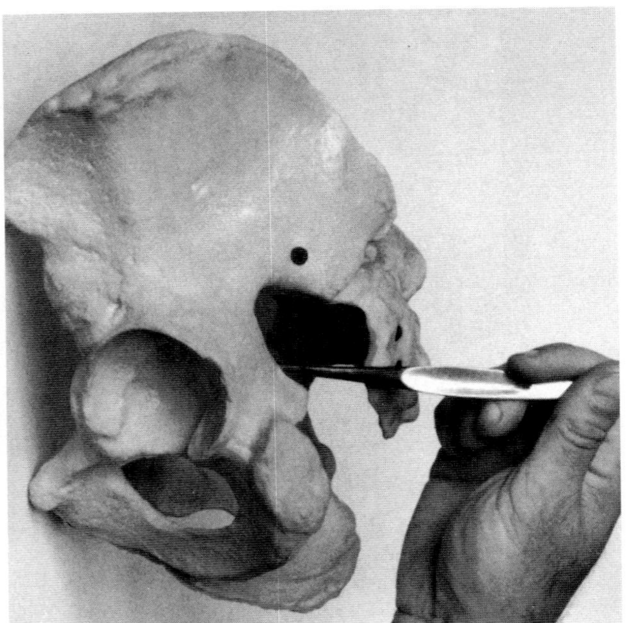

C

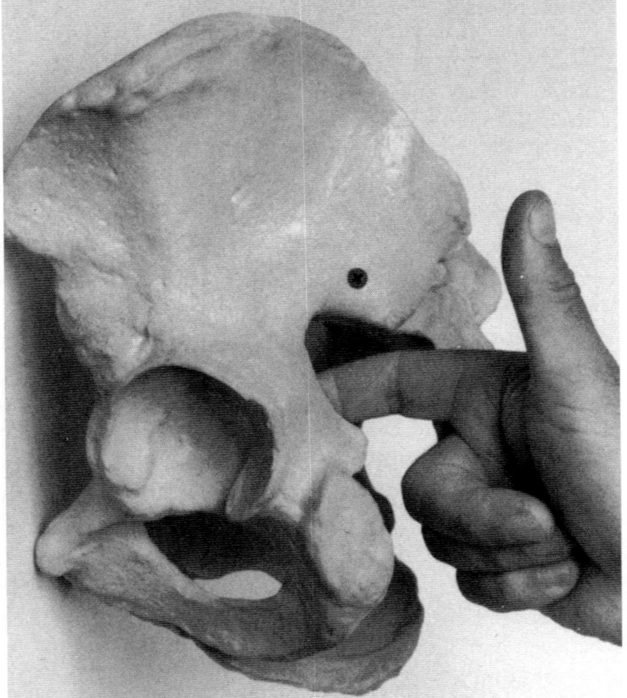

B

FIGURE 28-16. Inspection of the quadrilateral plate through a Kocher-Langenbeck approach. The quadrilateral plate may be inspected, if necessary, after dividing the insertion of the sacrospinous ligament from the ischial spine or after removing its insertion into the ischial spine with an osteotome **(A).** The surgeon should make certain that the structures in both the superior and the inferior gluteal notch are protected. Once the ligament has been released, a finger can be inserted to assess the adequacy of reduction of any fracture line along the quadrilateral plate **(B).** A periosteal elevator may also be used for this purpose **(C).**

weight-bearing surface of the acetabulum is necessary (high transtectal transverse or T-type fractures), osteotomy of the greater trochanter can be considered.

At this point, the entire posterior column can be visualized from the greater sciatic notch to the ischial tuberosity. The posterior articular surface of the femoral head usually can be easily visualized through the fractured posterior wall or column and a rent in the capsule is almost always seen. The hip capsule throughout the exposure should be preserved to as great an extent as possible to preserve the blood supply to the femoral head. Posterior wall and column fragments are identified and their edges debrided sharply. Intraarticular fragments can be removed at this point by distracting the hip joint using femoral traction with either a fracture table (Fig. 28-11) or a femoral distractor (Fig. 28-17). By internal rotation, the hip may be "redislocated" and washed of all small fragments of articular cartilage and bone (51).

After reduction of the hip joint and further exposure of the entire posterior column from the ischial spine to the greater sciatic notch, the fracture may be reduced and stabilized in an appropriate manner. Techniques from the posterior approach will depend on the specific fracture pattern, which is usually a posterior wall, posterior column, transverse, or T-type.

Posterior wall (Type A1) fractures are routinely thought of as simple fractures to treat. Unfortunately, this belief is incorrect, as their reconstruction is often complicated by significant comminution (71,140) or marginal impaction (Figs. 28-18 and 28-19) (38,70,140,141). These two entities make posterior wall fractures more difficult to treat, leading to among the poorest outcomes for all fractures of the acetabulum, especially when an associated posterior column or transverse fracture also is present (38,44,57,141). Marginal impaction of the articular surface is relatively common after a fracture of the posterior wall, occurring in 16% to 47% of cases, and usually associated with a posterior hip dislocation (38,70,140,141). As the femoral head dislocates, it not only fractures the posterior wall, but also implodes the articular surface. Impacted fragments are readily identified on the preoperative CT scan and when exposed at the time of surgery, are usually noted to be rotated 90 degrees so that the surgeon looks directly at the articular surface (Fig. 28-18). It is of paramount importance that large fragments be anatomically reduced at the time of surgery in order to maintain joint congruity.

After cleaning the joint of debris and stabilizing an associated column or transverse fracture, traction is released and the femoral head used as a template for the articular reduction. The medial aspect of each cortical wall fragment should be cleared of enough soft tissue to permit visualization of its reduction, while retaining as much of its capsular attachments as possible to preserve its blood supply. Extremely small and avascular fragments should be discarded. Next, any impacted articular fragments are gently elevated into a position congruent with the femoral head. The fragments must be derotated by gently teasing them up with an elevator until they are congruous with the femoral head (Fig. 28-19B). This invariably produces a metaphyseal defect underlying the articular fragment(s), which should be filled with autologous cancellous bone graft (easily obtained

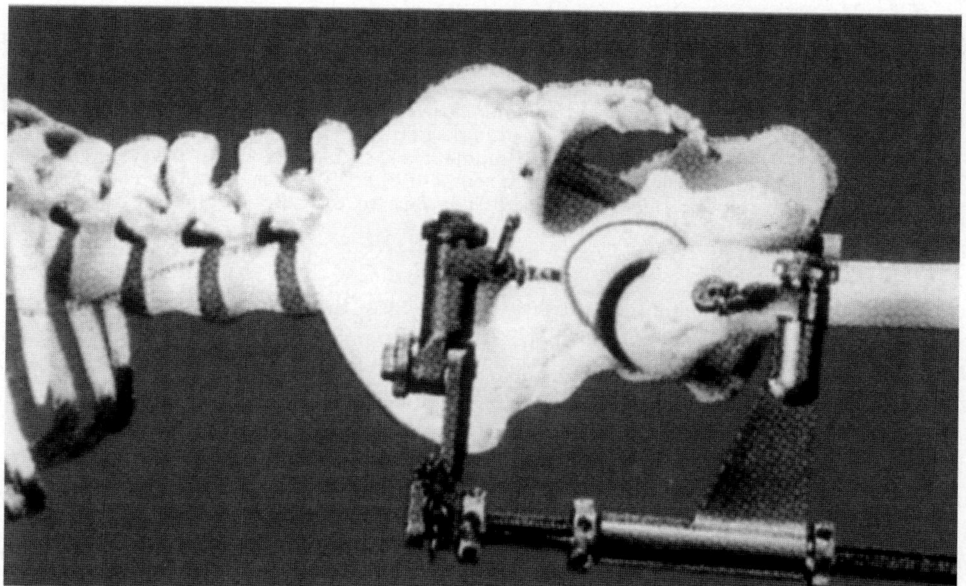

FIGURE 28-17. "Saw bones" pelvis in the prone position with femoral distractor applied to allow hip joint distraction. Note the Schanz screw in the sciatic buttress and the Schanz screw in the femur, placed through a small split in the vastus lateralis just distal to the greater trochanter. (From: Sledge CB, ed. *Master techniques in orthopaedic surgery: the hip.* Philadelphia: Lippincott-Raven, 1998, with permission.)

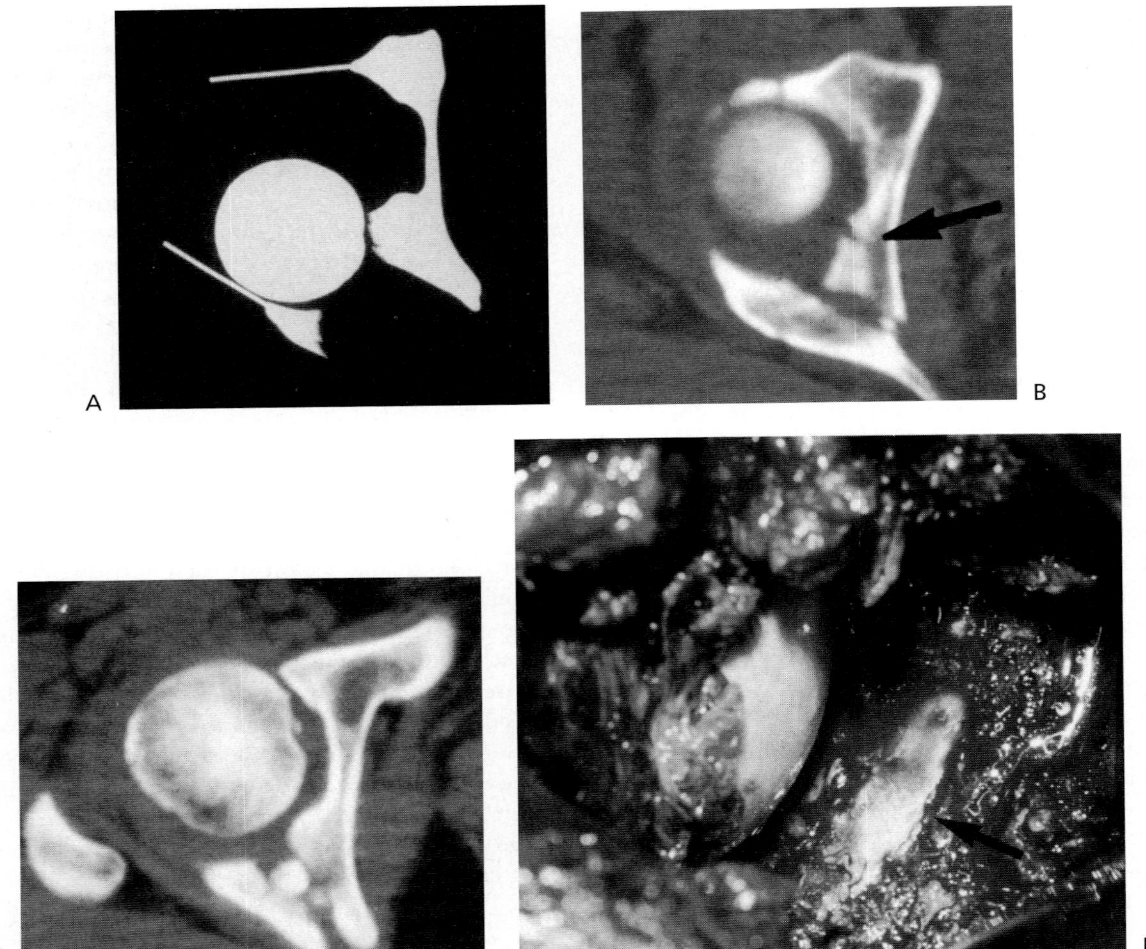

FIGURE 28-18. A: Drawing depicts a posterior dislocation of the hip. As the femoral head rotates out of the acetabulum, a segment of the articular surface is often impacted. This is clearly seen on computed tomography **(B)**, where a large fragment of articular cartilage has been impacted as the head dislocated. Even after reduction of the head, the fragment remains in the unreduced impacted position *(arrow)*. The impacted fragment drives the posterior wall fracture apart, and reduction cannot be achieved without first disimpacting the fragment **(C)**. The clinical appearance is typical. On exposing the hip joint, a segment of articular surface is rotated 90 degrees to its anatomic position. In this case, note the segment of articular cartilage. Normally it should lie adjacent to the femoral head and not in clear view of the surgeon through the Kocher-Langenbeck approach **(D)**.

through a small window in the greater trochanter) or other suitable material. In most instances, autologous cancellous bone graft material is then obtained through a small window in the greater trochanter and used to buttress the reduced marginal fragments (Fig. 28-19C). It is extremely difficult to get any form of internal fixation into these fragments (although bioabsorbable pins or small screws can be considered); therefore, the maintenance of their position is generally dependent on the bone graft and replacement of the main wall fragment on top. Unfortunately, marginally impacted fragments may be avascular and collapse in the postoperative period. The prognosis for the joint depends on how large these fragments are and whether good stability has been retained.

Next, the wall fragments are reduced and held in place by the Straight Ball Spike pusher, followed by provisional fixation with Kirschner wires. A 3.5-mm reconstruction plate is applied in the buttress mode over the reduced posterior wall and anchored to the ilium proximally and ischium distally. Underbending of this plate, in relation to the posterior wall, will aid in reduction of the construct and compress the fracture (Fig. 28-20). To best prevent fracture displacement, one or more lag screws (through or outside the plate) should be placed across the posterior wall into the posterior column. When the posterior wall is very comminuted, it is not possible to restore all the small articular fragments with individual lag screws. In this situation, as recommended by Jeffrey Mast (see Chapter 31), one can use spring hook plates (two-, three-,

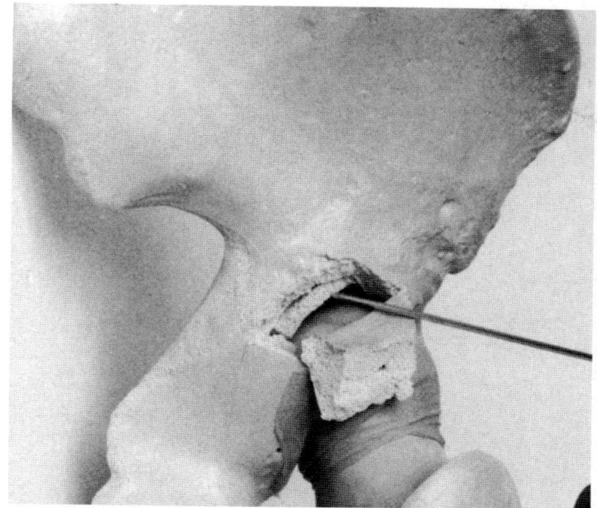

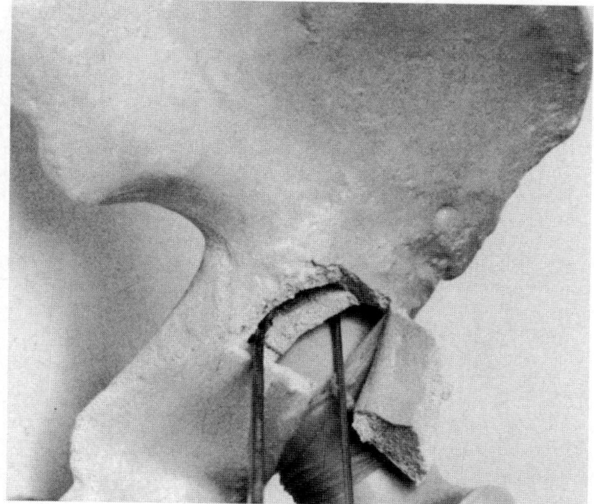

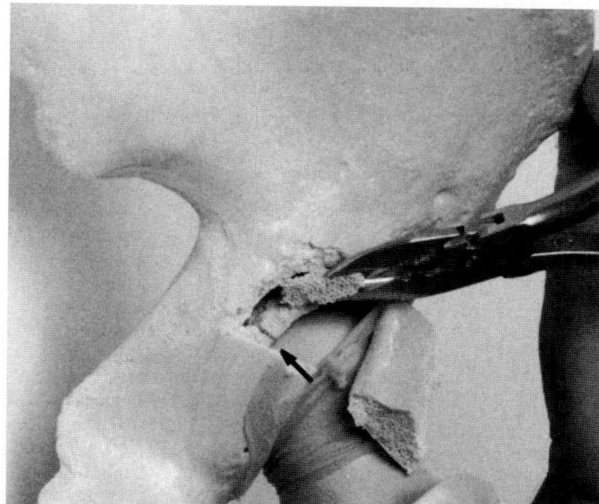

FIGURE 28-19. Reduction and fixation of a marginally impacted fragment of articular cartilage. **A:** Note the impacted fragment at the tip of the Kirschner wire. **B:** Using the femoral head as the pillar for reduction, the fragment is gently teased with an elevator. On some occasions impaction is so great that an osteotome is required to develop a plane. **C:** The fragment is held in place in the anatomically reduced position *(black arrow)* with a cancellous bone graft.

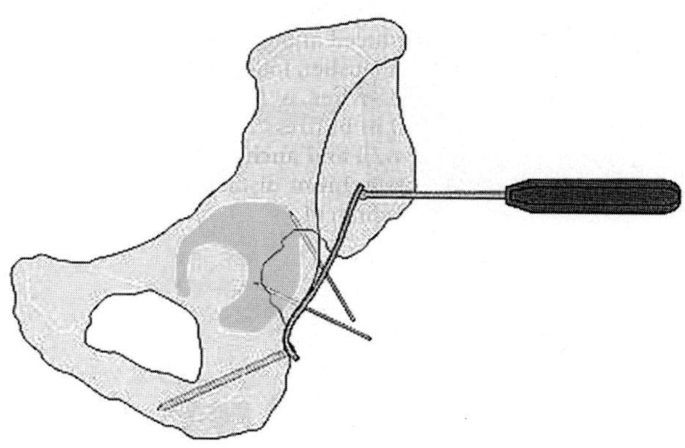

FIGURE 28-20. Posterior placement of an under-contoured (underbent) plate, during the reduction of a posterior wall fracture will direct compressive forces across the fragment(s), thus effecting a stable reduction. (From: Ruedi TP, Murphy WM, eds. *AO/ASIF principles of fracture management.* New York: AO Publishing, Thieme, 2000, with permission.)

or four-hole one-third tubular plates with their tips cut off through a hole and the newly created prongs bent downward to create small hooks) (45,54, 70,122,142,143). These plates are affixed in a loaded fashion underneath the posterior wall buttress plate more medially, but with the spring-loaded lateral hooks, providing a buttressing effect to the comminuted posterior wall (Fig. 28-21).

Fractures involving the posterior column (Type A2) generally result in posterior-medial displacement and internal rotation of the posterior column, as viewed from a posterior aspect. After debridement of the fracture and removal of all of the comminuted fracture fragments and/or organizing hematoma, posterior column fracture reduction is accomplished by correcting the rotation with a Schanz screw in the ischium, and the use of a pelvic reduction clamp in the greater sciatic notch to correct the medial displacement (Fig. 28-22). The gluteal neurovascular bundle can be damaged during this maneuver, and must be monitored. Alterna-

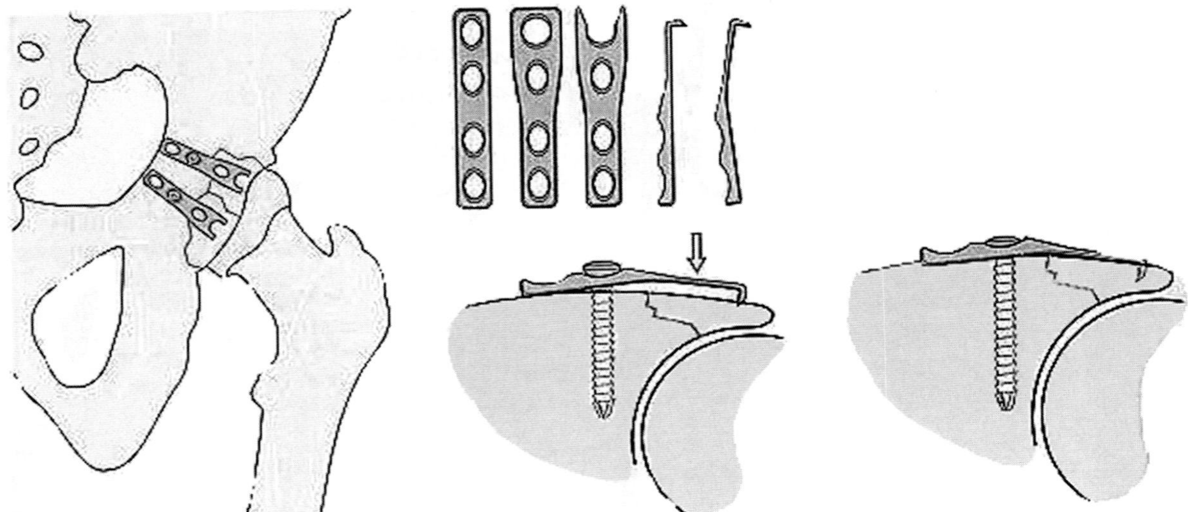

FIGURE 28-21. Spring hook plate technique for small posterior-wall fragments. (From: Ruedi TP, Murphy WM, eds. *AO/ASIF principles of fracture management*. New York: AO Publishing, Thieme, 2000, with permission.)

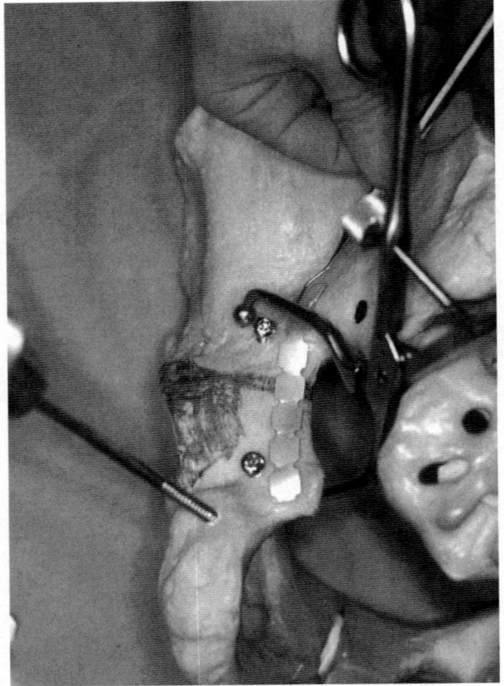

A

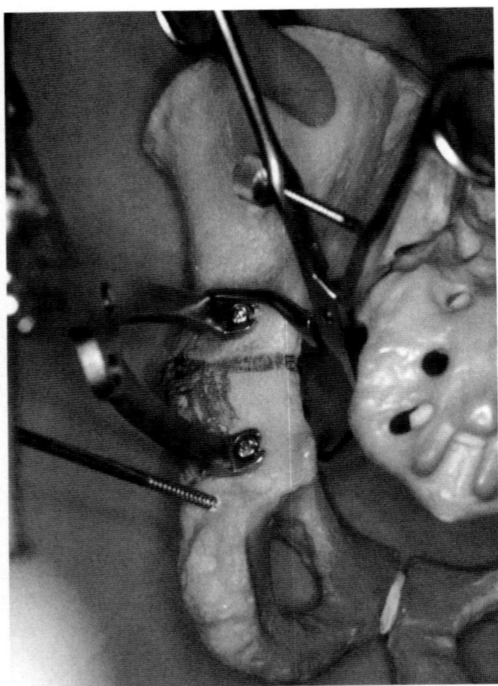

C

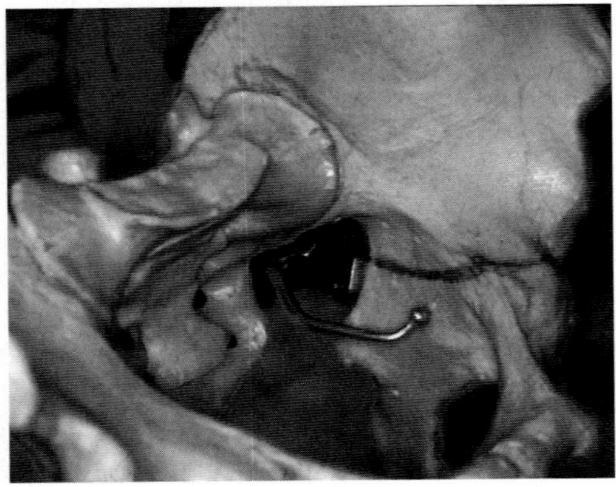

B

FIGURE 28-22. Model pelvis, in prone position, with a shaded diagram of a transverse with a posterior wall fracture. **A:** Posterior view demonstrating pelvic reduction forceps with pointed ball tips inserted into the greater sciatic notch, a Shantz pin placed in the ischium, and a screw in each major fragment to assist reduction. Also note the aluminum template placed where a contoured 3.5-mm reconstruction plate will be applied. **B:** Inner table view displaying proper orientation of the pelvic reduction forceps with pointed ball tips. **C:** Posterior view demonstrating the use of screw holding pelvic reduction forceps. (From: Bartlett CS, Helfet DL. The use of a single limited posterior approach and reduction techniques. *Semin Arthroplasty* 12:149, with permission.)

tively, the reduction is accomplished by screw-holding forceps applied to 4.5-mm bicortical screws inserted into each of the main column fragments. Care must be taken to position the screws away from the area of eventual plate placement. This clamp allows distraction, debridement, and compression of the fracture.

After reduction and provisional fixation with a Kirschner wire, direct visual inspection of the posterior fracture line best assesses displacement of the column, whereas rotation is best judged by digital palpation through the greater and lesser sciatic notches. A smooth quadrilateral surface is usually indicative of correct rotational alignment. When an accurate reduction has been confirmed, a 3.5-mm reconstruction plate is applied from the ischium to the ilium. A lag screw across the fracture, into the anterior column, prevents redisplacement. If combined with a posterior wall fracture, the posterior column reduction should be addressed first followed by double plating, one for the column and one for the wall, as necessary.

Transverse (Type B1) fractures require techniques similar to those used for posterior column fractures. However, although the retroacetabular fracture line in a transverse fracture may appear much the same as in the posterior column fracture, in these fracture types it is necessary to reduce not only the posterior column but also the anterior displacement and malrotation. Displacement can be controlled using the two-screw technique (Fig. 28-22C) with a screw-holding reduction clamp, as described for the posterior column fracture. The surgeon can use this clamp for distraction and debridement of the fracture line, all the way to the anterior column, and subsequently for manipulation and temporary reduction of the transverse fracture component. Rotation also can be controlled with either a Schanz pin in the ischium or pelvic reduction forceps with pointed ball tips placed into the sciatic notch. An elegant maneuver is to first secure a plate into one of the fracture fragments, and then to use the plate as a reduction tool.

After provisional fixation and inspection, stabilization is obtained with a 3.5-mm reconstruction plate applied to the medial border of the retroacetabular surface, and lag screw(s). This plate should be overcontoured to achieve compression of the anterior column segments as it is tightened down to the posterior column (Fig. 28-23). Undercontouring, as performed for posterior wall fractures, actually leads to distraction of the anterior column in transverse fractures. To prevent displacement of the anterior column, a posterior-to-anterior column lag screw is required for all transverse fracture types. This screw usually can be placed through the posterior buttress plate and must be oriented parallel to the quadrilateral surface to avoid joint penetration. Finger palpation along the quadrilateral plate aids in assuring correct position for the screw. This should be checked fluoroscopically on the operating table, specifically looking at the obturator oblique view to assess its position in the anterior column, and the iliac oblique view, to assure its extraarticular placement.

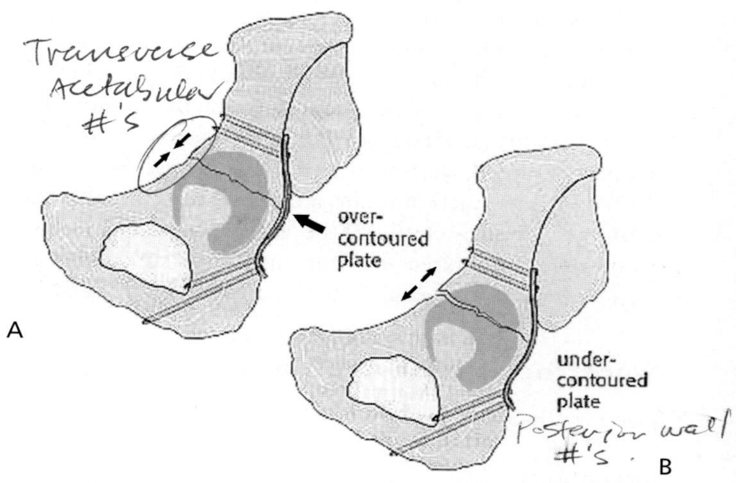

FIGURE 28-23. A: Posterior placement of an over-contoured (over-bent) plate during the fixation of a transverse fracture results in compressive forces over the anterior portion of the fracture and an optimal reduction. **B:** In contrast, placement of an under-contoured (under-bent) plate during the reduction of a transverse fracture will lead to distraction of the fracture anteriorly. (From: Ruedi TP, Murphy WM, eds. *AO/ASIF principles of fracture management.* New York: AO Publishing. Thieme, 2000, with permission.)

T-shaped (Type B2) fractures are among the most difficult of all fracture types to manage. It is a complex variant of the transverse fracture pattern, in which the inferior ischiopubic segment has been separated into anterior and posterior fragments by a vertical stem component. Because of this, it is impossible to control the separate anterior column fragment by direct manipulation of the posterior column fragment(s) when working through a posterior approach, except possibly by ligamentotaxis through nondisrupted joint capsule. Therefore, successful fixation of this fracture through a posterior approach is dependent on the surgeon's ability to obtain an indirect reduction of the anterior column and to confirm an accurate reduction by palpation of the anterior column and stem component through the greater sciatic notch. In order to achieve such a reduction, the surgeon must be familiar with the placement of instruments into the sciatic notch, and their use to manipulate the anterior column fragment after the provisional stabilization of the posterior column. For example, a small bone hook or pusher, gently introduced along the quadrilateral plate, can be used to derotate and pull the displaced portion of the anterior column posteriorly. This reduces this segment into the acute angle between the intact proximal anterior column and the reconstructed posterior column. Once an acceptable reduction has been accomplished, definitive fixation is achieved by the application of a posterior buttress plate and posterior to anterior lag screws as in transverse fractures. Care must be taken that implants for provisional or definitive fixation of one column do not cross into the opposite column, hindering or preventing its reduction (74). Care also must be taken to avoid intraarticular or intrapelvic placement of the lag screws.

The wound is closed in a meticulous fashion following completion of the operative procedure. The tendons of the piriformis and obturator internus muscles are reattached at the greater trochanter along with the remainder of the short external rotators. If a release of the gluteus maximus insertion has been required, this too is repaired at its insertion along the femur. Two suction drains are placed over the external rotators followed by closure of the iliotibial band and the fascia overlying the gluteus maximus muscle. A subcutaneous suction drain is inserted and the skin meticulously closed.

Transtrochanteric Approach

(See Fig. 28-24.)

Indications

The indications for the transtrochanteric approach are the same as those for the Kocher-Langenbeck, but this variation affords better visualization of higher transtectal, transverse, and T-type lesions.

Access

(See Fig. 28-24.) Access to the upper part of the posterior column into the greater sciatic notch is increased as compared to the standard Kocher-Langenbeck approach. Trochanteric osteotomy also allows visualization of the lateral aspect of the acetabular superior wall anteriorly to the anterior inferior spine of the ilium.

Position

This is the same as the Kocher-Langenbeck, with the lateral decubitus position more usual.

Advantages

This modification (osteotomy) extends the exposure to the anterior inferior iliac spine with improved visualization and access to the posterior column and superior aspect of the acetabulum (including the weight-bearing dome) (17,51, 82,124). Removal of the trochanter also removes much of the tension from the superior gluteal vessels and nerves and, thus, protects them. The standard Kocher-Langenbeck approach can be extended this way at any time should increased exposure be required.

Disadvantages and Dangers

The same neurovascular structures are at risk as in the standard Kocher-Langenbeck, except that increased stripping of the gluteus medius and minimus muscles leads to a significantly higher risk for abductor weakness and/or heterotopic ossification (51,111,137,144). Heterotopic ossification is often noted along the gluteus minimus and the debridement of any necrotic muscle here may decrease the risk of this complication (137). Furthermore, the unique disadvantages of this approach include the risk for nonunion of the trochanter. Also, the risk of avascular necrosis of the femoral head theoretically is increased by the interference with the

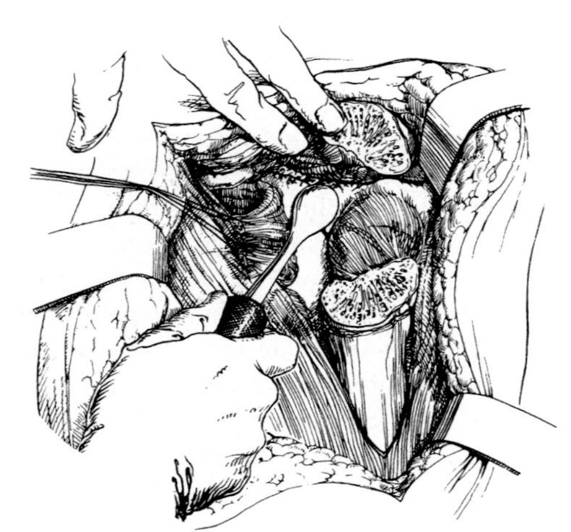

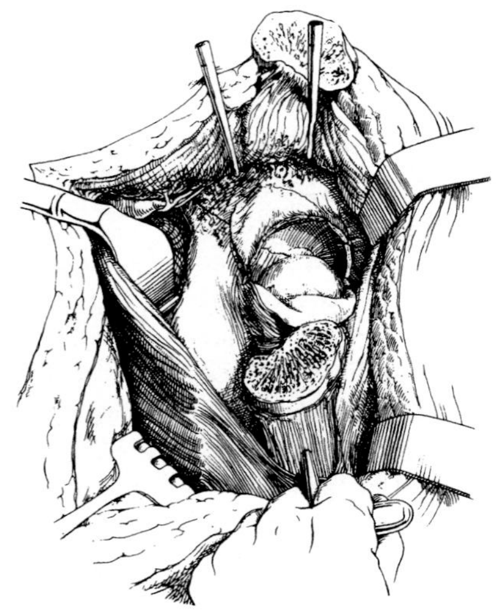

FIGURE 28-24. A: Osteotomy of the greater trochanter affords increased access to the superior portion of the posterior column and into the greater sciatic notch. It also allows visualization of the lateral aspect of the acetabular superior wall, in the area of the anterior inferior spine. Removal of the trochanter also diminishes the tension on the superior gluteal vessels and nerve. The initial approach is identical to the Kocher-Langenbeck. If, in the course of that exposure, the surgeon wishes increased access, the greater trochanter is predrilled and osteotomized as in **(A). B:** Access in the area of the greater sciatic notch anterior to the anterior inferior spine is increased. In this case the muscles are retracted with two Steinmann pins inserted into the lateral ilium. Note the superior gluteal vessels and nerve exiting the superior gluteal notch. In this drawing, the capsule has been elevated from the acetabular rim, allowing excellent exposure to the interior of the joint so that the articular fractures may be inspected.

posterior blood supply (98). Finally, visualization of most of the anterior column cannot be achieved except by looking into the hip joint or by palpating through the greater sciatic notch because this approach is still limited to the posterior column.

Surgical Technique

The skin incision is identical to that for the posterior Kocher-Langenbeck approach, except that the lateral portion is longer (51). If the standard Kocher-Langenbeck approach has been performed but the surgeon desires greater access, it is a simple matter to osteotomize the greater trochanter and gain access to the superior wall of the acetabulum and a portion of the anterior column. The anterior column can be stabilized only by retrograde screw fixation (it is impossible to use a plate); however, the superior weight-bearing surface of the acetabulum will be visualized laterally, and intraarticularly by division of the capsule and traction. For this approach, initially the technique is identical to that for the posterior Kocher-Langenbeck approach; then, the greater trochanter is predrilled to accept one or two 6.5-mm cancellous screws at closure and simply is cut using a Gigli saw. The Gigli saw is much safer and avoids the risk of sawing into the femoral head. At the time of closure, adequate fixation is obtained by two 6.5-mm cancellous lag screws (with or without tension band wires).

An alternative to the classic trochanteric osteotomy is to leave the origin of the vastus lateralis attached to the distal segment (17,124,145). The improved blood supply and stability afforded by this technique should minimize complications. When using this modification, fixation can be performed with 3.5-mm screws (17).

Anterior Iliofemoral Approach

(See Fig. 28-25.)

History

This approach is essentially a modification of the Smith-Petersen anterior approach to the hip, with stripping of the muscles off of the interior aspect of the pelvis.

Indications

Anterior column fractures and variants in which the main displacement is cephalad to the hip joint ("high" fractures)

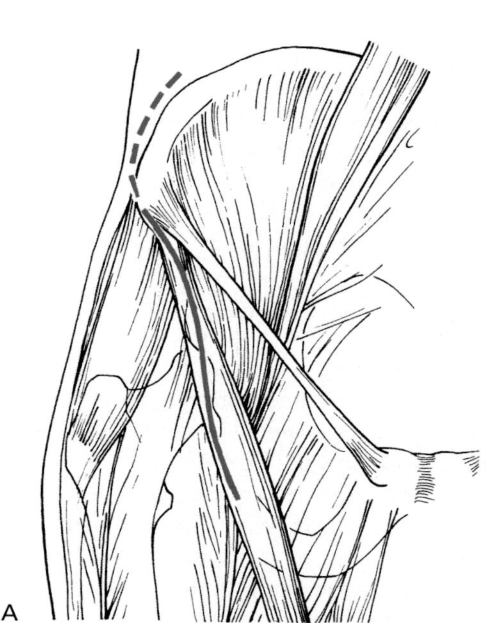

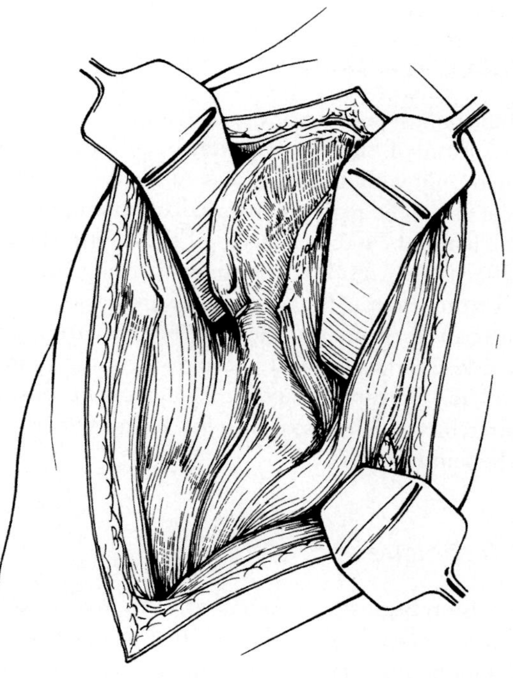

FIGURE 28-25. Iliofemoral approach. **A:** Skin incision. The posterior aspect of the incision would be 1 cm lateral to or 1 cm medial to the iliac crest and not over the bone itself. The distal limb may be as shown, along the lateral border of sartorius or following the line of the ilioinguinal approach. This is more versatile, as it allows the surgeon to switch to a more extensile ilioinguinal approach, if necessary. The interval to reach the deep muscles is between the sartorius medially and the tensor fascia femoris laterally. **B:** Deep dissection by removal of muscles from the outer, and often the inner, aspect of the pelvis. This approach allows easy access to the greater sciatic notch, and cerlage wires may be inserted with ease through this approach. The approach is often used in combination with the posterior Kocher-Langenbeck approach, when the surgeon prefers a combined approach, rather than a single extensile approach. (From: Schatzker J, Tile M. *The rationale of operative fracture care.* Heidelberg: Springer-Verlag, 1984, with permission.)

can be treated through this approach. Also, this is often the preferred anterior exposure when the surgeon desires simultaneous combined exposure of both the anterior and posterior column rather than a single extensile approach (72).

Access

(See Fig. 28-25.) Exposure of the anterior column is possible to the iliopectineal eminence by flexing and adducting the hip. Also, the lateral aspect of the iliac crest is accessible.

Position

The patient is placed in the supine position, unless combined with a posterior approach, in which case the "floppy lateral" position is used.

Advantages

This commonly used approach, known to most hip surgeons, requires no dissection of the femoral vessels.

Disadvantages and Dangers

Access to the anterior column of the acetabulum is very limited and fixation of the distal anterior column can be accomplished only with screws. Plates can be used only in the proximal area. The main neurovascular structure at risk is the lateral femoral cutaneous nerve of the thigh, which is often sacrificed with residual numbness causing minimal problems for the patient. If careless exposure passes medial to the iliopectineal eminence, then the femoral artery and vein are at risk. Careless exposure posteriorly in the vicinity of the sacroiliac joint can damage the L5 nerve root. Finally, excessive stretch on the iliopsoas muscle increases the risk of injury to the femoral nerve.

Surgical Technique

The skin incision begins 1 cm lateral or 1 cm medial to the iliac crest and is carried along the inguinal ligament in the fashion of a ilioinguinal approach, or occasionally, as noted in Fig. 28-25 in the interval between sartorius and tensor fasciae latae (51). The periosteum is raised from the iliac crest, and the iliopsoas muscle is stripped from the interior aspect of the ilium, posterior to the sacroiliac joint and the greater sciatic notch, both of which can be visualized easily. Stripping of the iliopsoas muscle is simple because the muscle is not attached to the interior aspect of the pelvis by Sharpey's fibers (51).

If access to the hip joint is desired, then the interval between sartorius and tensor fasciae latae may be developed by extending the dissection along the lateral aspect of the ilium. This requires stripping the lateral muscles by removing Sharpey's fibers and allows visualization of the anterior aspect of the capsule and the anterior inferior iliac spine. Further dissection medially along the anterior column is possible to the iliopectineal eminence. A portion of the capsule and direct head of the rectus may be raised to allow access to the interior aspect of the pelvis. For even greater access, the sartorius and inguinal ligament insertion may be divided 1 cm distal to the anterior superior spine, or an osteotomy of the spine performed. In this approach, the lateral cutaneous femoral nerve of the thigh almost always is sacrificed.

Anterior Ilioinguinal Approach

History

The ilioinguinal approach was developed and introduced by Letournel in the early 1960s (44,147,148) and has consistently produced good results in capable hands (42–44,122, 125,148). The problems with infection early on (with rates up to 30%) involved primarily the retropubic space of Retzius and were solved by moving the medial portion of the incision slightly proximal, placing drains in the retropubic space, and using prophylactic antibiotics (125). This approach creates three working portals or windows: The first is the internal iliac fossa bounded medially by the iliopsoas; the second is bounded by the iliopsoas and the femoral nerve laterally and the femoral vessels medially, giving access to the pelvic brim and quadrilateral space; and the third is medial to the femoral vessels, giving access to the superior pubic ramus and retropubic space of Retzius.

Indications

This approach is appropriate for all anterior lesions—anterior wall, anterior column, anterior with posterior hemitransverse—when access is required to the anterior aspect of the acetabulum distal to the iliopectineal eminence. Fractures proximal to the iliopectineal eminence may be approached by the anterior iliofemoral approach. The ilioinguinal approach also is frequently used by experienced hands to treat both-column fractures in which the posterior column component consists of a single large fragment. Finally, this approach is used for transverse, or T types, in which the rotation and displacement of the transverse limb is anterior.

Access

(See Fig. 28-26.) This approach offers direct visualization of the interior of the iliac wing, anterior sacroiliac joint, entire anterior column, and pubic symphysis.

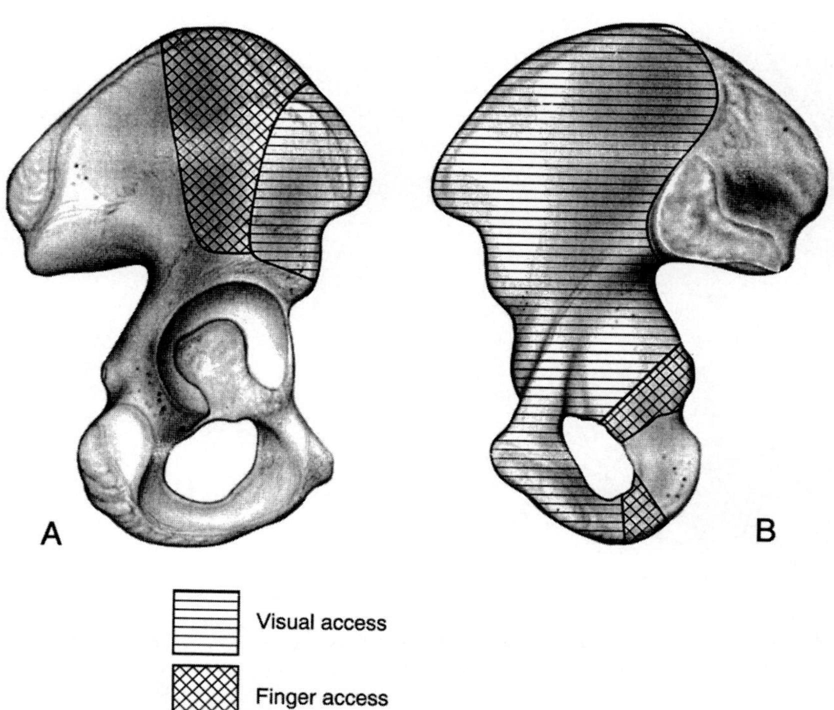

FIGURE 28-26. Access to the pelvis via the ilioinguinal approach, right side. **A:** The lateral (outer) bony pelvis. **B:** The medial (inner) bony pelvis. (From: Sledge CB, ed. *Master techniques in orthopaedic surgery: the hip.* Philadelphia: Lippincott-Raven, 1998, with permission.)

Position

The patient is placed in the supine position on a fluoroscopic table, supported on a bean bag and protected at all bony prominences. A support can be placed under the sacrum to aid in prepping and draping or under the contralateral buttock to improve visualization of the quadrilateral surface during the procedure. If a simultaneous combined anterior and posterior approach is being considered, then the "floppy" lateral position is used, which allows the patient to be rolled from front to back.

Advantages

Excellent access is afforded to the anterior and internal aspects of the entire pelvis and acetabulum. Also, heterotopic ossification is minimal because the iliopsoas muscle is only loosely attached to the ilium.

Disadvantages and Dangers

In its pure form, this approach is extraarticular with the reduction almost entirely by indirect means and performed outside the acetabulum through the three windows. Therefore, the presence of intraarticular fragments and the articular surface reduction cannot be visualized. Neither does the approach provide access to posterior wall fractures. A major disadvantage is possible damage to the femoral or other vessels, including laceration and thrombosis because of traction, or to the femoral nerves. Postoperative hernia also is a theoretical concern. The presence of a preexisting suprapubic catheter mitigates against the use of this approach because of concerns regarding infection. Other contraindications include abdominal distention, ileus, or other conditions that result in abdominal rigidity.

Femoral Vessels

The femoral vessels are at risk during mobilization of the vascular compartment off the iliopectineal fascia. They must be isolated with a wide ribbon Penrose drain and protected throughout the procedure (Figs. 28-27 through 28-31). The lymphatics in this area are often overlooked, which if disrupted can result in significant postoperative lymphedema (125). Leaving the conjoint tendon intact over their surface protects them from undue dissection and retraction.

Corona Mortis

A retropubic communication between the external iliac or deep inferior epigastric artery and the obturator, known as the corona mortis (44,149,150), may arise and extend over the anterior column in the area of the superior pubic ramus (Fig. 28-32). Alternatively, this vessel can represent the origin of the obturator artery from the external iliac system. Estimates of the prevalence of an anomalous origin of the obturator artery have ranged from 10% to 40% (44,48,122, 150). However, the higher end of this range is probably the more accurate figure. Teague and colleagues encountered retropubic anastomoses in 37% of their ilioinguinal exposures, with 43% of these patients having multiple vessels

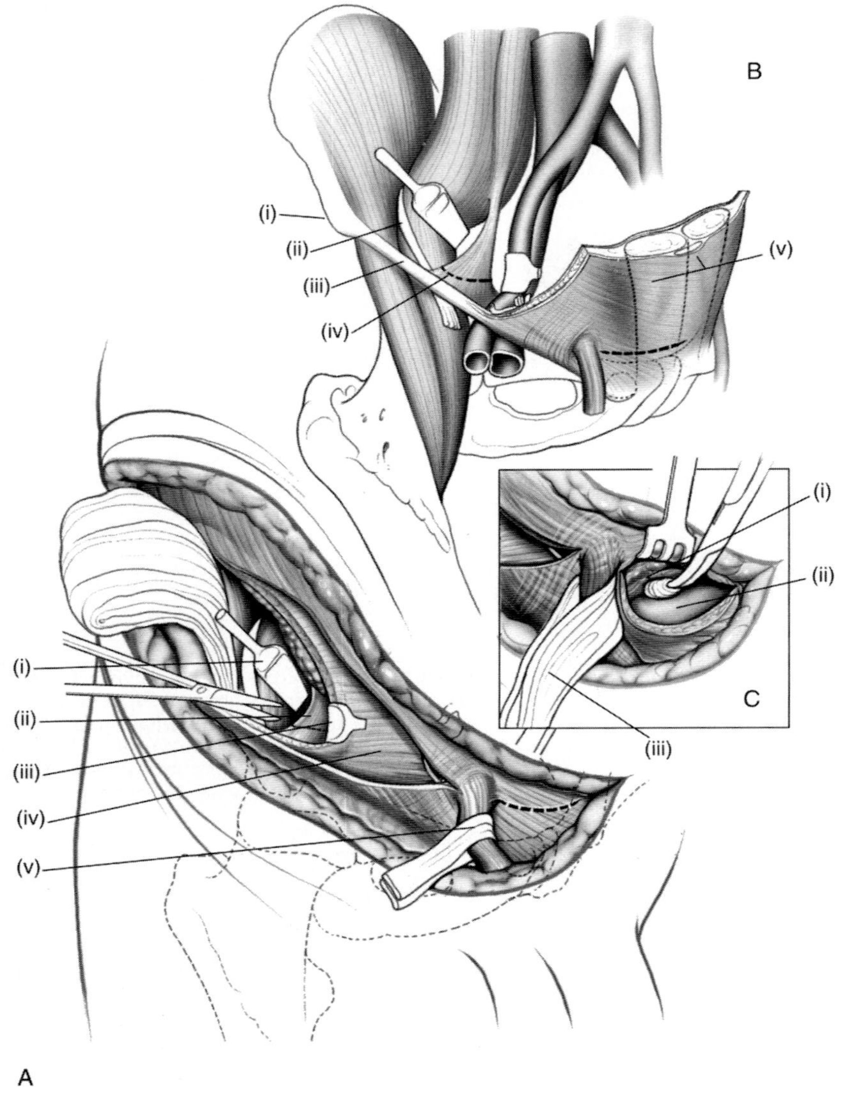

FIGURE 28-27. A: Incision of iliopectineal fascia: **(i)** Retraction laterally of the iliopsoas, femoral nerve, and lateral femoral cutaneous nerve; **(ii)** Incision of the iliopectineal fascia off the iliopectineal eminence; **(iii)** Medial retraction of the femoral vessels; **(iv)** Conjoint tendon overlying external iliac vessels; **(v)** Penrose drain around spermatic cord. **B:** Medial incision of rectus sheath: **(i)** anterior superior iliac spine; **(ii)** femoral nerve; **(iii)** inguinal ligament; **(iv)** iliopectineal fascia; **(v)** rectus. **C:** Exposure of superior pubis and symphysis: **(i)** bladder and space of Retzius; **(ii)** symphysis pubis; **(iii)** Penrose drain around spermatic cord. (From: Sledge CB, ed. *Master techniques in orthopaedic surgery: the hip.* Philadelphia: Lippincott-Raven, 1998, with permission.)

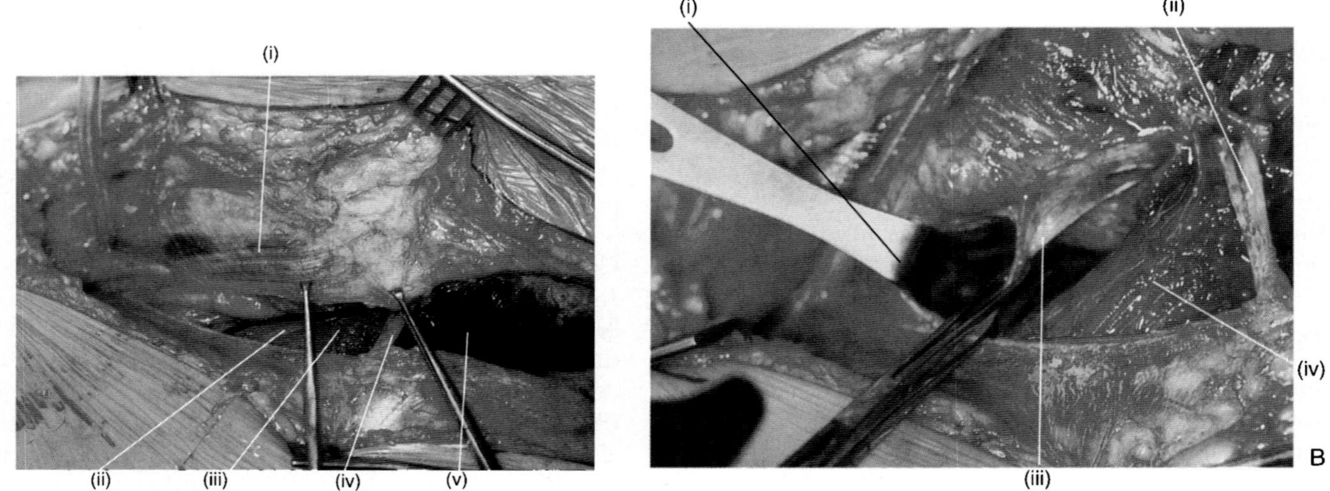

FIGURE 28-28. A: Release of external oblique and conjoint tendons, left side. **(i)** External oblique and conjoint tendons; **(ii)** femoral nerve; **(iii)** iliopsoas muscle; **(iv)** lateral femoral cutaneous nerve; **(v)** iliacus muscle mobilized off inner table of the pelvic wing. **B:** Excision of the iliopectineal fascia, left side. **(i)** Femoral vessels retracted and protected by blunt right angle retractor; **(ii)** lateral femoral cutaneous nerve; **(iii)** iliopectineal fascia; **(iv)** psoas muscle and femoral nerve. (From: Sledge CB, ed. *Master techniques in orthopaedic surgery: the hip.* Philadelphia: Lippincott-Raven, 1998, with permission.)

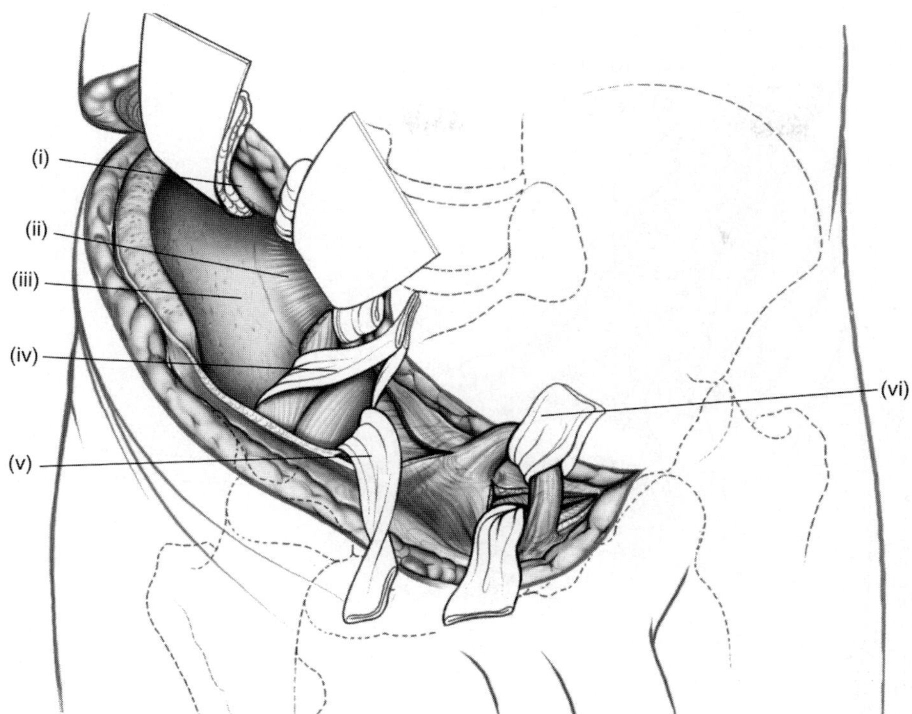

FIGURE 28-29. Lateral window of ilioinguinal, right side: **(i)** Iliopsoas muscle; **(ii)** sacro-iliac joint; **(iii)** internal iliac fossa; **(iv)** Penrose drain around iliopsoas, femoral nerve, and lateral femoral cutaneous nerve; **(v)** Penrose drain around femoral vessels; **(vi)** Penrose drain around spermatic cord. (From: Sledge CB, ed. *Master techniques in orthopaedic surgery: the hip.* Philadelphia: Lippincott-Raven, 1998, with permission.)

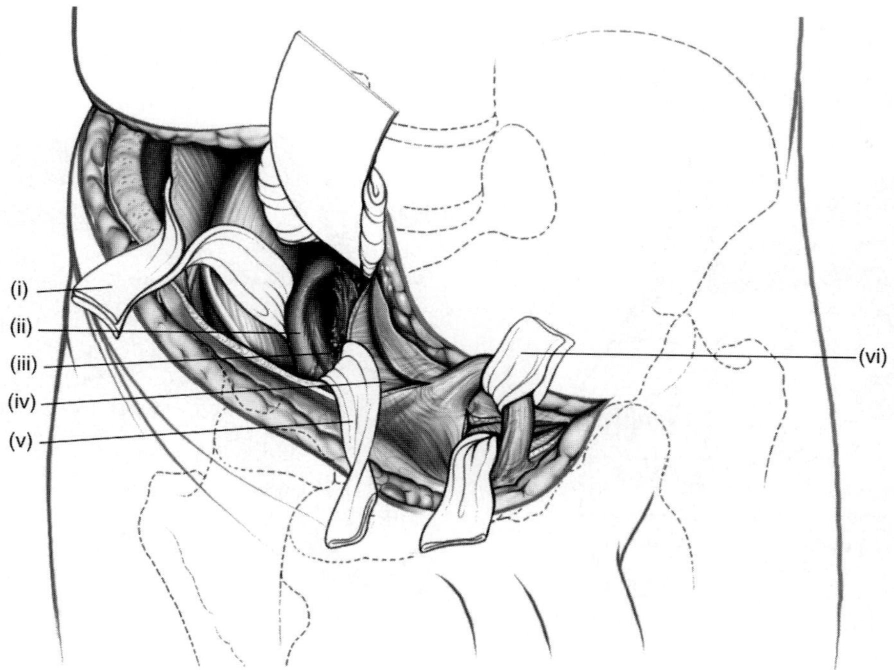

FIGURE 28-30. Middle window of ilioinguinal, right side: **(i)** Penrose drain around iliopsoas, femoral nerve, and lateral femoral cutaneous nerve; **(ii)** pelvic brim; **(iii)** iliopectineal fascia released down to iliopectineal eminence; **(iv)** femoral vessels protected by their overlying internal iliac muscle; **(v)** Penrose drain around femoral vessels; **(vi)** Penrose drain around spermatic cord. (From: Sledge CB, ed. *Master techniques in orthopaedic surgery: the hip.* Philadelphia: Lippincott-Raven, 1998, with permission.)

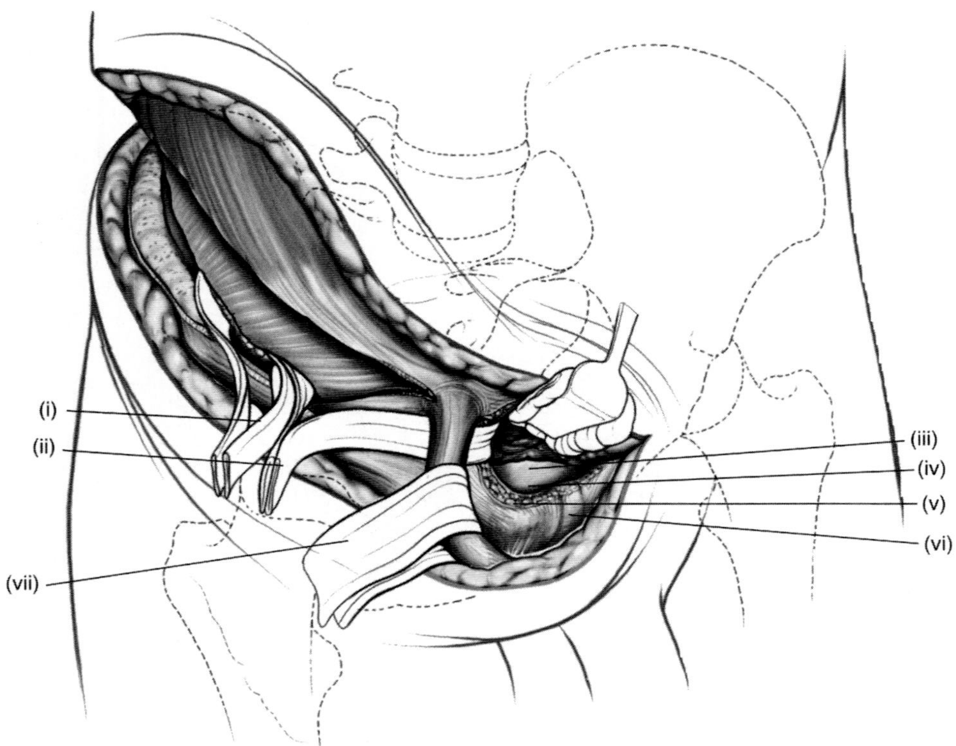

FIGURE 28-31. Medial window of ilioinguinal, right side: **(i)** Penrose drain around iliopsoas, femoral nerve, and lateral femoral cutaneous nerve; **(ii)** Penrose drain around femoral vessels; **(iii)** bladder and space of Retzius; **(iv)** pubis; **(v)** pubic tubercle and cut end of rectus muscle; **(vi)** symphysis pubis; **(vii)** Penrose drain around spermatic cord. (From: Sledge CB, ed. *Master techniques in orthopaedic surgery: the hip.* Philadelphia: Lippincott-Raven, 1998, with permission.)

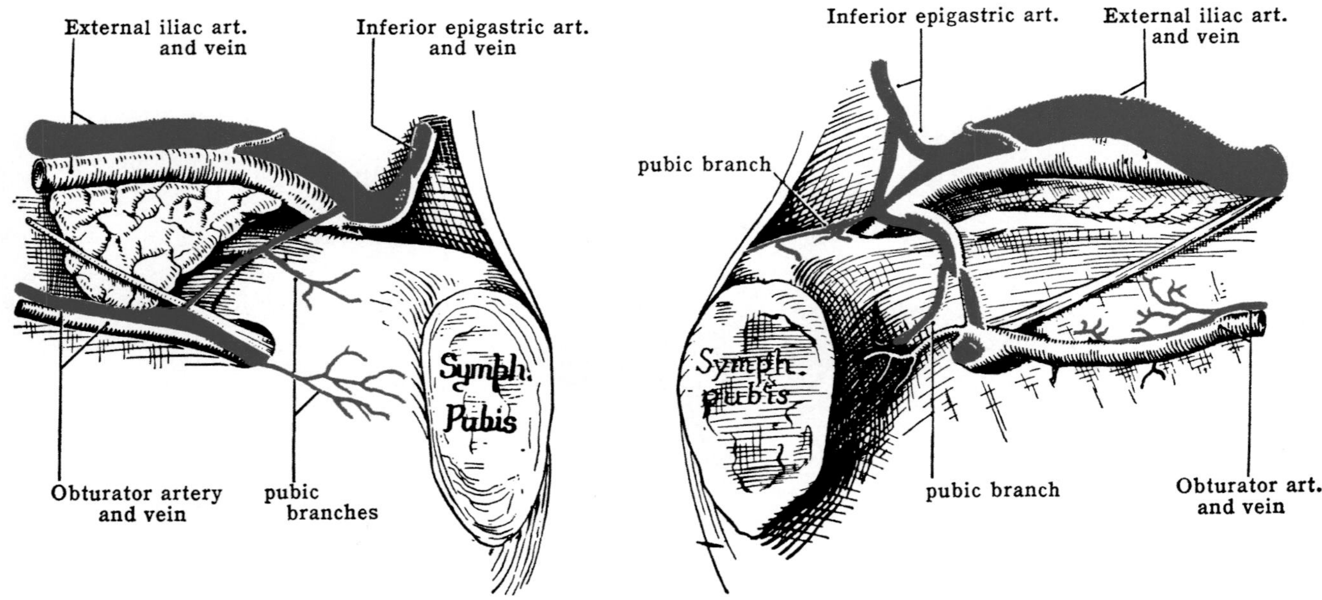

FIGURE 28-32. A: Behind the body of the pubis the pubic branch of the obturator artery forms an anastomosis with the pubic branch of the inferior epigastric artery. **B:** The obturator artery arises from the inferior epigastric via the pubic anastomosis. In a study of 283 limbs, the obturator artery arose from the internal iliac artery in 70%, from the inferior epigastric in 25.4%, and from both equally in 4.6%. (From: Anderson JE. *Grant's atlas of anatomy,* 8th ed. Baltimore: Williams & Wilkins, 1983, with permission.)

along the posterior superior aspect of the superior ramus (149). Furthermore, two cadaver studies have detailed a large number of both arterial and venous anastomoses, with arterial anastomoses in 34% and 43% of specimens, venous anastomoses in 70% and 59%, and both arterial and venous anastomoses in 20% and 27%, respectively (84% and 73% of the specimens had at least one venous or arterial connection of approximately ≥2 mm diameter) (149,150). That there appears to be a higher incidence of vascular connections based on cadaver studies is likely because of the impact of the fracture pattern with the potential disruption of some of these connections at the time of the injury.

Femoral Nerve

The femoral nerve is at risk during mobilization and excessive retraction of the iliopsoas muscle (Fig. 28-29). Hip flexion aids in relaxation of the iliopsoas muscle, minimizing the need for any undue retraction.

Lateral Femoral Cutaneous Nerve

Because of its position and variable anatomy (151,152), the lateral femoral cutaneous nerve is at risk when mobilizing the transversalis abdominus and internal oblique muscles off the inguinal ligament just medial to the anterior superior iliac spine. The nerve also can be stretched during mobilization and excessive retraction of the iliopsoas muscle. Patients should be warned preoperatively to expect this complication; approximately 35% develop loss of sensation and 5% develop meralgia parasthetica (151).

Inguinal Canal

An inadequate closure of the floor of the inguinal canal can lead to a direct hernia. To avoid this complication, a sound closure of the insertion of the transversalis abdominus muscle and the internal oblique muscle into the inguinal ligament is necessary. The contents of the spermatic cord are at risk during exposure of the external inguinal ring and should be carefully isolated and retracted with a Penrose drain (Figs. 28-27 and 28-33).

Obturator Neurovascular Structures

The obturator artery and nerve are at risk during exposure of the quadrilateral surface and must be protected with carefully placed retractors.

Surgical Technique

The cutaneous incision travels 1 cm medially or laterally along the anterior two thirds of the iliac crest in a curvilinear fashion toward the anterior superior iliac spine, where it then continues parallel to the inguinal ligament ending just beyond the midline at a point 2 cm above the pubic symphysis (Fig. 28-34).

The proximal aspect of the approach is exposed first by releasing the lateral insertion of the external oblique muscle in the avascular plane between its insertion and that of the abductor muscles (Fig. 28-35). A subperiosteal dissection is carried out elevating the abdominal musculature along with the iliacus muscle to expose the internal iliac fossa (Fig. 28-

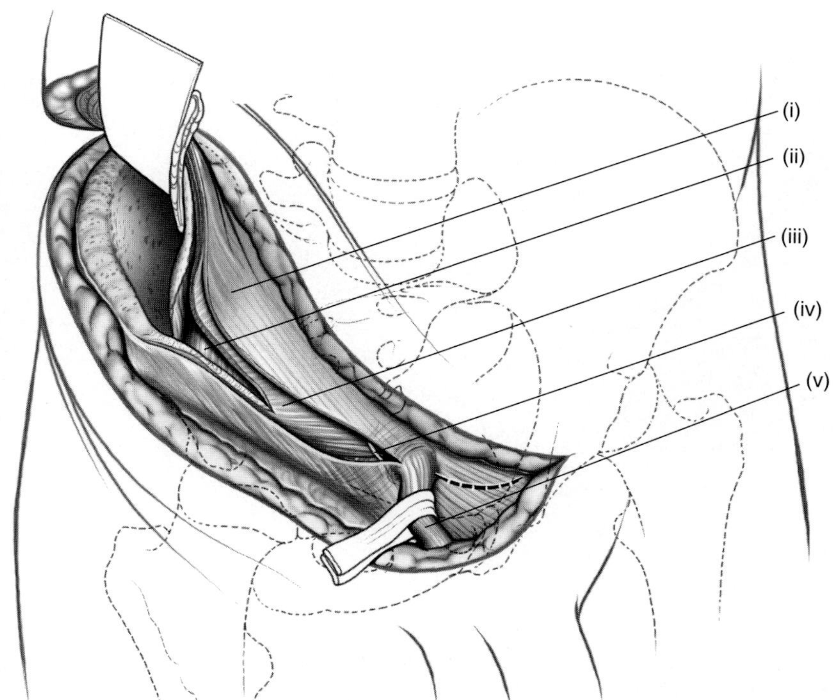

FIGURE 28-33. The inguinal exposure, right side: **(i)** External oblique; **(ii)** iliopsoas; **(iii)** conjoint tendon: internal oblique and transversalis fascia; **(iv)** ilioinguinal nerve; and **(v)** spermatic cord. (From: Sledge CB, ed. *Master techniques in orthopaedic surgery: the hip.* Philadelphia: Lippincott-Raven, 1998, with permission.)

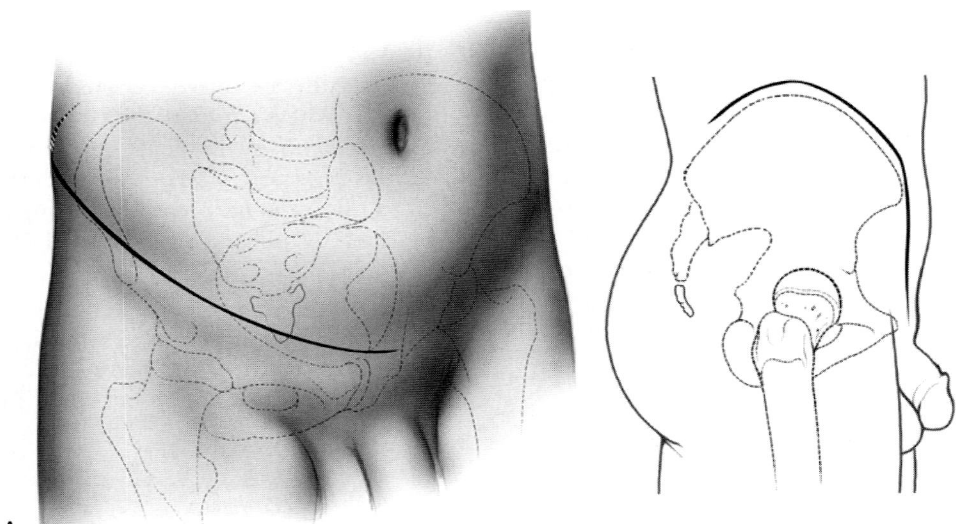

FIGURE 28-34. The ilioinguinal incision, right side. **A:** Obturator oblique view. **B:** Lateral view. (From: Sledge CB, ed. *Master techniques in orthopaedic surgery: the hip.* Philadelphia: Lippincott-Raven, 1998, with permission.)

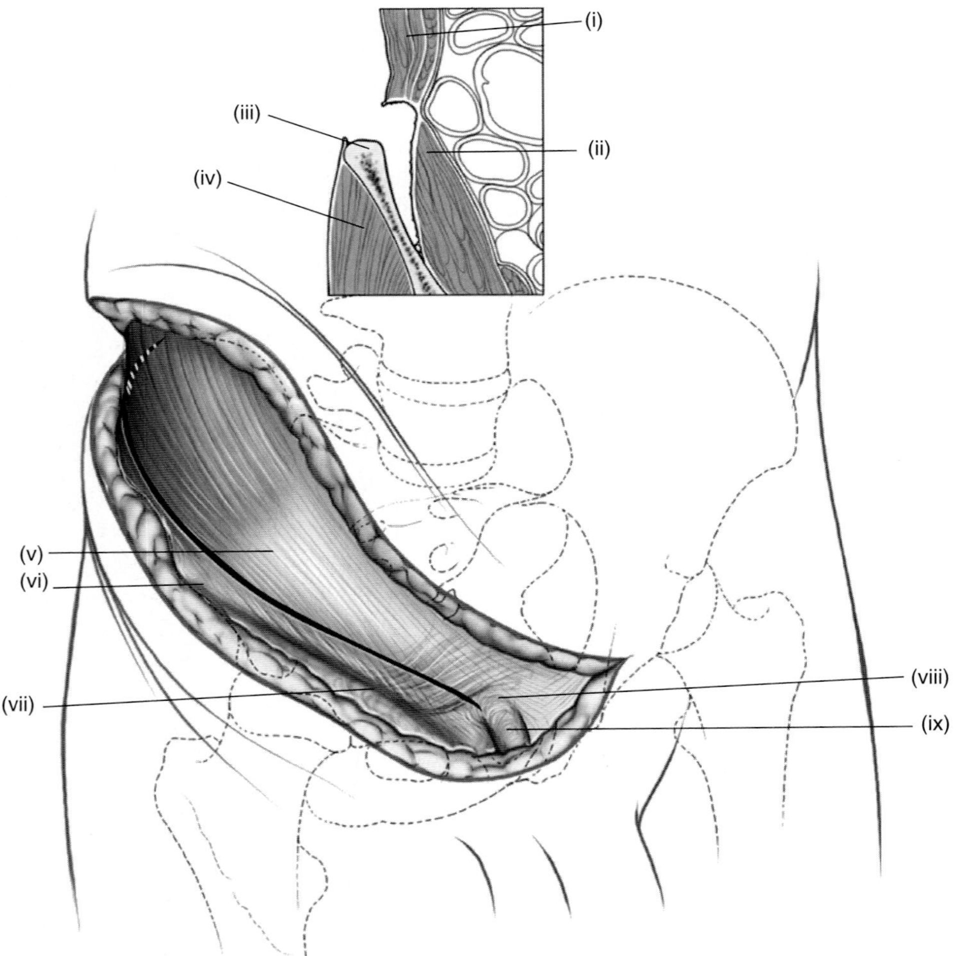

FIGURE 28-35. Exposure of iliac crest and external oblique muscle, right side. **(i)** Abdominal muscles freed from crest; **(ii)** iliacus; **(iii)** iliac crest; **(iv)** gluteus medius; **(v)** external oblique; **(vi)** anterior superior iliac spine; **(vii)** inguinal ligament; **(viii)** superficial inguinal ring; and **(ix)** spermatic cord. (From: Sledge CB, ed. *Master techniques in orthopaedic surgery: the hip.* Philadelphia: Lippincott-Raven, 1998, with permission.)

33). Dissection is easy in this area because no Sharpey's fibers connect the iliopsoas to the medial surface, except at the iliac crest (51). During this portion of the exposure, a nutrient artery often is encountered along the iliac fossa, which requires hemostasis. The dissection is carried posterior to the sacroiliac joint and inferior to the greater sciatic notch. Next, the iliac fossa is packed with sponges and attention directed to the inguinal portion of the dissection.

If the dissection is to be taken to the symphysis pubis (as is normally required), the external inguinal ring (the termination of the inguinal canal) and the structures exiting it must be identified, isolated, and protected using a Penrose drain (Fig. 28-33). These structures include the spermatic cord in the male, the round ligament in the female, the ilioinguinal nerve, and the genital branch of the genitofemoral nerve. Knowledge of these structures as well as the pertinent anatomy of the inguinal region is crucial to the next portion of the procedure.

The external oblique aponeurosis is the most superficial layer of the abdominal wall muscles and is encountered under the subcutaneous tissue. Medially, below the level of the umbilicus, it forms the superficial lamina of the rectus sheath. Distally, the termination of its aponeurosis forms the inguinal ligament, which is firmly attached to the iliac wing laterally and pubic tubercle medially. Inferiorly, the inguinal ligament rotates to a horizontal orientation (known as the "shelving border"), which forms the inferior wall of the inguinal canal (122). The internal oblique muscle lies deep to the external oblique and superficial to the underlying transversus abdominis. It takes its origin in part from the iliac crest and investing fascia of the iliopsoas. Its aponeurotic termination is medially continuous with the anterior layer of the rectus sheath and inferiorly fuses with the transversus aponeurosis forming the conjoint tendon (falx inguinalis) (122). The transversus abdominis is the deepest of the three abdominal wall flat muscles, with its fibers running horizontally forward, becoming aponeurotic and blending into the anterior rectus sheath medially. The conjoint tendon continues distally to merge into the shelving border of the inguinal ligament.

The external oblique aponeurosis is incised 5 mm from its insertion on the inguinal ligament from the anterior superior iliac spine to the external inguinal ring or just above the ring (Figs. 28-33 and 28-35). The inferior flap is gently retracted with Allis clamps in order to identify the conjoint tendon (internal oblique and transversalis abdominus muscles) and its distal insertion into the inguinal ligament. This exposes the structures in the inguinal canal, a triangular cavity that measures approximately 4 cm in the adult (122). The anterior wall is formed by the external oblique aponeurosis, the inferior wall by the shelving portion of the inguinal ligament, and the posterior wall by structures derived from the transversus abdominis (122). The deep inguinal ring is formed from a defect in the transversalis fascia. The spermatic cord (males) or round ligament (females) pass through this. The ilioinguinal nerve emerges from the lateral border of the psoas major muscle, extends forward on the iliacus, and pierces the transversus abdominis and internal oblique to traverse the inguinal canal (122). The genital branch of the genitofemoral nerve penetrates the deep ring to lie along the posterior aspect of the cord or round ligament.

A thickening of the endoabdominal fascia over the pelvic exit of the iliacus and psoas muscles (psoas sheath), known as the iliopectineal fascia, merges into the inguinal ligament and is the boundary between the true and false pelvis. This fascia serves as a major anatomic landmark for the next portion of the dissection as it separates the structures running under the ligament into two compartments: the lateral lacuna musculorum (iliopsoas, femoral nerve, and lateral femoral cutaneous nerve of the thigh) and the medial lacuna vasorum (external iliac vessels and lymphatics). Lateral to the iliopectineal fascia, while applying gentle tension on the inferior leaf of the external oblique, the conjoint tendon is incised from the inguinal ligament with a 2 mm cuff to facilitate the ease of its repair later (Fig. 28-33). Here, care must be maintained to avoid injury to the lateral femoral cutaneous nerve, which courses immediately beneath the conjoint tendon just medial to the anterior superior iliac spine (ASIS) (44,122,151,152). Hospodar and colleagues (152) recorded an average of 20 mm medial to the ASIS in 68 cadaver dissections. However, the location of the nerve is quite variable, with it traveling up to 4 cm or more medially and having a different course, such as passing through the inguinal ligament or sartorius muscle (151,152).

As the incision proceeds medially, the reflection of the iliopectineal fascia is encountered (Figs. 28-27, 28-28, and 28-33). Extreme care must be exercised, as the femoral vascular bundle lies just medial to this structure. Great care must be taken when exposing, elevating, and mobilizing the femoral vessels. The entire sheath should be freed and protected, including the lymphatics, so that postoperative edema does not become a problem. Also, massive thrombosis of the femoral artery or vein may occasionally occur with this approach. Because of these concerns and in contrast to the classical description (44,125) we prefer to leave the conjoint tendon intact over the femoral artery, vein, and lymphatics. This avoids any unnecessary dissection (Figs. 28-27A and 28-33) and protects these structures from undue traction.

Medial to the vessels, the conjoint tendon can be incised, if required, and the ipsilateral rectus abdominis muscle released 1cm from its anterior insertion from the pubic tubercle to the pubic symphysis (Figs. 28-27A,B and 28-31). This portion of the exposure allows access to the space of Retzius and the symphysis (Fig. 28-27C). It should be appreciated that in the presence of anterior pelvic ring injuries, one or both of the rectus abdominis muscles already may be avulsed off the pubic tubercle and ramus, in which case the bladder is at increased risk of iatrogenic injury during the exposure. Keeping the bladder decompressed with a Foley catheter lessens such risks. A final consideration is that an associated anterior pelvic ring injury might require fixation across the pubic symphysis necessitating a partial release of the contralateral rectus abdominis muscle.

The iliopectineal fascia must be isolated and excised in order to access the quadrilateral surface (Figs. 28-27A,B and 28-28). Laterally the iliopsoas muscle and the femoral nerve are carefully and bluntly separated off the iliopectineal fascia with a small elevator, blunt-tipped scissors, or hemostat, and mobilized with a 1-in. Penrose drain (not shown). The femoral vasculature and lymphatics are next delicately dissected off the iliopectineal fascia medially, maintaining these structures as a unit with the overlying conjoint tendon. Frequently, small vessels penetrate this fascia and require ligation. Once the iliopectineal fascia has been isolated and the adjacent structures gently retracted, it is divided down to the iliopectineal eminence and posteriorly along the pelvic brim to just anterior to the sacroiliac joint using scissors or a scalpel under direct visualization.

A broad Penrose drain then is passed around the femoral vessels, lymphatics, and the overlying conjoint tendon (Fig. 28-29). Dissection is carried out along the pelvic brim, under the femoral vessels and surrounding lymphatics, to expose the middle fossa (the quadrilateral plate) (Fig. 28-30). At this point, it is important to search for the corona mortis, a variable retropubic anastomosis, which should be ligated if identified (Fig. 28-32). There is normally an anastomosis between the inferior epigastric and the obturator artery, which must be ligated or clipped (51,83), but if the entire obturator artery crosses the column and is inadvertently divided disastrous consequences may ensue. When mobilizing the femoral vessels the surgeon should inspect the area under vessels in an attempt to identify such anomalous vessels (on average 6 cm from the symphysis but ranging widely) (150) in order to ligate them.

Access to the acetabulum through the ilioinguinal approach is now complete. Medial retraction of the iliopsoas muscle and femoral nerve allows access to the internal iliac fossa and anterior sacroiliac joint, the first (lateral) window of the ilioinguinal approach (Fig. 28-29). The second (middle) window is visualized by lateral retraction of the iliopsoas muscle and the femoral nerve and medial retraction of the femoral vasculature allowing access to the pelvic brim, the quadrilateral surface, and the posterior column (Fig. 28-30). The third (medial) window is exposed by lateral retraction of the femoral vasculature and lymphatics and allows access to the superior ramus and pubic symphysis (Fig. 28-31). The contents of the inguinal canal can be mobilized either medially or laterally as needed. The obturator vessels and nerves can be visualized through either the second or third window and require protection during exposure and reduction of the fracture. A limited subperiosteal exposure of the outer surface of the anterior iliac wing occasionally is needed in order to apply pelvic reduction clamps to control either the iliac wing fragments or the posterior column.

Reduction of the acetabular fracture should be performed in a stepwise fashion according to the preoperative plan. Unlike most other articular fractures, acetabular fracture reduction proceeds from the periphery toward the joint in a sequential fashion. Every step is critical to the outcome of the procedure, including an accurate reduction of all fracture fragments, since the articular surface is not directly visualized through this approach. Because peripheral malalignment can result in major articular incongruence (a major concern with this approach as the major portion of the articular reduction is by indirect means peripherally), reduction of each fracture segment must be performed painstakingly and exactly. Each fracture line should be carefully irrigated and debrided to remove hematoma and small fragments. The hip joint also is irrigated and loose fragments removed through the displaced portion of the articular fracture.

Both the exposure and the stabilization can be aided by hip flexion in order to relax structures crossing anterior to the hip joint. A Schanz screw inserted through the lateral aspect of the femur into the femoral head followed by distal traction also can be extremely helpful because it can facilitate fracture reduction through ligamentotaxis. This is especially useful in cases where the femoral head has protruded through the quadrilateral surface.

Reconstruction of anterior column with a posterior hemitransverse (Type A3) and both-column (Type C) fractures begins with reduction of the individual peripheral fracture fragments to portions of the intact pelvis. Working from the periphery toward the articular surface, fragments are sequentially reduced and provisionally stabilized. This process requires patience and a 3D understanding of the pelvic anatomy. The iliac crest portion of the fracture can be reduced with pointed reduction clamps, or specially designed pelvic reduction clamps then stabilized by any combination of lag screws or 3.5-mm reconstruction plates. It is often helpful to predrill a gliding hole prior to fracture reduction in order to assure optimal lag screw position in the thin cortical cap of the iliac crest. Screws also can be placed from anteriorly into the sciatic buttress.

For anterior column with a posterior hemitransverse fractures, the anterior column is next reduced to the intact iliac wing and temporarily stabilized with a Kirschner wire or 3.5-mm lag screw into the sciatic buttress through the lateral window of the ilioinguinal approach. Then through the middle window, any anterior wall fracture is reduced. Finally, any superior pubic rami and displaced pubic column fractures are reduced and provisionally stabilized through the medial window. For both-column fractures, the reconstruction must be performed perfectly, from the iliac crest to the symphysis pubis, in order to provide an anatomic template for subsequent reduction of the posterior

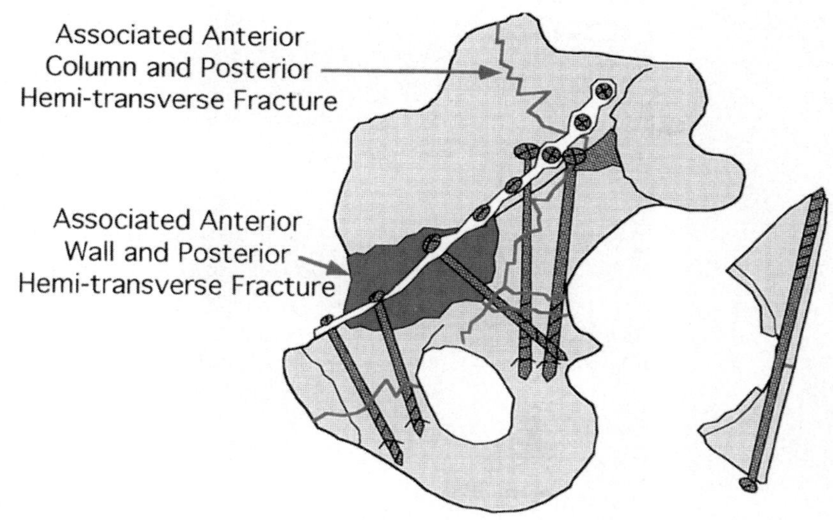

FIGURE 28-36. Example of contoured pelvic reconstruction plate, anterior screw placement, posterior screw placement, and posterior column lag-screw placement from an ilioinguinal approach, right side. (From: Sledge CB, ed. *Master techniques in orthopaedic surgery: the hip.* Philadelphia: Lippincott-Raven, 1998, with permission.)

column to the reduced anterior column. An incomplete anterior column fracture may require completion, to permit an adequate reduction. The anterior column segment is typically shortened and externally rotated. In order to reduce this segment to the intact iliac wing ("spur" sign) (see Figs. 28-28C and 28-43C), a significant amount of longitudinal traction is often required.

Definitive fixation of most fracture types involves a 3.5-mm reconstruction plate molded along the iliac fossa, across the iliopectineal eminence to the pubic tubercle and pubic column (Fig. 28-36). This should not cross the symphysis pubis unless there are associated ramus fractures, or if there is involvement of the symphysis pubis with an associated pelvic ring injury. This plate must be perfectly molded, otherwise its fixation to the pelvis can lead to malreduction of the acetabular fracture. The plate is stabilized to the internal iliac fossa, superior to the acetabulum, with 3.5-mm cortical screws, and medially to the pubic tubercle and ramus. Fixation within the thin central area of the iliac fossa should be avoided. In contrast, the sciatic buttress and quadrilateral plate, proximal to the acetabulum, provide the most optimal purchase for stabilization of the anterior column to the iliac wing and posterior column.

Following anatomic reduction and stabilization of the anterior column, the rotated and medially displaced posterior column is reduced to the restored anterior column. This is mandatory for both-column fractures and anterior column with a posterior hemitransverse fractures where the hemitransverse component is high, cutting into the greater sciatic notch. However, when the hemitransverse component of the later exits lower at the level of the ischial spine or lesser sciatic notch, the inferior segment can be difficult to manipulate and small amounts of displacement should be accepted, rarely mitigating for a supplemental posterior approach.

Reduction of the posterior column segment often requires lateral and anterior traction of the hip, via the Schanz screw in the femoral head, and specially designed pelvic reduction clamps. One tine of the clamp is placed on the outer surface of the ilium, through a small limited exposure, and the other tine is placed through the lateral or middle window of the ilioinguinal exposure onto the quadrilateral plate and/or posterior column (Fig. 28-37). A small supplemental bone hook, gently slid down the quadrilateral plate, can hook the ischial spine and pull the posterior column up to the anterior column. On reduction of the posterior column, 3.5-mm lag screws are inserted through the pelvic brim superior to the acetabulum into the posterior column (Fig. 28-38). Care must be taken to avoid intraarticular placement of these lag screws, which are often up to 110 mm in length. This requires a careful appreciation of the location of the acetabulum relative to the fixed pelvic landmarks (i.e., inferior to the anterior inferior iliac spine and under the iliopectineal eminence). To best prevent joint penetration, these screws should parallel the quadrilateral surface, aiming for the ischial spine (Fig. 28-39). From a more proximal starting point in the iliac fossa, one can aim for the ischial tuberosity, often obtaining fixation with long screws.

After completion of fracture reduction and fixation, drains are inserted into the space of Retzius (if it has been opened), over the quadrilateral surface, and along the internal iliac fossa. The rectus abdominus muscle is reattached to the pubis. The floor of the inguinal canal is repaired by suturing the conjoint tendons of the transversalis abdominis and the internal oblique muscles to the inguinal ligament

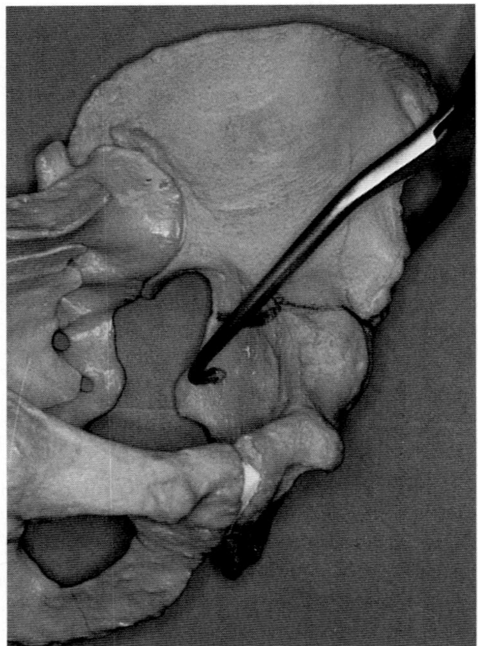

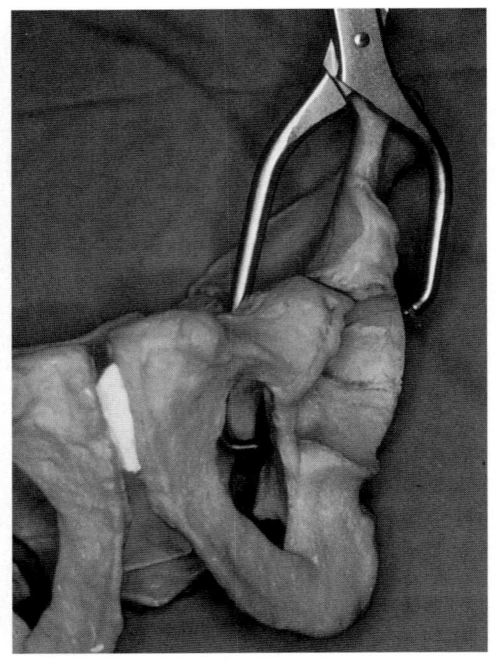

FIGURE 28-37. "Saw bones" left hemipelvis: using an offset large pelvic clamp (Synthes, Paoli, PA) to obtain reduction. The longer arm of the clamp is placed along the quadrilateral plate and the shorter arm inserted through an interval between the anterior inferior and anterior superior iliac spines to lie on the outer table of the iliac wing. **A:** Iliac oblique view. **B:** Obturator oblique view. (From: Sledge CB, ed. *Master techniques in orthopaedic surgery: the hip.* Philadelphia: Lippincott-Raven, 1998, with permission.)

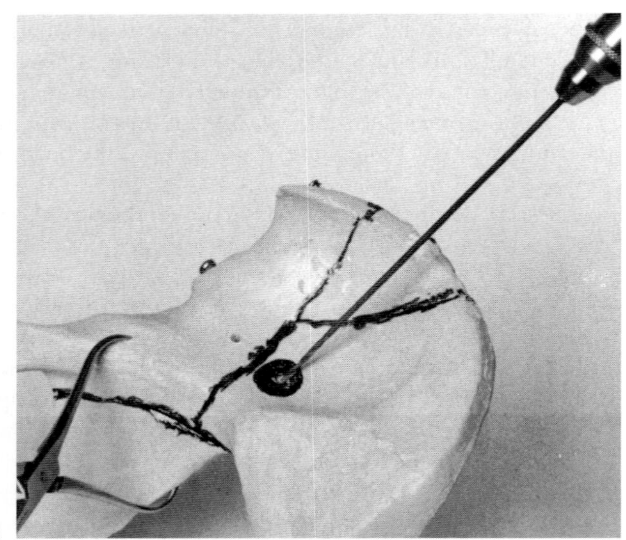

FIGURE 28-38. A: Posterior column lag screw. Note the entry point at the tip of the drill just anterior to the pelvic brim at the sacroiliac joint. A lag screw in this area tends to pull the posterior column up to the anterior column, thus reducing it; however, incorrect placement allows it to penetrate the joint. The posterior column must have provisional fixation with a pointed reduction clamp **(A)** or a cerclage wire **(B),** as seen in this case demonstrating a both-column fracture. An anterior column lag screw is noted fixing the anterior column to the posterior iliac fragment. **C:** The posterior lag screw is inserted.

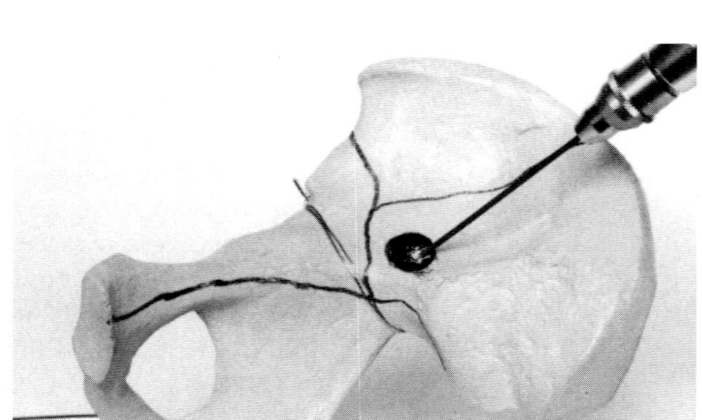

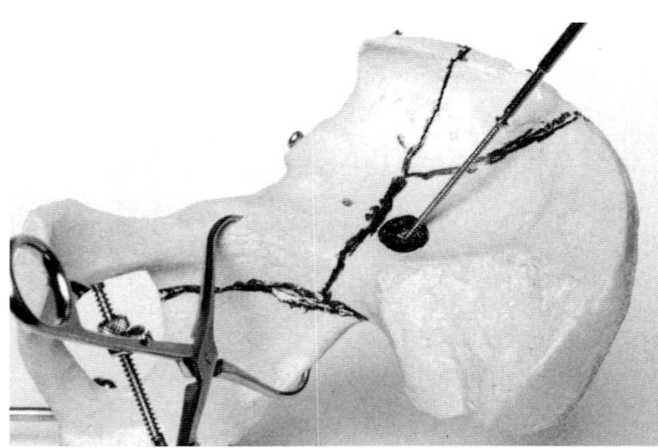

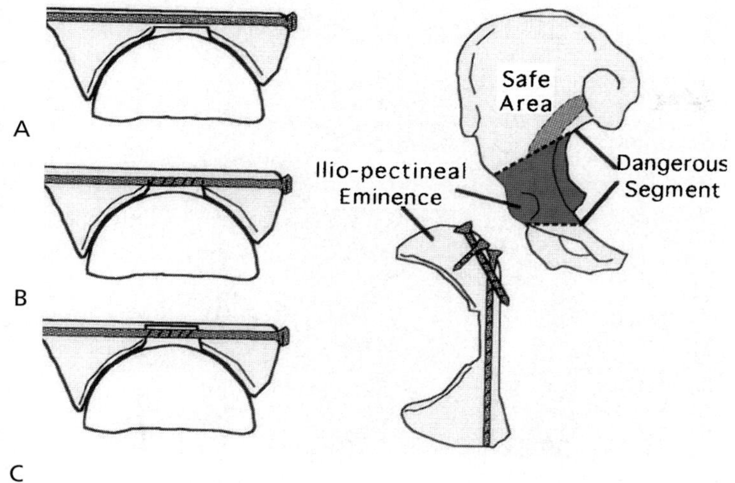

FIGURE 28-39. Safe and danger zones for anterior to posterior screw placement, right side. (From: Letournel E, Judet R. In: Elson RA, ed. *Fractures of the acetabulum,* 2nd ed, Chapter 22, New York: Springer-Verlag, 1993, with permission.) **A, B,** and **C** all represent safe screws parallel to the quadrilateral plate, yet variable relative to the cotyloid fossa.

with nonabsorbable sutures. The roof the inguinal canal is restored by repair of the external oblique aponeurosis and external inguinal ring, allowing passage of the spermatic cord in the male and the round ligament in the female. The external oblique muscle is then reattached to the inguinal ligament and the iliac crest using nonabsorbable sutures. A superficial suction drain is inserted, and the skin closed.

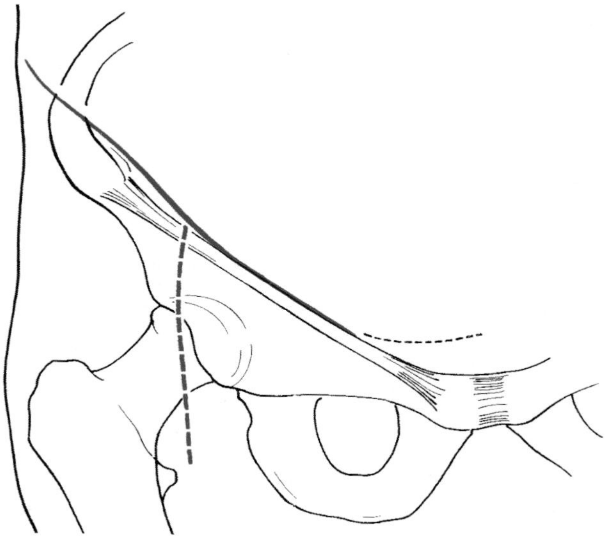

FIGURE 28-40. Ilioinguinal approach with T extension to allow intraarticular visualization of the hip joint. By developing the interval between the sartorius and tensor—the Smith-Petersen approach—with or without division of the conjoint insertion of the ilioinguinal ligament and sartorius, the anterior aspect of the hip joint can be approached, as noted in the iliofemoral approach. This combined approach affords a complete view of the medial surface of the pelvis through the ilioinguinal approach and the anterior aspect of the hip joint, as noted in the iliofemoral approach. This approach is valuable if cerlage wires are to be used for reduction techniques and also for the placement of the large clamps for reduction. (From: Schatzker J, Tile M. *The rationale of operative fracture care.* Heidelberg: Springer-Verlag, 1987, with permission.)

Modifications of the Ilioinguinal Approach

Several modifications of the anterior ilioinguinal approach are available, including distal, lateral, or even posterior extension (Figs. 28-40 and 28-41). It is advantageous that the decision to use them can be made either during preoperative planning or implemented during the operative procedure. The major disadvantage of these modifications is the stripping of lateral muscles with the risk of heterotopic ossification and the possibility of devascularization of articular fragments. Prophylaxis against heterotopic ossification is recommended. Additionally, the failure to maintain strict subperiosteal dissection can lead to injury of the sciatic nerve and superior gluteal neurovascular structures.

Occasionally, it may be desirable for the surgeon to visualize the hip joint intraarticularly. This can be accomplished easily by combining the ilioinguinal with the Smith-Petersen iliofemoral approach (see Figs. 28-40 and 28-60) (51). A vertical incision is made, starting at the anterior superior spine, and extended distally. The sartorius insertion to the anterior superior spine usually is predrilled and removed with a saw or osteotome, allowing access to the lateral aspect of the pelvis. The remainder of the approach is the standard iliofemoral one. This outer table exposure may be limited, but it allows the passage of cerclage wires, which is very valuable in reducing these fractures (51,148,152).

A second modification of the ilioinguinal involves a more limited extension of the lateral incision (Fig. 28-41) (148). This consists of limited elevation of the gluteus medius and minimus from the lateral aspect of the ilium, starting at the gluteal tubercle and continuing anteriorly to the interspinous notch and posteriorly to the greater sciatic notch. Care is

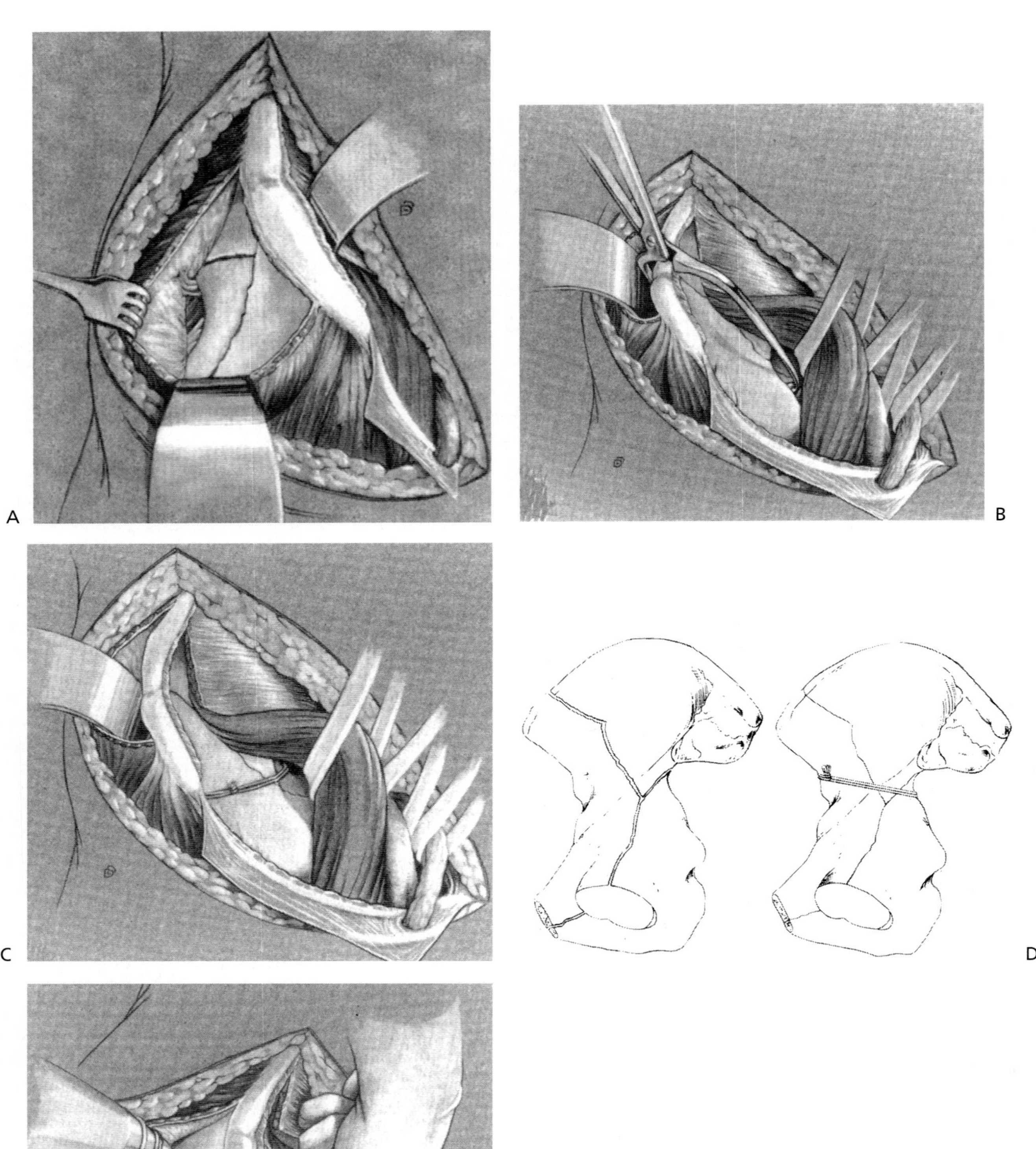

FIGURE 28-41. A: Exposure of lateral ilium after elevation of gluteus medius and minimus muscles. **B:** Temporary stabilization of fracture using pelvic damp on each side of the innominate bone. **C:** Position of cerclage wire through greater sciatic notch and interspinous notch. **D:** Model demonstrates cerclage wire as an aid to fracture reduction. **E:** Position of drill for lateral to medial lag screw placement. (From: Gorczyca JT, Powell JN, Tile M. Lateral extension of the ilioinguinal incision in the operative treatment of acetabulum fractures. *Injury* 1995;26(3): 207–212, with permission.)

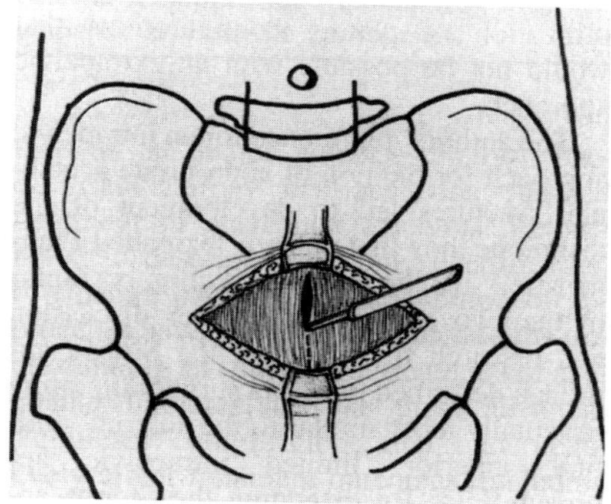

FIGURE 28-42. A transverse incision is made 2 cm above the symphysis. Anterior fascia is incised at the midline. Acetabular fracture fixation via a modified Stoppa limited intrapelvic approach. (From: Cole JD, Bolhofner BR. Description of operative technique and preliminary treatment results. *Clin Orthop* 1994;(305): 112–123, with permission.)

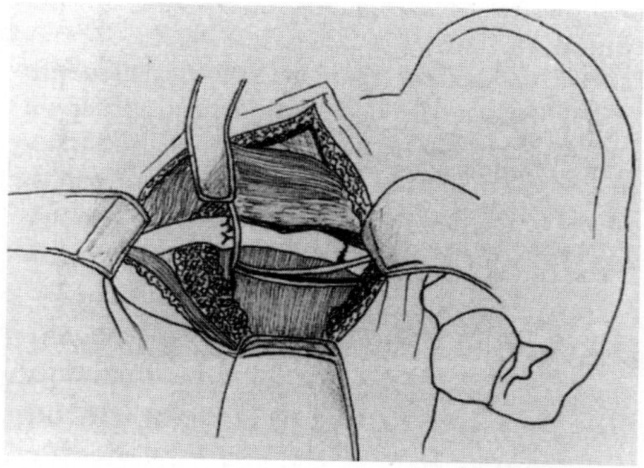

FIGURE 28-44. Anastomotic branch of the inferior epigastric and obturator vessels are visualized. Retraction of the rectus and external iliac vein is performed. (From: Cole JD, Bolhofner BR. Description of operative technique and preliminary treatment results. *Clin Orthop* 1994;(305):112–123, with permission.)

taken to preserve the attachment of the muscles to the iliac crest posterior to the gluteal tubercle. The periosteal elevator must maintain contact with the bone at all times in order to avoid injury to the sciatic nerve, superior gluteal nerve, and superior gluteal vessels as the subperiosteal dissection continues posteriorly. Through this approach, a pelvic clamp can be placed on each side of the innominate bone to aid reduction, and implants—including cerclage wire or lateral-to-medial lag screws—become possible (148).

For both-column fractures, which extend into the sciatic buttress or sacroiliac joint, the classical ilioinguinal approach provides inadequate visualization. As an alternative to extensile approaches in these cases, Weber and Mast (154) described another modification of the ilioinguinal approach, which incorporates the posterior approach to the sacroiliac joint. The patient is positioned on a radiolucent operating table with the affected side rotated up 45 degrees. By tilting the table down 45 degrees toward the affected side, the patient is thus oriented in the supine position and by rotating the table up 45 degrees, the patient reaches a lateral position that allows posterior exposure. The ilioinguinal portion of the procedure is performed as described. However, the incision along the iliac crest is carried more posteriorly to the posterior superior iliac spine, then directed straight inferiorly as described in the classic approach to the sacroiliac joint. After the dissection is carried through the subcutaneous tissue to the gluteus fascia, the gluteus maximus muscle is released from the posterior crest and sacrum. A subperiosteal dissection then is performed to the level of the fracture.

Modified Stoppa Approach

(See Figs. 28-42 through 28-48.)

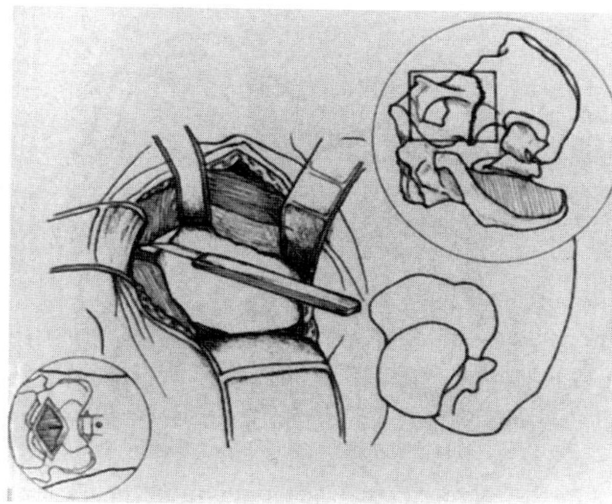

FIGURE 28-43. Elevation of the rectus insertion on the pubis. (From: Cole JD, Bolhofner BR. Description of operative technique and preliminary treatment results. *Clin Orthop* 1994;(305): 112–123, with permission.)

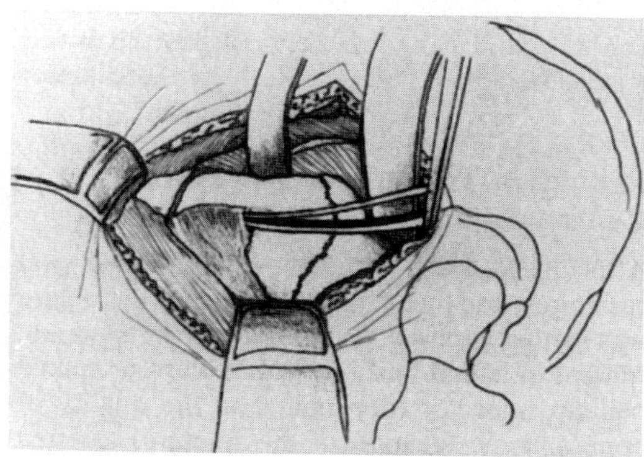

FIGURE 28-45. Elevation of the iliacus and psoas allows exposure of the iliac fossa. Elevation of the obturator internus exposes the medial wall and obturator fossa. Dissection medial to the sacroiliac joint allows exposure of the lateral sacral ala for Hohman retractor placement. (From: Cole JD, Bolhofner BR. Description of operative technique and preliminary treatment results. *Clin Orthop* 1994;(305):112–123, with permission.)

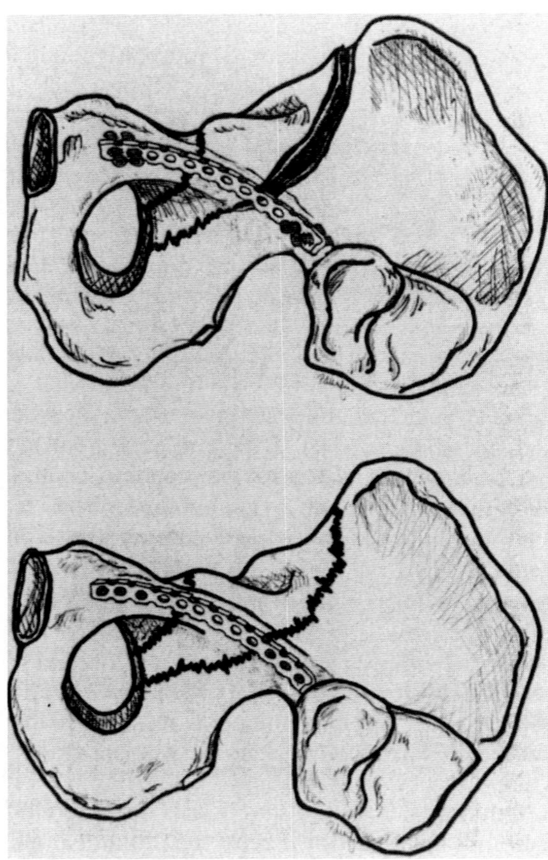

FIGURE 28-46. Anterior column with associated anterior wall fracture reduced with a brim reconstruction plate. (From: Cole JD, Bolhofner BR. Description of operative technique and preliminary treatment results. *Clin Orthop* 1994;(305):112–123, with permission.)

History

The anterior Stoppa surgical approach was originally described in the hernia literature (155,156). It has since been modified and promoted by Dean Cole and Brett Bolhofner for acetabular fracture surgery (83).

Indications

An alternative to the ilioinguinal or more extensile approaches, this exposure has led to good results when treating a variety of fracture types, including displaced anterior column or wall fractures, transverse fractures, T-shaped fractures, both-column fractures, and anterior column or wall fractures associated with a posterior hemitransverse component (83).

Access

This approach provides excellent visualization of the pelvic ring, including the medial wall, dome, and quadrilateral plate. Further posterior dissection with elevation of the external iliac vessels allows exposure of the sacroiliac joint and sacral ala.

Positioning

The patient is placed supine on a radiolucent operating room table. The entire lower abdominal and pelvic region as well as the entire hindquarter of the affected side is prepped and draped completely free. The surgeon assumes a position on the side opposite the fractured acetabulum.

Advantages

Excellent access is afforded to the anterior and internal aspects of the entire pelvis and acetabulum. Like the ilioinguinal and anterior iliofemoral approaches, this exposure can be combined with the Kocher-Langenbeck when required. Some advantages over the ilioinguinal approach

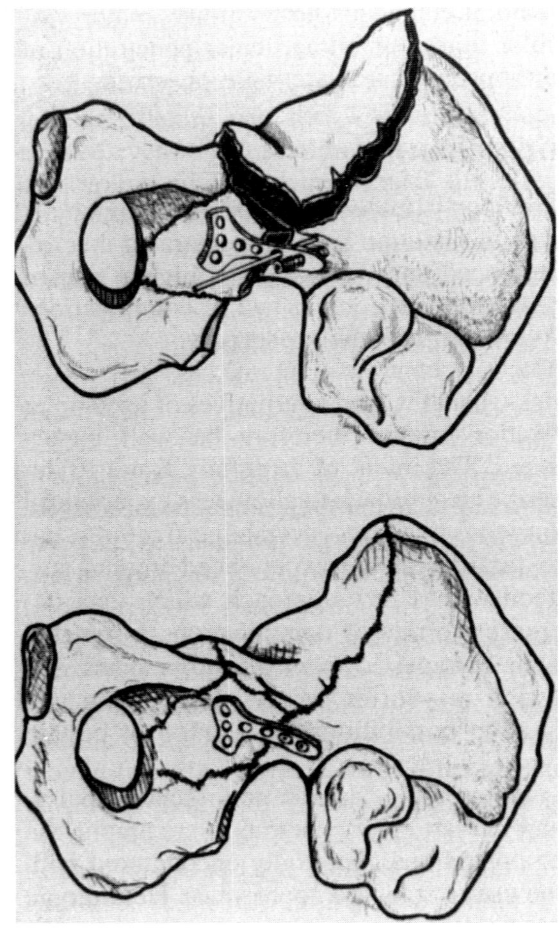

FIGURE 28-47. Large medial wall fracture fragment is reduced with a radius plate. (From: Cole JD, Bolhofner BR. Description of operative technique and preliminary treatment results. *Clin Orthop* 1994;(305):112–123, with permission.)

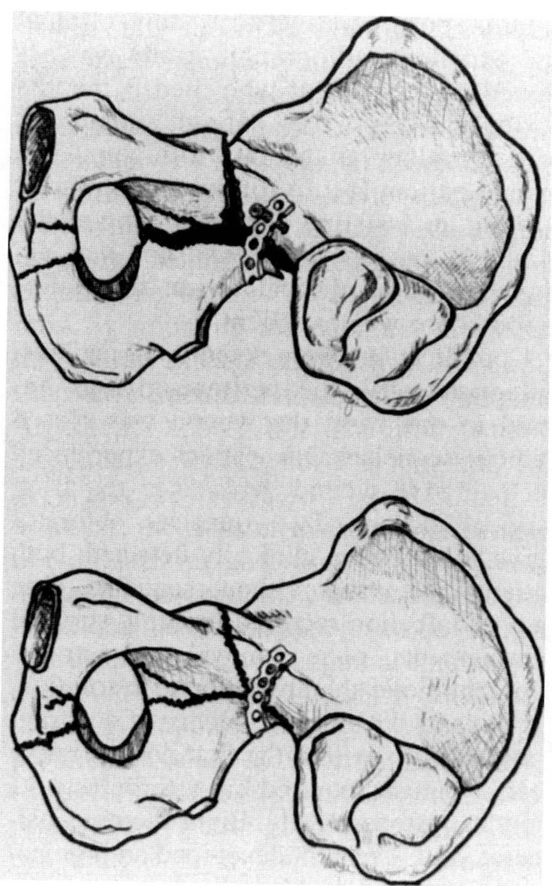

FIGURE 28-48. Posterior column fragment is reduced with a forked reconstruction plate. (From: Cole JD, Bolhofner BR. Description of operative technique and preliminary treatment results. *Clin Orthop* 1994;(305):112–123, with permission.)

include preservation of the lateral femoral cutaneous nerve, less direct surgical exposure of the femoral vascular structures, including the lymphatics, and better exposure of some fracture types, including those involving the medial wall of the acetabulum (83).

Disadvantages and Dangers

Like the ilioinguinal, this approach is essentially extraarticular, which does not provide direct visualization of posterior structures and requires indirect reduction maneuvers. Therefore, it should not be used in the presence of sciatic buttress comminution, fractures >3 weeks old, and fractures with pure posterior pathology. The presence of a preexisting suprapubic catheter mitigates against the use of the approach because of concerns regarding infection. Other contraindications include abdominal distention, ileus, or other conditions that result in abdominal rigidity. With the exception of the lateral femoral cutaneous nerve, the same structures are at risk as during the ilioinguinal approach. It is particularly important with this exposure to pay attention to the location of the obturator neurovascular bundle and the lumbosacral trunk at all times.

Surgical Technique

The surgical incision begins 2 cm superior to the symphysis pubis in a transverse fashion with the length extending approximately from the ipsilateral external inguinal ring to the contralateral external ring. The rectus abdominus muscle is split vertically from inferior to superior with care taken to stay extraperitoneal in the proximal portion (Fig. 28-42). Protecting the bladder, the rectus is retracted superiorly, with sharp dissection used to elevate the rectus to expose the symphysis body and superior pubic ramus (Fig. 28-43).

The rectus and neurovascular structures next are retracted laterally and anteriorly to protect them. The remainder of the surgical procedure is performed beneath the iliac vessels, femoral nerve, and psoas muscle. A plethora of vascular anastomoses are often encountered, the majority being communications of the inferior epigastric and obturator vessels (83). Anastomoses of the external iliac extending to the bladder and multiple nutrient vessels also are common. These are ligated as necessary with suture ligation or vascular clips. As with the ilioinguinal approach, this portion of the exposure places vascular structures at risk, particularly if a "corona mortis" is present. The initial vascular obstruction is an anastomotic branch between the inferior epigastric and the obturator vessel. This is always present but variable in size. Another common obstacle is the nutrient vessel branch from the iliolumbar artery, which is often severed by the fracture or torn during elevation of the iliacus. Prior to elevation of the posterior iliacus, this vessel should be clipped to avoid excessive hemorrhage. Large lymph nodes also may need to be retracted or excised as necessary to improve visualization. Despite these structures, appropriate placement of retractors provides adequate exposure (Fig. 28-44).

Further access is developed from anterior to posterior along the pelvic brim, sharply dividing and elevating the iliopectineal fascia superiorly and the obturator fascia inferiorly. Complete access to the sacroiliac joint can be obtained by working posteriorly. Elevation of the psoas muscle further exposes the sciatic buttress and posterior aspect of the pelvic brim. Exposure to the sacral ala is obtained with gentle retraction of the psoas and iliac vessels (Fig. 28-45).

With the exposure completed, flexion, rotation, abduction, adduction of the hip are possible through the freely draped limb; these improve visualization. Flexion, in particular, relaxes the retracted anterior structures. Limited tension on a sacral retractor just lateral to the lumbosacral trunk is recommended because the lumbosacral trunk and obturator nerves are tethered closely to the superior lateral corner of the obturator foramen.

Reduction techniques include medial-to-lateral pushing with a blunt or spiked ball tip impactor. A bone hook can be

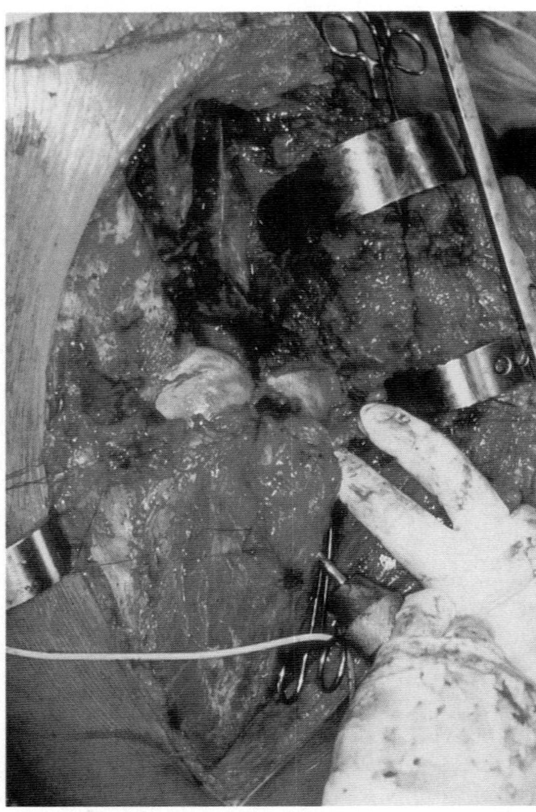

FIGURE 28-49. The extended iliofemoral approach for exposure of a comminuted left both-column acetabular fracture. The femoral head can be seen and there is a Schanz pin in greater trochanter, parallel with femoral neck. (From: Sledge CB, ed. *Master techniques in orthopaedic surgery: the hip.* Philadelphia: Lippincott-Raven, 1998, with permission.)

placed in the greater sciatic notch to elevate the posterior column. Lateral traction can be applied via a Schanz screw in the proximal femur. Longitudinal traction can be obtained through the use of a femoral distractor or a fracture table. Multiple plate configurations are possible, including a reconstruction plate contoured over the medial aspect of the pelvic brim and spring or hook plate constructs (Figs. 28-46 through 28-48) (83).

Extended Iliofemoral Approach

(See Figs. 28-49 through 28-57.)

History

Introduced by Letournel in 1974 (42,44), the extended iliofemoral approach is an anatomic approach that follows an internervous plane, reflecting anteriorly the femoral nerve-innervated muscles and posteriorly the muscles innervated by the superior and inferior gluteal nerves. The posterior flap is mobilized as a unit without damaging its major neurovascular bundle (Fig. 28-49) (44).

Indications

The approach is indicated for complex fracture patterns when a major extensile approach is required for the posterior and lateral aspects of the hemipelvis (as per triradiate), exposure of both the anterior and posterior columns are needed for acute both-column lesions (Type C), and for late reconstructive cases. It has particular value when fracture comminution extends into the sciatic iliac joint.

Access

This approach provides direct visualization of the entire outer aspect of the ilium, the posterior column and wall down to the ischium, and the hip joint (Fig. 28-50). With further devascularization and retraction of the iliopsoas and abdominal muscles medially, exposure of the internal aspect of the ilium also is possible.

Position

The patient is supported on a bean bag and placed in the lateral decubitus position on a radiolucent operating table. The hip is kept extended and the knee flexed throughout the procedure to minimize sciatic nerve injury.

Advantages

This is an excellent extensile approach to the entire hemipelvis, the outer wall of the ilium, and the posterior column and posterior wall.

Disadvantages and Dangers

The major technical limitation of the extended ilio-femoral exposure is access to the low anterior column (48), where the dissection becomes more difficult and dangerous medial to the iliopectineal eminence. In this area, the iliopsoas and iliopectineal fascia block the exposure with the more medial vascular structures at risk.

Heterotopic ossification (HO) is a complication of all the approaches to the outer aspect of the ilium with rates ranging from 18% to 90% (44,47,56,109,111,136). It is particularly common and severe after extensile approaches with a larger proportion of patients suffering functional limitations (44,47,56,109,134,136). For example, Letournel (44) reported its occurrence in 46% of his extended iliofemoral approaches as compared with 21% for all other approaches. (These rates were 69% and 24% prior to his use of prophylaxis, respectively.) Matta (47) noted a significant loss of motion in 20% of patients and Letournel (44) observed severe HO (Brooker III and IV) in 35% of patients treated by this approach within 3 weeks of injury. Even with prophylaxis, Alonso (134) encountered heterotopic ossifica-

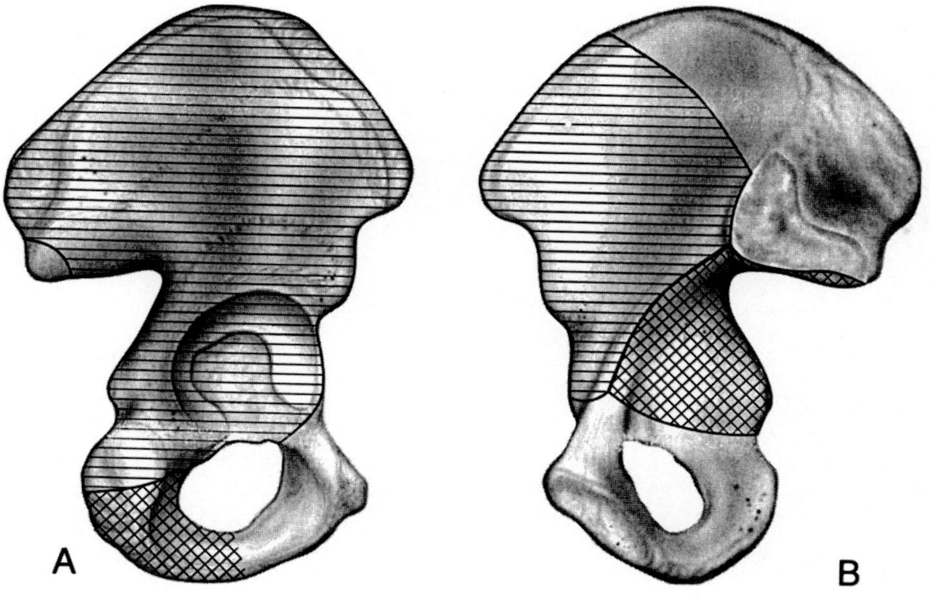

FIGURE 28-50. Access to the right pelvis via the extended iliofemoral approach. **A:** The lateral (outer) bony pelvis. **B:** The medial (inner) bony pelvis. (From: Sledge CB, ed. *Master techniques in orthopaedic surgery: the hip.* Philadelphia: Lippincott-Raven, 1998, with permission.)

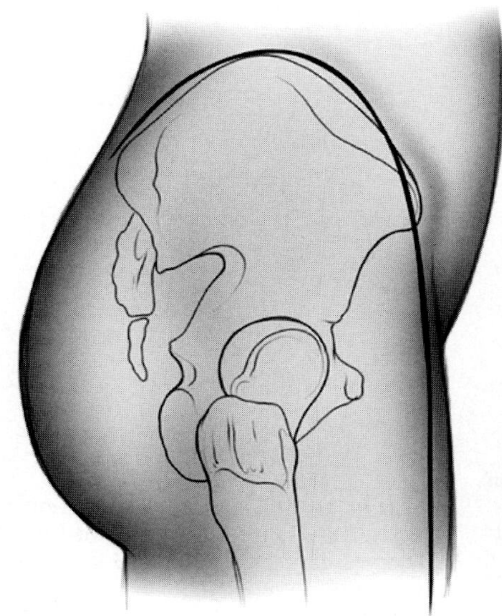

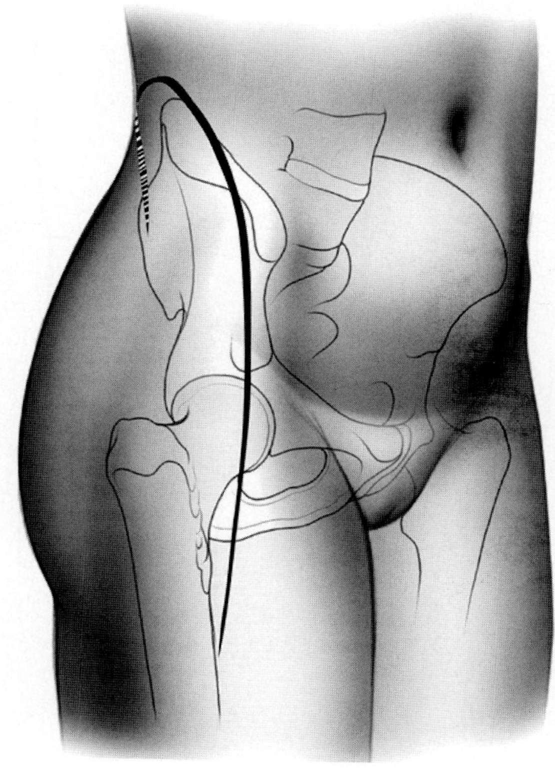

FIGURE 28-51. Skin incision. **A:** The inverted-J skin incision, right side. **B:** Anterolateral view: the inverted J skin incision with distal extension for the extended iliofemoral approach. (From: Sledge CB, ed. *Master techniques in orthopaedic surgery: the hip.* Philadelphia: Lippincott-Raven, 1998, with permission.)

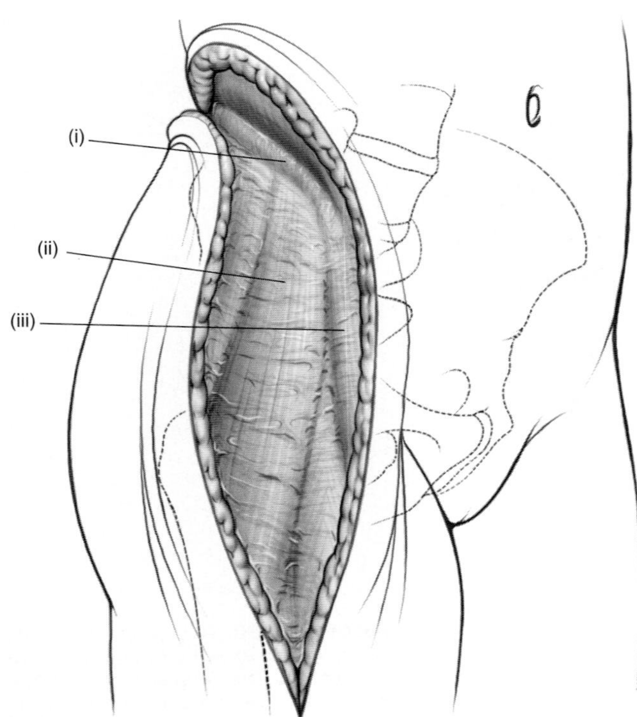

FIGURE 28-52. Exposure of right iliac crest and anterior distal limb. **(i)** Avascular "white line;" **(ii)** fascia covering tensor fascia lata muscle; **(iii)** fascia covering sartorius muscle. (From: Sledge CB, ed. *Master techniques in orthopaedic surgery: the hip.* Philadelphia: Lippincott-Raven, 1998, with permission.)

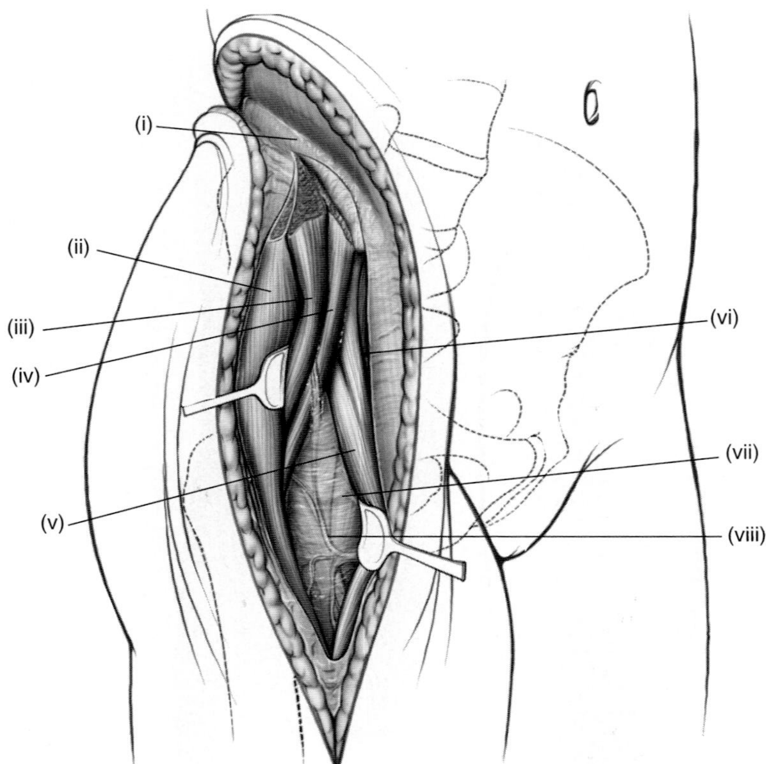

FIGURE 28-53. Subfascial reflection of tensor fascia lata and abductor muscle origins from right iliac crest. **(i)** Avascular "white line;" **(ii)** tensor fascia lata muscle; **(iii)** gluteus medius muscle; **(iv)** gluteus minimus muscle; **(v)** rectus femoris muscle; **(vi)** sartorius muscle; **(vii)** "no name" fascia covering vastus lateralis; **(viii)** ascending branch of the lateral femoral circumflex artery. (From: Sledge CB, ed. *Master techniques in orthopaedic surgery: the hip.* Philadelphia: Lippincott-Raven, 1998, with permission.)

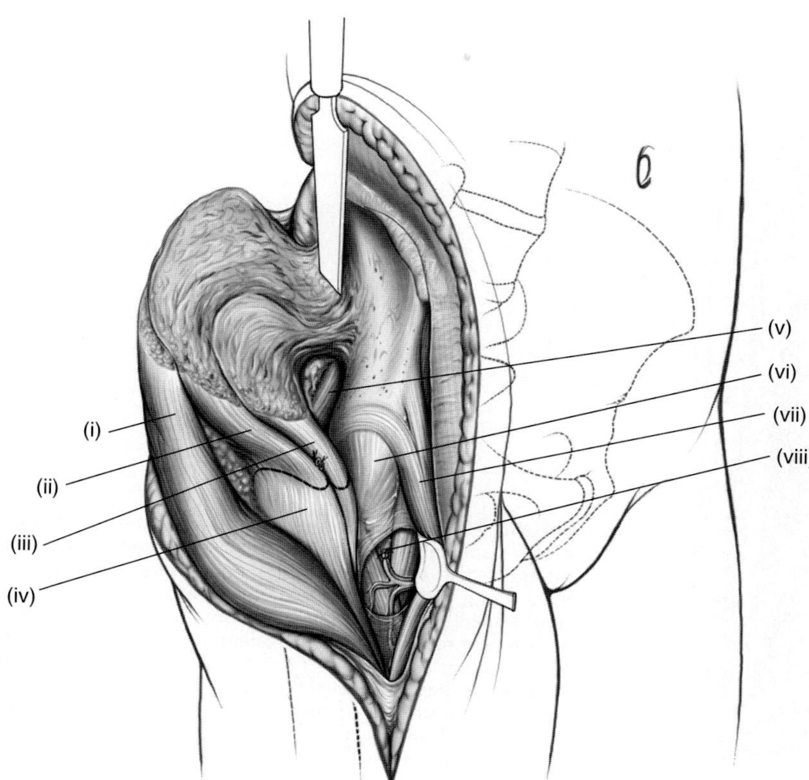

FIGURE 28-54. Proximally, the abductor and tensor fascia lata muscles have been stripped subperiosteally from the outer table of the right ileum. Distally, the ascending branch of the lateral circumflex artery has been ligated. The abductor insertions have been marked for release. **(i)** Tensor fascia lata muscle; **(ii)** gluteus medius muscle; **(iii)** gluteus minimus muscle; **(iv)** greater trochanter; **(v)** piriformis muscle; **(vi)** hip joint capsule; **(vii)** two heads of the rectus muscle; **(viii)** ligated ascending branch of the lateral femoral circumflex artery. (From: Sledge CB, ed. *Master techniques in orthopaedic surgery: the hip.* Philadelphia: Lippincott-Raven, 1998, with permission.)

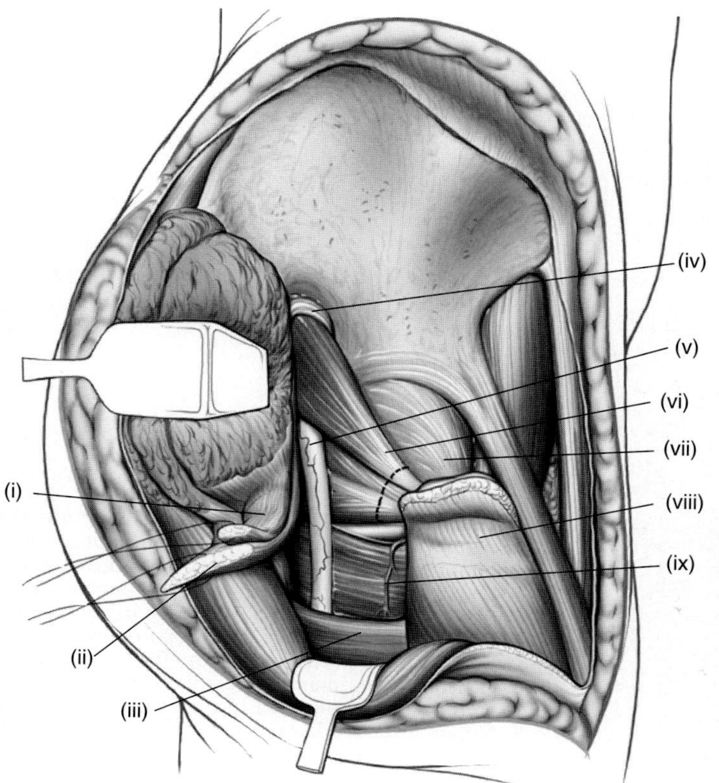

FIGURE 28-55. The abductors of the right hip have been tagged and their insertions into the greater trochanter released, allowing their muscle pedicle to be retracted to expose the sciatic nerve. The external rotators have also been marked for release. **(i)** Gluteus minimus tendon; **(ii)** gluteus medius tendon; **(iii)** gluteus maximus tendon; **(iv)** superior gluteal neurovascular bundle; **(v)** sciatic nerve; **(vi)** piriformis and conjoint tendons; **(vii)** hip joint capsule; **(viii)** greater trochanter; **(ix)** medial femoral circumflex artery overlying quadratus femoris. (From: Sledge CB, ed. *Master techniques in orthopaedic surgery: the hip.* Philadelphia: Lippincott-Raven, 1998, with permission.)

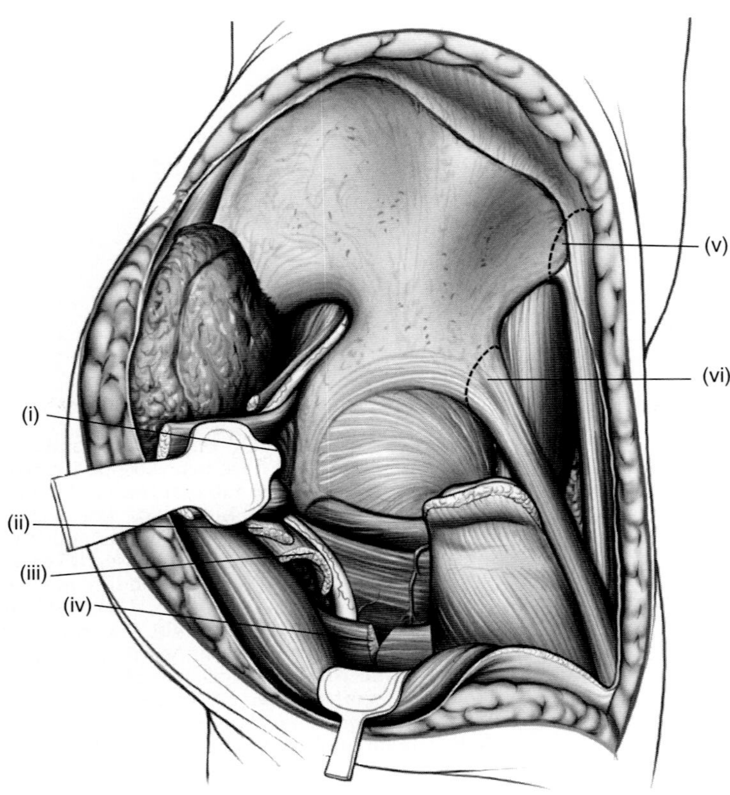

FIGURE 28-56. Retraction of right hip external rotator muscles and release of gluteus maximus insertion distally. Medially, the anterior superior and inferior iliac spines have been marked for either release or osteotomy. **(i)** Blunt Hohmann in lesser sciatic notch. The conjoint tendons have been positioned between the retractor and the sciatic nerve; **(ii)** gluteus minimus tendon; **(iii)** gluteus medius tendon; **(iv)** partial release of gluteus maximus tendon; **(v)** anterior-superior iliac spine and sartorius muscle origin; **(vi)** anterior-inferior iliac spine and direct head of rectus femoris muscle. (From: Sledge CB, ed. *Master techniques in orthopaedic surgery: the hip.* Philadelphia: Lippincott-Raven, 1998, with permission.)

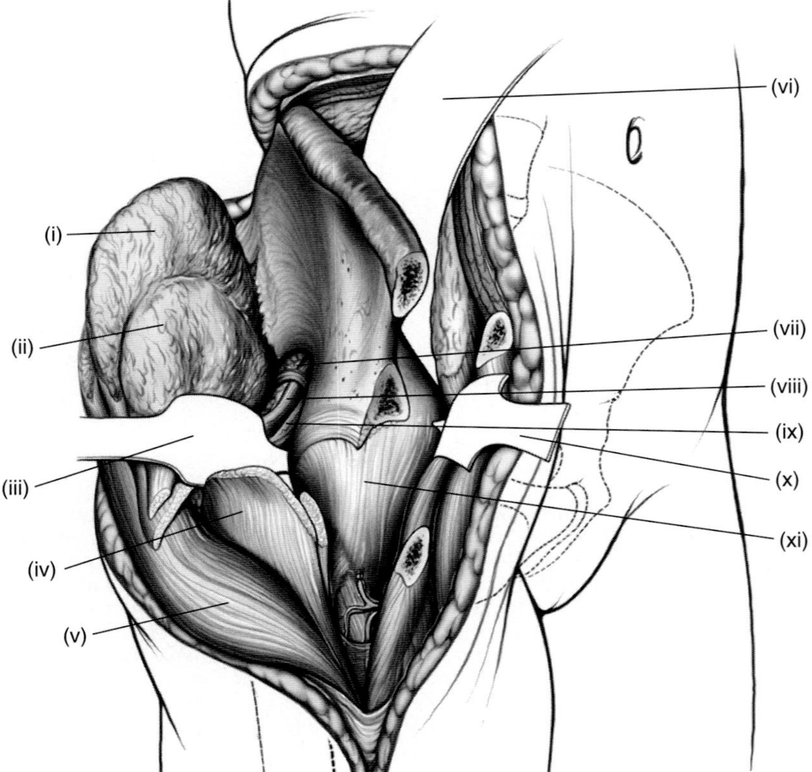

FIGURE 28-57. Maximal exposure of right acetabulum. **(i)** Gluteus medius muscle; **(ii)** gluteus minimus muscle; **(iii)** blunt Hohmann in lesser sciatic notch; **(iv)** greater trochanter; **(v)** tensor fascia lata muscle; **(vi)** malleable retractor under the iliacus muscle; **(vii)** superior gluteal neurovascular bundle; **(viii)** piriformis muscle; **(ix)** sciatic nerve; **(x)** spiked Hohmann retractor over the anterior capsule of the hip; **(xi)** hip joint capsule. (From: Sledge CB, ed. *Master techniques in orthopaedic surgery: the hip.* Philadelphia: Lippincott-Raven, 1998, with permission.)

tion in 86% of their patients and a 14% rate of Brooker III or IV HO. Therefore, an associated closed head injury might be considered a relative contraindication for this approach (48). Heterotopic ossification often is noted along the gluteus minimus and the debridement of any necrotic muscle in this location may decrease the risk of this complication (137).

Sciatic Nerve

As with all posterior approaches, the sciatic nerve is at risk during exposure of the posterior column and needs to be identified along the belly of the quadratus femoris muscle as in the Kocher-Langenbeck approach, then protected behind the conjoint tendon (Fig. 28-55). Traction along the nerve should be avoided by maintaining the hip extended and the knee flexed at all times.

Lateral Femoral Cutaneous Nerve

The lateral femoral cutaneous nerve is at risk during exposure along the anterior superior iliac spine. It also can sustain a traction injury during mobilization of the soft tissues. Patients should be warned preoperatively to expect this complication.

Superior Gluteal Neurovascular Bundle

As with the Kocher-Langenbeck approach, this neurovascular structure is at risk for injury. It is of particular concern during this approach because the entire abductor flap is mobilized around this pedicle (Fig. 28-55).

Abductor Muscle Flap Necrosis

A major concern is the vascularity of the large gluteus medius and gluteus minimus muscle flap. In this approach, all of the lateral muscles are detached from the ilium with the additional ligation of their anterior collateral supply from the inferior epigastric artery and are thus ultimately hinged on their only remaining blood supply: the superior gluteal pedicle. If this vessel has been damaged by the fracture or the surgical approach, then the hip abductors flap may be at risk for complete ischemic necrosis. Bosse and colleagues (134,158) have described this in detail and recommended preoperative arteriography for all acute cases. However, concerns regarding abductor muscle flap necrosis may be more theoretical than clinical (44,134,158). In over 400 acetabular fractures addressed with an extended iliofemoral approach by Letournel, Matta, Mast, and Martimbeau, there have been no reports of abductor flap necrosis (44). Alonso and colleagues (134) did not observe this complication using either an extended iliofemoral or triradiate approach in 59 cases of complex acetabular fractures.

Furthermore, massive abductor necrosis resulting from a superior gluteal artery injury combined with an extended iliofemoral approach is described based on animal and cadaver studies only (158,159). A recent canine study by Tabor and coworkers (158) has found that although necrosis of muscle and loss of mass does occur after the extended iliofemoral approach in the presence of gluteal vessel injury this does not appear to be functionally significant. In their study, none of the gluteal muscle flaps suffered complete ischemic necrosis. Thus, some collateral flow to the abductor muscles appears to be present and may increase in the presence of a superior gluteal vessel injury.

Femoral Neurovascular Structures

The iliopsoas muscle and the iliopectineal eminence lie at the medial extent of the extended iliofemoral approach. Further medial dissection without an ilioinguinal incision places the femoral neurovascular structures at great risk (Fig. 28-57).

Surgical Technique (Extended Iliofemoral Approach)

There are three main stages to the dissection (44): (a) Elevation of all the gluteal muscles with the tensor fascia lata; (b) division of the abductors and external rotators of the hip; and (c) an extended capsulotomy along the lip of the acetabulum. The end result is complete exposure of the outer aspect of the ilium and the whole posterior column inferiorly to the upper part of the ischial tuberosity. Furthermore, the approach can be extended to allow a limited exposure of the internal iliac fossa and the anterior column to the level of the iliopectineal eminence. Thus, simultaneous extensile exposure of both the anterior and posterior columns is possible, which permits direct visualization of their reduction and fixation (Fig. 28-49). As this approach creates significant soft-tissue flaps, it is important to keep them moist with wet sponges throughout the procedure.

The incision is in the form of an inverted J (Fig. 28-51A). It begins at the posterior-superior iliac spine and extends around the iliac crest toward the anterior-superior iliac spine. From here, the distal arm of the incision proceeds along the anterolateral aspect of the thigh for a distance of 15 to 20 cm (Fig. 28-51B) (44,48). There is a tendency for the surgeon to extend this more medially than desired. To avoid this, one should visualize a point 2 cm lateral to the superolateral pole of the patella. With the leg held in neutral rotation, this location is generally in line with the desired incision (44,48). As the incision is carried distally, a gentle curve posteriorly may be helpful in more obese patients (48).

The exposure begins in a stepwise fashion by first identifying the avascular fascial periosteal layer along the iliac crest between the abdominal muscle insertions and hip abductor origins and sharply releasing the tensor fascia lata muscle and the gluteus medius muscles subperiosteally from the outer aspect of the iliac crest (Figs. 28-52 and 28-53). Often it is easiest to start in the area of the gluteus medius tubercle where landmarks are more obvious, and to progress posteriorly and anteriorly from this point. Posteriorly, the strong fibrous origin of the gluteus maximus should be sharply released from the crista glutei (106). Under direct vision, the musculature along the external surface of the iliac wing is released in a subperiosteal fashion from the outer aspect of the iliac crest up to the superior border of the greater sciatic notch and anterosuperior aspect of the hip joint capsule, as in the Smith-Petersen incision (Fig. 28-54). Care must be taken to identify and protect the superior gluteal neurovascular bundle as it exits the greater sciatic notch.

Next, the distal limb of the incision is developed. In order to protect the lateral femoral cutaneous nerve and the majority of its branches, the incision is carried through the fascial sheath of the tensor fascia lata muscle (Fig. 28-53). Having incised the fascia overlying the tensor fascia lata muscle, the muscle belly is reflected off the fascia and retracted laterally to expose the fascia overlying the rectus femoris. The exposure stays lateral to the branches of the lateral femoral cutaneous nerve and therefore places them at minimal risk.

Small vessels from the superficial circumflex artery are divided and coagulated between the superior and inferior spines (44), the fascial layer overlying the rectus femoris muscle is divided longitudinally, and the reflected and direct heads of the muscle are retracted medially to expose the aponeurosis over the vastus lateralis muscle (Fig. 28-54), where a small vascular pedicle often requires coagulation (44). The aponeurosis over the vastus lateralis muscle can be divided longitudinally to expose the underlying ascending branches of the lateral circumflex vessels, which must be isolated and ligated. (Rarely, these vessels can be spared if a more limited exposure is acceptable.) Next, the thin sheath of the iliopsoas muscle is exposed and longitudinally incised, and an elevator used to strip the muscle from the anterior and inferior aspects of the hip capsule. At this point, any remaining musculature along the external surface of the iliac wing is released in a subperiosteal fashion, while protecting the superior gluteal neurovascular bundle as it exits the greater sciatic notch (Fig. 28-54). The exposure of the iliac wing is complete after the reflected head of the rectus femoris has been released from its insertion.

As described by Letournel (42), the posterior column is then exposed by dividing the insertions of the gluteus minimus, gluteus medius, and short external rotator muscles from the greater trochanter (Fig. 28-55). First, the gluteus minimus tendon is identified over the anterior portion of the greater trochanter, tagged, and transected, leaving a small 3- to 5-mm cuff for repair. The gluteus minimus muscle also has extensive attachments to the superior aspect of the hip capsule, which need to be released. Posteriorly and superiorly, the gluteus medius tendon, measuring 15 to 20 mm in length also is isolated, tagged, and transected, leaving a 3- to 5-mm cuff for repair. It is important to sequentially and carefully transect and tag these structures for subsequent reattachment. In contrast to sharply releasing the abductor and external rotator insertions into the greater trochanter as per Letournel (42), some have preferred to divide the greater trochanter to give equal visualization and ensure adequate reattachment (51).

After releasing the gluteus minimus and gluteus medius insertions onto the greater trochanter, the tensor fascia lata and gluteal muscles are held in continuity as a flap and reflected posteriorly to expose the external rotators. From this point, the posterior dissection is similar to the Kocher-Langenbeck. To decrease tension, the tendonous femoral insertion of the gluteus maximus muscle is identified, and transected with a cuff for repair. The sciatic nerve is identified and the tendons of the piriformis muscle, obturator internus muscle, and inferior and superior gemelli muscles are tagged and transected. The piriformis muscle is followed toward the greater sciatic notch and the obturator internus muscle to the lesser sciatic notch, where retractors can be inserted, allowing complete exposure to the posterior column of the acetabulum (Fig. 28-56). This completes the exposure of the posterior column and the lateral aspect of the iliac crest.

Although medial exposure of the anterior column is limited by the iliopsoas muscle and iliopectineal eminence, further access to the internal iliac fossa and acetabulum can be obtained by subperiosteal release of the sartorius and direct head of the rectus or by osteotomy of the superior and inferior iliac spines, respectively (Figs. 28-56 and 28-57). The insertion of the external oblique muscle on to the crest also can be subperiosteally released to reveal the inner table of the pelvis. The internal iliac fossa is then further exposed through subperiosteal dissection of the iliacus muscle. However, such extensile exposure of both the outer and inner tables of the iliac wing, especially in the presence of local fractures, increases the likelihood of iliac bone devascularization. Although such devascularization is rare, Matta (39) has warned of its occurrence, especially in associated both-column fractures. To avoid this potentially disastrous complication, he suggested leaving the direct head of the rectus femoris and anterior hip joint capsule attached to the anterior column at a minimum. The blood supply to the dome of the acetabulum also is at risk during dissection at the anterior inferior iliac spine (160).

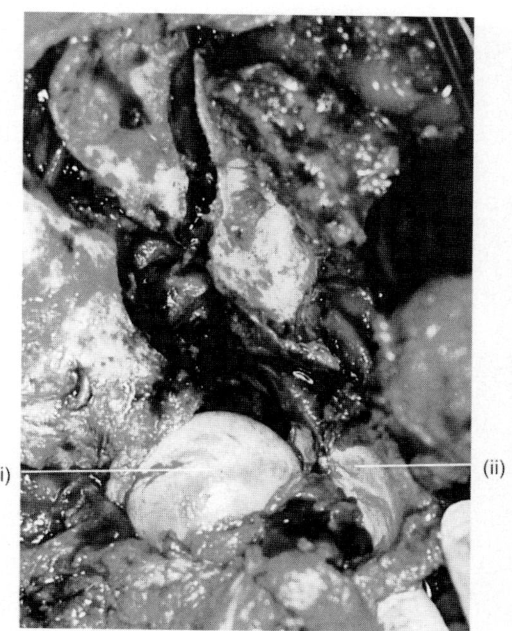

FIGURE 28-58. Close-up of acetabular joint exposure of patient. **(i)** Femoral head; **(ii)** loose articular fragment. (From: Sledge CB, ed. *Master techniques in orthopaedic surgery: the hip.* Philadelphia: Lippincott-Raven, 1998, with permission.)

Visualization of the acetabular articular surface can be performed with a marginal capsulotomy, leaving a cuff of tissue for repair followed by distraction of the hip joint with either a Schanz screw placed into the femoral head or with a femoral distractor (Figs. 28-49 and 28-58). At this point, the limits of the extended iliofemoral approach have been reached and reduction of the fracture fragments can now be completed according to the preoperative plan.

As in the ilioinguinal exposure, both column (Type C) fractures require sequential reconstruction from the periphery toward the acetabulum (Figs. 28-59 and 28-60). First, the iliac wing is stabilized with lag screws and/or 3.5-mm reconstruction plates. Next, and under direct visualization of the acetabular articular surface, the posterior column is reduced to the iliac wing by similar techniques as discussed in the section on the Kocher-Langenbeck approach. Prior to definitive reduction, a gliding hole can be inserted into the proximal aspect of the posterior column from superior to inferior, assuring the correct position of the gliding hole in the middle of the posterior column. Following reduction, it is then possible to insert a 4.5- or 3.5-mm cortical lag screw down the posterior column. Additional stabilization is accomplished with a 3.5-mm reconstruction plate molded to the posterior column.

With direct visualization of the acetabular articular surface, the anterior column can now be reduced and attached to the intact (or reconstructed) segment. Fixation is achieved with 3.5-mm lag screws inserted from the anterior-inferior spine into the sciatic buttress, anteriorly from the inner table or crest into the intact ilium and superior posterior column, and/or anterior column lag screws from the lateral aspect of the iliac wing. Generally, the latter requires insertion three finger breadths proximal to the superior aspect of the articular surface (4 to 6 cm), and one finger breadth posterior to the gluteal ridge on the outer aspect of the iliac crest (Figs. 28-61 and 28-62) (44,161). The lag screw is then angled from posterior-superior to anterior-inferior directly down the superior pubic ramus with the assistance of intraoperative fluoroscopy. Care must be taken to assure that this screw remains extraarticular and does not penetrate the anterior aspect of the superior ramus, in the area of the ilio-pectineal eminence where the femoral vasculature is closely adherent.

For T-shaped (Type B2) and the more comminuted variants, the anterior column may be reduced first with respect to the residual acetabular "roof" portion of the ilium (117). The screw holding forceps and 4.5-mm screws proximal and distal to the posterior column fracture improve distraction, debridement of the fracture surfaces, and reduction. A laminar spreader in the fracture site also is useful. For additional control, a Schanz screw is placed in the ischium, or a pelvic clamp in the greater sciatic notch. Definitive stabilization is similar to that described for the both-column fracture, with lag screw fixation of the two columns and a posterior buttress plate.

After completion of the operative repair, two deep suction drains are placed along the external surface of the iliac wing, posterior column, and vastus lateralis muscle. If the internal iliac fossa has been exposed, a third drain is placed here. A subcutaneously placed drain also should be considered. All drains should exit anteriorly. The hip capsule is repaired first, followed by reattachment of the tendonous femoral insertion of the gluteus maximus and the short external rotators. The tendons of the gluteus minimus and gluteus medius muscles are also sutured to their respective attachment sites on the greater trochanter with multiple sutures. Letournel has recommended five or six sutures for each tendon (44). Reattachment of the origin of the gluteal muscles and tensor fascia lata muscle to the iliac crest can be facilitated by hip abduction. If a medial exposure had been required, the origins of the sartorius and direct head of the rectus femoris muscles are reattached through drill holes (or by lag screws if osteotomies have been performed). This is followed by reattachment of the external oblique muscle along the iliac crest and repair of the fascia overlying the proximal thigh. Active hip abduction, any adduction, and flexion past 90 degrees should be avoided for 6 to 8 weeks.

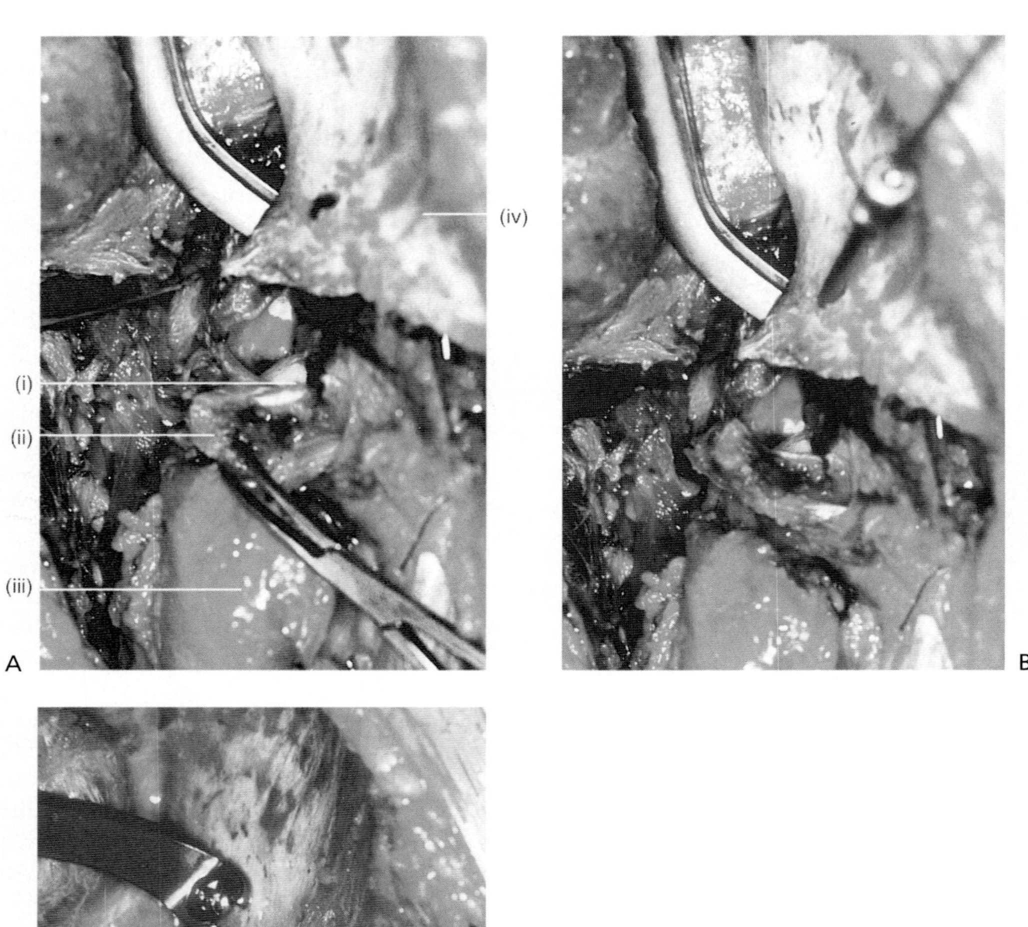

FIGURE 28-59. Reduction of an associated both-column right acetabular fracture. **A:** A laminar spreader is placed in the fracture site to expose the joint and allow debridement. **(i)** Femoral head in joint; **(ii)** superolateral dome fragment with capsular attachments; **(iii)** greater trochanter; **(iv)** intact iliac wing. **B:** The gliding hole is predrilled for the anterior to posterior column screw. **C:** A Farabeuf clamp affixed to screws is used to reduce the anterior column to the superolateral fragment, and a pelvic reduction clamp affixed to screws is used to reduce the anterior to the posterior column (posterior column portion not shown). (From: Sledge CB, ed. *Master techniques in orthopaedic surgery: the hip.* Philadelphia: Lippincott-Raven, 1998, with permission.)

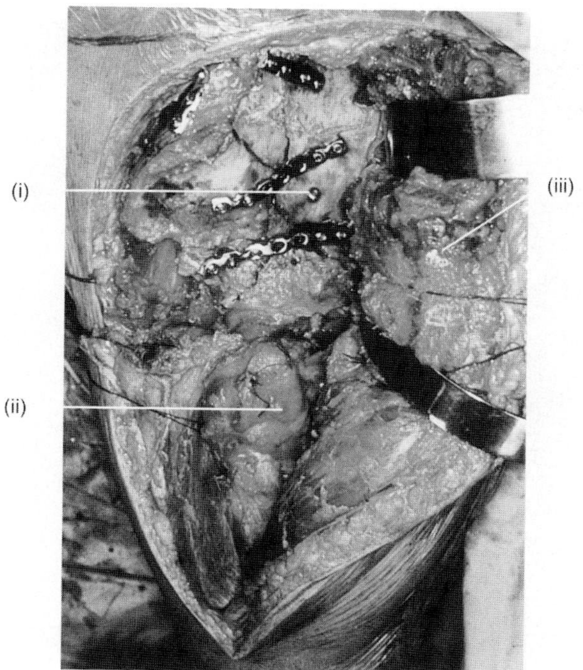

FIGURE 28-60. Reconstruction of comminuted left both-column acetabular fractures. Reconstruction proceeds centripetally from the periphery. **(i)** Anterior to posterior column lag screw; **(ii)** greater trochanter; **(iii)** abductor muscles and tensor fascia lata. (From: Sledge CB, ed. *Master techniques in orthopaedic surgery: the hip.* Philadelphia: Lippincott-Raven, 1998, with permission.)

Triradiate Approach

(See Fig. 28-63.)

History

This approach was developed and promoted by Mears (116,117). Most recently, a modified triradiate approach (MTRI) has been developed by the same surgeon, which preserves the abductor muscle attachment to the greater trochanter, avoids trochanteric osteotomy, and preserves the anterosuperior hip-joint capsule, including the contiguous origins of the indirect and direct heads of the rectus femoris (162).

Indications

The triradiate is an extensile approach to the posterior and lateral aspects of the hip for difficult transtectal transverse, T-type lesions, and both-column fractures with posterior wall involvement.

Access

(See Fig. 28-63.) Access is afforded to the entire posterior column and posterior wall area, and to the entire lateral aspect of the iliac crest, back to the iliac tubercle area or beyond. Visualization of these areas is valuable in high both-column fractures.

Position

The patient is placed in the lateral decubitus position.

Advantages

Compared with the standard Kocher-Langenbeck, access to the lateral wall of the ilium and to the posterior aspect of the ilium and ischium is markedly increased. Also, the approach allows a skin bridge across the iliac crest posteriorly, which preserves some blood supply to the gluteal muscles and therefore is theoretically safer than the extended iliofemoral approach.

Disadvantages and Dangers

If a careful surgical technique is not employed, particularly during the early portions of the exposure, then this approach can result in a higher rate of wound problems related to viability of the skin flaps. Of additional concern is a marked increase in heterotopic ossification as encountered with all approaches that strip the lateral muscles off the ilium. Furthermore, this approach may result in the division of the lateral cutaneous nerves to the thigh, a nuisance complication. The triradiate approach also is limited in that it leaves a segment of the gluteal musculature in place, preventing mobilization of the superior gluteal neurovascular bundle. This hinders access to the sacroiliac joint and posterior ilium adjacent to the posterior superior iliac spine (44). Finally, the disadvantages and dangers inherent to the Kocher-Langenbeck and transtrochanteric approaches also apply.

Surgical Technique

The incision is T- or Y-shaped (Fig. 28-63A), the posterior and inferior limbs exactly that of the posterior Kocher-Langenbeck, the anterior limb rising at the greater trochanter and moving anterior toward the superior spine of the iliac crest. If further access to the lateral aspect of the ilium is required, then the incision is carried posteriorly along the crest (Fig. 28-63A) until the most posterior fracture line is reached. Osteotomy of the greater trochanter, as previously described, affords access to the entire anterolateral aspect of the ilium. Anteriorly, the tensor muscle may be divided or the surgeon may dissect anterior to it between the tensor and the sartorius, exposing the anterior border of the gluteus medius (Fig. 28-63B,C) (51). This muscle, with the underlying gluteus minimus, is stripped from the lateral wall of the ilium (Fig. 28-63D). The blood supply is maintained by the superior gluteal vessels and by the muscular

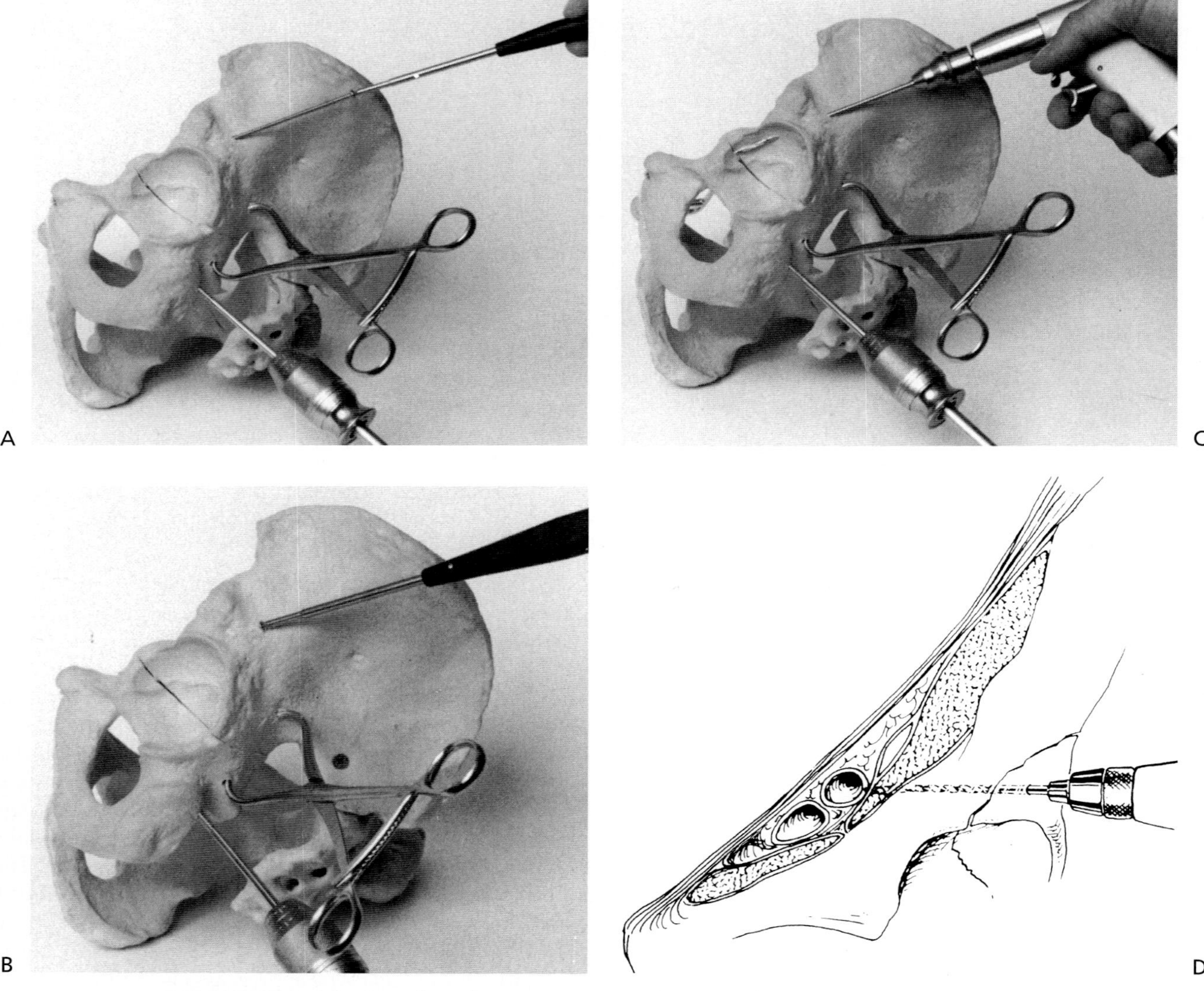

FIGURE 28-61. Anterior column lag screw. **A:** Note the point of insertion posterior to the anterior inferior spine. Remember the large mass of soft tissue (hip abductors) in this area. This screw can be inserted only with adequate retraction, and usually through an extensile approach. When it is accurately placed, excellent reduction and fixation of the anterior column may be achieved **(B).** Because of the thinness of the anterior column just proximal to the iliopectineal eminence (10 to 12 mm), it is not difficult for the drill bit—and the screw—to enter the hip joint **(C).** At the iliopectineal eminence the superior gluteal artery and vein are tethered tightly to the anterior column by the iliopectineal fascia and may be damaged by the drill bit penetrating anteriorly **(D).**

FIGURE 28-63. Triradiate transtrochanteric approach. **A:** Skin incision. Note that the anterior limb of the skin incision may be taken posteriorly to expose the iliac crest or anteriorly to expose the internal aspect of the pelvis. No skin flaps must be raised. All dissection must be carried through the skin and through the fascia for elevating the anterior flap. **B:** The tensor fasciae latae muscle is exposed without raising skin flaps. **C:** The anterior aspect of the tensor fasciae latae may be divided, or (preferably) the plane between the tensor fasciae latae and the sartorius is developed and the dissection carried out in that plane to the iliac crest. **D:** Removal of the greater trochanter exposes the lateral and posterior aspects of the ilium. At the superior aspect the muscle may be removed posterior to the fracture lines as noted. **E:** Capsulorraphy of the hip joint may be performed, or the capsule may be stripped from the lateral ilium. Great care must be taken to ensure that the fragments are not devitalized, and in many instances the capsule is left intact to ensure blood supply to the fragments. (Schatzker J, Tile M. *The rationale of operative fracture care.* Heidelberg: Springer-Verlag, 1987.)

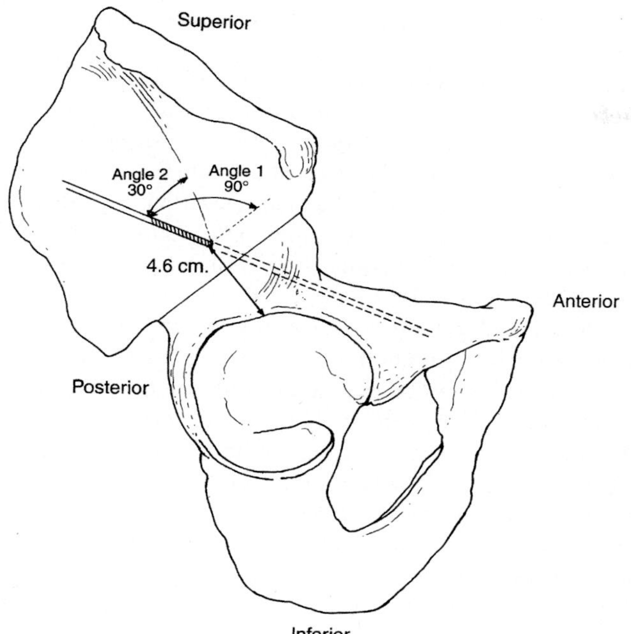

FIGURE 28-62. The angles of inclination for screw placement. Angle 1: The angulation between the longitudinal axis of the anterior column and the line connecting the apex of the sciatic notch and anterior interspinous notch measured in the sagittal plane. Angle 2: The angulation between the longitudinal axis of the anterior column and the posterolateral surface of the iliac wing measured in the transverse plane. (From: Ebraheim NA, et al. Anatomic basis of lag screw placement, in the anterior column of the acetabulum. *Clin Orthop* 339:202, with permission.)

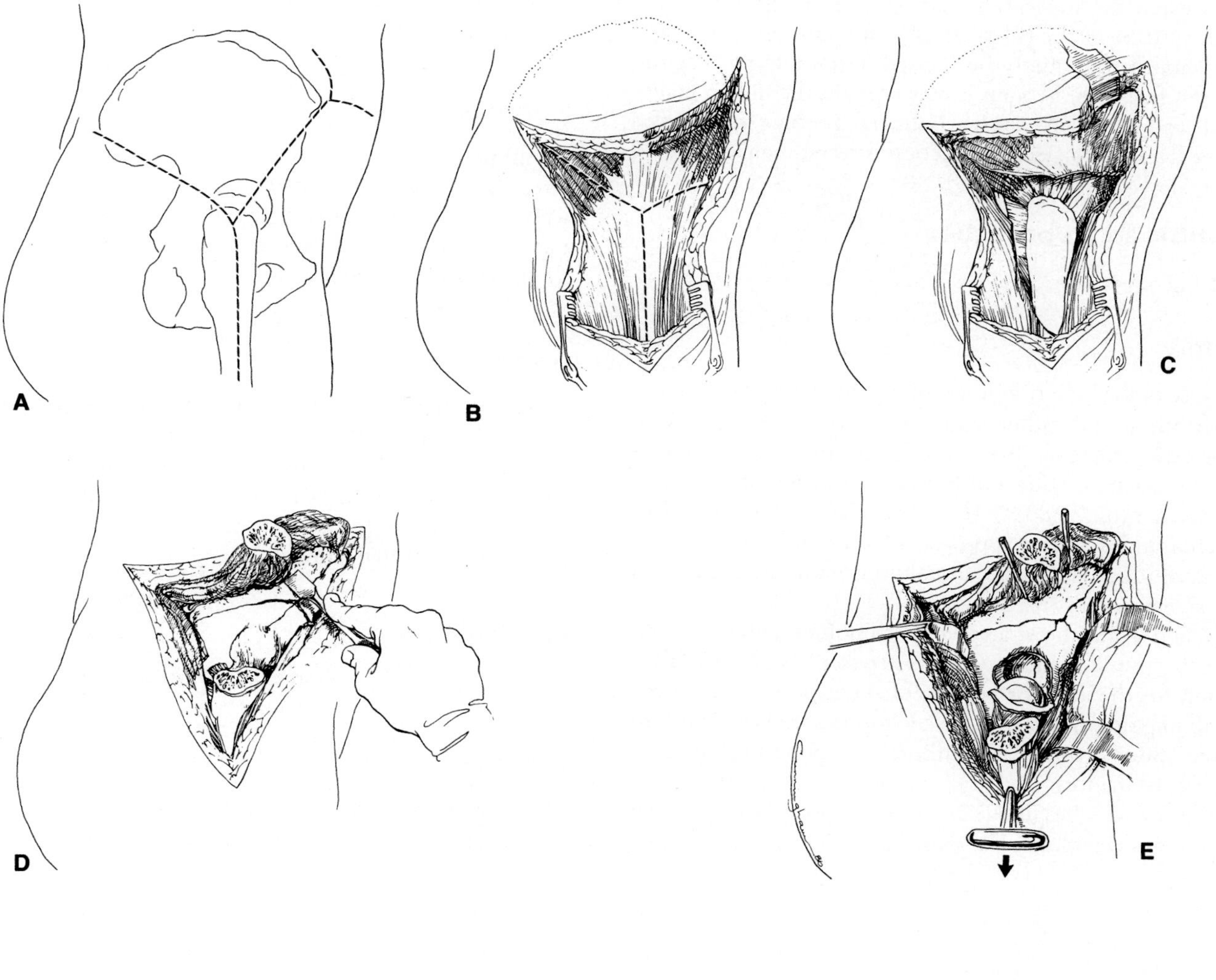

aponeurosis over the posterior aspect of the iliac crest (Fig. 28-63E).

Extreme care must be taken to ensure the viability of the skin flaps. The skin should not be undermined; the flaps should contain the underlying tensor fasciae latae muscle and fibrous layer (Fig. 28-63B). Skin necrosis should be avoided if this principle is adhered to strictly. Almost all acetabular fractures involving the posterior column may be approached by this incision, which affords excellent visualization of the fracture.

Ruedi (21) has described a modification of this approach: a straight incision beginning in the midportion of the iliac crest and extending 10 cm distal to the greater trochanter. The tensor fasciae latae is split to the level of the crest and opened like a book. The greater trochanter is then divided and the gluteus medius split to the greater sciatic notch. The advantage of this approach is that it allows easy access to the iliac crest when the crest is fractured, usually with the anterior column. Access also is provided to the posterior column.

If complete visualization of the anterior column is required, the anterior limb may be carried anteriorly and the iliopsoas removed from inside the pelvis; in fact, an ilioinguinal approach is possible. Great care must be taken to ensure preservation of the blood supply to all articular fractures when the muscles are stripped from the inner and outer surfaces of the pelvis. In this situation, the joint capsule should only rarely be incised, especially with both-column fractures, because it may contain the only remaining blood supply to the periarticular fracture fragments. Instead, an extraarticular reduction is recommended (51).

Combined Approaches

(See Fig. 28-64.)

History

Because of the high risk of morbidity, including heterotopic ossification and other complications of the extensile approaches, there has been a trend toward using simultaneous or staged anterior and posterior (Kocher-Langenbeck) approaches (62,72,83,85,107,128). The combination of an anterior and posterior approach allows simultaneous access to the anterior and posterior columns without resorting to an extensile exposure.

When using the strategy of a combined approach, frequently, the iliofemoral (Smith-Petersen) is all that is required for the anterior portion of the exposure. However, the ilioinguinal or even modified Stoppa approaches are also viable options, with some authors even preferring the routine use of the former (107).

Routt and colleagues (72) chose an iliofemoral approach for the associated anterior exposure (23 cases) when fractures involved the anterior column cephalad to the iliopectineal eminence, and an ilioinguinal approach (one case) when the anterior column portion of the fracture was more caudad or when access to the symphysis pubis was required for reduction and fixation. Using such simultaneous combined approaches, they were able to obtain an anatomic reduction in 88% of their cases. Complications included an incidence of iatrogenic nerve injury of 8% and an 8% incidence of significant functional limitation because of heterotopic ossification.

Moroni and colleagues (85) feeling that the disadvantage of operating on a patient in the lateral decubitus position (as required for a simultaneous approach) is more important compared to the benefit of being able to manipulate both the anterior and posterior columns simultaneously, recommend a staged combined approach. The most displaced and comminuted column is treated first with the ilioinguinal approach performed in the supine position and the Kocher-Langenbeck in the prone position. Following closure of the wounds, the patient is repositioned for the next portion of the procedure and the second approach performed. These authors reported that they achieved a satisfactory or anatomic reduction in 89% of cases. Complications included an incidence of iatrogenic nerve injury of 6%, significant wound drainage 17%, and 6% AVN. No patient demonstrated significant functional limitation because of heterotopic ossification.

Indications

Combined approaches may be used instead of a single extensile approach (triradiate, extended iliofemoral) when access to both columns is required. Thus, it is indicated for some transverse and T-type fractures (Type B) and both-column fractures (Type C).

Access

Posteriorly, access is gained to the posterior wall and posterior column, and if the greater trochanter is removed, to an even wider area. (See Transtrochanteric Approach.) Anteriorly, depending on the anterior exposure used, access may be gained to the entire anterior column, including sacroiliac joint to the symphysis pubis.

Position

The floppy lateral position is used, with no fixed supports.

Advantages

Excellent visualization is gained of the anterior and posterior aspects with less dissection than for the extensile approaches.

This should lead to fewer complications such as heterotopic ossification or neurovascular injury.

Disadvantages

The operator cannot see the entire fracture pattern through one approach. By placing the patient in the floppy lateral position, both the anterior and posterior exposures are compromised to some degree with respect to visualization (as opposed to a supine position for anterior exposures and a prone position for posterior approaches). Moving the patient back and forth from the supine to the prone position also makes reduction and fixation more difficult. Finally, simultaneous combined approaches have the potential to lead to excessive loss of blood and a higher rate of infection.

Surgical Technique

The techniques of both the anterior iliofemoral and ilioinguinal approaches already have been described, as has the posterior Kocher-Langenbeck, with or without trochanteric osteotomy. The techniques are exactly the same, only in this situation they are used together (Fig. 28-64).

TECHNICAL POINTS

Traction

Some traction is essential for the reduction of almost any acetabular fracture, but especially those with intact capsule or soft tissues. Without adequate traction, either by traction

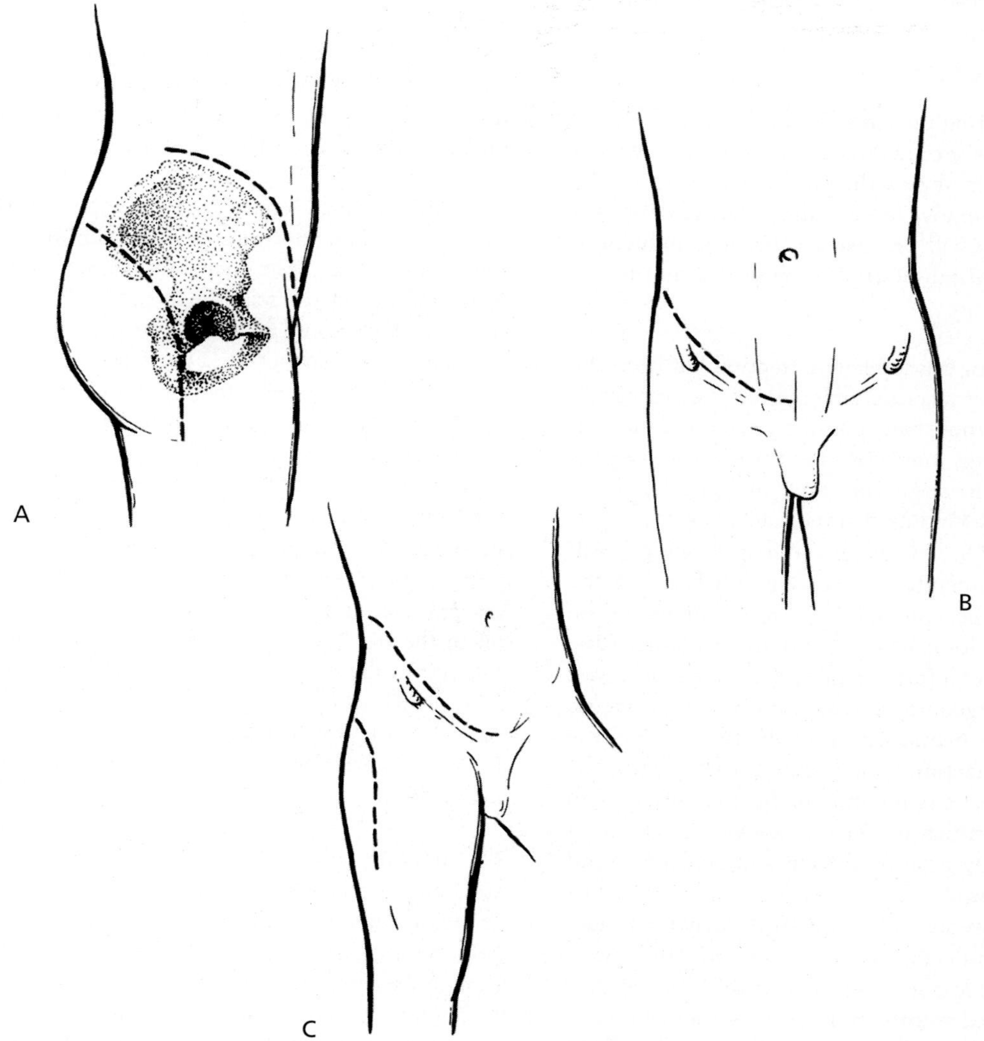

FIGURE 28-64. Diagram to show the incisions used for the combined approach in: **(A)** lateral decubitus position; **(B)** supine position; **(C)** floppy lateral position. (From Schmidt CC, Gruen GS. Related articles: nonextensile surgical approaches for two-column acetabular fractures. *J Bone Joint Surg (Br)* 1993;75(4):556–561, with permission.)

table or surgical assistants, anatomic reduction is virtually impossible to achieve. Traction may be achieved either preoperatively or intraoperatively.

Preoperative Traction

This is extremely important in polytrauma patients, because operative reduction may have to be delayed. Preoperative traction maintains the closed reduction of anterior or posterior dislocations in most instances, and with central displacement of the head distracts the articular cartilage of the head away from the jagged edges of the ilium. In particular, pressure necrosis can develop quickly; therefore, traction becomes important. Usually, traction should be applied with a supracondylar femoral pin. A trochanteric pin should never be used at this stage, because it could interfere with surgical approaches in the region of the greater trochanter.

Intraoperative Traction

In addition to facilitating the reduction, intraoperative traction also is useful to subluxate the femoral head from within the acetabulum. This allows the surgeon to inspect the articular surface and remove loose bodies or redundant ligamentum teres, which will prevent a concentric reduction. Intraoperative traction can be applied by several means.

Traction Table

The classic method for intraoperative traction has been the Tasserit ("Judet"-type) fracture table, which was especially designed for this purpose and permits lateral and skeletal traction as well as image intensification throughout the procedure. However, although this type of table has been deemed invaluable by Letournel and others as an intraoperative tool (38,39,44,68,125) its universal application is still a controversial recommendation and is usually based on the preference of the surgeon. In fact, unfortunately, the Tasserit table is no longer commercially available. One drawback to the use of a fracture table is that the assistance of an unscrubbed surgeon or a technician trained in its use is essential, to enable manipulation of the limb during the operation (51). If a traction table is used because that is the surgeon's preference, it is incumbent on that surgeon to choose a versatile one; that is, one that allows manipulating the limb in almost any position (prone, supine, lateral) and still permits fluoroscopy.

We and other surgeons (45,51,65,106) rarely use a traction table, for several reasons. First, we do not have a Tasserit table. Second, a fracture table with a central post may hinder unbridled fluoroscopic views intraoperatively. Third, fractures of the contralateral superior and inferior pubic rami preclude its use because the perineal post tends to increase the pelvic deformity (68). Fourth, the post occasionally hinders reduction. Fifth, specific complications have been associated with traction (e.g., pudendal nerve palsy). Sixth, the fracture table may limit full motion of the extremity (e.g., hip flexion with the ilioinguinal approach). Seventh, and most important, it is possible to achieve similar traction and limb positioning without the fracture table.

Therefore, we prefer to place the patient on a totally radiolucent table, which can rotate (Jackson, OSI in type) and drape the affected extremity "free," which allows full and unrestricted manipulation of the hip joint during surgery. During surgery, various means of intraoperative traction are available. (See Manual Traction.) Until the issue has been studied more rigorously, surgeon's preference dictates whether or not a traction table is used, but either way the patient must be intraoperative x-ray "visible."

Manual Traction

The alternative to the traction table is to apply traction directly to the femoral head by various means, such as a sharp hook placed around the greater trochanter, a corkscrew driven into the femoral neck, or with the femoral distractor applied to Schanz pins in the proximal femur and greater sciatic buttress (Fig. 28-65).

1. *Manual pull.* Traction can be applied to the limb with the patient in any position by direct pull through the thigh on the flexed knee. The knee should always be flexed, to prevent traction on the sciatic nerve, and with anterior exposures the hip should be flexed, to prevent traction on the femoral artery and nerves. Direct pull on the thigh by an assistant is not very effective in maintaining constant traction throughout the operative procedure, although its intermittent use can be very helpful.
2. *Corkscrew.* A corkscrew or large Schantz pin applied through the lateral femur into the femoral head and connected to a T-handle chuck can afford excellent traction, particularly in young individuals (Fig. 28-65A). The pin is inserted through a hole in the upper lateral femur, just distal to the trochanteric ridge, aiming along the edge of the calcar into the hard subchondral bone of the femoral head. The device often loosens during the procedure in older patients with porotic bone. There also is a theoretical possibility of interfering with the blood supply to the femoral head, although this would be extremely unlikely.
3. *Large, sharp hook.* A large, sharp bone hook (Fig. 28-65) may be placed in the fossa between the greater trochanter and the femoral neck, the same entry point used in closed femoral nailing. If the greater trochanter has not been removed, traction can be applied by splitting the tendon of insertion of the gluteus medius and placing the hook through it. Placement of the hook under direct visualization is extremely easy with surgical approaches that involve an osteotomy of the greater trochanter. The theoretical disadvantage, again, is interference with the blood supply to the femoral head, but the main blood supply is more posterior or medial; therefore, this would be extremely unlikely.

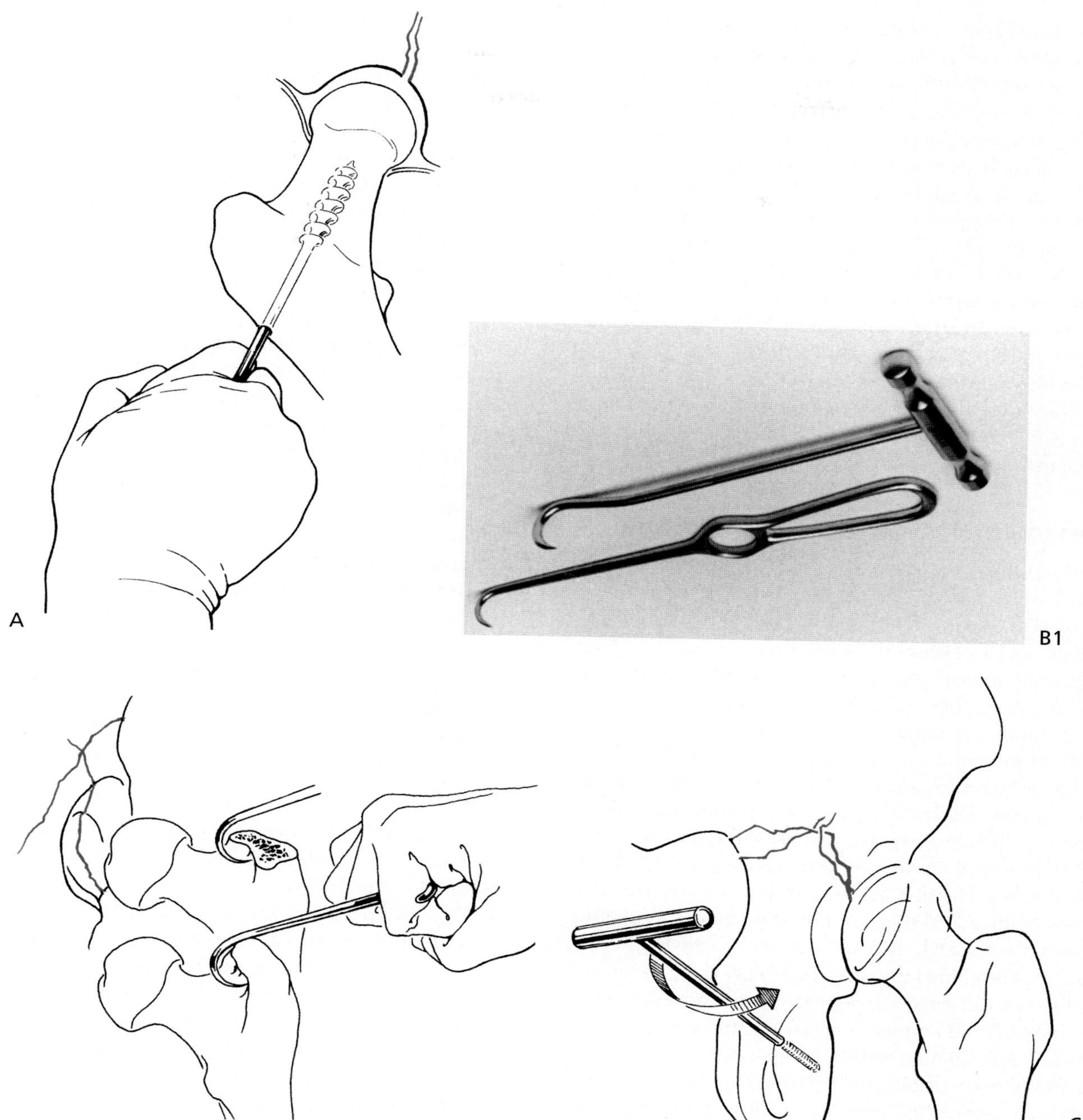

FIGURE 28-65. Intraoperative manual traction. Traction may be applied through the limb in any position, so long as the knee is flexed. This is not very effective; traction applied directly to the femur is more effective. These helpful hints bear remembering: **A:** A corkscrew inserted into the femoral head with a T handle allows direct traction. This is helpful with normal bone, although in osteoporotic bone the corkscrew may pull out. **B1,2:** A large, sharp hook inserted over the greater trochanter, should it be intact, or, alternatively, over the osteotomized distal end of the trochanter. This is an excellent form of traction. The hook has a T handle, and there is no potential for pull out, as the sharp end of the hook is inserted in extremely strong bone. **C:** Insertion of a Schantz pin with a T handle into the ischial tuberosity allows rotation of the posterior column and is an essential aid to reduction of transverse or T fractures. (Parts A and C from Schatzker J, Tile M. *The rationale of operative fracture care.* Heidelberg: Springer-Verlag, 1987, with permission.)

4. *Schantz pin(s).* A Schantz pin inserted into the medial portion of the ischial tuberosity and attached to a T-handle chuck (Fig. 28-65C) allows manipulation of the malreduced posterior column. This technique is particularly helpful when reducing transverse type fractures, especially in the lateral position. Pulling directly up toward the ceiling reduces the fracture line and rotating the Schantz pin can correct rotational deformities of the posterior column. It is virtually impossible to derotate the posterior column without this maneuver (52).

5. *The AO Universal Large Distractor (Synthes, Paoli, PA).* An elegant technique, and our preference, is to use this to distract and inferiorly subluxate the femoral head from the acetabulum (Fig. 28-17). Typically, its application involves the insertion of two 5-mm Schantz pins: one into the sciatic buttress proximally and another into the femur at the level of the lesser trochanter. Traction and limb positioning then can be "dialed in."

Assessment of Reduction and Fixation

Prior to closure, the reconstructed acetabulum should be assessed using visualization, palpation, and intraoperative radiographs to confirm that a satisfactory reduction has been achieved, and to ensure there has been no inadvertent intraarticular hardware placement. Because intraarticular hardware penetration can lead to rapid chondrolysis, it is imperative that the surgeon not leave the operating room until the absence of intraarticular hardware has been confirmed. Depending on the exposure used, the adequacy of the reduction of the posterior column to the anterior column is determined by digital palpation along the quadrilateral surface, either directly from within the pelvis or through the greater and lesser sciatic notches. Division of the sacrospinous ligament or osteotomy of the ischial spine is often required when palpating the reduction through the two notches (Fig. 28-16).

Range of motion of the hip with a finger along the quadrilateral surface can detect the presence of any crepitation in the joint, indicative of residual bony fragments or intraarticular hardware. Auscultation with a sterile stethoscope also has been shown to be efficacious (51,163). If possible, the quality of the reduction and presence of intraarticular hardware should be ascertained by inspection of the articular surface through the capsulorrhaphy and direct traction. Where visualization is not possible, a small blunt elevator can be inserted through the capsular incision, in an attempt to palpate a protruding screw and determine articular step off.

Intraoperative fluoroscopic anteroposterior and Judet views (obturator and iliac 45-degree oblique), are essential to ensure an adequate reduction of the columns and a concentric reduction of the articular surface. Fluoroscopy also is the most sensitive intraoperative means of confirming the proper extraarticular placement of hardware, especially the posterior to anterior lag screws (164–166). For example, intraarticular screw placement can be ruled out by directing the fluoroscopic view parallel to the quadrilateral surface, aiming down the lag screw. Along the posterior wall, intraarticular penetration of screws can be ruled out by orienting the C-arm to the iliac oblique view then rolling the C-arm further (and often the fracture table as well) with spot views until no hardware is observed in the joint.

We routinely obtain a CT scan on the fifth postoperative day. This allows a more critical evaluation of the fracture reduction and the identification of any residual intraarticular bone fragments or implants. Moed and coauthors (70) found that although 92 of 94 patients (98%) had reductions graded as anatomic after surgical stabilization of posterior wall fractures, postoperative CT of 59 patients revealed incongruity of >2 mm in 15% and fracture gaps of ≥2 mm in 75%. This may have implications with respect to studies, which have only evaluated fracture reductions with plain films, and might explain why some patients have gone on to poor results after seemingly anatomic reconstructions. One drawback of CT is that it has been noted to produce a high false-positive rate when detecting intraarticular screw placement (164). Follow-up with plain films for at least 2 to 5 years is recommended as radiographic results at 2 years more closely correlate with 10-year survival rates (167) and avascular necrosis can occur as many as 5 years after the initial injury (50).

OTHER SPECIAL TECHNICAL FACTORS: SURGICAL DISLOCATION OF THE FEMORAL HEAD FOR TREATMENT OF FRACTURES OF THE ACETABULUM

Introduction

The standard Kocher-Langenbeck approach is mainly used for posterior wall and column fractures and for certain transverse or T-shaped fractures and fracture dislocation patterns (44,47). Evaluation of fracture reduction predominantly relies on the extraarticular fracture lines of the retroarticular surface and palpation of the quadrilateral surface. A posterior capsulotomy and traction on the femur allows a limited insight into the hip joint (44). Intraarticular inspection is facilitated in the presence of posterior wall comminution and is limited in fracture patterns with small posterior rim fragments or an intact posterior wall. Fracture lines of the anterior column, such as in transverse or T-shaped fractures, are hardly visible; intraarticular visual control of reduction of comminuted posterior wall fractures is very restricted too. A limited exposure of the supraacetabular region may pose a further difficulty of the standard Kocher-Langenbeck approach in fractures with involvement of the anterosuperior dome area (44,82,144).

Based on a technique for safe surgical femoral head dislocation without the risk of avascular necrosis of the head (15), the presented modified approach to the hip extends exposure to the superior rim area and provides visualization of the entire hip joint for treatment of selected acetabular fractures (17,181). Surgical dislocation of the femoral head can be performed in either direction posteriorly or anteriorly, even in patients with a prior traumatic posterior fracture-dislocation. Exposure of the entire head and acetabulum allows for accurate assessment of anatomic reduction, safe extraarticular placement of fixation screws, complete removal of free fragments, and more accurate evaluation of cartilage damage. This has been found to be helpful, especially in comminuted posterior wall fractures, in transverse or T-shaped fractures alone or combined with posterior wall fragments. Of note, these fracture types are typically more difficult to treat and are among the ones with the least favorable results (44,47,182–185). In addition, this approach allows optimal protection of the posterior portion of the gluteus medius and minimus muscles during manipulations for reduction and fixation of the fracture (17).

Surgical Technique

Positioning

The patient is placed in a lateral decubitus position with padding of the uninvolved leg, on a regular operating table. No traction is applied to the involved leg. The surgeon is positioned at the back side of the patient.

Surgical Approach

A Kocher-Langenbeck type skin incision is used. The fascia lata is incised in line with the skin incision. The gluteus, maximus muscle fiber bundles are split carefully longitudinally. After longitudinal incision and dissection of the

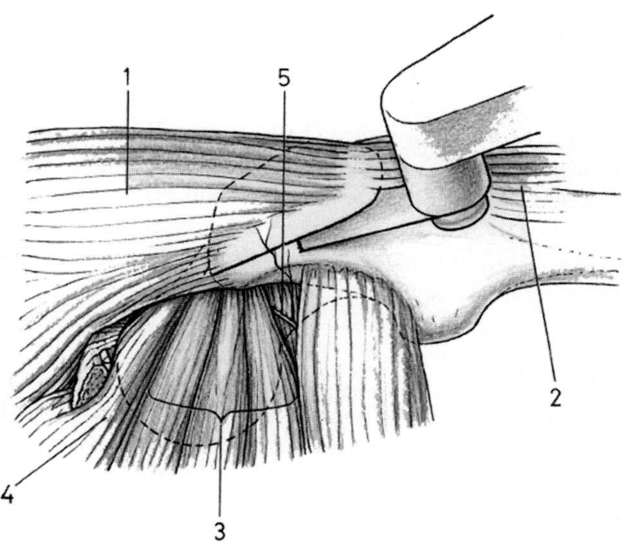

FIGURE 28-66. Digastric trochanteric osteotomy with the oscillating saw leaving the majority of the gluteus medius tendon cranially and the insertion of the vastus lateralis muscle caudally at the fragment; gluteus medius, muscle *(1);* vastus lateralis muscle *(2);* gemelli and obturator internus muscles *(3);* piriformis muscle *(4);* deep branch of medial femoral circumflex artery *(5).*

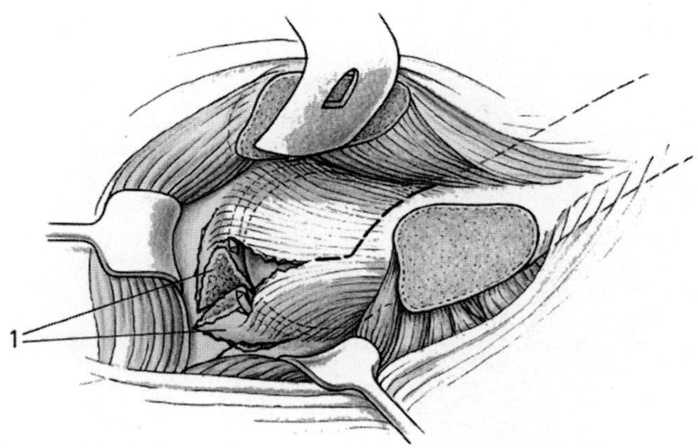

FIGURE 28-67. Exposure of the capsula and posterior-superior wall fragments *(1);* the capsulotomy *(dotted line)* is done as an extension of the traumatic capsular laceration, preserving the capsular attachments of the main rim fragments.

trochanteric bursa, the posterior border of the gluteus, medius muscle, and its tendinous insertion at the posterior-superior edge of the greater trochanter is exposed. In the same way the posterior-superior origin of the vastus lateralis muscle at the innomnate tubercle and femur has to be identified and mobilized over a distance of approximately 10 cm. With an oscillating saw a trochanteric osteotomy, with the vast majority of the gluteus medius muscle insertion and the entire origin of the vastus lateralis muscle attached to it (digastric osteotomy) is performed. Thereby, a small portion of the very posterior gluteus medius tendon insertion has to remain attached to the stable trochanteric portion in order to prevent the osteotomy from being too medial, and thereby risking damage to the deep branch of the medial femoral circumflex artery and/or its subsynovial ramifications (Fig. 28-66). After the osteotomy, these fibers are cut sharply, allowing the trochanteric fragment to be flipped anteriorly. The osteotomy runs lateral to the insertion of the short external rotators, which remain attached to the proximal femur. Some fibers of the piriformis muscle insertion remaining attached to the trochanteric fragment have to be cut close to the lifted trochanter to facilitate its flipping. The deep branch of the medial femoral circumflex artery remains protected, since the artery crosses posterior to the obturator externus tendon and runs cranially, anterior to the remaining external rotator muscles (Fig. 28-66). As a next step, the interval between the inferior border of the gluteus minimus muscle and superiorly to the piriformis muscle and tendon has to be identified and entered. Subsequent release of the origin of the gluteus minimus and vastus lateralis and vastus intermedius muscles from the underlying bone and capsule allows the trochanteric fragment to be mobilized further anteriorly. Positioning of the leg in progressive external rotation and flexion by an assistant facilitates this surgical step. Finally, the entire anterior and superior aspect of the capsule becomes fully exposed (Fig. 28-67).

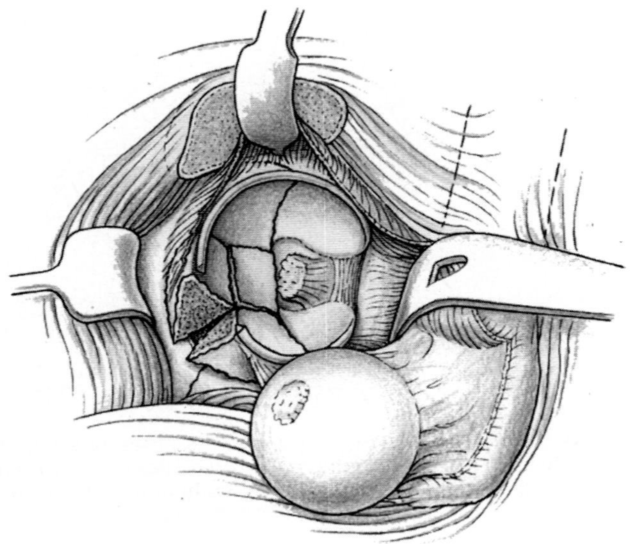

FIGURE 28-68. Complete intraarticular exposure after anterior surgical dislocation of the femoral head.

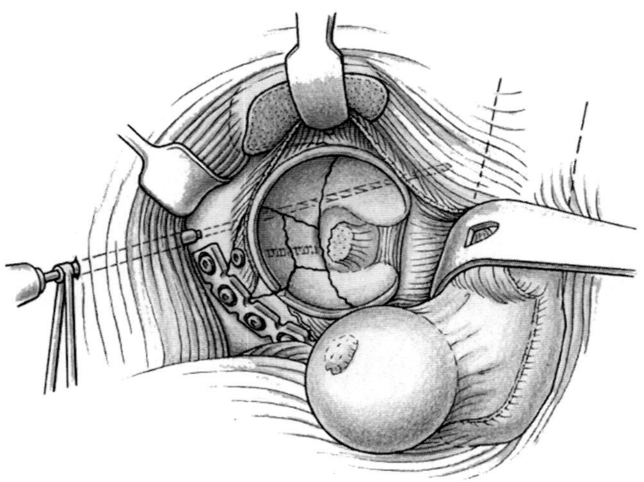

FIGURE 28-70. Placement of a long screw in the anterior column with an entry point posterior-superior to the acetabulum with the femoral head dislocated. Intraarticular screw placement can be excluded by visual control.

For complete joint visualization, an anterior and superior capsulotomy is performed and the femoral head is dislocated in the anterior direction. In cases with an intact capsule, the capsulotomy is done close to the acetabular rim cranially and posteriorly and is directed toward the proximal femur, anteriorly and inferiorly, thereby creating a Z-shaped opening (right side). Modification of the capsulotomy according to the wall fracture pattern may be needed and has to be done in a way that the remaining capsular attachments to the acetabular wall fragments are preserved. Care is taken not to damage the labrum. Through adduction and external rotation of the leg, the femoral head subluxates or can be dislocated anteriorly.

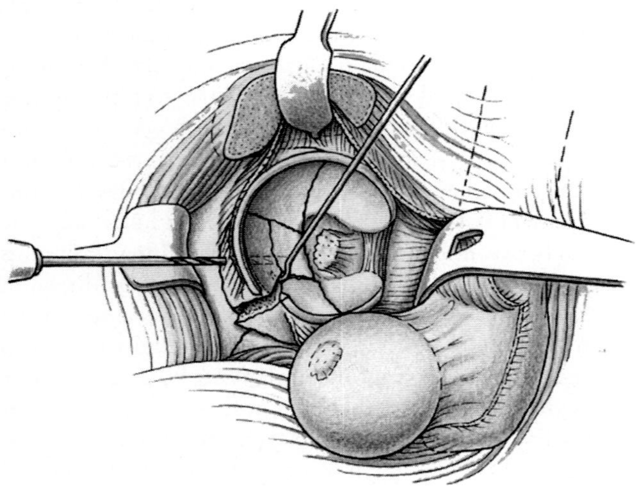

FIGURE 28-69. Visualization during reduction and screw fixation of free articular fragments or posterior-superior rim fragments with the femoral head dislocated.

For complete dislocation, the femoral head ligament has to be transected if it is still intact. A circumferential view of the acetabulum and a nearly circumferential view of the femoral head is obtained through this maneuver (Fig. 28-68). Comminuted posterior and superior wall fragments can be reduced and fixed with screws with the head dislocated (Fig. 28-69). In the same way, a long anterior column screw with an entry point posterior-superior directed to the upper pubic ramus can be placed under direct visual control to confirm extraarticular placement (Fig. 28-70).

Posterior dislocation of the femoral head can be done instead of or in addition to an anterior dislocation but the exposure of the acetabulum is more limited. For more extensile exposure of the retroacetabular area, the piriformis tendon may be released or the interval between gemellus inferior and obturator externus muscles can be entered. If the triceps coxae has to be released in addition a minimal distance of 2 cm to the posterior aspect of the greater trochanter should be maintained in order not to endanger the deep branch of the medial femoral circumflex artery (14).

Closure

After dislocation of the femoral head the round ligament is resected in order not to interfere with joint motion. The capsula is closed with 2.0 absorbable sutures. Care has to be taken not to tighten the capsula too much because this might compromise the femoral head perfusion by tension on the terminal arterial branches within the superior retinaculum (16). Transected tendons of the external rotators should be reattached. The refixation of the osteotomized, greater trochanter is achieved by two to three 3.5-mm, cortical screws. The rest of the wound is closed within layers after placement of a drain.

Aftertreatment

Weight-bearing is protected to 5 to 10 kg for 8 weeks. Flexion of the hip is restricted to 90 degrees. No muscle exercises are allowed. In cases with major muscle contusion or a previous history of heterotopic, ossification prophylactic treatment with oral indomethacin 75 mg per day is given for 3 weeks. Conventional radiographs are obtained 8 weeks after surgery. In the majority of cases the osteotomy of the greater trochanter is solidly healed at this point. Progressive weight bearing until full weight bearing is allowed through a further 2- to 3-week period. Active muscle exercises for regaining strength of the gluteus medius muscle are started. In cases where the osteotomy does not seem to be solidly healed, another 4-week period of protected weight bearing is recommended.

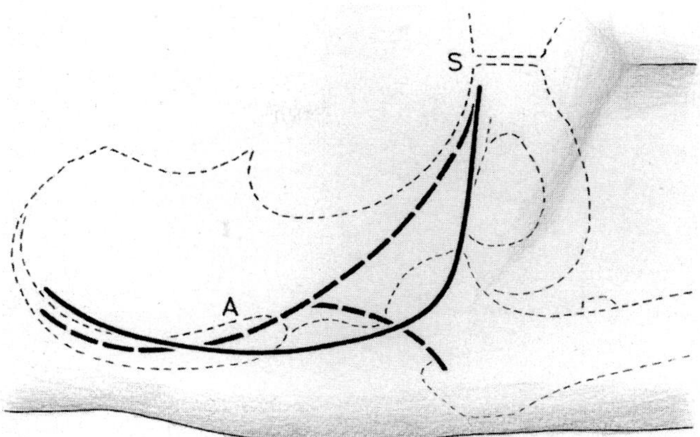

FIGURE 28-71. Curved skin incision *(black line)* for approach to the left hip joint. Triradiate shaped incision *(interrupted line)* with the inferior limb similar to a Smith-Petersen approach.

EXTENSION OF THE ILIOINGUINAL APPROACH

Introduction

The ilioinguinal approach for treatment of acetabular fractures has been popularized predominantly by Letournel (42,147). This approach uses three windows through intervals between muscles and blood vessels to access the anterior column of the pelvis. The posterior column is addressed indirectly mainly through the second window. Difficulties arise in low anterior column fractures and/or comminution of the anterior wall, in which exposure is generally limited by the iliopsoas muscle. Obesity may provide another significant obstacle for adequate exposure and fracture manipulation. Modification of the ilioinguinal approach by combining it with an extension such as a Smith-Petersen approach (186) seems beneficial in these selected cases (187). The extension exploits the internervous plane between the sartorius and rectus femoris muscles with the femoral nerve and the tensor fasciae latae and gluteus medius muscles with the superior gluteal nerve. An osteotomy of the anterior superior iliac spine and release of the rectus femoris muscle origins allows mobilization and medial retraction, especially of the iliopsoas muscle, which largely increases access through the first window and to the anterior wall. Furthermore, anterior access to the hip joint is provided with the option of intraarticular inspection and removal of intercalated or free intraarticular fragments. The surgical extension with osteotomy of the ASIS and mobilization of the muscles to the medial side also helps to decrease tension on the lateral femoral cutaneous nerve (LFCN), and thus decreases the rather frequent nerve damage with a classical ilioinguinal approach (151,152).

Surgical Technique

Positioning

A regular operating table is chosen and no traction is applied. The patient is placed in the supine position with the affected leg mobile, without any specific padding under the buttocks. Preferably, a radiolucent table is chosen in order to allow for an intraoperative imaging to judge the fracture reduction.

Surgical Approach

The lateral part of the incision starts at the same point at the junction of the posterior and middle third of the crista iliaca as originally described for the ilioinguinal approach, but runs initially almost vertical, staying laterally to the crista iliaca and ASIS. At approximately 5 cm distal and lateral of the ASIS the incision is curved medially at an angle of about 100 degrees toward the symphysis (Fig. 28-71). As an alternative an incision with three limbs can be used. This triradiate configuration of the incision includes the classical ilioinguinal skin incision connected with an additional longitudinal incision of about 12- to 15-cm length. The latter one meets the first incision immediately lateral to the ASIS and is directed distally and slightly laterally. The deep dissection through the first window is the same as for the classical ilioinguinal approach, with elevation of the iliacus muscle off the inner table of the iliac wing. At the ASIS this modified approach turns into the Smith-Petersen approach. The internervous interval is exploited between the sartorius and rectus femoris muscles with the femoral nerve (medially) and the tensor fascia lata and gluteal muscles with the superior gluteal nerve (laterally) (186). If needed, the second and the third window of the classical ilioinguinal approach are exposed in the usual way before proceeding with the Smith-Petersen extension. After that the first step of the extension is to develop the interval between the tensor fasciae latae and sartorius muscles. An osteotomy of the ASIS with the attached inguinal ligament and sartorius muscle is performed with a chisel. The osteotomized fragment has an approximate size of 2 × 1 cm, which should allow screw fixation at the end of the procedure. Thus, the LFCN is retracted medially with the sartorius muscle (Fig. 28-72).

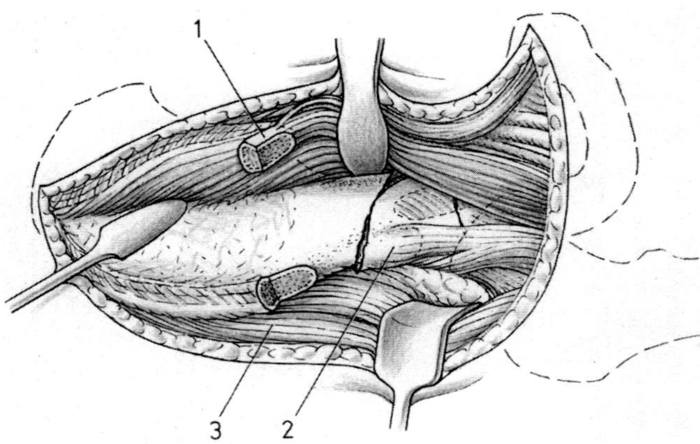

FIGURE 28-72. Medial retraction of the osteotomized anterior superior iliac spine *(1)* with attached sartorius muscle. Rectus femoris muscle still attached to the anterior inferior iliac spine *(2)*. Lateral retraction of the tensor fasciae latae muscle *(3)*.

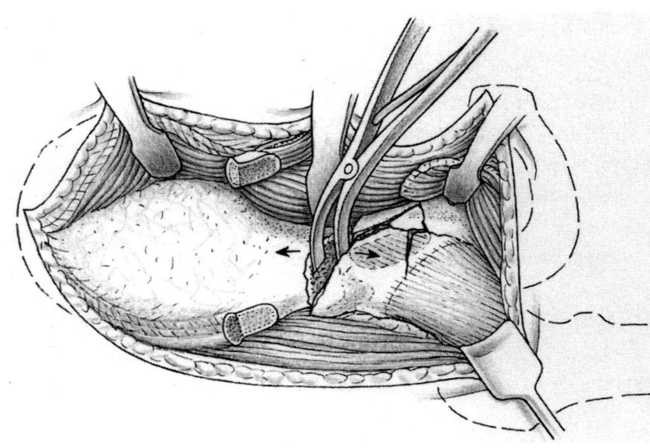

FIGURE 28-74. Spreading of the main fragments with a laminar spreader.

The straight and reflected head of the rectus femoris muscle are transected at the anterior inferior iliac spine (AIIS). Relaxing and retraction of the medial structures are obtained by placing the leg in moderate flexion with the help of a rolled-up towel or knee holder. Posterior to the rectus muscle and lateral to the iliacus muscle lies the iliocapsularis muscle, which covers the anterior aspect of the hip joint capsule. It has to be dissected sharply off the anterior capsule and reflected medially together with the main iliacus muscle (188). Opening of the iliopectineal bursa and medial retraction of the iliopsoas muscle allows abundant exposure of the entire anterior wall, including the iliopectineal eminence without stretching of the LFCN

There is excellent visualization and access to low fracture lines of the anterior column and separate or comminuted anterior wall fragments (Fig. 28-73), allowing anatomic reduction, especially when comminuted, and even buttressing with a small one-third tubular plate. Intercalated fragments, which may block reduction, can be extracted more easily from the fracture gap by using a laminar spreader. This even allows visualization of the femoral head and extraction of intraarticular fragments through the fracture gap (Fig. 28-74). There is easier access to fracture lines of the quadrilateral surface, which also can be reduced by placing one leg of a curved reduction clamp near the AIIS through the enlarged first window (Fig. 28-75). This is especially helpful in cases with comminution of the low anterior column and anterior wall, because it may become extremely difficult to get a firm grip with the reduction clamp through the second window in order to reduce the quadrilateral surface and posterior column. Digital control of reduction of the quadrilateral surface in the same way is facilitated through the enlarged first window. If needed, the abductors can be partially taken off the outer wing of the ilium subperiosteally. Occasionally, this may be necessary to judge fracture lines on the outside of the iliac wing, for placing a reduction clamp, or for improving access to the hip joint. In most cases, however, tunneling of the musculature between

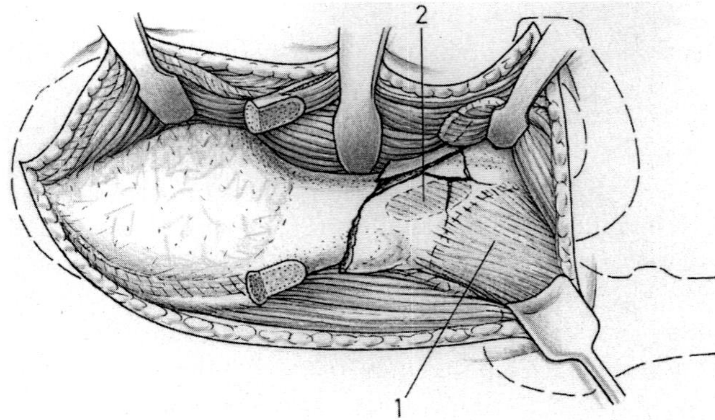

FIGURE 28-73. Exposure after detachment of the rectus femoris muscle and mobilization of the iliopsoas and iliocapsularis muscles medially; anterior aspect of the hip joint capsule *(1)*; iliopectineal bursa *(2)*.

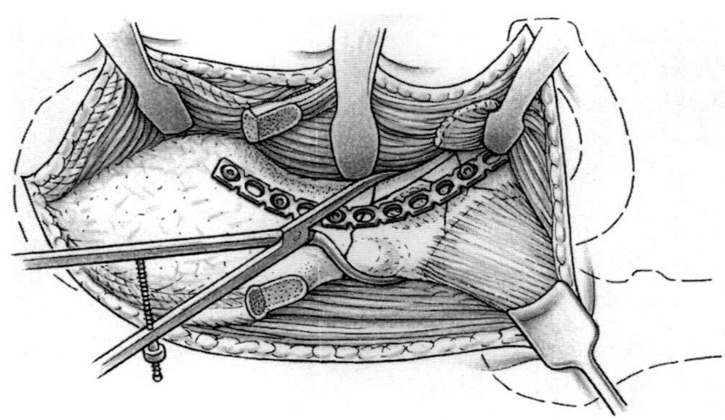

FIGURE 28-75. Reduction of the posterior column by placing one leg of a curved reduction clamp on the quadrilateral surface with the other leg placed around the anterior inferior iliac spine.

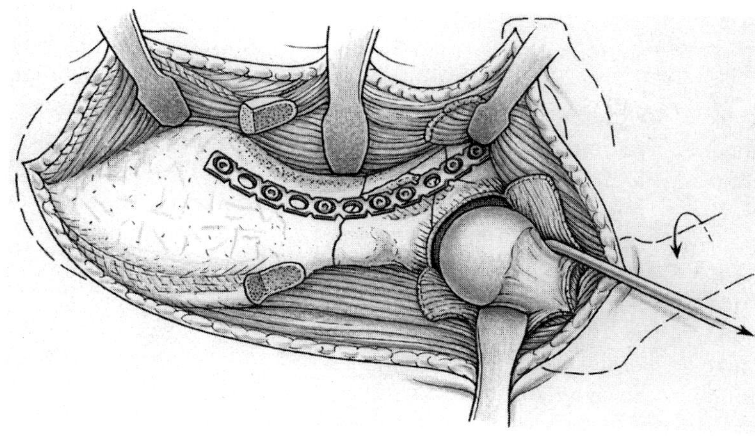

FIGURE 28-76. After a T-shaped capsulotomy, the femoral head can be subluxated with limited insight into the hip joint, or it can even be dislocated.

the ASIS and AIIS is sufficient, leaving the main origin of the tensor fasciae latae, gluteus medius and minimus muscles intact. The hip joint can be opened by a T-shaped capsulotomy. Subsequently, the femoral head can be subluxated by gentle traction with a bone hook placed just above the lesser trochanter on the femoral neck (Fig. 28-76). This does not endanger the deep branch of the medial circumflex artery, representing the main blood supply to the femoral head (14). Intraarticular access allows for assessment of the articular surfaces of both the femoral head and acetabulum, fixation or excision of free fragments, inspection of the labrum and intraarticular control of fracture reduction, and extraarticular placement of screws.

If not done prior to the Smith-Petersen part of the approach, the second and third windows of the ilioinguinal can be opened even now in the same way as originally described. To restore tension on the inguinal ligament for easier dissection, the osteotomized ASIS may be temporarily reattached with a small pointed clamp to its original position. After that the skin incision and further steps can be performed in the usual way.

Closure

The hip capsule is closed at the end of the procedure. The straight and the reflected origins of the rectus muscle are reattached, thereby using nonabsorbable transosseus sutures for the straight portion. The sartorius muscle is refixated with its ostetomized bony origin (ASIS) with a 2.7-mm screw. The remainder of the closure is in layers. Deep drains are left in place for 1 to 2 days.

Aftertreatment

Active leg raising is not allowed for the first 6 weeks to obtain uneventful healing of the reattached muscles. Protected weight bearing with 5 to 10 kg is maintained for 8 weeks. Prophylactic treatment by oral indomethacin or radiation may be considered in cases with major muscle contusion or a previous patient's history of HO.

POSTOPERATIVE MANAGEMENT

Deep infection is a devastating complication following fixation of acetabular fractures, with an incidence as high as 9% but probably nearer 4% to 5% (39,44,47,55,111). Because of such concerns, we advocate the routine use of prophylactic antibiotics, multiple suction drains in all recesses to prevent hematoma formation, surgical evacuation of hematomas, and if present, debridement of the Morel-Lavalle lesion over the greater trochanter (44,118). Drains are not discontinued until output has tapered to 10 to 20 mL per 8-hour shift, usually by 48 to 72 hours. Intravenous cefazolin is continued for a minimum of 48 to 72 hours and until the suction drains are removed. Serous drainage following pelvic surgery is not uncommon and often improves when range of motion activity, such as a continuous passive motion machine, is discontinued (51,72). However, if it persists beyond one week, formal wound exploration, drainage, and debridement should be considered. After lengthy procedures or more extensile approaches, or in the presence of persistent drainage, some have anecdotally noted that a longer duration of antibiotic treatment of up to 7 to 10 days may be of benefit (140).

The indications for prophylaxis for HO are controversial. Certainly, mild amounts of heterotopic bone often form after surgical reconstruction of the acetabulum in as many as 90% of patients (44,47,70,73,109–111,136,168–170). In most cases, its presence is of little functional significance. However, in approximately 5% to 14% of cases (39,59,72,116,168) but reportedly as high as 53% of cases (169), HO is substantial enough to cause significant restriction of hip motion; therefore, some form of prophylaxis is often desirable.

Various risk factors have been identified for HO, including the extended iliofemoral and Kocher-Langenbeck approaches; associated head, abdominal, and chest injuries; trochanteric osteotomy, T-type fractures, greater severity of articular damage, sciatic nerve damage, and male sex (81,82,110,121,136,168). Heterotopic bone formation is particularly common and severe with the extended iliofemoral approach because of stripping of the external surface of the iliac wing (44,56,57,109,128,136). In contrast, the ilioinguinal approach has the lowest incidence of HO (44,57). Although two studies have failed to note a correlation with the posterior Kocher-Langenbeck approach (110,136), Letournel observed significant heterotopic bone formation in 5%. Although this rate was not as great as that observed in his patients after the extended iliofemoral approach (14%), it was almost 10 times that seen after an ilioinguinal approach (0.6%) (44).

The most common forms of prophylaxis against HO are indomethacin (75 mg daily) (44,73,87,136,169–172) and low-dose radiation therapy (700 to 1,000 cGy in single or divided doses) (44,87,109,120,170,171,173–175), both of which have been shown to decrease the rate of significant HO formation after surgical treatment of acetabular fractures when given early. Although a recent prospective study found these two methods to be equally effective (171), another prospective study, which used CT to measure HO formation, has questioned the efficacy of indomethacin (168).

Our routine prophylaxis for all patients is indomethacin 25 mg orally three times daily (or 75 mg sustained release orally once daily) for 6 weeks if they undergo a Kocher-Langenbeck or extensile approach. Those patients for whom indomethacin is contraindicated are treated with low-dose radiation therapy, usually a single dose of 700 cGy. We do not routinely administer prophylaxis to patients who undergo fixation through an ilioinguinal approach unless a limited subperiosteal exposure of the outer cortex of the ilium was performed for insertion of pelvic reduction clamps.

As discussed, DVT remains a grave concern (see Chapter 9). Therefore, routine postoperative thromboembolism prophylaxis is recommended because of the high risk of DVT and its potential catastrophic sequela of pulmonary embolism (95,97). This includes sequential compression devices and pharmacologic therapy. A therapeutic level of coumadin with an international normalization ratio is efficacious, although low molecular weight heparin is gaining in popularity (51,87,95,176). However, the major downside of postoperative anticoagulation early on is hematoma formation. Also, the optimal duration of postoperative anticoagulation is unclear. Although full weight bearing and therefore absolute mobilization of the patient typically are delayed for at least 8 weeks, long-term anticoagulation with coumadin presents difficulties such as reliable monitoring and theoretical concerns such as bleeding complications. Our postoperative anticoagulation regimen includes compression boots while hospitalized, and 6 weeks of low-dose warfarin.

A protocol used by Fishmann and colleagues (177) has attempted to balance the desire to minimize postoperative hematoma formation while providing an adequate time window for postoperative anticoagulation in the pelvic trauma patient. Patients were routinely treated with knee-high graduated elastic stockings (TED) and external pneumatic compression devices preoperatively (EPC), with noninvasive screening being performed via duplex ultrasonography within a few hours of admission. The EPCs were worn at all times during the postoperative period except during physical therapy or nursing care. When the drains were removed (between 48 and 72 hours postoperatively) warfarin therapy was started with an initial dose of 7.5 mg and adjusted daily (twice weekly on discharge) to obtain a therapeutic index of 1.3 to 1.4 times control (international normalized ratio of 2:3). The EPCs were discontinued 2 days after this level of anticoagulation had been maintained. After discharge, the patients continued prophylactic warfarin therapy for 3 more weeks. Patients younger than 22 years of age did not receive postoperative warfarin. The authors reported that they significantly reduced their overall incidence of venous thrombosis from 27% to 3%, with a more modest decrease in the rate of proximal vein thrombosis from 3% to 12% to 2% (177). The rate of postoperative wound hematoma was only 1.5%, with a rate of nonfatal pulmonary embolism of 1%.

At the end of the operative procedure the surgeon must evaluate the osteosynthesis honestly. Rehabilitation may be instituted early if the patient is young, the bone good, and the internal fixation stable. This includes early mobilization with the patient encouraged to sit up and dangle within the first 24 to 48 hours following surgery. In some cases, Hamilton Russell traction also can be used for the first few days. To prevent stiffness in the hip joint, continuous passive motion (CPM) also has been used in the immediate postoperative period. Experimental studies by Salter and coworkers (178) suggest this has a marked beneficial effect on the joint. Some have also noted its application helpful in clinical experience (51). We do not routinely use CPM during the postoperative period, because we have not had difficulty regaining hip motion in this patient population. If CPM is to be used, the internal fixation must be stable lest the fragments become displaced and anatomic reduction lost.

After removal of the drains—usually by the third day—patients are allowed partial weight bearing (not more than 20 lbs) with the foot flat using crutches for 6 to 8 weeks. Range of motion exercises are also instituted, although some limitations may be set depending on the presence of significant posterior wall involvement and whether a trochanteric osteotomy was required. (In the case of an extended iliofemoral approach or a trochanteric osteotomy, active abduction is avoided for 6 to 8 weeks.) Strengthening exercises and gait training are initiated by the physical therapist. However, weight bearing is not advanced for 6 to 8 weeks. Acetabular fractures with a concomitant neurologic injury can pose a difficult rehabilitation problem, because of lack of motor activity or neurogenic pain, and frequently require treatment in conjunction with a pain management service. Careful follow-up care is mandatory. If the radiographs indicate good healing with no loss of the stable internal fixation, weight bearing usually can be advanced at 8 weeks, with full weight bearing achieved by 12 to 14 weeks.

A troublesome occurrence is the loss of reduction during the early postoperative period. This is especially true in elderly patients with osteopenic bone where it is important to adequately buttress the fractures (89,176,179,180). The stability of the internal fixation must be questioned for older patients, those with osteoporotic bone, and in cases of severe marginal impaction where there is concern about dislodgement of the fragments. In such cases, it is best to err on the side of caution before allowing the patient to ambulate. Some have recommended consideration of skeletal traction for a full 6 weeks (51). At that point, healing of the cancellous bone usually is adequate to begin the rehabilitation program. Early ambulation for this group of individuals is particularly dangerous, because loss of the anatomic reduction usually spells disaster for the joint. It is far better to risk the extra weeks of bed rest and minimize complications of thromboembolic disease by using anticoagulants, than to jeopardize the fracture by prematurely releasing the patient to a rehabilitation program.

CONCLUSION

The learning curve for the successful management of acetabular fractures is quite steep (44,50). However, a careful and complete preoperative assessment of the fracture pattern and displacement are invaluable in choosing the optimal approach to the acetabulum as well as the proper means of reduction and fixation. Every acetabular fracture has a specific character or personality, and thus, its treatment must be individualized.

REFERENCES

1. Chandler SB, Kreuscher PH. A study of the blood supply of the ligamentum teres and its relation to the circulation of the head of the femur. *J Bone Joint Surg* 1932;14:834–846.
2. Chung SMK. The arterial supply of the developing proximal end of the human femur. *J Bone Joint Surg* 1976;58-A:961–970.
3. Crock HV. A revision of the anatomy of the arteries supplying the upper end of the human femur. *J Anat* 1965;99:77–88.
4. Judet J, Judet R, Lagrange J, Dunoyer J. A study of the arterial vascularization of the femoral neck in the adult. *J Bone Joint Surg* 1955;37-A:663–680.
5. Sevitt S, Thompson RG. The distribution and anastomosis of the arteries supplying the head and neck of the femur. *J Bone Joint Surg* 1965;47-B:560–573.
6. Tucker F. Arterial supply to the femoral head and its clinical importance. *J Bone Joint Surg* 1949;31-B:82–93.
7. Wertheimer LG, Lopes SF. Arterial supply of the femoral head. *J Bone Joint Surg* 1971;53-A:545–556.
8. Trueta J, Harrison MHM. The normal vascular anatomy of the femoral head in adult man. *J Bone Joint Surg* 1953;35-B: 442–452.
9. Trueta J. The normal vascular anatomy of the human femoral head during growth. *J Bone Joint Surg* 1953;39-B:358–394.
10. Lanz J, Wachsmuth W. *Praktische Anatomie. Bein und Statik.* Berlin: Springer Verlag, 1972.
11. Ogden JA. Changing patterns of proximal femoral vascularity. *J Bone Joint Surg* 1974;56-A:941–950.
12. Theron J. L'artériographie dans les necroses primitves de la tΛte femorale. *Acta Orthop Belg* 1981;47:225–229.
13. Howe WW, Lacey T, Schwartz RP. A study of the gross anatomy of the arteries supplying the proximal portion of the femur and the acetabulum. *J Bone Joint Surg* 1950;32-A: 856–866.
14. Gautier E, Ganz K, Krügel N, et al. Anatomy of the medial femoral circumflex artery and surgical implications. *J Bone Joint Surg* 2000;82-B:679–683.
15. Ganz R, Gill TJ, Gautier E, et al. Surgical dislocation of the adult hip a technique with full access to the femoral head and acetabulum without the risk of avascular necrosis. *J Bone Joint Surg* 2001;83-B:1119–1124.
16. Nötzli HIP, Siebenrock KA, Hempfing A, et al. Perfusion of the femoral head during surgical dislocation of the hip: monitoring by Laser Doppler flowmetry. *J Bone Joint Surg* 2002;84-B: 300–304.
17. Siebenrock K, Gautier E, Ziran BH, et al. Trochanteric flip osteotomy for cranial extension and muscle protection in acetabular fracture fixation using a Kocher-Langenbeck approach. *J Orthop Trauma* 1998;12:387–391.
18. Bauer R, Kerschbaumer F, Poisel S. *Operative approaches in orthopaedic surgery and traumatology,* 1st ed. New York: G Thieme Verlag, 1987.
19. Hoppenfeld S, deBoer P. *Surgical approaches in orthopaedics: the anatomic approach,* 1st ed. Philadelphia: JB Lippincott, 1984.
20. Letournel E, Judet R. Vascular supply. In: *Fractures of the acetabulum,* 2nd ed. Berlin: Springer-Verlag, 1993:20–22.
21. Rüedi T, von Hochstetter AHC, Schlumpf R. *Surgical approaches for internal fixation.* Berlin: Springer-Verlag, 1984.
22. Bergoin M, Louis R. Vascularisation de l'os coxal. *Travaux de l'Institut d'Anatomie de Marseille Fasc* 1961;19:91–95.
23. Fischer LP, Noyer D, Gonon GP, et al. Vascularisation de l'os coxal. *Bull Assoc Anat* 1977;61:343–356.
24. Itokazu M, Takahashi K, Matsunaga T, et al. A study of the arterial supply of the human acetabulum using a corrosion casting method. *Clin Anat* 1997;10:77–81.
25. Katthagen BD, Spies H, Bachmann G. Arterial vascularization of the bony acetabulum. *Z Orthop Ihre Grenzgeb* 1995;133: 7–13.
26. Crock HV. *An atlas of vascular anatomy of the skeleton and spinal cord.* London: Martin Dunitz, 1996.
27. *Gray's anatomy,* 38th ed. London: Churchill Livingstone, 1995.
28. von Lanz T, Wachsmuth W. *Prakfische Anatomie.* Berlin: Springer-Verlag, 1984.
29. Beck M, Leunig M, Ellis T, et al. The acetabular blood supply. Implications to periactabular osteotomies, submitted.
30. Hempfing A, Leunig M, Notzli HP, et al. Acetabular blood flow during Bernese periacetabular osteotomy (PAO). An intraoperative study using Laser Doppler flowmetry, submitted.
31. Thomas G. Die arterielle Gefüssversorgung des Pfannendachgebietes beim Erwachsenen. *Arch Orthop Unfallchir* 1965;58: 300–305.

32. Damsin JP, Lazennec JY, Gonzales M, et al. Arterial supply of the acetabulum in the fetus: application to periacetabular surgery in childhood. *Surg Radiol Anat* 1992;14:215–221.
33. Ebraheim NA, Lu J, Biyani A, et al. Anatomic considerations of the principal nutrient foramen and artery on internal surface of the ilium. *Surg Radiol Anat* 1997;19:237–239.
34. Hijikata HS, Ogichi H, Macida H, et al. Treatment and prognosis of complication for rotational acetabular osteotomy. *Hip Joint* 1991;17:217–220.
35. Ninomiya S. Rotational acetabular osteotomy for the severely dysplastic hip in the adolescent and adult. *Clin Orthop* 1989; 247:213–216.
36. Leunig M, Siebenrock KA, Mahomed MN, et al. Bernese periacetabular osteotomy: technical aspects and clinical results. *Hip Int* 1999;9:119–126.
37. Leunig M, Siebenrock KA, Ganz R. Rationale of periacetabular osteotomy and background work. *J Bone Joint Surg* 2001;83-A: 438–448.
38. Letournel E, Judet R, Elson RAT. *Fractures of the acetabulum.* Berlin: Springer-Verlag, 1981.
39. Matta JM, Merritt PO. Displaced acetabular fractures. *Clin Orthop* 1988;230:83–97.
40. Judet R, Judet J, Letournel E. Fractures of the acetabulum: classification and surgical approaches for open reduction. Preliminary report. *J Bone Joint Surg (Am)* 1964;46:1615–1646.
41. Judet R, Lagrange J. La voie postero externe de gibson. *Presse Med* 1958;66(3):263–264.
42. Letournel E. Acetabulum fractures: classification and management. *Clin Orthop* 1980; 151:81–106.
43. Letournel E. *The Hip: Proceedings of the fifteenth open scientific meeting of The Hip Society.* St. Louis: CV Mosby, 1987: 157–180.
44. Letournel E, Judet R. *Fractures of the acetabulum,* 2nd ed. New York: Springer-Verlag, 1993.
45. Bartlett CS, Helfet DL. Acetabular fractures: evaluation, classification, treatment concepts, and approaches. In: Ruedi TP, Murphy WM, Colton CL, et al. *AO principles of fracture management.* New York: Thieme, 2000.
46. Matta JM. Acetabular fractures. *J Orthop Trauma* 2000;14(5): 377–378.
47. Matta JM. Fractures of the acetabulum: accuracy of reduction and clinical results in patients managed operatively within 3 weeks after the injury. *J Bone Joint Surg* 1996;78A:1632–1645.
48. Mayo, KA. Surgical approaches to the acetabulum. *Tech Orthop* 990;4(4):24–35.
49. Pennal GF, Davidson J, Garside H, et al. Results of treatment of acetabular fractures. *Clin Orthop* 1980;151:115–123.
50. Tornetta P. Displaced acetabular fractures: indications for operative and nonoperative management. *J Am Acad Orthop Surg* 2001;9(1):18–28.
51. Kellam JP, Tile M. Surgical techniques. In: Tile M, Burgess A, Helfet DL, et al. *Fractures of the pelvis and acetabulum.* Baltimore: Williams & Wilkins, 1995:355–396.
52. Heeg M, de Ridder VA, Tornetta P, et al. Acetabular fractures in children and adolescents. *Clin Orthop* 2000;14(376):80–86.
53. Kebaish AS, Roy A, Rennie W. Displaced acetabular fractures: Long-term follow-up. *J Trauma* 1991;31(11):1539–1542.
54. Matta JM, Anderson LM, Epstein HC, et al. Fractures of the acetabulum: a retrospective analysis. *Clin Orthop* 1986;205: 230–240.
55. Rowe CR, Lowell JD. Prognosis of fractures of the acetabulum. *J Bone Joint Surg* 1961;43(A):30–59.
56. Tile M, Kellam JF, Joyce M. Fractures of the acetabulum: classification, management protocol and results of treatment. *J Bone Joint Surg* 1985;67(B):173.
57. Matta JM. Fractures of the acetabulum: accuracy of reduction and clinical results. *J Bone Joint Surg (Am)* 1996;78:1632–1645.
58. Matta JM, Letournel E, Browner BD. Surgical management of acetabular fractures. *AAOS Instruct Course Lect* 1986;35: 382–397.
59. Matta JM, Mehne DK, Roffi R. Fractures of the acetabulum: early results of a prospective study. *Clin Orthop* 1986;205: 241–250.
60. Olson SA. The computerized tomography subchondral arc: a new method of assessing acetabular articular continuity after fracture (a preliminary report). *J Orthop Trauma* 1993;7(5): 402–413.
61. D'Aubigne RM. Management of acetabular fractures in multiple trauma. *J Trauma* 1968;8:333–349.
62. Goulet JA, Bray TJ. Complex acetabular fractures. *Clin Orthop* 1989;240:9–20.
63. Hak DJ, Hamel AJ, Bay BK, et al. Consequences of transverse acetabular fracture malreduction on load transmission across the hip joint. *J Orthop Trauma* 1998;12(2):90–100.
64. Heeg M, Ostvogel H, Klasen H. Conservative treatment of acetabular fractures: the role of the weightbearing dome and anatomic reduction in the ultimate results. *J Trauma* 1987; 27(5):555–559.
65. Helfet DL, Schmeling GJ. Management of complex acetabular fractures through single nonextensile exposures. *Clin Orthop* 1994;305:58–68.
66. Hofman AA, Dahl CP, Wyatt RWB. Experience with acetabular fractures. *J Trauma* 1984;24:750–752.
67. Malkani AL, Voor MJ, Rennirt G, et al. *Increased peak contact pressure following incongruent reduction of transverse acetabular fractures: a cadaveric model.* Presented at the 12th Annual Meeting of the Orthopaedic Trauma Association, Boston, September 27–29, 1996.
68. Matta JM. Operative indications and choice of surgical approach for fractures of the acetabulum. *Tech Orthop* 1986; 1(1):13–22.
69. Mayo KA. Fractures of the acetabulum. *Orthop Clin North Am* 1987;18(1):43–57.
70. Moed BR, Carr SE, Watson JT. Open reduction and internal fixation of posterior wall fractures of the acetabulum. *Clin Orthop* 2000;82(377):57–67.
71. Olson SA, Bay BK, Pollak AN, et al. The effect of variable size posterior wall acetabular fractures on contact characteristics of the hip joint. *J Orthop Trauma* 1996;10(6):395–402.
72. Routt MLC Jr, Swiontkowski MF. Operative treatment of complex acetabular fractures: combined anterior and posterior exposures during the same procedure. *J Bone Joint Surg (Am)* 1990; 72:897–904.
73. Ruesch PD, Holdener H, Ciarmitaro M, et al. A prospective study of surgically treated acetabular fractures. *Clin Orthop* 1994;305:38–46.
74. Tile M. Fractures of the acetabulum. *Orthop Clin North Am* 1980;11(3):481–506.
75. Tile M, Burgess A, Helfet DL, et al. *Fractures of the pelvis and acetabulum.* Baltimore: Williams & Wilkins, 1995.
76. Keith JE, Brashear R, Guilford B. Stability of posterior fracture-dislocations of the hip. *J Bone Joint Surg (Am)* 1988;70(5): 711–714.
77. Vailas JC, Hurwitz S, Wiesel SW. Posterior acetabular fracture-dislocations: fragment size, joint capsule, and stability. *J Orthop Trauma* 1989;29:1494–1496.
78. Tornetta P. Non-operative management of acetabular fractures. The use of dynamic stress views. *J Bone Joint Surg (Br)* 1999; 81(1):67–70.
79. Levine RG, Renard R, Behrens FF, et al. Biomechanical conse-

quences of secondary congruence after both-column acetabular fracture. *J Orthop Trauma* 2002;16(2):87–91.

80. Brueton RN. A review of 40 acetabular fractures: the importance of early surgery. *Injury* 1993;4:171–174.
81. Wright R, Barrett K, Christie MJ, et al. Acetabular fractures: long-term follow-up of open reduction and internal fixation. *J Orthop Trauma* 1994;8(5):397–403.
82. Bray TJ, Esser M, Fulkerson L. Osteotomy of the trochanter in open reduction and internal fixation of acetabular fractures. *J Bone Joint Surg* 1987;69-A:711–717.
83. Cole JD, Bolhofner BR. Acetabular fracture fixation via a modified Stoppa limited intrapelvic approach: description of operative technique and preliminary treatment results. *Clin Orthop* 1994;305:112–123.
84. Johnson EE, Matta JM, Mast JW, et al. Delayed reconstruction of acetabular fractures 21–120 days following injury. *Clin Orthop* 1994;305:20–30.
85. Moroni A, Caja VL, Sabato C, et al. Surgical treatment of both-column fractures by staged combined ilioinguinal and Kocher-Langenbeck approaches. *Injury* 1995;26(4):219–224.
86. Oransky M, Sanguinetti C. Surgical treatment of displaced acetabular fractures: results of 50 consecutive cases. *J Orthop Trauma* 1993;7(1):28–32.
87. Stannard JP, Alonso JE. Controversies in acetabular fractures. *Clin Orthop* 1998;353:74–80.
88. Helfet DL, Anand N, Malkani AL, et al. Intraoperative monitoring of motor pathways during operative fixation of acute acetabular fractures. *J Orthop Trauma* 1997;11(1):2–6.
89. Helfet DL, Borrelli JD Jr, DiPasquale TG, et al. Stabilization of acetabular fractures in elderly patients. *J Bone Joint Surg (Am)* 1992;74:753–765.
90. Helfet DL, Hissa EA, Sergay S, et al. Somatosensory evoked potential monitoring in the surgical management of acute acetabular fractures. *J Orthop Trauma* 1991;5(2):161–166.
91. Helfet DL, Schmeling GJ. Somatosensory evoked potential monitoring in the surgical treatment of acute, displaced acetabular fractures: results of a prospective study. *J Orthop Trauma* 1992;6:484.
92. Vrahas M, Gordon RG, Mears DC, et al. Intraoperative somatosensory evoked potential monitoring of pelvic and acetabular fractures. *J Orthop Trauma* 1992;6(1):50–58.
93. Geerts WH, Code KI, Jay RM, et al. A prospective study of venous thromboembolism after major trauma. *N Engl J Med* 1995;332(21):1448–1449.
94. Kudsk KA, Fabian TC, Baum S, et al. Silent deep vein thrombosis in immobilized multiple trauma patients. *Am J Surg* 1989; 158:515–519.
95. Montgomery KD, Geerts WH, Potter HG, et al. Thromboembolic complications in patients with pelvic trauma. *Clin Orthop* 1996;329:68–87.
96. Stickney JL, Helfet DL. Deep vein thrombosis prevention in orthopaedic trauma patients. *J Orthop Trauma* 1991;5(2): 227a.
97. Montgomery KD, Potter HG, Helfet DL. Magnetic resonance venography to evaluate the deep venous system of the pelvis in patients who have an acetabular fracture. *J Bone Joint Surg* 1995; (11):1639–1649a.
98. Montgomery KD, Potter HG, Helfet DL. The detection and management of proximal deep venous thrombosis in patients with acute acetabular fractures: a follow-up report. *J Orthop Trauma* 1997;11(5):330–336.
99. Carpenter JP, Holland GA, Baum RA, et al. Magnet resonance venography for the detection of venous thrombosis: comparison with contrast venography and duplex doppler ultrasonography. *J Vasc Surg* 1993;18:734–741.
100. Stannard JP, Riley RS, Alonso JE, et al. *Mechanical DVT prophylaxis.* Presented at the 15th annual meeting of The Orthopaedic Trauma Association. Charlotte, NC, 1999.
101. Morgan SJ, Stover MS, Stackhouse DJ, et al. *Magnetic resonance venography: interobserver variability in the identification of pelvic venous thrombosis.* Presented at the 15th annual meeting of The Orthopaedic Trauma Association. Charlotte, NC, 1999.
102. Stover MS, Morgan SJ, Bosse MJ, et al. *Prospective comparison of contrast enhanced computed tomography vs magnetic resonance venography in the detection of occult deep pelvic vein thrombosis in patients with pelvic and acetabular fractures.* Presented at the 14th annual meeting of The Orthopaedic Trauma Association. Vancouver, BC, 1998.
103. Harley JD, Mack LA, Winquist RA. CT of acetabular fractures: comparison with conventional radiography. *Am J Roentgenol* 1982;138:413–417.
104. Mack LA, Harley JD, Winquist RA. CT of acetabular fractures: analysis of fracture patterns. *Am J Roentgenol* 1982;138: 407–412.
105. Orthopaedic Trauma Association Committee for Classification. Fracture and dislocation compendium. *J Orthop Trauma* 1996; 10(Suppl 1):71–75.
106. Bartlett CS, Helfet DL. The use of a single limited posterior approach and reduction techniques for specific patterns of acetabular fractures. *Semin Arthroplast* 2001;12(3):144–161.
107. Schmidt CC, Gruen GS. Non-extensile surgical approaches for two-column acetabular fractures. *J Bone Joint Surg (Br)* 1993; 75(4):556–561.
108. Helfet DL, Schmeling GJ. The management of acute, displaced complex acetabular fractures using indirect reduction techniques and limited surgical approaches. *Orthop Trans* 1991;15: 833–834.
109. Bosse MJ, Poka A, Reinert CM, et al. Heterotopic ossification as a complication of acetabular fracture: prophylaxis with low-dose irradiation. *J Bone Joint Surg (Am)* 1988;70:1231–1237.
110. Ghalambor N, Matta JM, Bernstein L. Heterotopic ossification following operative treatment of acetabular fracture. *Clin Orthop* 1994;305:96–105.
111. Kaempffe FA, Bone L, Border JR. Open reduction and internal fixation of acetabular fractures: heterotopic ossification and other complications of treatment. *J Orthop Trauma* 1991;5(4): 439–445.
112. Leenen LPH, van der Werken C, Schoots FJ, et al. Internal fixation of open unstable pelvic fractures. *J Trauma* 1993;35(2): 220–225.
113. Senegas J, Liorzou G, Yates M. Complex acetabular fractures: a transtrochanteric lateral surgical approach. *Clin Orthop* 1980; 151:107–114.
114. Muller ME, Allgower M, Schneider R, et al. *Manual of internal fixation techniques recommended by the AO group.* New York: Springer-Verlag, 1991.
115. Reinert CM, Bosse MJ, Poka A, et al. A modified extensile exposure for the treatment of complex or malunited acetabular fractures. *J Bone Joint Surg (Am)* 1988;70(3):329–337.
116. Mears DC, Gordon RG. Internal fixation of acetabular fractures. *Tech Orthop* 1990;4(4):36–51.
117. Mears DC, Rubash HE. Extensile exposure of the pelvis. *Contemp Orthop* 1983;6:21–31.
118. Hak DJ, Olson SA, Matta JM. Diagnosis and management of closed internal degloving injuries associated with pelvic and acetabular fractures: the Morel-Lavallee lesion. *J Trauma* 1997; 42(6):1046–1051.
119. Garland D, Miller G. Fractures and dislocations about the hip in head-injured adults. *Clin Orthop* 1984;186:154–158.
120. Skura DS, Buchsbaum S. Prophylactic low-dose postoperative

irradiation for the prevention of heterotopic ossification in acetabular fractures. *Orthop Trans* 1992;16(1):221a..
121. Webb LX, Bosse MJ, Mayo KA, et al. Results in patients with craniocerebral trauma and an operatively managed acetabular fracture. *J Orthop Trauma* 1990;4(4):376–382.
122. Kottmeier SA, Farcy JPC, Baruch HM. The ilioinguinal aproach to acetabular fracture managment. *Op Tech Orthop* 1993;3(1):60–70.
123. Tornetta P, Reilly MC, Matta JM. Acetabular fracture/dislocation. *J Orthop Trauma* 2002;16(2):139–142.
124. Ebraheim NA, Wong FY. Sliding osteotomy of the greater trochanter. *Am J Orthop* 1997;26(3):212–215.
125. Matta JM. Operative treatment of acetabular fractures through the ilioinguinal approach:A 10-year perspective. *Clin Orthop* 1994;305:10–19.
126. Alonso JE, Davila R, Bradley E. Extended iliofemoral versus triradiate approaches in management of associated acetabular fractures. *Clin Orthop* 1994;(305):81–87.
127. Tabor OB, Bosse MJ, Greene KG, et al. Effects of surgical approaches for acetabular fractures with associated gluteal vascular injury. *J Orthop Trauma* 1998;12(2):78–84.
128. Sims SH, Kellam JF, Bosse MJ. *Planned simultaneous anterior and posterior approaches for the treatment of complex and malunited acetabular fractures.* Presented at the 12th annual meeting of The Orthopaedic Trauma Association. Boston, 1996.
129. Borrelli J. Intraneural sciatic nerve pressures relative to the position of the hip and knee: a human cadaveric study. *J Orthop Trauma* 2000;14(4):255–258.
130. Baumgaertner MR, Wegner D, Booke J. SSEP monitoring during pelvic and acetabular fracture surgery. *J Orthop Trauma* 1994;8(2):127–133.
131. Arrington ED, Hochschild DP, Steinagle TJ, et al. Monitoring of somatosensory and motor evoked potentials during open reduction and internal fixation of pelvis and acetabular fractures. *Orthopaedics* 2000;23(10):1081–1083.
132. Haidukewych GJ, Scaduto JM, Dipasquale TG, et al. *Iatrogenic nerve injury during acetabular fracture surgery: a comparison of monitored and unmonitored patients.* Presented at the 15th annual meeting of The Orthopaedic Trauma Association. Charlotte, NC, 1999.
133. Middlebrooks ES, Sims SH, Kellam JF, et al. Incidence of sciatic nerve injury in operatively treated acetabular fractures without somatosensory evoked potential monitoring. *J Orthop Trauma* 1997;11(5):327–329.
134. Bosse MJ, Poka A, Reinert CM, et al. Preoperative angiographic assessment of the superior gluteal artery in acetabular fractures requiring extensile surgical exposures. *J Orthop Trauma* 1989; 2(4):303–307.
135. Johnson EE, Eckhardt JJ, Letournel E. Extrinsic femoral artery occlusion following internal fixation of an acetabular fracture. A case report. *Clin Orthop* 1987;217:209–213.
136. Moed BR, Maxey JW. The effect of indomethacin on heterotopic ossification following acetabular fracture surgery. *J Orthop Trauma* 1993;7(1):33–38.
137. Russell GV, Rath EMS, Routt ML. Gluteus minimus debridement to prevent heterotopic ossification after acetabular surgery. In: *Surgery of the pelvis and acetabulum: the 4th international consensus.* Birmingham, AL, 1998.
138. Dickinson WH, Duwelius P, Colville MR. Muscle strength testing following surgery for acetabular fractures. *J Orthop Trauma* 1993;7(1):39–46.
139. Borrelli J, Goldfarb C, Ricci W, et al. Functional outcome after isolated acetabular fractures. *J Orthop Trauma* 2002;16(2): 73–81.
140. Saterbak AM, Marsh JL, Nepola JV, et al. Clinical failure after posterior wall acetabular fractures: the influence of initial fracture patterns. *J Orthop Trauma* 2000;14(4):230–237.
141. Brumback RJ, Holt ES, Poka A, et al. Acetabular depression fracture accompanying posterior fracture dislocation of the hip. *J Orthop Trauma* 1990;4(1):42–48.
142. Goulet JA. Comminuted fractures of the posterior wall of the acetabulum. *J Bone Joint Surg (Am)* 1994;76(10):1457–1463.
143. Mast JW, Ganz R, Jakob RP. *Planning and reduction techniques in fracture surgery.* New York: Springer-Verlag, 1989.
144. Heck BE, Ebraheim NA, Foetisch C. Direct complications of trochanteric osteotomy in open reduction and internal fixation of acetabular fractures. *Am J Orthop* 1997;26:124–128.
145. Chen WM, McAuley JP, Engh CA, et al. Extended slide trochanteric osteotomy for revision total hip arthroplasty. *J Bone Joint Surg (Am)* 2000;82(9):1215–1219.
146. Letournel E. Les fractures du cotyle. etude d'une series de 75 cas [French]. *J Chir* 1961;82:47.
147. Letournel E. The treatment of acetabular fractures through the ilioinguinal approach. *Clin Orthop* 1993;292:62.
148. Gorczyca JT, Powell JN, Tile M. Lateral extension of the ilioinguinal incision in the operative treatment of acetabulum fractures. *Injury* 1995;26(3):207–212.
149. Teague DC, Graney DO, Routt ML. Retropubic vascular hazards of the ilioinguinal exposure:a cadaveric and clinical study. *J Orthop Trauma* 1996;10(3):156–159.
150. Tornetta P, Hochwald N, Levine R. Corona mortis. *Clin Orthop* 1996;329:97–101.
151. De Ridder VA, de Lange S, van Popta J. Anatomic variations of the lateral femoral cutaneous nerve and the consequences for surgery. *J Orthop Trauma* 1999;13:207—211.
152. Hospodar PP, Ashman ES, Traub JA. Anatomic study of the lateral femoral cutaneous nerve with respect to the ilioinguinal surgical dissection. *J Orthop Trauma* 1999;13(1):17–19.
153. Schopfer A, Willet K, Powell J, et al. Cerclage wiring in internal fixation of acetabular fractures. *J Orthop Trauma* 1993;7:236.
154. Weber TG, Mast JW. The extended ilioinguinal approach for specific both column fractures. *Clin Orthop* 1994;305:106–111.
155. Stoppa RE. The treatment of complicated groin and incisional hernias. *World J Surg* 1989;13:545.
156. Stoppa RE, Rives JL, Warlaumont CR, et al. The use of dacron in the repair of hernias of the groin. *Surg Clin NA* 1984;64:269.
157. Juliano PJ, Bosse MJ, Edwards KJ. The superior gluteal artery in complex acetabular procedures:a cadaveric angiographic study. *J Bone Joint Surg (Am)* 1994;76:244.
158. Tabor OB, Bosse MJ, Greene KG, et al. *The effects of the abductor muscles of surgical approaches for acetabular fractures associated with gluteal vascular injury.* Presented at the 12th annual meeting of the Orthopaedic Trauma Association. Boston, September 27–29, 1996.
159. Reilly MC, Matta JM, Olson S, et al. *The superior gluteal artery in the extended ilio-femoral approach.*Presented at the 12th annual meeting of The Orthopaedic Trauma Association. Boston, 1996.
160. Chapman MH. *Effect of surgical approaches on the blood supply to the acetabulum.* Presented at: Surgery of the pelvis and acetabulum: the 3rd international consensus. Pittsburgh, 1992.
161. Ebraheim NA, Rongming X, Biyani A, et al. Anatomic basis of lag screw placement in the anterior column of the acetabulum. *Clin Orthop* 1997;339:200–205.
162. Mears DC, MacLeod MD. Acetabular fractures: TRI and MTRI approaches. In: Wiss DA, Thompson RC, eds. *Fractures: master techniques in orthopaedic surgery.* Philadelphia: Lippincott-Raven, 1998.
163. Anglen JO, Dipasquale TG. The reliability of detecting screw penetration of the acetabulum by intraoperative auscultation. *J Orthop Trauma* 1994;8:404–408.

164. Carmack DB, Moed BR, McCarroll K, et al. *Reliability of detecting screw penetration of the acetabulum using intraoperative fluoroscopy and computed tomography.* Presented at the 16th Annual Meeting of The Orthopaedic Trauma Association. San Antonio, TX, 2000.
165. Ebraheim NA, Savolaine ER, Hoeflinger MJ, et al. Radiological diagnosis of screw penetration of the hip joint in acetabular fracture reconstruction. *J Orthop Trauma* 1989;3(3):196–201.
166. Norris BL, Hahn DH, Bosse MJ, et al. Intraoperative fluoroscopy to evaluate fracture reduction and hardware placement during acetabular surgery. *J Orthop Trauma* 1999;13(6): 414–417.
167. Reilly MC, Matta JM. *The correlation between early radiographic results and long term clinical outcome following fracture of the acetabulum.* Presented at the 13th annual meeting of The Orthopaedic Trauma Association. Louisville, KY, 1997.
168. Matta JM, Siebenrock KA. Does indomethacin reduce heterotopic bone formation after operations for acetabular fractures? A prospective randomized study. *J Bone Joint Surg (Br)* 1997; 79(6):959–963.
169. Moed BR, Karges DE. Prophylactic indomethacin for the prevention of heterotopic ossification after acetabular fracture surgery in high-risk patients. *J Orthop Trauma* 1994;8(1): 34–39.
170. Moed BR, Letournel E. Low-dose irradiation and indomethacin prevent heterotopic ossification after acetabular fracture surgery. *J Bone Joint Surg (Br)* 1994;76(6):895–900.
171. Burd TA, Anglen JO. Indomethacin compared with localized irradiation for the prevention of heterotopic ossification following surgical treatment of acetabulum fractures. *J Bone Joint Surg (Am)* 2001;83(12):1783–1788.
172. McLaren AC. Prophylaxis with indomethacin for heterotopic bone. *J Bone Joint Surg (Am)* 1990;72(2):245–247.
173. Anglen JO, Moore KD. Prevention of heterotopic bone formation after acetabular fracture fixation by single-dose radiation therapy: a preliminary report. *J Orthop Trauma* 1996;10(4): 258–263.
174. Childs HA and coworkers. A prospective evaluation of the timing of postoperative radiotherapy for preventing heterotopic ossification following traumatic acetabular fractures. *Int J Radiat Oncol Biol Phys* 2000;47(5):1347–1352.
175. Slawson RG, Poka A, Bathon GH, et al. The role of postoperative radiation in the prevention of hetertopic ossification in patients with posttraumatic acetabular fracture. *Int J Radiat Oncol Biol Phys* 1989;17(3):669–672.
176. Mears DC. Surgical treatment of acetabular fractures in elderly patients with osteoporotic bone. *J Am Acad Orthop Surg* 1999;7(2):128–141.
177. Fishmann AJ, Greeno RA, Brooks LR, et al. Prevention of deep vein thrombosis and pulmonary embolism in acetabular and pelvic fracture surgery. *Clin Orthop* 1994;305:133–137.
178. Salter RB. The biological effect of continuous passive motion on the healing of full thickness defects in articular cartilage: an experimental investigation in the rabbit. *J Bone Joint Surg (Am)* 1980;62:1232.
179. Dipasquale TG, Paksima N, Helfet DL. Stabilization of acetabular fractures in the elderly patient: a 7-year outcome report. Presented at the 64th annual meeting of The American Academy of Orthopaedic Surgeons. San Francisco, 1997.
180. Spencer RF. Acetabular fractures in older patients. *J Bone Joint Surg (Br)* 1989;71(5):774–776.
181. Siebenrock KA, Gautier E, Woo AKH, et al. Surgical dislocation of the femoral head for joint debridement and accurate reduction of fractures of the acetabulum. *J Orthop Trauma* 2002; 16: 543–552.
182. Baumgartner MR. Fractures of the posterior wall of the acetabulum. *J Am Acad Orthop Surg* 1999;7:54–65.
183. Epstein HC, Wiss DA, Cozen L. Posterior fracture dislocation of the hip with fractures of the femoral head. *Clin Orthop* 1985;201:9–17.
184. Saterbak AM, Marsh JL, Brandser E, et al. Outcome of surgically treated posterior wall acetabular fractures. *Orthop Trans* 1997;21:627.
185. Upadhyay SS, Moulton A. The long term results of traumatic posterior dislocations of the hip. *J Bone Joint Surgery* 1981;63-B:548–551.
186. Smith-Petersen MN. Approach to and exposure of the hip joint for mold arthroplasty. *J Bone Joint Surg* 1949;3-IA:40-46.
187. Kloen P, Siebenrock KA, Ganz R. Modification of the ilioinguinal approach. *J Orthop Trauma* 2002;16:586–593.
188. Ward WT, Fleisch I-D, Ganz R. Anatomy of the iliocapsularis muscle. Relevance to surgery about the hip. *Clin Orthop* 2000;374:278–285.

29

COMPUTER-ASSISTED CLOSED TECHNIQUES OF REDUCTION AND FIXATION

DAVID M. KAHLER

INTRODUCTION

Formal internal fixation of acetabular fractures has traditionally required large surgical exposures. These exposures can be associated with significant complications, including infection, wound healing problems, major blood vessel or nerve injury, denervation or devascularization of the abductors, and heterotopic ossification. For the most part, these complications are related to the surgical exposure itself, rather than to the initial traumatic injury. Therefore, it seems reasonable to consider percutaneous stabilization of selected acetabular fractures in order to avoid exposing the trauma patient to the morbidity of an extensive surgical exposure.

The following groups of fractures may be amenable to minimally invasive surgical fixation.

1. Nondisplaced (1 to 3 mm) but potentially unstable fractures involving the weight-bearing dome. Transtectal transverse fractures with roof arcs measuring <45 degrees may fall into this category (1). Tornetta has recently provided a technique for stressing nondisplaced fractures under fluoroscopic guidance that helps to confirm potential instability in slightly displaced fractures (2). Percutaneous stabilization of these fractures may prevent late fracture displacement and allow beneficial early mobilization of the trauma patient.

2. Slightly displaced fractures (3 to 5 mm) with gap displacement that may be reduced with percutaneously placed lag screws. In the absence of translational displacement, certain anterior column, transverse, anterior column/posterior hemitransverse, and posterior column fractures can be adequately fixed with large diameter lag screws placed perpendicular to the fracture lines.

3. Displaced fractures (>5 mm) that fall into one of the preceding two categories following a closed reduction maneuver. Occasionally, transverse and column fractures with subluxation or dislocation of the femoral head may assume acceptable position following a maneuver to reduce the femoral head beneath the weight-bearing dome. The surgeon also may apply preoperative or intraoperative traction to improve the reduction. More recently, a distraction frame that applies lateral traction through both greater trochanters has been used to reduce hip subluxation prior to fixation in transverse and posterior column fractures. The surgeon also may potentially reduce selected anterior column fractures with Schanz pin joysticks placed in both iliac wings, and hold the reduction with a temporary external fixator during percutaneous fixation.

4. Displaced both-column fractures with good secondary congruity. In the both-column fracture that has medialized with gap displacement but good secondary

congruity, the fracture can be stabilized *in situ* with two cannulated screws placed into the anterior and posterior columns. This can prevent further fracture displacement, and eliminates the need for prolonged traction or restricted mobilization of the patient. Reduction sometimes can be improved with the bilateral distraction frame. Percutaneous stabilization allows the elderly patient with the typical geriatric both-column fracture to be mobilized immediately; the hip later may be reconstructed, if necessary, by elective total hip arthroplasty after the patient's medical status is optimized.

5. Displaced acetabular fractures in morbidly obese patients. In this situation, the trauma surgeon may be willing to accept somewhat greater final fracture displacement than usual, as the perceived risk of surgical complications related to a formal surgical exposure is increased. Precise percutaneous lag screw placement may provide some reduction and stabilize the fracture adequately to allow mobilization, while minimizing risks related to an extensile surgical exposure. It may be more prudent to accept 3 mm of articular displacement in a very large patient than to strive for an anatomic reduction through an extensive open exposure.

Fractures of the posterior wall of the acetabulum are rarely amenable to percutaneous reduction and fixation. Given the anatomy of the sciatic nerve in close proximity to the fracture fragment, it is difficult to safely place percutaneous screws across posterior wall fractures without risking nerve injury. Open reduction also is usually necessary to adequately debride the hip joint and reduce marginal impaction. The unstable posterior wall fracture/dislocation remains an indication for formal open reduction and internal fixation using a buttress plate, with or without supplemental lag screw or spring plate fixation.

The surgeon contemplating percutaneous fixation of any acetabular fracture must be mindful that these techniques have not yet been validated in randomized clinical trials. The early clinical results of percutaneous fixation have been extremely encouraging, both in decreasing hospital stay and morbidity in longitudinal studies, and in case reports for selected fractures (3–5). Although patients generally will opt for less invasive surgical techniques when given a choice, they should be informed that this technique is currently viewed as an experimental procedure. These techniques should be performed only by experienced acetabular fracture surgeons, in the event that a change in surgical plan and conversion to an open procedure is necessary. A thorough knowledge of the nuances of pelvic osseous and soft-tissue anatomy is necessary to plan trajectories and safely place percutaneous screws; advanced appreciation of radiographic anatomy is essential when relying on nonstandard fluoroscopic projections to provide guidance. The surgeon always must be prepared to revert to a formal open approach in the event of inadequate imaging or inadequate reduction for percutaneous technique. It is unlikely that an inadequately reduced fracture treated with percutaneous technique ever has a better outcome than a well-reduced fracture treated with standard open technique, in the absence of complications related to the approach.

EARLY EXPERIENCE

Percutaneous acetabular fracture fixation was first performed under computed tomography (CT) guidance by placing the patient into a standard CT scanner (6). In this technique, both the patient and the rest of the operating room (scrub nurse, instruments, bean bag, anesthesiologist, surgeon, and radiologist) were brought into a standard CT suite. Patients were rolled into the lateral position and the CT gantry angled perpendicular to the fracture. The patient was prepped and draped in the usual fashion, and run back and forth into the scanner to identify appropriate starting points and trajectories for screws. Additional CT images were obtained after placing needles and later guidewires along the path of intended fixation, prior to placing the actual implant (cannulated screw). Final screw position and reduction of the fracture by lag screw technique could be confirmed easily with final CT images (Fig. 29-1). Twenty-five patients were treated using this technique from 1990 to 1995 (7). The majority of the fractures stabilized with this technique were anterior column, transverse, and combination (anterior column/posterior hemitransverse) patterns, and were usually stabilized using two or three large-diameter 7.0- or 7.3-mm cannulated screws. Using lag screws placed perpendicular to the plane of fracture displacement, average preoperative displacement of 7 mm was reduced to 2 mm. For patients with isolated injuries, average hospital stay postfixation was 2 days. Three patients with residual displacement of 5 to 8 mm eventually went on to total hip replacement, and were considered failures in patient selection. In the remaining patients for whom a minimum of 2-year follow-up was available, the average self-administered hip score (8) was 89 out of 100 possible points. This series helped to define the indications for minimally invasive acetabular fracture fixation, and also provided support for continued clinical use of the technique.

CT-guided technique had several obvious limitations. There were concerns regarding the performance of an invasive procedure in a room that was not designed for this purpose, and in fact, one screw out of the 60 placed became infected and required late removal. In addition, screws had to be placed in plane with the CT gantry; this limited the possible screw trajectories, as the gantry can only be angled about 20 degrees before contacting the patient. Reduction maneuvers and traction could not be easily applied inside the CT scanner. For these reasons, only 16% of acetabular fractures admitted to the author's institution during the study period could be treated using this technique. Even when proficiency had been gained, the procedure often re-

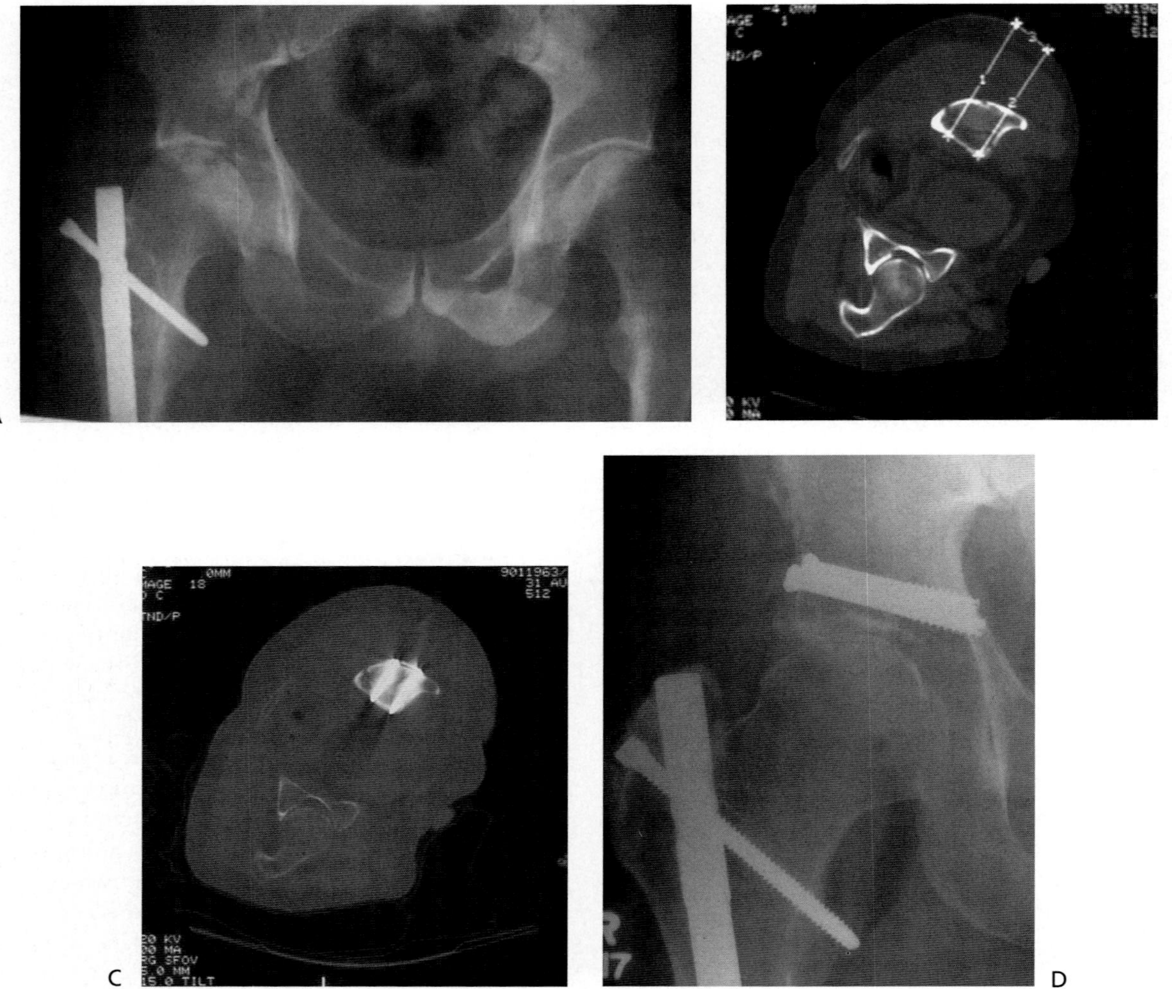

FIGURE 29-1. A: This shows a slightly displaced transverse acetabular fracture in a multiply traumatized patient. The fracture is transtectal and there is 7-mm gap displacement. **B:** This shows planned trajectories for two cannulated lag screws placed perpendicular to the fracture line. **C:** This shows the final position of the two screws with some compression across the fracture. **D:** This is the radiographic result at two-year followup, with a healed fracture and congruent hip joint.

quired more than 45 minutes for each screw inserted. Patients were also exposed to significant doses of radiation during the procedure, as up to 45 individual CT slices per screw were sometimes required for accurate placement. The radiation exposure is equivalent to approximately 250 chest radiographs (Agarwal SK, unpublished data, 1998).

Standard C-arm fluoroscopy (without relying on cross-sectional CT imaging) is sometimes sufficient for percutaneous placement of screws about the pelvis and acetabulum. The biggest limitation of this technique is that imaging is available in only one plane at a time. The surgeon must position the implant in one view, and then obtain additional images in other planes for "trial-and-error" placement of guidewires or screws. Significant operating room time is expended while the fluoroscopy technician positions the c-arm to supply views in multiple planes, both during and after implant placement. Although most orthopedic surgeons are comfortable with this technique for hip fractures and intramedullary nailing, this procedure exposes both the patient and surgeon to significant radiation doses. When working around the complex anatomy of the pelvis, an erroneous first pass of the guidewire potentially can have disastrous consequences when relying on only one planar image at a time for guidance.

For all of these reasons, it became clear that we had to search for a new technology that would allow minimally invasive acetabular fracture fixation to be brought back to the operating room, while also allowing more versatile screw trajectories with less radiation exposure and greater first-pass accuracy. The advent of computer-assisted orthopedic surgery provided this technology.

COMPUTER-ASSISTED ORTHOPEDIC SURGERY (IMAGE-GUIDED SURGERY)

Computer-assisted orthopedic surgery (CAOS) makes use of stored imaging data to provide guidance during surgical procedures. Patient-specific imaging data are harvested using conventional technique (CT or fluoroscopy) and stored on a computer workstation. The computer system can then track special surgical instruments relative to the stored imaging data, providing the surgeon with information about the position of the instruments and implants relative to the patient's anatomy.

Orthopedic surgeons are experienced in minimally invasive techniques using two-dimensional (2D) video output during either arthroscopy or C-arm fluoroscopy. CAOS takes this a step further, by providing access to either a three-dimensional data set (3DCT guidance) or multiple simultaneously displayed stored fluoroscopic images (virtual fluoroscopy). For both techniques, most current image-guided surgery systems use an optical tracking system (digital camera array and digitizer) to follow both the position of the patient and special surgical instruments during the course of the procedure (Fig. 29-2). The predicted position of the surgical instruments is then displayed on a computer monitor relative to the position of the stored images. This process is known as surgical navigation. In the author's experience, optimal accuracy is provided by tracking the drill guide used to place guidewires for cannulated screws, rather than by tracking the drill itself. The two basic types of computer guided surgery systems (3DCT versus virtual fluoroscopy) each have unique advantages and disadvantages when applied to orthopedic trauma.

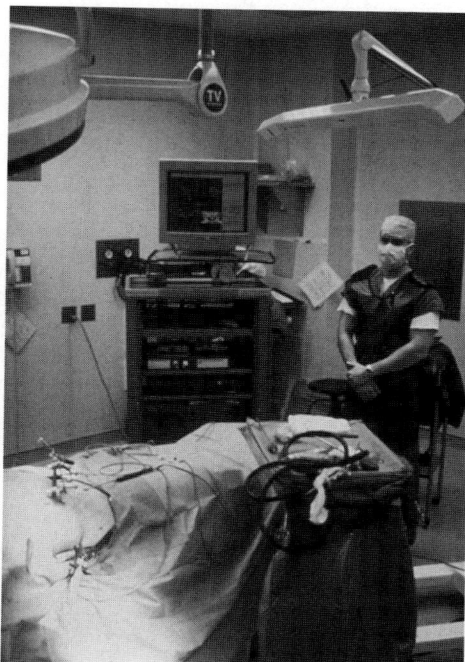

FIGURE 29-2. Typical operating room setup for image-guided surgery. In this first generation system, the camera is at upper right, and looks down to the surgical field where several image-guided instruments are visible. The workstation is visible in the background. A computer mouse provided the surgeon interface in early systems.

The first 3DCT systems were used in intracranial neurosurgery in the late 1980s. These systems rely on a stored patient-specific CT data set to build a virtual model of the patient's anatomy. Surgical plans or trajectories may be devised and stored preoperatively. Through a process known as registration, the surgeon would then match the patient's anatomy to the virtual model. The computer could then display the position of instruments such as probes or drill guides relative to the virtual model. A 3DCT system became available for spine surgery in the early 1990s (Stealth Station, Sofamor-Danek, Memphis, TN). With minor software and instrument modifications, this system was first adapted for pelvic and acetabular fracture fixation in 1996. Approval for clinical use was granted in 1997 following accuracy validation in a cadaver study (9,10).

Virtual fluoroscopy (fluoroscopic navigation) was refined and approved for clinical use in 1999. Before this time, the distortion inherent in analogue C-arm images prevented their use in surgical navigation. Software algorithms were developed for powerful computer workstations that allowed them to rapidly warp the C-arm images to make them optically correct and allow their use for guidance. The surgeon uses a standard C-arm unit to harvest multiple 2D images in the operating room. A camera tracks the position of the C-arm unit during image acquisition and the images are warped, stored, and displayed on a workstation. Up to four individually stored images may be displayed at any one time. The camera can then track special instruments and display their position relative to each of the stored images. The arrival of virtual fluoroscopy greatly broadens the potential applications of CAOS in orthopedic trauma. Computer-assisted technique now may be applied to essentially any procedure that traditionally relies on intraoperative fluoroscopy for guidance.

In general, orthopedic surgeons have been relatively slow to embrace computer-assisted technology, primarily, it seems, owing to concerns about cost and complexity of the systems. Many surgeons remain unaware of the fact that these systems and software packages are now commercially available, although several hundred such systems have been installed in hospitals in the United States. The European orthopedic community appears to be adopting the use of these systems more quickly than surgeons in the United States. In 1998, a jointly sponsored National Institutes of Health (NIH)/AAOS workgroup convened to define CAOS and identify potential applications that warranted research support. CAOS, or image-guided surgery, was defined as the use of either a 3D data set or multiple stored 2D images to define and execute a surgical plan using real-time surgical navigation. Orthopedic trauma (pelvis and acetabulum), spine surgery, and total joint arthroplasty were identified as the key potential impact areas for this new technology.

Three-Dimensional (Computer-Based) Versus Two-Dimensional (Fluoroscopy-Based) Surgical Navigation for Pelvic and Acetabular Fractures

The 3DCT-based CAOS systems proved to be very versatile in planning novel screw trajectories for pelvic fracture fixation, and also proved to provide exceptional accuracy during execution of the preoperative plan. Surgical plans could be defined and stored preoperatively by identifying precise entry and target points for screws on the virtual 3D model. The preoperative planning software helped to define safe pathways for screw placement in many applications about the pelvis. Early work showed that this technology provided sufficient accuracy to place both iliosacral screws and percutaneous screws for fixation of the acetabular columns (Fig. 29-3) (9,11). In actual clinical use for posterior pelvic ring fixation, both operative time and fluoroscopic time were significantly reduced when compared to standard fluoroscopic technique, and there were no screw malpositions noted (11).

Although 3DCT guidance remains a powerful clinical tool, the applications of this technology in fracture care were relatively limited, as a 3D model had to be "built" using CT data obtained prior to surgical fracture reduction. The model could not be easily updated to provide guidance for fixation following fracture reduction. In general, fractures could be stabilized using 3DCT guidance only if they were minimally displaced, or if a closed reduction could be obtained and maintained with an external fixator prior to obtaining the preoperative CT scan (Fig. 29-4). As such, this technology found only limited utility in selected applications about the pelvis and acetabulum (5,9–11). It could not be easily adapted to long bone applications, or to any application where bone fragments would be manipulated after the CT scan was performed. Nonetheless, the experience gained in performing percutaneous fixation of selected acetabular fractures proved invaluable in later adapting the newer virtual fluoroscopy systems to percutaneous fixation. The screw pathways defined in clinical cases from 1997 to 1999 are still used in the newer virtual fluoroscopy applications.

With the advent of virtual fluoroscopy in 1999, images could be harvested and stored in multiple planes, during and after operative fracture reduction or implant placement. The need for the time-consuming "registration" step is eliminated in this newer technology. In addition, the virtual model could be updated easily at any point during the procedure by simply obtaining new images. The surgeon may be well away from the surgical field during image acquisition, and there is no radiation exposure to patient or surgeon during surgical navigation. The development of virtual

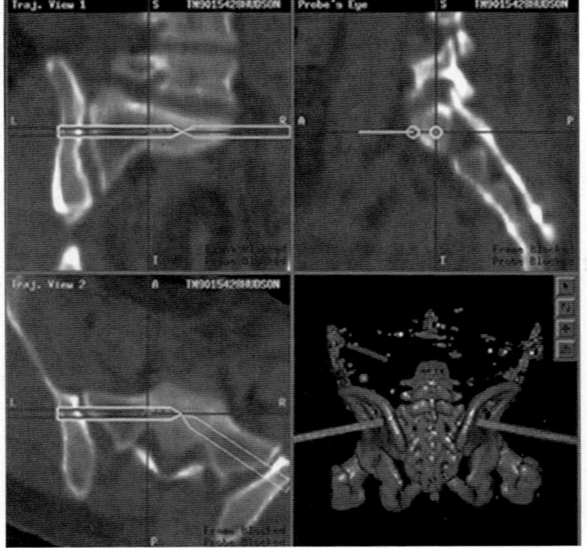

A

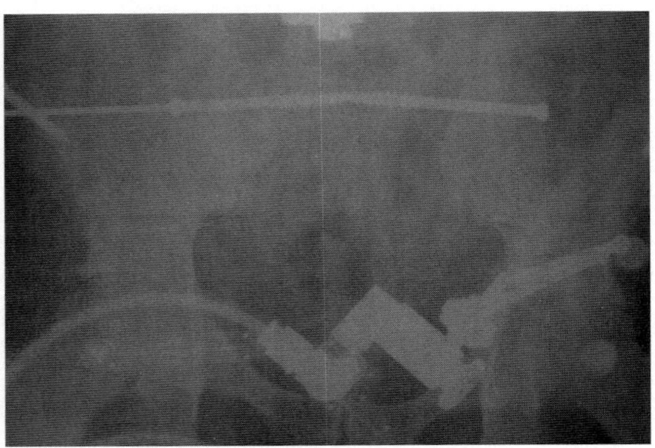
B

FIGURE 29-3. A: This shows the screen output with stored surgical plans for placement of bilateral iliosacral screws for stabilization of bilateral sacroiliac joint disruptions, following closed reduction with an external fixator. The 3DCT model is visible at lower right, and the navigation views show the planned path of screw placement in two orthogonal planes. A third plane is perpendicular to the path of the screw. The 3DCT technique provided exceptional accuracy. **B:** This shows tip-to-tip accuracy in screw placement intraoperatively. This patient also had percutaneous stabilization of a transverse acetabular fracture with lag screws.

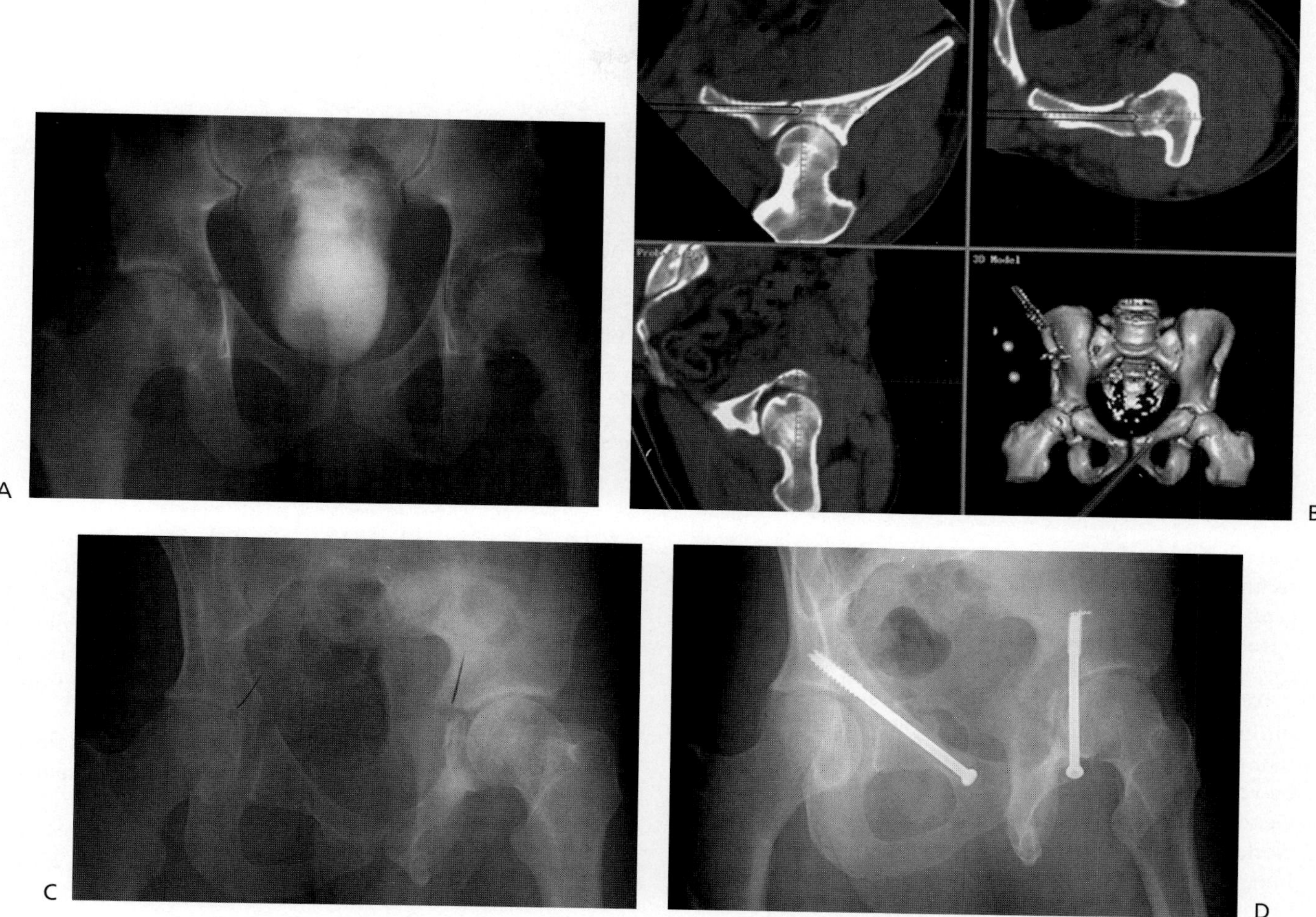

FIGURE 29-4. In this patient, 3DCT technique has been used to stabilize bilateral transverse acetabular fractures using retrograde anterior column screws. **A:** This shows the initial injury anterior-posterior pelvis. **B:** This depicts the screen interface with surgical plan and drill guide shown relative to the three-dimensional model. **C,D:** These show the degree of reduction possible with a precisely placed percutaneous lag screw.

fluoroscopy has expanded the applications of CAOS to essentially all procedures that have traditionally required intraoperative fluoroscopy for fracture reduction or positioning of implants. For the first time, CAOS techniques could be applied to routine long bone fracture management, and were no longer limited to spine and pelvic applications (Table 29-1) (12).

Newer angle/distance features in the software packages facilitate planning and execution of osteotomies for joint realignment and correction of deformity. The systems have proven to be well suited to a variety of pelvic and acetabular fracture applications, including minimally invasive techniques that were first made possible by the 3DCT technology. The newest systems are entirely surgeon driven, using a touch screen interface that eliminates the need for an unscrubbed assistant or technical support staff (Fig. 29-5). Replacement of the previous mouse driven (or so-called "shout

TABLE 29-1. EXAMPLES OF POTENTIAL APPLICATIONS OF VIRTUAL FLUOROSCOPY IN ORTHOPEDIC SURGERY

Iliosacral screws
Anterior or iliac pelvic ring disruption
Acetabular fracture
Femoral neck fracture
Intramedullary nailing: starting point, fracture reduction, and freehand locking
Osteotomies of long bones and pelvis
Slipped capital femoral epiphysis
Epiphyseodesis
Biopsy or ablation of skeletal neoplasms

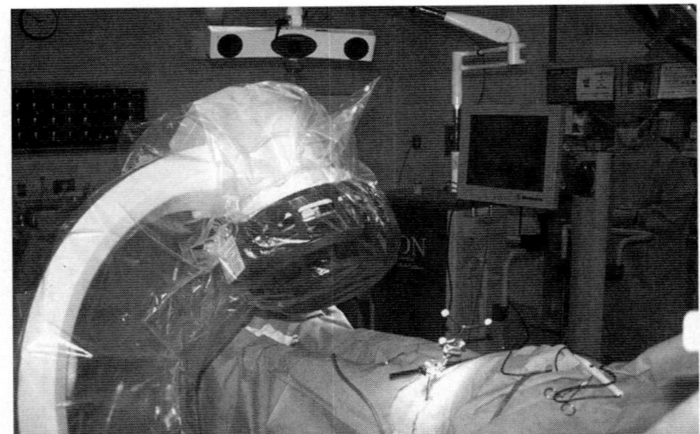
A

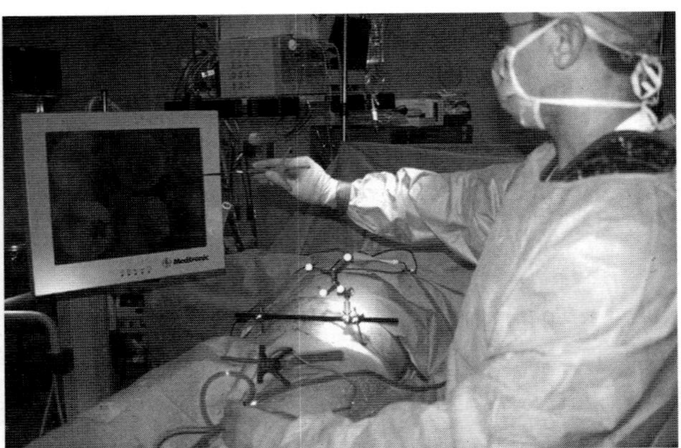
B

FIGURE 29-5. A modern virtual fluoroscopy system in use (iON-FluoroNav, Medtronic/Smith and Nephew, Memphis, TN). A reference frame has been attached to an anterior pelvic fixator, and the C-arm has been retrofitted with a calibration target that allows the camera to track the C-arm. The touch screen interface seen at right is more surgeon-friendly than the previous mouse-driven interface. The surgeon is manipulating navigation images using a sterile stylet.

and click") interface has led to improved acceptance of this technology in the operating room, both on the part of surgeons and nursing staff. In the author's practice, the newer virtual fluoroscopic navigation has now essentially replaced the 3DCT technology.

When using virtual fluoroscopy for surgical navigation during implant placement, it is essential that the surgeon take the time to harvest adequate images. The surgeon must be very familiar with radiographic anatomy in a variety of customized oblique imaging planes, particularly when working around the pelvis and the columns of the acetabulum. Image quality in pelvic applications sometimes is compromised by patient obesity, bowel gas, or retained intraabdominal contrast. In many applications, it is difficult logistically to obtain the two ideal orthogonal images perpendicular to the path of intended drilling and fixation, leading to increased reliance on nonstandard oblique radiographic projections. In all applications, the surgeon must have the diligence to ensure that the images are adequate to safely proceed. In the event that adequate fluoroscopic images cannot be obtained, the surgeon must have the discipline to abandon the surgical navigation and use an alternative method. The surgeon then has the responsibility to either proceed with formal open reduction, or consider 3DCT technique at a separate operative sitting.

Surgeons are often quick to note several obvious drawbacks in choosing CAOS over standard technique. Those wishing to use this technology must invest some time in learning to use the interfaces and software. The surgeon, scrub nurse, and assistants also must learn to operate without obstructing the digital camera's view of the operative field. The operating room must be large enough to accommodate the computer system and camera, as well as the C-arm unit. Cables connecting the two units may interfere with mobility of personnel and equipment in the operating suite. There is inevitably some setup time involved in interfacing the system with the C-arm and placing a reference array on the patient prior to obtaining images. In the author's experience, this process adds 10 to 15 minutes at the start of the surgical procedure. Although this time is essentially always recouped during the procedure by gaining increased first pass accuracy, many surgeons still find the setup time objectionable.

CAOS equipment and instruments are costly, and financial considerations will likely hinder widespread acceptance in the short term. Nonetheless, the technology offers substantial potential benefits, including improved accuracy, decreased operative time, and decreased invasiveness. However, the greatest benefit may lie in decreasing the orthopedic surgeon's reliance on intraoperative ionizing radiation for guidance during surgery. Radiation exposure to the surgeon's body and hands is essentially eliminated using CAOS techniques.

Iliosacral Screws (Posterior Pelvic Ring Disruption: SI Joint, Sacral, or Crescent Fracture)

This application is particularly well suited for virtual fluoroscopy. The surgeon initially reduces the pelvic ring using closed methods (traction, external fixator, or Schanz pin joystick), and confirms adequate reduction with C-arm images. It is helpful to maintain the reduction with either a temporary external fixator or a 2.8-mm wire passed from the ilium into the sacral ala. Multiple images then are harvested and stored on the computer workstation. Up to four images are used; the author prefers to use anterior-posterior (AP), inlet, outlet, and oblique lateral views for intraoperative guidance. The trajectory feature is used to identify the optimal starting point on the skin, and the drill guide is passed bluntly down to the ilium. The ideal trajectory into the center of the S1 body is chosen in all four views, and a guidewire is drilled to the appropriate depth using the trajectory length feature. Confirmatory images are obtained, and the cannulated screw is then passed over the guidewire. In the author's experience, fluoroscopic time is reduced by over 50%, total surgical time (including setup) is decreased, and the first pass of the guidewire has been acceptable in nearly every case. Rare instances of intraosseous pin deflection have been observed, and mandate that confirmatory images be obtained prior to actually passing the screw over the guidewire. There have been no complications or screw malpositions noted in over 30 individual screw placements using virtual fluoroscopic technique (13).

Pelvic Ring Disruption

Bony disruption of the pelvic ring often may be managed using percutaneous technique, provided that an acceptable reduction can be obtained and maintained during imaging. It has not yet proven possible to safely stabilize a pure symphyseal disruption percutaneously. Nonetheless, it has often been possible to stabilize many osseous anterior and posterior ring injuries using large-diameter cannulated screws. This usually is done in the supine position using a retrograde anterior column screw for the anterior ring, and an "LCII screw" for the posterior ring.

The retrograde screw starts just inferior and lateral to the ipsilateral pubic tubercle, and courses through the superior pubic ramus across the fracture and just anterior/superior to the hip joint. A 7.3-mm screw usually can be used in male patients; safe passage of this screw sometimes is impossible in female patients, and the surgeon must be prepared to perform an open reduction in such cases. Obturator/outlet and iliac/inlet views are helpful, although standard Judet views may be adequate for navigation. A true AP always is used to provide initial orientation in almost all applications.

The LCII screw starts at the anterior inferior iliac spine, passing through the broad column of bone just above the acetabulum, coursing above the sciatic notch, and terminating near the posterior iliac spine adjacent to the sacroiliac joint. Standard Judet and inlet views are used for this screw, although an image should optimally be obtained in line with the planned trajectory of the screw as well.

SCREW TRAJECTORIES FOR SPECIFIC ACETABULAR FRACTURE PATTERNS

In general, anterior column, posterior column, transverse, and anterior column/posterior hemitransverse fractures are best suited for percutaneous technique, provided an acceptable closed reduction or lag screw reduction can be performed. Both-column fractures with good secondary congruity also can be stabilized *in situ,* particularly in elderly patients. It has not yet been possible to safely reduce and stabilize posterior wall fractures with percutaneous technique. Excluding posterior wall fractures, almost 50% of acetabular fractures at the author's home institution are now treated percutaneously, and clinical outcomes are being monitored.

The High Anterior Column Acetabular Fracture

These coronal plane fractures traverse the superior weight-bearing dome of the acetabulum, exiting through the iliac wing. Abdominal and gluteal muscle forces frequently cause significant displacement. The anterior fracture fragment, including a variable portion of the weight-bearing dome, typically is displaced cephalad, but may be reduced by application of longitudinal traction. The fragment usually is externally rotated and sometimes medialized as well. Schanz pin joysticks are used to manipulate the fracture, and reduction is maintained by application of a temporary external fixator. Reduction is assessed using Judet iliac and obturator oblique views. In the event of an unsuccessful closed reduction with an external fixator, a limited lateral window ilioinguinal exposure provides sufficient access for improvement of reduction.

For virtual fluoroscopic navigation, four individual radiographic projections are stored on the image guided surgery workstation. AP, inlet, and Judet views provide sufficient information for safe screw placement; the obturator oblique Judet view may be angled cephalad or caudad so that the C-arm is oriented in line with the intended path of screw placement. A true lateral of the pelvis often is helpful as well, but is difficult to obtain in the obese patient. The fracture is stabilized using two 7.3-mm cannulated screws passed over 2.8-mm guidewires placed just inferior to the anterior superior iliac spine. The first screw is similar to the LCII screw, and the second starts at the anterior-inferior iliac spine and is angled toward the ischial spine (Fig. 29-6). During the past 10 years, the author has stabilized over 20 high anterior column fractures using this technique. There has been no case of loss of reduction or development of arthrosis to date. The average postsurgical hospital stay for patients with isolated injuries treated percutaneously has been 2 days.

Transverse Acetabular Fractures

Nondisplaced fractures with worrisome roof arcs, and displaced fractures reducible with lateral traction are amenable to percutaneous internal fixation. A lateral traction (distraction) external fixator may be applied using Schanz pins placed in both greater trochanters. Residual gap displacement often is reducible using a lag screw placed perpendicular to the fracture line. True AP and true lateral views usually are sufficient for lag screw placement. Additional screws may be placed into the anterior column using antegrade or retrograde technique, and into the posterior column using retrograde technique through the ischial tuberosity (Fig. 29-7).

A

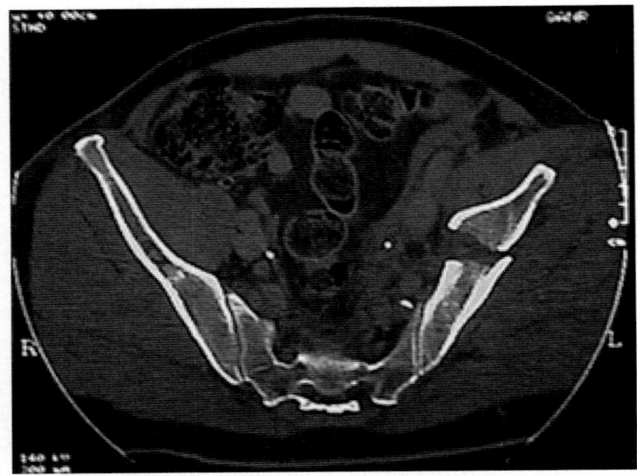

B

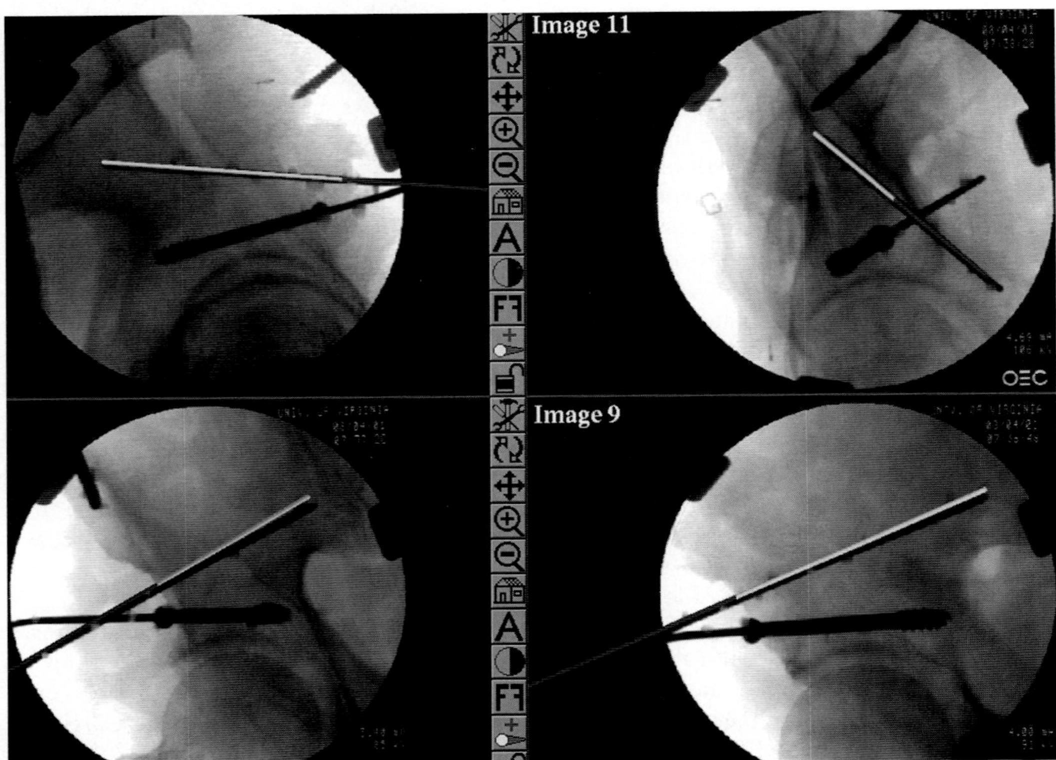

FIGURE 29-6. A: Typical fracture displacement in the high anterior column acetabular fracture. The fracture is reduced intraoperatively with a temporary external fixator. Two screws placed in standard trajectories then are used to stabilize the fracture. **B:** In the navigation views, the drill guide is shown, and the predicted trajectory is superimposed on the actual position following guidewire placement.

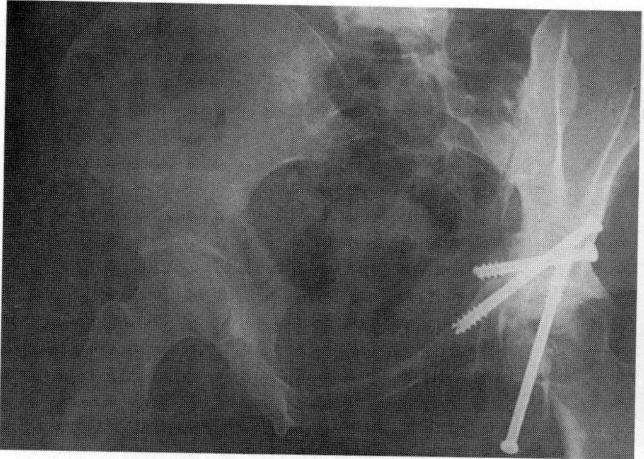

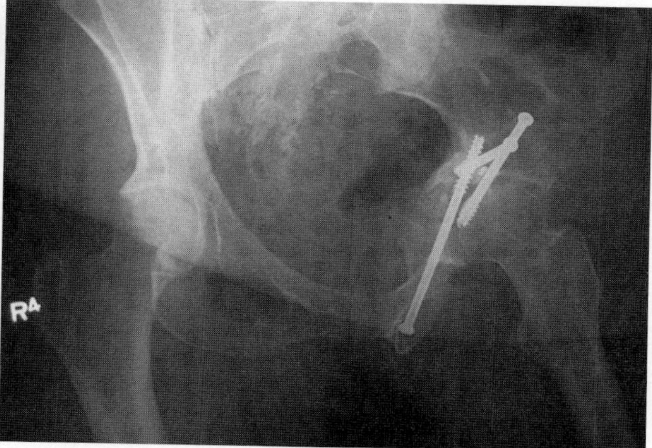

FIGURE 29-7. Judet views of a transverse acetabular fracture nonunion stabilized with a lag screw, an antegrade anterior column screw, and a retrograde posterior column screw.

The ideal radiographic views for surgical navigation are still evolving, but in general the surgeon should strive to obtain two orthogonal views perpendicular to the intended path of fixation. Anterior column/posterior hemitransverse fractures are stabilized with a lag screw and an LCII screw.

Posterior Column Fractures

Fractures of the posterior column usually are associated with subluxation or dislocation of the femoral head. Occasionally, an acceptable closed reduction can be obtained by simply reducing the hip dislocation, or by applying a distraction frame (Fig. 29-8). The fracture may be stabilized by placing a long cannulated screw from just inferior to the anterior inferior iliac spine, angled behind the hip joint to engage the region of the ischial spine (Fig. 29-9).

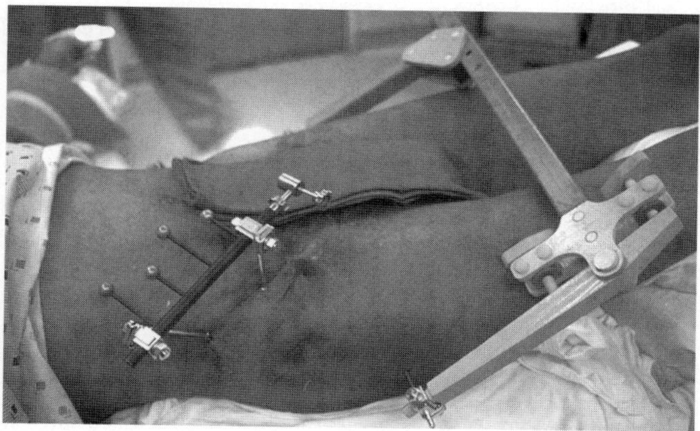

FIGURE 29-8. A radiolucent distraction frame is used to reduce a posterior column fracture by applying lateral traction through pins placed in both greater trochanters. In this case, a registration frame for three-dimensional computed tomography guided fixation also has been placed.

REDUCTION OF RADIATION EXPOSURE TO PATIENT AND SURGEON

Ionizing radiation exposure is probably an under appreciated risk for both trauma surgeons and trauma patients. Reduction of radiation exposure to patient and surgeon is a tangible advantage of using computer-assisted technique, rather than standard fluoroscopy, for placement of fixation screws. One minute of intraoperative fluoroscopy about the pelvis is equivalent to about 40 mSv (4 Rads, 4,000 mRem) of radiation, or approximately equivalent to 250 chest x-rays or a CT scan of the pelvis. The careful surgeon absorbs very little direct radiation during fluoroscopic imaging, but is still subject to scatter from the patient's anatomy; the patient absorbs most of the radiation dose. In actual practice, surgeons frequently place their hands in the radiation beam, especially during fracture reduction and freehand locking of intramedullary nails. The Occupational Safety and Health Administration's guidelines recommend no more than 50 rem per year of hand exposure, and this corresponds to only 12 minutes of fluoroscopy time per year (14). It is quite possible for an orthopedic surgeon to exceed this threshold.

Measurable health effects can occur at much lower doses of radiation. For example, air travel above 30,000 feet results in a slight increase in background radiation exposure owing to reduced atmospheric absorption. Career high-altitude airline pilots receive about 3 to 6 mSv of radiation over environmental background (0.6 to 2.0 mSv) per year, or about twice the dose received by the general population. This small additional radiation dose would be equivalent to about 10 to 15 seconds of fluoroscopy about the pelvis or hip. It is distressing to note that pilots have a fivefold increase in myeloid malignancies and a threefold increase in skin cancers when compared to the population at large (15). Although the skin cancer risk may be related to increased

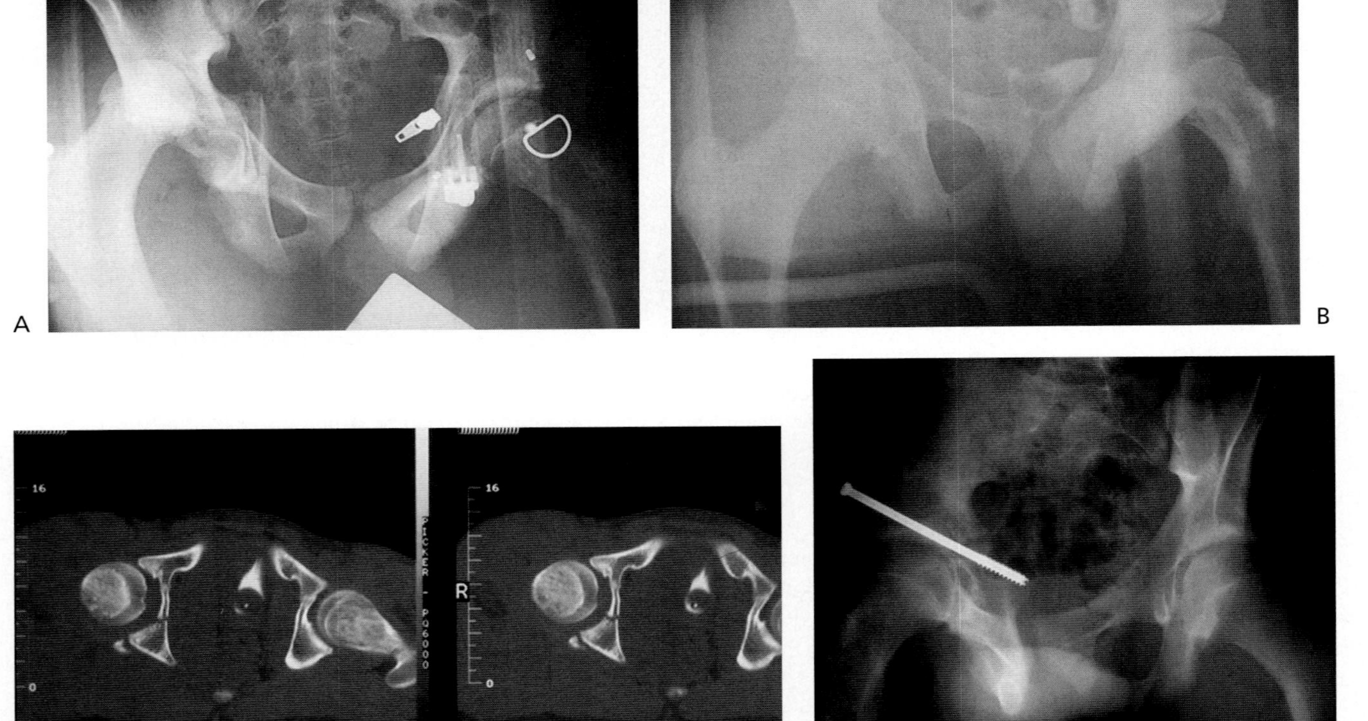

FIGURE 29-9. A: A displaced posterior column fracture dislocation in a multiply traumatized young skier. **B,C:** These figures show a radiograph and computed tomography post reduction. **D:** The fracture was stabilized with a single long lag screw.

sun exposure, increased background radiation exposure is felt to be responsible for the hematopoietic malignancies.

CONCLUSION

Virtual fluoroscopy, a new development in the field of CAOS, has numerous potential applications in the field of orthopedic trauma. Using this technique, cannulated screws may be precisely placed within the pelvis using only a few individual fluoroscopic images. Despite the need for specialized equipment and instruments, this technology has the potential to greatly decrease the orthopedic surgeon's reliance on intraoperative ionizing radiation during the performance of minimally invasive surgery.

REFERENCES

1. Olson SA, Matta JM. The computerized tomography subchondral arc: a new method of assessing acetabular continuity after fracture (a preliminary report). *J Orthop Trauma* 1993;7:402–413.
2. Tornetta P III. Nonoperative management of acetabular fractures: the use of dynamic stress views. *J Bone Joint Surg Br* 1999; 81-B:67–70.
3. Parker PJ, Copeland C. Percutaneous fluoroscopic screw fixation of acetabular fractures. *Injury* 1997;28:597–600.
4. Starr AJ, Reinert CM, Jones AL. Percutaneous fixation of the columns of the acetabulum: a new technique. *J Orthop Trauma* 1998;12(1):51–58.
5. Zura RD, Kahler DM. Case report: a transverse acetabular nonunion successfully treated with computer-assisted percutaneous internal fixation. *J Bone Joint Surg* 2000;82-A:219–224.
6. Gay SB, Sistrom C, Wang G-J, et al. Percutaneous screw fixation of acetabular fractures with CT guidance: preliminary results of a new technique. *Am J Radiol* 1992;158:819–822.
7. Kahler DM, DeGrange D, Wang G-J. *Percutaneous fixation of selected acetabular fractures using computed tomographic (CT) guidance.* Presented at American Academy of Orthopedic Surgery annual meeting. Atlanta, GA, February 24, 1996.
8. Johanson NA, Charlson ME, Szatrowski TP, et al. A self-administered hip-rating questionnaire for the assessment of outcome after total hip replacement. *J Bone Joint Surg Am* 1992;74: 587–597.
9. Kahler DM, Zura R. Evaluation of a computer-assisted surgical technique for percutaneous internal fixation in a transverse acetabular fracture model. *Lecture Notes Comput Sci* 1997;1205: 565–572.
10. Kahler DM. Computer-assisted fixation of acetabular fractures and pelvic ring disruptions. *Tech Orthop* 2000;10(1):20–24.

11. Kahler DM, Mallik K. Computer-assisted iliosacral screw placement compared to standard fluoroscopic technique. *Comput Aid Surg* 1999;4(6):348.
12. Kahler, DM. *Virtual fluoroscopy: a tool for decreasing radiation exposure during femoral intramedullary nailing.* Poster presentation, American Academy of Orthopedic Surgery annual meeting, San Francisco, March, 2001.
13. Kahler DM, Mallik K, Tadje J. *Computer-guided percutaneous iliosacral screw fixation of posterior pelvic ring disruption compared to conventional technique.* Presented at Fifth North American Program on Computer-Assisted Orthopedic Surgery, Pittsburgh, July 7, 2001.
14. Mehlman CT, DiPasquale TG. Radiation exposure to the orthopedic surgical team during fluoroscopy: "how far away is far enough?" *J Orthop Trauma* 1997;11(6):392–398.
15. Gundestrup M, Storm HH. Radiation-induced acute myeloid leukaemia and other cancers in commercial jet cockpit crew: a population-based cohort study. *Lancet* 1999;354:2029–2031.

30

FLUOROSCOPIC-ASSISTED CLOSED TECHNIQUES OF REDUCTION AND FIXATION

ADAM J. STARR

INTRODUCTION

> . . . I will have no man in my boat, said Starbuck, who is not afraid of a whale.
>
> Herman Melville, *Moby Dick or, The Whale*

The techniques of percutaneous screw fixation of pelvic ring disruptions have been well described (1–4). Percutaneous methods are beneficial because they offer stability with limited dissection, and a decreased risk of soft-tissue complications. Closed reduction and percutaneous screw fixation of disrupted sacroiliac joints or sacral fractures is now an accepted form of treatment (1,2). Percutaneous screw fixation of fractures of the posterior portion of the iliac wing also has been reported, with acceptable results (3). Similarly, percutaneous fixation of fractures of the anterior pelvic ring has been described (4), and this technique is in use in several centers.

Percutaneous screw fixation of acetabular fractures is a technique in its infancy. To date, reports concerning percutaneous stabilization of acetabular fractures have been confined to descriptions of the repair of nondisplaced or minimally displaced fractures (5–7), stabilization of a well-aligned acetabular fracture nonunion (8), or the use of the technique as an adjunct to traditional open reduction and internal fixation (9,10).

The experience with percutaneous screw fixation of acetabular fractures at our institution began with the treatment of nondisplaced or minimally displaced fractures (7). These procedures were carried out to prevent fracture displacement, or to allow weight bearing in patients who had contralateral lower extremity injuries that precluded weight bearing. As our familiarity with the percutaneous technique increased, we applied it to certain displaced acetabular fractures (11).

CAVEAT

Percutaneous stabilization of acetabular fractures is not a procedure to be undertaken lightly. The technique relies on fluoroscopy to ensure safe placement of guidewires in the bone. The surgeon must be aware that what he cannot see can hurt his patient. In spite of the small incisions employed, the risks to the patient are quite great. Errant screw placement, errant clamp placement, or inability to adequately reduce, judge, or stabilize the fracture can all lead to disastrous consequences for the patient. Knowledge of the three-dimensional (3D) anatomy of the pelvis and surrounding structures is required if the procedure is to be carried out safely.

In addition, it must be noted that percutaneous screw fixation of acetabular fractures still should be considered ex-

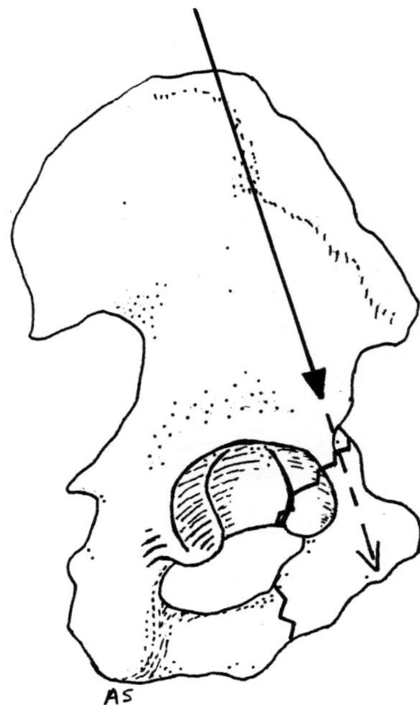

FIGURE 30-1. Pathway for placement of the anterior column screw. Antegrade or retrograde placement is possible. Retrograde placement is usually simpler, unless the patient is obese. In obese patients, the contralateral thigh gets in the way of the surgeon's hand, and prevents correct placement of the guidewire. During placement of the anterior column guidewire the femoral nerve, artery and vein are at risk. Also, the round ligament or spermatic cord can be damaged.

perimental surgery. The exact indications, complications, and long-term results are not yet known. For this reason, the use of this procedure probably should be confined to surgeons experienced in acetabular fracture surgery, who can recognize the potential complications posed by the technique, as well as its potential benefits.

SCREW PATHWAYS AND FLUOROSCOPIC VISUALIZATION

There are several screw pathways that have proven to be consistently useful in the percutaneous treatment of acetabular fractures. These pathways, and the fluoroscopic views used to exploit them, are described here.

Anterior Column Screw

The anterior column screw can be placed in an antegrade or retrograde fashion (Fig. 30-1). Each direction makes use of the same fluoroscopic views to ensure safe placement of the guidewire (Figs. 30-2 and 30-3). Usually, retrograde placement is easier. However, in obese patients the contralateral thigh may get in the way of the surgeon's hand, and make retrograde screw placement difficult.

Posterior Column Screw

The starting point for the posterior column screw guidewire is at the ischial tuberosity (Fig. 30-4). The wire then passes up the ischium behind the acetabulum (Fig. 30-5). The hip and knee are held in a flexed position to draw the sciatic nerve away from the tip of the ischium, and allow palpation of the tuberosity.

LC-2 Screw

This screw was first used to stabilize "crescent" fractures or lateral compression Type 2 pelvic ring disruptions (3). It is also useful for stabilizing fractures of the acetabulum that involve the iliac wing, such as anterior column or both-column fractures (Figs. 30-6 to 30-9). The guidewire for

A

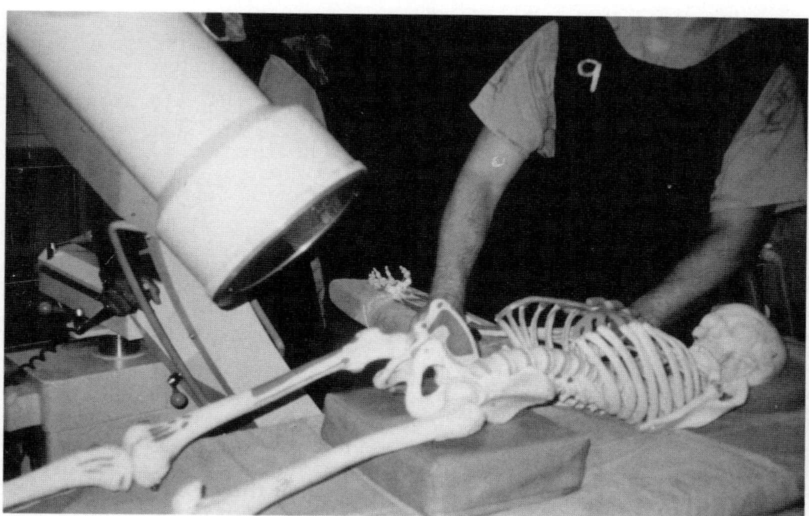

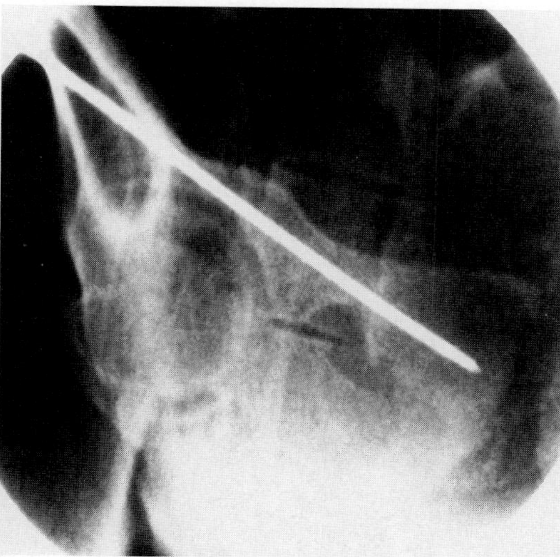

B

FIGURE 30-2. A: C-arm position for the outlet-obturator view. **B:** This view is used to ensure that the anterior column screw guidewire does not penetrate the acetabulum or exit the anterior column superiorly. (From: Starr AJ, Reinert CM, Jones AL. Percutaneous fixation of the columns of the acetabulum: a new technique. *J Orthop Trauma* 1998;12:51–58, with permission.)

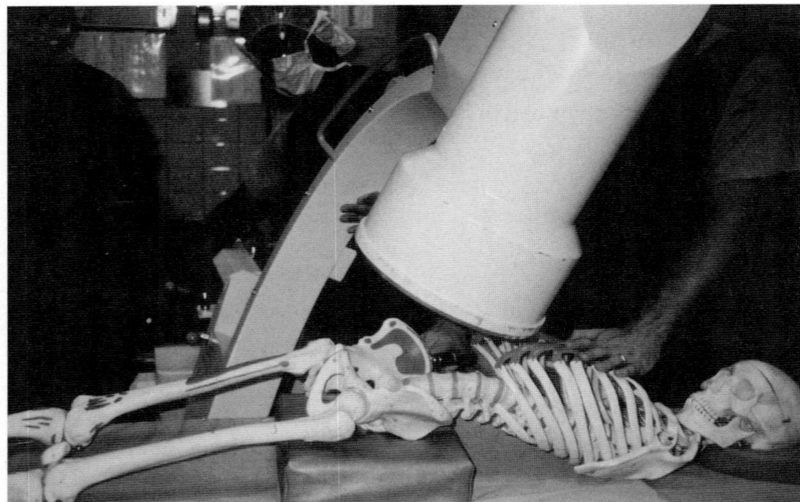

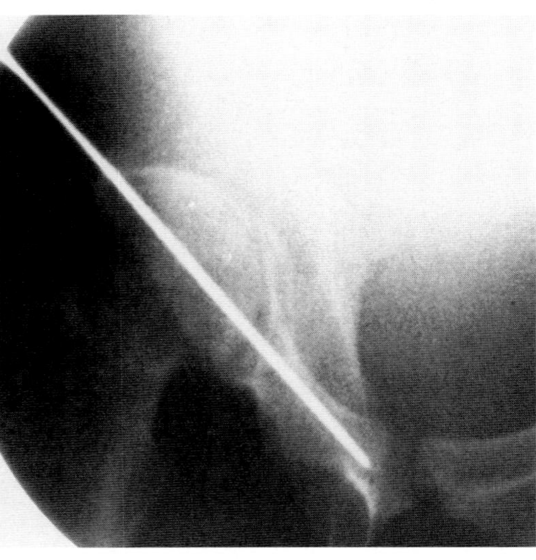

A B

FIGURE 30-3. A: C-arm position for the inlet-iliac view. **B:** This view is used to ensure that the anterior column screw guidewire does not exit the superior pubic ramus either anteriorly, toward the femoral neurovascular structures, or posteriorly toward the bladder. (From: Starr AJ, Reinert CM, Jones AL. Percutaneous fixation of the columns of the acetabulum: a new technique. *J Orthop Trauma* 1998;12:51–58, with permission.)

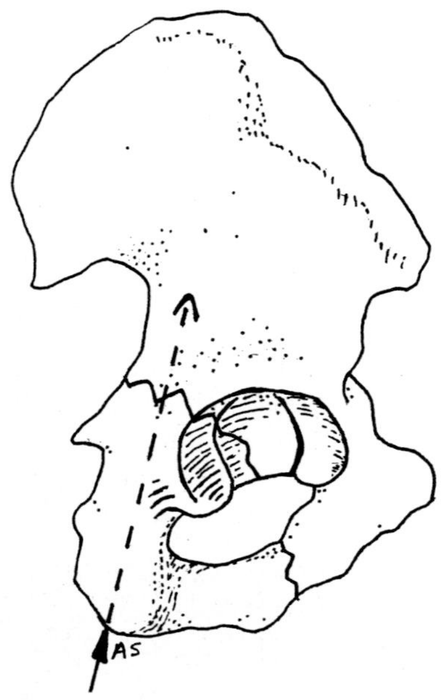

FIGURE 30-4. Pathway for placement of the posterior column screw. The sciatic nerve and all the structures that exit the greater sciatic notch are at risk. Hip flexion relaxes the sciatic nerve, and draws it away from the starting point at the ischial tuberosity.

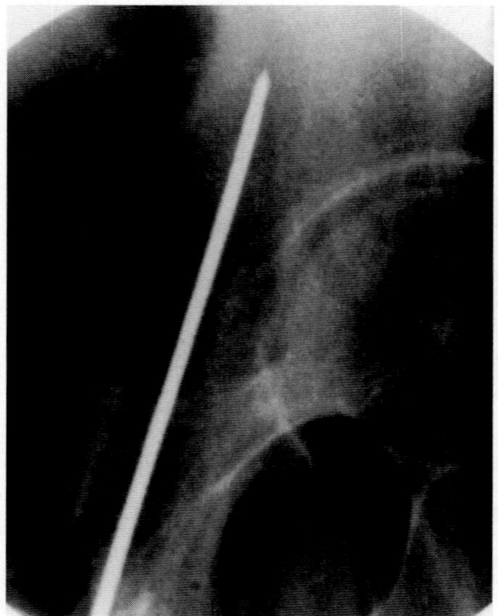

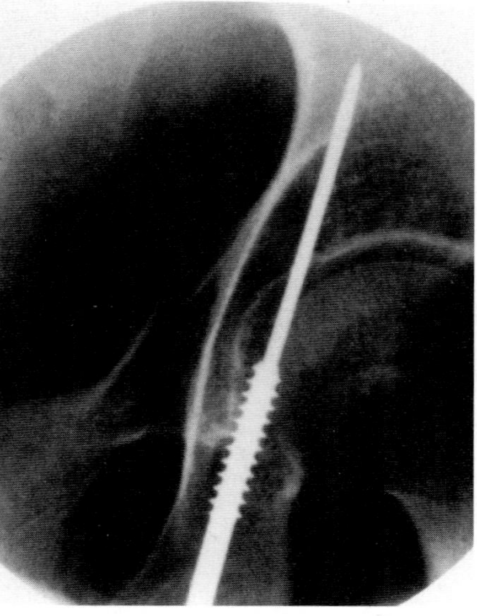

A, B

FIGURE 30-5. Posterior column screw guidewire placement. **A:** The iliac oblique view is used to ensure that the guidewire remains posterior to the acetabulum and does not enter the greater sciatic notch. **B:** The anterior-posterior view of the pelvis is used to ensure that the guidewire does not exit the medial or lateral cortices of the ischium. (From: Starr AJ, Borer DS, Reinert CM. Technical aspects of limited open reduction and percutaneous screw fixation of fractures of the acetabulum. *Op Tech Orthop* July 2001, with permission.)

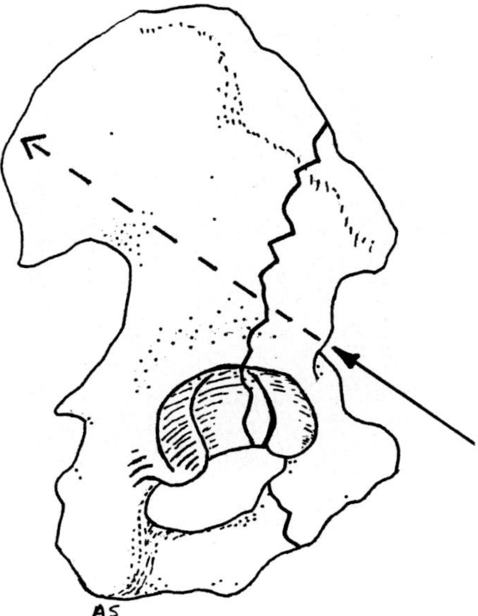

FIGURE 30-6. Pathway for placement of the "LC-2 screw." (From: Starr AJ, Borer DS, Reinert CM. Technical aspects of limited open reduction and percutaneous screw fixation of fractures of the acetabulum. *Op Tech Orthop* July 2001, with permission.)

A

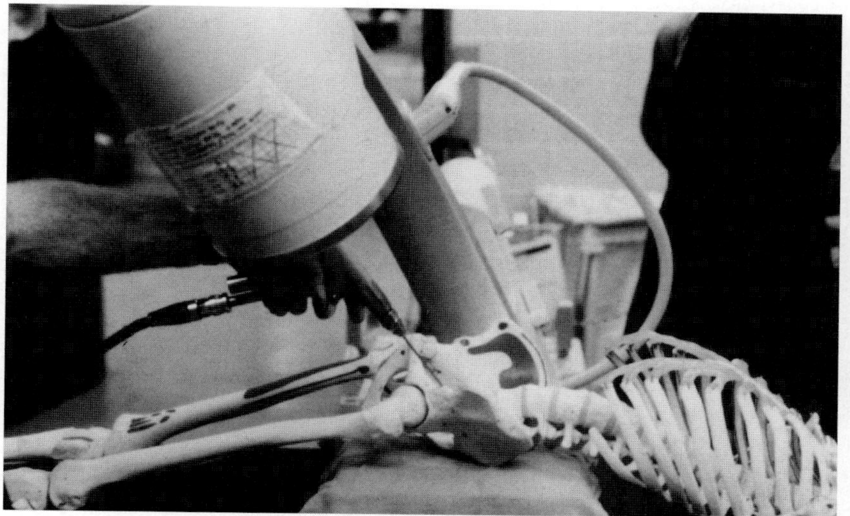

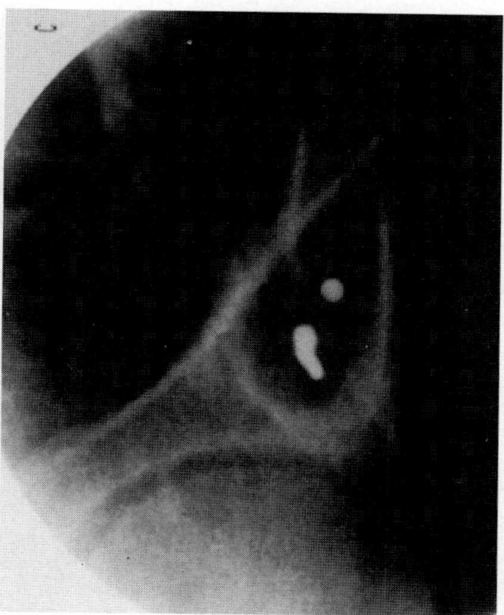

B

FIGURE 30-7. A: C-arm position to start the LC-2 screw. **B:** This position is used to visualize the "tube" of bone the guidewire will pass down. The guidewire starts at the anterior inferior iliac spine and heads toward the posterior inferior iliac spine. (From: Starr AJ, Walter JC, Harris RW, et al. Percutaneous screw fixation of fractures of the iliac wing and fracture dislocations of the sacro-iliac joint (OTA types 61-B2.2 and 61-B2.3, or Young-Burgess "Lateral Compression Type II" pelvic fractures). *J Orthop Trauma* 2002;16:116–123, with permission.)

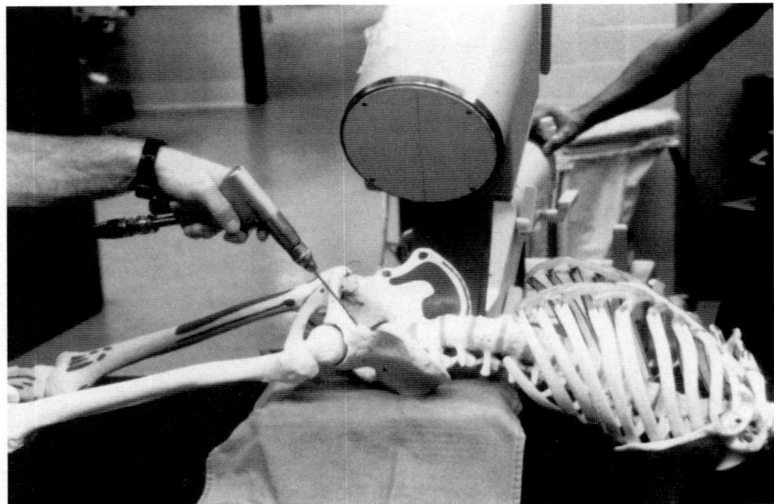

A

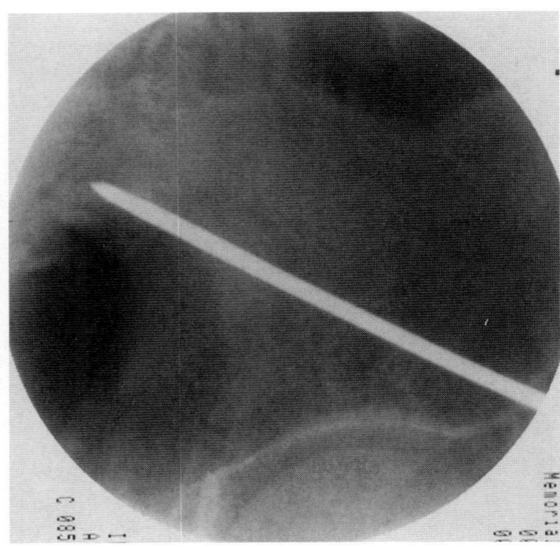

B

FIGURE 30-8. C-arm position to obtain an iliac oblique view **(A),** to watch the LC-2 guidewire pass above the greater sciatic notch **(B).** At bottom, the notch is visible at about the 8 o'clock position, whereas the acetabulum and femoral head are visible at about the 4 to 6 o'clock positions. (From: Starr AJ, Walter JC, Harris RW, et al. Percutaneous screw fixation of fractures of the iliac wing and fracture dislocations of the sacro-iliac joint (OTA types 61-B2.2 and 61-B2.3, or Young-Burgess "Lateral Compression Type II" pelvic fractures). *J Orthop Trauma* 2002;16:116–123, with permission.)

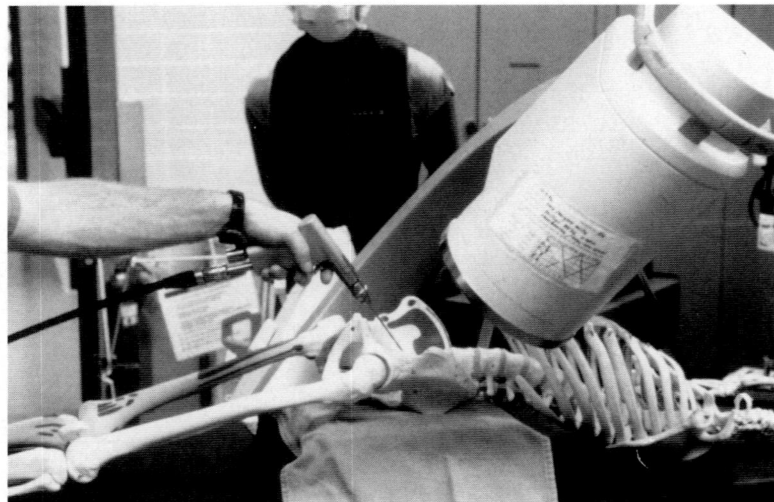

A

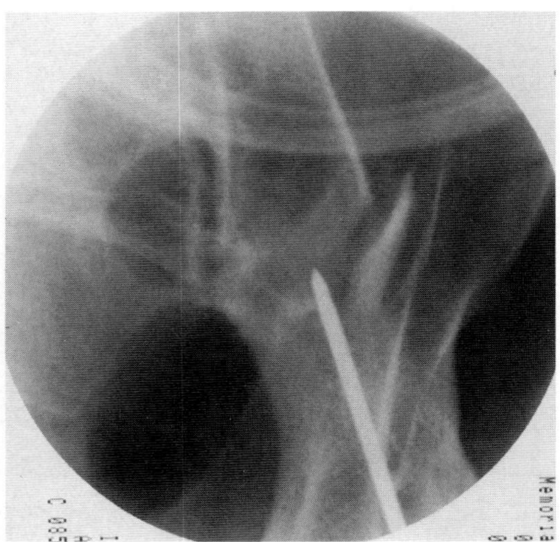

B

FIGURE 30-9. C-arm position **(A)** to ensure that the LC-2 screw guidewire remains centered between the inner and outer cortices of the ilium **(B)** as it moves toward the posterior inferior iliac spine. As it nears the posterior portion of the ilium, the guidewire skirts the sacroiliac joint, visible at bottom. (From: Starr AJ, Walter JC, Harris RW, et al. Percutaneous screw fixation of fractures of the iliac wing and fracture dislocations of the sacro-iliac joint (OTA types 61-B2.2 and 61-B2.3, or Young-Burgess "Lateral Compression Type II" pelvic fractures). *J Orthop Trauma* 2002;16: 116–123, with permission.)

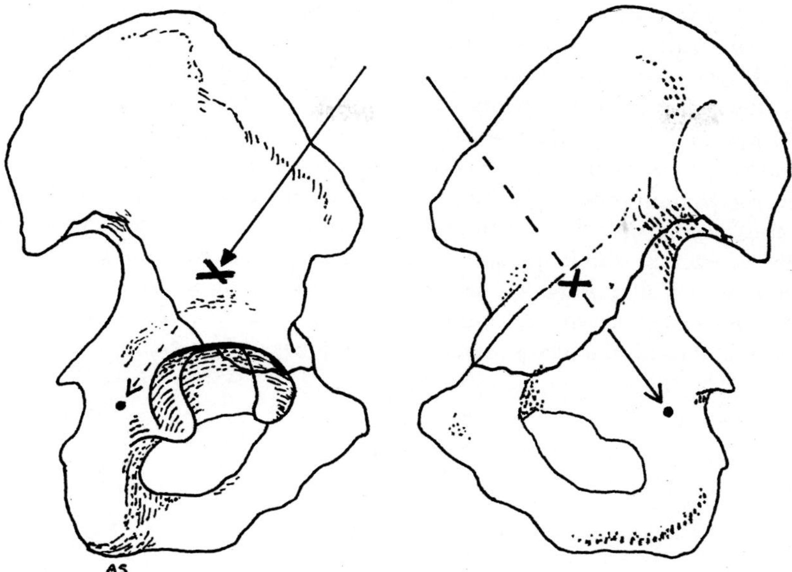

FIGURE 30-10. Pathway for placement of the "magic screw." (From: Starr AJ, Borer DS, Reinert CM. Technical aspects of limited open reduction and percutaneous screw fixation of fractures of the acetabulum. *Op Tech Orthop* July 2001, with permission.)

this screw is placed from the anterior inferior iliac spine toward the posterior inferior iliac spine, or vice versa.

Magic Screw

This screw can be used to hold the quadrilateral plate in a reduced position. The guidewire is started on the oblique surface of the iliac wing, at a point proximal and posterior to the acetabulum. The wire should exit the bone through the inner cortex of the quadrilateral plate, at or near the ischial spine (Fig. 30-10). During passage of the guidewire, the anterior-posterior (AP), inlet, and iliac oblique views are used to ensure that the guidewire does not penetrate the acetabulum, or go past the quadrilateral plate into the true pelvis.

SURGICAL INDICATIONS

Surgeons who attempt this technique soon discover that seeing the fracture is not the problem. The various fluoroscopic views can be learned fairly quickly, and fracture anatomy usually is clearly visible with the use of the fluoroscope. The problem lies in obtaining an acceptable reduction. Bringing the acetabulum into an acceptable position, and then maintaining that reduction until percutaneous screws can be passed across the fracture is not simple.

It is difficult to achieve anatomic reduction of "complex/associated" (12) acetabular fractures using this method. Closed manipulation of the hip or limited open techniques are not yet sufficient to perfectly align fractures with multiple fragments. Thus, this technique should not be used if a perfect reduction is required, and a complex/associated fracture pattern is present.

Because of this limitation, the use of this technique in young patients is restricted to those with "simple" fracture patterns, as defined by Letournel (12). Simple fracture patterns can sometimes be reduced using closed or limited open techniques. The judgment as to whether or not a fracture can be reduced with closed or limited open methods depends on the surgeon's experience. Assessment of the fracture under anesthesia is very useful. Markedly displaced fractures sometimes are dramatically improved with simple longitudinal traction. Further manipulation in the operating room may be all that is necessary to bring the joint to an acceptable position (Fig. 30-11). If preoperative radiographs reveal a simple fracture that may be amenable to closed or limited open reduction techniques, the current practice at our institution is to offer this option to the patient, with the understanding that failure of these methods will immediately be followed by a traditional open approach.

Elderly patients appear to tolerate imperfect reduction better than young patients (13). Thus, this technique has broader indications for use in the elderly, even if a complex fracture is present. The limited dissection, shortened surgical time, and scant blood loss make this technique particularly attractive in elderly patients who are not good candidates for a lengthy open procedure (Fig. 30-12). Patients in this age group also are good candidates for hip arthroplasty should they go on to develop posttraumatic arthritis after the percutaneous procedure.

Additionally, there are some instances where traditional open reduction and internal fixation techniques seem doomed to failure in elderly patients. Cases with severe comminution can be difficult to repair in older patients, because osteopenic bone does not hold screws well. Similarly, femoral head injury can lead to posttraumatic arthritis, even if a perfect reduction of the acetabulum is obtained (12).

Total hip replacement after failed open reduction and internal fixation of an acetabular fracture is difficult, and has results that are poorer than those seen after primary total hip replacement (14). In cases with severe acetabular comminution and osteopenia, or where femoral head injury is present, the percutaneous technique may be a useful way to preserve bone stock for later total hip arthroplasty without resorting to a large open procedure. Fracture stabilization with percutaneous screws alleviates pain and allows patient mobilization, both important considerations in elderly patients. It also allows improvement of fracture alignment to make later hip replacement simpler. Hip arthroplasty after percutaneous screw fixation of an acetabular fracture is relatively straightforward. The percutaneous approach does little damage to the surrounding soft tissues. So, the dense, contracted scar commonly seen after a traditional open technique is not an issue.

A

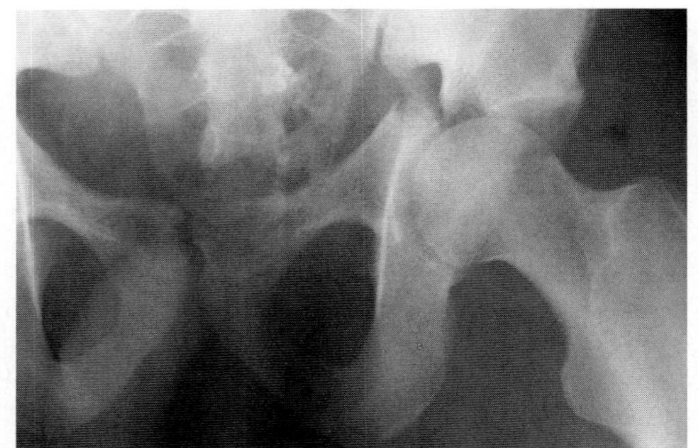

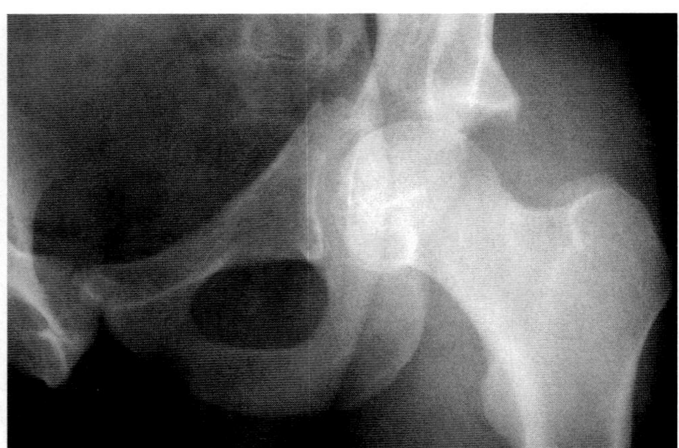

B

C

FIGURE 30-11. A–C: Anterior-posterior, obturator, and iliac oblique views of a 20-year-old man injured while riding a jet ski. He sustained a transverse acetabular fracture and ipsilateral fractures of the femur and patella. He was treated with open reduction and internal fixation of his patella, retrograde intramedullary nailing of the femur, and limited open reduction and percutaneous screw fixation of his acetabular fracture. Traction on the hip after femoral nailing markedly improved the alignment of the acetabular fracture. The modified pelvic reduction clamp was used to reduce the remainder of the displacement of the caudal fracture fragment.

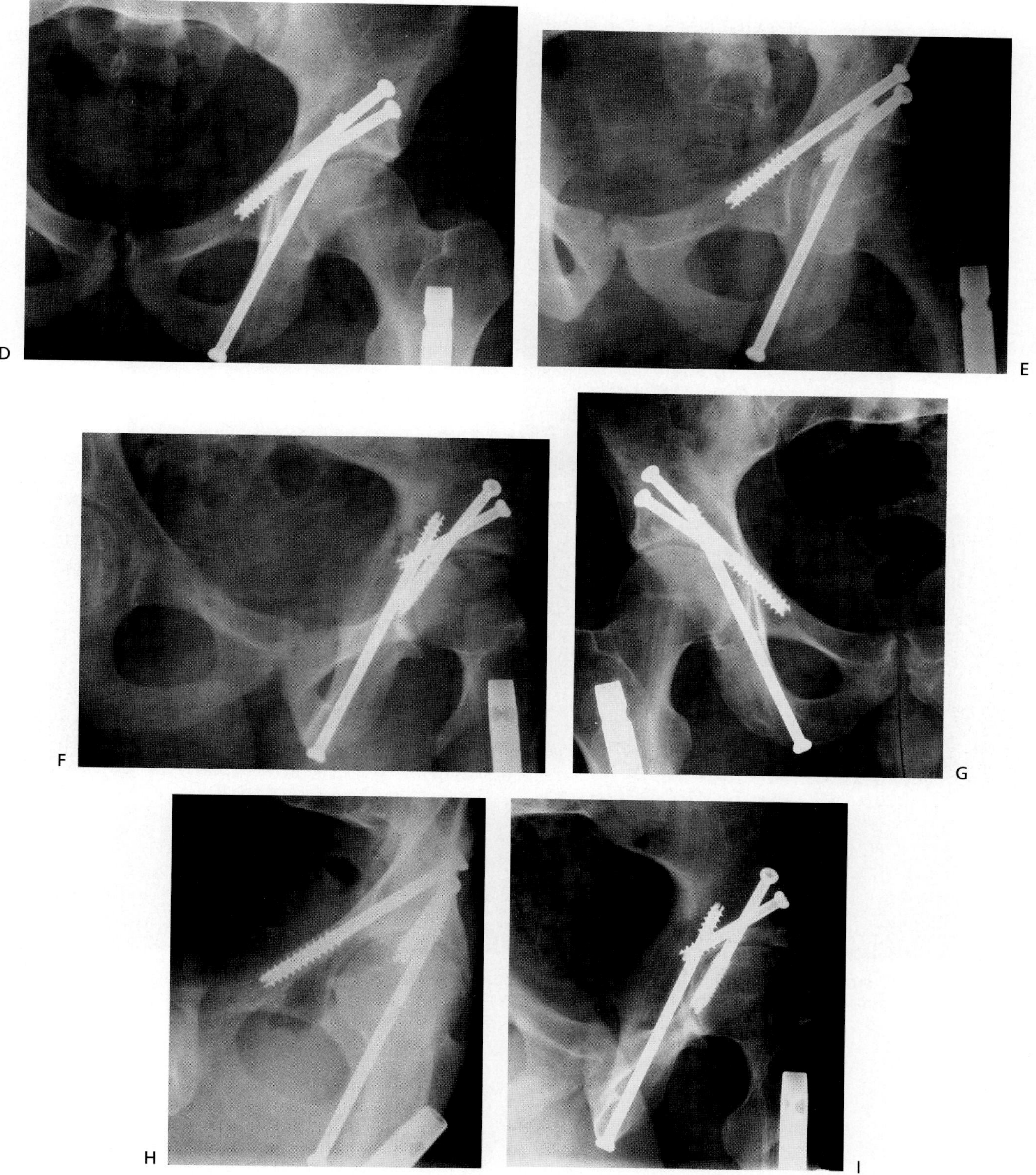

FIGURE 30-11. ***(continued)*** **D–F:** Reduction was maintained with anterior and posterior column screws, and a magic screw. **G–I:** His Harris Hip Score is 100 and his function is excellent at 2 years. He has returned to riding his jet ski.

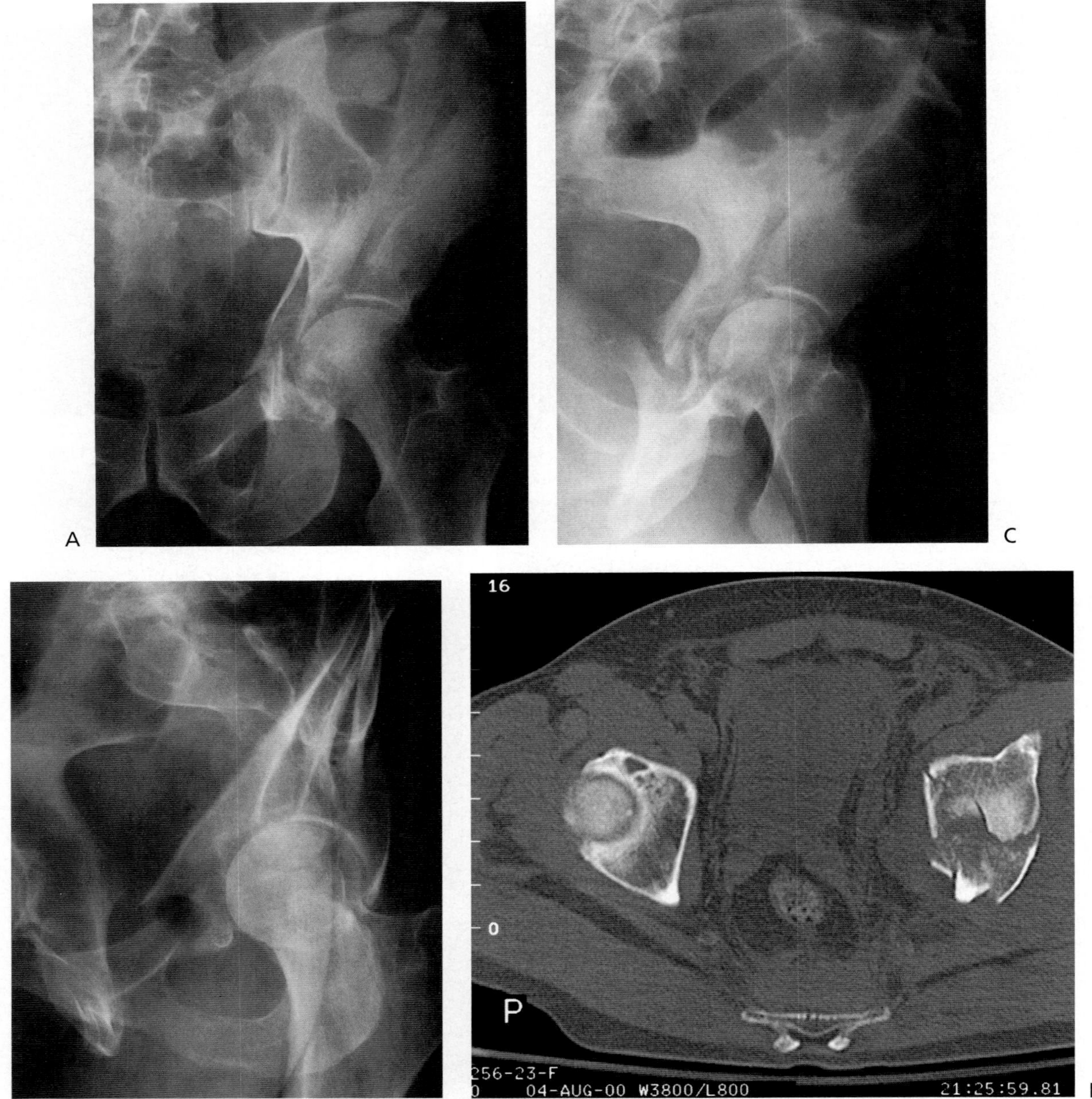

FIGURE 30-12. A–D: Anterior-posterior, obturator, and iliac oblique views, and a computed tomography scan of a 64-year-old man injured in a fall.

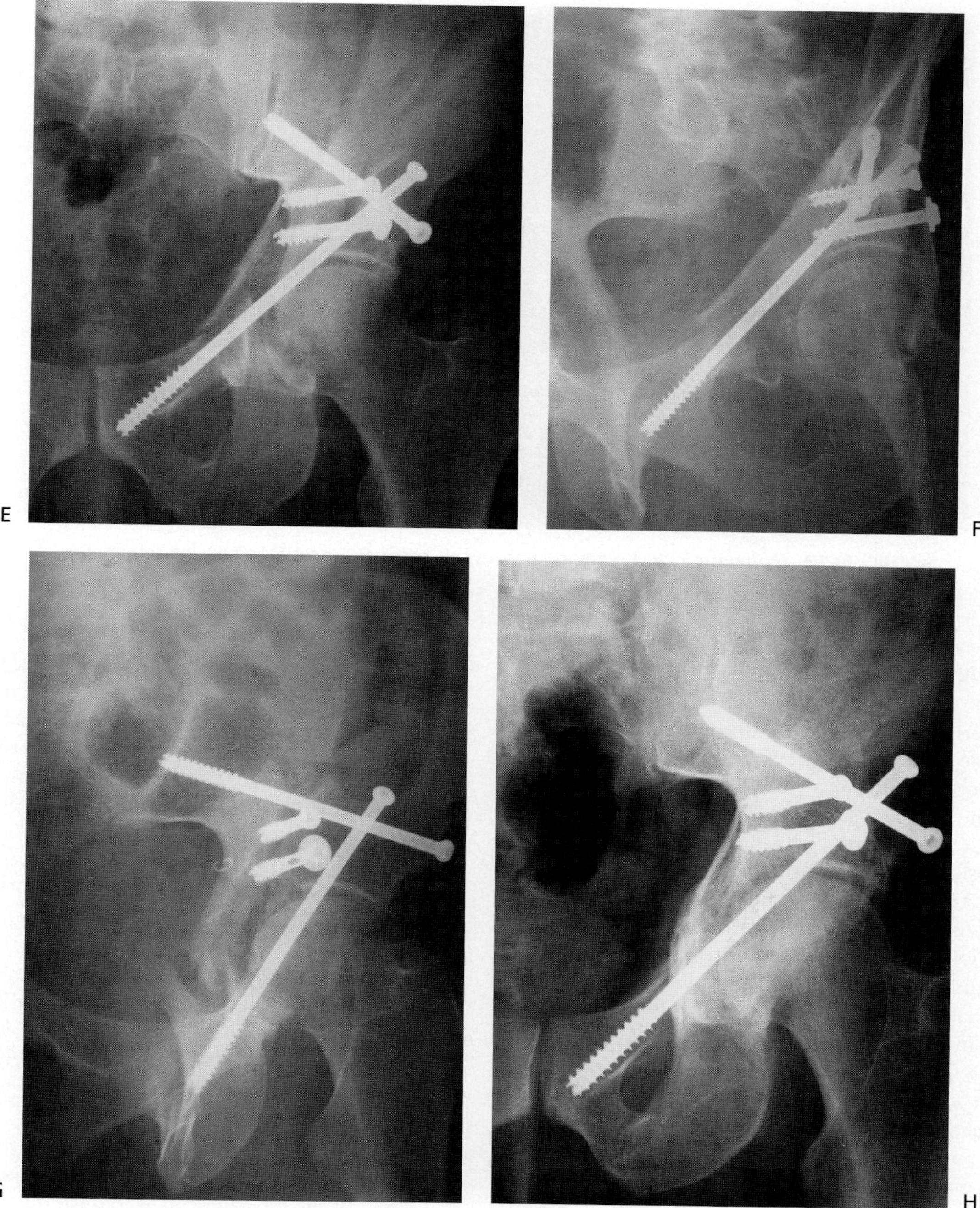

FIGURE 30-12. ***(continued)*** **E–G:** The patient's both-column acetabular fracture was treated with limited open reduction and percutaneous screw fixation. Although his reduction is by no means anatomic, it did afford him prompt relief of pain, and allowed mobilization. The patient had minimal blood loss (approximately 50 mL) during the procedure. The patient was pain free at 6 months, returned to work as a farmer, and had a Harris Hip Score of 91.

(Figure continues)

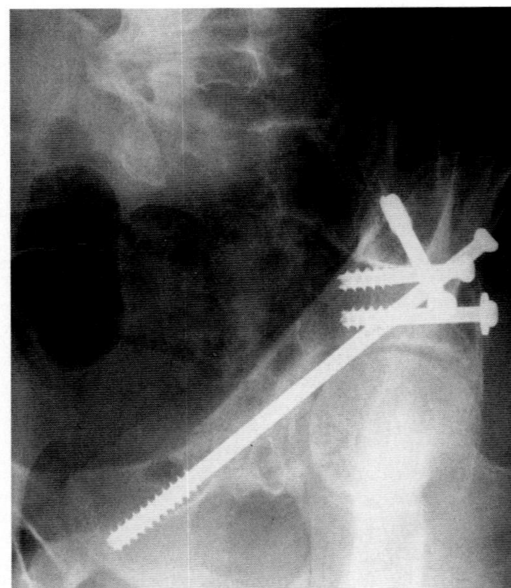
I

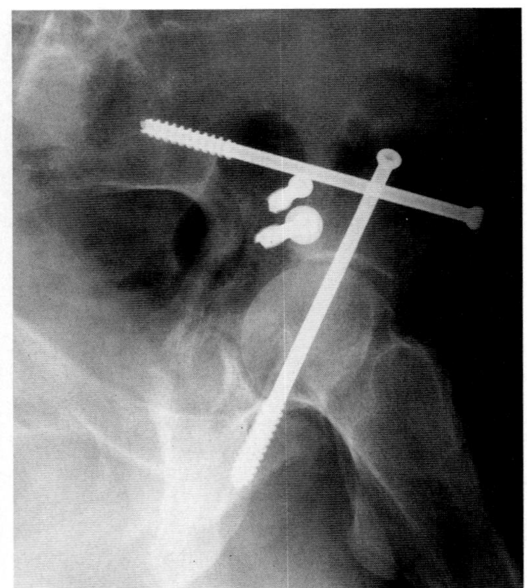
J

FIGURE 30-12. ***(continued)*** **H–J:** Radiographs reveal complete fracture union, and remodeling of the fracture.

REDUCTION MANEUVERS

Surgery is performed on a radiolucent operating table. Knowledgeable, skilled fluoroscopy personnel are essential. The fluoroscopy technician's understanding of the bony anatomy of the pelvis must be equal to that of the surgeon, if the procedure is to be successful.

Supine positioning is used most commonly. The lower abdomen and the ipsilateral leg are draped free to allow manipulation of the fracture. Chemical paralysis of the patient makes reduction easier. Nitrous oxide anesthetic should not be used, because the gas will enter the bowel and make fluoroscopic visualization of the fracture difficult. In addition, the surgeon must be sure no contrast material is in the bowel, because it can obscure bony details during surgery.

Reduction is judged with fluoroscopy. The surgeon can assess the adequacy of reduction achieved by using the image intensifier and multiple oblique views.

No single maneuver reduces all fractures of the acetabulum. Under fluoroscopic control, various motions are tried, to see what works best at bringing the fracture back into alignment. Internal or external rotation of the hip, abduction of the hip, traction on the leg—all may be useful in realigning the pieces of the acetabulum. Closed reduction relies on intact attachments of soft-tissue structures around the hip. The hip capsule, ligament of Bigelow, and origin of the hip adductor muscles are all useful in achieving a reduction. Chemical paralysis lessens the deforming forces of the patient's muscles. Reduction soon after injury increases the chances of success. As with other fractures, delay in treatment beyond a few days allows organization of the fracture hematoma, which makes closed reduction impossible.

In many fractures, the caudal fragments are driven medially, pushed inward by the femoral head as it hits the acetabular surface. Thus, external rotation of the hip, and traction on the thigh, can sometimes improve fracture alignment. However, each fracture has to be assessed individually to discover the maneuver that best reduces the fragments into an acceptable position.

LIMITED OPEN REDUCTION

In some cases, instruments placed through stab wounds or limited surgical exposures may be used to improve reduction. In every instance, the surgeon must be aware of structures that lie in the path of percutaneously placed tools. Anyone unfamiliar with the 3D anatomy of the pelvis should not attempt this procedure.

Several devices are useful in improving fracture alignment. A ball-spike placed through a stab wound over the lateral aspect of the hip can be used to push the iliac wing into a better position. Blunt dissection through the abductor musculature allows the surgeon to place the ball-spike directly against the iliac wing. Pressure then can be applied to the iliac wing to improve the alignment of the ilium in relation to the other fracture fragments. This maneuver can be useful in reduction of both-column fractures, or fractures involving the anterior column. Similarly, a joker placed medial to the sartorius muscle can be used to push down on the pecten pubis, to improve the alignment of the anterior column. The joker can be placed through a small incision made directly over the anterior inferior iliac spine. A small Cobb elevator can be used for the same purpose. In each case, blunt dissection with a hemostat is used to create a pathway, which allows direct contact with the bone. It is relatively simple to reach the pecten pubis in this manner, but the surgeon must be aware at all times of the proximity of the femoral vessels and nerve. This reduction maneuver is helpful in the reduction of fractures with comminution of the area around the pecten, or along the anterior portion of the brim of the pelvis.

The injury mechanism that creates the fracture often results in medial displacement of the quadrilateral plate. Thus, it is sometimes necessary to bring the quadrilateral plate back under the iliac wing. A modified pelvic reduction clamp (Fig. 30-13) can be used to achieve this result. The long, straight tine of the clamp is placed through a stab wound just proximal and medial to the anterior superior iliac spine. While the hip is flexed to relax the iliopsoas, the tine of the clamp is passed down the inner cortex of the iliac wing, over the pelvic brim, and down along the medial surface of the quadrilateral plate. As the tine passes down the surface of the quadrilateral plate, the fracture is felt. Usually, the caudal fragment of bone is displaced medially. The tine is lifted over the fracture, then seated on the flat surface of the quadrilateral plate distal to the fracture. Passage of the long, straight tine is observed with fluoroscopy. Both the AP and iliac oblique views are useful. The AP view reveals how far past the pelvic brim the tine has passed, whereas the iliac oblique view reveals the position of the tine on the quadrilateral plate. It is important not to place the tine of the clamp into the greater sciatic notch. Frequent use of the iliac oblique view prevents this occurrence. Once the medial tine is seated, the outer tine of the clamp is passed through the abductor muscles and is seated in the supraacetabular region in the cephalad fragment of bone. Closing the clamp brings the caudal fragment lateral, thus reducing the fracture.

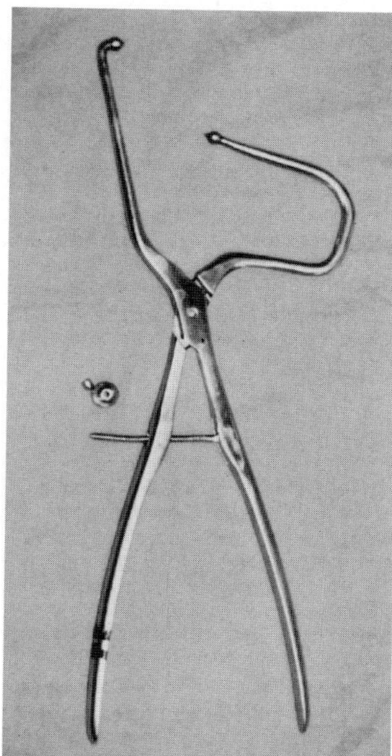

FIGURE 30-13. Modified pelvic reduction clamp. The long, straight tine is passed down the inner cortex of the ilium, over the brim of the true pelvis, and down the surface of the quadrilateral plate. Once the inner tine is seated distal to the fracture, the outer tine is passed through the hip abductor muscles and is seated in the supraacetabular region on the cephalad fragment of bone.

CANNULATED SCREW GUIDEWIRES AND WIRE GUIDES

Extra-long guidewires (350-mm lengths) for large fragment cannulated screws are necessary to reach the pelvis through the surrounding soft tissues (Fig. 30-14). Smaller diameter screws can be used, but extra-long guidewires, or long drill bits, are necessary in every case. Old cannulated screwdrivers with broken hex heads are used to place the guidewires. These broken screwdrivers' tips are sharpened down to produce a cannulated point. The point can be seated against the bone, which facilitates placement of guidewires along the oblique surfaces of the pelvis.

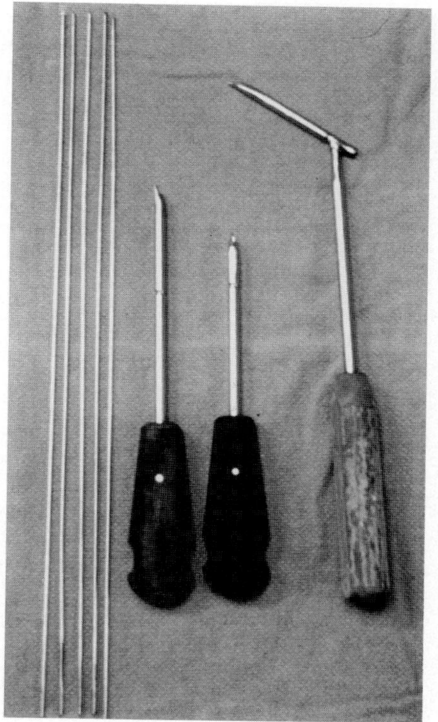

FIGURE 30-14. Instruments. Extra-long guidewires *(far left)* are necessary to penetrate the thick soft-tissue envelope surrounding the pelvis. Cannulated screwdrivers are used to create guidewire positioning devices with sharpened tips. The one at far right has an offset neck, to keep the surgeon's hand from under the fluoroscopic beam. (From: Starr AJ, Borer DS, Reinert CM. Technical aspects of limited open reduction and percutaneous screw fixation of fractures of the acetabulum. *Op Tech Orthop* July 2001, with permission.)

COMPLICATIONS

We noted three complications in a series of 21 patients treated with this technique (11). One young patient had a transient femoral nerve palsy. The modified pelvic reduction clamp passing underneath the iliacus and psoas muscles likely caused this. Tension on these muscles probably stretched the nerve. The femoral nerve lies anterior to the interval between these two muscles, and is at risk for injury during clamp placement down the quadrilateral plate. Fortunately, the nerve recovered, and the patient returned to his job as a construction worker.

Additionally, two elderly patients had minor losses of reduction after surgery. Both of these patients ambulated without assistive devices. Both patients went on to heal, and both had a good result. Because this technique probably sees the most use in elderly patients, it seems likely that loss of reduction is the most common complication encountered. The osteopenic bone that predisposes old patients to have these fractures in the first place is also the culprit in this frustrating setback.

ACKNOWLEDGMENTS

I would like to acknowledge my partners, Drake S. Borer and Charles Reinert, from UT Southwestern Medical Center in Dallas, and Alan L. Jones, from Shock Trauma in Baltimore. None of these techniques would have been possible without the efforts of these three men.

REFERENCES

1. Routt ML Jr, Kregor PJ, Simonian PT, et al. Early results of percutaneous iliosacral screws placed with the patient in the supine position. *J Orthop Trauma* 1995;9:207–214.
2. Routt ML Jr, Simonian PT, Mills WJ. Iliosacral screw fixation: early complications of the percutaneous technique. *J Orthop Trauma* 1997;11:584–589.
3. Starr AJ, Walter JC, Harris RW, et al. Percutaneous screw fixation of fractures of the iliac wing and fracture dislocations of the sacro-iliac joint (OTA types 61-B2.2 and 61-B2.3, or Young-Burgess "Lateral Compression Type II" pelvic fractures). *J Orthop Trauma* 2002;16:116–123.
4. Routt MLC, Simonian PT, Grujic L. The retrograde medullary superior pubic ramus screw for the treatment of anterior pelvic ring disruptions: a new technique. *J Orthop Trauma* 1995;9:35–44.
5. Gay SB, Sistrom C, Wang GJ, et al. Percutaneous screw fixation of acetabular fractures with CT guidance: preliminary results of a new technique. *AJR* 1992;158:819–822.
6. Parker PJ, Copeland C. Percutaneous fluoroscopic screw fixation of acetabular fractures. *Injury* 1997;28:597–600.
7. Starr AJ, Reinert CM, Jones AL. *Percutaneous fixation of fractures of the acetabulum.* Paper presented at Surgery of the Pelvis and Acetabulum: Third International Consensus. Pittsburgh, October 5–11, 1996.
8. Zura RD, Kahler DM. A transverse acetabular nonunion treated with computer-assisted percutaneous internal fixation. A case report. *J Bone Joint Surg (Am)* 2000;82:219–224.
9. Brown GA, Willis MC, Firoozbakhsh K, et al. Computed tomography image-guided surgery in complex acetabular fractures. *Clin Orthop Rel Res* 2000;(370):219–226.
10. Starr AJ, Reinert CM, Jones AL. Percutaneous fixation of the columns of the acetabulum: a new technique. *J Orthop Trauma* 1998;12:51–58.
11. Starr AJ, Borer DS, Reinert CM, et al. *Early results and complications following limited open reduction and percutaneous screw fixation of displaced fractures of the acetabulum.* Paper presented at the Orthopaedic Trauma Association 16th Annual Meeting. San Antonio, TX, October 12–14, 2000.
12. Letournel E, Judet R. *Fractures of the acetabulum.* New York: Springer-Verlag, 1981.
13. Helfet DL, Borrelli J Jr, DiPasquale T, et al. Stabilization of acetabular fractures in elderly patients. *J Bone Joint Surg (Am)* 1992;74:753–765.
14. Templeman DC, Olson S, Moed BR, et al. Surgical treatment of acetabular fractures. *Instruct Course Lect* 1999;48:481–496.

PART D. TECHNIQUES OF REDUCTION AND FIXATION FOR ACETABULAR FRACTURES: OPEN METHODS

31

TECHNIQUES OF OPEN REDUCTION AND FIXATION OF ACETABULAR FRACTURES

JEFFREY W. MAST

INTRODUCTION

Fracture reduction is always the challenging step of bone surgery. Knowledge of the mechanism of the fracture, the region of the bone fractured, as well as the muscles attached to the various fragments aid the surgeon in understanding residual displacements.

As with long bones, fractures of the pelvis involving the acetabulum also have characteristic displacements, depending on the fracture type. This chapter deals with techniques of reduction that are of proven utility.

POSTERIOR WALL FRACTURES

Posterior wall fractures are approached through a posterior approach. The Kocher-Langenbeck exposure is most commonly used. A Judet table is used and the patient is placed in the prone position in the methods taught by Letournel.

Posterior wall fractures can be very demanding technically. They are frequently not a single fragment, and the comminution may be intraarticular or extraarticular. Large wall fragments may be split or fissured longitudinally, making both reduction and fixation more difficult.

Because of the close relationship of the sciatic nerve to the external rotators of the hip, the difficulty encountered in the reduction of the wall fracture is the lack of safe space to use standard clamps to secure the reduction while fixation is applied.

In addition, the ascending branch of the medial femoral circumflex artery is in close relationship to the tendon of the obturator externus muscle on its way to the femoral head. It courses proximally, diving under the obturator internus tendon on its way to piercing the posterior capsule. Thus, the main blood supply to the head may be injured unless special attention is used in the dissection.

Consequently, special instruments are necessary to reduce the displaced wall fragments. The "piccador" is a ball-spiked tipped rod that can be used to push against the fractured wall, forcing the fragments into reduction and holding them there until a Kirschner wire can be drilled across the fragment to fix it in the reduced position.

Instruments that are helpful also are pointed reduction forceps of various shapes and angulations. In addition, clamps whose limbs may be attached to screw heads inserted into the fracture fragments are frequently valuable. The Farabeuf clamp and pelvic reduction forceps are commonly used examples of these devices (Fig. 31-1).

In my opinion, one of the most valuable reduction tools is the plate used as a clamp (Fig 31-2). This technique is particularly useful because there is limited space to use a clamp. In general, a short three-hole plate is used. It is attached to the intact bone through a screw placed through the second hole, the empty hole of the plate. Its projecting end is adjusted so that it overlaps the displaced fragment, tightening the screw, causing the plate to be lagged to the bone. The end of the plate overlapping the displaced fragment clamps the fragment at the same level as the intact bone. Sometimes a small instrument, called a dental pick, is needed to toggle

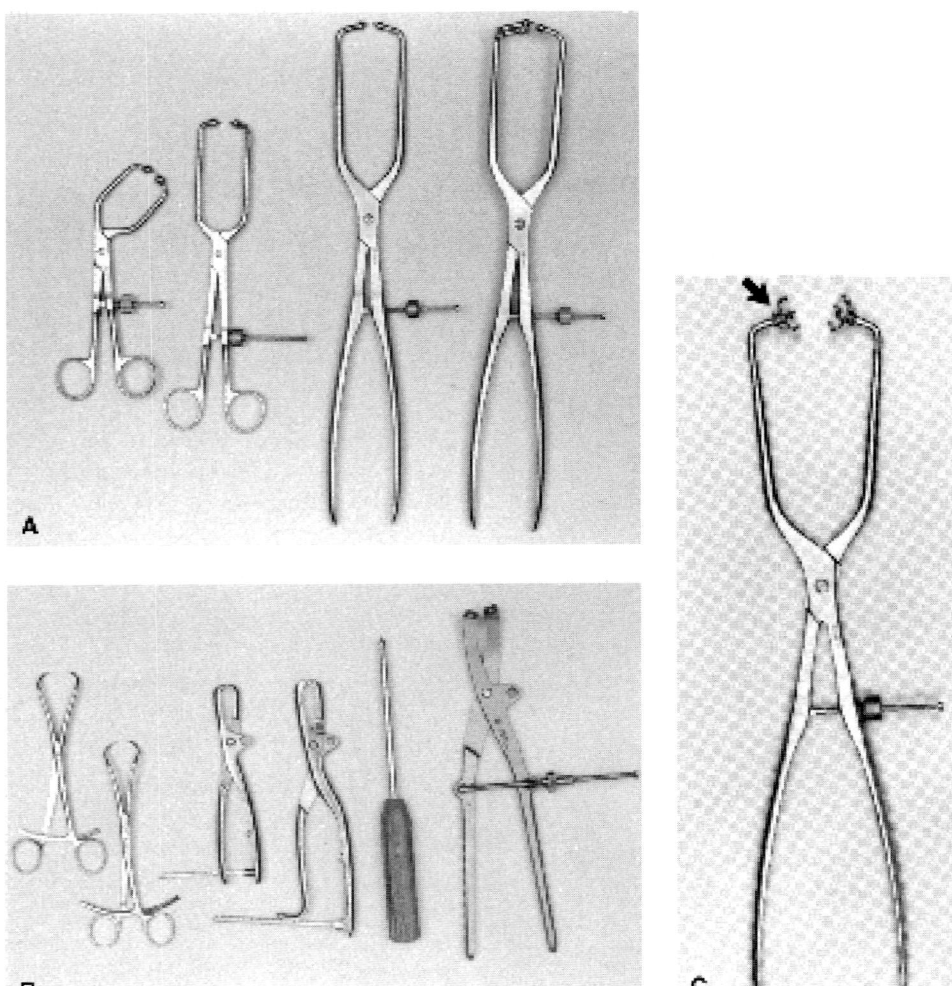

FIGURE 31-1. A–C: Special clamps and the ball spike pusher to help with reduction in the acetabulum. Clamps include the large and small offset clamp, the single-pronged and double-pronged clamp to fit over the iliac crest, pointed reduction clamps, Farabeuf clamps in two sizes, and pelvic reduction clamps. Note also the ball spike pusher, which is invaluable in reducing small fragments of the acetabular wall and for pushing on the iliac crest. All of these clamps and the ball spike pusher can be fitted with a spiked disc *(black arrow)* that fits over the ball to prevent the spike from sinking into osteoporotic bone.

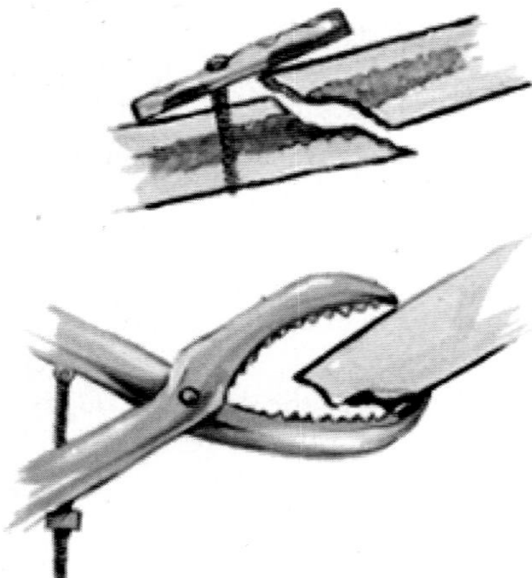

FIGURE 31-2. The plate as a clamp: Note how the plate overlapping the near side of an oblique fracture acts as one jaw of the clamp and the one on the far side of the fracture acts as the other jaw. The screw in the plate acts as the threaded spindle to tighten the jaws.

the fragment as the pressure is applied by the end of the plate. This helps to facilitate the fit of the fragment as the reduction force is applied by the end of the plate.

Reduction of the fragments is influenced by the position of the hip when posterior wall fragments have labral and capsular attachments. *Hip extension and external rotation* usually are required to replace the fragments back in their beds. One has to remember that capsular attachments that we desire to preserve are influenced by the same forces following reduction and fixation. Accordingly, if the fragments are not well fixed, flexion and internal rotation may redisplace these fragments by pulling them out from under their fixation. The reduction may be lost, and—just as important to the outcome—the bared fixation may now contact the femoral head cartilage, causing wear and eventual destruction of the articular surface.

Most fractures of the posterior wall are associated with posterior dislocations of the hip. Letournel has pointed out that what happens to the capsule of the hip joint at the time of fracture of the posterior wall, associated with a posterior dislocation of the hip, has an effect on the displacements found at surgery.

Impaction of the articular segment is unlikely when the capsule is ruptured in association with a dislocation and a posterior wall fracture. However, when the capsule is still attached to the displaced wall fragment, there is a high possibility of finding marginal impaction inside the socket.

Marginal impaction complicates the reduction of the posterior wall fragment (Fig. 31-3). Before reducing the wall, the impacted articular surface must be accurately disimpacted and the fragments reoriented in their anatomic position using the reduced femoral head as a template.

Restoration of the joint surface can be difficult, depending on the degree of impaction. The technique involves taking a small osteotome several millimeters above the impacted fragment, and driving the blade of the osteotome into the compressed cancellous bone behind the fragment. It is necessary to undercut the impacted fragment along its entire length. Gently, the impacted fragment is bent into its proper orientation using a curved osteotome as a lever. The

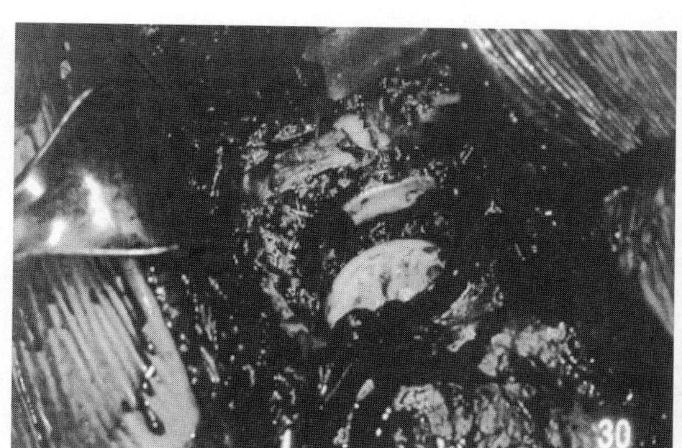
A

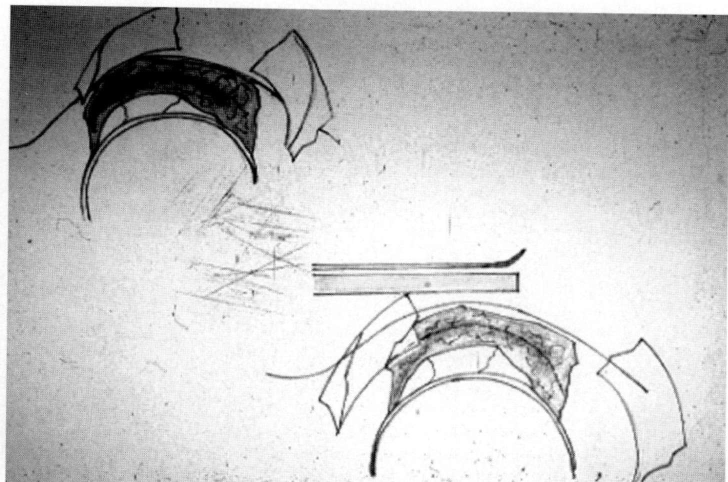
B,C

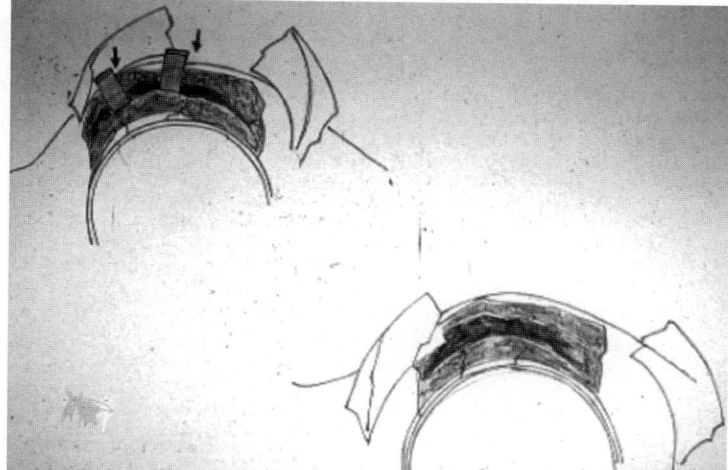
D,E

FIGURE 31-3. A: Typical impaction of the posterior articular surface seen in posterior wall fractures with an intact capsule attached to the wall fragment (From Ref. 1). **B:** Marginal Impaction. Small osteotomes, such as Lambotte's, may be used to cut above the area of impaction as illustrated. **D,E:** The osteotomes are worked above the impaction prizing it down using the femoral head as a template. This creates a gap above the reduced impaction.

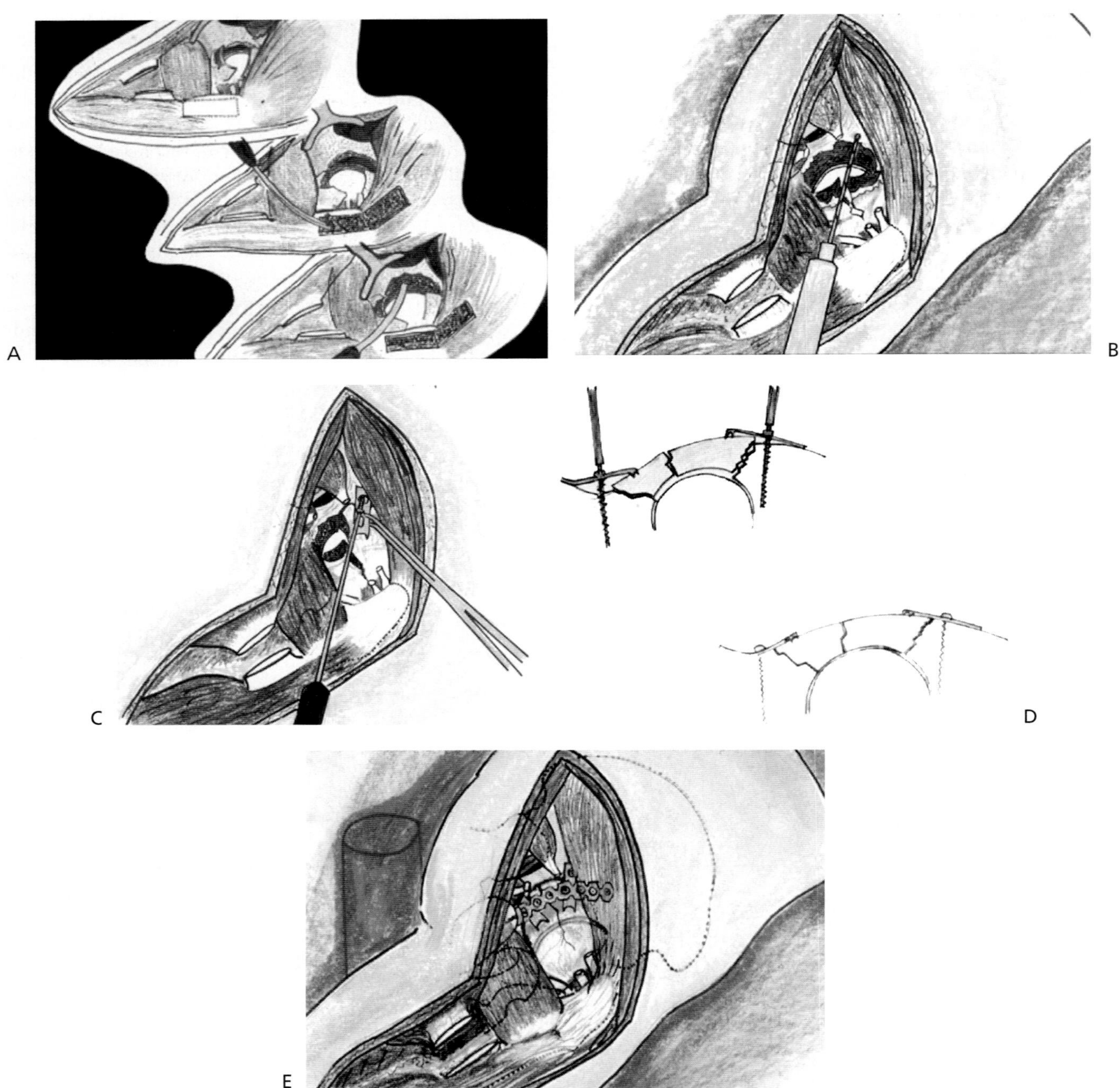

FIGURE 31-4. A: Bone graft may be obtained from the trochanter, which is windowed, the cancellous bone is harvested and used to fill the defect above the reduced impaction. **B:** Temporary fixation is then carried out using a plate as a clamp. **C:** As the screw is tightened, the plate clamps down on wall fragment providing provisional stabilization of the wall fragment. **D:** *(top)* Use of a spring plate to reduce *(bottom)* posterior wall fragments. **E:** The buttress plate is contoured and placed over the "spring plates," reinforcing the fixation of the posterior wall.

object is to slowly bend the fragment into position without breaking it. The bone graft then is impacted into the secondary void created by articular disimpaction.

In another instance, with posterior dislocation of the femoral head, the posterior wall fracture with its intact capsular attachments may result in the wall fragments becoming incarcerated in the socket. The posterior fragments are displaced posteriorly with the femoral head, but become anterior in position relative to the head, which is fully displaced into the dislocation cavity, because they are tethered by the capsule.

An intraarticular incarceration occurs with the reduction of the dislocation as the fragments are pushed into the socket by the force of reduction of the femoral head. The capsular attachments remain intact, but now exist between the interior of the socket and the "reduced" femoral head. The capsular attachments to these fragments are what make their management difficult, because extracting these fragments from the joint without re-dislocating the hip is difficult. With the patient prone on the Judet table, distraction forces can be applied through the leg that subluxate the ball in the socket. This allows removal of the incarcerated fragments, although they may be difficult to extract even with this advantage.

As a general rule, small fragments may be fixed with spring plates after reduction, and posterior wall fragments must be buttressed by a plate fixed to the proximal and distal aspects of the intact posterior pelvic bone (Fig. 31-4). This buttress plate must make solid contact with the wall fragment and protect it from redisplacement. The screws must be oriented so as to not enter the joint. This can be facilitated by a guide pin placed before reduction in the intact bone, which defines the medial extent and orientation of the joint.

Another method sometimes employed is to drill the hole in the wall fragment for lag screw fixation prior to reduction. The location of the drill hole can be verified as central in the fragment and its extraarticular orientation confirmed. In this way the extraarticular position of the screw can be assured by examining the fractured surface of the wall fragment.

Actually, this is a situation in which there is an advantage to have the patient free in a lateral position, because the head may be readily dislocated. The "trochanteric flip" is the most favorable surgical approach (Fig. 31-5). In this case, the fragments and their capsular attachments may be extracted from the joint easily (Fig. 31-6).

Posterior Column Fractures

Posterior column fractures can include transitional forms between extensive posterior wall and pure posterior column.

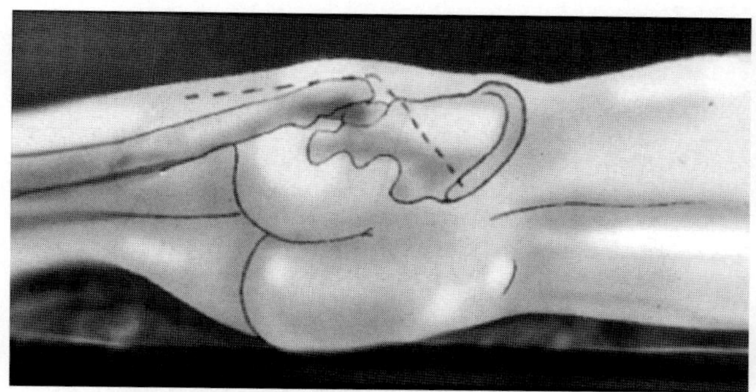
A

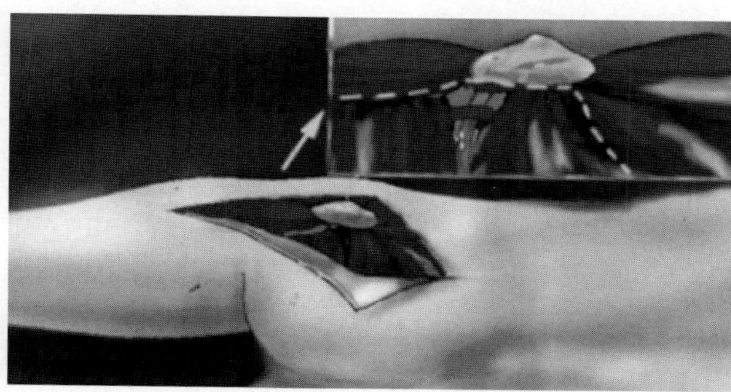
B

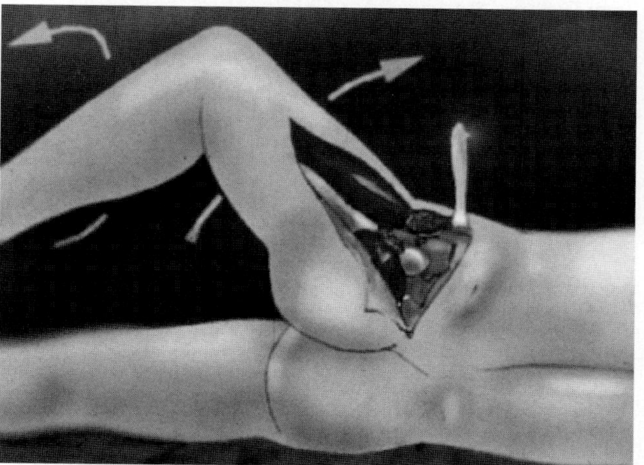
C

FIGURE 31-5. The trochanteric flip technique. **A:** A Kocher-Langenbeck or Gibson skin incision is made. The patient is stabilized in the lateral position. **B:** After incising the aponeurosis of the tensor fascia lata and retracting it posteriorly, the posterior aspect of the vastus lateralis and gluteus minimus is mobilized from posterior to anterior after incising the fascia. **C:** A trochanteric osteotomy is made from posterior to anterior and the mobilized muscles, along with the trochanter, are displaced anteriorly by flexing, abducting, and externally rotating the leg. The anterior capsule is opened and the hip dislocated anteriorly by external rotation.

As Letournel has described, column fractures occur in the frontal plane, and the characteristic posterior column fracture consists of a fracture that is high (at the level of or including the angle of the greater sciatic notch), and may be associated with an additional fracture of the posterior wall. The column fracture usually is posterior medially displaced and rotated about the vertical axis inwardly.

The surgical approach is posterior, and the position of the patient is prone. The Judet table is beneficial; the Farabeuf clamps as well as pelvic reduction forceps (also called Jungbluth clamps) are valuable. They may be attached by screws such that one jaw is attached to the posterior column fragment and one jaw to the intact posterior pelvis. In addition, a Shantz screw with a T-handle is inserted into the column fragment (usually the ischium), and used as a lever to control the rotation. The pelvic reduction forceps can be used to distract or compress and/or to displace the column anteriorly or posteriorly. Control of the posterior column reduction is confirmed by inserting a finger into the greater sciatic notch and palpating the oblique fracture line as the Schantz pin is manipulated, varying the rotation of the fragment.

The surgical problem that presents is how to obtain preliminary fixation so that the reduction aides may be removed from the bone to allow definitive fixation. This is another situation in which a three-hole reconstruction plate may be used as a clamp to provide temporary fixation. After approximating the fractured bone surfaces with the pelvic reduction clamps, the plate is attached to the unstable fragment with a single screw. The edge of the plate is oriented to overlap the stable part of the bone. By tightening the screw, the plate end presses down on the intact portion, preventing further displacement of the posterior column. The bulky reduction clamps may be removed. The plate controls the fragment, even though no definitive fixation has been applied. Fine tuning of the position of the fragment is still

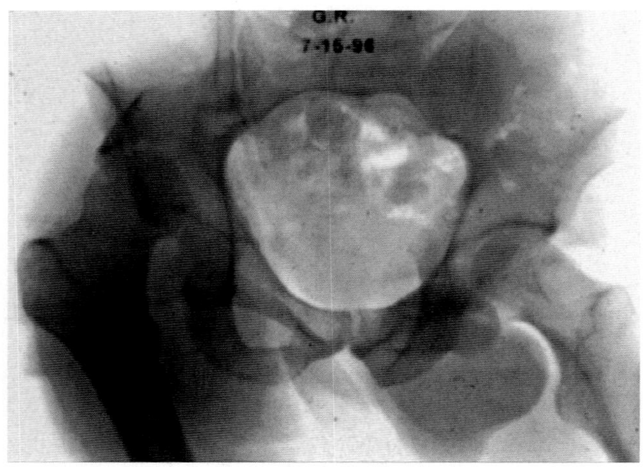

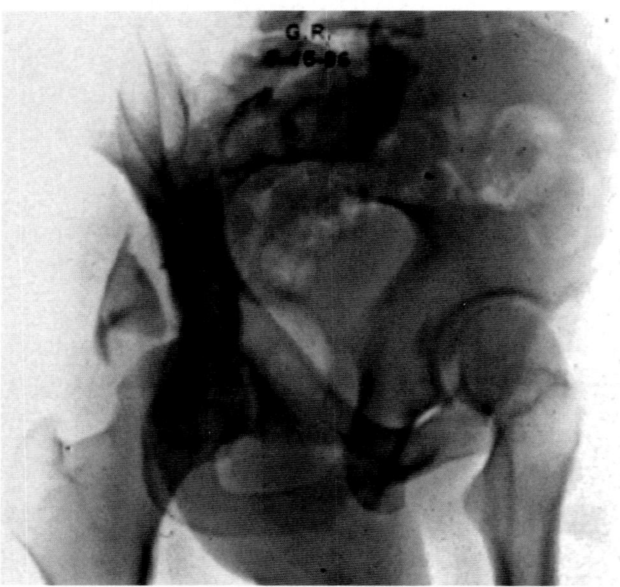

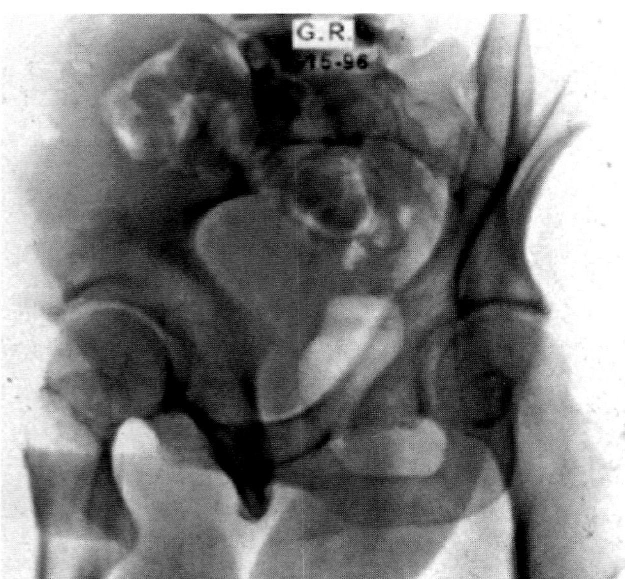

FIGURE 31-6. Case of posterior dislocation using trochanteric flip approach. **A:** Posterior wall fracture that is very superior in location. Note the decrease in the shadow of the source. **B:** This is a good indication for the trochanteric flip surgical approach. **C:** Iliac oblique view of same case.

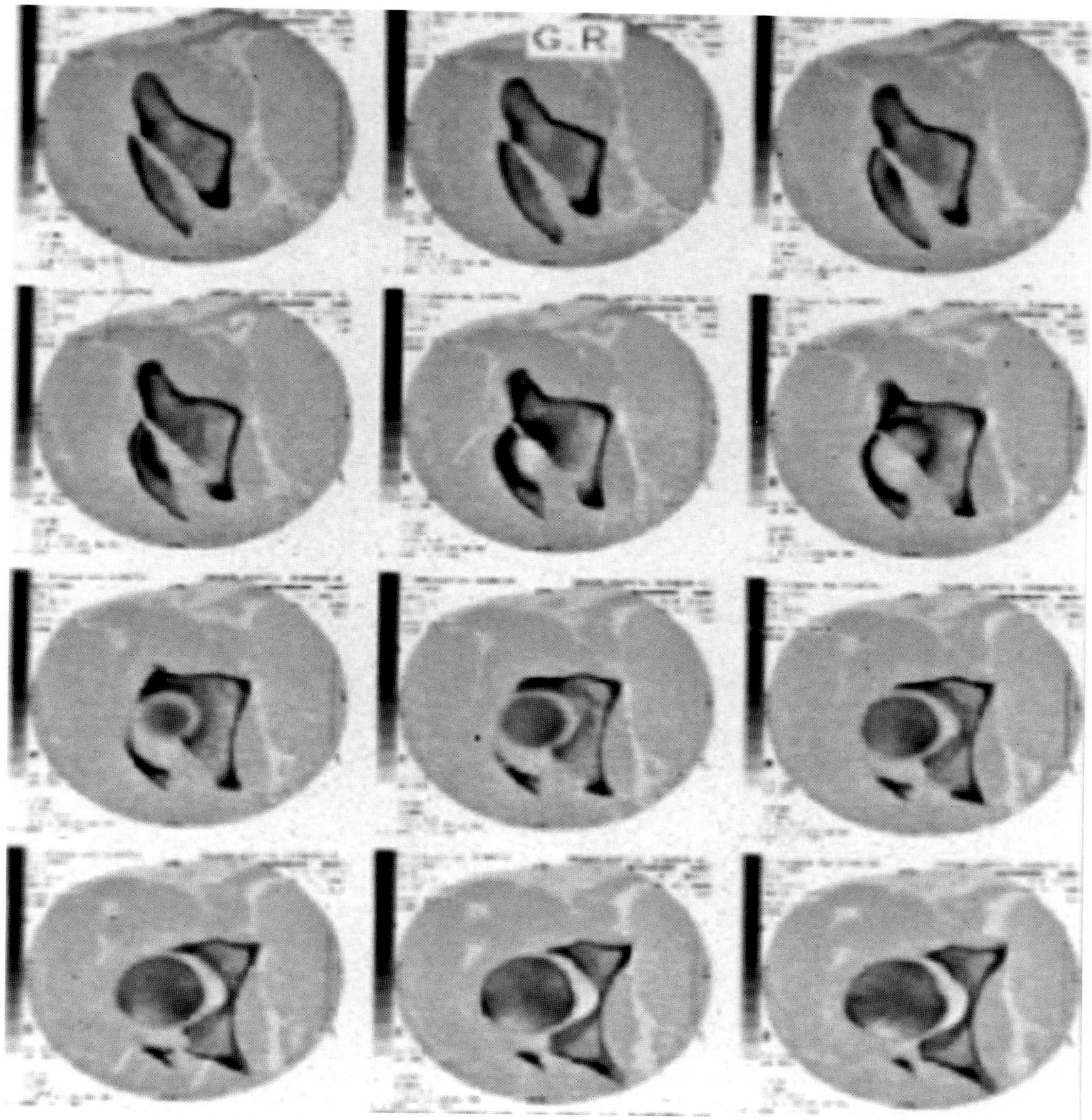

FIGURE 31-6. ***(continued)*** **D:** Computed tomography scan showing very superior location of the wall fracture in roof of the joint.

(Figure continues)

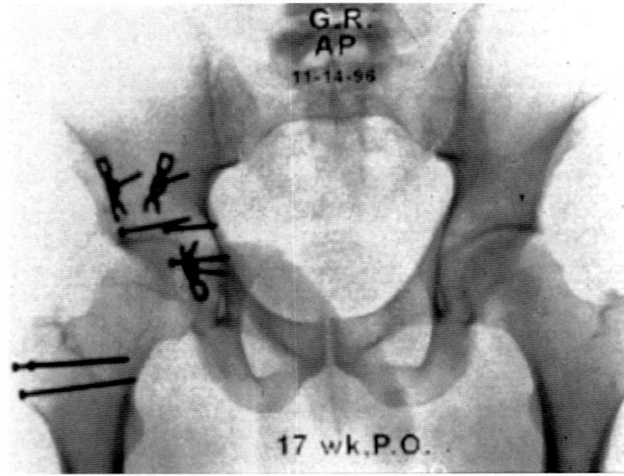

FIGURE 31-6. ***(continued)*** **E:** Fixation with multiple small spring plates and lag screws. **F:** Postoperative iliac oblique view. **G:** Postoperative obturator oblique view.

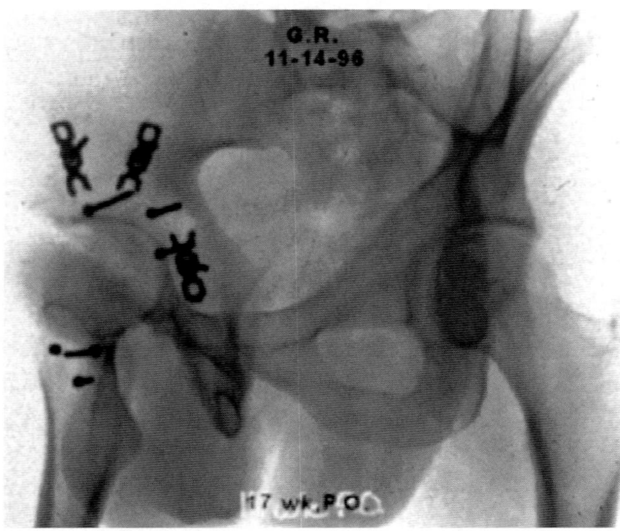

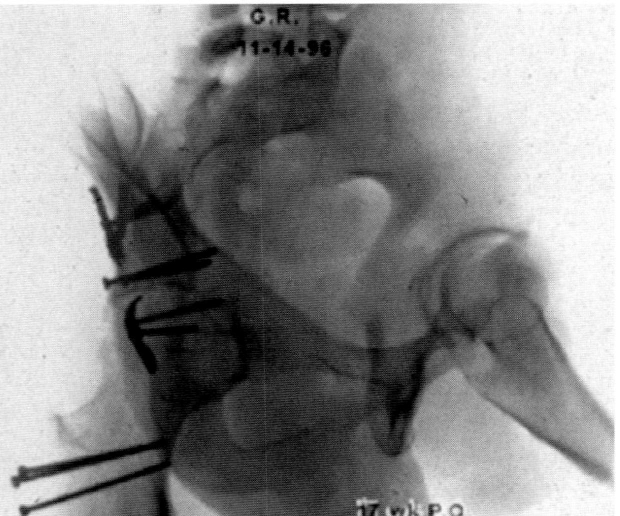

possible because of this. When reduction is anatomic, the definitive fixation may be achieved with a well-contoured plate that crosses the main fracture line of the posterior column, the screws of which fix the oblique fracture line across the quadrilateral plate by passing from posterior to anterior.

When posterior column fractures are associated with posterior wall fractures (Fig. 31-7), the area of contact between the major main fragments may be decidedly decreased. Notwithstanding, the posterior column must be first brought into reduction (Fig. 31-8). The reduction can be confirmed by inspecting the intraarticular surface within the joint through the defect in the wall; then the wall fragment is fit into the remaining defect and fixed with screws. The technique described in the preceding becomes even more helpful in these circumstances, and may be augmented by the use of 2-mm Kirschner wires for temporary fixation. The ball-spiked pusher is useful to manipulate the wall and hold it closely approximated until it can be fixed by screws and buttressed by a plate that also fixes the posterior column fracture.

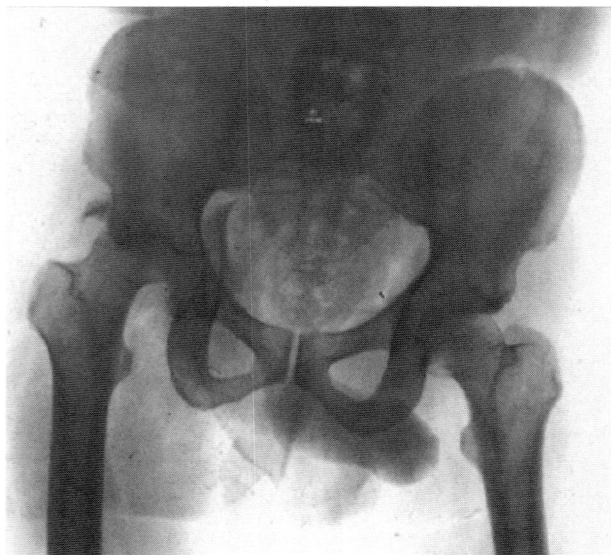

FIGURE 31-7. Posterior column–associated posterior wall fracture associated with a dislocation of the femoral head.

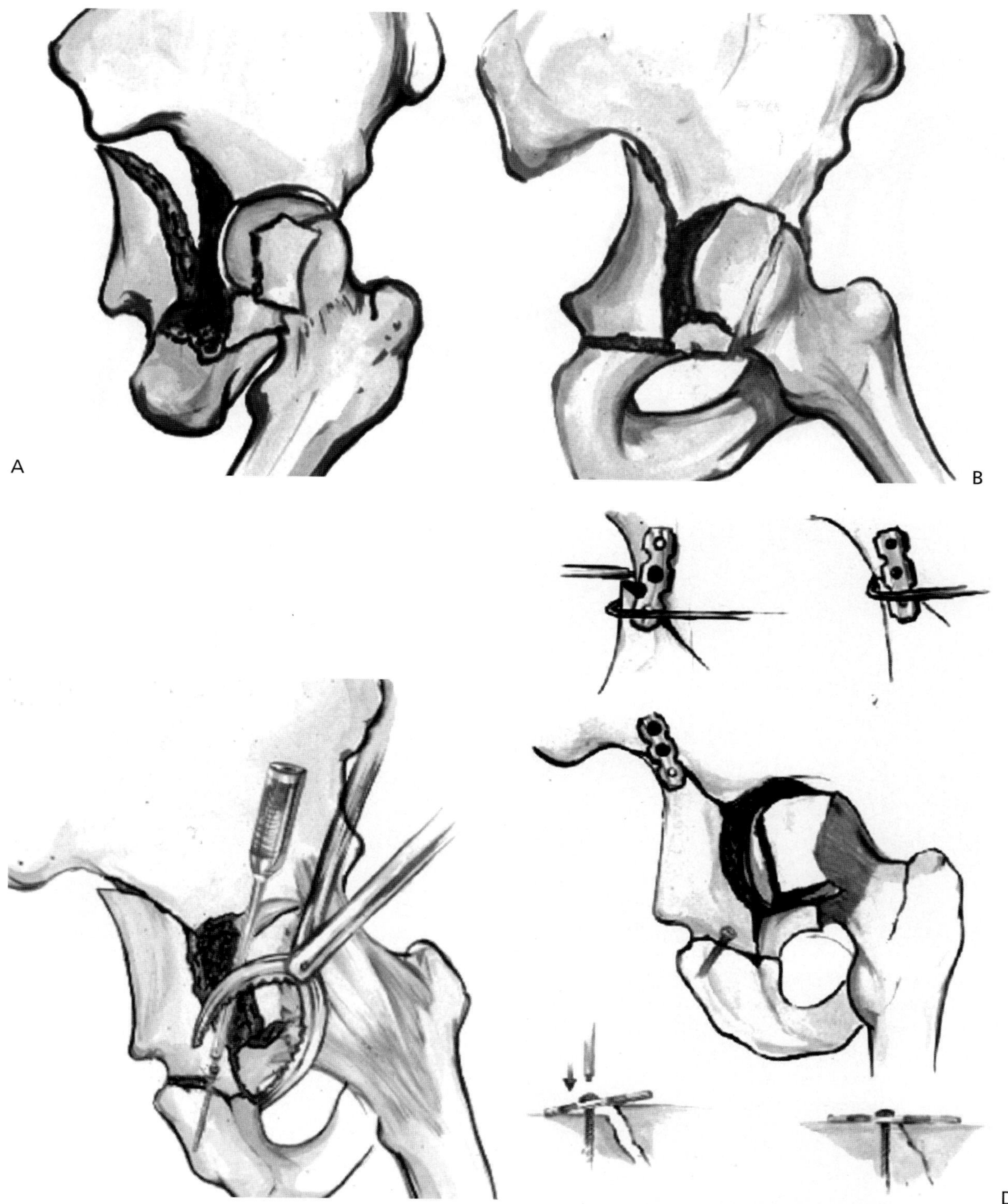

FIGURE 31-8. Posterior column, posterior wall technique of reduction and fixation. **A:** Transitional fracture extended posterior wall. Posterior wall–associated posterior column with femoral head dislocation. **B:** Drawing of a transitional fracture pattern between extended posterior wall, posterior column–associated posterior wall. **C:** Preliminary reduction of the difficult inferior fracture with pointed reduction clamps and fixation of the gain achieved with a screw. **D:** Reduction of the upper end of the fracture may be facilitated by a small three-hole plate that pushed the fracture into reduction. It is attached by a screw to the fragment displaced away from the surgeon.

(Figure continues)

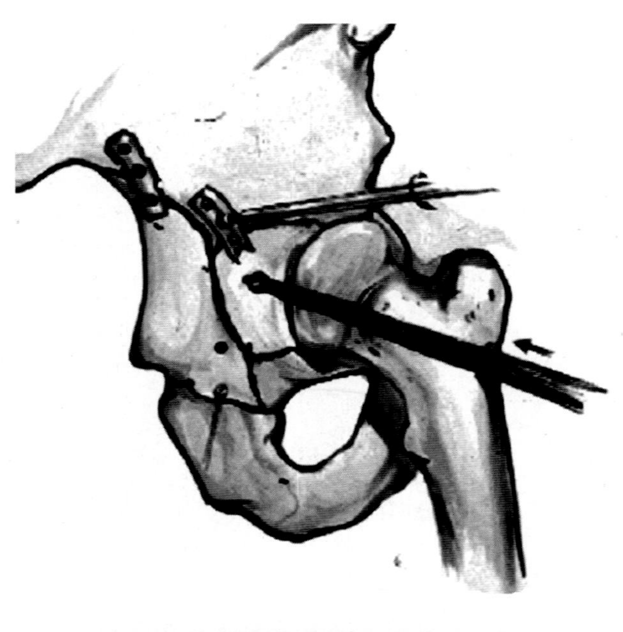
E

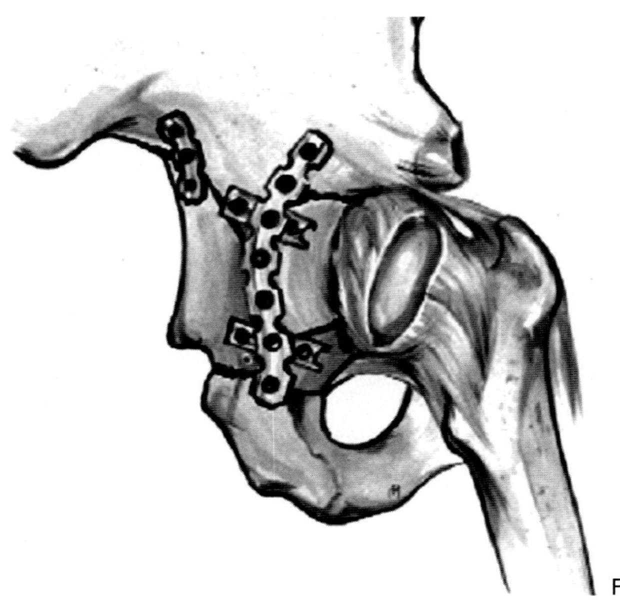
F

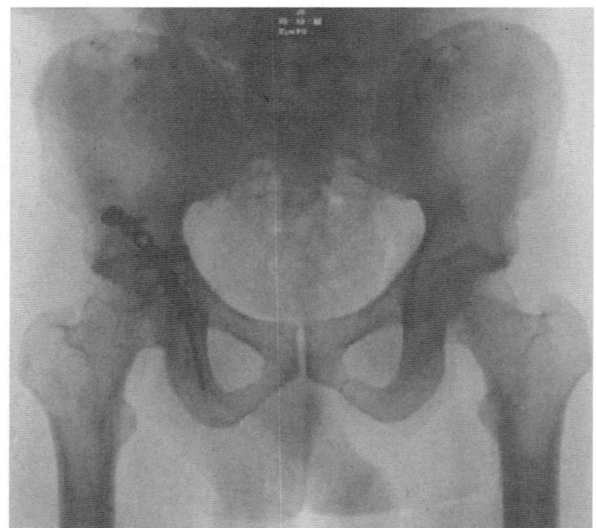
G

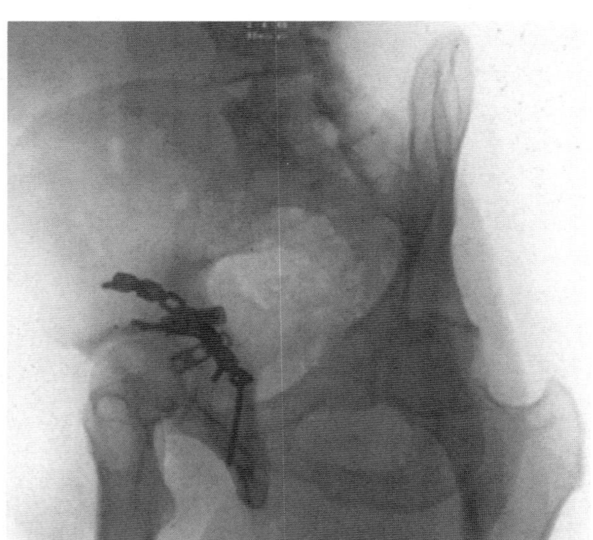
H

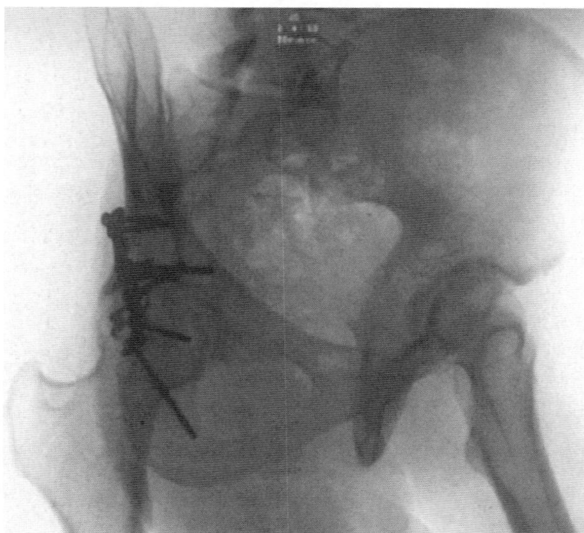
I

FIGURE 31-8. ***(continued)*** **E:** The piccador is used to hold the wall fragment into position as a spring plate provides preliminary fixation. **F:** Final fixation including buttress plate along the posterior column overlying the two spring plates. **G:** Fixation of the posterior column posterior wall fracture similar to the illustration, including a posterior buttress plate and two small spring plates. **H:** Iliac oblique. **I:** Obturator oblique.

Anterior Wall Fracture

An anterior wall fracture essentially is a segmental fracture of the anterior column that includes the anterior segment of the acetabulum. Externally, it is comprised of the anterior lip and varying amount of the quadrilateral plate. The anterior articular facet and a variable portion of the acetabular fossa are involved on the inner surface.

The surgical approach used is the anterior ilioinguinal, or sometimes the anterior Smith-Petersen approach. The difficulties presented with this fracture are twofold. First, although itself a rare fracture pattern, it is most common in elderly persons, frequently as a result of relatively low-energy violence. The bone involved commonly is osteoporotic. Second, the fracture lines exit in the region below the femoral vessels and iliopsoas muscle. Further, the extension of the fracture frequently involves the quadrilateral plate, which descends into the true pelvis from the pelvic brim. These circumstances lead to difficulty in exposure and visualization of the fracture lines and its bony landmarks.

Reduction of the fracture becomes difficult under these circumstances. The femoral head is dislocated anterior-medially. Frequently, there is a medial impaction of the medial portion of the roof of the acetabulum.

The Judet table may be very advantageous in fractures in which there is marginal impaction. The head can be centered under the roof using a combination of longitudinal traction and lateral traction applied through the trochanter. This may be verified by the use of the image intensifier. The displacement in wall fracture can be exaggerated and the marginal impaction can be treated through the displaced wall fragment using the reduced femoral head as a template for the reduction of the impacted articular fragments. The disimpacted fragments are supported by cancellous bone graft, which may be combined with demineralized bone matrix to give it a puttylike consistency to facilitate its application to the defects.

The wall fracture must be reduced following successful reduction of the impaction, with the femoral head centered below the roof of the remaining articular segment of the intact anterior column. Of course, there are clamps available for this purpose. The angled fibular clamps and the pointed reduction forceps are well adapted for use along the pelvic brim. Rectangular pointed reduction forceps may be used between the quadrilateral plate and the unbroken pelvis. One point is placed on the quadrilateral plate surface, while the other is placed on the external surface of the bone just lateral to the anterior inferior iliac spine. The wall fragment can be reduced in this way.

However, the plate that must be used to buttress the fragment cannot be applied while the clamps holding the reduction are in location, because they interfere with the optimal plate position on the pelvic brim.

Consequently, it is more effective to precontour a pelvic reconstruction plate and slide it under the vessels and iliopsoas, centered along the pelvic brim. Next, it is screwed to the body of the pubis distal to the exit of the distal fracture line, and affixed with screws along the pelvic brim on the proximal side of the fracture. Tightening the screws exerts a clamping effect on the wall fracture. Because there are no screws as yet fixing the wall fragment, minor changes in the reduction can be carried out with a ball-spiked pusher, or the mentioned clamps. When reduction of the wall is satisfactory, definitive screws may be applied through the plate, completing the stabilization. When the quadrilateral plate is a separate fragment or is comminuted, longer screws may be needed to fix or buttress this thin bone plate. Sometimes the screws must pass very medial in the acetabular fossa. Occasionally, a thin plate (e.g., a one-third tubular plate), is prepared by flattening it between two hammers and then bending it acutely so that one limb projects beneath the pelvic brim plate and one limb projects against the quadrilateral plate to buttress it.

Anterior Column Fractures

This fracture group requires an anterior approach; the ileoinguinal approach is required because the fracture extends to the pubic symphysis and the ischiopubic ramus. The fracture of the anterior column is displaced anteriorly and medially. Usually there is a fracture of the quadrilateral plate if the femoral head penetrates the pelvis, and the deformity of the acetabulum is such that the pelvic brim is displaced anteriorly and rotated externally around its long axis. To the contrary, the quadrilateral plate fragment is rotated internally. This leaves a significant gap in the fracture just inferior to the pelvic brim. The head is easily visible in the fracture deformity. Mears has called this the "barroom door" deformity, although it is more akin to the swing doors depicted in old-fashioned Western saloons.

In actuality, the displacement is easier to appreciate in the region of the joint. To varying degrees the fracturing forces may dissipate as the fracture propagates more proximally. In high fractures of the anterior column, at the level of the iliac crest, the displacement may be minimal and the fracture line incomplete. In such circumstances there may be plastic deformation of the bone; the first step of reduction may be to "complete" the partial fracture in the wing.

The Judet table is useful in these situations. We usually need longitudinal traction, combined with lateral traction through a stout Schantz screw inserted through the trochanter into the femoral neck. This combination helps to centralize the femoral head in the remaining portion of the joint.

Some hip flexion can be added to facilitate the exposure. This relaxes the psoas muscle and allows exposure of the internal iliac fossa to the pubic symphysis. Again, plate application is helpful as a reduction tool. A short reconstruction plate may be placed with a screw in the intact posterior portion of the anterior column fragment. The short plate position should be selected with anticipation for the location of the pelvic brim plate that is to be used for definitive fixation. The terminal portion of the plate is allowed to overlap the displaced proximal portion of the anterior column. Any residual shortening can be eliminated with combined traction and the use of a 7-mm Hohmann as a "pry bar" in the apex of the proximal fracture line. Additionally, if the fragment is large enough, a "joystick" (a 4.5-mm Schantz screw) may be inserted into the fragment in the area of the anterior superior spine and used to derotate the displaced column fragment.

The screw in the plate is tightened when the length has been regained and the rotation and curvature of the column approximated. Powered by the tightening of the screw, the empty overlapping plate end, like the jaw of a clamp, presses the proximal fragment end into an improved relationship with the major pelvic fragment.

Small corrections are easy following provisional stabilization of the anterior column. Either they may be made with pointed reduction clamps used distally along the pubic ramus, or the "setting" screw may be loosened slightly and a small hook used to improve the rotation of the fragment, regaining the proper curvature of the pelvic brim. After the reduction is improved, the set screw in the plate is tightened again, clamping the end of the plate once more on the proximal end of the anterior column fracture.

Once the column fracture is reduced, definitive fixation is provided by the application of a pelvic reconstruction plate. The plate must be accurately contoured to the pelvic brim.

The essential fixation screws of the pelvis start coming into play with anterior column fractures. These fix the broken anterior column fracture to the unbroken posterior column fracture.

Four long screws that traverse the acetabular trabecular system are essential to the surgeon. These screws should be practiced on plastic pelvic bones until their orientation and relationships to the landmarks around the acetabulum are second nature.

1. *Anterior anterior column to posterior anterior column.* The core hole for this screw is started just medial to the center of the anterior inferior iliac spine and is directed in a posterior direction hugging the inside curvature of the innominate bone. The screw is long and exits in the vicinity of the posterior superior iliac spine.

2. *Anterior column to posterior column.* The core hole for this screw is started along the pelvic brim, through the reconstruction plate or just lateral to it, at distance of 2 cm lateral to the margin of the SI joint and at a level of the anterior superior iliac spine. The hole is drilled in the direction of or slightly anterior to the ischial spine.

3. *Posterior anterior column to anterior anterior column.* This screw is not needed to fix a pure anterior column fracture, but is used frequently to fix the anterior portion of a "T," or transverse fracture. The core hole is started on the posterior slope of the rounded prominence of the anterior pillar of the acetabulum, about a thumb-breadth above the roof of the joint. The drill is oriented toward the inside of the inside concave curvature of the pelvic brim and aimed at the distal body of the pubis.

4. *Posterior anterior column to posterior column.* This screw is rarely useful because it is only easily accomplished on the extended iliofemoral approach. The core hole is made from the external surface of the external iliac wing to the posterior column. To accomplish this, the drill hole has to be started with the point almost perpendicular to the entry surface. Once the hole is started, the drill is brought almost tangent to the external iliac surface and in the direction of the iliac spine.

Obviously, many screw directions are needed to solve the problems of fracture fixation under the circumstances of different fracture configuration in various anatomic regions of the acetabulum. The osseous anatomy must be understood to be successful (1).

Before moving on, it should be recognized that many high anterior column fractures are associated with a fracture fragment that comprises the superior wall of the acetabulum. This fragment actually extends quite far posteriorly, but not to the full extent of the posterior acetabular surface or the greater sciatic notch.

This superior wall fracture is interesting because the displacement usually is greatest along its spiked tip away from the joint. That the acetabular labrum is intact maintains the peripheral relationship with the edge of the acetabulum. This fact helpfully gives a solution to a difficult situation, because reduction proximally along the extraarticular fracture lines may be relied on to produce reduction at the joint surface.

How can we reduce the superior wall fracture associated with the anterior column fracture? Most important, the fragment is found with high anterior column fractures. The fracture line that breaks the crest may be traced externally to the apex of the superior wall fracture. The periosteal elevator encounters the cancellous surface of the displaced superior wall fragment because of the displacement of the fragment. Dissection above the cortical surface of the displaced fracture allows exposure of the four fracture edges. Manipulation of the displacement sometimes involves opening or separating the anterior column fragment and correcting the displacements with a dental pick. Alternatively, a small Hohmann retractor tip can be inserted between the fracture surfaces and used as a lever. In this way it should be possible to fit the chevron fragment into its negative defect with a pointed reduction forceps. If this can be accomplished, the articular reduction also should be accurate, because the acetabular labrum is intact and attached to the periphery of the articular fragment.

Fixation of this fragment can be accomplished with a spring plate attached to the intact wing fragment, by a lag screw placed from inside the internal iliac fossa to the external iliac surface, or percutaneously from the anterior fragment to the intact ilium behind the anterior column fracture.

Transverse Fractures

As discussed, transverse fractures can be divided into transtectal, juxtatectal, and infratectal, depending on the relationship of the transverse fracture line to the roof of the acetabulum. This influences the surgical approach, which in turn determines which instruments can be used for reduction.

Letournel carefully described the displacement of the transverse fractures. He described two major displacements of the ischiopubic segment. It is all mitigated by the fact that the pubic symphysis is attached to the ischiopubic fragment. From the reference of a vertical axis through the pubic symphysis, there is an inward rotation, which is greater posterior than anterior, and appears to be an inward rotation of the ischiopubic segment on the anterior-posterior (AP) projection. About an axis more horizontal, from the posterior point of fracture in the greater sciatic notch to the pubic symphysis, the pelvic brim is tilted inward and the ischial tuberosity is tilted outward. The pubic symphysis may be abnormally distorted because of these displacements. Likewise, there may be a contrary rotation of the iliac fragment such that it is rotated outward and associated with an inferior disruption of the SI joint. The femoral head may appear dislocated between the two fragments in a "central" or medial direction in such a case.

Reduction Techniques

The patient is operated on the Judet table in the prone position in the instance of a juxtatectal- or infratectal-transverse fracture. The Kocher-Langenbeck surgical approach is used. Pelvic reduction clamps (Fig. 31-9A), a Schantz screw with a "T-handled" chuck (Fig. 31-9B), and a small three-holed pelvic reconstruction plate are useful instruments.

After fracture exposure, the pelvic reduction forceps are applied to the two fragments such that each leg of the clamp is attached to each fragment by means of a 4.5-mm screw (Fig. 31-10). Anticipation is required in order that the screws are in proper orientation such that the fracture fragments are in approximately in the same planar orientation when the clamp is applied and the screws tightened.

A 4.5- or 5-mm Schantz screw is inserted into the ischium, at or just proximal to the tuberosity (Fig. 31-11A,B) parallel to the frontal plane and posterior to the proximal femur. With these instruments in place, gentle distraction of the transverse fracture line is carried out using the clamp in a distraction mode. The fracture surfaces are cleaned, and the rotation can be adjusted using the Shantz screw. Control of the rotation of a transverse fracture is obtained by inserting the finger through the greater sciatic notch and palpating the fracture line as it courses the quadrilateral surface. The displacement can be influenced either through pushing or pulling on the Shantz screw (Fig. 31-11C,D). These offsets can also be eliminated by the force exerted through the screw fixing the pelvic reduction clamp to the fragments. This is particularly true for the leg on the ischiopubic fragment. If the screw in the limb of the clamp on the "intact" iliac fragment is snugged down, then tightening the screw in the leg of the clamp on the ischiopubic fragment elevates the fragment and improves the displacement. In addition, small angulations can be produced and the reduction can be further improved by rocking or torquing the clamp.

Once more, however, there is little room for additional fixation devices. There is little space to accomplish the definitive fixation of plate and screws with the clamps in place.

This is another situation in which a plate used as a clamp may be used to provide provisional fixation, so that the large space-occupying reduction aids may be removed (Fig. 31-12). Well-placed Kirschner wires fixing the two fragments may as well be used to provide temporary fixation.

In all of these circumstances, a search for loose bodies or marginal impaction should be carried out dealing with these aspects of the injury in a logical order before definitive fixation is carried out.

Transtectal transverse fractures present a more difficult problem, because the displacement of the fracture occurs in the "weight-bearing" portion of the joint. According to Letournel, an extensile approach is indicated because of this.

In many cases an extended iliofemoral approach is indicated; however, some cases may be done through the trochanteric flip (digastric approach), a surgical exposure described by the French surgeon Courtpied. If this is the case, then the tactic and instruments used are very similar to those used with the juxtatectal and infratectal patterns of the fracture (Figs. 31-5 and 31-6).

There is a much larger exposure with the extended approach. This allows the use of larger reduction instruments, such as the Jungbluth forceps, "king tongs" clamps, and asymmetric reduction forceps (Fig. 31-13).

The reason for the extended surgical approach is to have access to the anterior and posterior portion of the acetabular joint surface in the region of the roof. In the high forms of the transverse fracture the rupture of the bone extends across this critical area. The joint capsule is opened so that the intraarticular surface may be visualized. This is possible with either the extended iliofemoral approach, or the trochanteric flip surgical exposure.

The reduction may be facilitated by the use of pointed reduction forceps. One clamp is positioned anteriorly with a point secured to the anterior column posterior to the anterior inferior spine of the pelvis. The other point is secured on the pelvic brim just distal to the iliopectineal eminence. This clamp may be used to close the anterior fracture gap. Confirmation of reduction is controlled by viewing the anterior fracture line through the joint.

The posterior portion may be reduced using a clamp straddling the fracture as it crosses the posterior column. The Jungbluth pelvic reduction forceps are helpful in this position, or again a second pointed reduction forceps may be used.

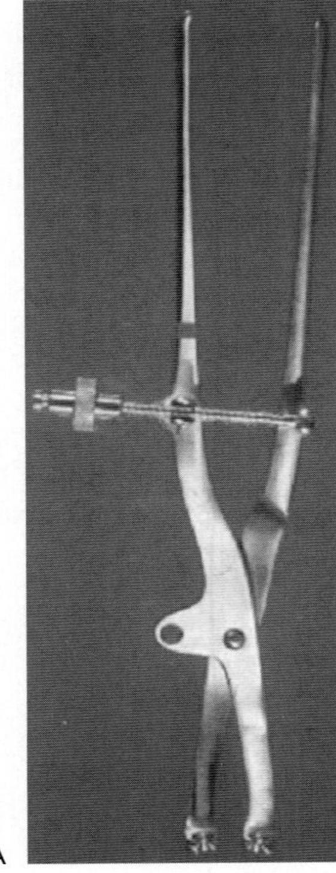

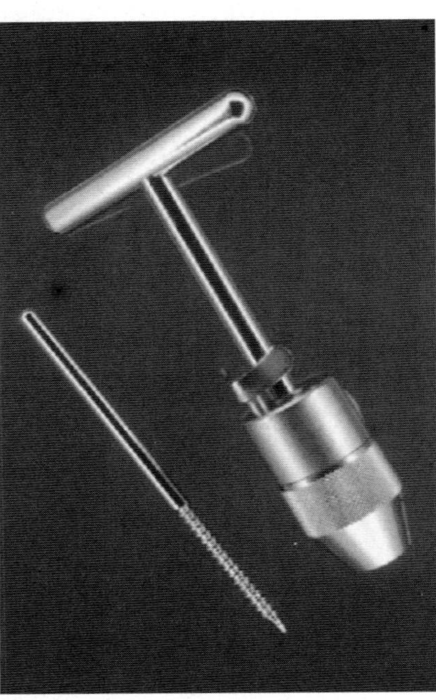

FIGURE 31-9. **A:** Pelvic reduction forceps. **B:** Schantz screw "T"-handled chuck.

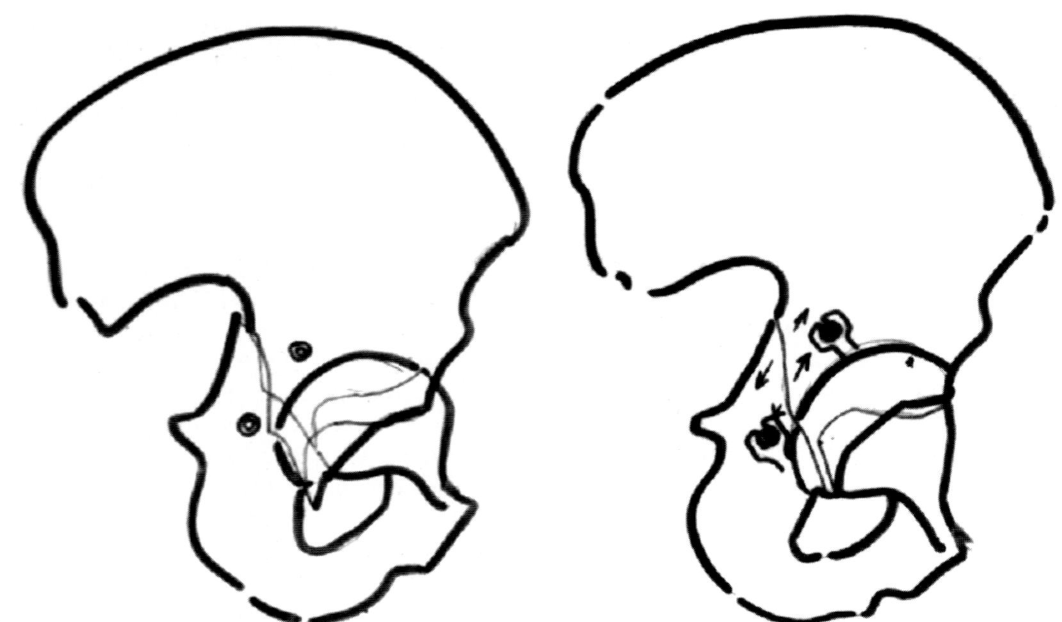

FIGURE 31-10. Technique of application of pelvic reduction clamp. **A:** Diagrammatic illustration of the use of the pelvic reduction forceps. Screws are placed on both sides of the fracture. **B:** The ends of each leg of the clamp are attached to the bone with the screws. Distraction or compression can be carried out to reduce the fracture.

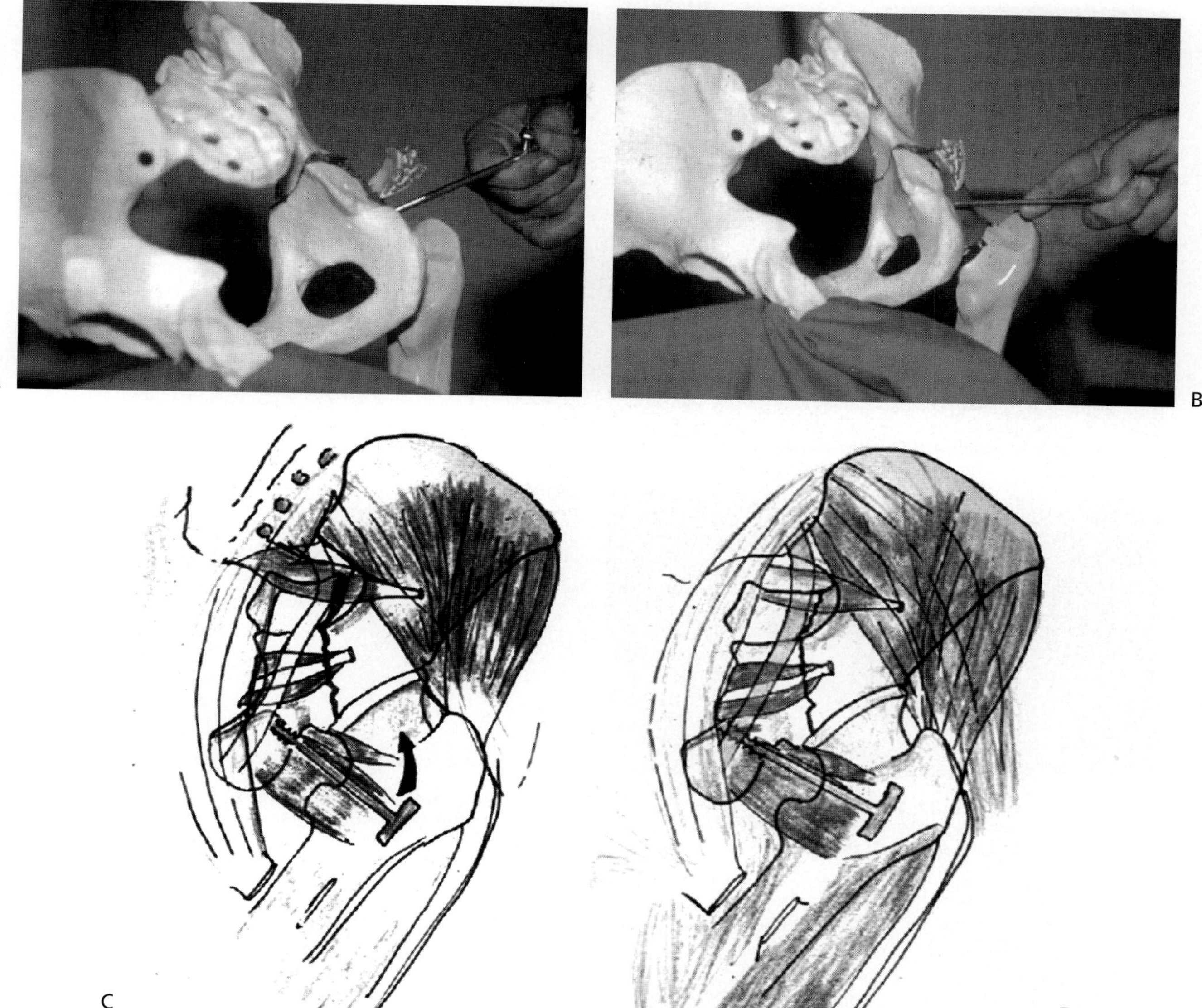

FIGURE 31-11. Schantz screw into ischium to control rotation. **A:** The Schantz screw is inserted into the ischium and used to control the rotational displacement of the ischiopubic fragment. **B:** The reduction can be verified by palpation of the fracture with the index finger. **C:** Diagram of how this maneuver is accomplished through the Kocher-Langenbeck approach. **D:** After rotational reduction.

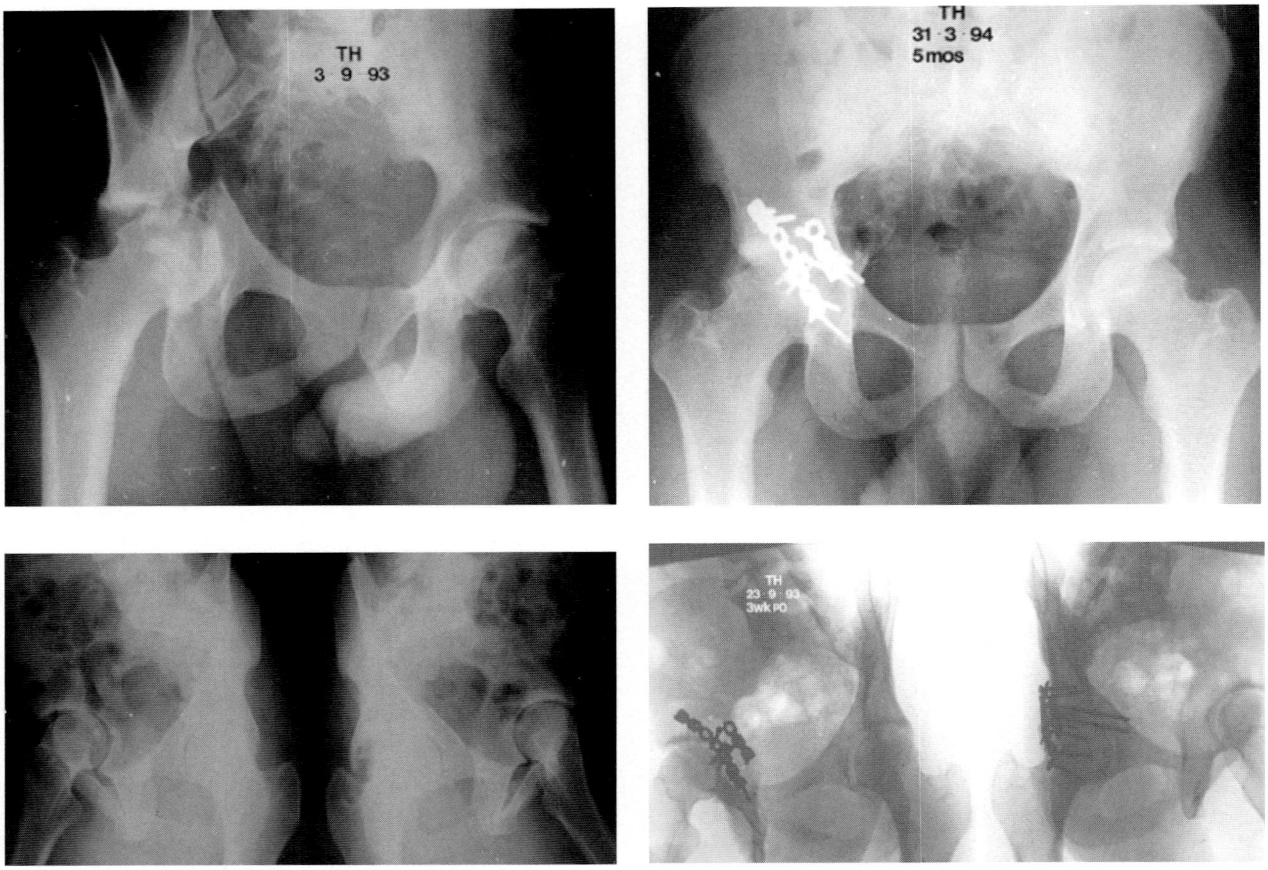

FIGURE 31-12. **A:** Illustrative case of juxtatectal transverse fracture. **B:** Iliac and obturator oblique views. **C:** Front view of the juxtatectal transverse fracture, after reduction and fixation. **D:** Iliac and obturator oblique views.

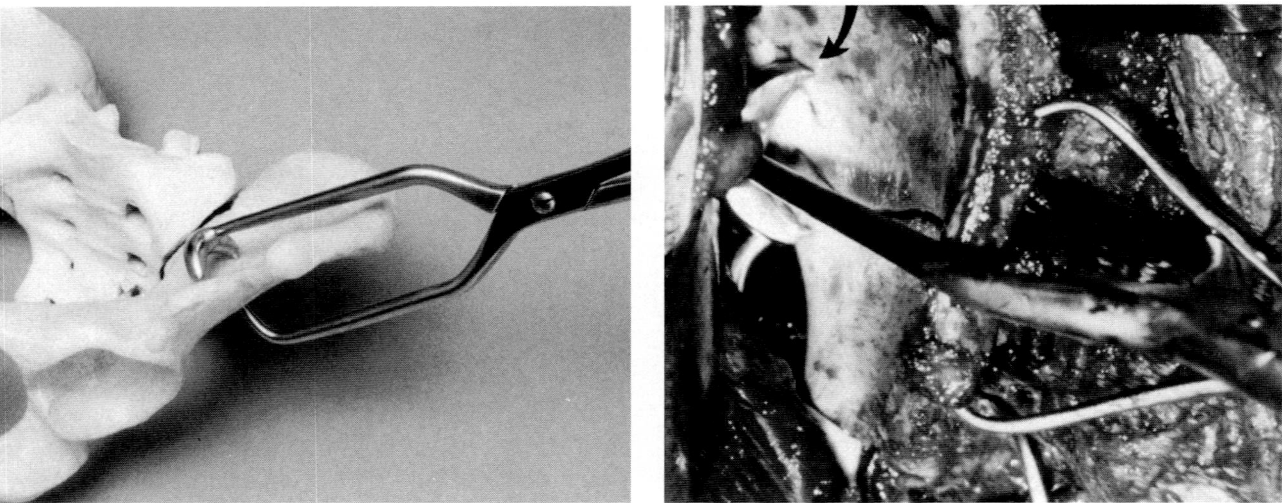

FIGURE 31-13. Demonstration of clamp position. **A:** The double-pronged pelvic reduction forceps (Queen tongs) is used to compress the anterior column against the ilium in the both-column fracture. Also, the large single-pronged clamp may fit over the iliac crest and can be used to reduce the columns where the muscles have been stripped from both sides of the ilium, as in the iliofemoral approach. **B:** The intraoperative photograph shows the position of this clamp over the iliac crest in a both-column fracture. Note also the use of the pointed reduction clamps to hold the fracture along the iliac crest as the large clamp is being tightened. *(continued)*

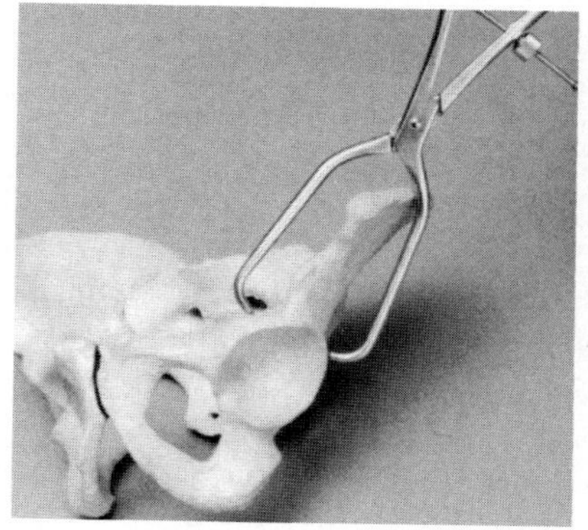

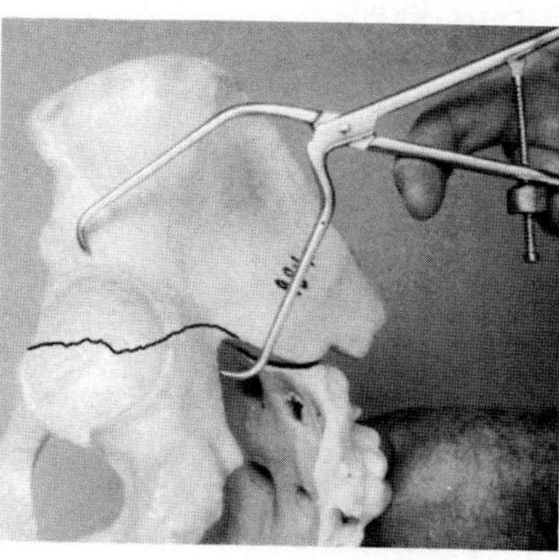

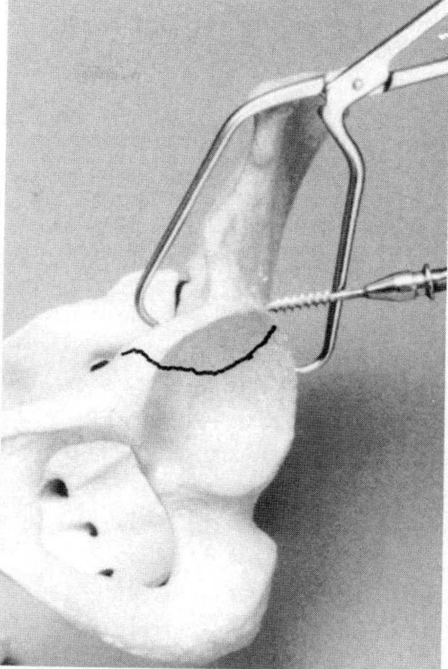

C,D E

FIGURE 31-13. *(Continued).* **C:** The offset clamps may be used through the greater sciatic notch **(D)** to hold a transverse fracture or posterior column fracture, as this case demonstrates the insertion of an anterior column lag screw **(E).**

Fixation is provided by a long screw after reduction of the anterior portion of the transverse fracture is accomplished. This screw starts a thumb breadth above the rim of the joint on the posterior slope of the external contour of the anterior pillar of the acetabulum and is directed from posterior to anterior to the pubic tubercle.

Fixation of the posterior aspect of the transverse fracture generally is carried out with a contoured reconstruction plate, as described in the discussion of fractures of the posterior column.

THE ASSOCIATED FRACTURES

Essentially, the surgical tactic in most of the associated fractures is to convert the related fracture to a simple type through reduction and fixation of the dominant associated lesion.

For example, in the anterior column–associated posterior hemitransverse fracture, the surgical approach is to the anterior column moiety (anterior ilioinguinal) and the reduction of the anterior column fracture is carried out. The reduction maneuvers follow the same order described for fractures of the anterior column. However, having reduced and fixed the anterior column portion, there remains a displaced posterior column fracture with which to contend. This is a unique situation: It is important to know how to gain full benefit of the exposure. The use of the Judet table is an asset because the approach to the bone has been anterior and what is left to reduce and fix is posterior.

Posterior Column–Associated Posterior Wall

Extended posterior wall fractures are transitional in type to this fracture association. In many cases, the displacement of the posterior column is not as large as when a posterior column fracture exists as a single entity (Figs. 31-7 and 31-8).

The lesions are posterior; therefore, the surgical approach is posterior. The patient is operated in the prone position on the Judet table. A large Steinman pin is placed in the distal femur.

After fracture exposure, Farabeuf forceps may be used by placing screws in the posterior column fracture and intact ilium. Using the screw head-holding ends of the forceps, the posterior column fracture may be manipulated into a reduced position. Occasionally, because the site of distal extension of the fracture is into the dense soft tissue in the inferior aspect of the ischium, the ischium must be carefully exposed, the soft tissues removed, and a clamp inserted from the posterior surface of the inferior posterior column fracture through the obturator foramina to the intact opposite side of the esteem. The inferior aspect of the fracture thereby can be closed tightly. The proximal limb of the fracture—which is usually at the level of, or includes a portion of the angle of the greater sciatic notch—is reduced with a small bone hook or the Farabeuf clamp. This is yet another situation where a small three-holed 3.5-mm reconstruction plate used as a clamp may be of value in affording temporary fixation. The reduction of the joint surface can be inspected by viewing the fractured articular surface through the defect in the posterior wall before its reduction. The reduction of the posterior wall fracture then proceeds as described.

Reduction of the posterior column is more difficult under these circumstances, because of the reduced fracture surfaces available for reduction owing to the associated wall fracture.

Transverse Associated with Posterior Wall

As described under the pure transverse fractures, the choice of surgical approach is influenced by the level of the transverse fracture in relation to the acetabular roof. Therefore, most of these fractures may be approached and reduced through the Kocher-Langenbeck or extended iliofemoral approach. The reduction of the transverse fracture is less difficult in many cases, because the displacement of the transverse fracture may not be as large with the presence of the wall fracture. In many cases, there may be only minor displacement of the transverse fracture. Nevertheless, these fractures may be exceedingly difficult, particularly if the transverse fracture is displaced and the posterior wall moiety is extended in nature.

Fractures with extended posterior wall comminution may demand two approaches. In this regard, evaluation of the two-dimensional computed tomography scan is helpful. To be noted is the level and displacement of the transverse fracture line, along with the fragmentation of the posterior wall fracture. With the transverse fracture displaced, reduction of the extensively fragmented posterior wall is extremely difficult because the landmarks between the ischiopubic fragment and the rest of the innominate bone may be absent owing to the extensive nature of the wall fractures.

Under these circumstances, the transverse component of the fracture may be approached anteriorly (Fig. 31-14). It is essentially a two-fragment fracture and may be exposed and reduced from a portion of the ilioinguinal surgical approach, although fixation with a plate from just lateral to the SI joint to the pubic symphysis may require the use of all four windows.

The wound is closed once restoration of the pelvic ring is accomplished. The patient is then placed in the prone position and reduction and fixation of the extensive posterior wall fracture is accomplished as described (Fig. 31-15).

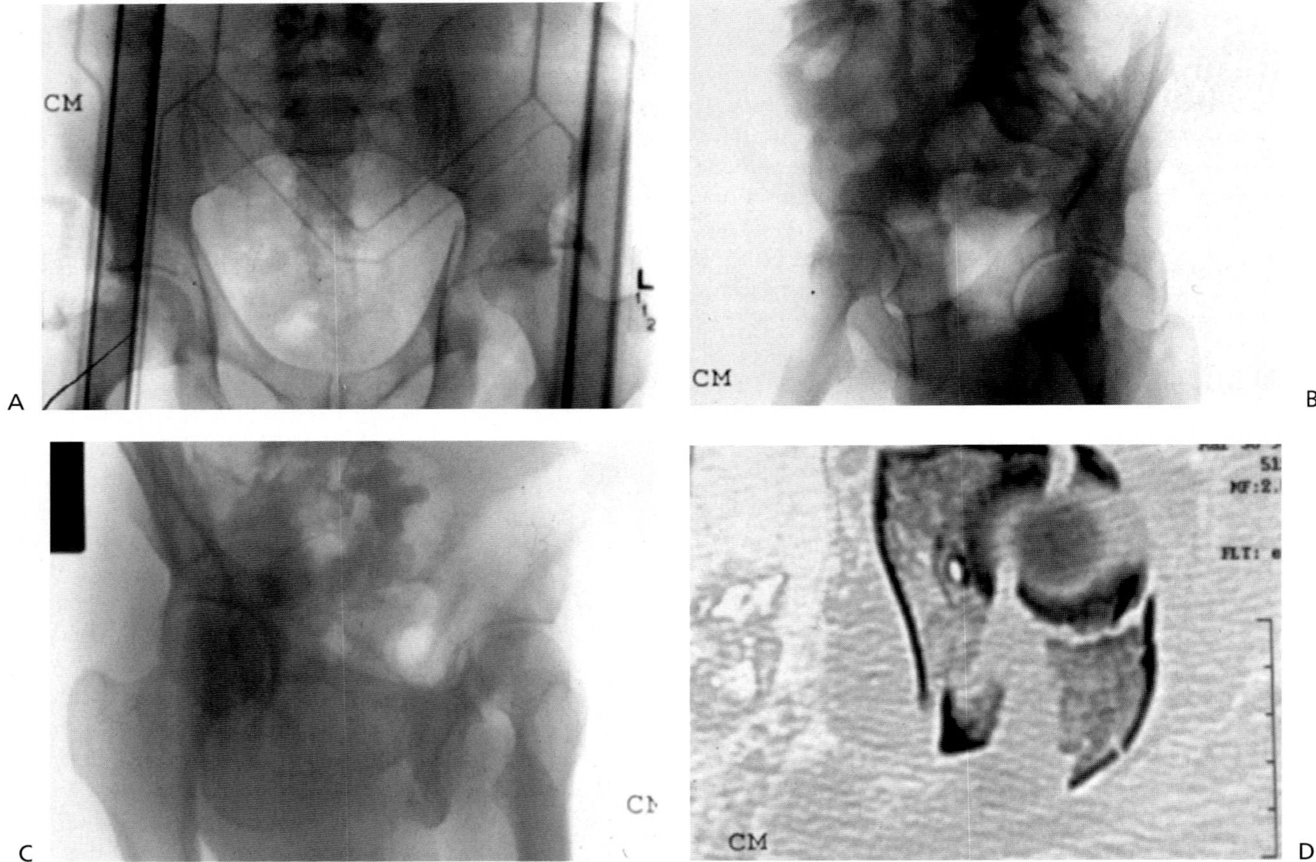

FIGURE 31-14. **A:** Transverse and posterior wall fracture operated through trochanteric-flip approach. (Case courtesy of Keith Mayo.) **B:** Obturator oblique. **C:** Iliac oblique view. **D:** Computed tomography scan that illustrates the transtectal level of the transverse fracture line.

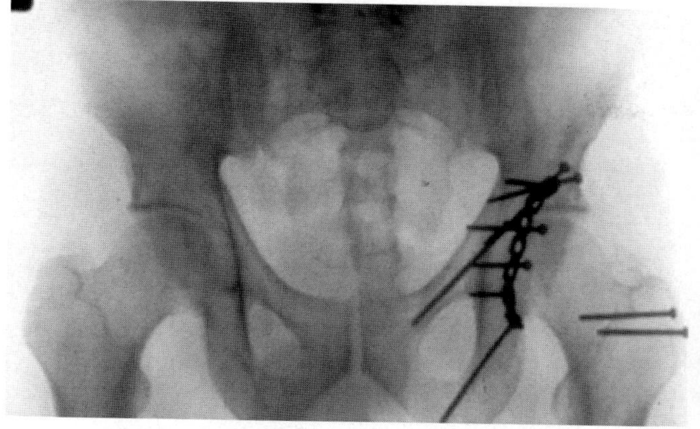
E

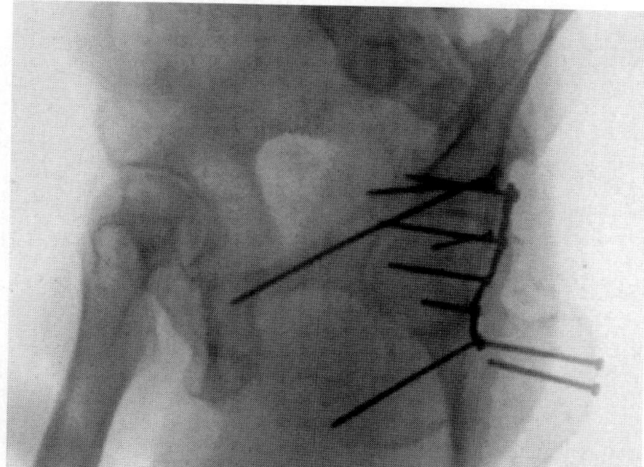
F

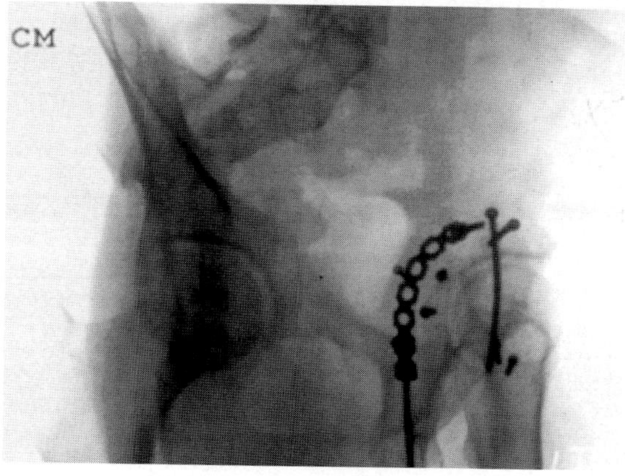

G

FIGURE 31-14. ***(continued)*** **E:** Through this approach it is possible to both reduce the fracture as described and to apply the plate and screws, including the long screws along the anterior column and the long dimension of the ischium. **F:** Obturator oblique. **G:** Iliac oblique.

T-Shaped Fractures

These fractures are among the most difficult to manage. The transverse component of the "T" determines the choice of approach. Transtectal transverse fracture lines require an approach that gives access to the anterior and the posterior articular surface of the acetabulum so that the intraarticular fracture displacements can be perfectly reduced. Thus, the extended iliofemoral or trochanteric flip surgical approaches may be used, because both give access to the anterior portion of the joint. They also allow access to the anterior wall area as far distal as the iliopectineal eminence, which does not allow the use of a pelvic brim plate, but does allow manipulation of the anterior column fracture with pointed reduction forceps. Fixation with carefully placed screws from the posterior aspect of the anterior column across the transverse intraarticular fracture component to the anterior column on the distal side of the fracture.

Fractures that have juxtatectal or infratectal transverse fracture components usually demand the use of the Kocher-Langenbeck approach. The question that arises is, which portion of the "T" should be reduced first? Emile Letournel recommended reducing the posterior column first. This portion of the fracture usually was reduced with the use of Farabeuf forceps and two screws, one placed in each fragment, as has been mentioned for the reduction of pure posterior column fractures following reduction of the posterior column.

The residual displacement of the anterior column was assessed by digital palpation of the fracture through the greater sciatic notch and along the quadrilateral plate surface. In this approach, pointed clamps need to be carefully inserted through the notch to the anterior column on its posterior extent. The image intensifier may be employed to confirm the reduction, or palpation of the reduction with the finger along the quadrilateral plate may be carried out. Fixation of the anterior column portion of the "T" is from a screw(s) directed from posterior to anterior, usually just medial to the angle of the greater sciatic notch. In some instances where the anterior fracture is low, these screws pass through the fossa acetabularis and must be checked carefully to be sure that they avoid contact with the femoral head.

The other alternative is to reduce the anterior column first, using clamps once again through the greater sciatic notch. Before the reduction of the posterior column is reduced, the articular displacement and reduction may be controlled through the joint. The displacement of the posterior column and addition of a capsulotomy allow intraarticular control of the fracture. This is particularly true when using the Judet table because traction may be added and the femoral head may be pulled away from the joint surface to

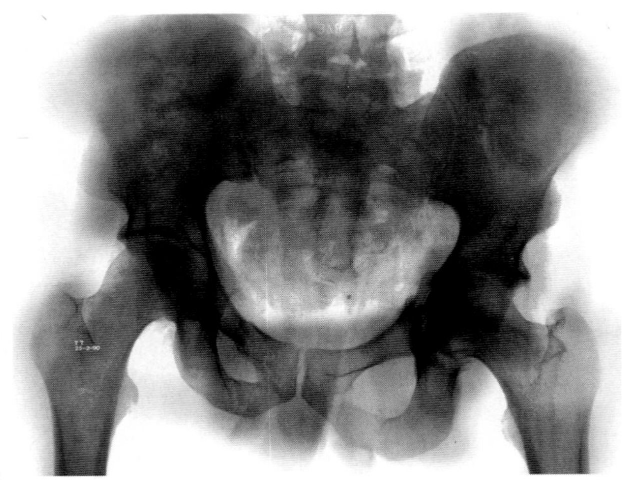

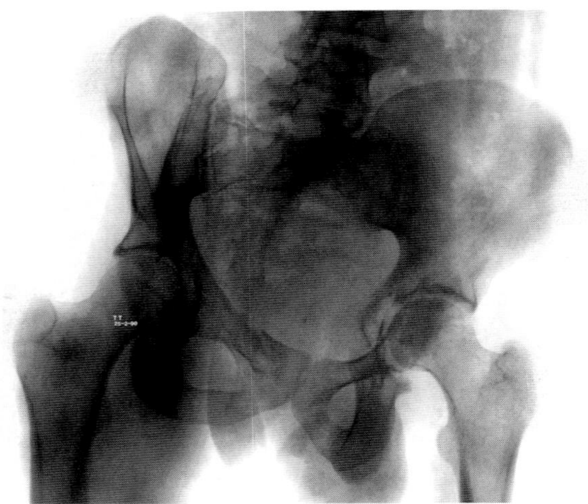

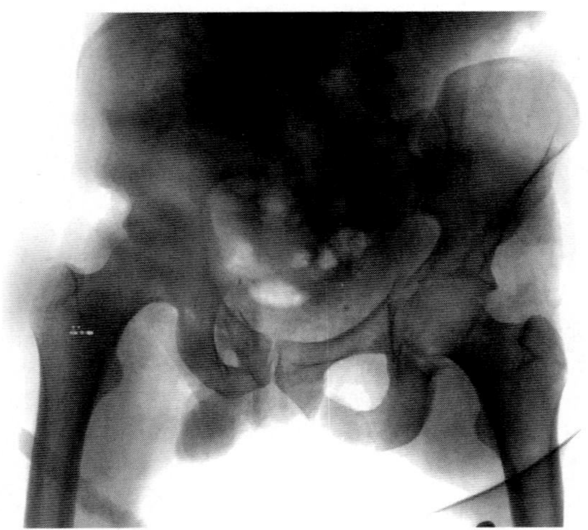

FIGURE 31-15. Combined approaches for transverse fracture **A:** Such a case is illustrated in the following example. An infratectal transverse fracture that was approached by consecutive ilioinguinal and Kocher-Langenbeck approaches. Comminution of the posterior wall–associated severe marginal impaction were hallmarks of the injury. **B:** Poor quality iliac oblique shows that the transverse moiety is very low posteriorly. **C:** Poor obturator oblique shows the simple fracture presentation along the low anterior column, Femoral head is subluxed medially **(D1–4).**

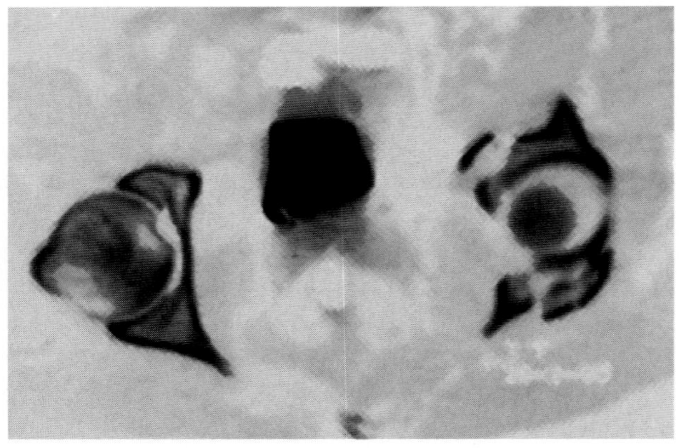

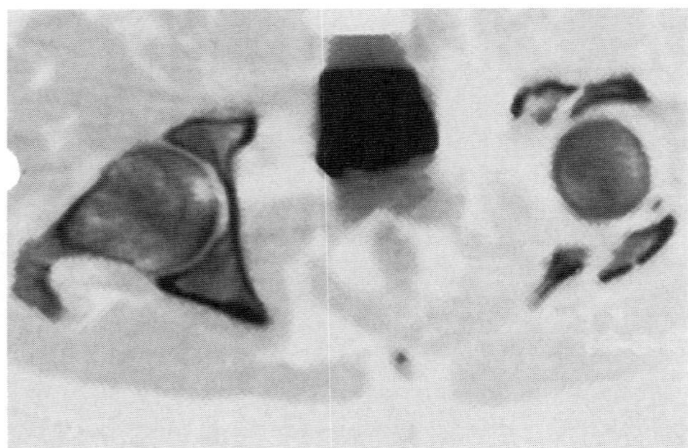

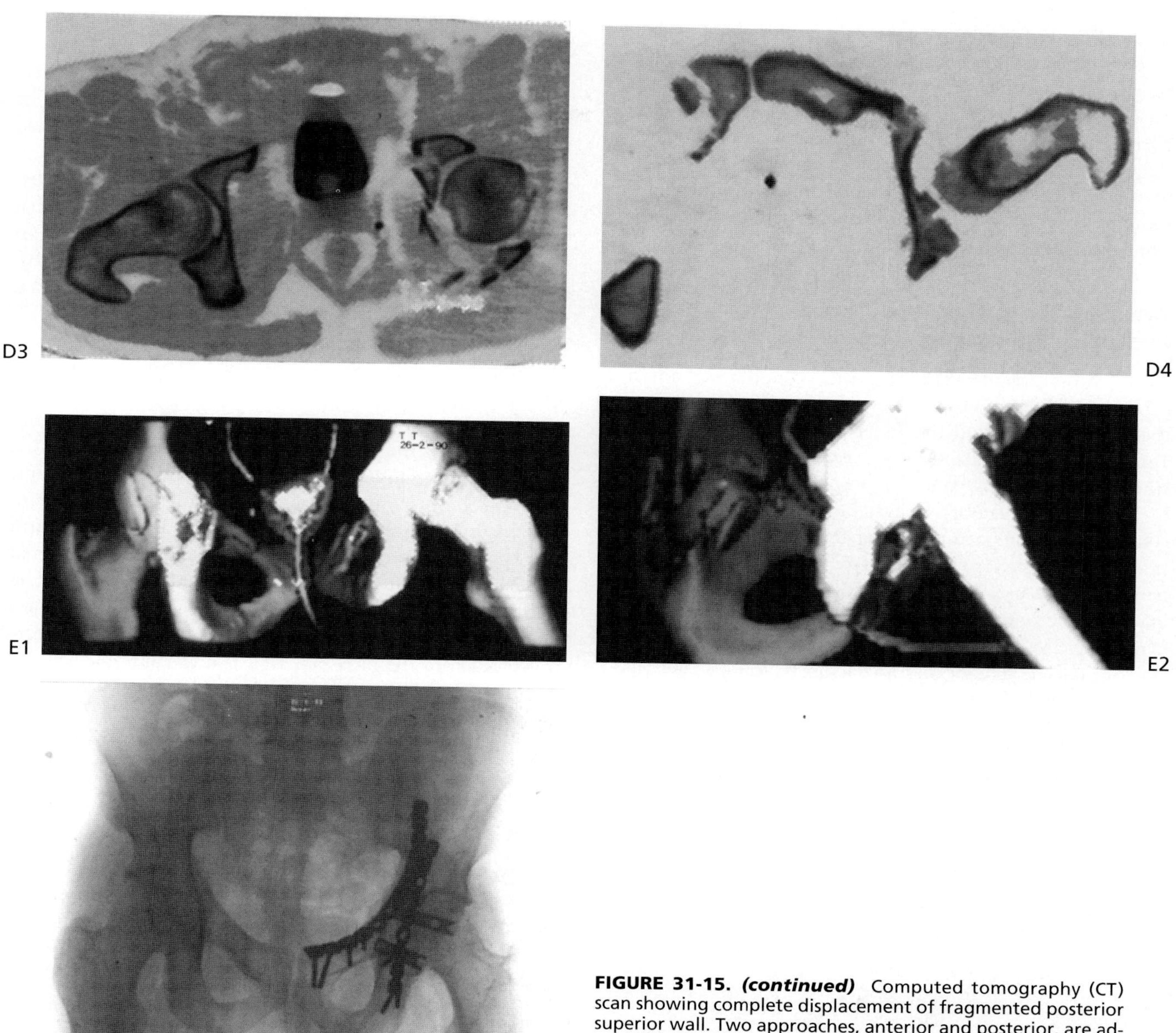

FIGURE 31-15. ***(continued)*** Computed tomography (CT) scan showing complete displacement of fragmented posterior superior wall. Two approaches, anterior and posterior, are advantageous **(E1,2).** Three-dimensional CT reconstruction shows the posterior medial problem. **F:** Result after anterior followed by posterior approach.

enable the surgeon to control the fracture surfaces. Once the anterior portion of the "T" is reduced, it may be temporarily fixed with Kirschner wires. Permanent fixation is obtained by screws placed in the same way as before, just lateral to the greater sciatic notch and from posterior to anterior parallel to the quadrilateral plate. Reduction of the posterior column then is carried out as described. Fixation with a plate also should provide a few screws that not only stabilize the posterior column, but also fix the anterior column fracture.

Anterior Column–Associated Posterior Hemitransverse

This group of fractures (Fig. 31-16A) is approached anteriorly through the ilioinguinal exposure with the patient in the supine position on the Judet table. Both longitudinal and lateral traction are set up as valuable adjunctive measures to facilitate the reduction (Fig. 31-16B).

In general, the femoral head follows the displaced anterior column fracture in fractures sharing the characteristics of anterior column posterior hemitransverse fractures. The posterior hemitransverse usually is not markedly displaced. They frequently exhibit moderate comminution at the junction of the hemitransverse fracture with the anterior column along the pelvic brim. The anterior column fracture typically is externally rotated along its long axis; it is shortened and medially displaced. A piece of articular cartilage still connected to the intact portion of the iliac wing remains in the posterior medial aspect of the joint (Fig. 31-16A). longitudinal traction, usually with the leg slightly flexed, neutralizes the shortening effect, so that with a tool such as a 7-mm Hohmann retractor, the proximal wing-like extension of the fracture located in the internal iliac fossa along the pelvic brim may be levered into reduction. The rotation of the wing can be controlled by a Schantz pin inserted between the cortical tables of the fragment.

Lateral traction applied through a Shantz screw inserted through the trochanter may be used to correct the medial subluxation of the femoral head, bringing it into an anatomic relationship to the acetabulum (Fig. 31-16B). With the head no longer in a protrusio position, the normal curvature of the pelvic brim may be restored (Fig. 31-17).

Once more, temporary fixation with a three-hole plate as described holds this proximal portion of the anterior column fracture temporarily in a reduced position. Then it can be "fine-tuned" by using pointer reduction forceps at other locations along the anterior column.

Finally, a relatively long curved pelvic reconstruction plate can be precontoured and placed on the pelvic brim. The plate is secured distally to the body of the pubis, and having accurately reduced the pubic ramus to its normal curvature, the plate is secured to a second point along the pubic branch. Proximally, the plate—usually 14 holes long—is secured by screws to the bone proximal to the terminal reach of the proximal aspect of the anterior column fracture. Seating this plate along the pelvic brim has the additional effect of completing the reduction of the anterior column portion of the fracture. All fixation at this point is into the anterior column.

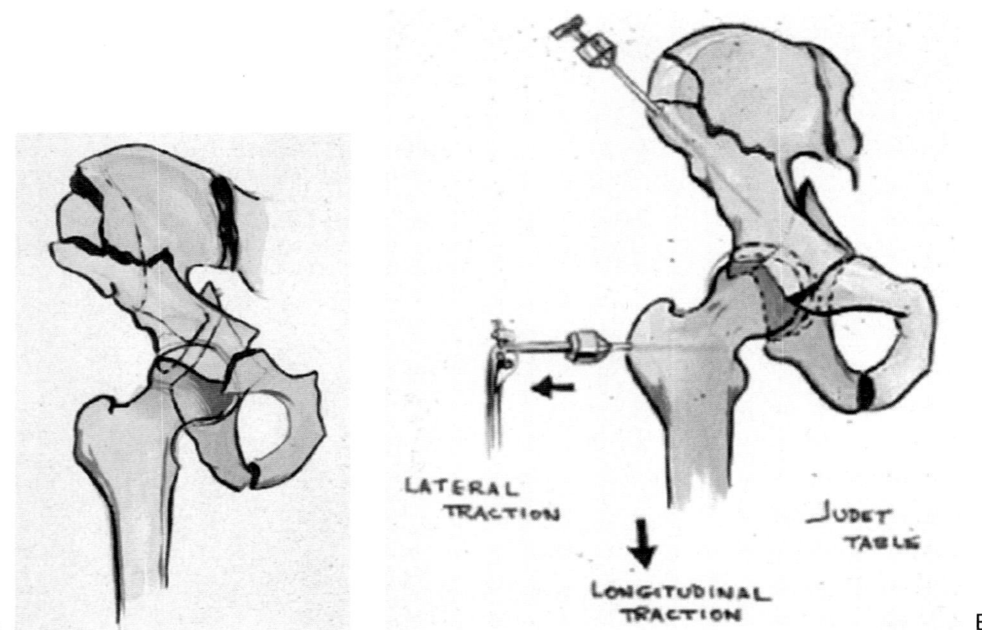

FIGURE 31-16. A: Diagram of anterior column posterior hemitransverse fracture. **B:** Arrangement of devices used to apply forces to reduce the fracture with the Judet table, and an additional Shantz screw in the anterior column fragment.

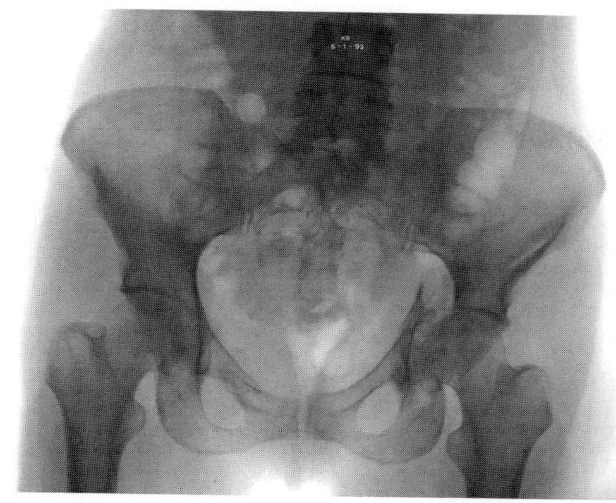

FIGURE 31-17. A: Anterior column posterior hemitransverse fracture allowing illustration of the methods used for reduction. **B:** Obturator oblique radiograph. **C:** Illustration of anterior column posterior hemitransverse fracture. **D:** Reduction and fixation starts with the wedge fragment.

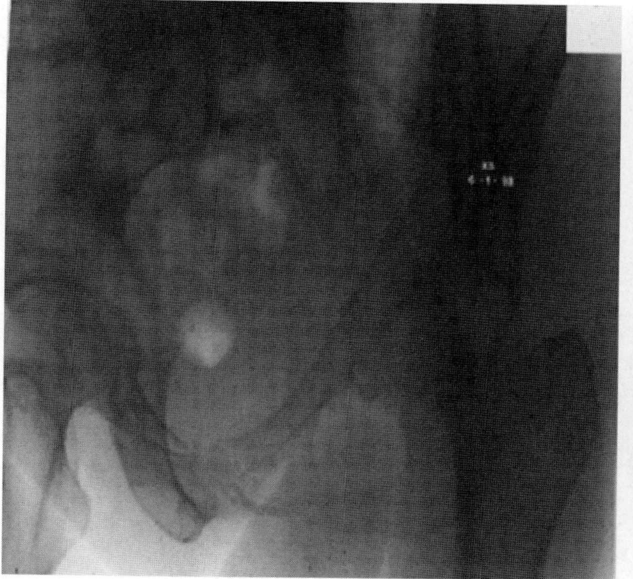

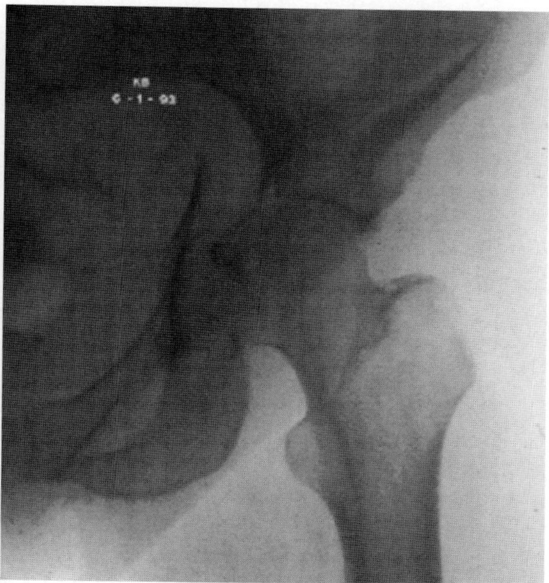

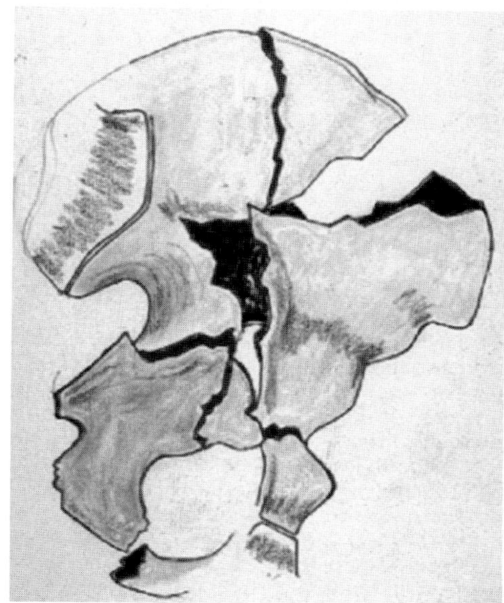

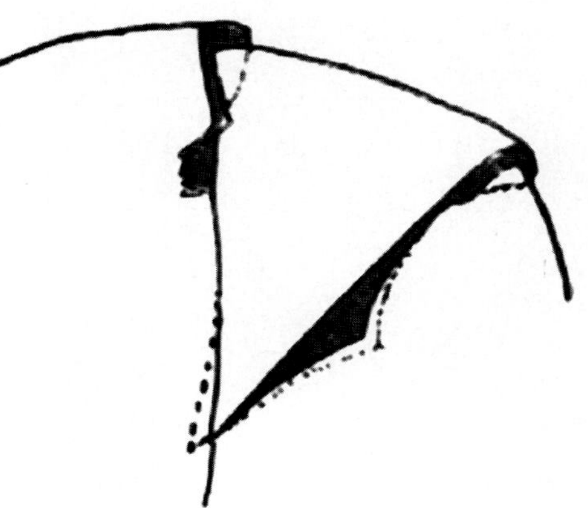

(Figure continues)

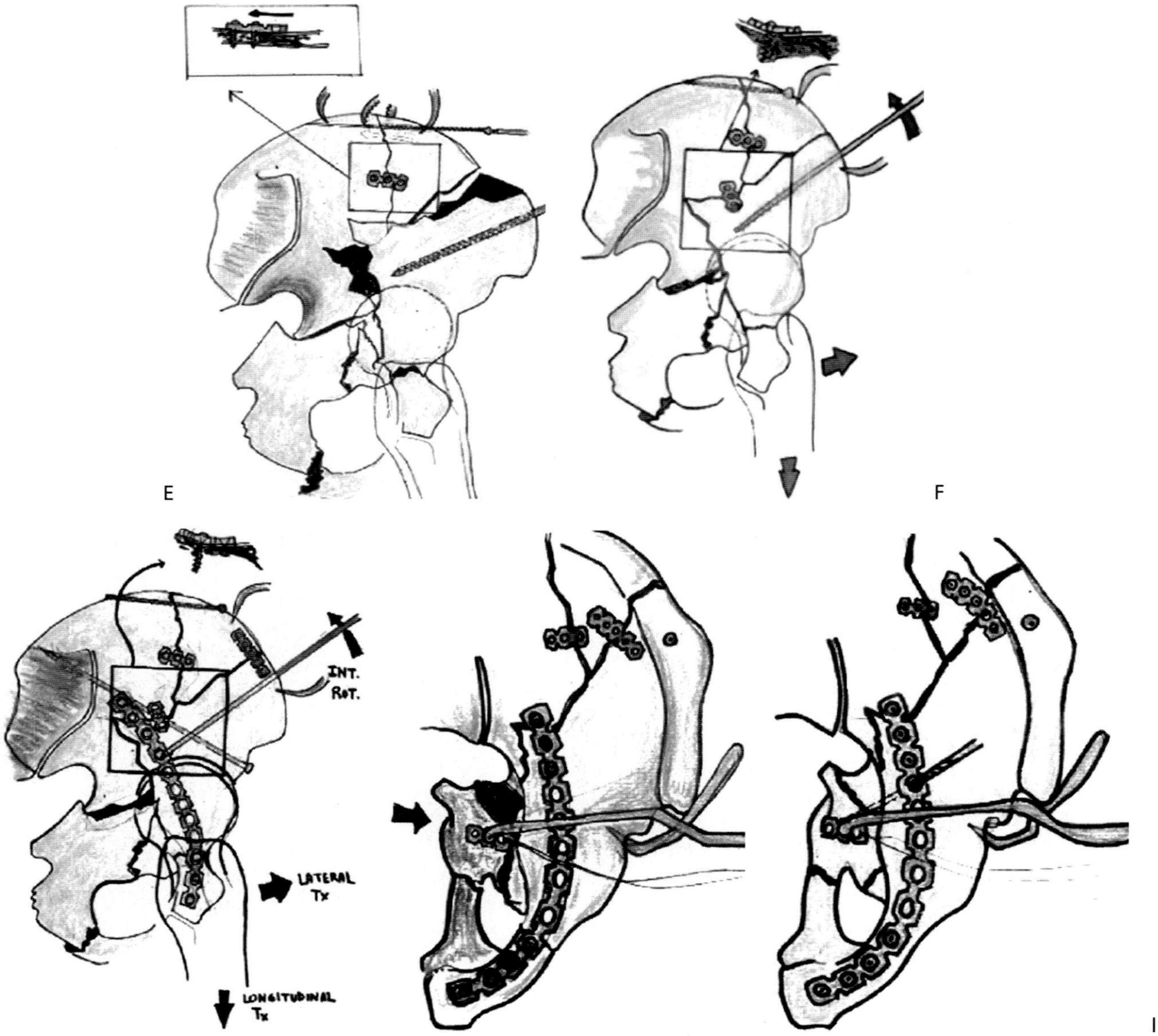

E

F

INT. ROT.

LATERAL Tx

LONGITUDINAL Tx

G, H

I

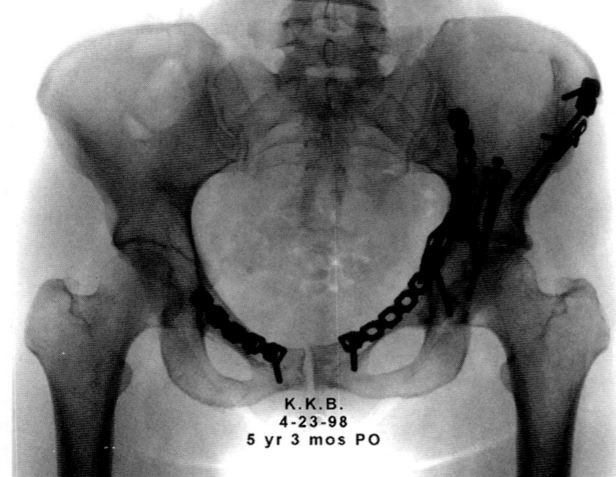

J

FIGURE 31-17. ***(continued)*** **E:** The essential reduction of the wing is made through the first window starting with the wedge fragment; the reduction is effected by pointed reduction and aided by a plate used as a clamp. **F:** After reduction of the wedge fragment, the anterior column is reduced with a "joystick" in the major anterior wing fragment and fixed temporarily with a small plate used as a clamp. The arrows signify the direction of forces provided by the Judet table through traction. **G:** The pelvic brim plate is applied through the first, second, and third windows. **H:** The reduction of the posterior column is made through the second window with the fracture table, or the first window without. In this case the hip may be flexed to relax iliopsoas. **I:** Reduction of the posterior column with the asymmetric reduction forceps with fixation with screws.

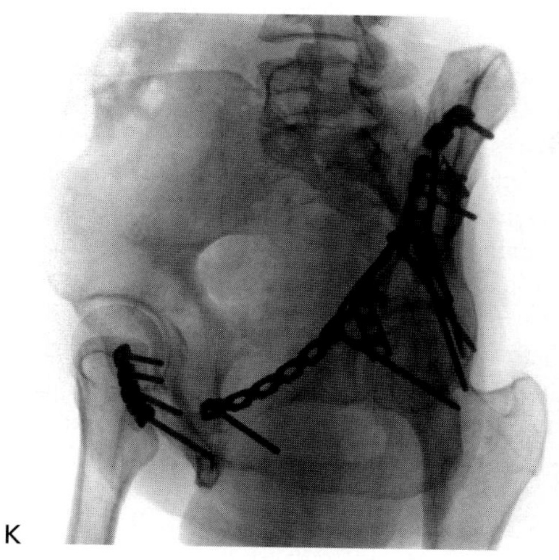

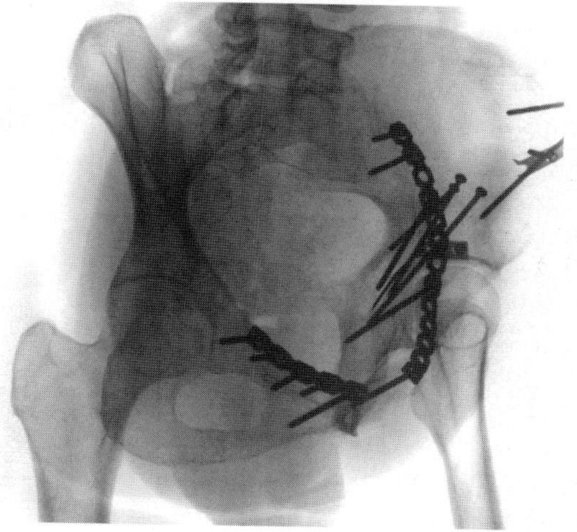

FIGURE 31-17. *(continued)* J: Anterior-posterior pelvis postoperatively showing fixation montage. **K:** Fixation seen in obturator oblique. **L:** Iliac oblique view showing fixation of the fracture.

Reduction of the posterior column from the front is the next step to be accomplished. Inspection of the quadrilateral plate is carried out through either the first or second windows of the ilioinguinal approach. It is here that one appreciates the posterior column fracture and its displacement.

The lateral traction is checked to make sure that there is no residual medialization of the head. This is confirmed by checking once more with the image intensifier on the AP projection. Following these steps, the asymmetric reduction forceps are carefully introduced through the first, or more frequently, the second window. One point of the clamp is placed against the displaced posterior column fragment, while the other point is placed against the external surface of the reconstructed anterior column. The clamp is manipulated and closed. This reduces the posterior column fracture underneath and in alignment with the anterior column. Confirmation of the reduction is obtained by digitally examining the fracture along the quadrilateral surface. Additionally, the image intensifier is used to verify the restoration of the radiologic landmarks of the acetabulum.

Fixation of the posterior column is carried out by long screws directed from anterior to posterior, which may be inserted through the pelvic brim plate or slightly lateral to it. These screws provide fixation of the posterior column.

Both-Column Fractures

These fractures are common and are similar to "T," anterior column, and posterior hemitransverse fracture types. They often exhibit relatively marked displacements. The one thing they have in common is that in all cases, the acetabulum is not attached to the ipsilateral SI joint—a so-called floating hip.

The most common surgical approaches used for this fracture are extensile because of the need to expose the innominate bone above the acetabulum. In the Letournel experience, this means the ilioinguinal and extended iliofemoral approach: two approaches that are performed sequentially rather than simultaneously.

Another extensile approach, the "triradiate" exposure, was popularized by Dana Mears (2). It is not unlike the extended iliofemoral approach except that it requires a trochanteric osteotomy and is not so handy when it comes to the manner by which access to the iliac crest is obtained. Dealing with the muscle belly of the tensor fascia lata also is not as facile.

Reduction of the elements of a both-column fracture are not different than those that have been discussed, except that the "spur sign"—the pathonomic radiographic evidence of a both-column fracture—must be reduced. The "spur sign" is created by the medialization of the acetabulum in relationship to the intact iliac wing. Reduction of the medialized socket can be the most difficult portion of the case, because it is sometimes incarcerated behind and medial to the intact portion of the iliac wing.

The patient is placed in the lateral position on the Judet table if the extended iliofemoral approach is used. One may exert lateral as well as longitudinal traction with this table. This is an important feature because the medial displacement of the acetabulum can be influenced by the lateral force exerted by the padded perineal post against the proximal thigh. This, together with the longitudinal traction, helps to decrease the displacement of the joint. Surgical access is possible to the entire external surface of the bone, including the area of the "spur" sign, with the wide exposure afforded by the extended approach. The wing fractures posterior to this fracture line must be accurately reduced and fixed before an attempt is made to lateralize the acetabulum at the level of the spur sign.

Reduction of the important displacement may be achieved in conjunction with the table and the pelvic reduction forceps attached to the intact portion of the iliac wing and the medialized acetabular fragment. Sometimes a

Hohmann retractor, its tip placed in the fracture line, may be used to lever the joint segment laterally.

If operating through the extended approach, this fracture line may be controlled along the external surface of the bone. Clamps and levers may be used to lateralize the articular segment, and provisional stabilization secured by the use of a short plate attached by screws to the fragment containing the articular segment. The plate extension overlaps the wing fragment and prevents the acetabulum from redisplacing medially. The "spur" remains reduced.

Definitive fixation in the form of lag screws or plates then can be contoured and applied so as to maintain the reduction until fracture regeneration has occurred, the ilioinguinal approach to both-column fractures is used when the posterior column is a single fragment without comminution and the ipsilateral SI joint is not involved. If the SI joint were involved, classically one would elect the extensile approach because the SI joint can be exposed, reduced, and fixed through such an exposure.

The fracture table is employed with the ilioinguinal approach with both longitudinal and lateral traction. Additionally, Hohmann retractors used as levers, as described, may be useful. The asymmetric reduction forceps—one point against the medially displaced articular segment and one point on the outside surface of the intact wing segment—may be used to decrease or eliminate the displacement. Additionally, joysticks help to overcome rotational displacement, and short plates are used as described earlier to hold reduction gains incrementally until final reduction has occurred.

Palpation of the fracture lines along the quadrilateral plate and scrutiny of the fracture lines across the pelvic brim indicate successful correction of the displacement of the spur sign. Because these bony surfaces are at approximately 90 degrees to one another, they also give an indication as to the overall reduction.

Another alternative surgical approach to the both-column fractures that may be valuable in fractures is an anterior ilioinguinal approach, but it has some features that would indicate an extended iliofemoral approach. These are fractures that have a pattern that is more displaced medially than laterally, yet fractures of the posterior column are without comminution.

Elements that seem to contraindicate the ilioinguinal approach are involvement of the sciatic buttress or ipsilateral

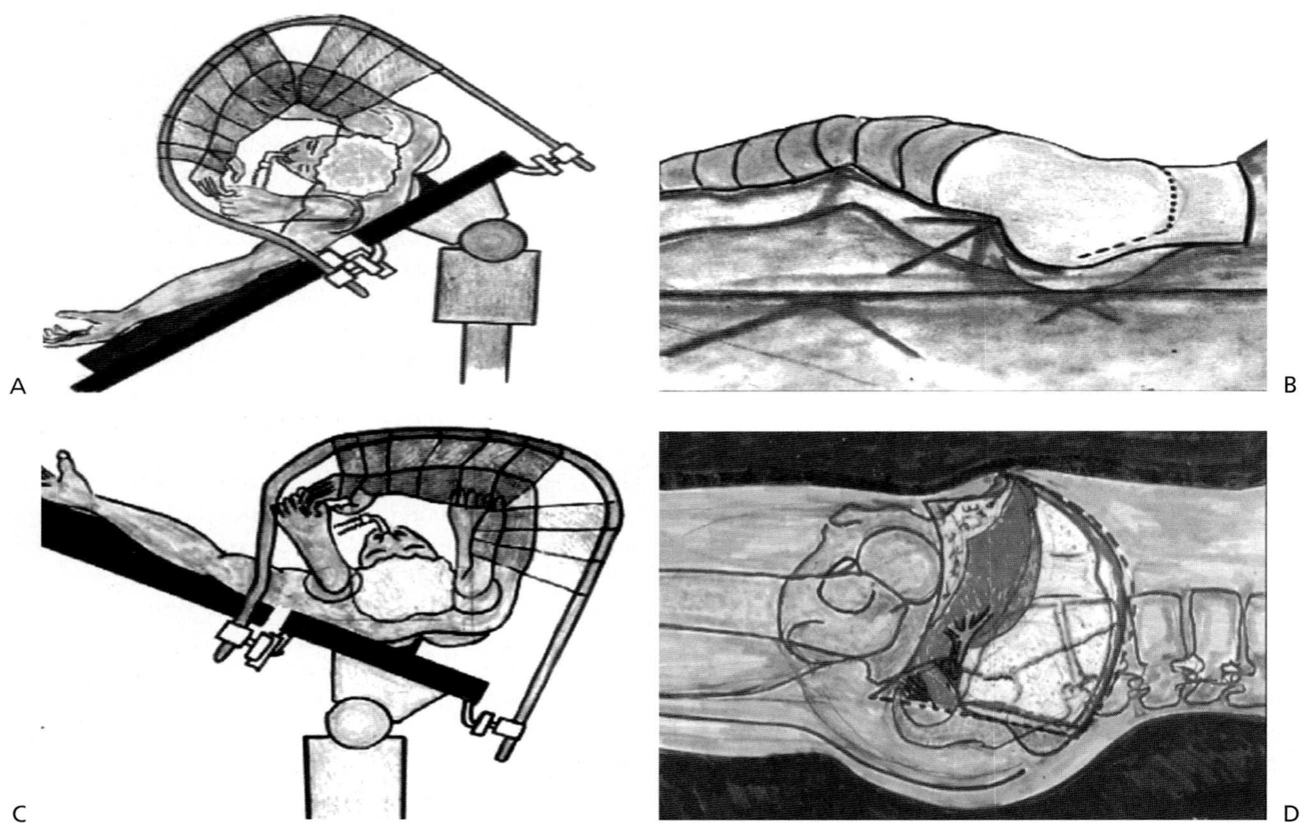

FIGURE 31-18. A: Extended ilioinguinal approach for both-column fracture. **B:** After draping, it allows an extended posterior-lateral surgical approach. **C:** The other position of the table allows the patient to be in the supine position. **D:** The posterior portion of the surgical approach, taking down the glutei. The superior gluteal vessels are seen coning out of the greater sciatic notch.

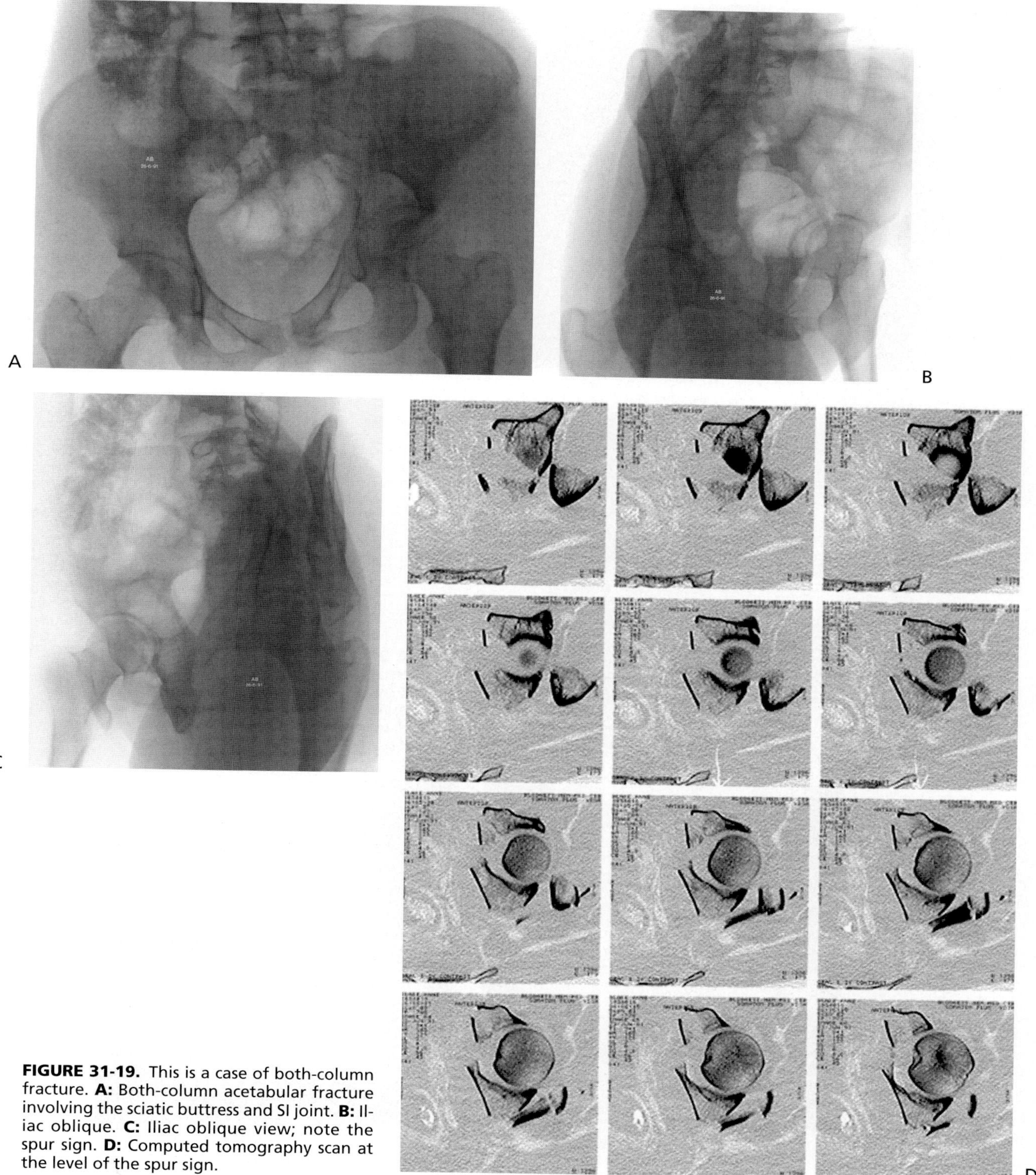

FIGURE 31-19. This is a case of both-column fracture. **A:** Both-column acetabular fracture involving the sciatic buttress and SI joint. **B:** Iliac oblique. **C:** Iliac oblique view; note the spur sign. **D:** Computed tomography scan at the level of the spur sign.

(Figure continues)

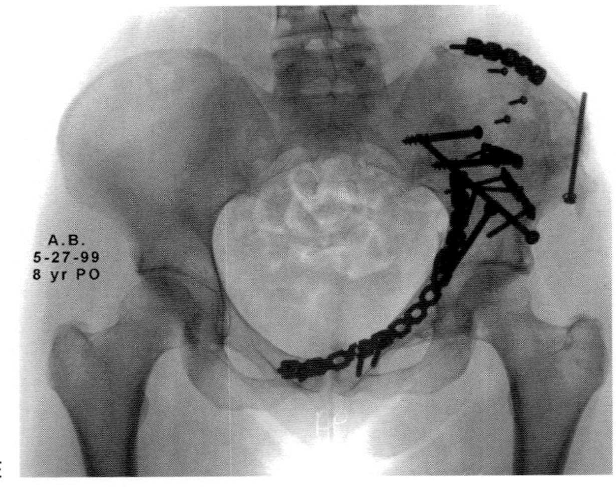

E

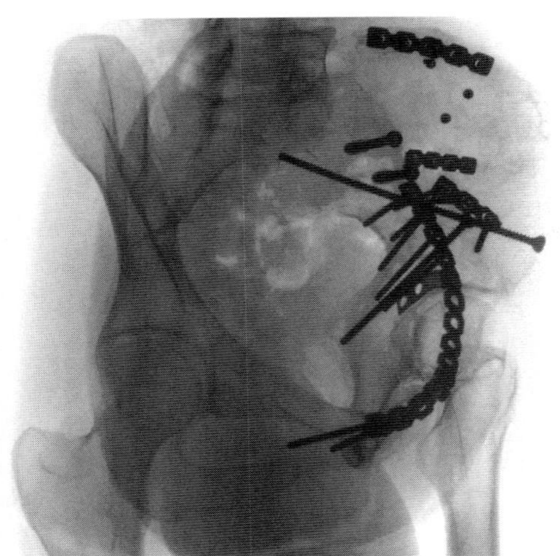

F

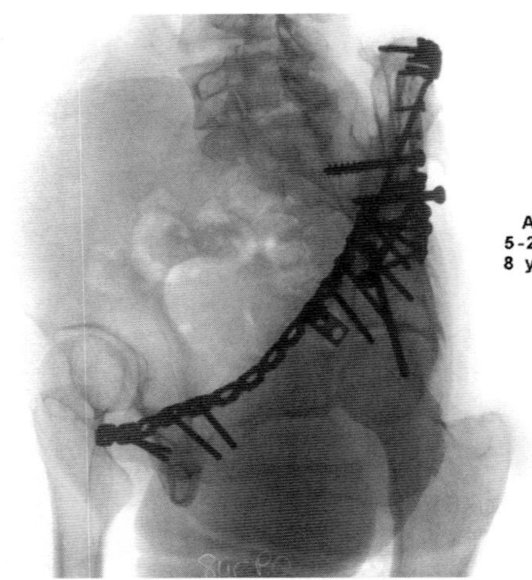

G

FIGURE 31-19. ***(continued)*** **E:** Postoperative anterior-posterior view; **F:** Postoperative iliac oblique view. **G:** Postoperative obturator oblique view. **H:** Clinical photograph anterior view of scar. **I:** Clinical photograph posterior view of scar.

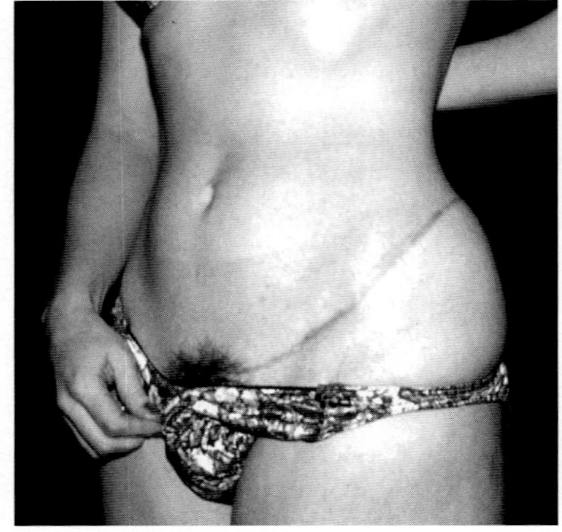

H

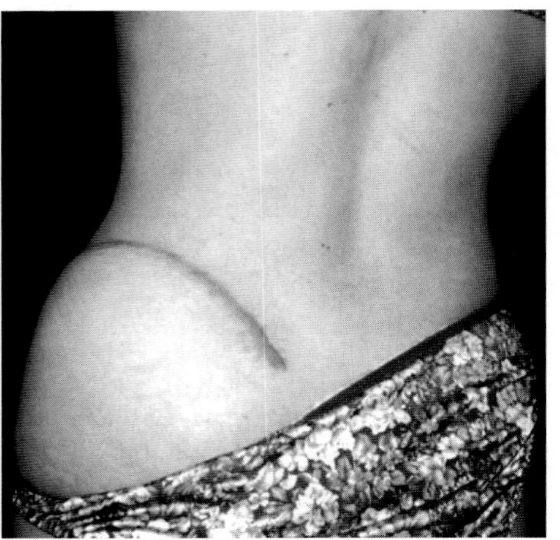

I

SI joint. The extended ilioinguinal approach may be useful in cases such as these.

The extended ilioinguinal approach combines the posterior approach to the SI joint with the ilioinguinal approach. The difficulty of the approach is found in the need for careful setup of the patient on the table. The patient is positioned 45 degrees oblique on the table and stabilized with a deflatable "bean bag" supported by kidney rests (Fig. 31-18). The table must be able to tilt mechanically so that the patient is lateral in one extreme and supine in the other. The approach is to the posterior innominate bone to the level of the gluteus medius tubercle, and then anterior and intrapelvic along the anterior wing and pubic arch. This gives access to the posterior ilium and sciatic buttress along the angle of the greater sciatic notch in addition to the anterior wing of the anterior column, pelvic brim, quadrilateral plate, and pubic ramus to the tubercle and symphysis. In this approach one does not take the anterior circumflex vessels, so that vascularity through collateral circulation is not disturbed, even though an extended exposure is carried out and high fractures through the sciatic notch may be approached. This is a potential problem discussed by some with the extended iliofemoral. The other feature that is valuable is that by being able to turn the table so that the patient is in the supine position, the effect of gravity on the medially displaced articular segment is neutralized, which makes reduction of the "spur" easier to accomplish.

Useful instruments are the pelvic reduction forceps posteriorly and pointed reduction forceps along with the asymmetric reduction forceps used in the ilioinguinal portion of the approach to reduce the posterior column (Fig. 31-19).

CONCLUSION

The surgical treatment of acetabular fractures, including both reduction and fixation, rests on the ability of the surgeon to diagnose the fracture type through standard x-rays and CT scans. Having done so, the appropriate surgical approach can be selected. Letournel believed that most of the fractures of the acetabulum can be treated through one approach. He maximized the effectiveness of this approach by using the Judet extension table.

This discussion centers on the usual methods employed in overcoming the displacements of the fractures described in the groups defined by Letournel (1). Most of these basic maneuvers are those that Letournel used in treating over 1,000 fractures of the acetabulum in his remarkable career.

Every year, many new ideas are introduced by enthusiastic surgeons who are beginning their careers in pelvic surgery. We have all shared in the enthusiasm of self-discovery. It was always a humbling experience to describe one of these new innovations to Letournel. He would listen politely, go to his box of retired instruments, and pull out an old but similar instrument that he had greeted with enthusiasm years before, and that had been retired because it had just not proved to be of enough value. In short, the basics as experienced over the years by Letournel (1) as well as the principles he taught, were the legacy that he gave us.

REFERENCES

1. Letournel E. *Judet fractures of the acetabulum,* 2nd ed. Berlin: Springer-Verlag, 1993.
2. Mears DC, MacLeod MD. Surgical approaches: triradiate and modified triradiate. In: Wiss DA, ed. *Master techniques in orthopaedic surgery: fractures.* New York: Lippincott-Raven, 1997:701–728.

PART D. TECHNIQUES OF REDUCTION AND FIXATION FOR ACETABULAR FRACTURES: OPEN METHODS

32

CERCLAGE WIRES

MARVIN TILE

Cerclage wires have a limited role to play in the surgical management of acetabular fractures (1). Their primary role is in the reduction of fractures, especially high transverse and both-column types, although in some circumstances they have been used as the primary form of fixation (2). However, as fixation devices they are mainly used as adjuncts to more stable forms of fixation.

Cerclage wires are inserted through the greater or lesser sciatic notch, and greatly help the reduction of some fractures in the right circumstance (Fig. 32-1) (1,2). This technique is especially useful when the fracture line extends high into the greater sciatic notch, no matter the type (Fig. 32-2). This is true of high posterior column fractures that extend up into the upper part of the notch, transverse fractures that have an anterior or posterior limb that is high (Fig. 32-2), and both-column fractures, when tightening the wires often achieves anatomic reduction of the fracture with traction on the femoral head (Fig. 32-3). In most instances the wire may be retained, to help maintain the reduction while using more stable fixation. Inserting the wire is relatively easy, although obviously access must be available to both sides of the ilium. The sciatic nerve is protected by a sciatic nerve retractor, blunt Holman retractor placed at the greater sciatic notch, or special Rang retractors designed for passage of a Gigli saw in an innominate osteotomy. The technique is similar to the use of a Gigli saw in the innominate osteotomy of Salter. A no. 18 wire, often doubled, can be passed through the notch; then the fracture is reduced and the wire is tightened anteriorly in the region of the anterior inferior spine (Fig. 32-1).

In some instances the cerclage wire can be passed through the inferior gluteal notch (Fig. 32-4). In these cases the wire tends to constrict the capsule unless the anterior limb of the wire is higher than the anterior inferior iliac spine. It can, in fact, be entered through a drill hole superior to the anterior inferior spine, in order to prevent constriction of the capsule.

The wire can be a time-saving device, just as it can be in other fracture situations in the body. For example, a 39-year-old woman who had a both-column fracture suffered a saddle pulmonary embolism after exposure of the entire fracture (Fig. 32-4). The anesthetist wished us to abort the case, because he feared the patient would die on the table. We inserted cerclage wires through both the lesser and greater sciatic notches, tightened the wires, and achieved virtually anatomic reduction. There was time for only minimal screw fixation definitively. The patient was awakened and placed in traction. She survived and has an excellent result to this date.

In the proper instances, this technique may simplify reduction and fixation of difficult fractures.

REFERENCES

1. Schopfer A, Willett K, Powell J, et al. Cerclage wiring in internal fixation of acetabular fractures. *J Orthop Trauma* 1993;7:236.
2. Kang CS. *A new fixation method of acetabular fractures.* Presented at SICOT Meeting. Munich, Germany, August 16–21, 1987.

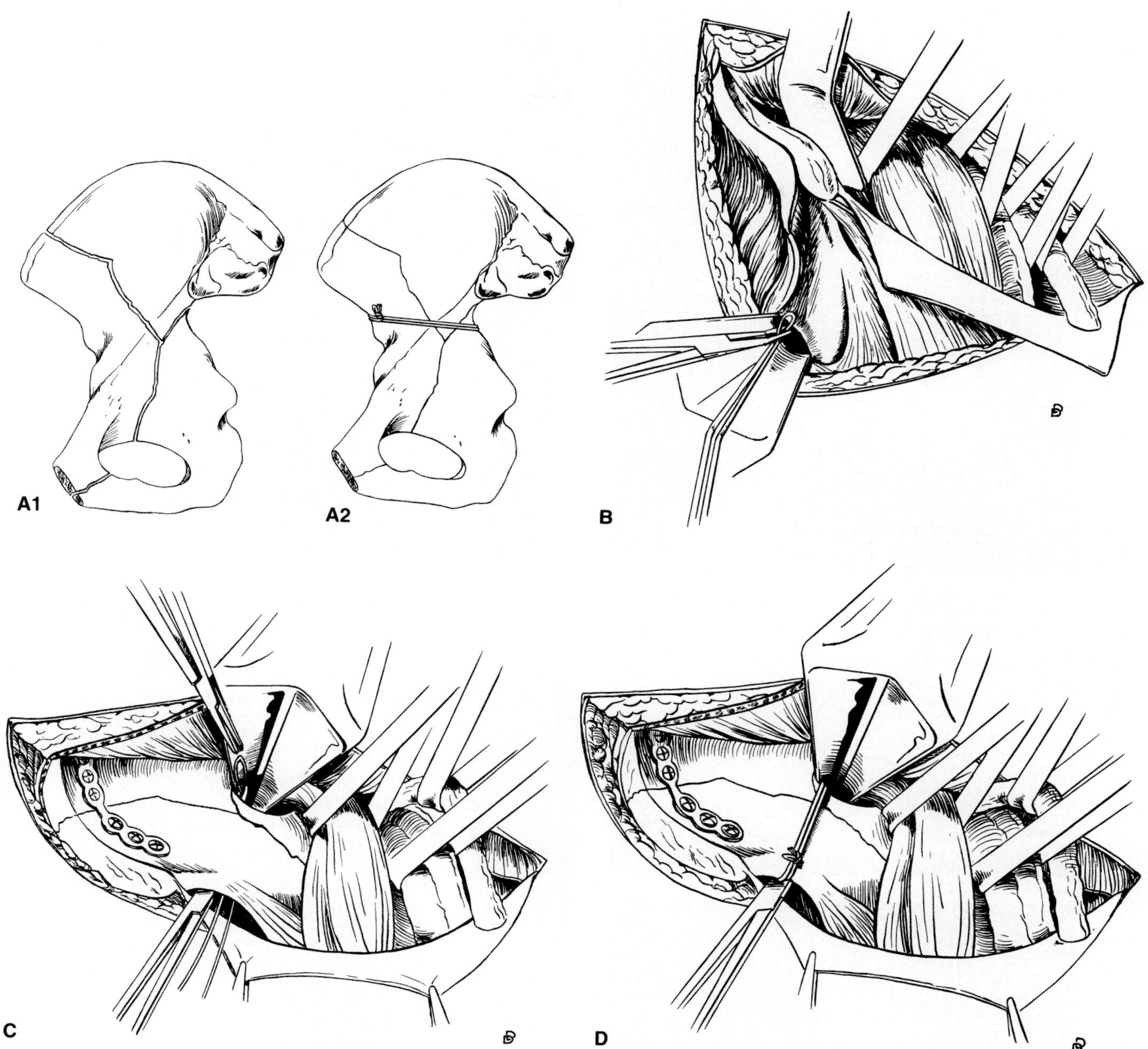

FIGURE 32-1. Use of cerclage wires for reduction and temporary fixation. **A:** A both-column acetabular fracture *(A1)* was reduced and fixed with a double-loop cerclage wire from the greater sciatic notch to a point just cephalad to the anterior inferior spine *(A2)*. The technique of insertion of the wires is as follows. **B:** Both the medial and lateral aspects of the ilium are exposed to the greater sciatic notch. One exposure, usually the medial one, must be large; the opposite one may be small. **C:** Insertion of Rang retractors through the notch protects the sciatic nerve. The fracture must be reduced temporarily with clamps to safely pass the wire, in this case on a long, right-angled (Mixter) clamp. The iliac fracture was previously fixed with a curved plate. The wire secures the posterior column. The approach in this case is the ilioinguinal one but modified to allow lateral exposure of the greater sciatic notch. **D:** The final appearance of the wire in place through the first window of the ilioinguinal approach.

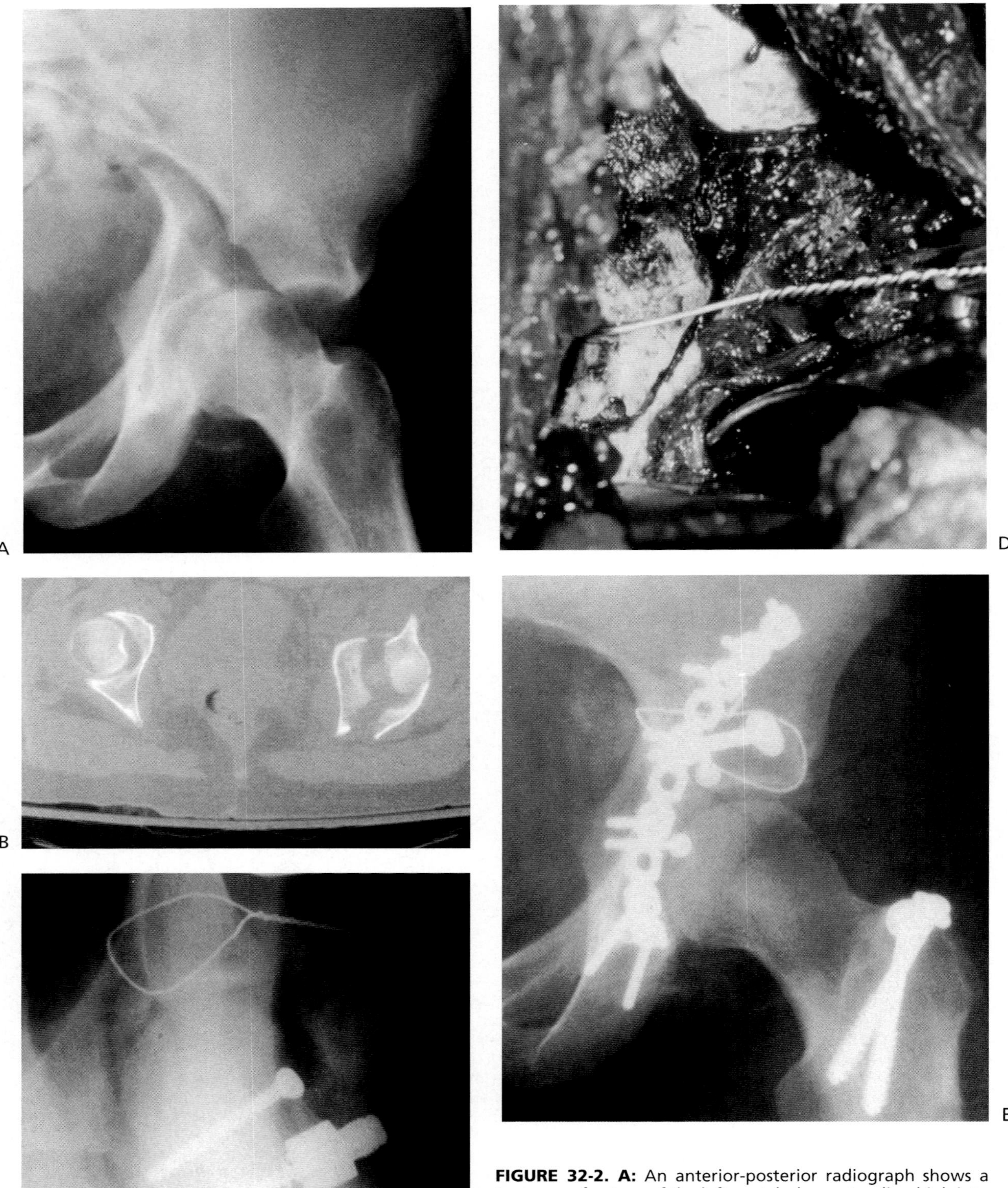

FIGURE 32-2. A: An anterior-posterior radiograph shows a transverse fracture of the left acetabulum extending high into the superior gluteal notch. This is an excellent indication for the use of the cerclage wire, as a technique for both reduction and fixation. **B:** Computed tomography shows the classic appearance of a transverse fracture. **C:** An 18-gauge wire was passed through the greater sciatic notch *(black arrow)* and tightened. Note the anatomic reduction achieved with the wire alone. **D:** The position of the wire through the greater sciatic notch is seen in the intraoperative photograph. Stability was achieved with the wire in place and the addition of intrafragmental screws and a posteriorly placed reconstruction plate held by screws. The procedure was performed through a triradiate approach that allowed access to both sides of the ilium for insertion of the wire. **E:** Note the anatomic reduction. An excellent outcome was achieved in this case.

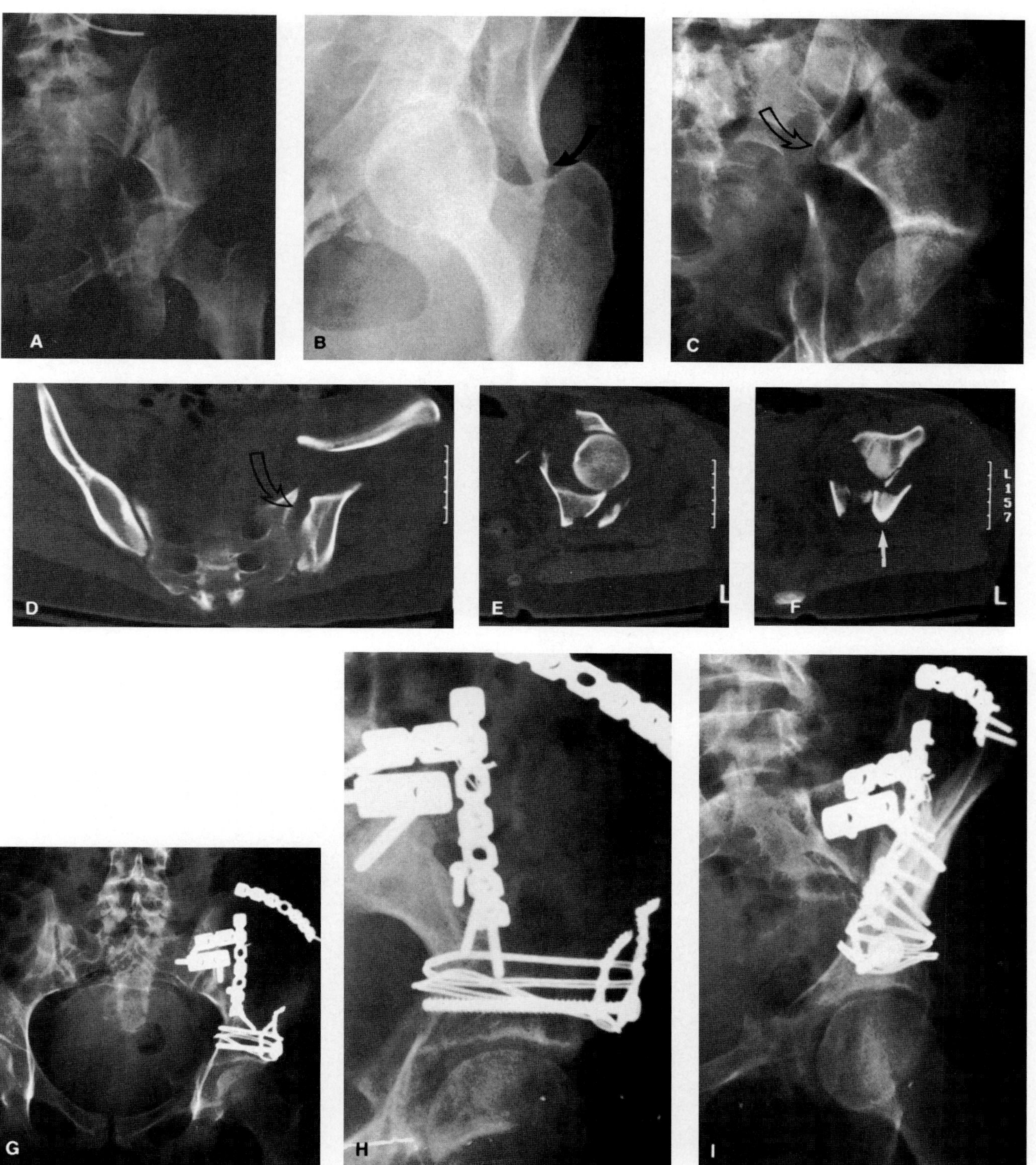

FIGURE 32-3. Use of cerclage wires in both-column fractures. **A:** Anterior-posterior radiograph exhibits a typical Type C3 both-column fracture in a 28-year-old woman. Note that the iliac portion of the fracture enters the sacroiliac joint. **B:** The pathognomonic spur sign is noted on the obturator oblique view *(black arrow),* and sacroiliac joint involvement in the iliac oblique view **(C). D:** The typical appearance of the both-column fracture is visible on computed tomography, which also exhibits sacroiliac joint involvement, the coronal split **(E,F). F:** This shows the typical appearance of the spur sign *(white arrow).* **G,H:** Note the use of two (18-gauge) double cerclage wires to bring the anterior and posterior columns together and the anterior column to the ilium. **I:** Anatomic reduction was obtained and held with plates, including two plates across the sacroiliac joint anteriorly.

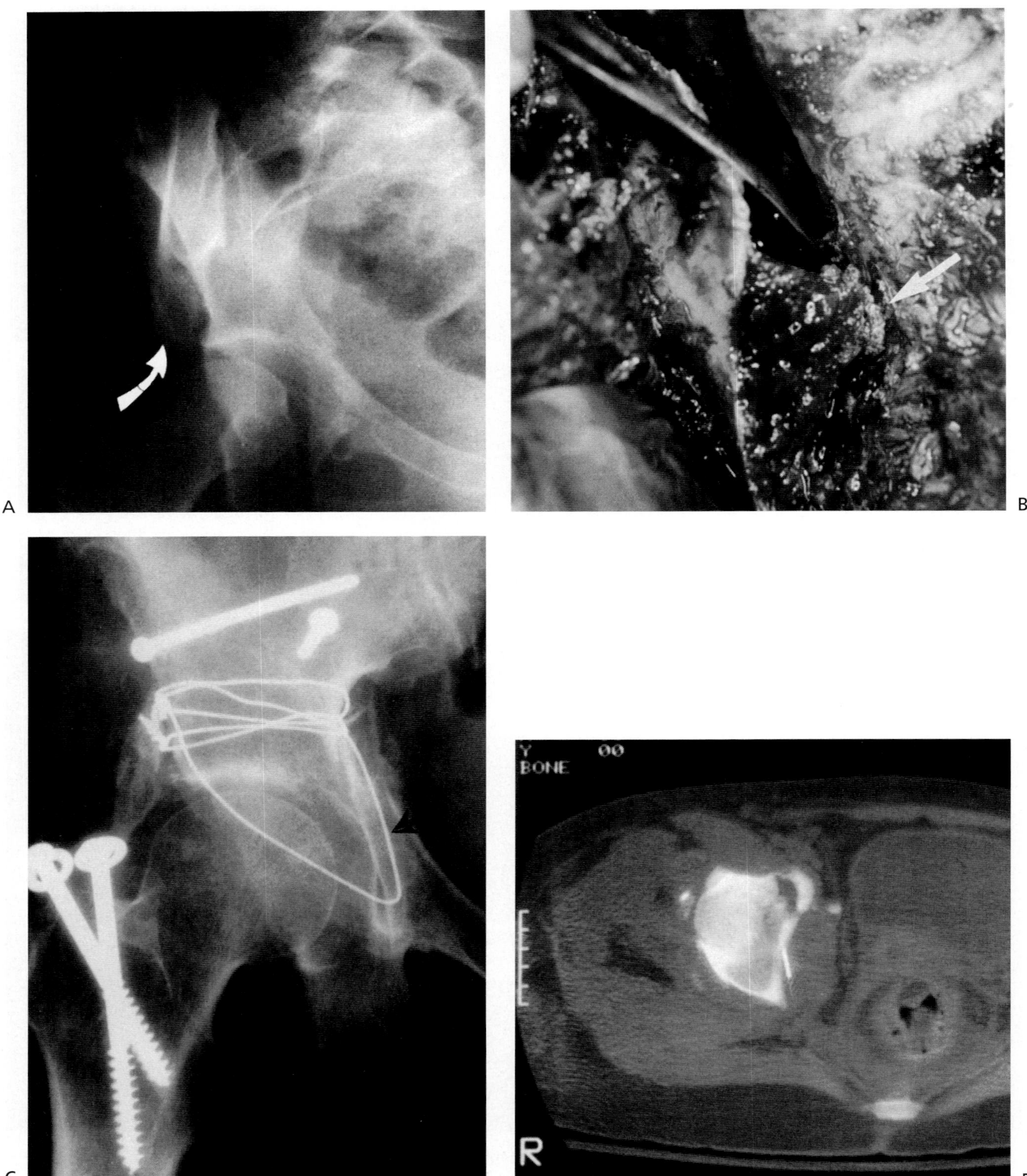

FIGURE 32-4. Cerclage wires as a time-saving device. A young woman developed a saddle pulmonary embolus just after the clinical exposure had been made through an anterior ilioinguinal approach. **A:** A classic both-column fracture with incongruity is noted, the spur sign denoted by the *white arrow.* **B:** The clinical photograph shows the displaced anterior column *(white arrow).* **C:** Because of life-threatening pulmonary problems, two cerclage wires were placed through the greater sciatic notch and one through the lesser notch *(black arrow),* and two interfragmental screws were inserted. This reduction proceeded extremely quickly. The patient survived and has an excellent clinical result with slight heterotopic ossification. **D:** Note the reduction achieved in the postoperative computed tomography and the position of one section of the wire.

33

EXTRAPERITONEAL FIXATION

EERO HIRVENSALO

INDICATIONS

Central protrusion of the femoral head through the quadrilateral surface often needs special attention. The comminution can be marked. This phenomenon is seen in many fracture patterns, including anterior column, transverse, T-type, or both column fractures (Table 33-1). It is important to recognize that there might be an impacted large articular fragment of the central dome that needs to be reduced to achieve an anatomic joint surface.

A direct intrapelvic extraperitoneal access to the central quadrilateral area gives an option to reduce the fragments situated in the most central and cranial part of the acetabulum. Moreover, it is possible to establish fixation through this true medial window (Fig. 33-1).

APPROACH

The extraperitoneal approach (Stoppa or midline approach) for the acetabular region is created through a 15-cm long low midline incision. A transverse Pfannenstiel incision is justified for cosmetic reasons but it does not allow enough space to operate on the lateral aspect of the inside pelvis. Blunt preparation along the visceral side of the superior ramus reveals the roof of the obturator foramen. The psoas muscle and femoral neurovascular structures are gently elevated. The iliopectineal fascia is cut to enhance the elevation of these structures. The fracture hematoma is cleaned from the quadrilateral area. A retractor is placed carefully under the posterior margin of the ischium. It should not be placed too cranially into the sciatic notch to avoid injuring the gluteal vessels and sciatic nerve. The obturator nerve and vessels can be pushed medially with the retractor. This gives a direct view of the fracture at the central acetabular as well as the medial periacetabular area.

REDUCTION AND FIXATION TECHNIQUES

Anterior Column Fracture with Central Comminution

(See Fig. 33-2.) The anterior column fragment and the fragments of the most central part of the quadrilateral surface can be gently displaced in order to evaluate the intraarticular status. Traction on the affected extremity is necessary. The impacted fragments can be reduced and the joint can be cleaned of any smaller loose bodies. Usually, especially in osteoporotic cases, bone grafting is needed to stabilize the fragment and thereby hold the reduced joint surface in the right position. Whenever the anterior column fracture extends to the iliac fossa a separate lateral approach along the iliac crest can be done to accomplish the fixation of the supraacetabular part.

The fixation can be planned on the quadrilateral area after cleaning and reduction of the acetabular and periacetabular fragments. The drill bit should be protected not to cause any visceral lesions. Self-tapping screws and powered screwdrivers are used.

The low anterior column fracture is fixed along the pelvic brim with a reconstruction plate. The quadrilateral surface is best covered by a one-third tubular plate placed as a spring plate perpendicular to the anterior column plate. Any thicker plate is difficult to place in the deep pelvic area. Moreover, the insertion of the screws in oblique direction is easier with thin plates. Because of the visualization of the entire quadrilateral area the plate can be fixed on both ends; that is, also into the posterior column. This gives extra stability to the osteosynthesis. A reducing force to the quadrilateral area can be created to

TABLE 33-1. INDICATIONS FOR EXTRAPERITONEAL FIXATION

Fractures involving the quadrilateral surface, especially with comminution and central protrusion of the femoral head:
Anterior column
Anterior column plus posterior hemitransverse
T fracture
Transverse fracture
Both-column fracture

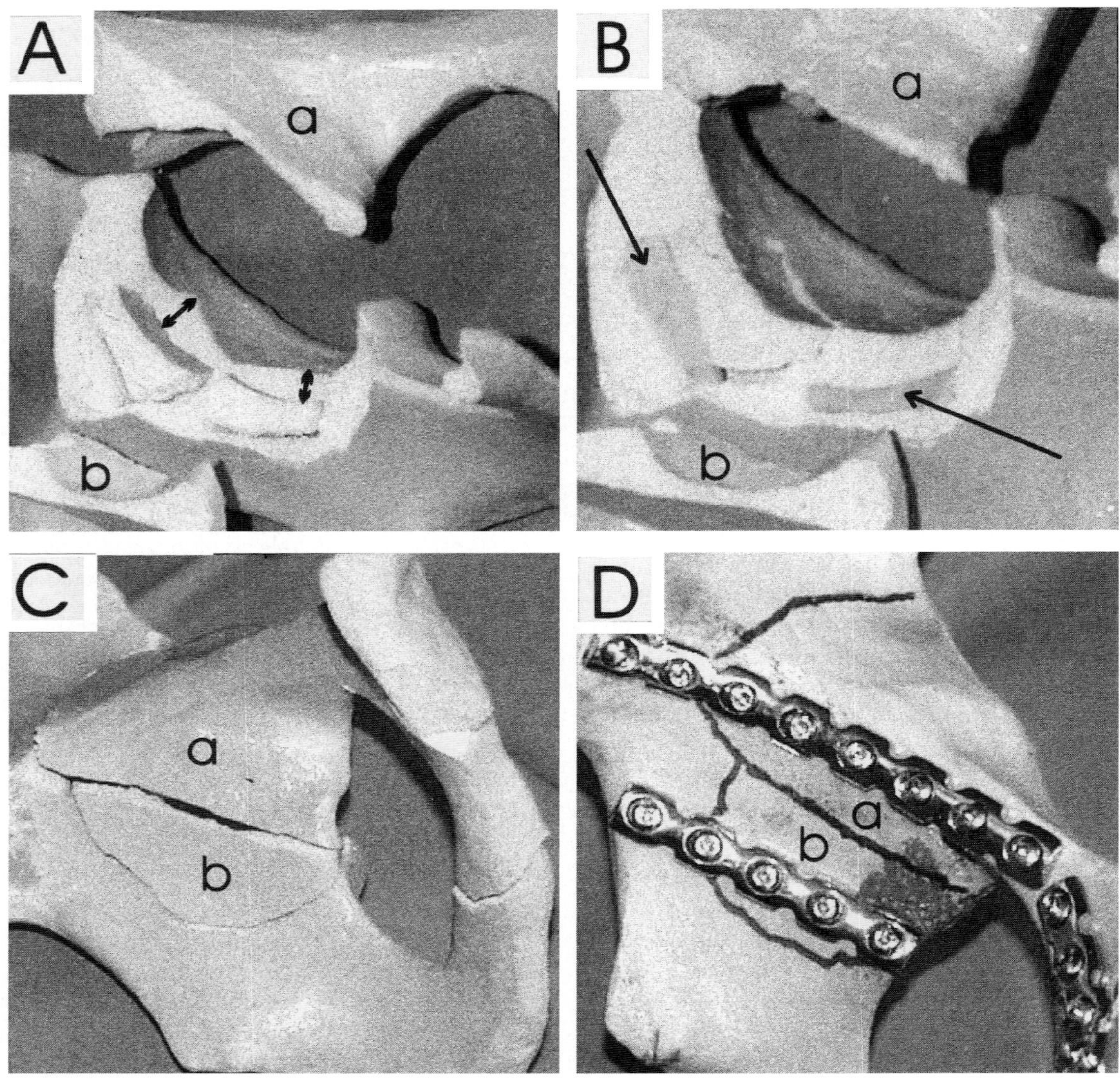

FIGURE 33-1. The technical figures on the plastic model show the extraperitoneal, intrapelvic (iliac) view during the operation. **A:** The central protrusion of the femoral head (missing in the figure) causes not only fragmentation on the quadrilateral bone but also comminution of the subchondral bone *(arrows).* **B:** In the operation the main fragments—anterior roof *(a)* and central fragment *(b)*—are elevated and the defects are filled with cancellous bone *(arrows).* **C:** The covering bone fragments around the quadrilateral surface *(a,b)* are reduced. **D:** The final situation after fixation.

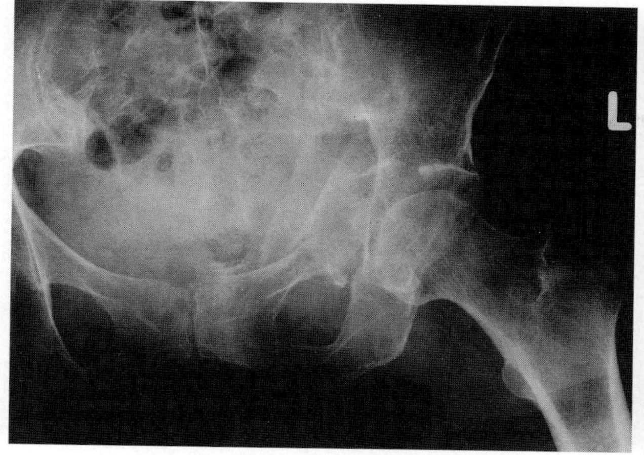

A

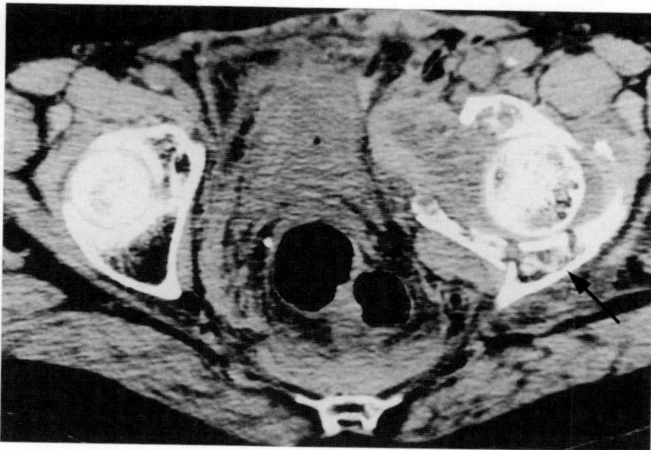
B

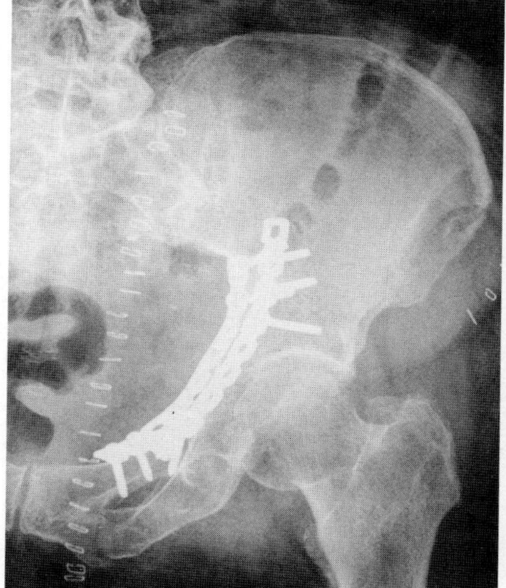
C

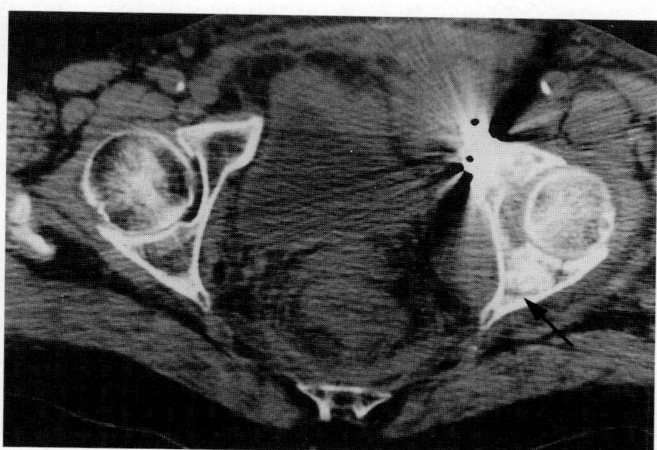
D

FIGURE 33-2. A 70-year-old woman sustained an anterior column with posterior hemitransverse fracture of the left acetabulum after falling on stairs. **A:** Anterior-posterior view (AP) shows a typical central acetabular comminution of an elderly patient. **B:** Computed tomography (CT) view reveals a markedly displaced posterior intraarticular fragment *(arrow).* The reduction of the comminuted intraarticular fragment was secured with bone grafting through the medial window on the quadrilateral surface. A lower medial incision and extraperitoneal approach only were necessary. The postoperative AP view **(C)** and especially the CT view **(D)** show the fragment in correct position after cancellous bone grafting *(arrow).*

resist the central protruding force of the femoral head by slight over-bending of the plate.

T-, or Transverse-Type Fractures

(See Fig. 33-3.) Two or occasionally three plates can be attached to the quadrilateral surface across the fracture lines. The anterior plate is placed on the pelvic brim. One plate is placed on the lower aspect of the quadrilateral area. Actually, this plate lies on the medial aspect of the posterior column. Care has to be taken to insert this plate accurately, below the point of the central acetabular area to avoid entering the joint with screws. Usually, especially in female patients, the dorsal part of the quadrilateral surface turns somewhat medially. In these cases the insertion of the screws is possible even in the most dorsal area of the medial surface. On the other hand, in some male patients the dorsal part of the quadrilateral surface may turn somewhat laterally. In these cases extraperitoneal dorsal fixation is not possible.

Both-Column Fractures

(See Fig. 33-4.) In both-column types, the fixation of the anterior column and the central quadrilateral area are

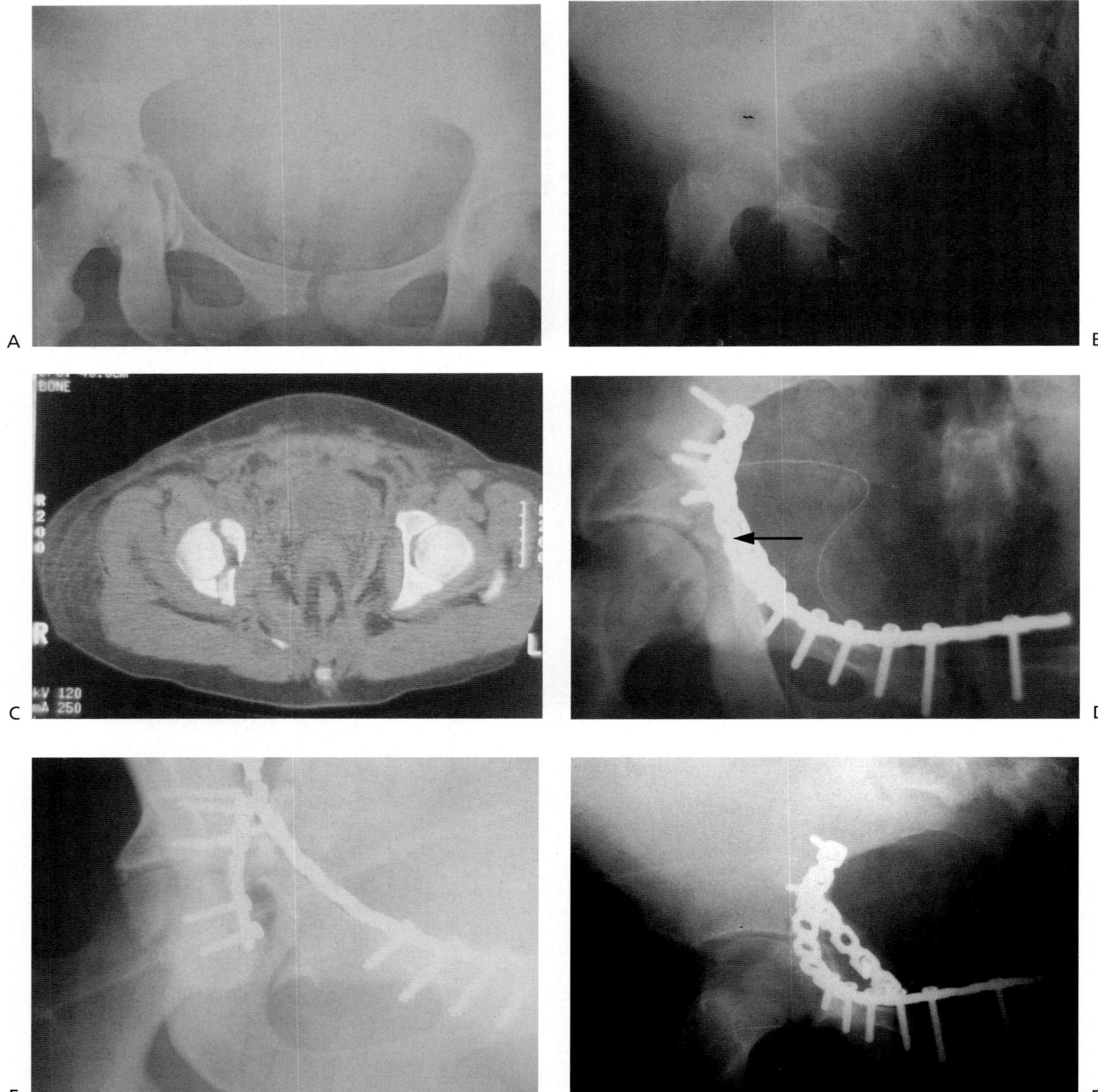

FIGURE 33-3. A 21-year-old woman sustained a T-type fracture in a falling accident. **A:** Preoperative anterior-posterior (AP) view. **B:** Iliac-view. **C:** Computed tomography scan demonstrate the oblique and slightly comminuted central acetabular area. Reduction of the main fragments as well as the small central fragment was carried out extraperitoneally through the low midline incision. Direct view on the quadrilateral area was prepared. **D:** The postoperative AP view shows a nearly anatomic position of the small central fragment indicated with an arrow. **E:** The iliac view demonstrates the position of the two medial plates. **F:** The shorter plate has been placed near the lower edge of the quadrilateral surface just above the ischial spine in order to fix the posterior column. No further exposures were needed.

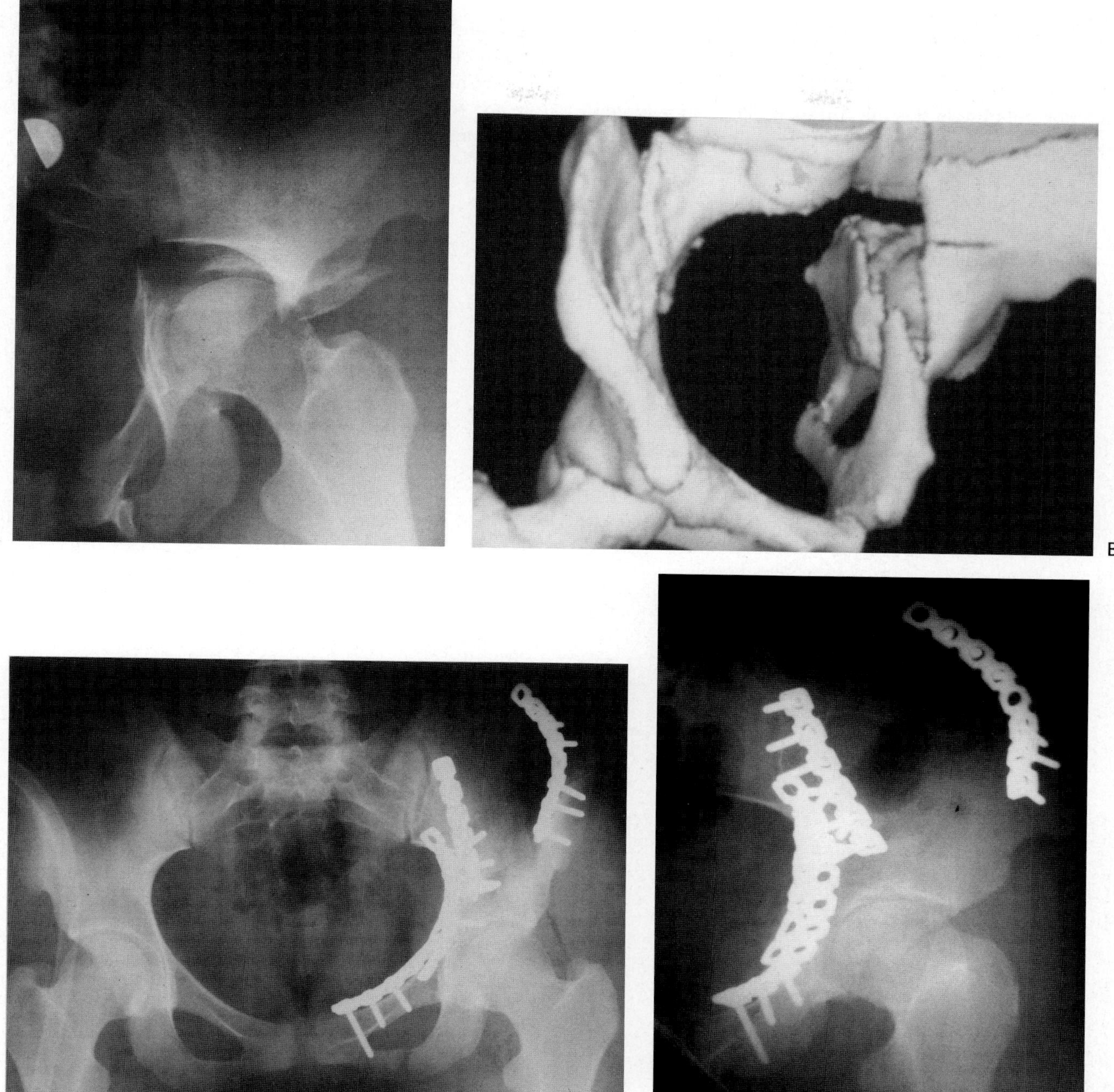

FIGURE 33-4. A 27-year-old woman sustained a both column fracture in a car accident. **A:** Preoperative anterior-posterior (AP) view and especially the three-dimensional iliac view demonstrate four separate fragments affecting the roof of the acetabulum. **B:** The quadrilateral component is solid and displaced medially together with the posterior column. The reduction was made through a lateral incision (upper anterior column) and through a low midline incision (lower anterior column and posterior column) extraperitoneally. **C:** The right position of the acetabular block was first secured with the two lateral plates through the lateral approach, AP view. The lower anterior column and the posterior column fractures were fixed with the two medial plates. **D:** The lower plate lies on the quadrilateral surface, seen most medially on the iliac view.

reduced and fixed first as described in the preceding. The reduction and fixation of the fracture of the posterior column are usually done through a separate Kocher-Langenbeck approach. Occasionally, however, the fixation of the posterior column is possible through the extraperitoneal exposure. A prerequisite for fixation is an anatomic position of the posterior column. Therefore, it is very important not to insert the screws to the posterior structures if the posterior column is not reduced. In these cases the comminuted central area is secured with a spring plate that is not fixed to the posterior column. Good preoperative planning is of great value in these cases.

34

USE OF BONE SUBSTITUTES

VICTOR A. DE RIDDER
S. DE LANGE

INTRODUCTION

The use of bone substitutes in acetabular fractures is uncommon. In a limited number of fractures cancellous or cortical bone can be used to fill a void, especially in a weight-bearing zone such as the posterior or superior part of the acetabulum.

The substitution of cancellous bone by a bone substitute in a compressed bone mass along a fracture is common practice, particularly if the bone is osteoporotic. The tibial plateau or the calcaneal fracture often is reconstructed, leaving a void in the osteoporotic bone mass to be filled with a cancellous bone graft or bone substitute.

Many bone substitutes have been developed, and many publications support the efficacy of the use of bone substitutes.

Cancellous bone grafting of a void after reconstruction of a comminuted and impacted posterior wall fracture of the acetabulum has shown good results and is standard treatment practice (1–4). However, these fractures remain a problem in older patients (5). The results of these impacted posterior wall fractures appear to be related to the age of the patient. In particular, the results in patients more than 60 years old have been less than optimal because of osteoporotic bone, impaction, and comminution in our patients. Several publications have discussed the difficult treatment of acetabular fractures in elderly patients with various results (5,6).

Letournel and Judet support good results in elderly patients. Their results were even better in the 70- to 79-year-old group than in the 60- to 69-year-old group. They attributed this to not enough numbers for an adequate statistical analysis for age groupings (2).

Collapse of the grafted posterior wall was observed in our older patient population, mostly within 6 months. Lower density of the cancellous bone graft of the posterior wall in these patients, and comminution of the posterior wall combined with impaction of the osteoporotic bone are considered main reasons for the poor stability and poor results.

Important technical feature of the bone replacement materials include both biologic and mechanical factors.

The biological materials and substances can possess osteogenic, osteoconductive, or osteoinductive activity, or combinations of these three activities. Osteogenic materials contain living mesenchymal cells capable of differentiating into osteoblasts. Through its structure, an osteoconductive material provides a receptive scaffold to facilitate new bone formation. An osteoinductive material can be defined as one that provides a biologic stimulus that induces mesenchymal cells to differentiate into osteoblasts.

CLINICAL STUDY

We have assessed the clinical utility of an *in situ* setting, high compressive strength, remodelable, calcium phosphate bone cement to fill the void after the standard osteosynthesis of the impacted posterior wall in older patients (7). As an example of these substances we have used Norian SRS and Biobon (8–10), and in this study only Norian SRS (Norian Corp., Cupertino, CA).

A prospective protocol was initiated in 1993. The inclusion criteria were a comminuted posterior wall fracture of the acetabulum with impaction of the underlying cancellous bone and a minimum age of 60 years. Exclusion criteria were previous operations of the pelvis, metabolic bone disease, local bone pathology (e.g., cancer and osteomyelitis), and severe osteoporosis inhibiting operative reconstruction, defined with the Singh classification and the visual aspect of the width of the pelvic cortex.

Between 1993 and 1999, 42 patients were treated for a posterior wall fracture of the acetabulum. Sixteen patients were more than 60 years old. Of these, six were excluded:

two were previously operated on the pelvis, two showed metastatic processes in the pelvis and acetabulum, and two had severe osteoporosis and previous fractures. These excluded patients were treated nonoperatively.

Ten patients were enrolled and treated. Informed consent was obtained of every patient. Average age was 71 years old (range 62 to 77). Six patients were female, four male. All had a posterior dislocation with impaction and comminution of the posterior acetabular wall and some degree of osteoporosis. The impaction and comminution was located at the posterior-superior region in four patients, posterior in three and posterior-inferior in three patients. Each comminuted fracture had between two and four major fragments. No intraarticular loose fragments were found on the computed tomography (CT) scan or during operation. All dislocations were reduced under general anesthesia within 6 hours of presentation. The impaction and comminution were diagnosed preoperatively with plain radiographs, the three Judet radiographic views and CT scan. CT scans were particularly useful to determine the extent of the impaction and create operative plan.

The reconstruction was performed through a Kocher-Langenbeck approach in a prone position on the traction table with electromyographic and somatosensory evoked potentials monitoring. The impacted chondral plate along with attached cancellous bone was elevated and the posterior wall reconstructed. In each case this resulted in a void of more than 1 cm^3. Rigid internal fixation was performed with a combination of plates and screws. The subchondral cancellous bone void in the posterior wall was filled with Norian SRS through a screw hole or small cortical gap using a 10- to 12-gauge needle after all internal fixation was in place. The volume of SRS used varied from 1.5 to 4.5 cc. The void was identified before replacement of the posterior wall cortex and filled with the Norian SRS paste without any pressure (Figs. 34-1 through 34-4).

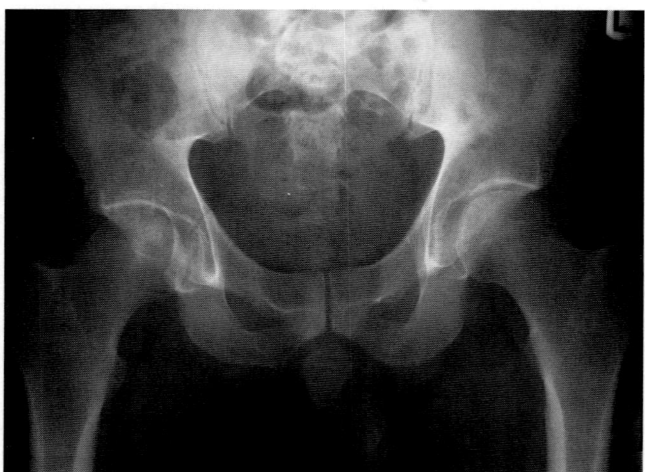

FIGURE 34-1. A patient with a posterior wall fracture on plain x-ray.

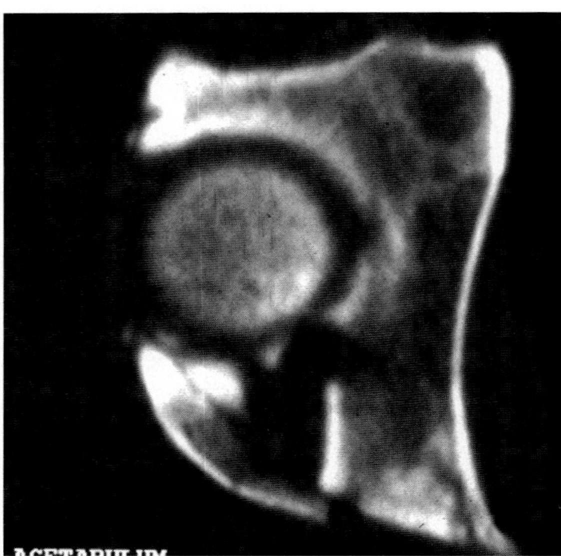

FIGURE 34-2. Posterior wall fracture and impaction on computed tomography scan.

The paste can leak into the joint if a defect is present in the articular surface; before hardening it has to be removed and the joint rinsed. Kopylov (11) reported Norian SRS paste injected into the carpal joint. It was not removed and resolved in time without adverse effects.

All patients began physical therapy and started partial weight bearing with two crutches within 1 week of surgery. Mobilization was increased to full weight bearing within 6 weeks. Between 6 to 12 weeks, one crutch was used as a stabilization aid and to enhance a feeling of safety in these older patients.

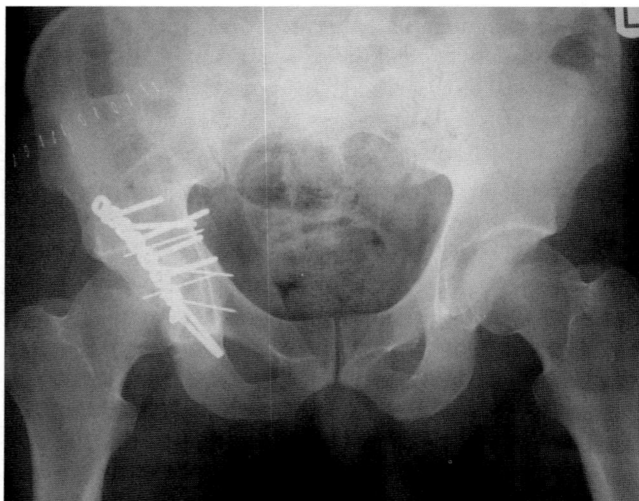

FIGURE 34-3. Posterior wall fracture and impaction on plain x-ray after reconstruction with plates and screws, and the void filled with skeletal repair system (SRS).

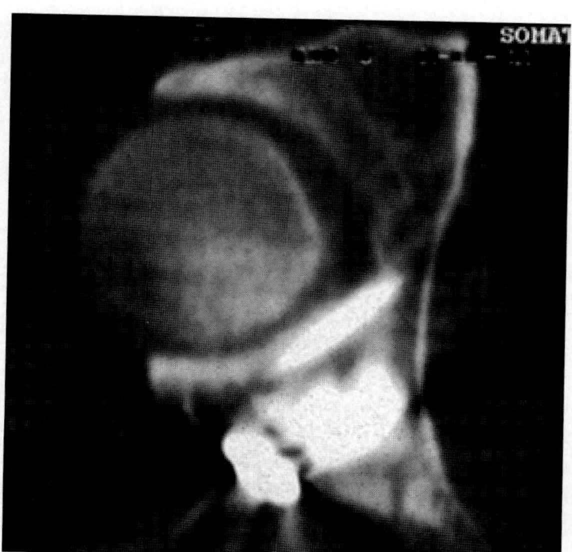

FIGURE 34-4. Posterior wall fracture and impaction on computed tomography scan after reconstruction with plates and screws, and the void filled with SRS.

After 6 and 12 weeks, 6 and 12 months, and 2 years the patients were seen at the outpatient clinic. Physical examination and plain radiographs were recorded. Pain, function, and radiographic results of the hip joint were graded using the d'Aubigne scoring system (1–6). CT scans were performed in all patients at 2 weeks and after 6, 12, and 24 months postoperatively. After 6 and 12 weeks, 6 and 12 months and 2 years the patients were seen at the outpatient clinic. Physical examination, plain radiographs, and d'Aubigne scores were assessed.

Norian SRS is an injectable, *in situ* setting, isothermic, calcium phosphate bone cement that cures *in vivo* to form carbonate apatite with chemical and physical characteristics similar to the mineral phase of bone (12). Calcium and phosphate source powders are mixed with a phosphate buffer solution to form an injectable material of paste-like consistency that conforms to fill the bone defect. It hardens within minutes, and achieves its maximum compressive strength of 55 mPa by approximately 12 hours. The reaction occurs at physiologic temperature and pH. Once mixed, the cement has a working time of 5 minutes at ambient temperature. Setting of the cement is temperature sensitive and begins to set within 2 to 3 minutes following injection into the bone void. During the 10-minute setting time, while the product hardens, all movements or manipulations should be avoided so as not to disturb the crystallization of Norian SRS (11,13–18). In the posterior wall fracture voids, the void is surrounded by a stable osteosynthesis; thus, the 10-minute setting time is sufficient to crystallize the carbonate apatite.

Ten patients have been treated with this protocol using Norian SRS cement to fill the void of the posterior wall of the acetabulum, and completed more than 2 years of follow-up. To compare the results of this study group we also examined previous patients conventionally treated in our hospital with a posterior wall acetabulum fracture.

The preoperative and postoperative care was identical to all previous posterior wall acetabulum fractures treated in this institution. The patients in the SRS group were discharged after 10 to 14 days to a rehabilitation facility, on average after 13 days. One patient had a superficial wound infection, none a deep infection. No patients had venous thromboses, or pulmonary or urinary problems. No neurologic problems were diagnosed preoperatively or postoperatively. The time to discharge, in-hospital rehabilitation, and pain medication were identical, the duration of the operation was the same as in the previous non-cement group of patients on average. Blood loss was in both groups the same, average 250 mL (150 to 500 mL).

After discharge the cement group improved functionally quicker than the conventional group of patients. Return to normal range of motion was on average within 5 weeks (range 4 to 6 weeks) compared to an average of 8 weeks (6 to 10 weeks), scored with the d'Aubigne points system (19). Full weight bearing without pain and aid of a crutch occurred within 10 weeks (8 to 11 weeks) in the cement group as compared to an average of 14 weeks in the conventional group (12 to 16 weeks). Return to daily activities and previous sporting activities (walking, golf, and tennis) were also about 4 weeks shorter, average of 22 and 26 weeks for the two groups.

The d'Aubigne scores were good in six patients (16 to 17 points) and excellent in four patients (18 points) in the SRS group after 6 months and remained unchanged through the 2-year outpatient clinic follow-up period.

The plain and Judet radiographic views were only helpful to determine narrowing of the joint space, which occurred in four patients (12 to 16 d'Aubigne points) between 6 and 12 months postoperatively. No further changes were observed during the 2-year plus radiographic and CT follow-up.

The CT scan shows the posterior wall accurately. A perfect reduction and reconstruction with a totally filled void was seen in six patients postoperatively. The remaining four patients showed a slight gap or an articular step-off of 1 to 2 mm. Six-, 12-, and 24-month CT examination revealed two patients with a collapse of the posterior wall. Ingrowth of cancellous bone was noted at the interface of bone and the SRS.

Posterior wall (PW) fractures of the acetabulum are seen in PW, PW/posterior column, PW/transverse, PW/T-shaped fractures. Poor clinical results of the posterior wall fracture of the acetabulum are probably caused by impaction, comminution, posterior dislocation femoral head, subchondral tear, and stripping of the posterior wall and femoral head, resulting in avascular necrosis, ischemia of the chondral plate, ischemia of fragments of the posterior wall, mechanical instability, and many other problems. The prognosis of the posterior wall fractures has been the subject of many discussions in recent publications (3,4,5,7,10,11, 20–27).

The single most important factor is probably the vascularization of the fragment of the posterior wall, either attached to the capsule or part of the impacted cancellous wall. If the posterior wall reconstruction is relatively unstable, then the revascularization of the ischemic fragments could be hindered.

Those factors that ultimately affect fracture construct stability may be avoided if regions of crushed cancellous bone resulting from the injury can be structurally augmented following fixation with conventional ORIF.

Good stability with no collapse has been reported in younger patients with good bone density following augmentation of the posterior wall with dense cancellous bone from the greater trochanter. In these younger patients, vascularization of the fragment is less compromised and revascularization more rapid than in the older patients studied in this investigation. Additionally, in aged patients, cancellous bone is of lower density; therefore, it offers insufficient structural support to augment the posterior wall (28).

Bone grafting has potential problems, including donor site morbidity and complications with autografts and potential transmission of viral disease with allografts. Methacrylate bone cement may cause thermal damage to surrounding bone and soft tissues and cannot be replaced by host bone. Injectable bone cement that hardens *in situ* to form a carbonated apatite similar to the mineral phase of bone provides mechanical strength for stabilization through healing of the fracture by filling of the cancellous bone defect. In addition to the mechanical advantage gained from filling irregular bone voids, the high compressive strength of this cement allows more rapid rehabilitation and mobilization of the patient (11,18,29).

EXPERIMENTAL STUDIES

Bone grafting or stabilization with intramedullary methylmethacrylate has been used to restore anatomy and stability. The implantation of Norian SRS cement in the cancellous bone defect has theoretical advantages compared to conventional methacrylate cement. Norian SRS cement is crystallographically and compositionally similar to the mineral phase of bone. This has been postulated as the reason for its replacement by bone through a remodeling process that involves osteoclastic resorption, similar to that by which native bone remodels (13,15). Norian SRS cement–augmented fracture patients improved functionally more rapidly than conventionally treated patients, which corroborates the biomechanical advantage of cement augmentation reported by Seleem and Tile in a cadaveric study in which similar fractures were evaluated biomechanically (25). They compared the stability of the impacted acetabular fragment supported with autogenous bone graft versus calcium phosphate cement in an *in vitro* biomechanical study.

Six unembalmed pelves, providing two paired hemipelvic specimens were used. Intact subchondral bone deformation in the side of the planned impacted fragment was recorded by a guidewire with a serrated tip that passed through a cannulated screw from the inside of the pelvis to the subchondral bone of the acetabulum.

Loads were applied through the femur by MTS machine with the hip joint in 60 degrees flexion, and 10 degrees adduction. Displacement of the subchondral bone was recorded by an LVDT fixed to the other end of the guidewire. Axial forces of 100 N (10 cycles), 250 N (1,010 cycles), and 750 N (10 cycles) were applied through the femur. Following intact testing, an impacted acetabular fragment in the posterior column of each hemipelvis was created and underlying cancellous bone was removed to create a defect. Two lag screws and a reconstruction plate fixed the posterior wall fracture. In one hemipelvis, the fragment was supported by autogenous cancellous bone graft. On the contralateral side, the fracture void was prepared in the same way. Norian SRS was injected in a retrograde fashion, completely filling the subchondral void. The results showed statistically significant differences ($p < 0.05$) in the mean displacement between carbonated apatite cement specimens and bone graft specimens at 100 N ($p < 0.05$), 250 N ($p < 0.002$), and 750 N ($p < 0.0004$). Significantly less displacement of the impacted acetabular fragments augmented with this cement was observed than when the fragments were augmented with cancellous bone graft. They concluded that carbonated apatite cement (Norian SRS) offered immediate mechanical integrity to the impacted fragment and remained stable. Improved construct stability and long-term remodeling of the underlying cement may improve clinical outcome.

Norian SRS can be injected following ORIF to form-fill these comprised regions. It hardens to an ultimate compressive strength of 55 mPa. Its ability to withstand compressive forces gives structural augmentation improving the fracture construct integrity.

CONCLUSION

Under the prospective protocol employed, this series of ten patients with an impacted and comminuted posterior wall with a cancellous bone defect larger than 1 cm^3, had good clinical results. Only two patients with a collapse of the posterior wall were seen, no adverse effects of the use of SRS were noted. The results and complications were comparable with other series of operatively treated patients (2,3,26,27). The mobilization and rehabilitation were rapid, the patients started partial weight bearing with two crutches within 1 week. They felt safe and had little pain, resulting in more rapid rehabilitation than observed in comparable patients treated conventionally. Return of function with less joint stiffness resulted in higher d'Aubigne scores.

A large number of synthetic bone substitutes have been developed during the last three decades. These materials have extensively been tested in animal studies with respect to biocompatibility, incorporation in bone, osteoconduction, and resorption. Calcium phophate ceramics, in particular hydroxyapatite, are the most widely used bone substitutes for the treatment of bone defects. In a prospective randomized trial the performance of hydroxyapatite was similar to autograft in the treatment of tibial plateau fractures in terms of radiographic healing and functional outcome. By using bone substitutes, the donor operation of autograft and associated morbidity can be prevented. The first generation of hydroxyapatite-based materials is not resorbable, but recently resorbable calcium phosphate cements have become available. These materials have been shown in animal experiments to be resorbed by osteoclasts as part of the normal bone remodeling process.

These promising early results represent limited clinical experience in treating these difficult acetabular fractures. The problem remains complex and is probably caused by a combination of trauma of the vascularization of the acetabulum and femoral head, and mechanical instability.

However, a high strength, isothermic, calcium phosphate cement susceptible to the native remodeling process that can be injected through screw holes or small cortical windows following ORIF, hardens rapidly at body temperature, and offers significant compressive strength appears appropriate for structural augmentation of a region of compromised cancellous bone in acetabular fractures. As an example of these substances we have used Norian SRS and Biobon.

The rapid return to daily life activities or work is a major goal for the treatment of acetabular fractures. An improved construct of the posterior wall allows for shorter immobilization time, earlier use of the hip joint, and reduced risk of limb stiffness.

REFERENCES

1. Baumgaertner MR. Fractures of the posterior wall of the acetabulum. *J Am Acad Orthop Surg* 1999;7(1):54–65.
2. Letournel E, Judet R. *Fractures of the acetabulum,* 2nd ed. Berlin: Springer-Verlag, 1993.
3. Matta JM, Meritt PO. Displaced acetabular fractures. *Clin Orthop* 1988;230:83–97.
4. Rommens PM, Gimenez MV, Hessmann M. Posterior wall fractures of the acetabulum: characteristics, management, prognosis. *Acta Chir Belg* 2001;101(6):287–293.
5. Mears DC. Surgical treatment of acetabular fractures in elderly patients with osteoporotic bone. *J Am Acad Orthop Surg* 1999; 7(2):128–141.
6. Helfet DL, Borrelli J Jr, DiPasquale T, et al. Stabilization of acetabular fractures in elderly patients. *J Bone Joint Surg Am* 1992;74(5):753–765.
7. Ridder De VA, Lange de S, Kerver AJH, et al. Posterior wall acetabular fractures: augmentation of comminuted and impacted cancellous bone with Norian SRS, a carbonated apatite cement. *Eur J Tr* 2002 (*in press*).
8. Boer FC den. Enhancement of bone repair with recombinant human osteogenic protein-1. Thesis, University of Amsterdam, 2001.
9. Knaack D, Goad MEP, Aiolova M, et al. Resorbable calcium phosphate bone substitute. *J Biomed Mater Res (Appl Biomat)* 1998;43:399–409.
10. Patka P, Haarman HJThJ, Bakker FC. Bottransplantaten en botvervangende materialen. *NTVG* 1998;142(16):893–896.
11. Kopylov P, Jonnson K, Thorgren KG, et al. Injectable calcium phospate in the treatment of distal radial fractures. *J Hand Surg* 1996;21B: 6:768–771.
12. Keith J, Brashear HR, Guilford WB. Stability of posterior fracture-dislocation of the hip. *J Bone J Surg (Am)* 1988;70:711–714.
13. Constantz BR, Ison IC, Fulmer MT, et al. Skeletal repair by in situ formation of the mineral phase of bone. *Science* 1995;267:1772,1796–1799.
14. Elder SH, Frankenburg EP, Yetkinler DN, et al. *Biomechanical evaluation of calcium phosphate cement-augmented repair of unstable intertrochanteric fractures.* 43rd Annual Meeting, Orthopaedic Research Society. San Francisco, 1997.
15. Frankenburg EP, Goldstein SA, Bauer TW, et al. Biomechanical and histologic evaluation of a calcium phosphate cement. *J Bone J Surg (Am)* 1998;80A(8):1112–1124.
16. Frankenburg EP, Patil PV, DeBano CM, et al. A four and one half year follow-up of a bioresorbable bone cement in a canine metaphyseal model. *Trans ORS* 1999;516.
17. Kiyoshige Y. Bone cementing of distal radial fractures in the elderly. In: Saffar P, Cooney WP, eds. *Fractures of the distal radius.* London: Martin Dunitz, 1995:84–88.
18. Kofoed H. Comminuted displaced Colles' fractures. Treatment with intramedullary methylmethacrylate stabilisation. *Acta Orthop Scand* 1983;54:307–311.
19. d'Aubigne RM, Cauchoix J, Ramadier JV. Evaluation: chifree de la fonction de la hauche. Application a l'etude des resultants des operations mobilisatries de la hauche. *Rev Orthop* 1949; 35:541–548.
20. Brumback RJ, Holt ES, McBride MS, et al. Acetabular depression fracture accompanying posterior fracture dislocation of the hip. *J Orthop Trauma* 1990;4:42–48.
21. Olson SA, Bay BK, Chapman MW, et al. Biomechanical consequences of posterior wall acetabular fractures and repair. *J Bone J Surg (Am)* 1995;77:1184–1192.
22. Olson SA, Bay BK, Pollak AN, et al. The effect of variable size posterior wall acetabular fractures on contact characteristics of the hip joint. *J Orthop Trauma* 1996;6:395–402.
23. Rowe CR, Lowell JD. Prognosis of fractures of the acetabulum. *J Bone J Surg (Am)* 1961;43:30–59.
24. Saterbak AM, Marsh JL, Brandser E, et al. Outcome of surgically treated posterior wall acetabular fractures. *OTA* 1996.
25. Seleem OA, Hearn TC, Yetkinler DN, et al. Stability of impacted acetabular fragment following augmentation with bone graft or calcium phosphate cement. *J Biomech* 1998;31(1):66.
26. Vailas JC, Hurwitz S, Wiesel SW. Posterior acetabular fracture-dislocations: fragment size, joint capsule, and stability. *J Trauma* 1989;29:1494–1496.
27. Wright R, Barrett K, Christie MJ, et al. Acetabular fractures: long-term follow-up of open reduction and internal fixation. *J Orthop Trauma* 1994;8:397–403.
28. Jowsey J. Bone morphology: bone structure. In: Sledge CB, ed. *Metabolic diseases of bone.* Philadelphia: WB Saunders, 1977: 41–47.
29. Lotz JC, Hu SS, Chiu DFM, et al. Carbonated apatite cement augmentation of pedicle screw fixation in the lumbar spine. *Spine* 1997;22:2716–2723.

35

INTRAOPERATIVE EVALUATION

MICHAEL A. TERRY
DAVID L. HELFET

There are a number of methods described to evaluate both fracture reduction and hardware placement. These include: direct visualization, palpation, auscultation, assessment of crepitus during manipulation, intraoperative radiologic assessment, intraoperative arthroscopy, postoperative arthroscopy, and postoperative radiologic assessment. The difference between methods that evaluate reduction and hardware placement intraoperatively and those that do so postoperatively is an important one. Although surgeon feedback and learning from postoperative evaluation may be obtained, any adjustments in hardware placement or reduction required after a postoperative evaluation necessitate a second operative procedure.

Direct visualization of reduction and hardware placement is ideal when possible. It allows intraoperative evaluation and is simple to perform. However, effective visualization is not only approach-dependent, it also depends on the fracture and location of hardware, necessitating a decision regarding distraction or dislocation of the femoral head and/or extending the surgical dissection. However, both of these present additional risks, especially to the blood supply to the femoral head and acetabulum.

Palpation includes intraoperative palpation of fragments and articular surfaces for incongruity or hardware and feeling for crepitus with range of motion of a joint. The latter is especially useful with digital palpation of the quadrilateral plate, which can be readily accomplished from anterior or posterior. The limitations of palpation are similar to those of visualization.

Auscultation of the hip joint has been described with (1) and without (2) the use of a stethoscope. This technique involves listening for sounds created by rough articular fragments that are poorly reduced or intraarticular hardware. This has been found to be highly reliable by some authors and is performed intraoperatively. Anglen and DiPasquale reported 100% sensitivity, specificity, and accuracy of their technique in the hands of the originators (1). Although they demonstrated excellent results from this technique in inexperienced users, they recommend at least one practice session using this method with a cadaver prior to its use in the operating room. The limitations of auscultation include determining what exactly is causing the audible sound and therefore, what hardware or fracture fragment needs to be adjusted.

Intraoperative radiography includes plain x-ray images, fluoroscopy, and arthrography. Plain film x-ray allows good visualization for the views that are obtainable, but it can be difficult to obtain various images with plain films because of the difficulties associated with patient positioning and the x-ray machine itself. Another drawback of plain film radiology is the amount of time spent taking the films and waiting for them to be developed and returned. Ebraheim and coworkers determined that the cross table lateral and Judet iliac views were more helpful than the anterior-posterior (AP) or Judet obturator views in determining screw placement. They suggested arthrography as an adjunct to plain film or fluoroscopic imaging if the joint space is poorly visualized (3).

Fluoroscopy can be used intraoperatively and produces images immediately. More views usually can be obtained using a fluoroscopy machine because it may be draped and positioned in the sterile field. The image quality found in fluoroscopy generally is considered inferior to plain films, but it continues to improve and the time convenience and additional views obtainable make this method very useful. Norris and coworkers showed a 100% correlation of intraoperative fluoroscopic images and plain films and were able to obtain adequate imaging of the acetabulum 95% of the time. They described fluoroscopy as safe, effective, easy to use, and reliable (4). Carmack and coworkers determined that fluoroscopy and computed tomography were equally accurate for determining intraarticular screw penetration (5). They also found that obtaining an axial image of the screw was as sensitive and specific as obtaining a tangential image when attempting to determine intraarticular placement of hardware.

All intraoperative imaging techniques can be limited by overlying bowel gas, obesity, intraabdominal contrast from previous studies in the multitrauma patient, drapes, patient position, and the operating room table.

Hip arthroscopy has been used during the initial procedure or in subsequent procedures to evaluate the joint after acetabular fracture (6–8). This allows direct inspection of the articular surfaces without dislocation of the joint. However, the entire joint surface is not visualized. Other limitations of arthroscopy include potential iatrogenic articular surface damage, fluid extravasation with potential compartment syndrome (8), and the time used in its set up and performance. Another critical issue with arthroscopy, palpation, and direct visualization is that hardware can penetrate the subchondral bone and not be noted because it is not completely through the cartilage. This can result in false-negative examinations with these types of evaluations.

Postoperative imaging of the hip using computed tomography (CT) scanning has long been considered the gold standard for evaluation of the reduction of acetabular fractures and hardware placement (2,3). Postoperative plain film evaluation with AP, lateral, and Judet views is used in addition to CT. Comparisons have demonstrated the postoperative CT scan is more specific if used at 1-mm slice thickness and 1-mm intervals when compared to 4-mm slice thickness and 3-mm intervals (5). The major limitation with any postoperative radiologic evaluation is that any changes that must be made as a result of these evaluations will result in a second operative procedure.

Because there are limitations associated with each type of evaluation, our protocol for reduction and hardware evaluation includes many of the preceding techniques. During the operative procedure, direct inspection, auscultation (without a stethoscope) and palpation are invaluable tools for the operating surgeon. We also use intraoperative fluoroscopy during hardware placement and reduction. Prior to removing the patient from the operating room, plain films (AP pelvis/Judet oblique views) are evaluated in orthogonal planes to check reduction and hardware placement. We do not routinely use arthrography and do not recommend arthroscopy with any acute fractures of the acetabulum. Postoperative CT scans then are reviewed prior to the patient's discharge from the hospital. This protocol uses multiple modes of evaluation intraoperatively to allow immediate correction of intraarticular hardware or malreduction. The postoperative protocol also allows a final evaluation using the "gold standard" (i.e., CT) prior to the patient's departure from the hospital.

REFERENCES

1. Anglen JO, DiPasquale T. The reliability of detecting screw penetration of the acetabulum by intraoperative auscultation. *J Orthop Trauma* 1994;8(5):404–408.
2. Letournel E, Judet R. *Fractures of the acetabulum,* 2nd ed. New York: Springer-Verlag, 1993.
3. Ebraheim NA, Savolaine ER, Hoeflinger MJ, et al. Radiological diagnosis of screw penetration of the hip joint in acetabular fracture reconstruction. *J Orthop Trauma* 1989;3(3):196–201.
4. Norris BL, et al. Intraoperative fluoroscopy to evaluate fracture reduction and hardware placement during acetabular surgery. *J Orthop Trauma* 1999;13(6):414–417.
5. Carmack DB, et al. Accuracy of detecting screw penetration of the acetabulum with intraoperative fluoroscopy and computed tomography. *J Bone Joint Surg Am* 2001;83-A(9):1370–1375.
6. Glick JM, et al., Hip arthroscopy by the lateral approach. *Arthroscopy* 1987;3(1):4–12.
7. Glick JM. Hip arthroscopy using the lateral approach. *Instr Course Lect* 1988;37:223–231.
8. Bartlett CS, et al. Cardiac arrest as a result of intraabdominal extravasation of fluid during arthroscopic removal of a loose body from the hip joint of a patient with an acetabular fracture. *J Orthop Trauma* 1998;12(4):294–299.

PART E. SURGICAL MANAGEMENT OF SPECIFIC ACETABULAR INJURY TYPES

36

SURGICAL MANAGEMENT OF A TYPES: A1, A2, A3

DAVID J.G. STEPHEN

TYPE A: PARTIAL ARTICULAR FRACTURES, ONE COLUMN OR WALL

A1: Posterior Wall Fractures

(See Fig. 36-1.) Posterior wall fractures occur in association with a posterior hip dislocation as a result of a posterior directed force. This mechanism commonly occurs when the flexed knee strikes the dashboard in a motor vehicle collision (1). Although this fracture has always been thought of as simple as compared with other acetabular types, it is far from a simple fracture. The prognosis must be guarded because of the relatively high incidence of posttraumatic degenerative arthritis leading to total hip arthroplasty (2). The factors that are associated with a poor result include posterior wall comminution (A1-2 fractures), marginal impaction (A1-3), an extended posterior wall fragment (especially superior), and articular damage to the femoral head. The general principles of the management of this specific fracture also apply to any of the other fracture types that involve the posterior wall.

Surgical Approach

Kocher-Langenbeck

Inspection and protection of the sciatic nerve are essential. In cases of large, displaced posterior wall fragments or irreducible posterior dislocations, care must be taken when incising the iliotibial band as the sciatic nerve, or the femoral head can be directly beneath the path of the scalpel. Often the best place to identify the sciatic nerve is along the posterior border of the quadratus femoris. However, to avoid damage to the medial circumflex artery, and thus decrease the risk of osteonecrosis, care must taken with dissection in the interval between the short external rotators and the quadratus femoris (3). With this surgical exposure, all soft-tissue attachments to the posterior wall must be retained, including the comminuted fracture. If increased visualization of the superior aspect of the acetabulum is required, a posterior portion of the abductors can be cut, the greater trochanter can be osteotomized, or the abductors can be taken in a tendinous sleeve with a smaller portion of the greater trochanter—the "trochanter slide."

Position

Prone or Lateral Decubitus

The position becomes surgeon preference. The prone position is preferred by some because it allows gravity to keep the hip reduced, and thus facilitates reduction of the fragment. The patient also can be positioned prone on a fracture table to allow in-line traction throughout the procedure, to distract the femoral head from the acetabulum. The lateral position allows access to the anterior aspect of the acetabulum in cases in which conversion of the Kocher-Langenbeck to an extensile approach, such as a triradiate or combined approach, is required.

Reduction Techniques

The posterior wall fragments with the attached soft tissue must be turned back, like the cover of a book, exposing the underlying femoral head. The capsule invariably is torn; the tear usually extends outward from the posterior wall segment. Some surgical extension of the capsular tear should be made, to afford better visualization of the hip. The capsulorrhaphy must be made at the acetabular side of the hip, just beside the acetabular labrum (3 to 5 mm), or, alternatively, the capsule may be elevated from the side wall and sutured back to bone at the conclusion of the case.

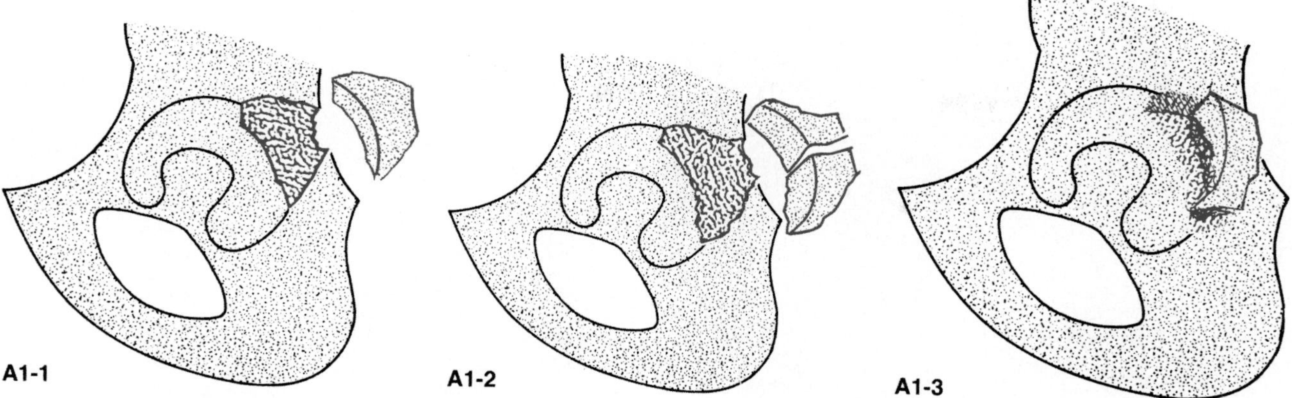

FIGURE 36-1. Posterior wall fractures. The posterior wall fractures, described in Chapter 25 are classified further into those with a single posterior wall fragment (A1-1), those that have multiple posterior wall fragments (A1-2), and those that are associated with marginal impaction (A1-3).

Severe comminution of the posterior wall (A1-2) or marginal impaction (A1-3) creates special problems of reduction and fixation (Fig. 36-1). These conditions should be anticipated from adequate preoperative assessment, including computed tomography (CT) and/or three-dimensional CT (3DCT). The entity of marginal impaction (i.e., when the intact articular cartilage surface of the remaining acetabular joint surface has been impacted or compressed) may be present (Fig. 36-2). This makes final reduction difficult to achieve and leaves a major joint incongruity. This usually can be visualized on CT, particularly before reduction of the posterior wall. If, as the surgeon visualizes the relationship between the femoral head and the intact portion of the acetabular rim, there is a gap between the articular surface of the acetabulum and the femoral head, then marginal impaction exists (Fig. 36-3A). This marginal impaction should be elevated, taking care to maintain the cancellous bone under it intact (Fig. 36-3B). This should be supported by cancellous bone graft or cortical strut, to aid in maintenance of the elevation of the marginally impacted fracture fragment (Fig. 36-3C). Failure to recognize and deal with these marginally impacted fragments can prevent anatomic reduction of the posterior wall fragment, but most importantly can change the contact pressures across the hip joint. Once elevated, the defect can be filled with autogenous graft from the greater trochanter

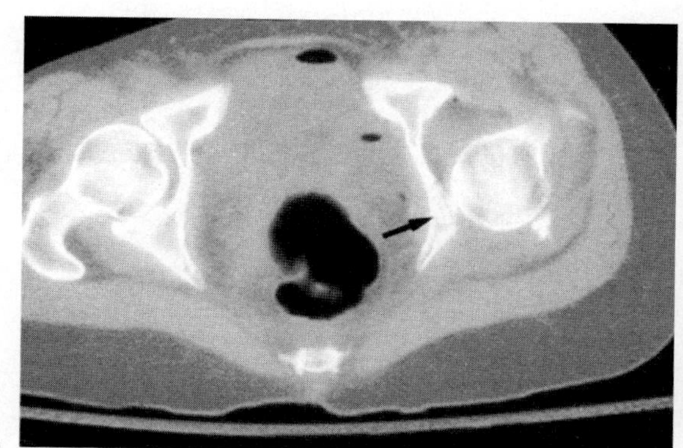

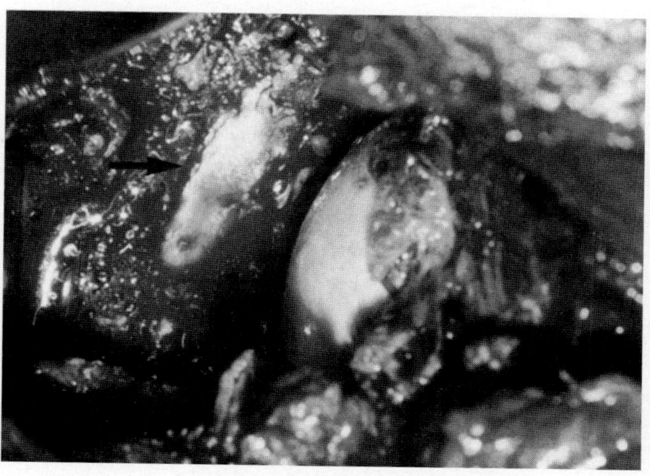

FIGURE 36-2. Marginal impaction of the articular surface. **A:** Axial computed tomography shows a posterior dislocation. Note that the femoral head in the dislocated position is impacting a portion of the articular surface of the acetabulum *(black arrow)*. The normal position of that fragment is approximately 90 degrees to its position, if one compares that area of the articular surface with a normal right hip. **B:** The appearance at surgery. The *black arrow* points to the marginally impacted fragment, which is rotated 90 degrees from its normal position adjacent to the femoral head. In this particular case, the impaction was so great that it was virtually impossible to find the fracture line under the impacted fragment at surgery 12 days following injury.

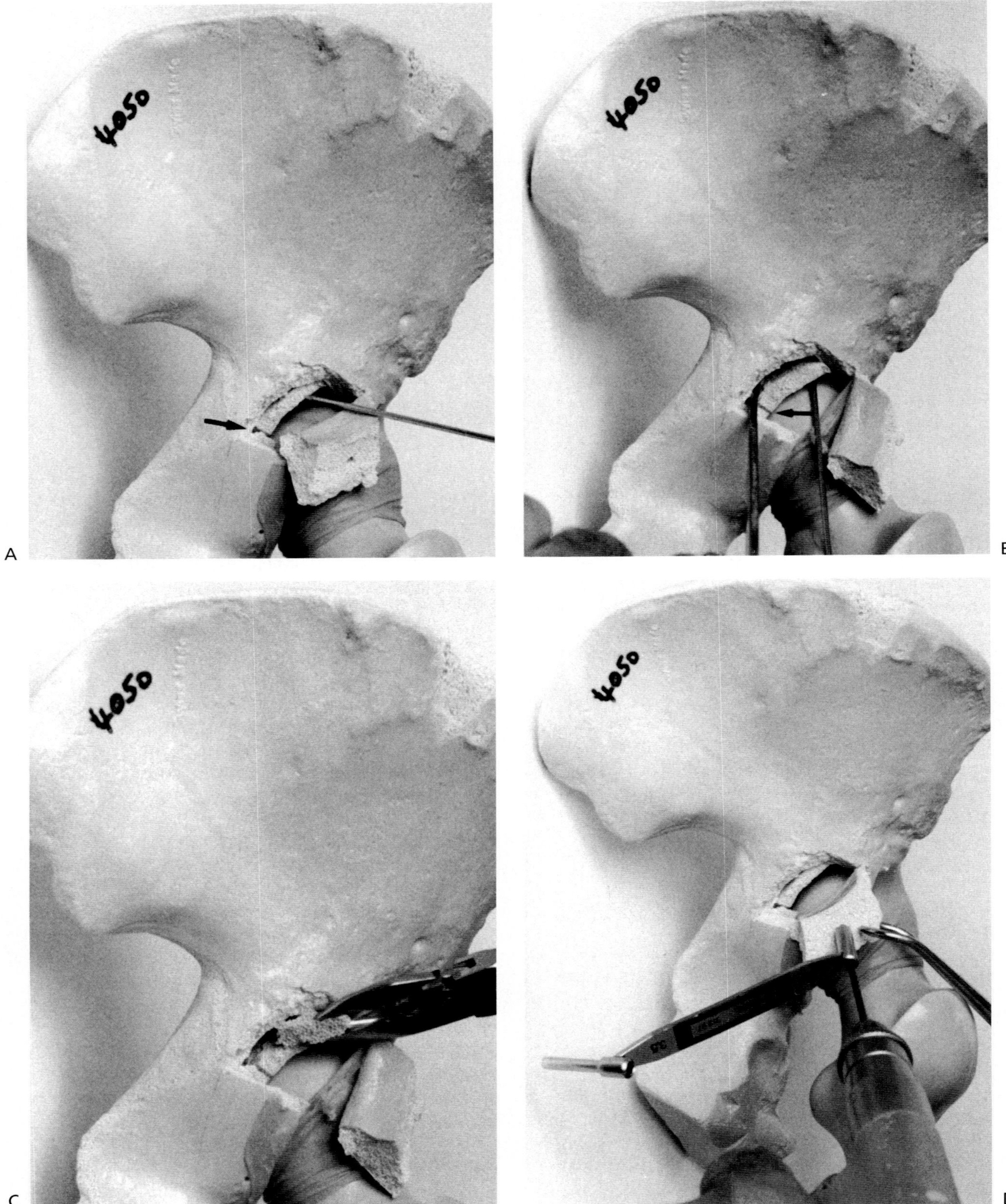

FIGURE 36-3. Marginal impaction. Reduction and fixation techniques involving the impaction and the posterior wall. **A:** Photograph demonstrates the marginally impacted fragment at the tip of the Kirschner wire. **B:** The fragment was gently teased back into its anatomic position using an elevator. The position is tested to verify anatomic reduction by palpating the joint, demonstrated by the Kirschner wire. The *black arrow* indicates the anatomic reduction of the fragment. **C:** Maintenance of reduction requires a cancellous bone graft to contour the femoral head, counteracting the tendency toward displacement after insertion of the bone graft. **D:** Predrilling the posterior wall fragment after reduction ensures that the posterior lag screw does not enter the joint.

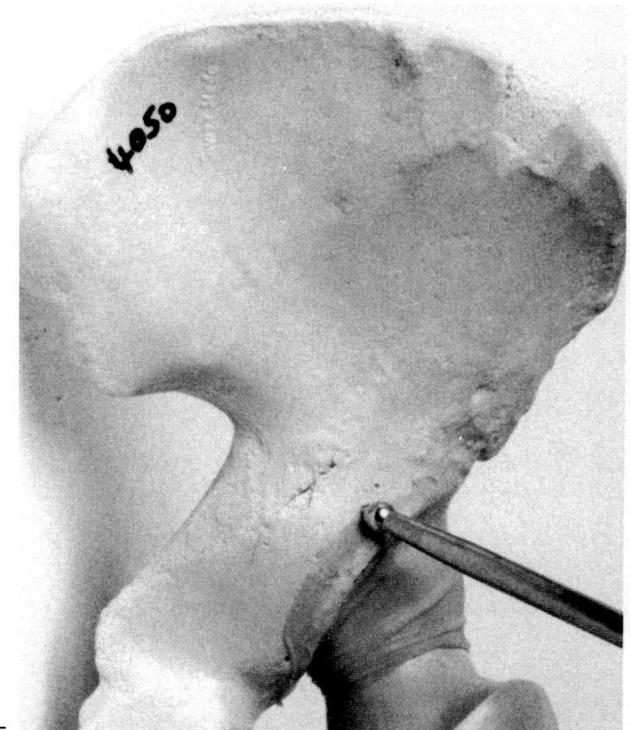

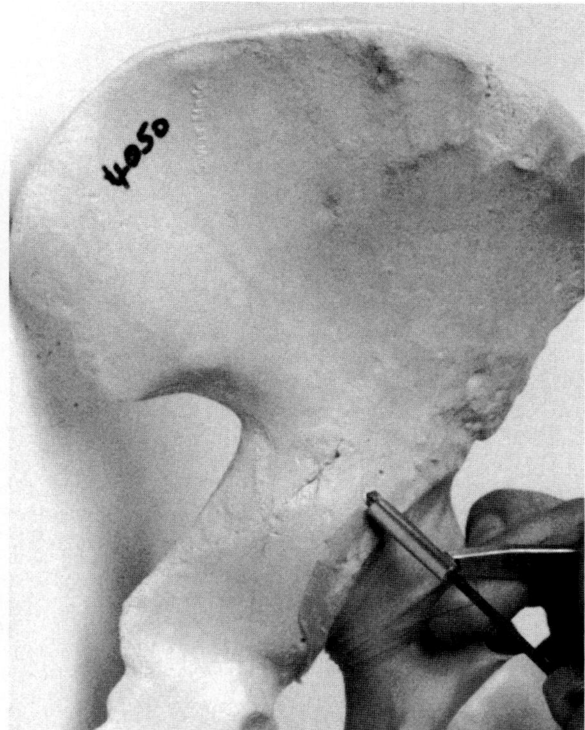

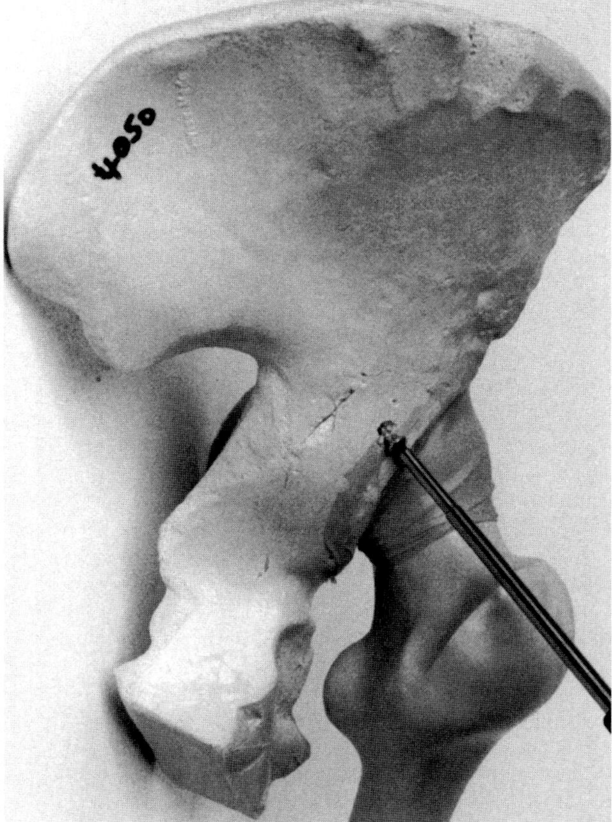

FIGURE 36-3. *(continued)* E: The posterior wall can then be reduced anatomically and held with a ball spike impactor, an invaluable instrument in pelvic surgery. **F:** After predrilling and reduction, the thread holes are drilled, making certain that the drill bit enters the same predrilled hole and thus ensuring that it does not enter the joint. **G:** Insertion of the lag screw is essential. This applies interfragmental compression to the fragment, ensures early union, and prevents displacement of the fragment. Attempts are made to buttress plate these fragments alone (Fig. 36-4).

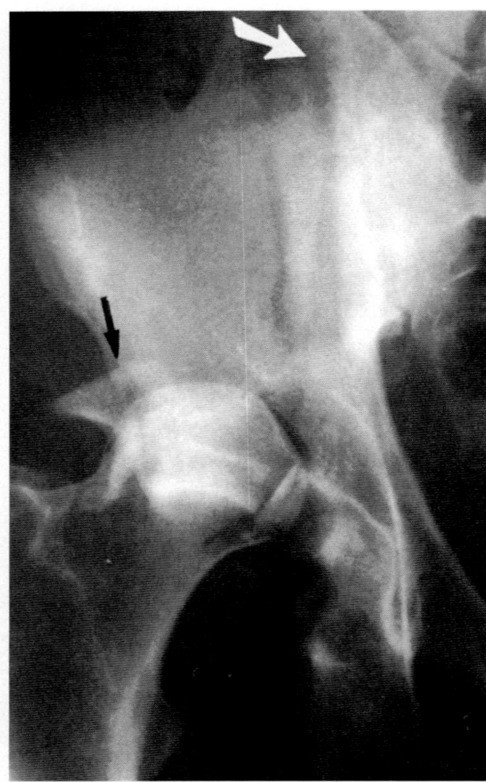

A

FIGURE 36-4. The importance of lag screws for posterior wall stability. **A:** Anterior-posterior radiograph demonstrates posterior dislocation of the hip. The *black arrow* shows the large posterior wall fracture. Note also the shearing fracture through the ilium to the crest *(white arrow)*. **B:** Fixation was performed through a transtrochanteric Kocher-Langenbeck approach. The iliac fracture was fixed with interfragmental compression and plates. The posterior wall fracture, however, was fixed, not with lag screws, but with only a buttress plate. Thus, there was no inherent stability in the posterior wall fragment. **C:** Six weeks after fixation the femoral head began to move into a position of subluxation. There was no evidence of sepsis. The subluxation occurred because the posterior wall fragment, having no support, gave way.

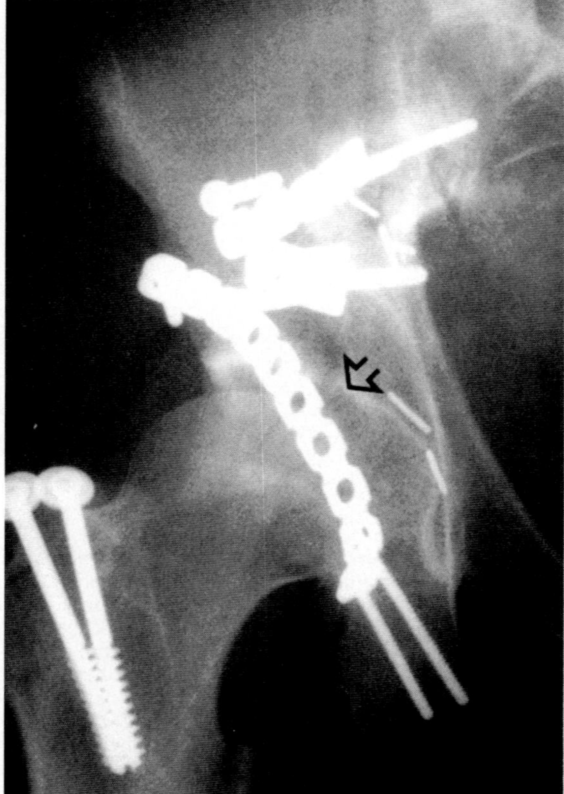

B

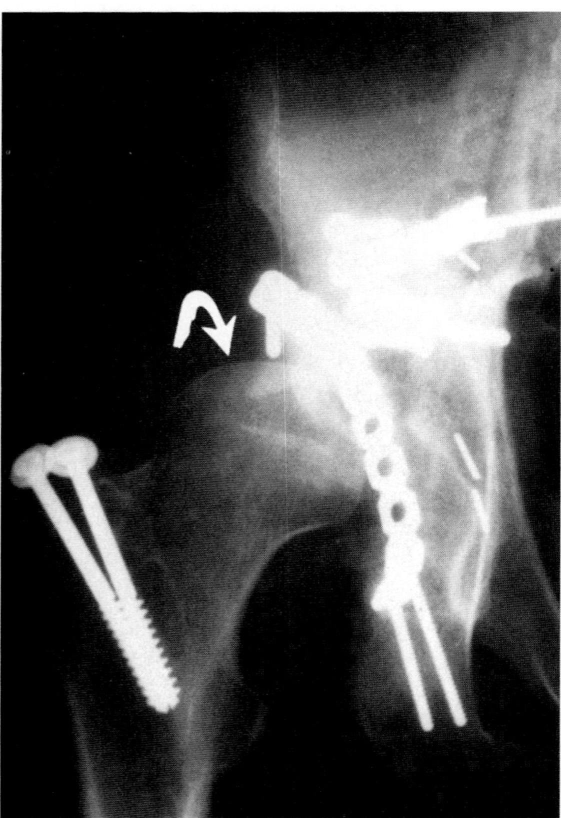

C

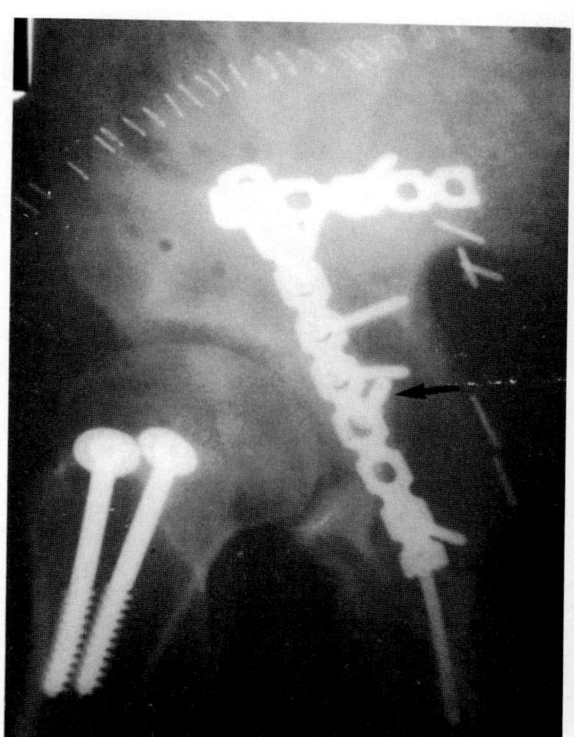

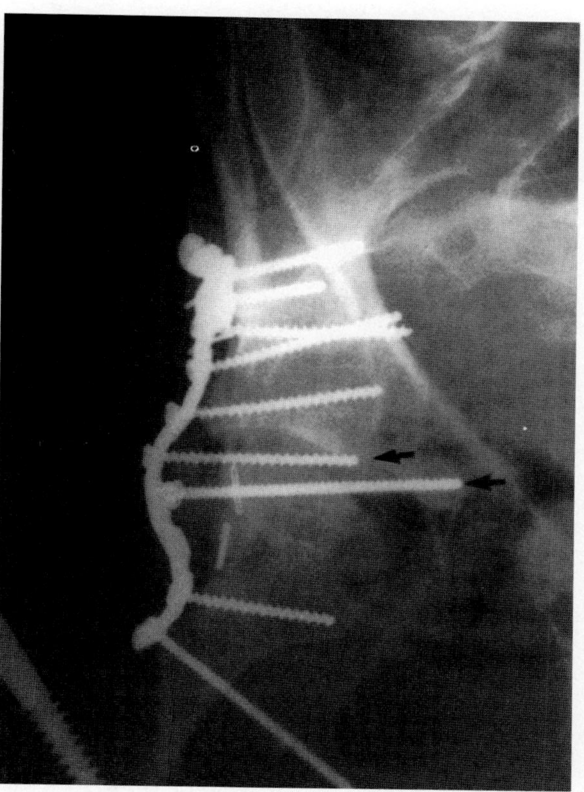

FIGURE 36-4. ***(continued)*** **D,E:** External and internal rotation views of the hip following secondary surgery. The surgery was difficult. One long lag screw was used to fix the fragment, and other lag screws were placed through the plate and into the fragment *(black arrows)*. When possible it is essential to use lag screws to prevent this complication.

or bone graft substitute. The disimpacted intraarticular fragments are sometimes large and unstable enough to require fixation. Often they are amenable to only minifragment screws (1.5- to 2.0-mm screws).

It is imperative that the edges of the fracture, particularly at the acetabular rim, be precisely cleaned to ensure anatomic reduction. The reduction is obtained by gentle longitudinal traction along the femoral neck, and slight abduction of the leg to relax the abductor musculature. The posterior wall fracture fragment can be wedged into place, ensuring reduction along its posterior column line and particularly at its two joint fracture line areas. Reduction is facilitated by the use of the ball spike impactor (Fig. 36-3E).

Fixation Techniques

Before reducing the fracture fragment itself, the surgeon should visualize and inspect the joint surface and its orientation. This allows appropriate placement of screws for fixation. Predrilling the glide holes through the unreduced fragment, working from inside outward, ensures they are properly placed away from the articular surface and centered in this fragment (Fig. 36-3D). The wall is then reduced and the thread holes are drilled (Fig. 36-3F). All drill holes for screws through the posterior wall fracture fragment must be placed parallel or diverging from the joint (Fig. 36-3G). This ensures that the threads and screws stay out of the joint.

Another option is to use temporary fixation with smooth wires. Once the fracture has been reduced, it is impossible to see into the joint, therefore, *intraoperative fluoroscopy* is useful to identify and rule out intraarticular hardware. Once satisfied that there is no intraarticular hardware, the wires can be replaced by lag screws. Either 3.5 cortical lag screws or partially threaded 4.0 screws can be used. Depending on the degree of comminution, the size of the fragment, and the quality of bone, the addition of washers to the lag screws can help to prevent cut out of the lag screws.

Occasionally, the posterior wall fracture fragment is a small rim that nevertheless holds articular cartilage. These fragments may be too small for typical fixation with 3.5- or 4.0-mm screws. Thus fixation with 2.7-mm screws and/or one-third tubular plate fashioned into a "spring" plate may be indicated. When possible, screws must be placed into the posterior wall fragments directly, to prevent displacement (Fig. 36-4A–E).

It is mandatory, with all posterior wall fracture fragments, that a plate be applied if early ambulation is anticipated (Fig. 36-5). This buttress plate neutralizes the forces directed onto

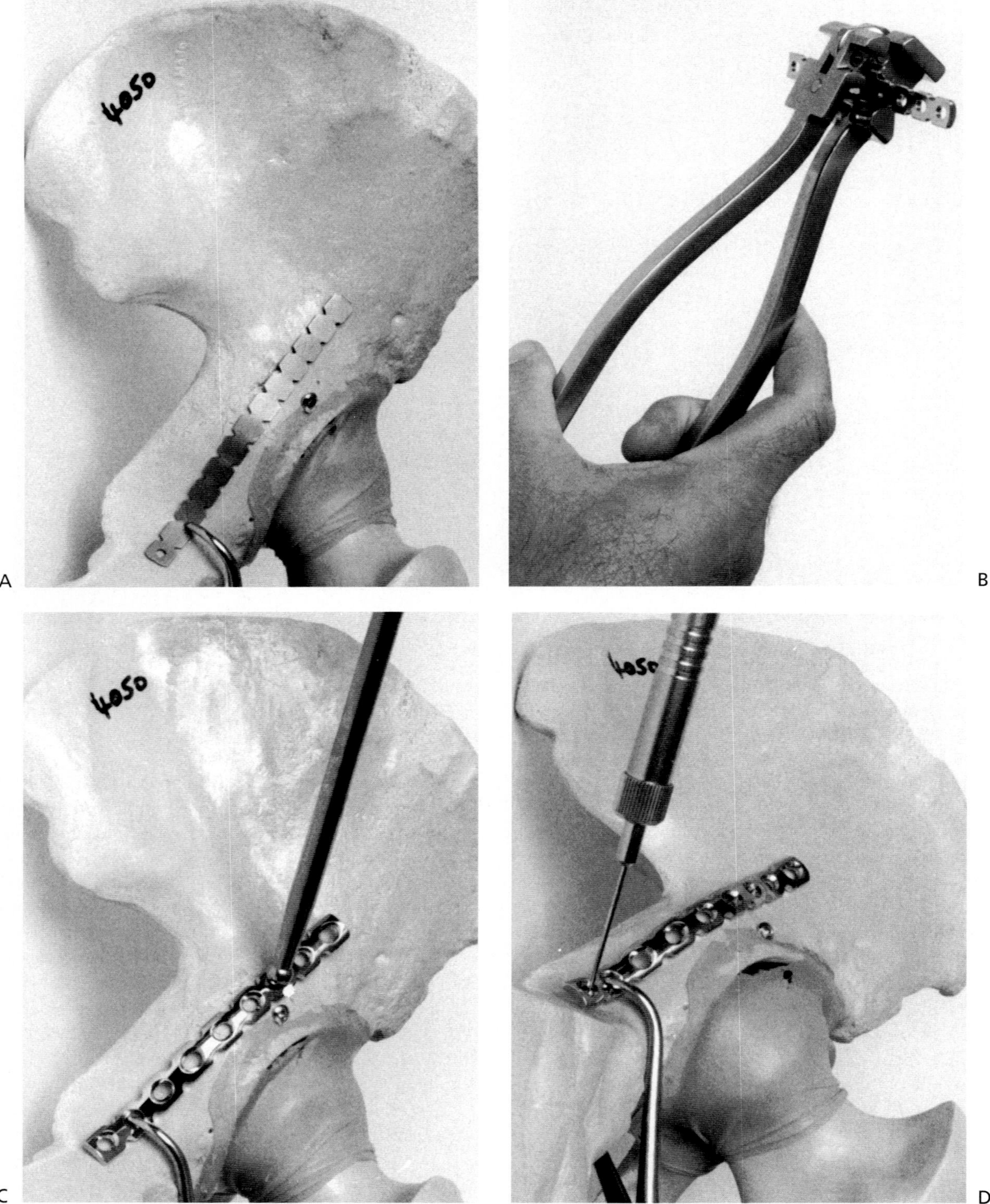

FIGURE 36-5. Buttress plate on the posterior column. **A:** The template is placed along the posterior column to fit the contour of the bone. Note that it crosses the main body of the posterior wall fracture, which was previously fixed with an intrafragmental screw. The distal portion will be anchored in the ischial tuberosity, the proximal portion in the hard bone just superior to the acetabulum. **B:** The 3.5-mm reconstruction plate, the implant of choice, is contoured to fit the template. This particular plate can be contoured in two planes using the bending pliers. **C:** The first screw is inserted, anchoring the plate to the proximal ilium. **D:** The important long screw into the ischial tuberosity is noted by the depth gauge. Note the direction along the ischial tuberosity. Often a 50-mm screw can be placed into this screw hole.

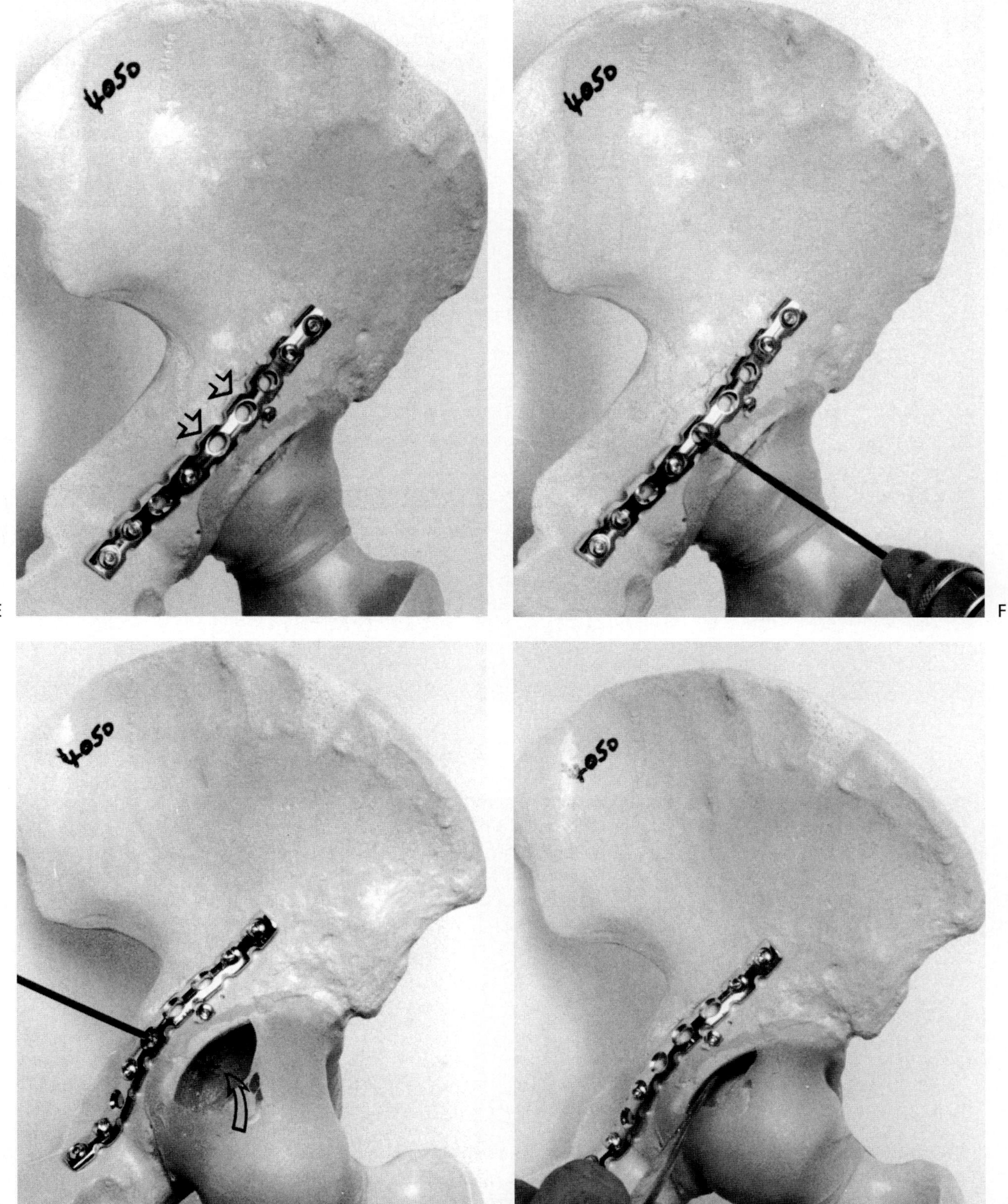

FIGURE 36-5. ***(continued)*** **E:** The plate is in position along the posterior column, buttressing the posterior wall. If screws are to be placed into the fourth and fifth holes of this nine-hole plate, great care must be taken to be certain that the screws diverge from the joint. **F:** The drill bit is aimed away from the joint, to be certain that the posterior column is not perforated intraarticularly, as noted in **(G).** At the end of the plating procedure the posterior column must be inspected, either by direct vision through the capsulorrhaphy incision or by using a Howorth elevator to be certain that there is no metal in the joint **(H).**

this posterior wall and tends to prevent redisplacement. The plate should be well molded to the posterior column, anchored at the ischial tuberosity by at least two screws, and in the hard bone superior to the acetabulum (Fig. 36-5A–C). It is important to place this buttress plate accurately over the main portion of the posterior wall fragment, but at the same time staying outside the margin of the hip joint. Also, if two plates are required in associated types, one plate may be anchored in the sciatic buttress superiorly (Fig. 36-5D–F). Again, all drill holes must diverge from the joint, especially those in the center of the plate, to avoid penetrating the articular surface (Fig. 36-5G,H). Again, intraoperative fluo-

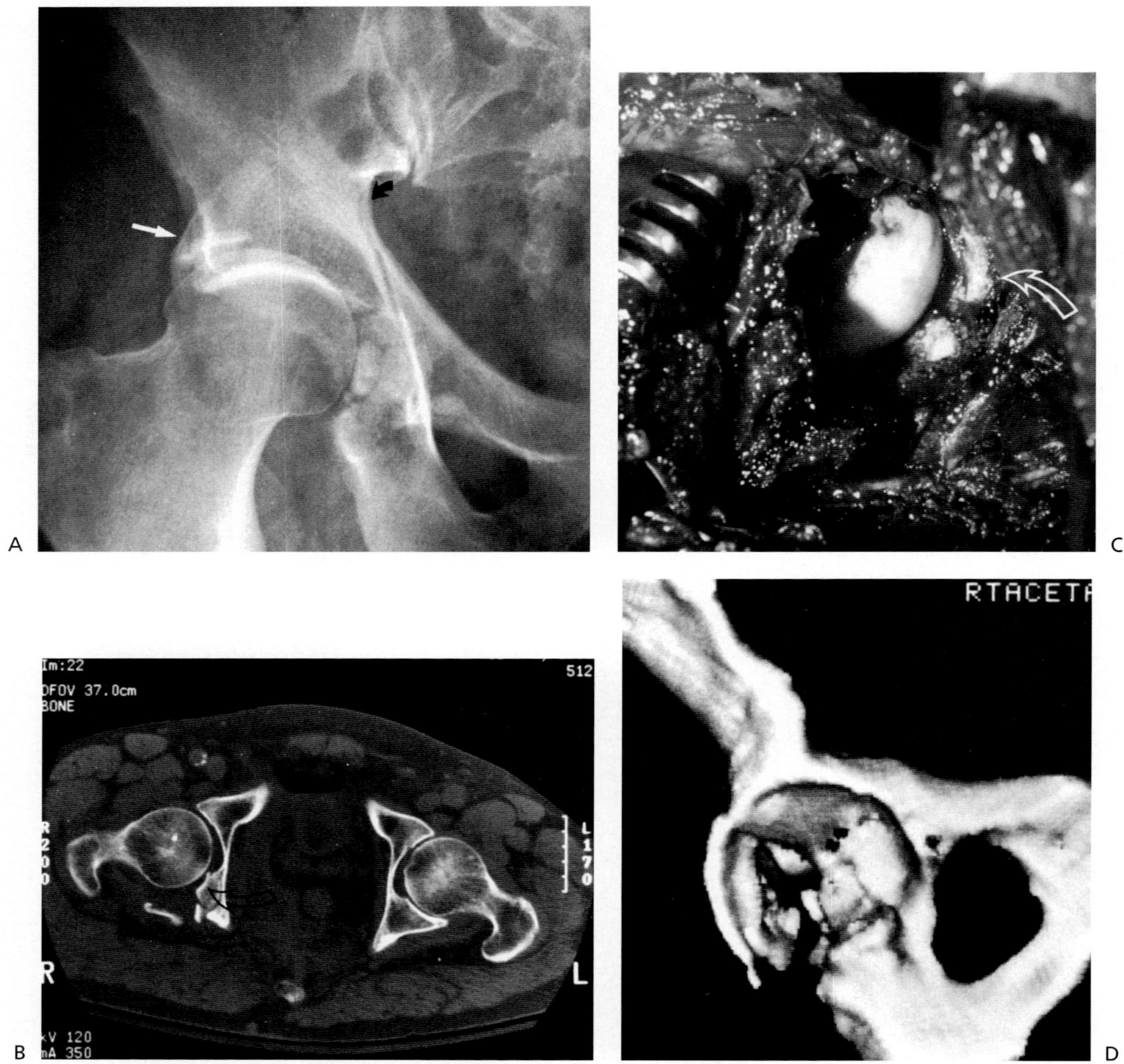

FIGURE 36-6. A: Anteroposterior radiograph of the right hip shows a posterior dislocation associated with a posterior wall fracture *(white arrow).* Note also that there are multiple fragments of the posterior wall along the joint margin and an associated transverse fracture *(black arrow).* **B:** Computed tomography performed after reduction of this dislocation clearly shows the marginally impacted fragment *(black arrow).* **C:** The clinical photograph shows the relation of the impacted fragments to the femoral head. Note that there are two impacted fragments that, through the posterior approach, are rotated 90 degrees. They should be facing the articular surface of the femoral head rather than "looking out'"' directly at the surgeon *(white arrow).* **D:** The three-dimensional computed tomography with the head subtracted shows the large posterior wall fragment that has the potential for instability and comminution, best seen from the posterior view **(E).**

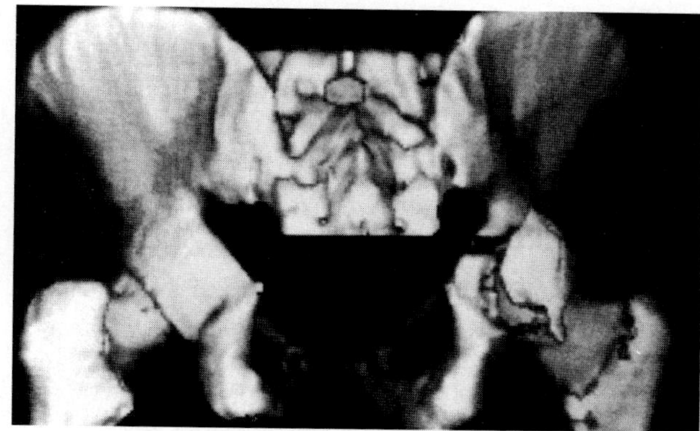

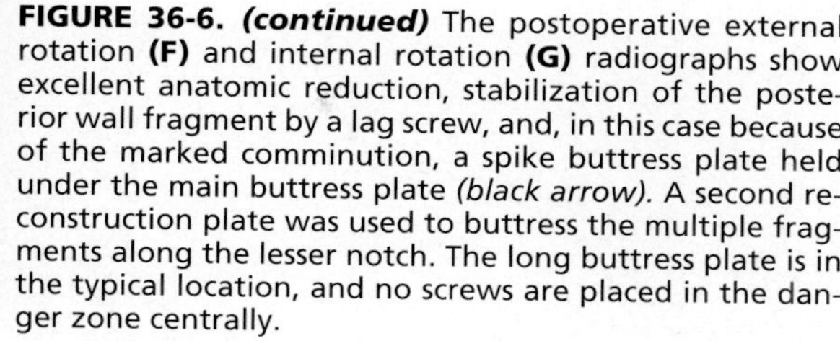

FIGURE 36-6. ***(continued)*** The postoperative external rotation **(F)** and internal rotation **(G)** radiographs show excellent anatomic reduction, stabilization of the posterior wall fragment by a lag screw, and, in this case because of the marked comminution, a spike buttress plate held under the main buttress plate *(black arrow)*. A second reconstruction plate was used to buttress the multiple fragments along the lesser notch. The long buttress plate is in the typical location, and no screws are placed in the danger zone centrally.

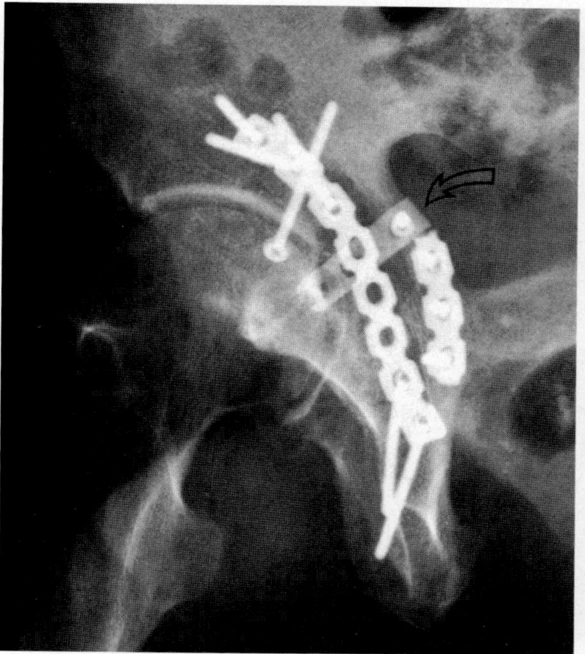

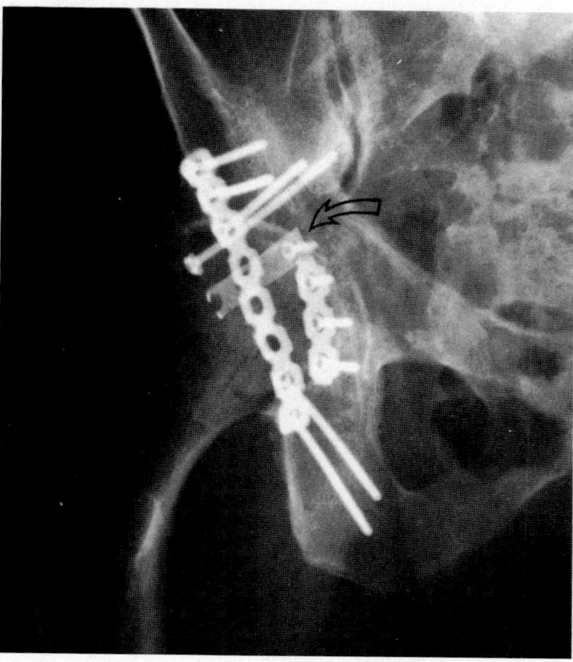

roscopy helps to ensure the hardware is extraarticular. A typical example of a complex multifragmented posterior wall fracture associated with an undisplaced transverse fracture fixed in an appropriate way with lag screws, two plates, and a spring plate is shown in Fig. 36-6.

A2: Posterior Column Fractures

(See Fig. 36-7A.) Isolated posterior column injuries are rare and usually are associated with a posterior dislocation of the hip. More commonly, the posterior column fracture is associated with a posterior wall fragment (A2-3) (Fig. 36-7C). Typically, the posterior column fractures through the obturator foramen into the greater sciatic notch (A2-2), but occasionally the fracture is limited to the ischium (A2-1) (Fig. 36-7B).

The fracture is usually displaced posteriorly, medially, and in internal rotation, as the posterior column rotates about the ischial tuberosity. As the femoral head is driven through the posterior column and fractures it, it tends to open up the posterior column like a swinging door, moving posteriorly into the pelvis. The superior gluteal vessels and nerve can be at risk with displaced fragments.

Surgical Approach

Posterior Kocher-Langenbeck

Osteotomy of the greater trochanter is helpful if more visualization is required for the ischial type (A2-1) or the associated types (A2-3), or if the wall fragment extends high in the greater sciatic notch.

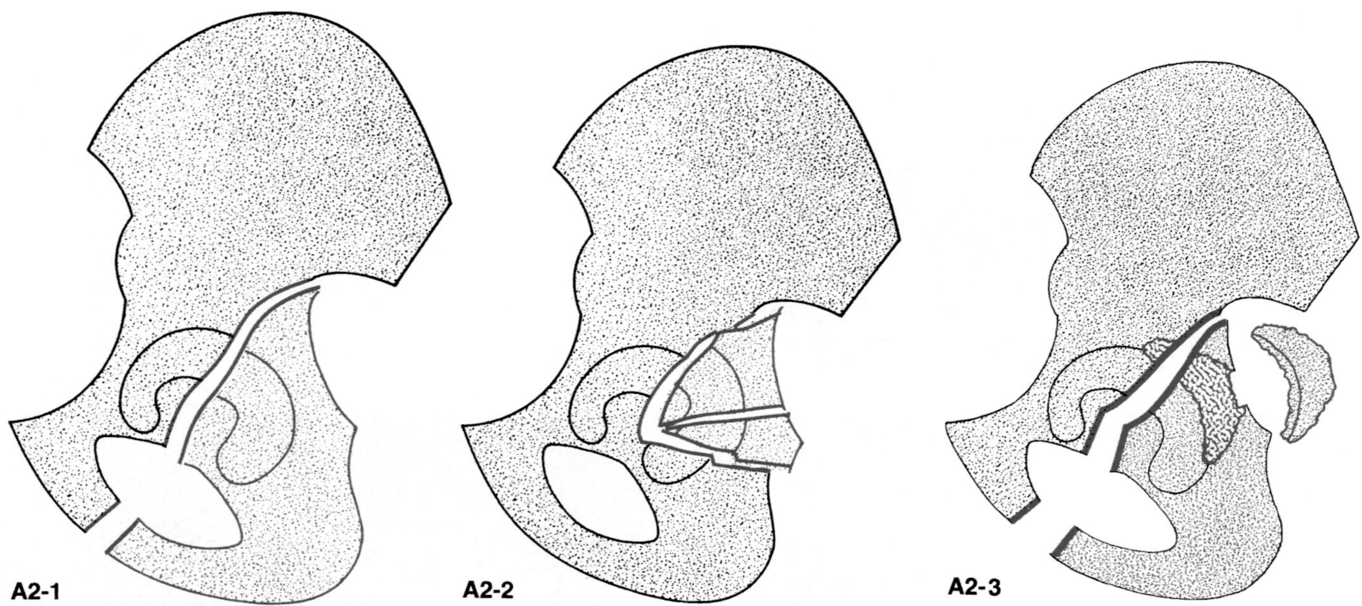

FIGURE 36-7. Posterior column fractures, Type A2 is further subdivided. The typical posterior column fracture (A2-2) is seen in the drawing, but subtypes include a posterior column fracture limited to the ischium (A2-1) and those associated with a posterior wall fragment (A2-3).

Position

Prone or lateral decubitus.

Reduction Techniques

During reduction, rotation of the posterior wall fragment must be corrected. The simplest way to do this is to place, into the ischial tuberosity, a 5-mm Schantz screw on a T-handle or some form of reduction pin to act as a handle for rotational control (Fig. 36-8A,B). With this in place and with exposure through the greater and lesser notch by removal of the sacrospinous ligaments (either by blunt or sharp dissection or osteotomy of the ischial spine) (Fig. 36-8C), the medial fracture line can be palpated inside the pelvis, along the quadrilateral plate, to determine the adequacy of the reduction (Fig. 36-8D,E). This also may be accomplished by externally lifting and rotating the posterior column fragment.

This reduction may be further facilitated by using the specially devised pointed reduction clamps, as described (Fig. 36-9A,B). Several types are available: standard pointed reduction clamps and offset pointed clamps that can be inserted onto the medial wall of the posterior column and then over the acetabulum onto the superior rim. External rotation also can be accomplished by clamping the jaws together, thus aiding reduction. This reduction also must be confirmed by inspecting inside the joint on the posterior column and by palpating the medial wall. Occasionally, using pelvic reduction forceps with screws affixed to the posterior column above the ischial tuberosity and to the superior portion of the iliac wing above the acetabulum also facilitates reduction (Fig. 36-9C,D).

For associated posterior wall and the posterior column fractures (A1), reduction of the posterior column component should be carried out first. This allows for articular visualization of the reduction and makes it easier to control the posterior column and apply fixation. Occasionally, this is not possible, and with some fractures it is easier to fix the posterior wall fracture fragment to the posterior column and then reduce the posterior column anatomically.

The hamstring muscles act as the major deforming force of the posterior column because of their origin from the ischial tuberosity. This may occur when the hip is flexed, pulling the posterior column fracture into a tilted position. It is advisable to reduce such fractures with the hip extended and the knee flexed 90 degrees. This allows maximum exposure posteriorly and removes the deforming force of the hamstrings.

Fixation Techniques

Once anatomic reduction has been obtained and the fracture is provisionally fixed with Kirschner wires and the reduction is confirmed radiographically, definitive fixation may proceed. The posterior column should be fixed with lag screws, which are usually easy to insert. The glide hole may be drilled before reduction, to ensure its proper placement (Fig. 36-10A). Once lag screw fixation has been obtained, the posterior column is buttressed by a 3.5-mm reconstruction plate from the ischial

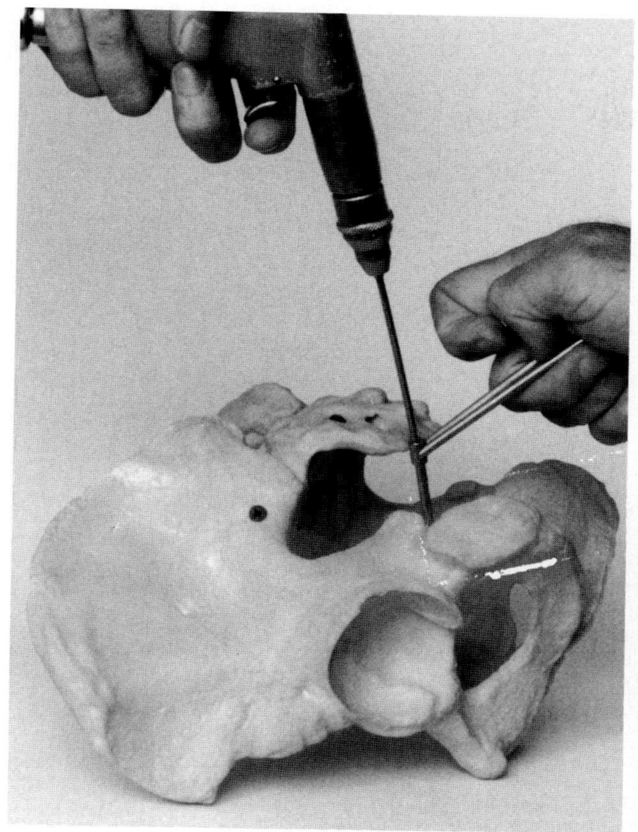
A

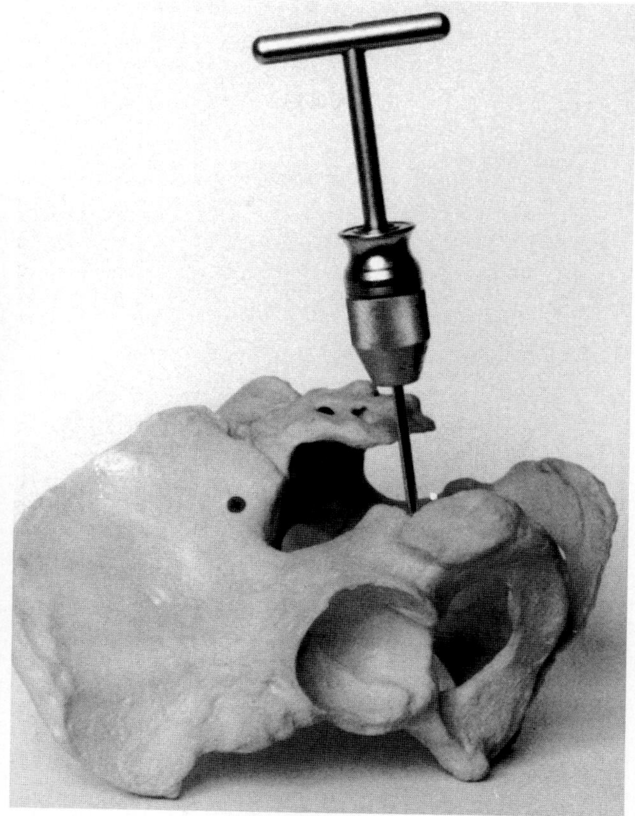
B

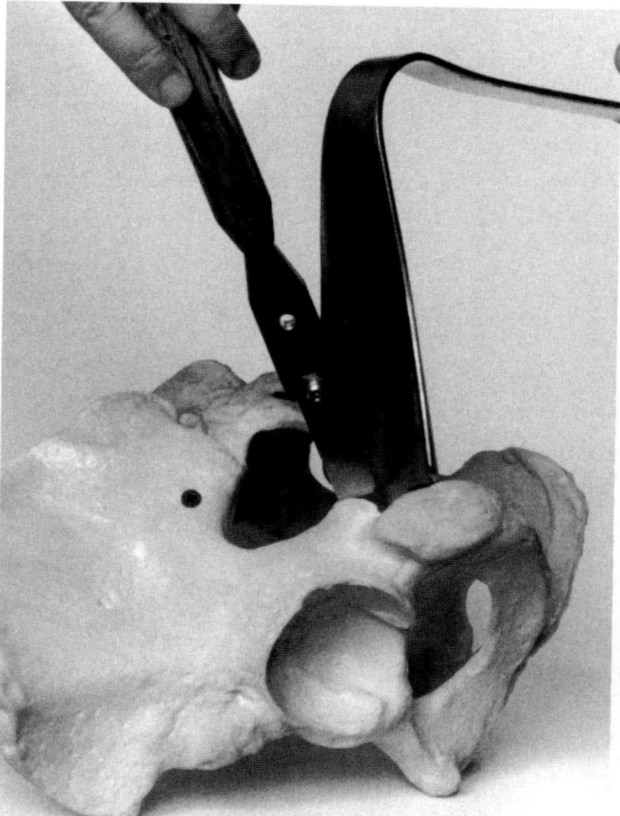
C

FIGURE 36-8. Reduction and fixation of a posterior column fracture. **A:** Drilling the hole with the 3.2-mm bit for insertion of the 5-mm Schantz screw just medial to the ischial tuberosity. **B:** This allows rotation of the posterior column fracture. This method of reduction is also invaluable for transverse fractures fixed posteriorly. **C:** To gain access to the quadrilateral plate to assess reduction, the sacrospinous ligament can be cut at its insertion or, preferably, a sharp osteotome can be used to osteotomize the ischial spine.

(Figure continues)

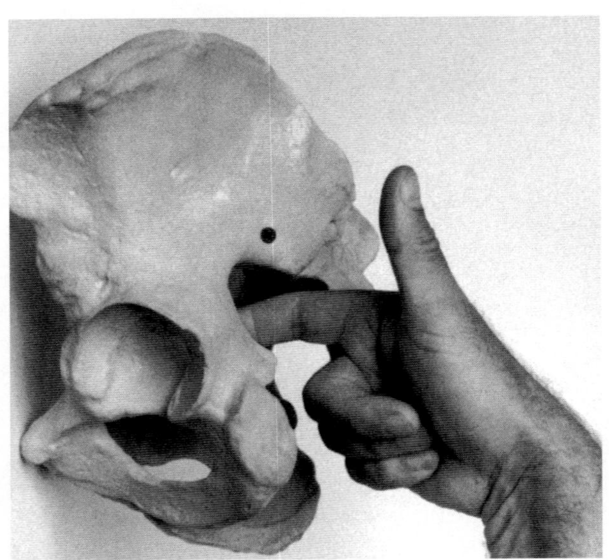

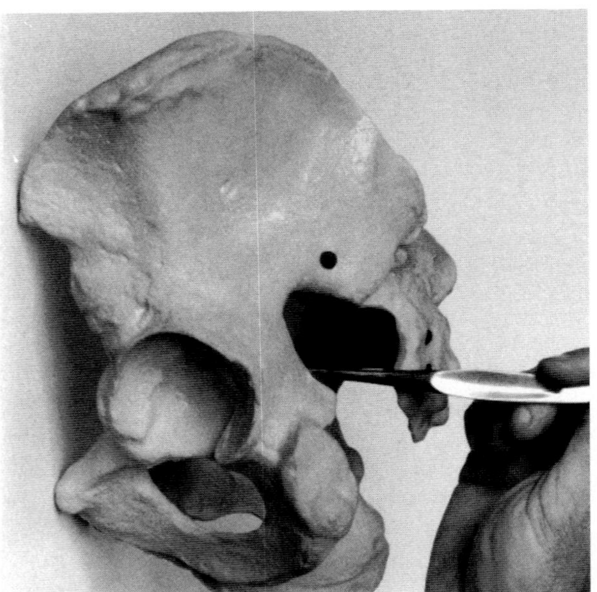

FIGURE 36-8. ***(continued)*** **D,E:** Following removal by osteotomy or division of the sacrospinous ligaments, an examining finger or a Howorth elevator can be inserted along the quadrilateral plate to assess reduction of the posterior column or transverse fracture.

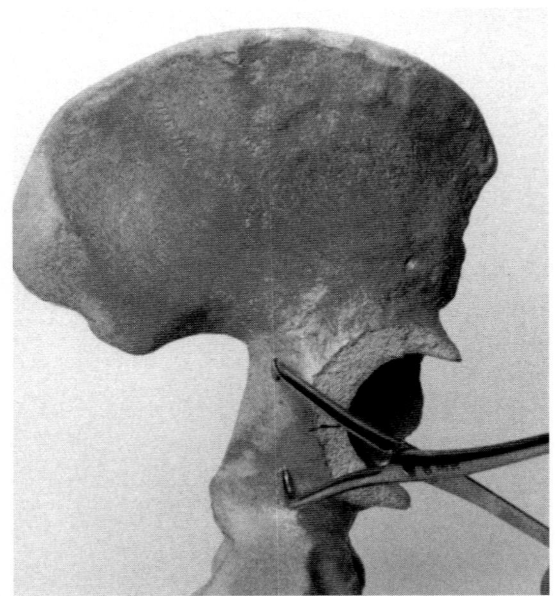

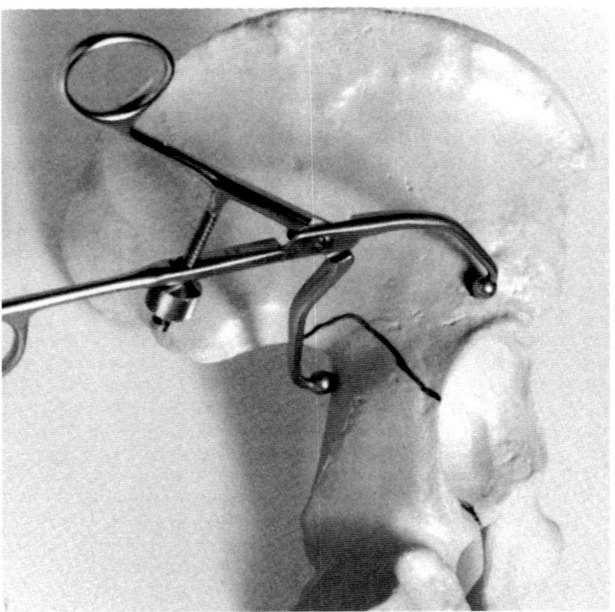

FIGURE 36-9. Posterior clamps for use on the posterior column. **A:** The standard pointed reduction clamps may be used to temporarily fix the posterior column, as noted. Occasionally, 2-mm drill holes should be made in the proper location, so that the points may be inserted. **B:** Offset clamps can be invaluable in this location with insertion through the greater sciatic notch onto the medial wall of the acetabulum and the other point in the proximal fragment, as noted.

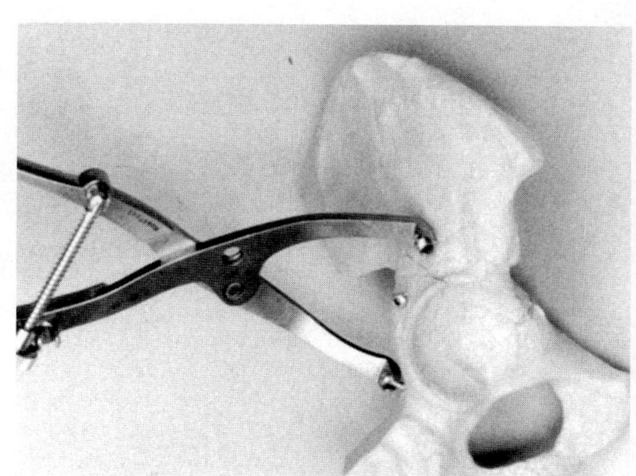
C

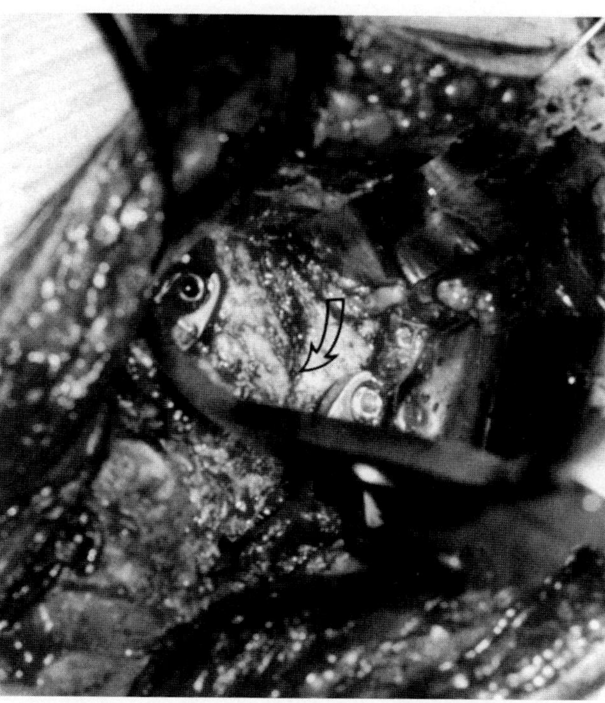
D

FIGURE 36-9. ***(continued)*** **C:** Although bulky, pelvic reduction clamps may be invaluable in some cases. **D:** Clinical photograph shows the pelvic reduction clamp compressing a posterior column fracture *(black arrow).*

tuberosity to the superior aspect of the acetabulum, taking care to keep screws out of the joint (Fig. 36-10B–D).

For associated posterior column and posterior wall fractures (A2-3), the same techniques are used (Fig. 36-11). Readers should refer to the preceding section on the complexity of the wall fragments, which may be comminuted or marginally impacted (Figs. 36-2 and 36-3). The sequence of reduction is to reduce, and fix the column first, then proceed with fixation of the posterior wall (after elevating any impacted fragments).

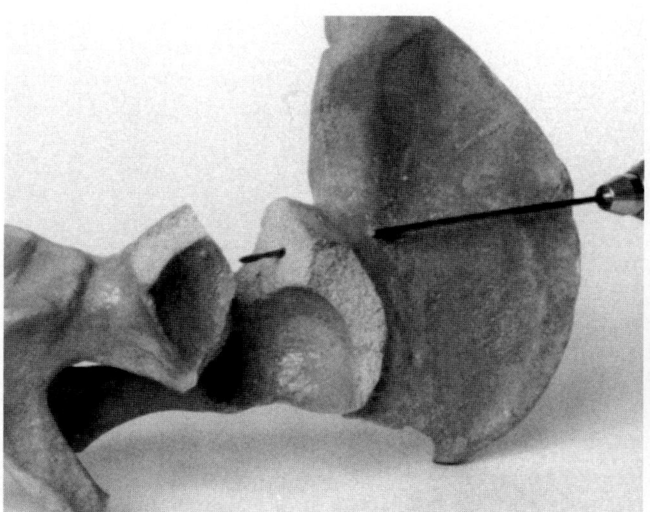
A

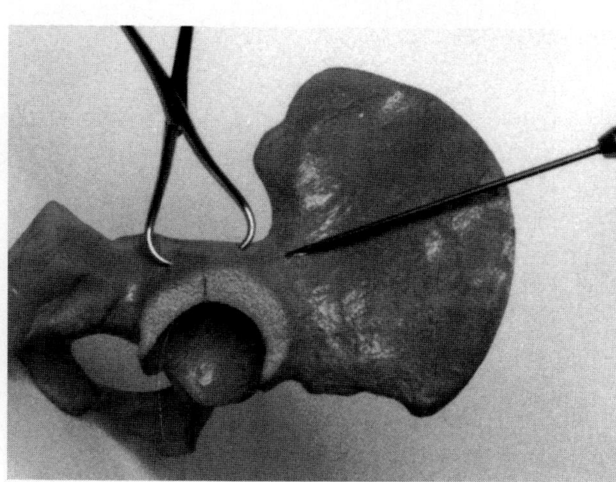
B

FIGURE 36-10. Lag screw fixation of posterior column. **A:** To avoid penetrating the joint, a glide hole should be drilled first with the fracture unreduced. Depending on what incision is used, the glide hole may be drilled with a 3.5-mm drill proximally or distally. **B:** The posterior column fracture is reduced and held with a pointed reduction clamp. Using the tap sleeve, the 2.5-mm drill bit is used to complete the hole in the posterior fragment.

(Figure continues)

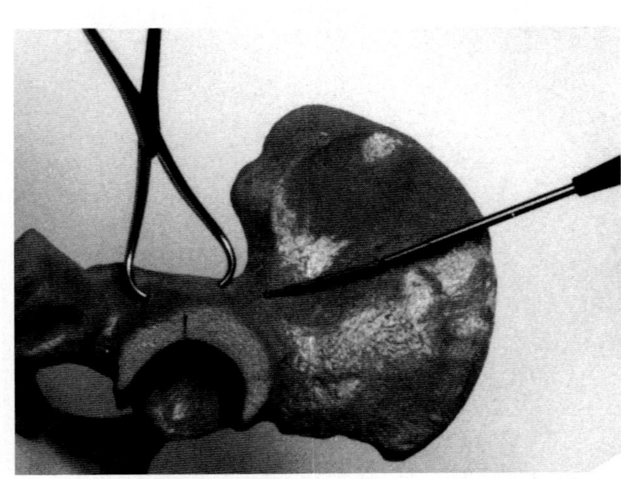

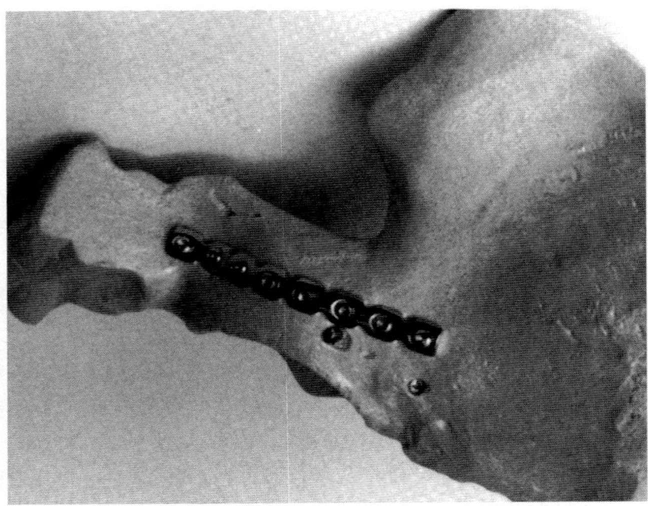

FIGURE 36-10. ***(continued)*** **C:** The lag screw is inserted, usually with a washer. **D:** The posterior wall fragments are reduced and held with intrafragmental screws. The posterior wall and posterior column are buttressed with a typical 3.5-mm reconstruction plate.

A3: Anterior Column or Anterior Wall Fractures

(See Fig. 36-12.) Isolated anterior wall fractures (A3-1) are uncommon and almost always are associated with anterior dislocation of the hip. Anterior wall fractures are more often associated with anterior column fractures or the interesting variant of the T fracture, the associated anterior with posterior hemitransverse fracture (B3). Isolated fractures of the anterior column (A3-2, A3-3) are, in fact, very common, but generally are less clinically significant than the posterior types. The isolated anterior column fracture was thought to be rare, but with the introduction of routine CT for pelvic trauma, many laterally placed superior pubic ramus fractures of the pelvis in lateral compression (B-type pelvis) enter the joint distally. Thus, the comprehensive classification differentiates high anterior column fractures (A3-3), which are clinically significant, from low ones (A3-

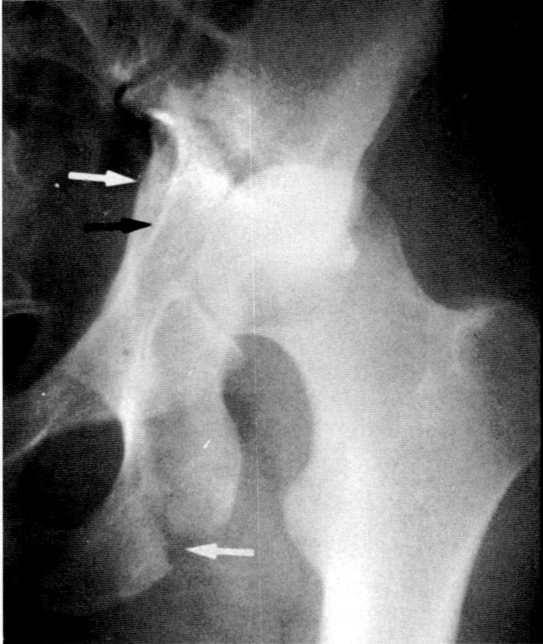

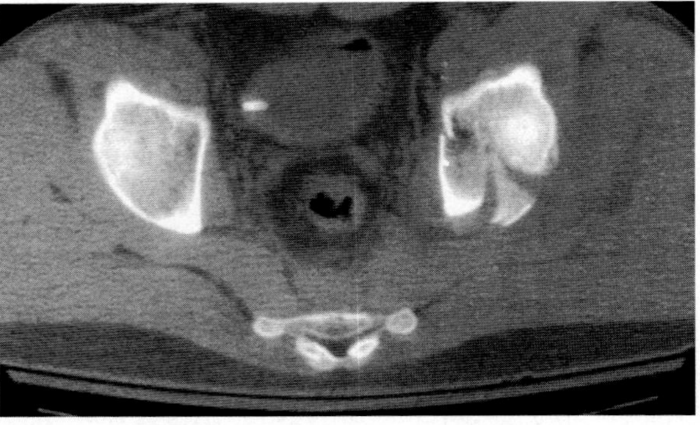

FIGURE 36-11. A typical posterior column-posterior wall fracture with internal fixation. **A:** Anteroposterior radiograph demonstrates the posteriorly dislocated hip and the posterior column-posterior wall fracture associated with it. The intact iliopectineal line indicates an intact anterior column *(black arrow)* and the displaced posterior column with the distal limb through the ischial tuberosity *(white arrows).*

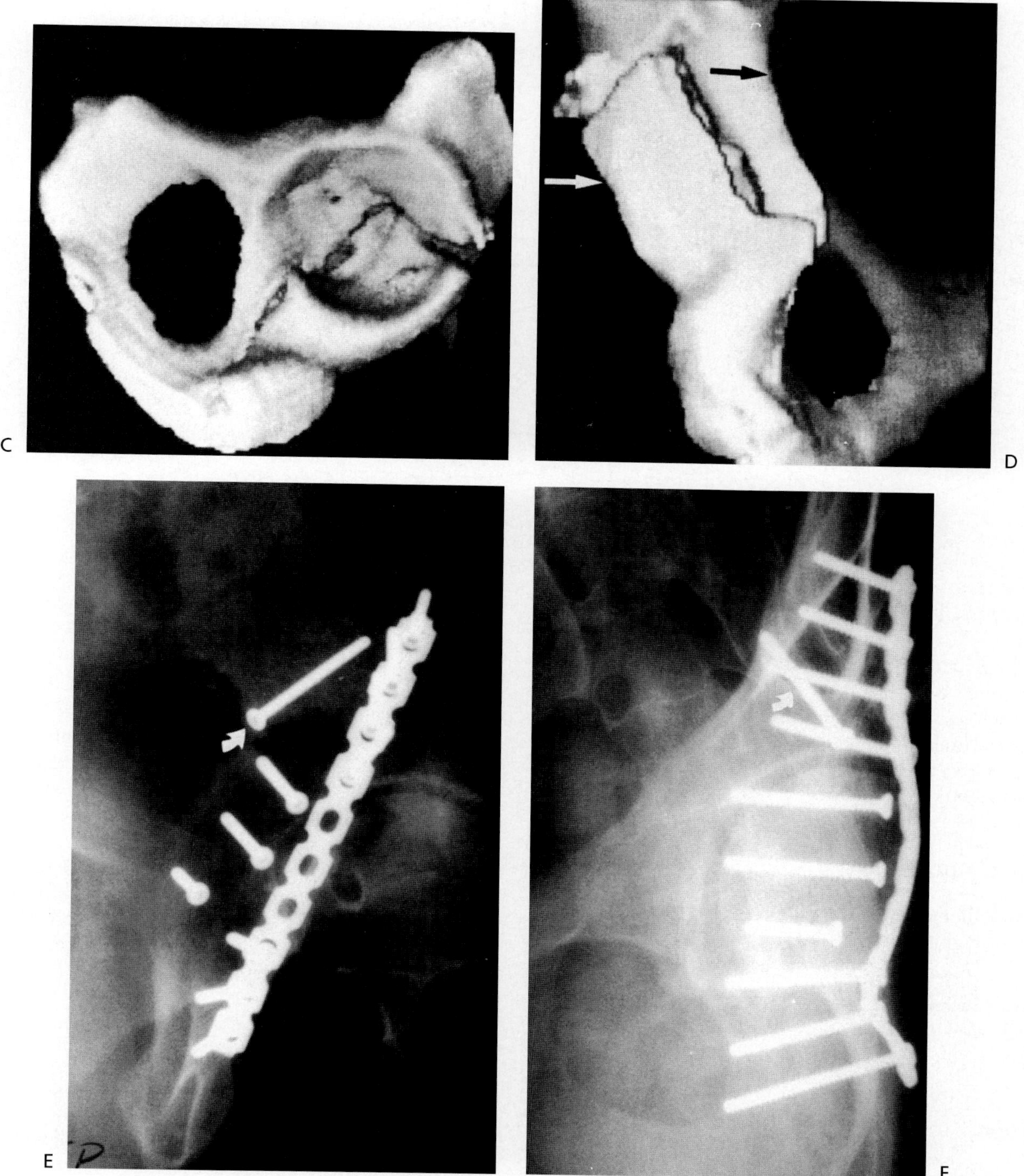

FIGURE 36-11. ***(continued)*** Computed tomography **(B)** and especially the three-dimensional computed tomography **(C,D)** clearly show the intact anterior column and displaced posterior column-posterior wall combination. Anatomic reduction was obtained; the posterior wall fracture was fixed with three interfragmental screws and the posterior column with a lag screw directed distal to proximal and a buttress plate, as noted in the external oblique radiograph **(E)** and the internal oblique view **(F).** The lag screw is noted with a *white arrow.*

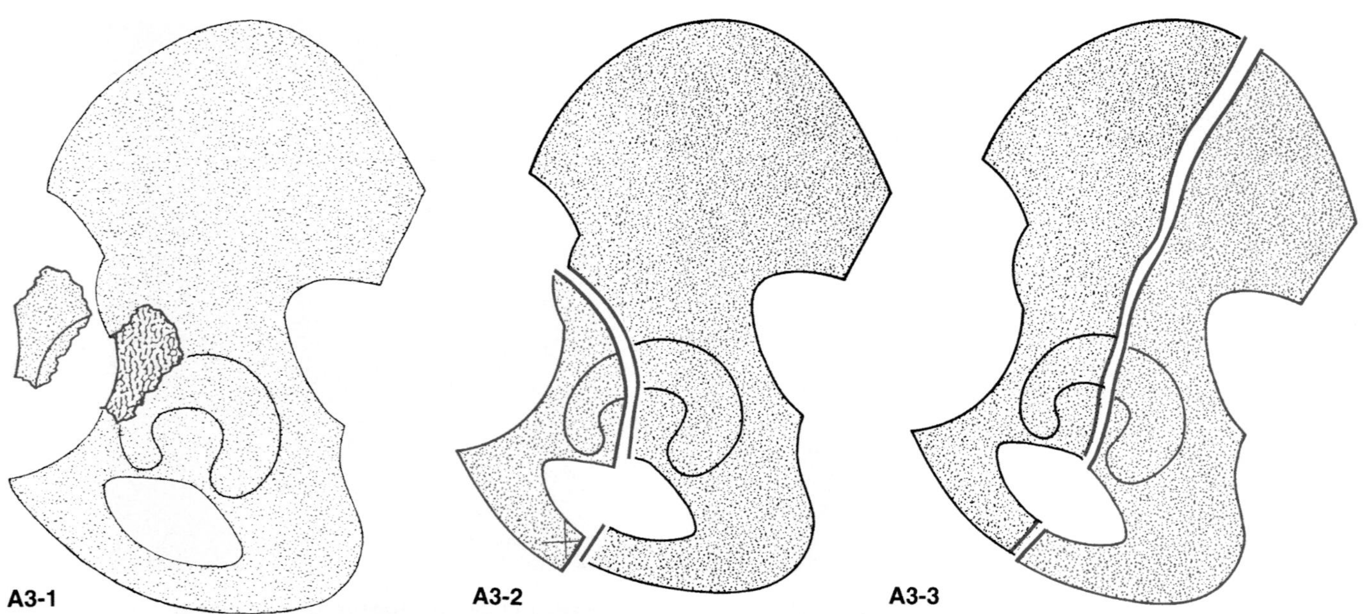

FIGURE 36-12. Type A3 anterior column anterior wall fractures. These may be further subdivided into isolated anterior wall fractures (A3-1), and fractures of the anterior column, which may be high, extending to the iliac crest (A3-2) or low, exiting below the crest (A3-3).

2), which usually do not cause significant incongruity. These can usually be managed nonoperatively with the expectation of a good result (D. Helfet, personal communication, 1993).

Surgical Approach

Anterior Iliofemoral (Smith-Petersen)
Only for high types (A3-3).

Anterior Ilioinguinal
For all other types including fractures of the wall (A3-1, A3-2).

Position

The correct position is supine.

Reduction Techniques

Anterior column fractures are relatively easy to reduce. They are usually exposed through an iliofemoral or ilioinguinal approach, and can be anatomically reduced by examining the fracture lines along the iliac wing and crest. Reduction is facilitated by the use of the large pointed clamps and other special clamps, including pelvic reduction clamps (Fig. 36-13A). Muscle attachments play a major role in displacement of these fracture fragments. The anterior superior spine has attached to it the sartorius and the inferior spine, the rectus femoris. These have a tendency to cause the fracture to be displaced outward and downward and tend to rotate it internally. Despite muscle relaxation, if the fracture fragment is still difficult to reduce, division of the tendon of rectus femoris and/or sartorius, if this was not done during the approach, may be necessary to facilitate the reduction.

Fixation Techniques

Fixation is usually accomplished by an interfragmental compression screw placed from the anterior inferior spine to the posterior iliac wing (Fig. 36-13B,C). This is all within thick cancellous bone, and excellent fixation can be obtained. A second screw can be placed across the top of the iliac crest if the fracture is high in the anterior column and extends out to the iliac crest above the anterior superior spine (Fig. 36-13D,E).

The screw fixation of the anterior column usually should be buttressed by a 3.5-mm reconstruction plate, either curved or straight. One or two plates usually suffice, as noted on the drawing (Fig. 36-13F) and the clinical cases (Fig. 36-14). If

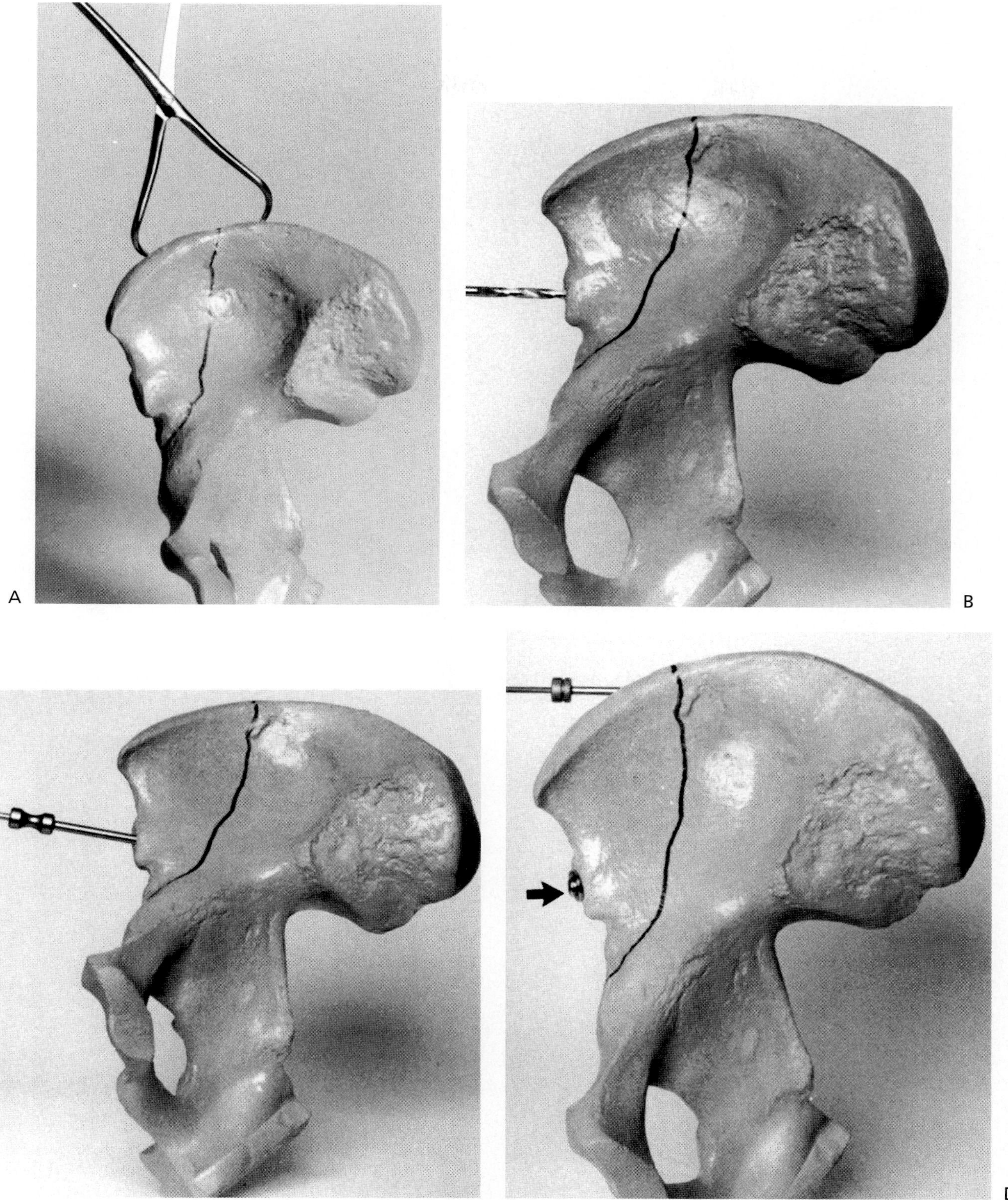

FIGURE 36-13. Reduction and fixation of the anterior column. **A:** A pointed reduction clamp temporarily fixes the anterior column fracture. **B,C:** Drilling the glide hole for insertion of a T guide into the glide hole and completion of the drilling from the anterior column into the posterior sciatic buttress with a 3.2-mm guide drill bit. **D:** Note the position of the 4.5-mm lag screw, which has excellent purchase in the bone of the sciatic buttress *(black arrow).* Also note the drilling of a guide hole for the insertion of a 3.5-mm lag screw at the iliac crest *(white arrow).*

(Figure continues)

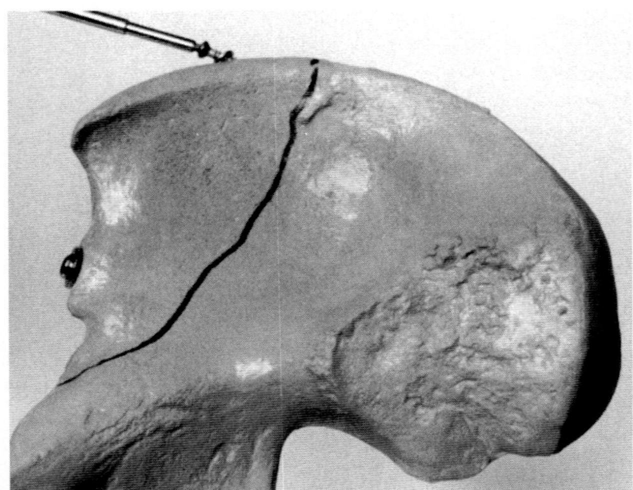

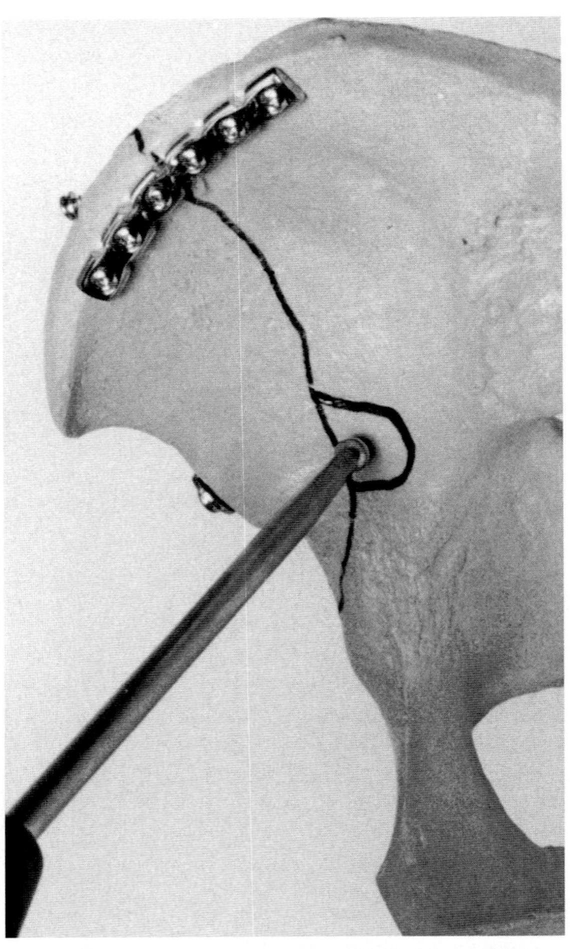

FIGURE 36-13. ***(continued)*** **E:** A 3.5-mm lag screw is inserted along the iliac crest. **F:** An alternative to fixation is a 3.5-mm plate, which is especially useful if the surgeon is concerned about the strength of the bone. Note also the insertion of a lag screw into a fragment of sciatic buttress. Reduction and fixation of this fragment is especially important in fixation of both-column fractures.

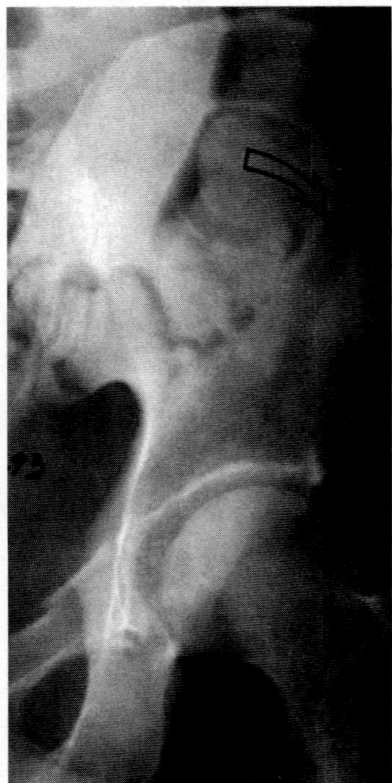

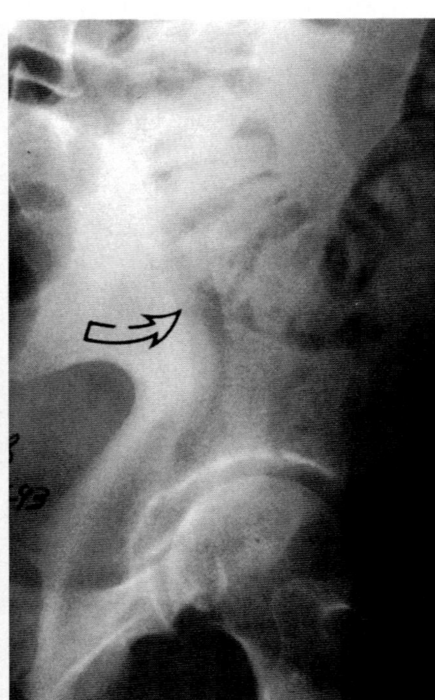

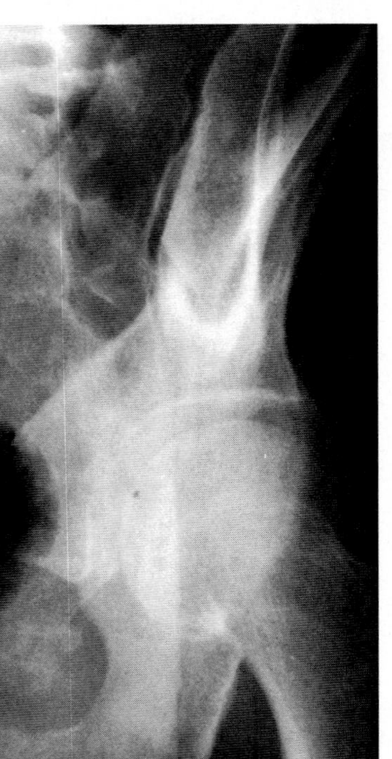

FIGURE 36-14. Anterior column fixation. **A:** Anterior-posterior (AP); **B:** Iliac oblique; and **C:** Obturator oblique radiographs of a high anterior column fracture *(black arrow)*.

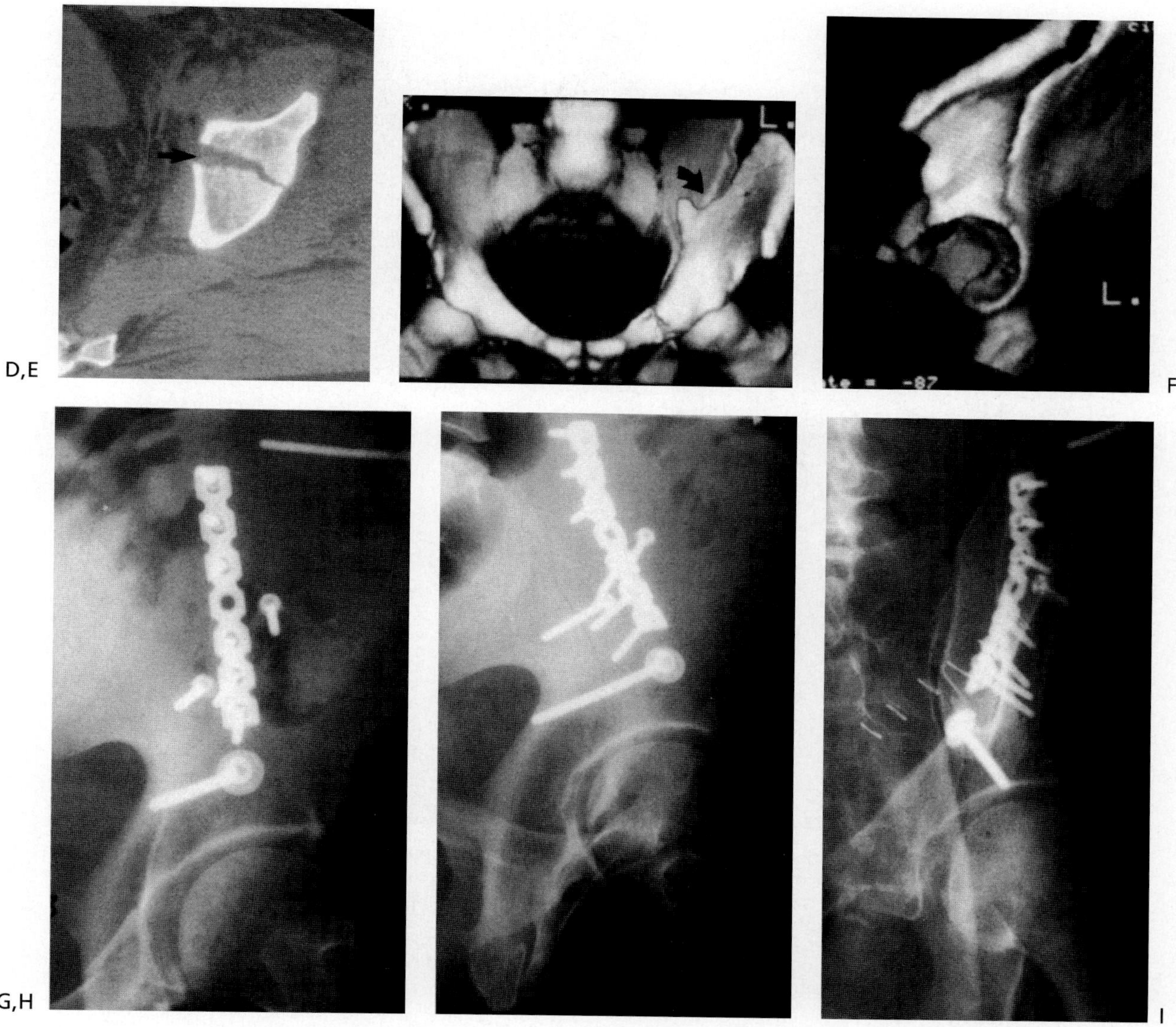

FIGURE 36-14. ***(continued)*** The amount of displacement at the joint level in the coronal plane is better seen on the axial computed tomography **(D)** and three-dimensional CT **(E,F).** Fixation in this case consisted of a typical AP lag screw, secondary lag screws, and a buttress plate **(G–I).**

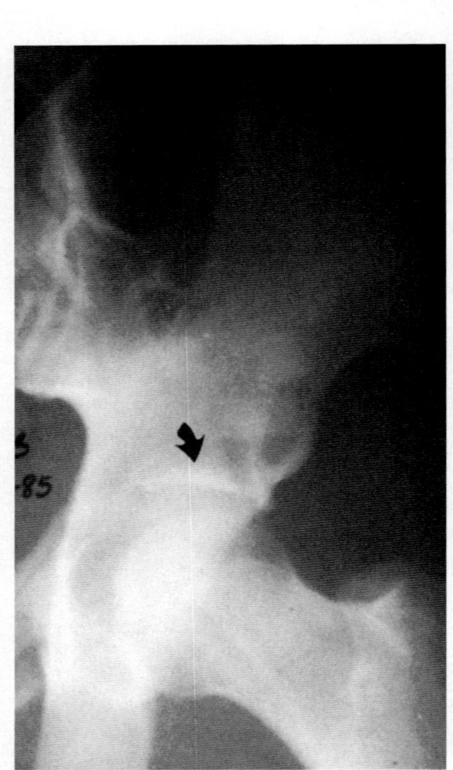

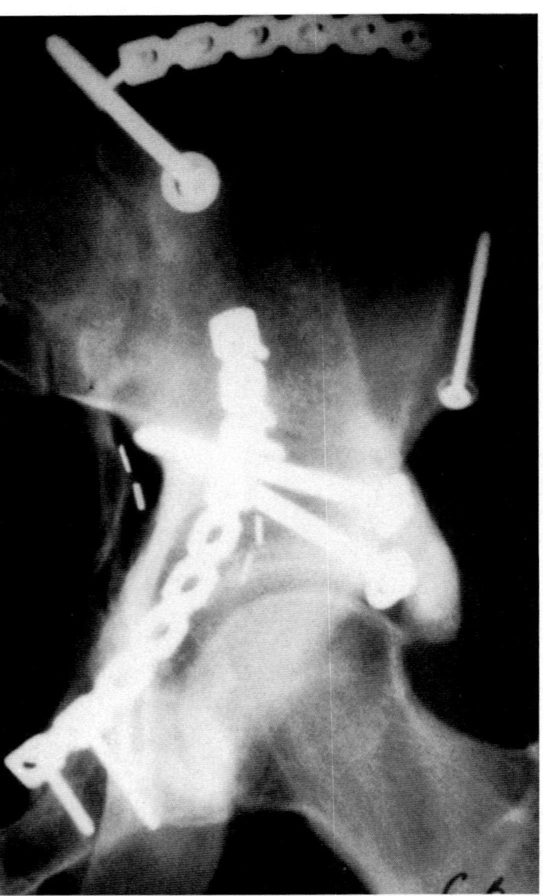

FIGURE 36-15. A: Anterior-posterior (AP) radiograph shows an anterior column fracture with displacement of the roof of the acetabulum. **B:** On a postoperative radiograph 5 years after internal fixation. Note the two AP lag screws, the buttress plate, and lag screw along the iliac crest, and the anterior column plate extending distal to the hip joint. On occasion, this plate is required to serve as a buttress over to the symphysis pubis. Note the osteophyte on the femoral head and the heterotopic ossification, which in this case did not limit motion, and the restoration of the dome to its anatomic position.

the fracture is low and involves the anterior wall fragments, the buttress must extend along the anterior column to the symphysis pubis (Fig. 36-13) as seen in the clinical cases (Fig. 36-15). Lag screw fixation directly into an anterior wall fragment must be done with great care, to avoid penetrating the joint. Predrilling before fixation may be used, as in the posterior wall.

REFERENCES

1. Tile M. *Fractures of the pelvis and acetabulum.* Baltimore: Williams & Wilkins, 1984.
2. Letournel E, Judet R. *Fractures of the acetabulum.* Berlin: Springer-Verlag, 1993.
3. Matta JM. Surgical treatment of acetabular fractures. In: Browner BD, Jupiter JB, Levine AM, et al., eds. *Skeletal trauma.* Philadelphia: W.B. Saunders, 1992.

PART E. SURGICAL MANAGEMENT OF SPECIFIC ACETABULAR INJURY TYPES

37

SURGICAL MANAGEMENT OF B TYPES: B1, B2, B3

DAVID L. HELFET

INTRODUCTION

Type B fractures (Fig. 37-1), including the transverse or T types, with or without posterior wall involvement, and the anterior with posterior hemitransverse, are among the most difficult to manage. If, as is often the case, such fractures are produced by significant forces and energy, the shearing force often damages the articular surfaces, and gross displacement and often instability results. Reduction may be very difficult to achieve, especially for T-type fractures, the latter for which an anatomic reduction is obtained in only 60% of cases, even in the most expert hands (1).

In the transverse and T types, the ilium is often externally rotated through a stable open-book type of sacroiliac disruption (Fig. 37-2). In attempts at reduction of these types, internal rotation of the proximal iliac fragment is required. No fixation of the sacroiliac joint is required if the sacroiliac joint is stable and has normal posterior support. When the transverse fracture is high (especially transtectal), the femoral head often impinges on the edge of the proximal fragment medially (Fig. 37-2). If left, the femoral head articular cartilage wears very rapidly and is unacceptable. Realigning the femoral head under the small remaining intact acetabular dome is easy, but hard to maintain without restoring the reminder of the displaced acetabulum (i.e., surgically); therefore, skeletal traction with enough weight to decompress the femoral head from the intact acetabular edge is necessary until expeditious surgery can be coordinated.

B1: TRANSVERSE FRACTURES

Surgical Approach

Type B1: Pure Transverse Fractures

The decision of surgical approach should be dependent on the level (i.e., the height) of the transverse fracture as well as its obliquity (i.e., on which side it is highest or involving more of the weight-bearing portion of the acetabulum), displacement, and rotation. Those highest anteriorly, with most displacement and involvement anteriorly, should be approached through an ilioinguinal approach and similarly posteriorly. The smaller the remaining intact articular surface of the dome the greater the difficulty in reducing these through single anterior and posterior approaches. Some have advocated dual or extensile approaches, but a posterior approach with a trochanteric flip osteotomy might be the ideal approach for such a fracture. This allows adequate exposure of the posterior column, dome, and articular surface (see Chapters 28 and 31). Clearly, late cases, or those you would consider the most difficult based on surgical experience, routine use of dual approaches, or even the extensile approach may be indicated. Clearly, those beyond 21 days may be best treated by an extensile approach.

The Transverse Fracture with an Associated Posterior Wall Fragment

A standard Kocher-Langenbeck approach is all that is indicated in the majority of these cases. However, if the transverse

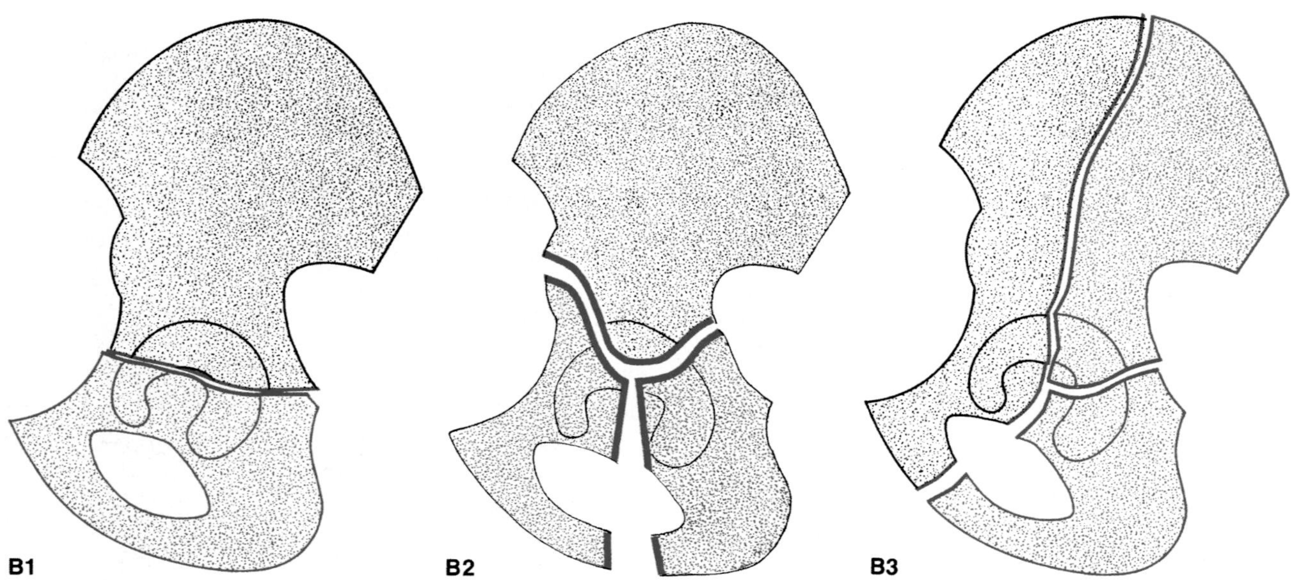

FIGURE 37-1. Type B partial articular fractures of the acetabulum include pure transverse fractures (B1), T-fractures (B2), and anterior plus posterior hemitransverse fractures (B3). All of these fractures are commonly associated with an acetabular wall fragment.

component is very high or there is additional significant anterior displacement/rotation, a limited lateral window of the ilioinguinal may be indicated to achieve a stable anatomic reduction. Because of the posterior wall component, rarely is it necessary to gain additional access to the articular surface of the dome other than what can be achieved by elevating underneath the intact abductors. However, a Kocher-Langenbeck with an additional trochanteric flip and dislocation of the femoral head may be the approach of choice in rare cases with additional dome comminution of displacement.

Position

The patient should be in the prone position for the Kocher-Langenbeck approach to be efficacious with transverse-type fractures. This allows the position and pull of the extremity to help reduce the inferior portion of the transverse component. A Kocher-Langenbeck approach in the lateral position is not the same, nor is the reduction and fixation that can be achieved through the approach the same.

The supine position should be used in an ilioinguinal approach; and the lateral decubitus position in combined or extensile approaches.

Reduction Techniques

This is discussed more fully in Chapter 31. The method of reduction depends not only on what approach is chosen, but also on the particular fracture pathoanatomy; therefore, very careful evaluation of the fracture pattern on plain radiographs and computed tomography (CT) is essential to determine the obliquity and displacement of the transverse component and whether there is any wall involvement (Fig. 37-3). This is necessary to determine not only the correct approach, but also the appropriate method of reduction and where or from which side the essential lag screws can be inserted. The ideal is an anatomic reduction of any acetabular fracture and because of the forces, compression with lag screws across the fracture will prevent displacement of any intraarticular component. Occasionally, owing to the obliquity of the fracture, interfragmentary compression from standard approaches causes shear and displacement—not compression. This, too, needs to be taken into account during the reduction maneuver. The planning and use of antishear or antiglide plates can then allow subsequent lag screw efficacious use.

The majority of these transverse type fractures are approached through the standard Kocher-Langenbeck approach with the patient in the prone position. The intraoperative view is of a displaced posterior column, the difference being that the inferior fragment has part of the anterior column and wall attached. The reduction is much more difficult, however, because the support of an intact anterior column was not available. To achieve such a reduction, adequate exposure with a full Kocher-Langenbeck approach in the prone position is essential, assuring access from the greater sciatic notch to the ischium and digital access to the quadrilateral plate both through the greater and

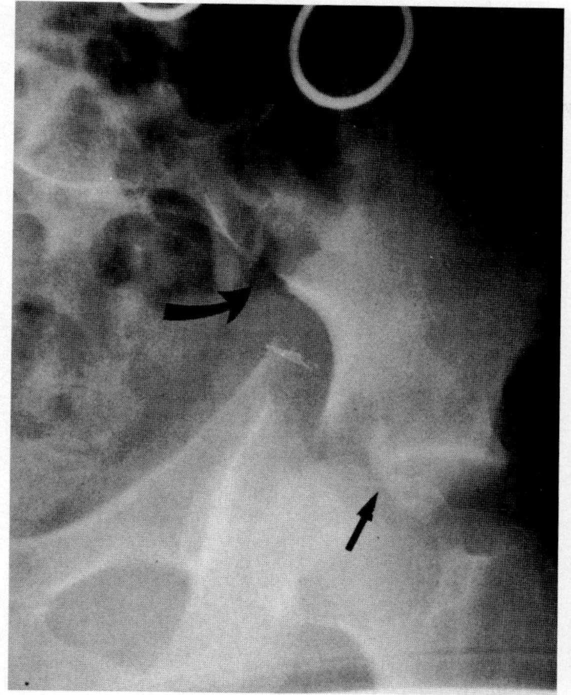

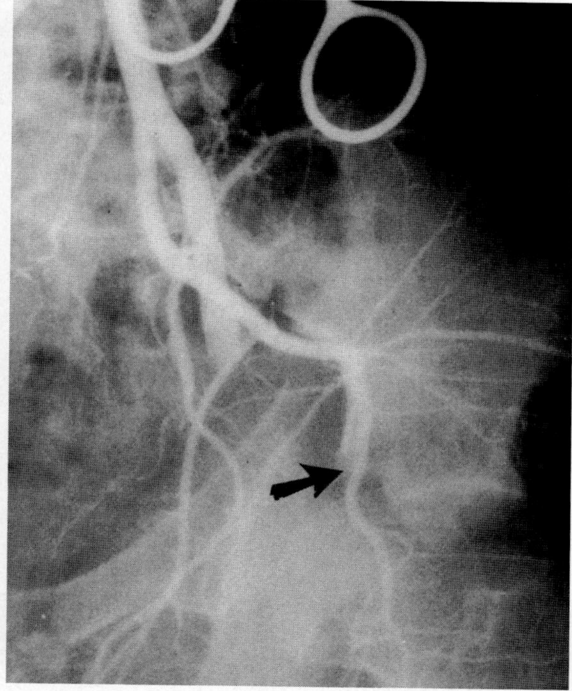

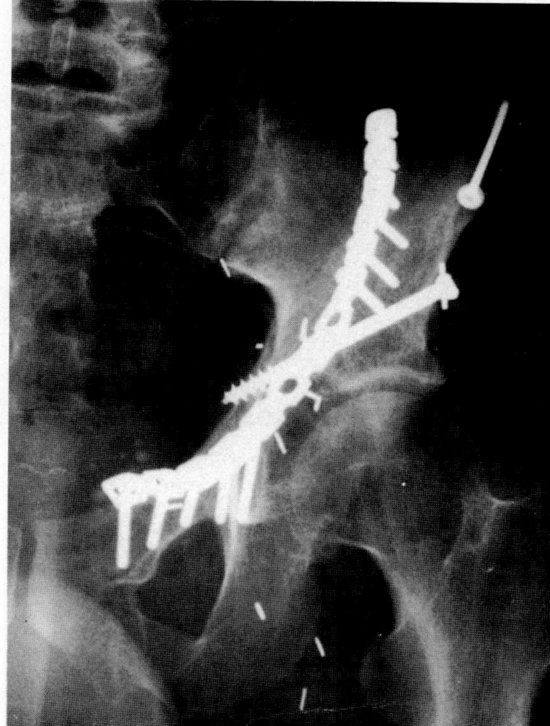

FIGURE 37-2. Type B1 transverse fracture exhibits external rotation of the proximal fragment. **A:** On the anteroposterior radiograph of a typical B1 transverse fracture with central displacement of the femoral head, note the marked external rotation of the iliac fracture through the sacroiliac joint, which is wide open anteriorly *(black arrow).* Note also the impingement of the femoral head on the sharp edge of the acetabular fragment *(straight arrow).* **B:** Arteriogram indicates an intimal tear in the internal iliac artery. **C:** Anterior-posterior radiograph shows the fixation of this transverse fracture through a modified ilioinguinal approach. Note the lag screw and the anterior plate fixation. The anterior approach was chosen because of a vascular injury, which was repaired at the same operative procedure.

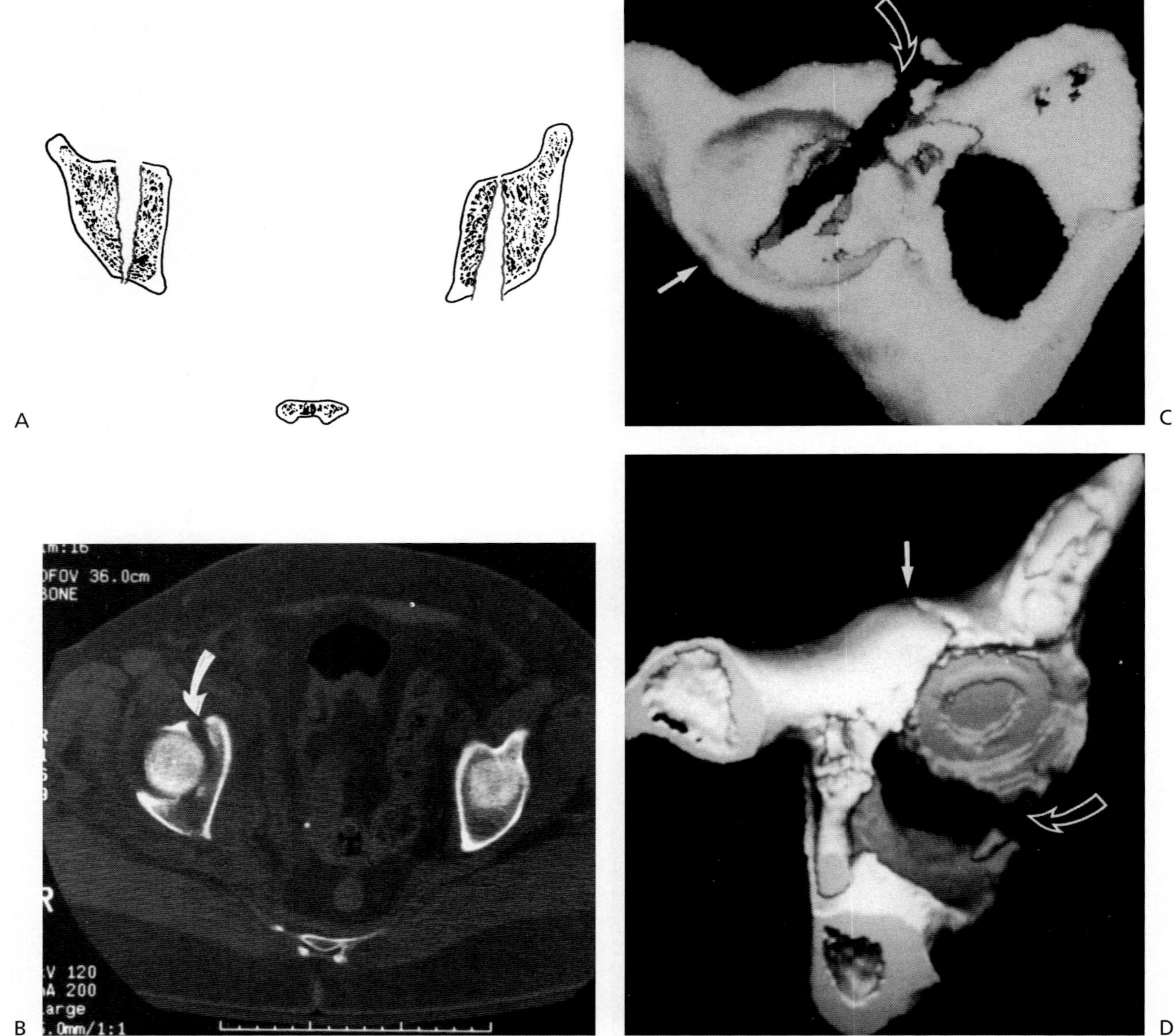

FIGURE 37-3. In a transverse fracture, the choice of the incision is dictated by the rotation of the fracture. **A,B:** In general, the fracture may be rotated so that there is a gap anteriorly or a gap posteriorly. **C:** This is further noted on the three-dimensional computed tomography, where the gap is clearly anterior *(curved arrow),* the fracture being hinged on the posterior column *(straight arrow).* Contrast this to the situation in **(D),** where the opening is through the posterior column *(curved arrow)* and hinged anteriorly *(white arrow).* For the lesion in **(C)** an anterior approach is indicated, for **(D),** a posterior approach.

lesser sciatic notches. This allows the insertion of a finger or a clamp into the inner aspect of the pelvis, affording control of the distal fragment both for displacement and rotation.

The forces necessary to create reduction of the displaced transverse fragment of the acetabulum mandates control of medial displacement and shear through the obliquity of the fracture. This is accomplished via placing a pelvic reduction clamp through the greater sciatic notch and reducing the displaced fragment to the intact ilium. Rotation is controlled with a Schantz pin in the ischium. A Jungblutt reduction clamp on either side of the fracture is most useful to help control displacement and rotation. In addition, a small reduction plate often is required not only to help with reduction, but also for temporary fixation. Traction through the femoral head is essential in order to use the femoral head and intact capsule, when possible, to supplement the reduction forces. Traction could be accomplished manually, with a femoral distractor and/or a fracture table. (See Chapter 31 for further details in the discussion of the reduction techniques.)

Posterior Approach for Pure Transverse Fractures

This approach is indicated when the displacement, rotation, or greatest involvement of the articular portion of the acetabulum is posterior. As in all patterns, if interfragmentary compression with a posterior column lag screw is planned, then the glide hole should be drilled prior to reduction. If this proves impossible, then the posterior column is reduced with the help of one of the following: (a) traction, (b) a Jungblutt pelvic reduction clamp, (c) a Schantz pin in the ischium, (d) special clamps, and (e) a small three- or four-hole reconstruction plate molded across the posterior column to help achieve and temporarily maintain reduction. Alternatively, Kirschner wires can be used, depending on the obliquity of the transverse fracture, to hold the reduction temporarily. A definitive posterior plate of the 3.5-mm reconstruction type extending from the sciatic buttress across the posterior column to the ischium is mandatory to obtain a stable reduction. Care should be taken to assure that the plate is overbent in order to avoid opening up of the fracture anteriorly with plate fixation.

Small posterior or anterior displacements can be corrected with the plate by pulling the displaced fragment to the plate helping the posterior column reduction. Minor correction of rotation can still be accomplished even though the plate has been applied with one screw on either side by digital palpation along the quadrilateral plate and inserting a pelvic reduction clamp into the greater sciatic notch onto the quadrilateral plate to assure the reduction, especially of rotation anteriorly of the inferior segment. Once aligned, lag screws should be inserted from posterior to anterior from just lateral to the greater sciatic notch, paralleling the quadrilateral plate into the anterior column (Fig. 37-4). Obviously, these are fraught with potential complications anteriorly referable to the neurovascular structures (see Chapter 39).

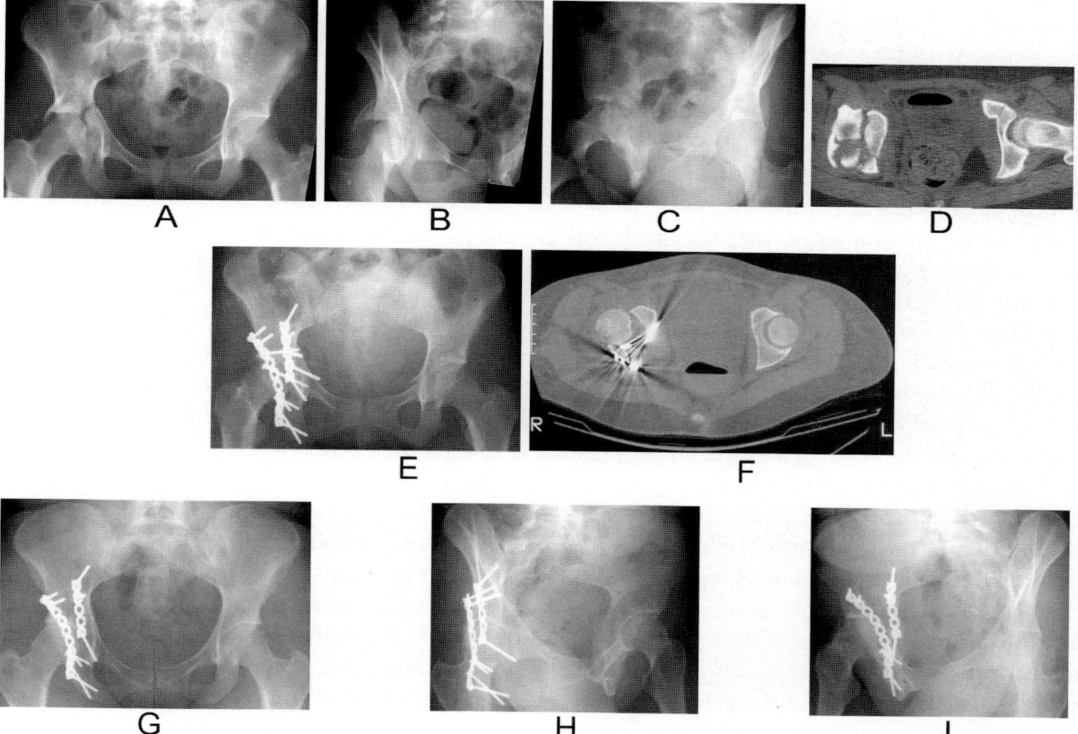

FIGURE 37-4. A 13-year-old female was involved in a high-speed motor vehicle accident as a restrained back seat passenger. Her injuries included a blunt right-sided thoracic trauma with an ipsilateral ischial T-type fracture of the acetabulum and associated posterior wall fracture. After stabilization of her general condition 48 hours after the accident, she was taken to the operating room where ORIF was performed through a Kocher-Langenbeck. Routine postoperative CT scan revealed intraarticular hardware needing removal. The patient returned at 10 years for follow-up with a normal gait and x-rays demonstrating excellent maintenance of the joint space, no evidence of avascular necrosis or posttraumatic arthritis, and no evidence of hardware loosening/breakage or heterotopic ossification. **A–C:** Anteroposterior and Judet films demonstrating a right-sided T-type acetabular fracture with associated posterior wall fracture. **D:** CT images of the acetabulum demonstrating the transverse aspect of the fracture and the posterior lesion. **E:** Postoperative film illustrates an anatomic reduction. **F:** Postoperative CT scan reveals presence of intraarticular hardware. **G–I:** Radiographs at 10 years illustrating a healed T-type acetabular fracture with associated posterior wall fracture.

An alternative lag screw is from the posterior ilium to the anterior column. The ideal starting point is just posterior to the gluteal ridge, three finger-breadths above the articular surface of the acetabulum. In the standard Kocher-Langenbeck approach this would have to be done percutaneously through the abductor muscles with fluoroscopic control. This screw has a small acceptable window in the anterior column; it is of concern is that the drill bit and/or screw may penetrate the joint or alternatively exit just beyond the iliopectineal eminence, hence injuring the femoral vessels. Such lag screws should be inserted with extreme care and not without experience. Some have recommended the use of the oscillating drill attachment to protect the soft tissues in case of cortical bone perforation. My own recommendation is to use a standard drill and continuously feel bone on the opposite side of the drill to assure no extraosseous penetration. Obviously, this posterior to anterior column screw is much easier to perform with an extensile approach.

Some transverse fractures begin in the infratectal or juxtatectal region posteriorly and extend superiorly into the inner pelvis, producing a very high spike of bone on the inner aspect of the pelvis where the posterior and anterior columns meet. The application of an offset pelvic clamp through the greater sciatic notch with one tine on the spike and the other on the superior aspect of the lateral portion of the iliac ring often reduces this fracture. Sometimes this is difficult or impossible through a posterior approach. If such is the case, especially if comminuted, it may be possible to insert a plate as a buttress for the reduction clamp in the greater sciatic notch, giving the moment of action of the tine of the clamp greater distribution. Also keeping the Jungblutt clamp on and controlling rotation and displacement at the time of the final fracture reduction also might be advantageous when such difficulty is encountered. If impossible, only the posterior column should be fixed anatomically, the wound should be closed, and a separate anterior exposure of the lateral window of the ilioinguinal should be used to reduce the high anterior spike with an antishear buttress plate.

Other transverse fracture types may be oblique in the opposite direction, so the use of the clamps must vary depending on the fracture type. There is also obliquity of the fracture in the medial lateral direction, which also may change the exact position of the application of the pelvic reduction clamp. Clearly, one has to "play" with traction, the rotation control through the ischium, and various pelvic reduction plates and lag screws to afford the reduction.

Anterior Ilioinguinal Approach

If the main displacement and rotation is anterior and this involves the greater portion of the articular surface of the acetabulum, then the anterior ilioinguinal approach is used. This allows direct reduction of the anterior spike of bone and its provisional fixation with Kirschner wires and/or a temporary reduction plate. Again, reduction of the posterior column has to be done indirectly, that is, through visualization and the feel of a finger along the quadrilateral plate, from the pelvic brim to the ischial spine. This is accomplished through the first or second windows of the ilioinguinal approach. One of the large pelvic reduction clamps may be required to control the displacement and rotation of the posterior column, even though the anterior column is well reduced. Again, traction may be mandated and can be accomplished through a Schantz pin from the trochanter into the femoral neck and head. If necessary, fluoroscopy can be used to assess the quality of reduction and temporary reduction can be maintained into the posterior column with Kirschner wires.

Transverse Fractures with Posterior Wall Involvement and/or Displacement

This fracture is the most common of the transverse types. It is almost always associated with the posterior hip dislocation.

Surgical Approach

The best approach is the posterior Kocher-Langenbeck routinely and only rarely an associated trochanteric flip osteotomy for greater access to the bone. At first glance it may appear to be a more difficult fracture to reduce because of the posterior wall, but in actual fact the displaced posterior wall allows easier access into the hip joint to assess the quality of the reduction, especially rotation, and allows visualization to assure that fixation from back to front is extraarticular.

Position

The recommended position is prone on a radiolucent table.

Reduction Techniques

These are similar to the transverse but with greater visualization and access to the joint during the reduction maneuvers. Attention is directed to reducing the posterior wall components following reduction and fixation of the transverse component, visualized intraarticularly. Traction through the femoral head, femoral distractor, or fracture table assures that all fragments are out of the joint with visualization and debridement, especially those nestled in the fovea. An inspection of the femoral head is possible at the same time. Marginal impacted fragments are realigned to the intact femoral head by releasing the traction and using osteotomes and bone graft, as previously described in Chapters 28 and 31. Posterior wall fragments are reattached sequentially, maintaining their capsular attachments temporarily with Kirschner wires. Prior to closure of the posterior wall it is important to determine the angle for lag screw fixation. Standard buttress plating is accomplished with a 3.5-mm reconstruction plate and additional spring plates as indicated, depending on fracture size and type. Lag screws should be inserted through the plate, if possible, but independently if not traditionally stabilized or significant posterior fractures.

Fixation Techniques

(See Fig. 37-5.)

Posterior Approach

If possible, it is best to use a posterior column lag screw, usually predrilling the glide hole. The column is then buttressed with a posterior 3.5-mm reconstruction plate from the sciatic buttress to the ischium with slight overcontouring.

A plate contoured for the posterior aspect of a transverse fracture must be "overcontoured," to provide a small gap between the plate and the posterior aspect of the acetabular surface. As the plate is tightened, it compresses the anterior aspect (Fig. 37-5G,H). With juxtatectal or lower transverse fractures posteriorly it is sometimes difficult to control the posterior column, especially when there is a high shear angle to the fracture. A 3.5-mm reconstruction plate that has been contoured to the inferior fragment of the posterior column then is applied and reduction is accomplished through the plate using a tenaculum or pointed reduction clamp and a unicortical drill hole in the iliac wing. Once the fracture has been reduced, the plate can be affixed to the bone with other screws. Because the plate is flexible, the screws tend to force the plate to take on the contour of the bone. This must be done very carefully and the fracture reduction must be watched to assure that the plate is not too rigid and displace the fracture fragment itself. If this occurs, this technique cannot be used as the method of fixation, only as one of reduction.

Posterior wall fractures should all be buttressed with plates, ideally, 3.5-reconstruction plates, but for smaller or

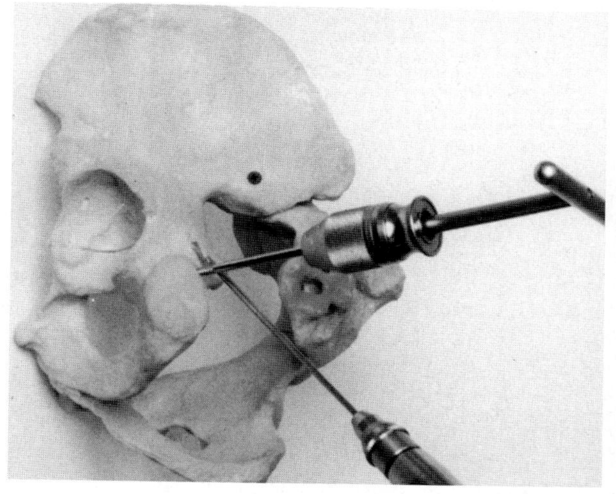

A

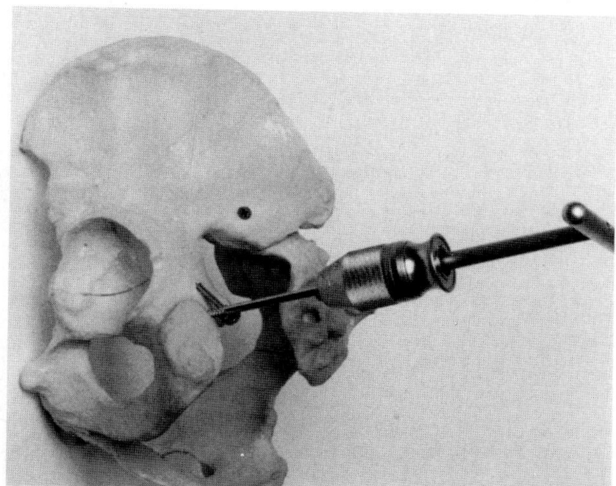

B

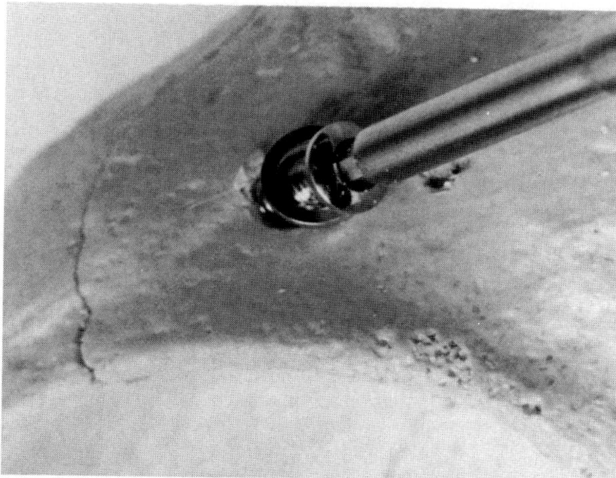

C

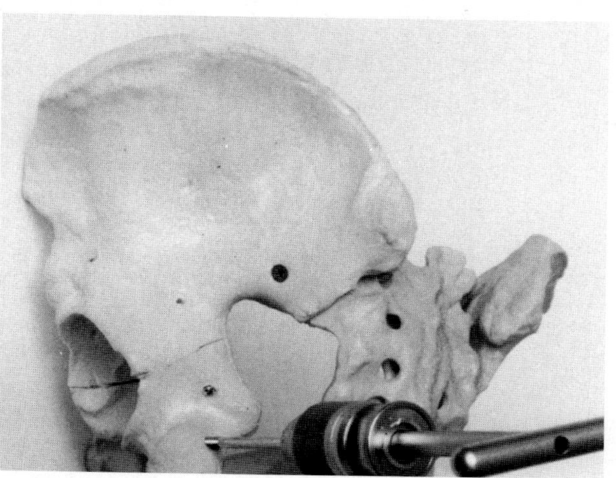

D

FIGURE 37-5. A: Posterior column fixation with lag screw and buttress plate. Reduction was aided by the Schantz pin in the ischial tuberosity. For illustration, a posterior reduction clamp has been removed. The glide hole is made in the distal fragment with a 3.5-mm drill bit. This can be done with the fracture reduced or unreduced. The tap guide is inserted and a 2.5-mm drill completes the hole. **C,D:** The posterior column lag screw immediately adjacent to the hard bone of the sciatic buttress is inserted.

(Figure continues)

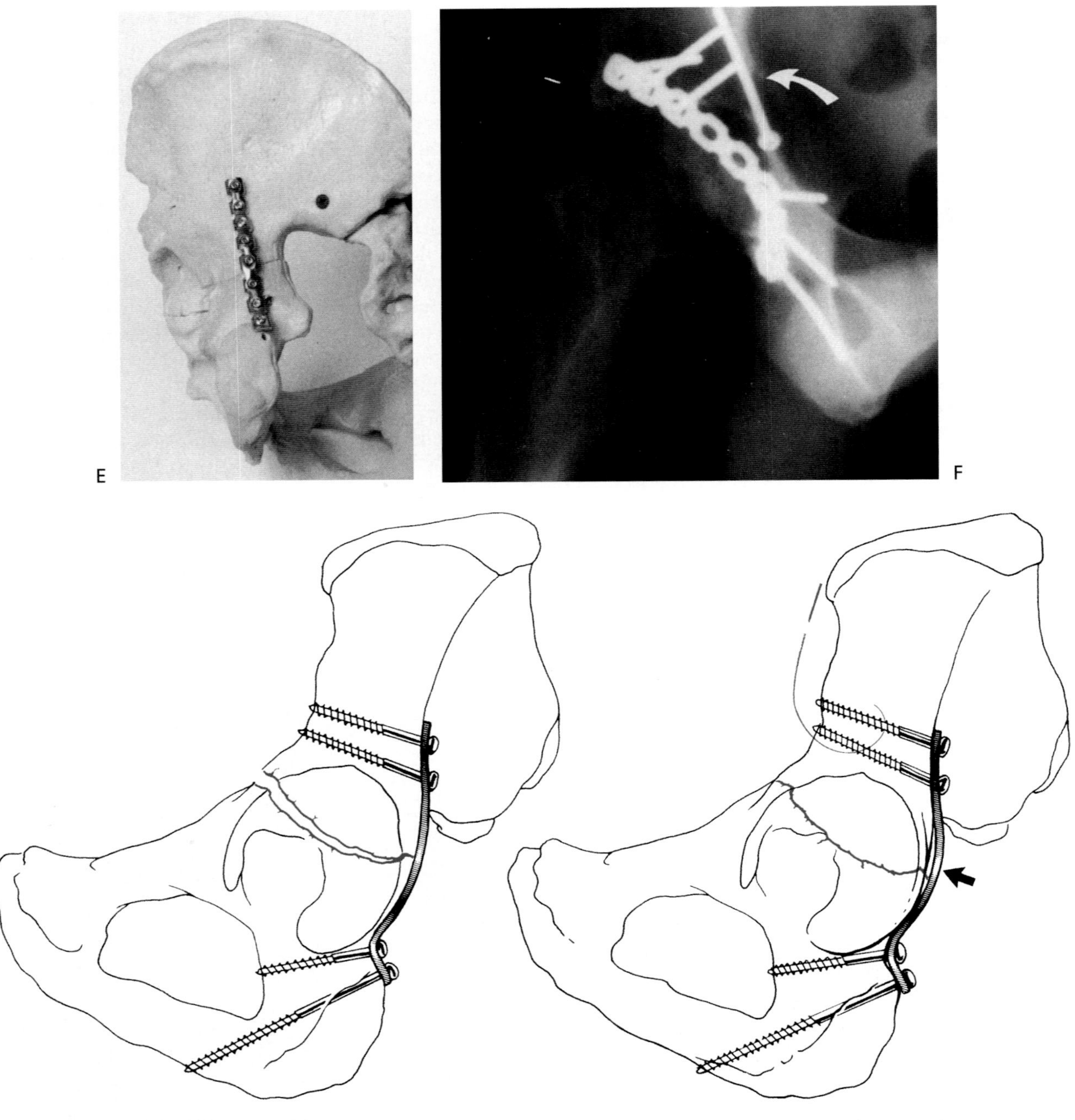

FIGURE 37-5. ***(continued)*** **E:** A well-molded buttress plate completes the posterior fixation of this transverse fracture. **F:** The position of the posterior column lag screw immediately adjacent to the hard bone of the sciatic buttress is seen in the anterior-posterior postoperative radiograph *(white arrow)*. Note also the posterior column buttress plate in this transverse fracture. **G:** Diagram demonstrates the adverse consequences of improper molding of the posterior column plate. The plate has been applied adjacent to the posterior column. The anterior column will be displaced when the screws are tightened. **H:** When the screws are tightened in this case, the fracture is compressed rather than distracted because the plate has been properly molded *(black arrow)*.

more peripheral wall fractures pointed one-third tubular "spring plates," as popularized by Mast, are the buttress of choice. Lag screws should be used for all fragments, posterior wall or column, whenever possible. Fixation of the anterior column to the posterior column through the Kocher-Langenbeck is accomplished by inserting screws from the sciatic buttress along the quadrilateral plate into the anterior column, or alternatively percutaneously from the iliac wing to the anterior column. Both of these are potentially dangerous, the latter even more so because of the increased length of the screws and the less digital control. Clearly, the drill bit or screw may penetrate the joint or, even worse, perforate the root of the pubic ramus and injure the femoral vessels. When inserting the screw from just lateral to the top of the greater sciatic notch along the quadrilateral plate into the anterior column, with the patient prone in the Kocher-Langenbeck approach, a finger along the quadrilateral plate will allow digital palpation of the drill oscillating just parallel to the quadrilateral plate. With gentle drilling, feeling bone at the end of the drill, it is possible to palpate when the drill penetrates the cortex of the anterior column. This should be accomplished with 3.5-mm screws, preferably two from posterior to anterior. Obviously this mandates the anterior column fracture being high enough in the front to allow fixation of the superior aspect of the fracture through this approach. Alternatively, more distal anterior fixation can be obtained from posterior through the previously described posterior to anterior lag screw (Fig. 37-4A). If the surgeon is inexperienced with these techniques or encounters any difficulty, it is safer not to use this form of lag screw anterior column fixation, but rather to perform an additional direct anterior approach and use visual anterior fixation techniques.

A Word of Warning

Failure to adequately fix the transverse fracture with a lag screw or screws, holding it only with a posterior buttress plate, may allow the transverse fracture to displace (Fig. 37-6). Therefore, when possible, posterior and/or anterior lag screw fixation is used on the transverse component (Fig. 37-7).

Anterior Approaches

Fixation is accomplished with lag screws from anterior to posterior, starting on the pelvic brim above the iliopectineal eminence and aiming along the quadrilateral plate for the posterior ischial spine. This should be inserted with digital palpation along the quadrilateral plate, but also understanding the outer anatomy and the safe zone for anterior to posterior screw insertion (see Chapters 28 and 31). In addition a 3.5-mm reconstruction buttress plate molded along the pelvic bone and ilium is mandatory.

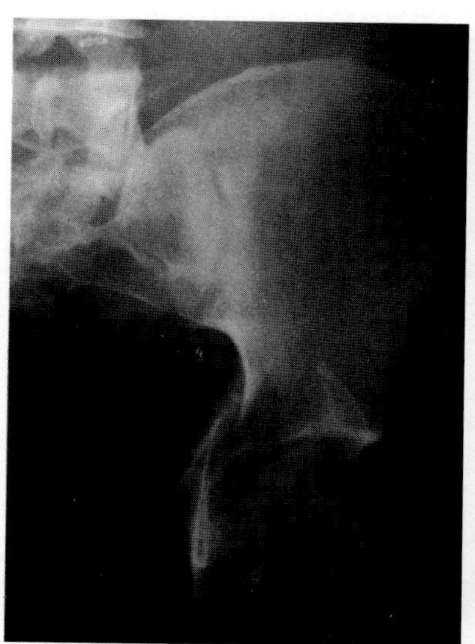
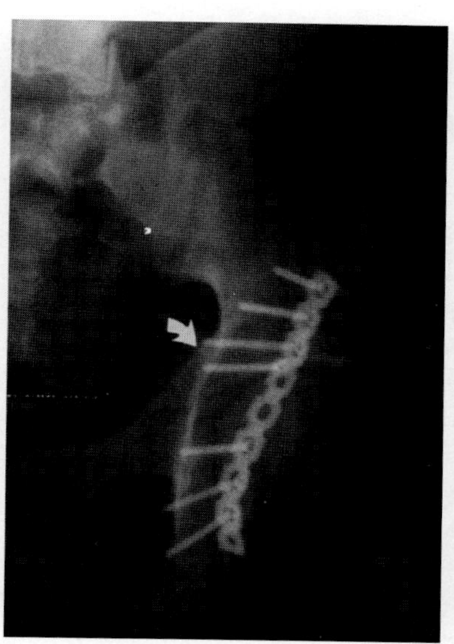
A,B

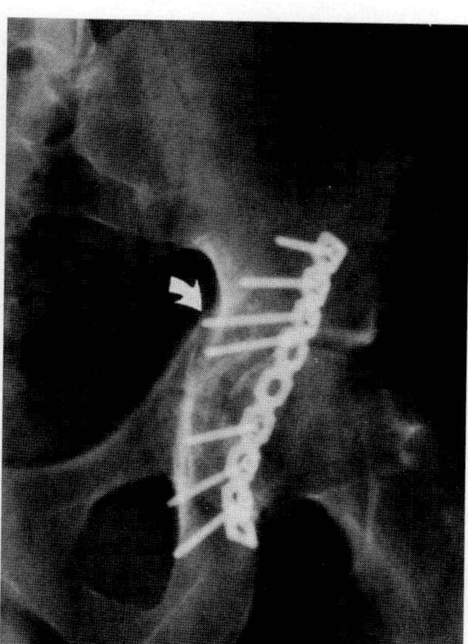
C

FIGURE 37-6. Plate fixation alone could lead to secondary redisplacement. **A:** Anterior-posterior radiograph shows a transverse fracture of the acetabulum with a small posterior wall fragment. The posterior wall fragment was fixed with a single lag screw, and a reconstruction plate was used to buttress the fracture. No lag screw was used across the posterior column or through the anterior column. **B:** Anatomic reduction of both the anterior and posterior column is denoted by the *white arrow.* In the early postoperative period it became obvious that the distal fragment of this transverse fracture had shifted. **C:** Note now that both the ilioischial and iliopectineal lines have shifted medially *(white arrow).* To prevent this, some other form of fixation, such as a posterior column lag screw described previously, an anterior column lag screw, or cerclage wires, is needed.

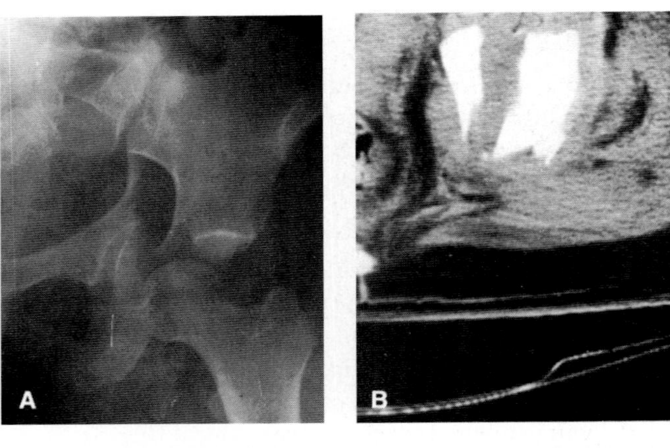

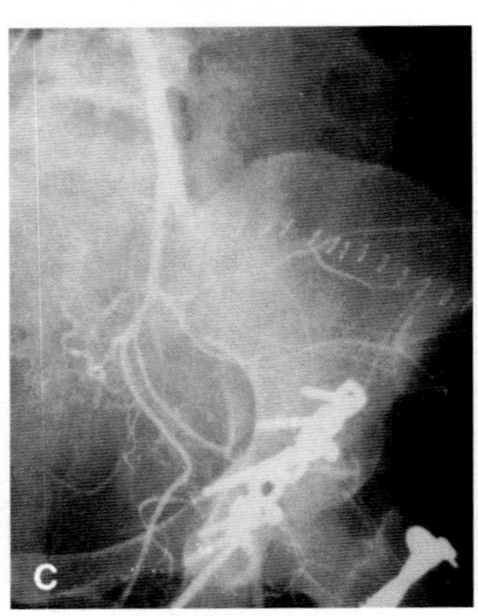

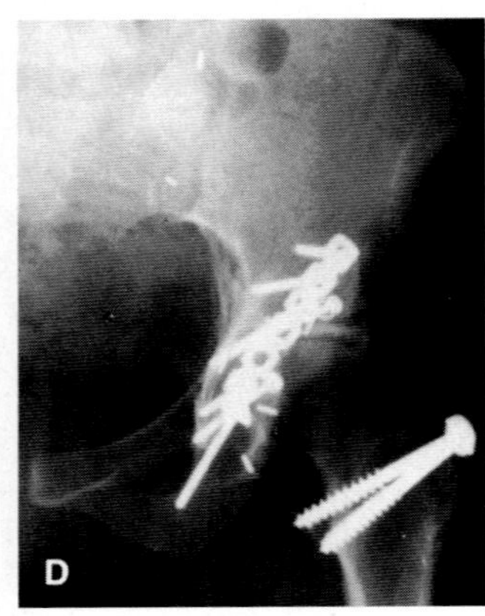

FIGURE 37-7. Transverse fracture fixation with posterior buttress plate and anterior column lag screw. Dangers of arterial injury: **A:** Anterior-posterior radiograph indicates a markedly displaced high-energy transverse fracture of the left acetabulum. **B:** Computed tomography of the left hip shows the displacement and the nature of this transverse fracture. **C:** Fixation was through a posterior Kocher-Langenbeck approach with removal of the greater trochanter. Excellent reduction and fixation was obtained with a posterior buttress plate and an anterior column lag screw. No untoward event was noted during surgery. Postoperatively, it was noted that the patient had no pulse in her left leg. Angiography revealed injury to the femoral artery. Immediate arterial reconstruction was performed and revascularization was achieved. **D:** Postoperative radiograph demonstrated healing in excellent anatomic position. The position of the anterior column lag screw is noted. The danger of penetration into femoral vessels with the drill bit cannot be overstated. An oscillating drill is recommended for this procedure.

B2: PARTIAL ARTICULAR FRACTURES (T-TYPE)

(See Fig. 37-8.) T-type fractures, especially those produced by a high-energy insult, are the most difficult fracture patterns with which to deal. The results of nonoperative care of this fracture pattern have been dismal. Conversely, it is the most difficult pattern for which to achieve an anatomic reduction; therefore, often the results of operative care also may be less than perfect (1,2). It is useful to think of the fracture as two distinct types: a posterior column fracture, with or without a posterior wall fracture, plus a separate anterior column fracture. Clearly, in this pattern, because the columns are separated from each other, reduction and fixation of one column do not ensure reduction of the other (Fig. 37-9A). If the T is regarded as two separate column fractures, an anterior and a posterior one, all of the techniques previously described for such lesions are applicable, depending on what approach is used (i.e., anterior or posterior). The difficult aspect is to reduce the opposite, nonvisualized column via indirect means (if dual or extensile approaches are not used). Therefore, from a posterior approach, the surgeon may use a posterior buttress plate and

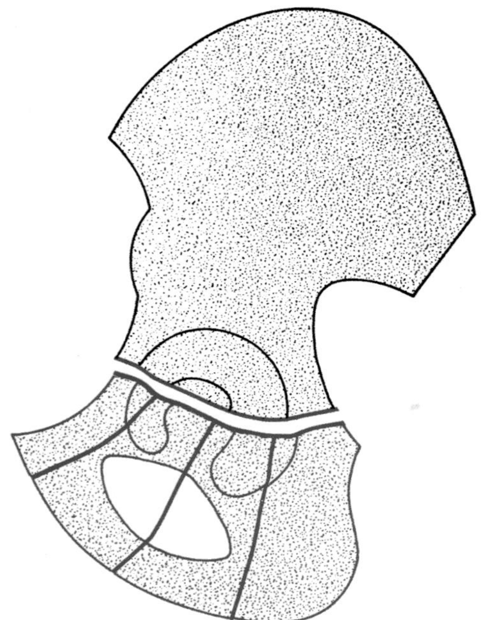

FIGURE 37-8. B2, T-type fractures. Note that the limb of the T most often exits through the obturator foramen and, less commonly, anteriorly through the pubis or posteriorly through the ischium.

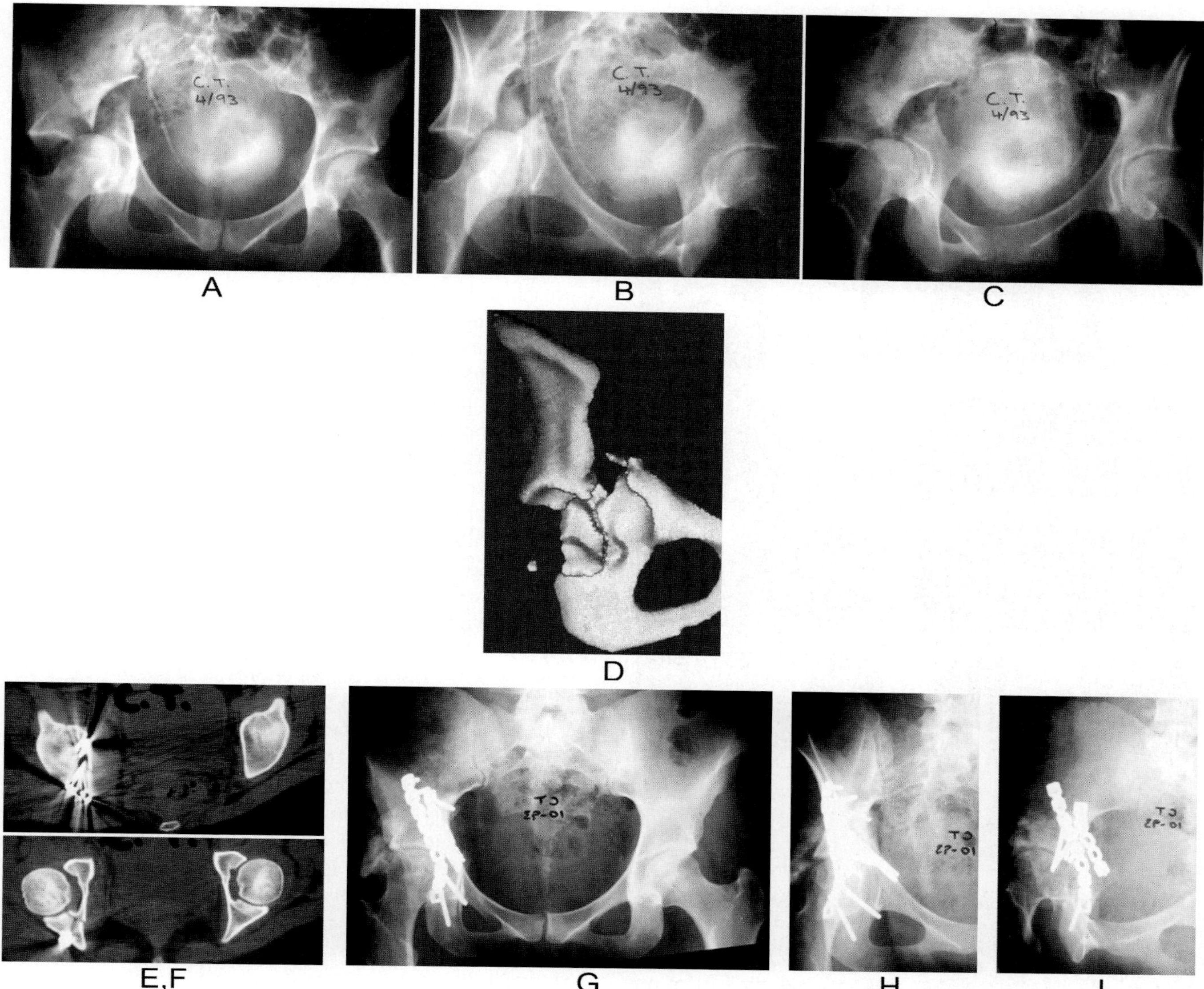

FIGURE 37-9. A 29-year-old female was a restrained driver of a motor vehicle involved in a high-speed, head-on collision. Radiographs obtained in the emergency room revealed a T-type fracture of the acetabulum. The patient was placed in tibial traction and transferred to our care for definitive management. ORIF was performed through a Kocher-Langenbeck approach. At 6 months following surgery the patient returned for followup with favorable clinical and radiological results. **A–C:** Anterioposterior and Judet injury radiographs illustrate a T-type fracture of the acetabulum. **D:** CT scan and three-dimensional reconstruction images. **E,F:** Postoperative CT reveals reduction of the fracture without evidence of intraarticular hardware. **G–I:** Postoperative x-rays taken six months following surgery illustrate a healed T-type acetabular fracture and preserved joint space. She was noted to have asymptomatic Brooker Type II heterotopic ossification that did not warrant excision.

then anterior column lag screws to reduce the anterior column. These can be put down parallel to the quadrilateral plate (Fig. 37-9); from an anterior approach, the reverse: an anterior buttress plate and then lag screws from anterior to posterior from the pelvic rim. Some have advocated cerclage wires as a helpful reduction technique, especially if the posterior column is fractured high into the greater sciatic notch. These fractures should be treated only by the most experienced surgeons under the "most ideal" circumstances, and they require careful preoperative assessment and planning to determine the best surgical approach and techniques for direct and indirect reduction and subsequent fracture stabilization (Fig. 37-10).

Surgical Approach

All surgical approaches, single, combined, and extensile, have been used for the treatment of displaced acetabular

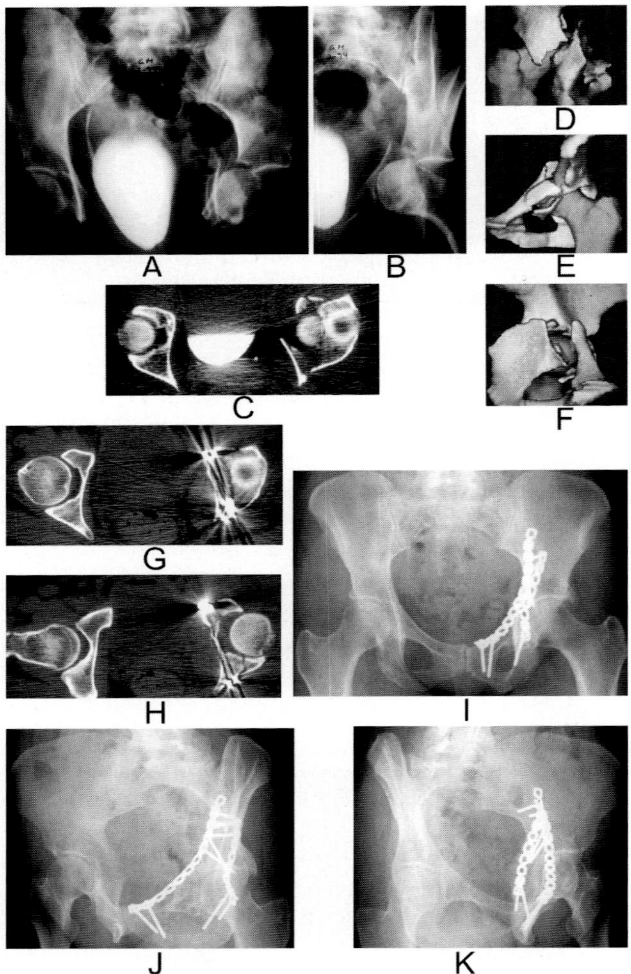

FIGURE 37-10. A 44-year-old female was a restrained driver of an automobile struck on the driver's side door by a truck. Anatomic reduction of the posterior column using a pelvic reconstruction plate was achieved through a Kocher-Langenbeck approach. As anterior reduction was not ideal, the patient was turned to a supine position for a sequential ilioinguinal approach and reduction and plating with a 3.5-mm pelvic reconstruction plate of the anterior portion of the T-type fracture. At 5 years follow up, the patient had an excellent clinical and radiographic result. **A,B:** Anterioposterior and obturator oblique injury films reveal a left displaced T-type acetabular fracture. **C:** CT scan outlines the transverse and vertical components of the fracture. **D–F:** 3D CT-reconstruction images illustrate medial displacement of the T-Type fracture with associated comminution of the anterior wall. **G,H:** Postoperative CT images confirm reduction of the fracture without evidence of intraarticular hardware. **I–K:** Radiographs at 5 years demonstrate anatomic reduction and preservation of the joint space without evidence of heterotopic ossification or avascular necrosis.

T-fractures. Ideally one would like to be able to see both the anterior and posterior column and an intraarticular view of the acetabulum at the same time. The extended iliofemoral or other extensile approaches allow this but not without paying a price of increased morbidity. Single anterior/posterior approaches with indirect anatomic reduction of the opposite nonvisualized column is ideal.

The most appropriate approach can be determined only after careful study of the pattern. Access to both columns directly or indirectly usually is necessary, unless the anterior column component is so far distal that it can be ignored. Access to the posterior column almost always is required. Initially the decision should be based on the fracture type itself. The level of the transverse component is probably the most important determinant of approach. The more displaced or the higher involvement in the obliquity of the transverse component would mandate that being the side for initial approach and reduction. Very often, however, an intraarticular view is necessary in order to get an anatomic reduction of the high or transtectal fractures. Recently, the combination of a Kocher-Langenbeck approach with a trochanteric flip made this possible without a transtectal approach. Clearly, most T-fractures with displacement have greater posterior than anterior displacement, and the approach of choice is the Kocher-Langenbeck.

Another factor that should be taken into account is the vertical limb. If it is an ischial T, as opposed to an obturator T, then a posterior approach is mandated. The status of the walls is the final issue to be addressed relative to the fracture itself. Obviously, if there is a posterior wall with a T, then a posterior approach is necessary in order to also reduce the wall. In fact, a displaced posterior wall makes intraarticular visualization easier from the Kocher-Langenbeck approach. Clearly, many patient factors and surgeon and institution assessment have to be included in this decision. If the surgery is done within the first 7 to 10 days, indirect reduction of the opposite column may be possible. If not, and especially for late cases, an extensile approach is mandated very often. Obviously, associated injuries and patient size might affect the decision. To do indirect reduction of the nonvisualized column mandates experience, the use of an array of pelvic clamps and reduction techniques, and intraoperative fluoroscopy. Ligamentotaxis with positioning of the femoral head intraoperatively definitely is useful, either via fracture table or femoral distractor.

The final determination as to the approach depends on the experience of the surgical team. Without a doubt, the approach used, extensile or not, should be the one that gives the surgeon the best option of obtaining an anatomic reduction. Emile Letournel advocated the preceding philosophy, that is, a single approach. Others more recently have advocated dual approaches simultaneously. Clearly, this so-called "floppy lateral" does not allow the full benefit of either the prone Kocher-Langenbeck or the supine ilioinguinal approach, but it has gained favor among those with less experience because it does allow access to both the outer landmarks of the anterior and posterior columns. Nevertheless, it does not address the shear fracture in the high transverse or transtectal fractures without a trochanteric osteotomy. The disadvantages of these combined approaches is the floppy lateral position itself and the fact that their routine use precludes learning or obtaining the experience in the single approaches for these or other complex fractures.

Position

The prone position is best if using the Kocher-Langenbeck approach. The supine position is best if using the ilioinguinal approach. The lateral position is best if using the extensile approach. The prone lateral position is best if using the Kocher-Langenbeck approach with trochanteric flip approach. The lateral position is best if using the combined approach.

Reduction and Fixation Techniques

By definition, a T-fracture has part of the acetabular articular surface still attached to the intact ilium. The philosophy must mandate reducing one column to the intact ilium anatomically and then bringing the other column to that. Emile Letournel recommended reducing the posterior column first. This is especially so when performing extensile or Kocher-Langenbeck approaches. Attention should be directed to thinking about lag screws prior to reduction so that posterior column lag screw gliding hole is drilled first. To reduce the posterior column, the same techniques should be used as advocated by Mast. The use of the Jungblutt reduction clamp is very helpful, with care being taken to assure that the screw placement for the clamp proximally and distally will not preclude your ability to palpate reduction through the greater sciatic notch, nor to apply a temporary short plate to hold the reduction if a posterior column lag screw is not possible. The two columns should be reduced, palpating in the greater and lesser sciatic notches as necessary, using a Schantz pin in the ischium to control rotation and, if necessary, using one of the offset clamps in the greater sciatic notch to afford the reduction. Once reduced, stabilize temporarily with a three-hole 3.5-mm reconstruction plate or, if there is room, use a definitive posterior column plate from the ischium all the way to the lateral border of the greater sciatic notch. Next, attention must be paid to reducing the anterior column into the reduced posterior column, again with palpation along the quadrilateral plate. Then it is possible to insert lag screws from back to front, just anterior to the border of the greater sciatic notch and angled along the quadrilateral plate to the iliopectineal eminence or just anterior. These are 3.5-mm cortical lag screws. However, even from a posterior approach, it may be advantageous sometimes to reduce the anterior column while visualizing it through the displaced posterior column. This is especially so if there is a displaced posterior wall. If it is impossible to reduce indirectly the opposite column after reducing one column, care should be taken to assure that no hardware or provisional fixation is impaling the opposite column or preventing its reduction.

Intraarticular visualization becomes easier, especially for the transtectal type fracture if there is a displaced posterior wall fracture, especially significant, associated with the T-fracture. The sequence would be posterior column, then anterior column, and only then posterior wall. Each one is described in the preceding.

Then the lateral or the first two windows of the ilioinguinal approach might be used if the major displacement is anteriorly and especially high anteriorly. Again, the anterior column would be reduced as described previously and stabilized temporarily with a Kirschner wire or a small 3.5-mm reconstruction plate. Then a definitive 3.5-mm reconstruction pelvic brim plate would be used and subsequent reduction using the pelvic reduction clamp of the displaced posterior column and stabilized with anterior to posterior 3.5-mm lag screws from the pelvic brim into the posterior column as described.

Whatever technique is used, careful evaluation and location of the hardware is mandated fluoroscopically prior to closure. This mandates repeating the anterior/posterior fluoroscopic view and the Judet views and, if still concerned, aiming the fluoroscopy down the path of the screw. The use of combined approaches simultaneously gives you the ability to visualize each column's reduction but it makes assessment of the complete fracture, especially in the mid-portion of the quadrilateral plate, harder because of the position of the patient. Reduction of the outer anatomy of the columns might not translate to a perfect reduction of the joint; this must be assessed on an individual basis, either fluoroscopically or by visualization of the joint through the fractured wall or via direct capsulotomy.

Clearly for late cases, the T acetabular fracture is the hardest fracture to reduce when displaced, and mandates careful take-down of the early healing, front, back, and intraarticular. An extensile approach with a trochanteric osteotomy is mandated for this. Then the posterior column is the easiest column to reduce and stabilize through such an extensile approach. Only then should the anterior column be reduced and stabilized as described. It is also possible with the extensile approach to insert an anterior column screw from superior and lateral to the acetabulum, on the other aspect of the iliac wing, into the anterior column as described. With the insertion of such a lag screw it is possible through the extensile approach to visualize the joint and to also maintain the reduction of the anterior column with a pointed reduction clamp of the iliopectineal eminence and on the lateral wing of the ilium.

B3: ANTERIOR COLUMN WITH POSTERIOR HEMITRANSVERSE FRACTURES

Partial Articular

(See Fig. 37-11.) Type B3 fractures are really a form of T-fracture with anterior displacement of the femoral head

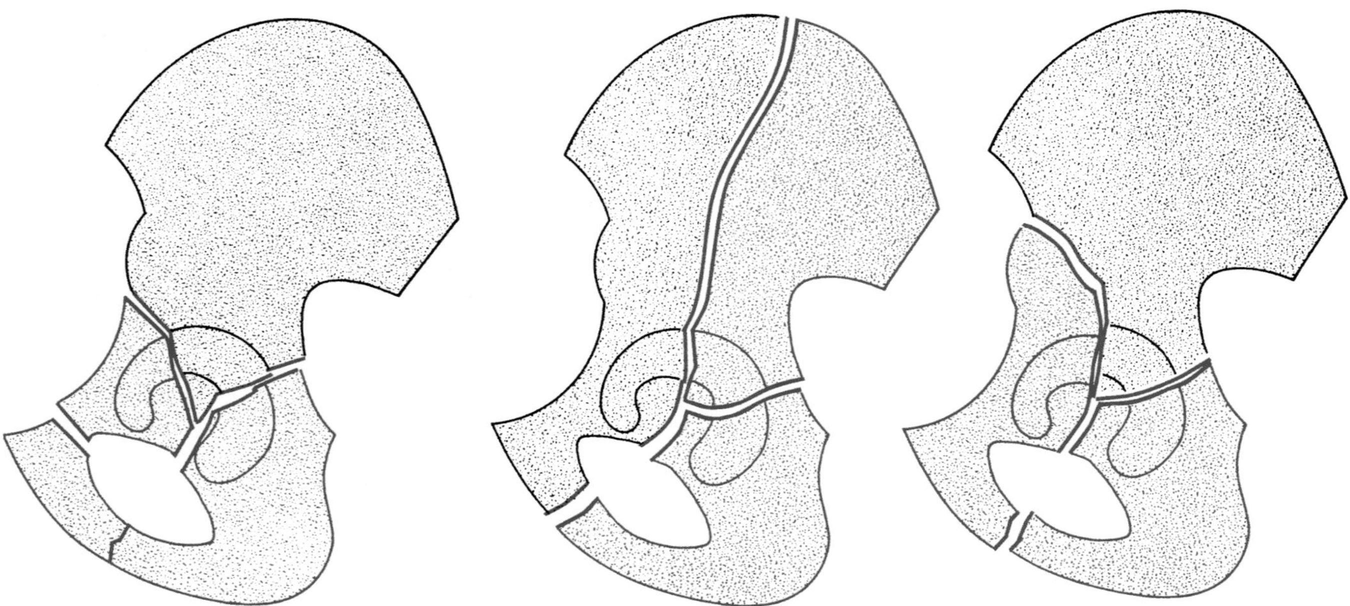

FIGURE 37-11. Type B3 anterior with posterior hemitransverse fracture. This is a type of T-fracture in which the displacement is anterior.

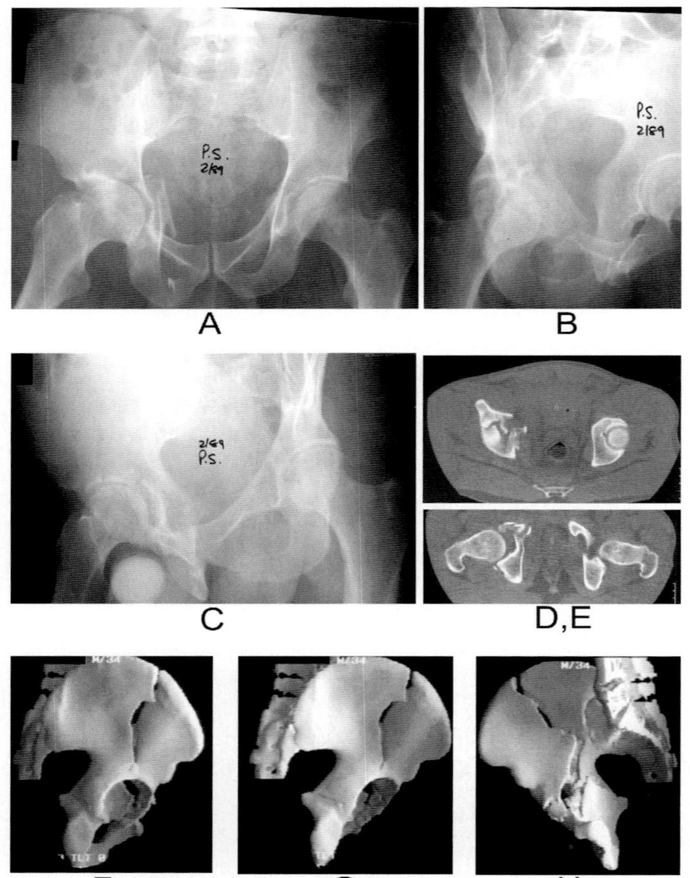

FIGURE 37-12. A 34-year-old male was a passenger in an automobile and sustained a right-sided anterior column posterior hemitransverse acetabular fracture. ORIF was performed using an ilioinguinal approach. The patient returned for follow-up at 2 years after ORIF. He was noted to have an excellent clinical and radiographic result without evidence of either avascular necrosis or degenerative arthritis of the hip joint. **A–C:** Anteroposterior and Judet injury radiographs demonstrate a right-sided anterior column posterior hemitransverse acetabular fracture. **D–H:** CT and three-dimensional reconstruction images of the acetabulum demonstrating the fracture pattern.

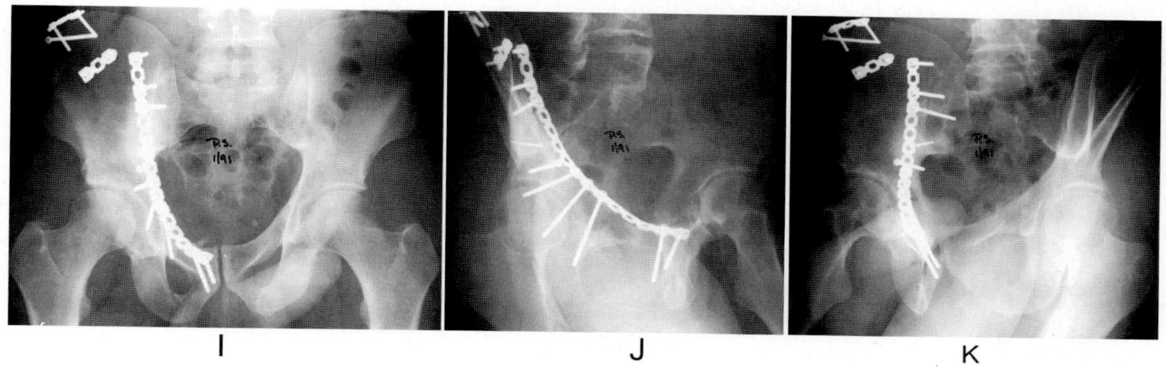

FIGURE 37-12. ***(continued)*** **I–K:** Radiographic images at 2 years follow-up show a healed anterior column with posterior hemitransverse acetabular fracture with excellent preservation of the hip joint space.

and an anterior column or anterior wall fragment. Because the posterior column is usually an undisplaced stable fracture in this configuration, the technical problems are virtually identical to those of anterior column or anterior wall fractures.

Surgical Approach

The surgical approaches of choice are the anterior ilioinguinal or rarely, for a high anterior column lesion, the anterior iliofemoral.

Position

The recommended position is supine, unless the posterior column is displaced or unstable, in which case the lateral position is used.

Reduction Techniques

Reduction techniques are identical to those for a T-fracture, anterior column and anterior wall fractures, and unstable posterior columns.

Fixation Techniques

Fixation is the same as for a T-fracture, anterior column and anterior wall fractures, and unstable posterior columns (Fig. 37-12A–G).

REFERENCES

1. Letournel E, Judet R. *Fractures of the acetabulum.* Berlin: Springer-Verlag, 1993.
2. Matta JM. Surgical treatment of acetabular fractures. In: Browner BD, Jupiter JB, Levine AM, et al, eds. *Skeletal trauma*, pp. 1181–1222, Philadelphia: WB Saunders, 1992.

PART E. SURGICAL MANAGEMENT OF SPECIFIC ACETABULAR INJURY TYPES

38

SURGICAL MANAGEMENT OF C TYPES: BOTH COLUMNS

KEITH A. MAYO

INTRODUCTION

Among the associated fracture patterns discussed in Chapter 25, both-column fractures are initially the most difficult to understand. This category encompasses a relatively diverse group of injuries linked by a common dissociation of the anterior and posterior columns and loss of any articular connection to the intact ilium. These patterns produce a free-floating acetabulum, to varying degrees based on displacement. Medial and superior displacement of the columns with the femoral head produces an en face view of the intact ilium on the obturator oblique radiograph, which Letournel termed the "spur sign" (see Chapter 25). Detailed analysis of the fracture patterns within this group is critical for all steps in the treatment pathway, from surgical approach choice to reduction and fixation strategies.

The most useful primary distinction among these fractures is the morphology of the iliac extension of the anterior column component.

Figure 38-1 shows a variant in which the iliac fracture extends to the crest, demarcating a single large anterior column fragment. This type of extension to the crest is the predominant pattern in all clinical series (1–3), but a wide variability exists in the number and complexity of secondary fracture planes within the anterior column (Fig. 38-2).

Figure 38-3 depicts a less common pattern where the iliac fracture exits anteriorly between the superior and inferior iliac spines. The level and orientation of the posterior column fracture pattern component also must be carefully studied. In most cases the posterior column fracture exits in the cranial portion of the greater sciatic notch, whereas obliquity in the coronal plane is more variable. Other important injury variants include patterns where there is fracture involvement of the sacroiliac joint, segmental involvement of the posterior column (Fig. 38-4) or significant displacement of an associated posterior wall component (Fig. 38-5). Radiographic diagnosis of these injuries can be taxing and should use all the plain radiographic and computer tomography imaging modalities discussed in Chapter 26. This analysis must include not only detailed study of fracture morphology, but also displacement and congruency assessment, which forms the basis of decisions on surgical intervention as discussed in Chapter 27.

SURGICAL APPROACH CHOICE

Fracture pattern is the predominant consideration in surgical approach choice. The majority of both-column fractures are optimally managed via an ilioinguinal approach. It is pivotal to remember that joint reduction via this approach lacks direct articular assessment possible via other approaches. It is based on sequential anatomic reductions building from the periphery of ilium toward the joint, evaluated by correction of extraarticular displacements and supplemented by intraoperative imaging. When this strategy appears unrealistic on the basis of careful *preoperative* planning, approach alternatives must be considered.

The first step in this sequence is perfect reduction of the anterior column to the intact ilium. The most common errors in this reduction are rotational, with failure to restore the normal concavity of the internal iliac fossa (Fig. 38-6). This critical initial malreduction compounds with subsequent reduction of secondary anterior column and posterior column fracture components, ultimately dooming the reconstruction to varying degrees of surgical secondary congruence that

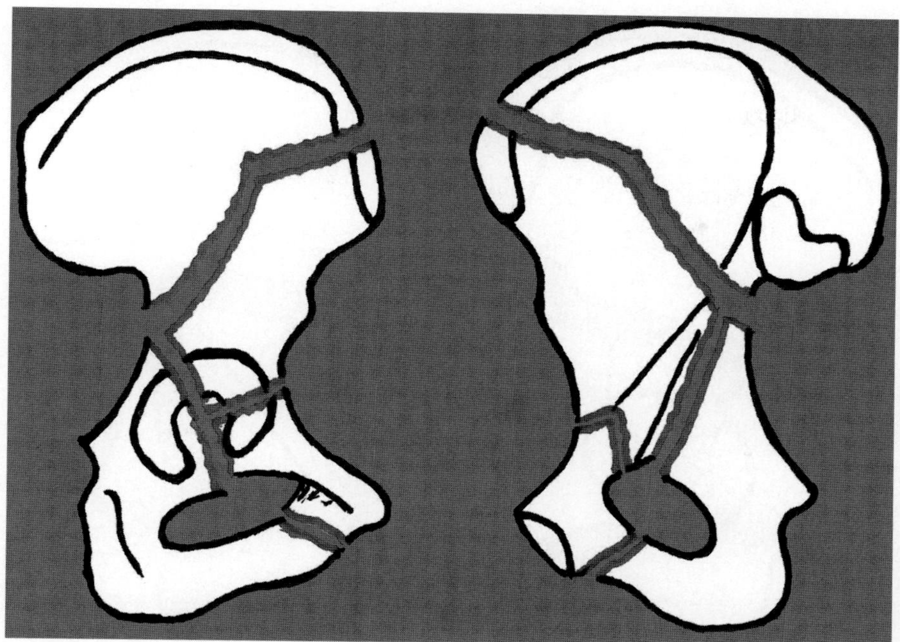

FIGURE 38-1. Both-column fracture with anterior column extension to the iliac crest. The inferior anterior column secondary fracture is frequently minimally displaced and the posterior column is a single large segment.

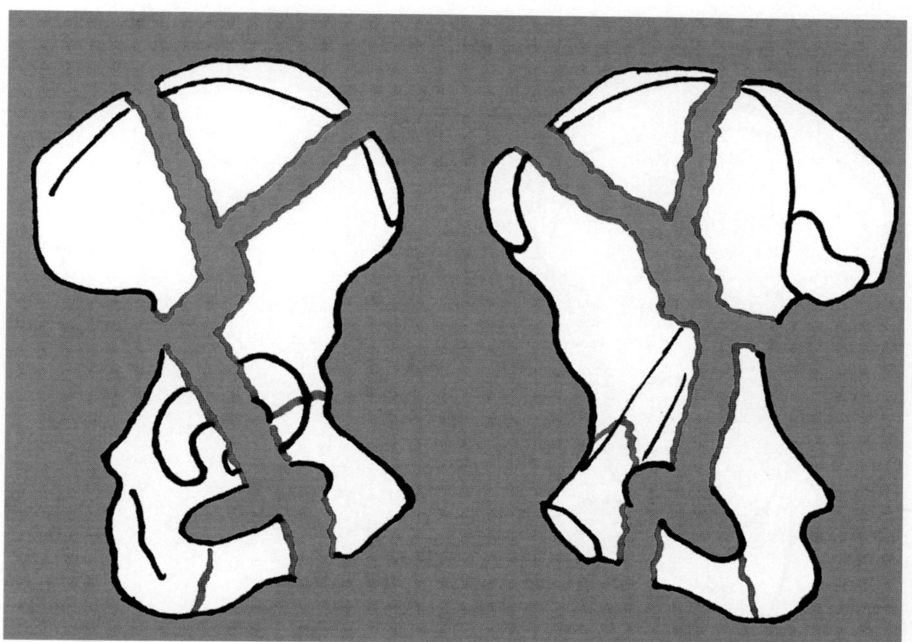

FIGURE 38-2. A more complex fracture pattern with intercalary iliac component.

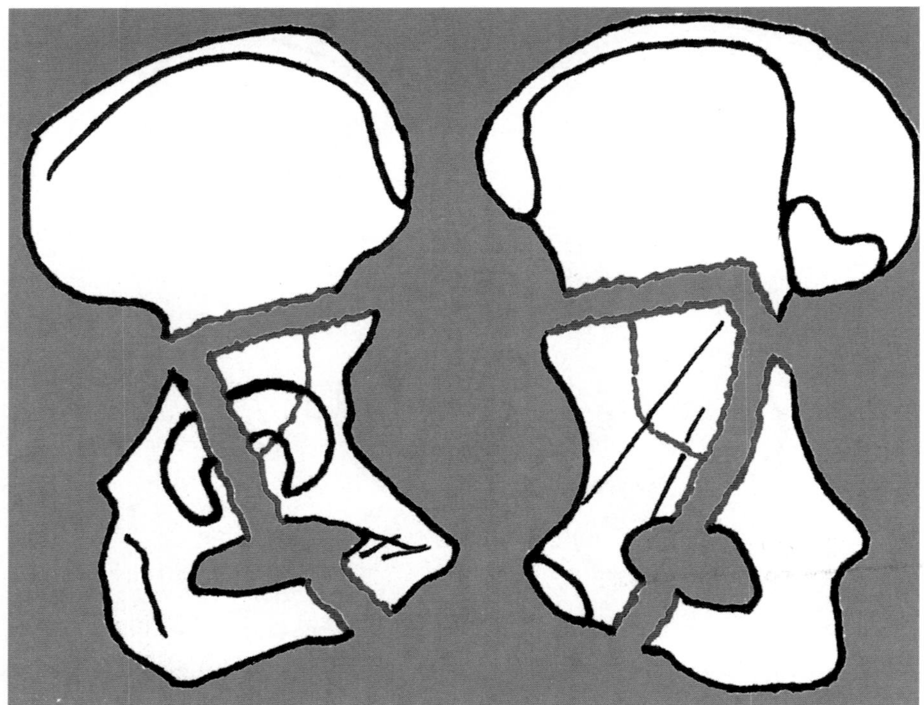

FIGURE 38-3. The anterior column component exits between the anterior superior and inferior iliac spines in this both-column variant.

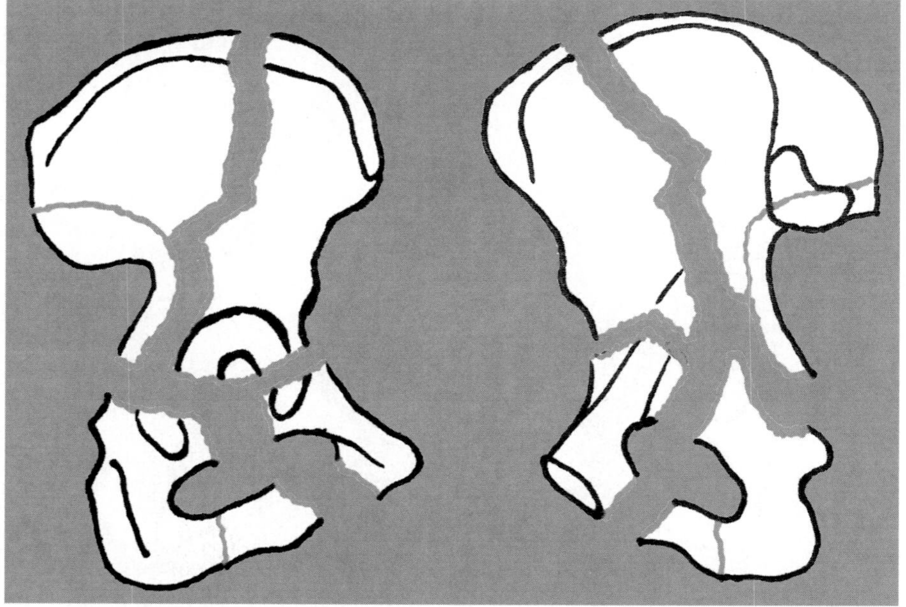

FIGURE 38-4. Problematic both-column variant with fracture demonstrating inferior SI joint and segmental posterior column involvement. Displacement of these secondary fractures is widely variable.

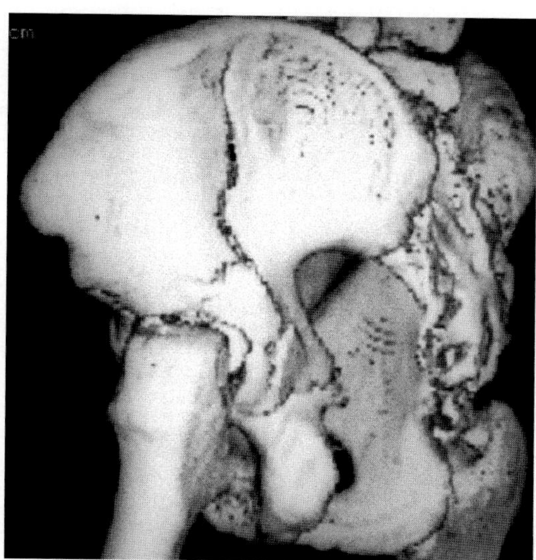

FIGURE 38-5. Rotational malrotation of the anterior column caused by failure to adequately assess the lateral (external iliac) portion of the reduction. This can be accomplished with minimal additional exposure from ilioinguinal approach.

have been shown not to provide durable outcomes. Both iliac comminution, and posterior extension of the anterior column fracture leaving a small intact iliac segment, can increase the complexity of anterior column reduction.

Control and reduction of the posterior column via the ilioinguinal approach can be compromised by segmental posterior column involvement and patterns that involve the inferior aspect of the sacroiliac joint. Atypical patterns that involve significant posterior wall moieties or marked articular comminution also present special challenges.

Table 38-1 outlines the utility of approach alternatives with regard to critical fracture pattern variables. Sequential ilioinguinal and Kocher-Langenbeck approaches should be planned for whenever possible but can be improvised when reduction/fixation of the opposite (posterior) column proves untenable. In this setting, anterior implants must be carefully positioned to not impede subsequent reduction maneuvers from the secondary posterior approach. Dual approaches provide simultaneous exposure of both columns, but can compromise optimum exposure and reduction possibilities of each. This usually represents excessive surgical dissection and morbidity in relation to a single carefully planned and executed approach. Extensile approaches include the extended iliofemoral and triradiate. These provide the best surgical visualization of most difficult injury patterns. However, they are attended by clearly higher complication rates and morbidity in most clinical series. Contrasting the two approaches, the extended iliofemoral appears to offer better exposure with equivalent complication rates.

The extended ilioinguinal (4) (see Chapters 28 and 31) and modified Stoppa (5) (see Chapters 28 and 33) warrant special discussion because of their relative obscurity. The extended ilioinguinal combines external iliac exposure from the posterior superior iliac spine to the gluteus medius tubercle with a standard ilioinguinal exposure from the medius tubercle anteriorly and medially. This is particularly useful for fractures involving the sacroiliac joint. Patient positioning and draping require careful attention to detail and its utility tapers rapidly with increasing patient size (obesity).

The modified Stoppa (see Chapters 28 and 33) and ilioinguinal provide similar access and utility when used for the treatment of both-column fractures. The modified Stoppa can be conceptualized as an expanded medial window of the ilioinguinal combined with a secondary incision along the crest to provide a portion or the entire lateral win-

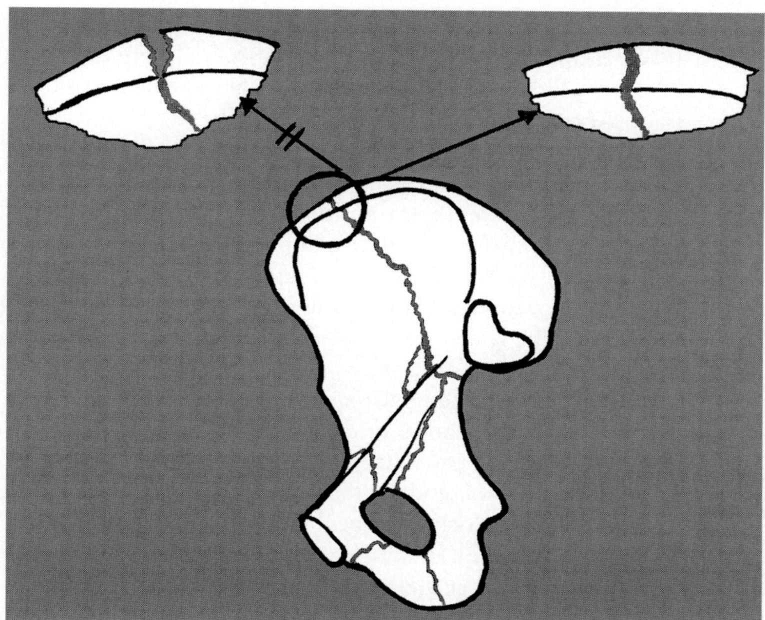

FIGURE 38-6. Three-dimensional computed tomography reconstruction of a transitional both-column fracture variant with segmental posterior wall component.

TABLE 38-1. BOTH-COLUMN ACETABULAR FRACTURES: APPROACH DETERMINATION FACTORS

Anatomic Factors	Ilioinguinal Approaches	Extended Approaches	Extensile Stoppa	Sequential/Dual	Modified Ilioinguinal
(Typical) Anterior column extends to crest Posterior column one segment	++++			++	+++
Iliac comminution	++		++	+	++
Posterior iliac anterior column extension (small intact iliac segment)	++	++	++		+
Segmental posterior column			+++	+	+
Significant posterior wall component			++	++++	
Fracture involves inferior sacroiliac joint	+	+++	+++		+
Articular comminution			+++		

dow of the ilioinguinal. In reality the distinction has continued to blur as we have become more facile at developing different portions of the ilioinguinal tailored to specific fracture patterns. The use of implants continues to differ significantly between these approaches, as is discussed later.

Surgeon specific experience with a given approach may either expand or contract the range of indications. Likewise, host factors such as age, pelvic ring soft tissue injury and comorbidities may impact approach choice. Extensile approaches are generally avoided in older patients because of increased surgical morbidity and longer convalescence. Presence of gluteal or trochanteric crush injury (Fig. 38-7) may warrant pushing the limits of the ilioinguinal or modified Stoppa approach as does coexisting significant head injury with its high risk of heterotopic ossification.

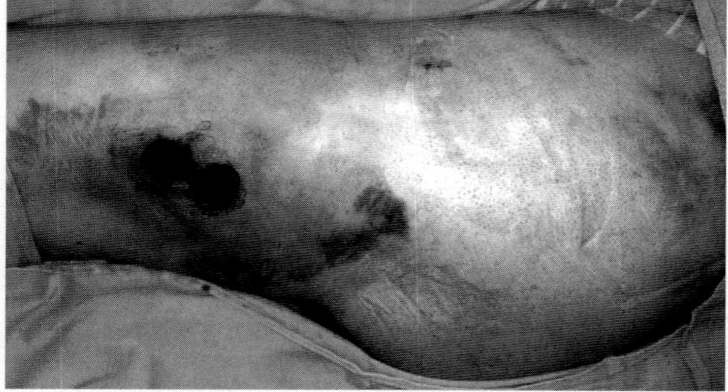

FIGURE 38-7. Trochanteric crush injury with secondary full thickness skin loss complicated this closed degloving (Morel-Lavalee) injury. These lesions can limit the safe use of posterior and extensile approaches in some fracture patterns.

OPERATING ROOM LOGISTICS/PATIENT POSITIONING

Intraoperative imaging needs should be anticipated and whenever possible C-arm fluoroscopy units should be positioned opposite the side of injury prior to surgical prep and draping. Operating room personnel traffic should be kept to a minimum. Because the majority of both-column fractures are operated through the ilioinguinal approach, routine skeletal muscle paralysis should be used until abdominal wall closure has been completed at the end of the procedure. Positioning obviously varies with approach chosen and table availability as well as surgeon preference. Derivatives of the Judet table (Fig. 38-8) have clear advantages for the standard approaches (Kocher-Langenbeck, ilioinguinal, extended iliofemoral). The table is a primary reduction aid via the use of distal and lateral traction. The use of other fracture extension tables has limited utility for these injuries because of design and safety issues. When the Judet table is unavailable, the optimum positioning for the ilioinguinal is illustrated in (Fig. 38-9). A completely radiolucent table is desirable. An advantage of this set-up is the increase in hip mobility, particularly in flexion. This increases the exposure through the lateral wound interval and also provides easier access through the second wound interval between the neural and vascular compartments. Traction in this setting is provided using manual or distractor force through a percutaneously placed proximal femoral Schanz screw. This logistical scenario is useful for the modified Stoppa as well. Use of sequential Kocher-Langenbeck or extensile approaches requires prone or lateral decubitus positioning that can be achieved on either the Judet table or a standard radiolucent table (Fig. 38-10) with the leg prepped and draped free.

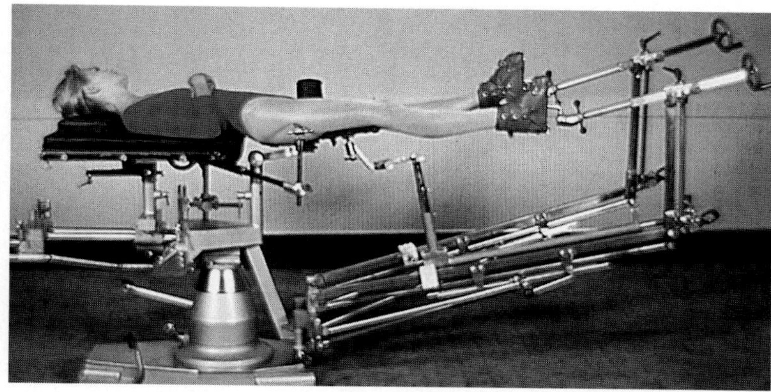

FIGURE 38-8. Supine positioning for the ilioinguinal approach demonstrated on an early Judet table. (Courtesy of Joel Matta.) Derivatives of this table are now difficult to find, but newer designs are forthcoming that incorporate the advantages of distal and lateral traction in multiple positions as well as improved imaging capabilities.

REDUCTION AND FIXATION

Acetabular fracture surgery is an instrumentation- and implant-intensive endeavor. Nonetheless, initial reduction strategies for both-column fractures rely on relatively simple distal and lateral traction. In most cases the capsular attachments to both columns are intact and provide an indirect realignment, particularly when this can be achieved in the acute setting before clot and granulation tissue become an impediment. This provides one of the rationales for interim skeletal traction pending definitive surgical treatment. Incomplete fractures (Fig. 38-11) can limit the effect of traction, because they typically represent a stable fracture displacement. These patterns most often involve the anterior column extension to the crest. The anterior column is hinged at the crest and is displaced along the pelvic brim cranially and posteriorly, thus frequently overlapping the intact ilium. This deformity can be difficult to overcome, even with the use of large tong reduction clamps that span the ilium from the displaced portion of the pelvic brim to the intact (lateral) supraacetabular surface. Additional use of a Schanz screw placed in the area of the anterior inferior iliac spine may be of help as a manipulation aid. Occasionally, it may be necessary to complete this fracture at the crest to fa-

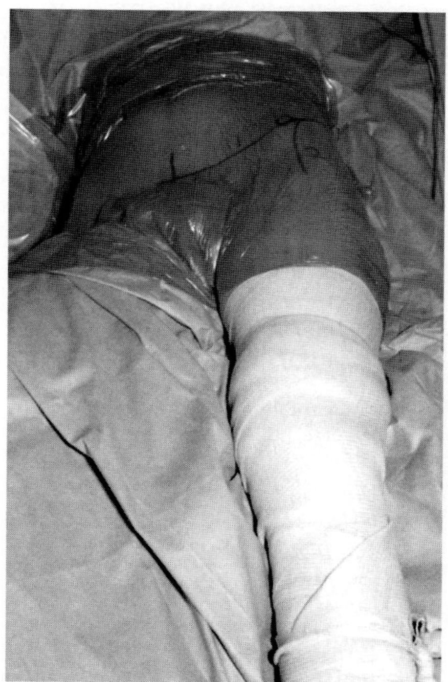

FIGURE 38-9. Alternative supine positioning for the ilioinguinal approach on a radiolucent table with the lower abdomen and involved hindquarter prepped into a single contiguous field.

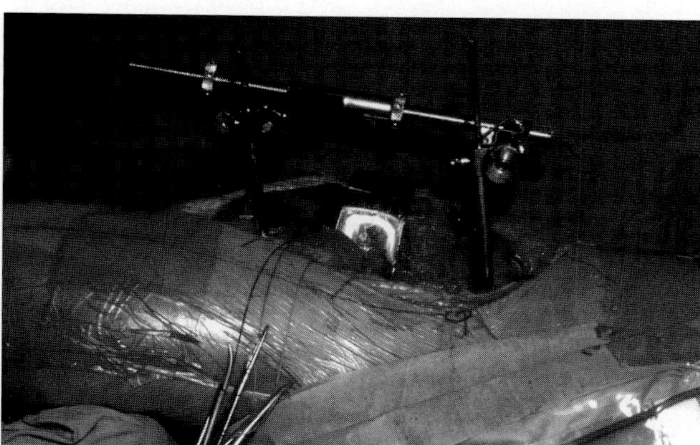

A

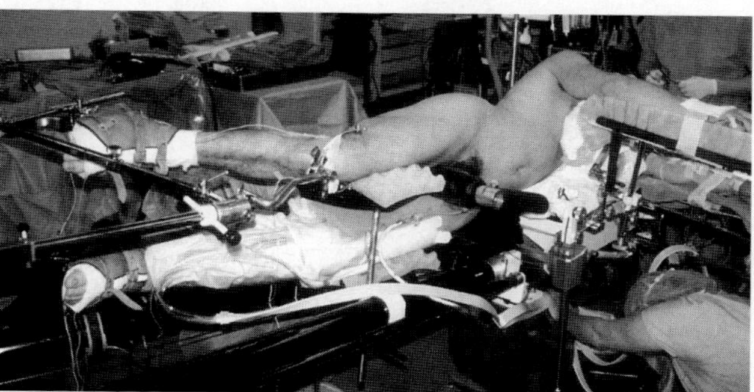

B

FIGURE 38-10. A: Lateral positioning for the extended iliofemoral approach with the hindquarter prepped free and distractor applied for longitudinal traction. **B:** Alternative positioning for the extended iliofemoral approach on the Tasserit (Judet) table utilizing distal and lateral traction.

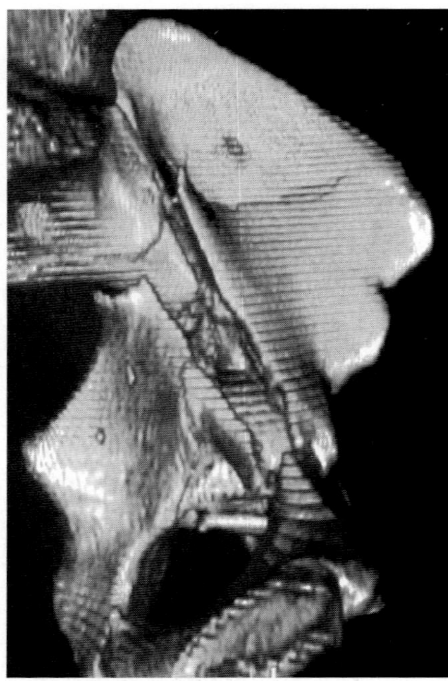

FIGURE 38-11. Both-column fracture with incomplete iliac extension. It may be necessary to complete this fracture in some cases.

cilitate an anatomic reduction. Although the incomplete fracture is usually oblique, the osteotomized extension can be made perpendicular to the crest. It is usually helpful to predrill the crest for tangential lag screw fixation prior to carrying out the osteotomy with a narrow chisel. This pattern then can be managed as the more typical complete anterior column extension to the crest. As noted, rotational malreduction must be avoided; this requires a limited external iliac exposure at the crest for full assessment. Temporary stabilization with clamps and/or Kirschner wires then is replaced with lag or position screws, depending on fracture obliquity. Perimeter reconstruction plates also can be used for fixation, but must be very carefully contoured to avoid a secondary malrotation.

In concert with the iliac crest reduction, placement of a precontoured pelvic brim plate, either temporary or definitive, is an effective strategy. A single screw placed near the fracture margin into the intact ilium in the area of the sciatic buttress acts as a clamp initially. Ultimately the plate can act as a buttress as well as an extended washer for screws placed into the posterior column. Plate reduction techniques for these injuries also have been addressed in Chapter 31. Alternately, the anterior column can be reduced at the pelvic brim with a tong clamp or picador and held with temporary wire fixation followed by short lag screws across the fracture obliquity just lateral to the brim. Once an anatomic reduction of the anterior column has been achieved, this fixation can be augmented by supraacetabular anterior to posterior lag or position screws (Fig. 38-12). The typical implants used in the

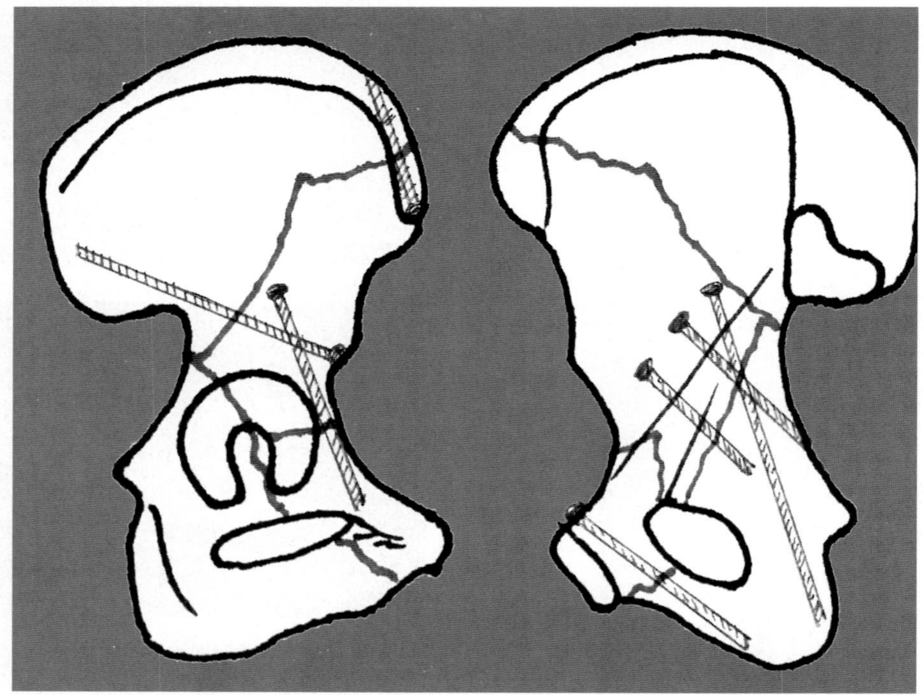

FIGURE 38-12. Schematic representation of the location of typical lag or position screws used to stabilize the anterior and posterior column components of the both-column fracture.

majority of acetabular fractures are 3.5-mm variants. Self-tapping screws with slightly larger heads are useful and malleable reconstruction plates are the norm. Larger implants are reserved for cases of significant osteoporosis, but should be readily available if needed. Recently introduced locking plates hold some promise for this group.

After the primary anterior column fracture has been reduced and stabilized, attention is then turned to reduction of the posterior column that is usually medially displaced and rotated. Once again traction provides the initial reduction force. The final posterior column reduction can be achieved by a variety of methods. Clamps from the quadrilateral surface to the internal iliac fossa or external iliac surface (Fig. 38-13) can be placed from any of the three wound intervals of the ilioinguinal approach or corresponding exposure for the modified Stoppa approach. Other methods include manipulation with a small bone hook placed into the lesser sciatic notch or cerclage wire passed around the innominate bone through the greater sciatic notch via a limited external iliac exposure (see Chapter 32). Imaging assessment of the reduction using multiple projections is helpful at this point to confirm an anatomic joint profile. Screw fixation of the posterior column is then carried out from the reconstructed pelvic brim, preferably through the previously placed plate discussed in the preceding. The trajectory of these screws is adjusted based on the coronal plane obliquity of the posterior column fracture. For patterns where the fracture is relatively horizontal, these screws can be long and placed down the full length of the column. As fracture obliquity increases, the screw starting point may have to be moved lateral to the pelvic brim to facilitate an exit on the quadrilateral surface.

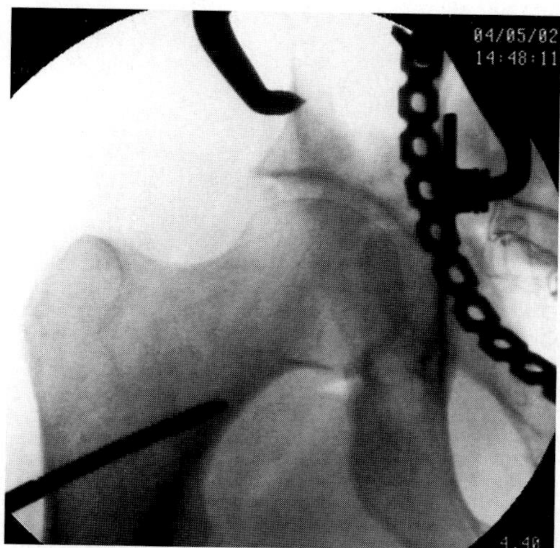

FIGURE 38-13. One of the reduction strategies for the posterior column. The anterior column has been temporarily reduced and buttressed with a pelvic brim plate. An asymmetric clamp has been placed through the first window of the ilioinguinal approach, spanning from the external ilium just lateral to the anterior inferior iliac spine to the quadrilateral surface. This clamp corrects the medial displacement and rotation of the posterior column prior to fixation from the internal iliac fossa.

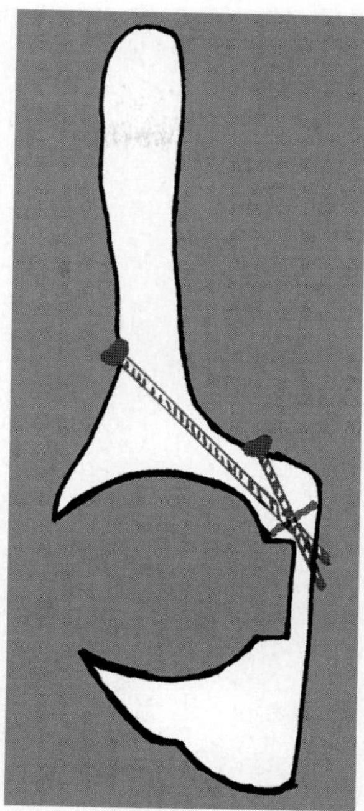

FIGURE 38-14. Posterior column fracture orientation dictates screw starting point and trajectory. As the fracture becomes progressively more oblique, screw placement moves lateral and the path is altered to exit the quadrilateral surface. Proximity to the joint also critically affects this position.

In some cases, the screws may need to be placed percutaneously from an external iliac starting point to obtain the optimum orientation (Fig. 38-14). Whenever possible, screw placement through the cotyloid fossa should be avoided because of the relative imprecision of imaging verification of articular safety in this location.

Following completion of the posterior column fixation, remaining low anterior column and pubic fractures are reduced and stabilized to the pelvic brim plate. Final adjustments to the plate contour can be made *in situ.*

Quadrilateral surface comminution can be addressed with spring plates (see Chapter 31) if needed. However, often this portion of the fracture pattern is primarily useful as an aid in assessing posterior column reduction and is structurally not a critical component of the internal fixation construct. In these cases, oblique lag or position screws from the internal iliac fossa just lateral to the pelvic brim plate are adequate.

A typical reduction sequence for a both-column fracture amenable to treatment via an ilioinguinal approach is depicted in Fig. 38-15. A wide spectrum of injuries can be operated through the ilioinguinal. Figures 38-16 and 38-17 depict relatively straightforward and more complex variants within this spectrum.

The modified Stoppa approach represents an alternative to a full ilioinguinal approach for some fracture patterns. An example of this treatment approach is represented in Fig. 38-18.

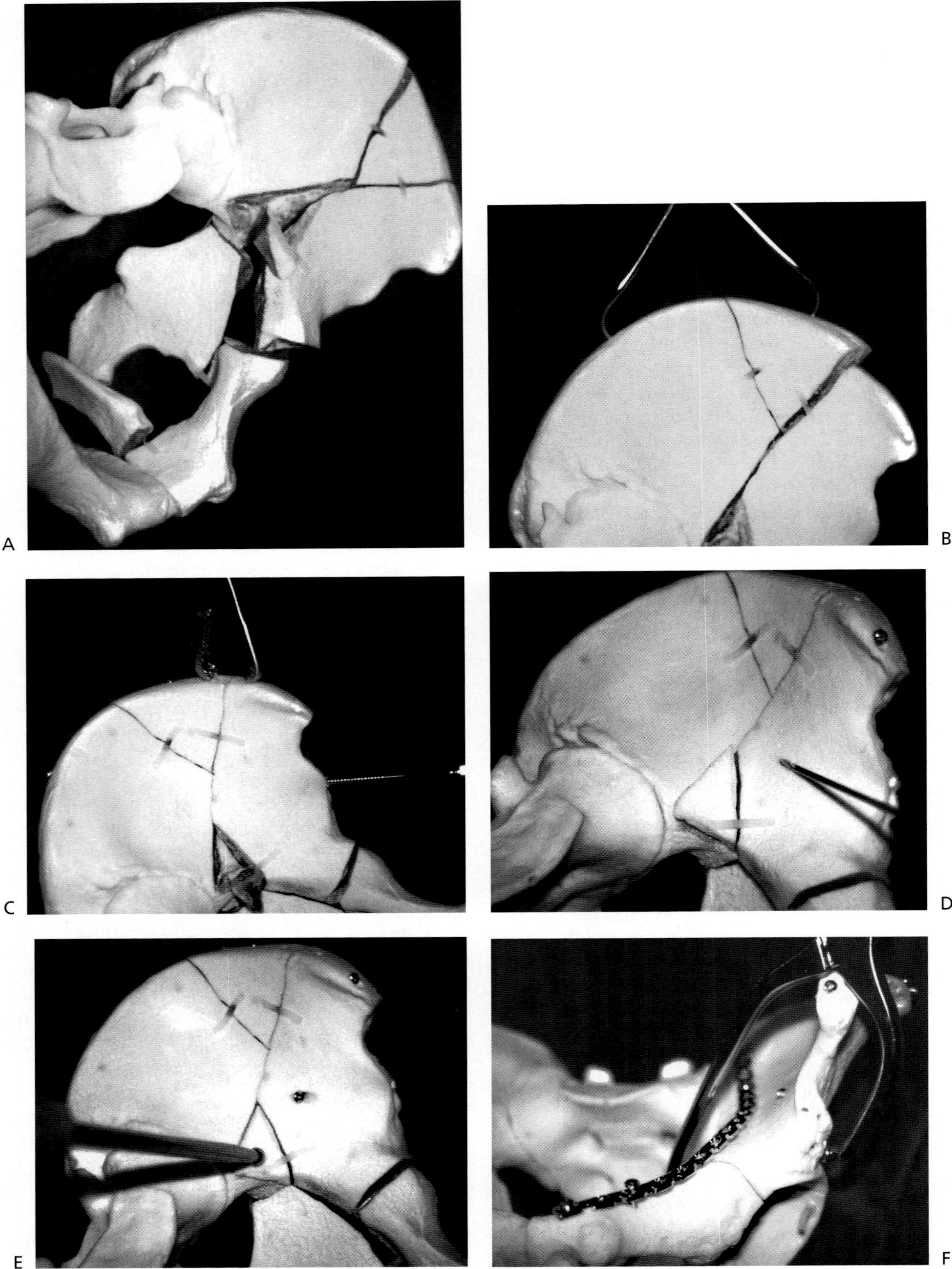

FIGURE 38-15. A: Fracture pattern. **B–E:** Sequential reconstruction of the anterior column.

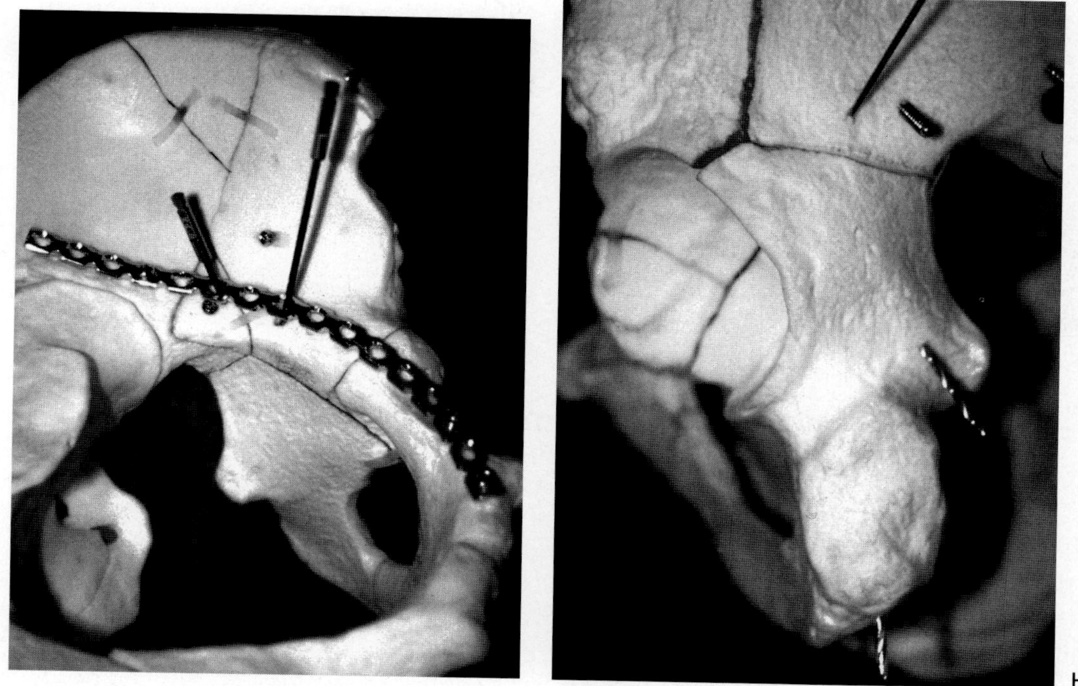

FIGURE 38-15. ***(continued)*** **F,G:** Reduction and fixation of the posterior column. **H:** Drill/screw trajectories for posterior column fixation.

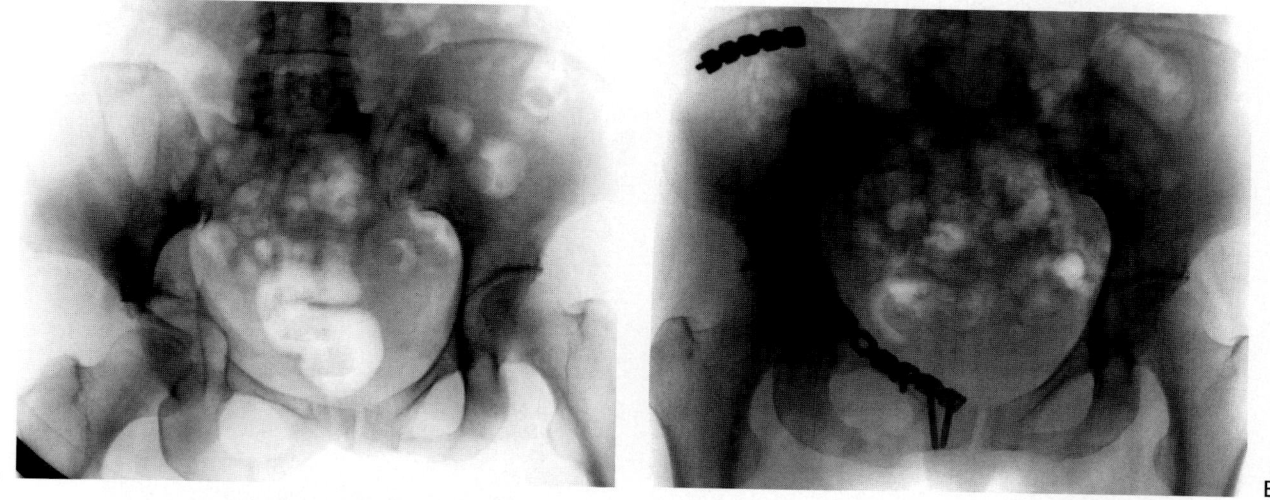

FIGURE 38-16. Preoperative **(A)** and postoperative **(B)** radiographs of 56-year-old woman with a both-column fracture consisting of single large anterior and posterior column components. Anatomic reconstructions should be expected in this setting.

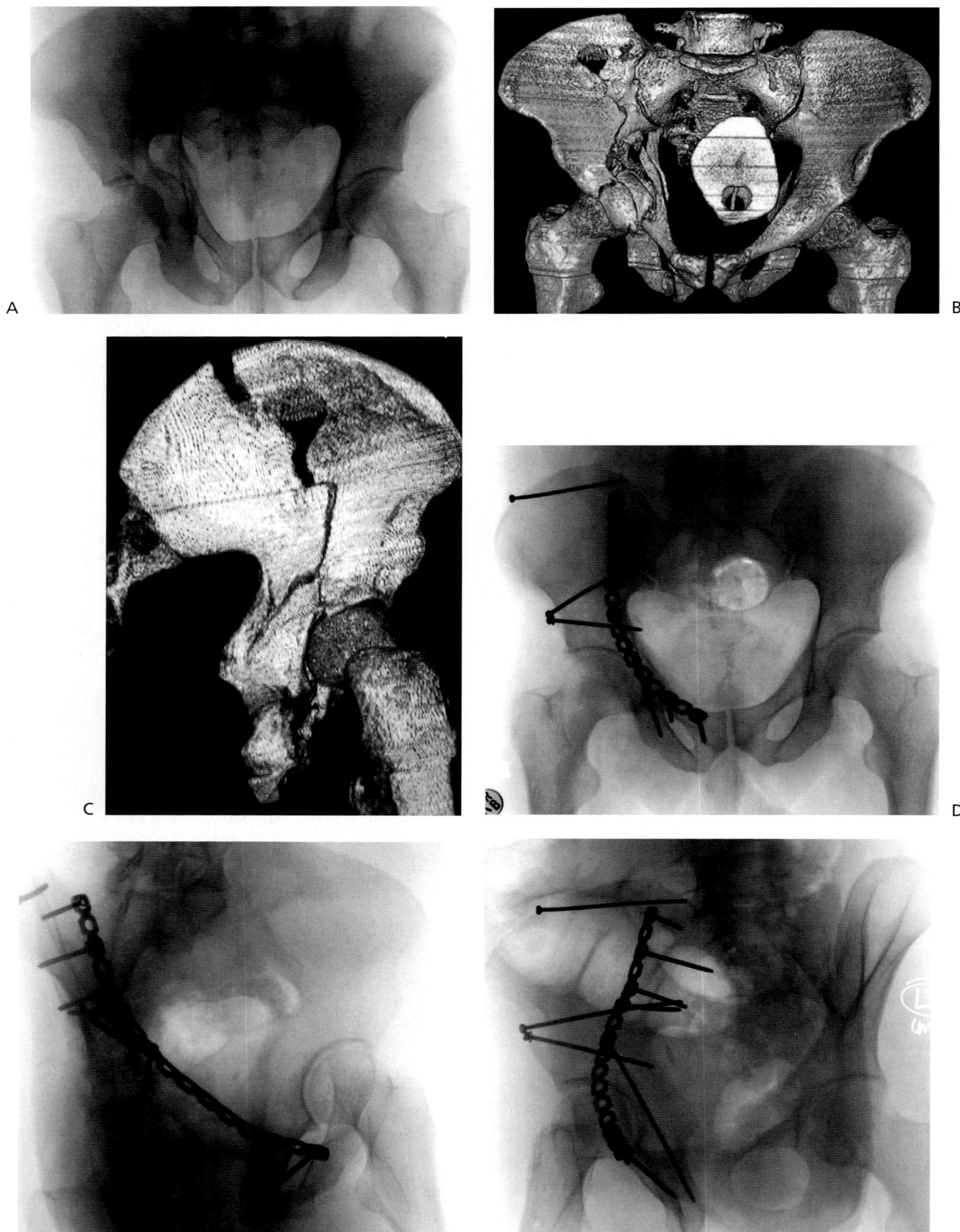

FIGURE 38-17. A–F: Complex fracture pattern in 19-year-old severely head injured man. The anterior column fracture extends very far posterior and there is a significant posterior wall fracture. Because of the head injury this fracture was operated through the ilioinguinal approach alone, achieving a relatively good indirect reduction of the posterior wall. The reduction is not anatomic, as the subtle surgical secondary congruence demonstrates.

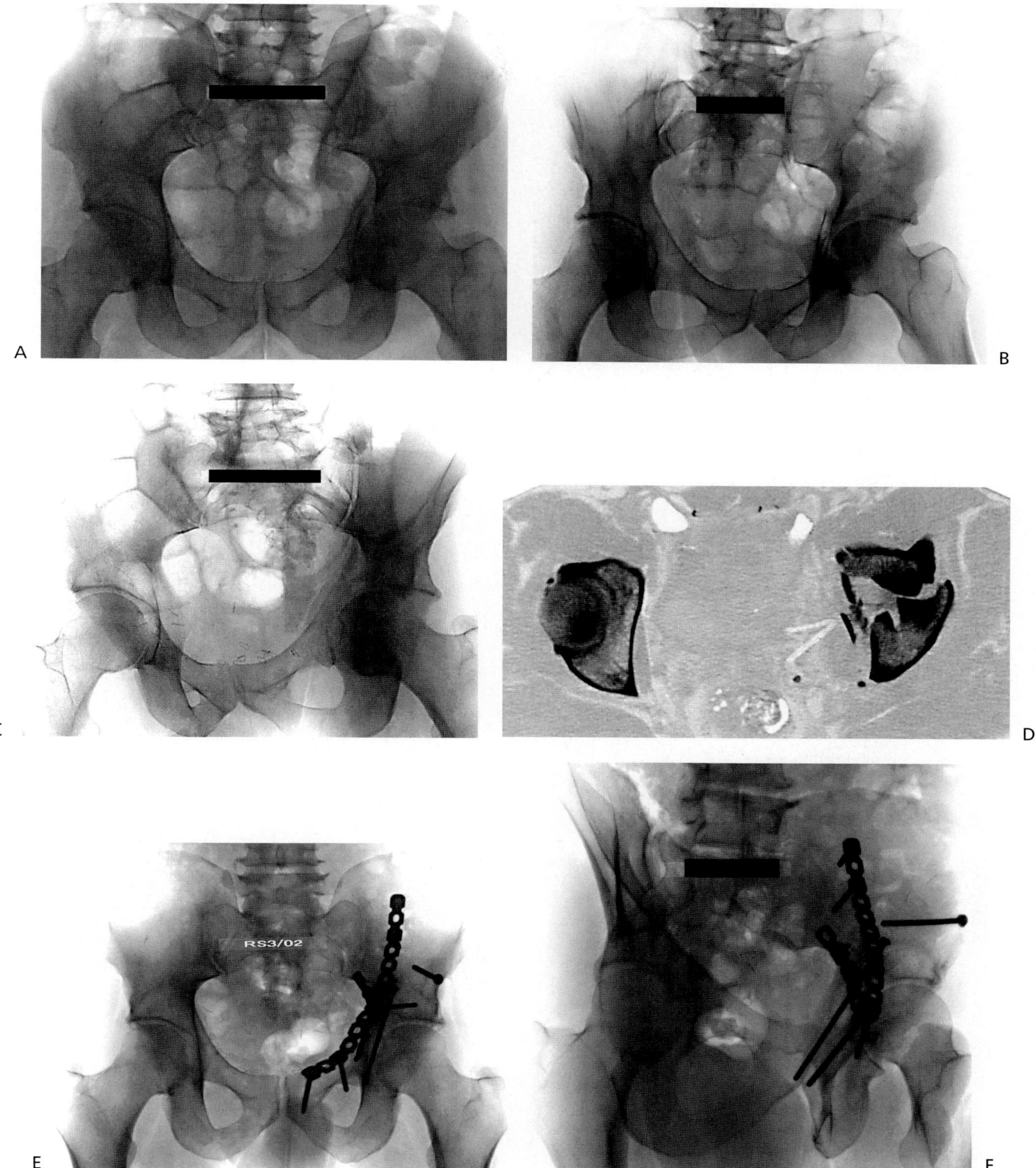

FIGURE 38-18. A–G: Transitional associated anterior/posterior hemitransverse fracture operated using a Stoppa approach and first window ilioinguinal counter incision. The quadrilateral plate buttress fixation is only possible via this approach. (Courtesy of Bret Bolhofner.)

(Figure continues)

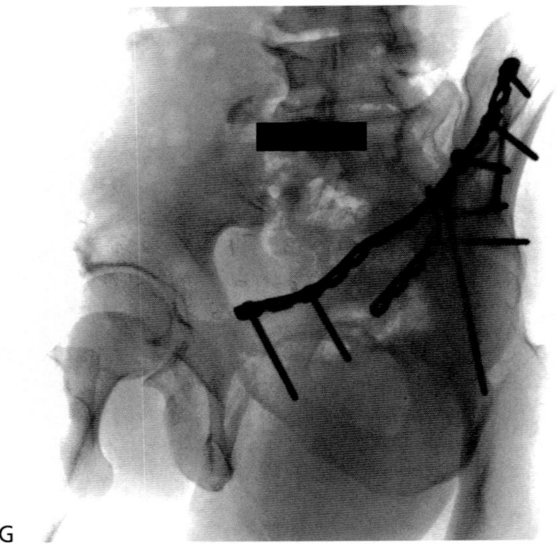

G

FIGURE 38-18. *(continued)*

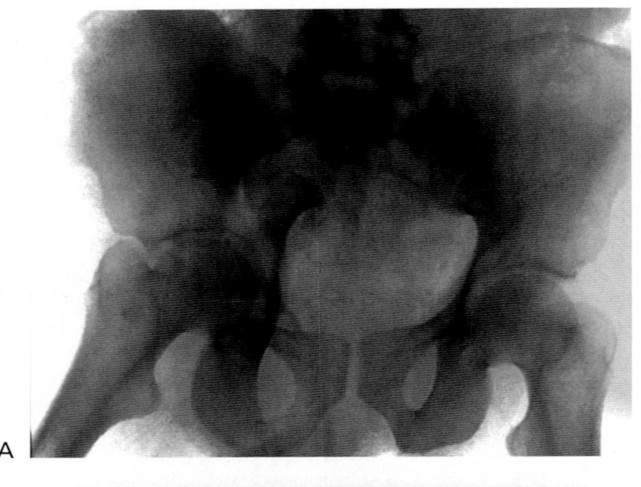

A

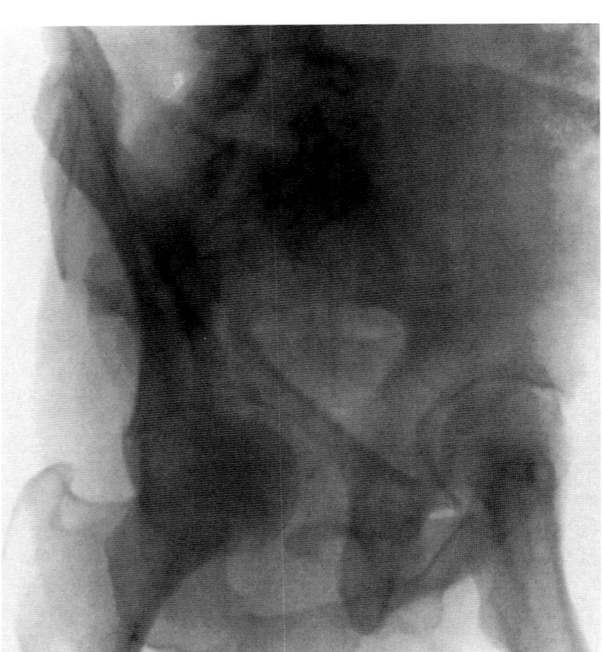

B

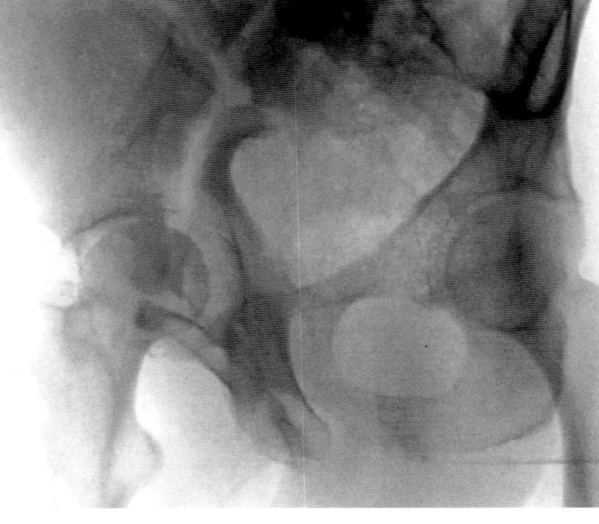

C

FIGURE 38-19. A–E: An extended ilioinguinal approach was used to treat this 54-year-old construction worker who sustained a both-column fracture with important involvement of the inferior aspect of the ipsilateral SI joint.

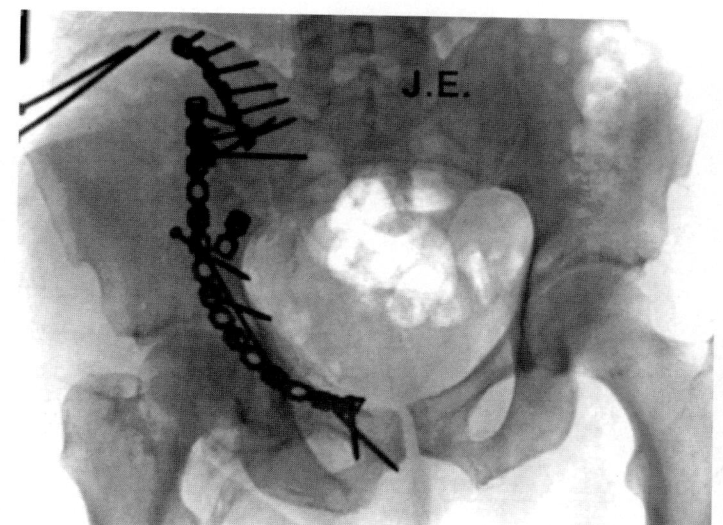

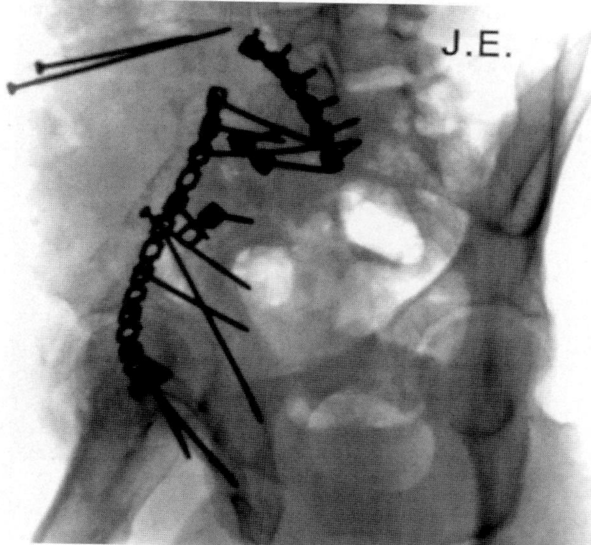

FIGURE 38-19. ***(continued)***

As noted, fracture patterns that involve the inferior sacroiliac joint present a special challenge. Figure 38-19 shows an example of this type of injury managed via the extended ilioinguinal approach.

The extended iliofemoral approach remains useful for complex patterns such as that seen in Fig. 38-20. This injury combines a relatively posterior anterior column extension with a segmental posterior column pattern and a displaced posterior wall. The extensile approach allows simultaneous visualization of all injury elements as well as direct articular reduction control.

An alternative to the extensile approaches in many cases is the sequential ilioinguinal, the Kocher-Langenbeck approach. An example of this surgical tactic is shown in Fig. 38-21.

CONCLUSION

Associated both-column fractures represent a demanding spectrum of injury subgroups. Rigorous preoperative diagnostic evaluation, operative tactic planning, and a thorough

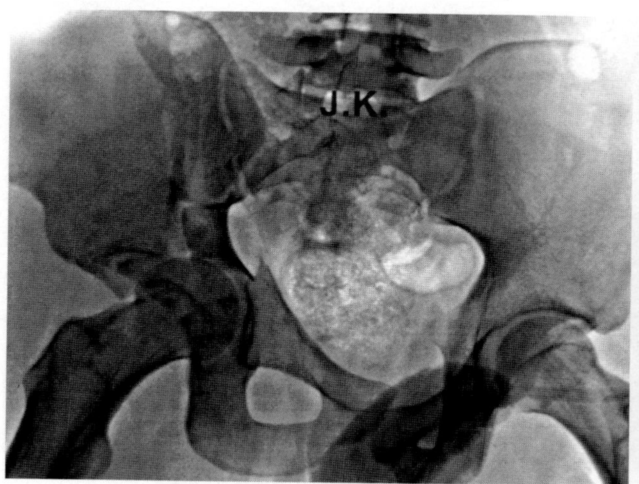

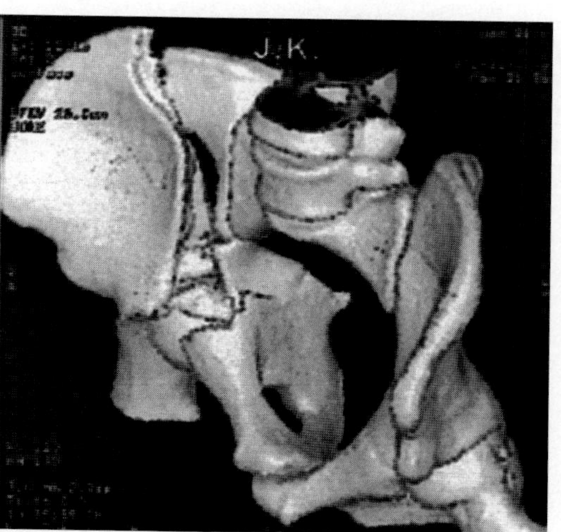

FIGURE 38-20. A–F: The fracture pattern in this 28-year-old man has two complicating factors. Segmental posterior column injury extending to the cranial margin of the greater sciatic notch and an associated posterior wall component led to extended iliofemoral approach.

(Figure continues)

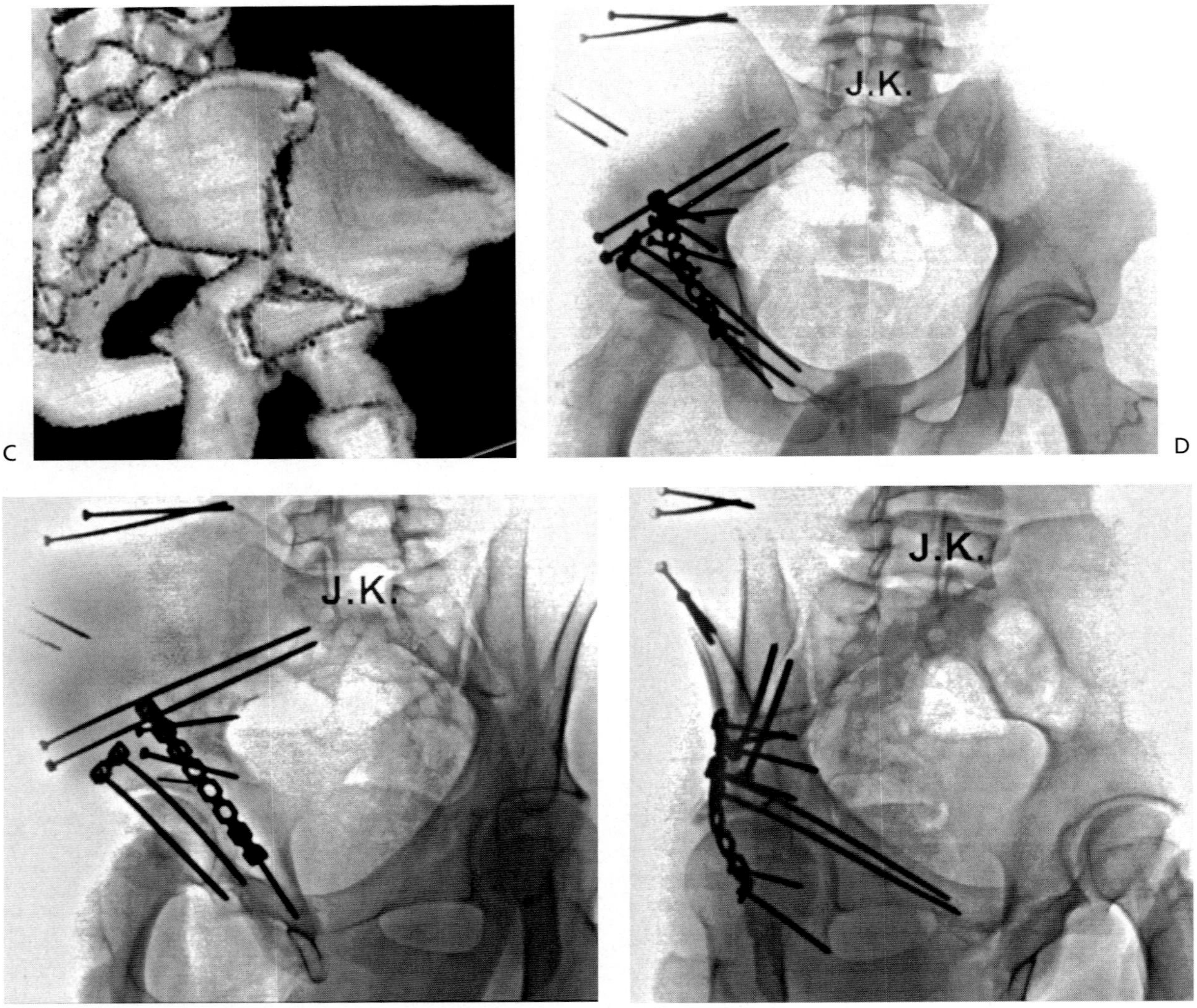

FIGURE 38-20. ***(continued)***

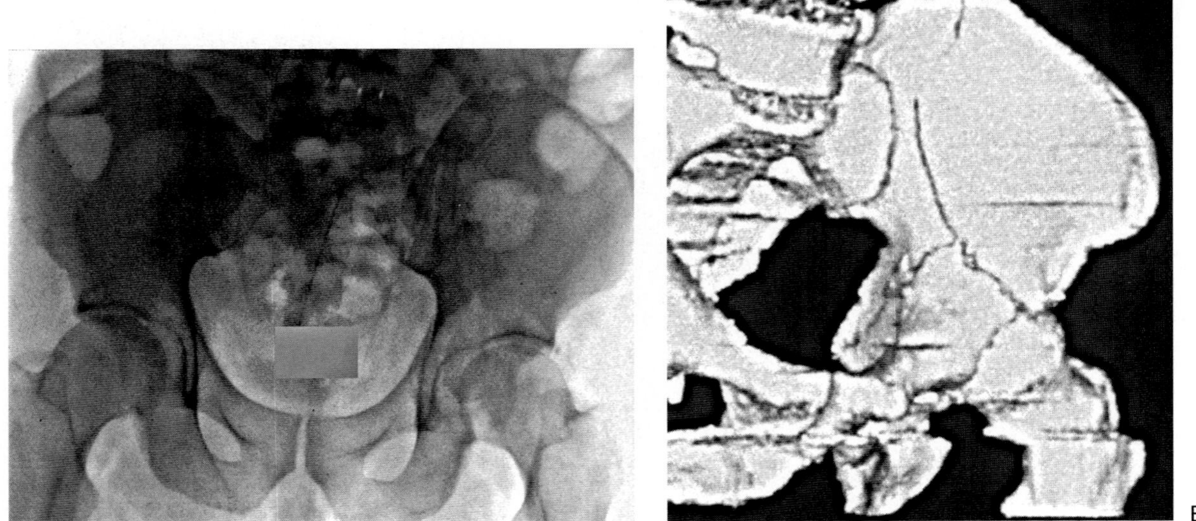

FIGURE 38-21. A–H: This obese 32-year-old man sustained a fracture with a comminuted posterior wall component and modest but significant anterior column displacement. This was operated using sequential partial ilioinguinal (first window) and Kocher-Langenbeck approaches.

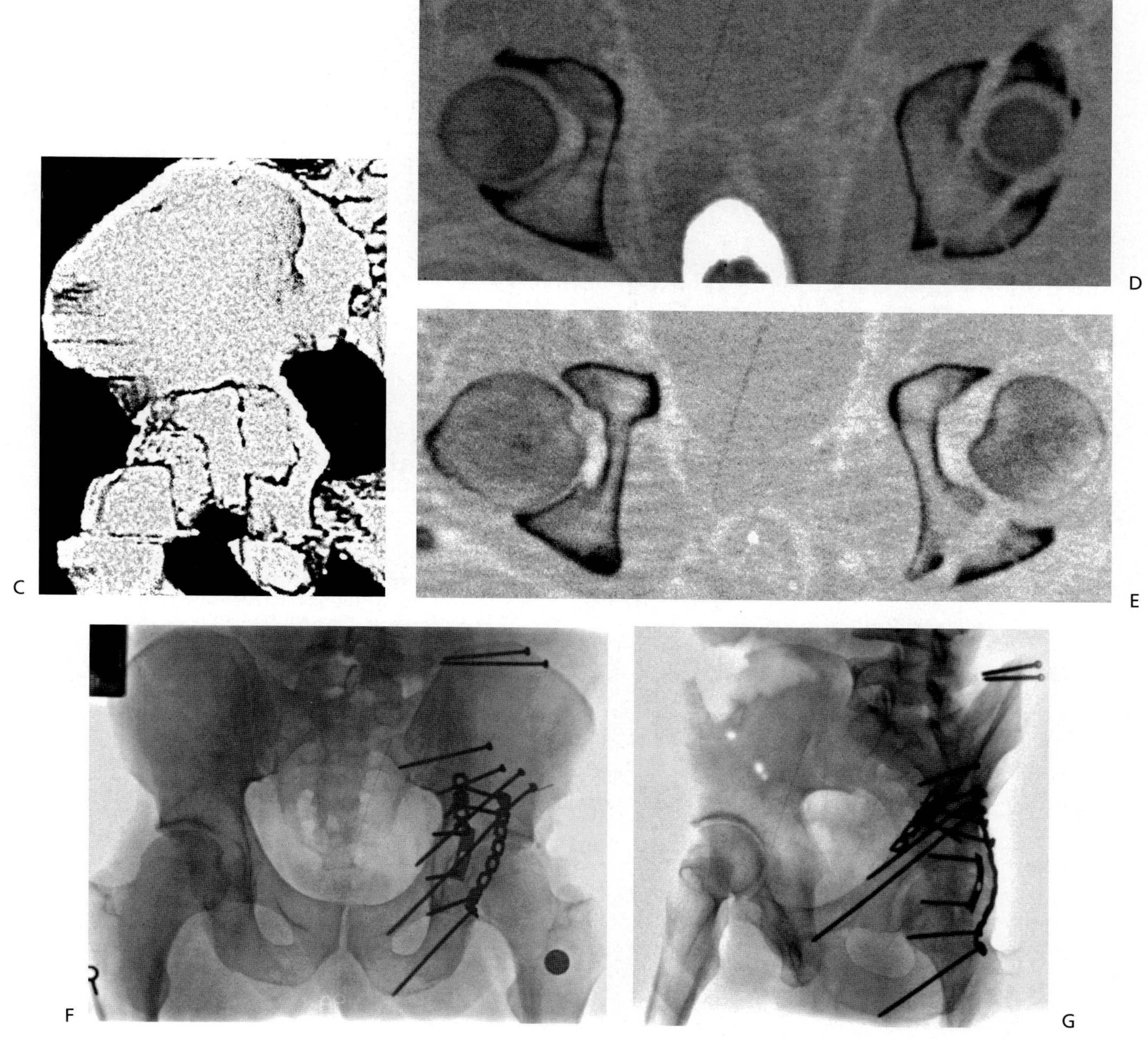

FIGURE 38-21. *(continued)*

(Figure continues)

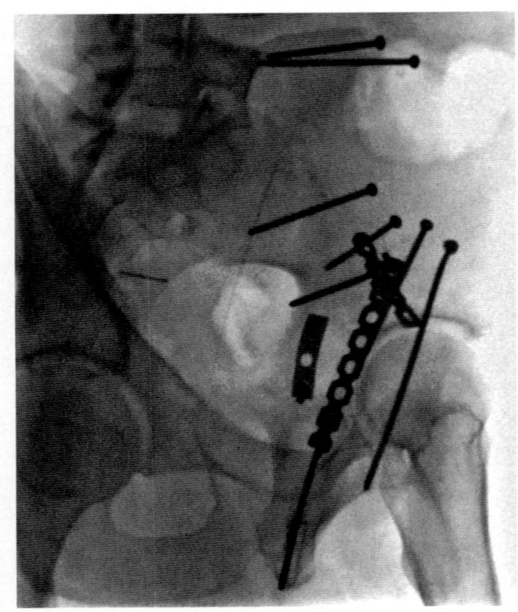

FIGURE 38-21. ***(continued)***

knowledge of the various approach alternatives are required for successful treatment outcomes.

REFERENCES

1. Letournel E, Judet R. *Fractures of the acetabulum.* Berlin: Springer-Verlag, 1993.
2. Matta JM. Accuracy of reduction and clinical results in patients managed operatively within three weeks after the injury. *J Bone Joint Surg (Am)* 1996;78(11):1632–1645.
3. Mayo KA. Open reduction and internal fixation of fractures of the acetabulum: results in 163 fractures. *Clin Orthop* 1994;(305): 31–37.
4. Weber TG, Mast JW. The extended ilioinguinal approach for specific both-column fractures. *Clin Orthop* 1994;(305):106–111.
5. Cole JD, Bolhofner BR. Acetabular fracture fixation via a modified Stoppa limited intrapelvic approach. Description of operative technique and preliminary treatment results. *Clin Orthop* 1994; (305):112–123.

39

EARLY COMPLICATIONS OF ACETABULAR FRACTURES

GREGORY J. SCHMELING
THOMAS J. PERLEWITZ
DAVID L. HELFET

INTRODUCTION

Displaced acetabular fractures generally represent high-energy injuries with the potential for multisystem involvement and significant morbidity and mortality. Successful outcomes are predicated on achieving an anatomic reduction of the weight-bearing surface of the acetabulum, concentric reduction of the femoral head, and avoidance of complications. In this chapter we address the complications related to an acetabular fracture and its treatment. Identification, management, and avoidance of these complications can significantly improve long-term patient outcomes (For early complications, see Table 39-1; for late complications, see Table 40–1).

DEATH

The reported prevalence of mortality associated with acetabular fracture surgery ranges from zero to 3.6% (1–13). Letournel and Judet reported 13 deaths in 569 cases (2.3%) (4). Seven of 13 were in patients 60 years or older, representing a mortality rate of 5.7% for that group. The most common cause of death was massive pulmonary embolism (4 of 13). The inclusion of two patients with unexplained circulatory collapse, presumably from undiagnosed pulmonary emboli, results in an incidence of thromboembolic events nearing 50% (6 of 13). In a series of 100 patients, Helfet and Schmeling reported two fatal pulmonary emboli after induction of anesthesia but before the surgical incision (2). Both of these patients were more than 15 days out from their initial trauma at the time they were transferred for management of their acetabular fractures.

THROMBOEMBOLISM

Pulmonary emboli remain one of the most significant complications associated with treatment of acetabular fractures. The prevalence in acute acetabular fractures ranges from 1% to as high as 5%. The latter rate is from the series reported by Helfet and Schmeling and includes two deaths after induction of anesthesia (2). The incidence of fatal pulmonary embolism is not well described nor accurately related to the incidence of deep vein thrombosis (DVT).

The incidence of clinically apparent DVT ranges from 2.3% to 5% in the acetabular fracture literature (1–6,8–13). The overall incidence of DVT in polytrauma patients with

TABLE 39-1. EARLY ACETABULAR COMPLICATIONS

Series	Cases (No.)	Mortality (%)	DVT (%)	Pulmonary Embolism (%)	Neurologic[a] (Sciatic) (%)	Infection (%)	Failure of Fixation (%)	Malreduction (%)
Letournel and Judet[b]	569	2.3	3	2.1	12/6	4.2	1	26
Matta et al.[c]	43	NR	NR	2	18/9	9	NR	NR
Matta[d]	226	NR	NR	NR	3	4	NR	6
Matta[e]	259	NR	NR	NR	12	5	3	8
Mears et al.[f]	100	1	5	1	16/3	4	1	4
Goulet et al.[g]	31	NR	NR	NR	NR	3	NR	6.5
Reinert et al.[h]	20	NR	NR	NR	5	5	NR	0
Kaempffe et al.[i]	55	NR	NR	NR	16	10	NR	NR
Routt et al.[j]	108	NR	NR	3	5	3	NR	4
Helfet et al.[k]	84	0	6	4	31/6	0	2	9.5

[a] Preoperative/postoperative sciatic nerve injury.
[b] Letournel E, Judet R. *Fractures of the acetabulum,* 2nd ed. Berlin: Springer-Verlag, 1993.
[c] Matta JM, Anderson LM, Epstein HC, et al. Fractures of the acetabulum: a retrospective analysis. *Clin Orthop* 1986;205:230–240.
[d] Matta JM. *Immediate and long term results of surgical treatment of acetabular fractures.* Presented at the first International Symposium on Surgical Treatment of Acetabular Fractures. Paris, May, 1993.
[e] Matta JM. Fractures of the acetabulum: accuracy of reduction and clinical results in patients managed operatively within three weeks after injury. *J Bone Joint Surg* 1996;78-A:1632–1645.
[f] Mears DC, Rubash HE, Sawaguchi T. Fractures of the acetabulum. The hip. *Proceedings of the thirteenth open scientific meeting of the hip society.* St. Louis: CV Mosby 1985: 95–113.
[g] Goulet JA, Bray TJ. Complex acetabular fractures. *Clin Orthop* 1989;240:9–20.
[h] Reinert CM, Bosse MJ, Poka A, et al. A modified extensile exposure for the treatment of complex or malunited acetabular fractures. *J Bone Joint Surg* 1988;70-A:329–337.
[i] Kaempffe FA, Bone LA, Border JR, et al. Operative fixation of displaced acetabular fractures: a retrospective review. *Orthop Trans* 1988;12:527.
[j] Routt MLC Jr, Swiontkowski MF. Operative treatment of complex acetabular fractures: combined anterior and posterior exposures during the same procedure. *J Bone Joint Surg* 1990;72-A:897–904.
[k] Helfet DL, Schmeling GJ. Management of acute, displaced acetabular fractures using indirect reduction techniques and limited approaches. *Orthop Trans* 1991;15:833–834.
NR, not recored.

lower extremity injuries is nearly 60% when vascular testing is used (14,15). The actual subclinical incidence of DVT associated with acetabular fractures is likely much higher than has been previously reported.

What is really worrisome is that none of the patients in the series of Helfet and Schmeling (2) had any clinical evidence of DVT. In fact, one of those who sustained a fatal pulmonary embolus had negative venous Doppler and lung perfusion scans 2 days prior to her demise. This seems to implicate the pelvic and internal iliac vessels as sources of the embolus. Routine methods of screening are inadequate for identification of thrombosis in these vessels. Magnetic resonance imaging (MRI) venography has been shown to be superior to contrast venography when evaluating patients with an acetabular fracture for DVT (16).

There is now consensus that some form of DVT prophylaxis is indicated as part of the treatment of patients with acetabular fractures (see Chapter 9). However, consensus is lacking as to the method of prophylaxis that is most efficacious yet confers the lowest perioperative risks. Letournel and Judet (4) have used heparin, coumadin, and, recently, low molecular-weight heparin. Coagulation studies are monitored daily. The heparin or low molecular weight heparin is used for the first 8 to 12 days, and then the patient was switched to coumadin for a total of 75 days. The DVT prophylaxis was stopped if the patient became ambulatory sooner.

Helfet and Stickney (17) completed a prospective study comparing the use of intermittent compression stockings (ICS) preoperatively with ICS plus subcutaneous heparin preoperatively or coumadin postoperatively. ICS have an effect on the clotting mechanism other than the mechanical one, or they activate fibrinolytic mechanisms (18). In addition, all of these patients were studied with noninvasive Doppler vascular evaluation on admission, preoperatively, and postoperatively (19–24). One hundred fourteen patients were entered in the study. The incidence of DVT in those patients with ICS alone was 16.8%, and in the anticoagulation group it was 1.8%. This study supports the use of ICS with some form of chemical anticoagulation in preventing DVT in patients with lower extremity trauma. However, it does not address the issue of preventing fatal pulmonary embolism.

Fishman and coworkers (25) performed a prospective nonrandomized study examining a protocol for DVT and pulmonary embolism prophylaxis in operative management of pelvic and acetabular fractures. There were 197 patients with 203 fractures (148 acetabular, 55 pelvic, two cases of bilateral acetabular fractures, four cases of combined acetabular and pelvic fractures). The protocol involved noninvasive screening of the lower extremities preoperatively, venal caval filters, mechanical antithrombotic devices intraoperatively and postoperatively, and chemical prophylaxis with warfarin for 3 weeks following removal of surgical drains. There was a 6% incidence of preoperative incidence of DVT and a 3% incidence of postoperative DVT. There was one fatal preoperative pulmonary embolism (0.5%) and two nonfatal postoperative pulmonary emboli (1%). Although the authors concluded that their protocol was efficacious statistical significance between groups was not demonstrated.

We currently recommend that all patients with acetabular fractures be treated with an intermittent compression device plus a form of chemical anticoagulation (subcutaneous heparin, low molecular weight heparin, coumadin) preoperatively and postoperatively. Coumadin is used only postoperatively. The coagulation value should reach 1.5 times normal. Screening for thrombosis may be indicated (color Doppler ultrasonography or venography) before surgical reconstruction.

Patients with a postoperative pulmonary embolism or DVT (proximal) are treated with full chemical anticoagulation (heparin/coumadin or low molecular weight heparin/coumadin). If additional injuries are such that anticoagulation is contraindicated, a vena cava filter is warranted. If the DVT is distal to the trifurcation of the popliteal artery, low molecular weight heparin is used and the patient is followed with sequential color Doppler ultrasound evaluations. Should proximal propagation be demonstrated, the clot is treated with full chemical anticoagulation. If no propagation is seen, the patient can be treated either with further observation low molecular weight heparin.

The problem treatment groups are those with a preoperative proximal DVT (demonstrated clinically or on vascular testing) or a pulmonary embolism. Many of these patients have additional injuries that may preclude anticoagulation therapy. Performing pelvic surgery on a fully anticoagulated patient would be contraindicated. Preoperative use of vena cava filters has proved most efficacious in this patient population (26).

Selected patients with a preoperative DVT may be fully anticoagulated with heparin, reversed immediately preoperatively, and anticoagulation resumed postoperatively. However, because propagation of the initial clot could occur during surgery, we recommend preoperative use of a vena cava filter for documented proximal DVT in these patients. Obviously, the decision to use anticoagulation alone in patients at high risk for thrombosis or a vena cava filter in the preoperative treatment of proximal thrombosis must be individualized for each patient.

What is to be done about the patient who is transferred to your hospital several days postinjury if DVT prophylaxis has not been initiated pretransfer? In this case, we recommend color duplex Doppler ultrasonography or an MRI venogram. If findings are negative, the patient is placed on routine prophylaxis as outlined in the preceding. The patient is treated with low molecular weight heparin and placement of a Greenfield filter is considered if positive for a proximal thrombus. Postoperatively the patient is treated with chemical anticoagulation.

A preoperative DVT distal to the trifurcation of the popliteal artery is treated like the postoperative one. Without evidence of propagation of the clot proximally, surgery could proceed as planned. Anticoagulation could be added postoperatively, as needed.

The issue of thromboembolism in trauma patients continues to be a subject of close scrutiny in many trauma centers. Hopefully, further experience with noninvasive testing of the pelvic venous system will make detection of a thrombus easier. Prospective studies are currently evaluating such regimens for their efficacy and safety in trauma patients.

INFECTION

The reported rate of deep infections following acetabular fracture surgery ranges from 0% to 10% (1–6,8–13). In two large series, the prevalence was higher early on, when the operative team was less experienced (4,8). This was owing primarily to incomplete understanding of the pathologic anatomy and to "errors of surgical approach, leading to long surgical procedures, which were followed by several bad infections" (4). The addition of perioperative antibiotics reduced the infection rate to 1% in Letournel and Judet's last 400 cases (4). Similarly, Matta reported a 9% prevalence in his initial series of 43 patients (6,27,28) but this decreased to 3% in his subsequent review of 98 patients.

In Letournel and Judet's series, the infection rate with the Kocher-Langenbeck approach was 4.1% (13 of 314) (4). As they were developing the ilioinguinal approach, the infection rate was an alarming 13.2%; however, with a "better understanding of the approach, precautions to preserve the lymphatics, and the use of antibiotics," the incidence decreased markedly (5%, 8 of 158). Helfet and Schmeling reported no infections in a series using either the Kocher-Langenbeck or the ilioinguinal approach (2).

One would expect that extensile exposures, with their significant soft-tissue dissection and prolonged operative time, would have a higher infection rate than the single anterior or posterior approach. The extensive subperiosteal dissection involved in the extended exposures potentially creates devascularized bone and soft tissue as well as potential spaces for hematoma formation. Bosse and coworkers raised our awareness of the potential problem with extensile acetabular fracture exposures in patients with a superior gluteal artery injury (29). During the extended iliofemoral exposure the gluteus medius and gluteus minimus are elevated off the outer table of the ilium, and their insertion is released from the greater trochanter. The only remaining blood supply to the gluteus medius and minimus muscles is from the superior gluteal vessels. Preoperative injury to this vessel and the use of the extended iliofemoral exposure may result in devascularization of the entire abductor muscle mass and subsequent tissue necrosis. This is a devastating complication. Bosse and coworkers recommend preoperative angiography for fractures involving the greater sciatic notch when an extensile exposure is planned.

However, this problem has only been demonstrated in dogs and cadavers. Letournel and Judet reported no incidences of flap necrosis in their series (4). Reilly and associates (30) used a doppler to assess flow in the superior gluteal artery during open reduction and internal fixation of 41 acetabular fractures involving the posterior column using the extended iliofemoral exposure. The average displacement of the sciatic notch component of the injury was 2.5 cm. Flow was found in 40 of 41 patients. There was no flap necrosis and all patients had some abductor function. Routine preoperative angiography for extended exposures is not indicated.

Neither Letournel and Judet (4) or Matta (6,27,28) have reported significant infection or wound complication rates with the use of the extended iliofemoral exposure. Reinert and coworkers reported an infection rate of 5% with his modification of the extended iliofemoral exposure (11). Mears, with the triradiate exposure, had an infection rate of 4% (9). The significance of preoperative injury to the superior gluteal vessels relative to wound complication rates and infection when an extended exposure is utilized is still unclear (Fig. 39-1). Owing to the experience gained in the pioneering work of Letournel, Judet, and Matta, most subsequent reports using their extended exposures note infection rates of 3% or less.

Other factors that predispose to wound infection are skin necrosis and hematoma formation. The prevalences of skin necrosis and hematoma formation in Letournel and Judet's series were 1.8% and 7.7%, respectively (4). Both of these complications can lead to infection. Recognition of the Morel-Lavallée skin injury is essential (Fig. 39-1B). This injury is closed internal degloving that leads to avulsion of the fat from the underlying fascia. The result is an avascular cavity filled with hematoma and liquified fat. This injury generally lies over the greater trochanter but may be found in the flank or lumbar region. It is a severe injury that devascularizes several soft-tissue planes. Hak and associates (31) reviewed 24 cases and presented a treatment protocol. Nearly 50% of the patients had positive cultures obtained from the lesion. They recommended debridement before or during acetabular fracture surgery. Even so, there was still a 13% incidence of infection. Postoperative hematomas must be viewed as potential sources of infection, and the mainstay of treatment remains perioperative prevention (hemostasis, suction drains, early evacuation, and debridement when they occur).

Prophylaxis

Careful preoperative screening of patients for any focus of infection is essential, especially for polytrauma patients who have been recumbent in traction. The source of any fever, leukocytosis, or abnormal urinalysis must be identified and adequately treated before surgery. If possible, the Foley catheter should be removed a few days before surgery.

Operating through damaged or contaminated soft tissue is to be avoided. This is especially important with crush injuries that require posterior approaches. Kellam and coworkers reported a 25% prevalence of skin slough in posterior pelvic approaches in patients following crush injuries (32). Morel-Lavallée lesions over the trochanter should be evacuated before posterior or extensile approaches are undertaken.

For patients with combined pelvic and acetabular fractures who required external fixation in the acute phase, the fixator must be removed and the soft tissues over the iliac crest allowed to heal before an anterior approach is attempted. Similarly, pin tract problems following injudicious use of trochanteric traction bolts may preclude timely surgery (Fig. 39-2). Meticulous prepping and draping help to prevent contamination from the perineal region. Careful handling of the soft tissues and respect for the biology of bone by the surgeon is necessary to avoid additional devitalization as a result of the surgical procedure. Intermittent and copious irrigation of the operative wound with saline or antibiotic irrigation solutions throughout the procedure helps remove contamination and debris. Prophylactic antibiotics should be administered and then continued for at least 48 hours after surgery. Antibiotics should be continued until the drainage ceases if there is excessive serous drainage from the wound postoperatively. Multiple suction drains should be used to prevent hematoma formation and eliminate potential dead spaces. Significant postoperative hematomas require urgent surgical irrigation and debridement.

Treatment

The identification of an acute postoperative wound infection demands urgent and aggressive surgical exploration. All devitalized infected tissue must be excised. Appropriate empiric antibiotic treatment should be initiated once surgical cultures have been obtained. Involvement of the hip joint must be assumed and carefully ruled out. The prognosis for salvage of the joint is guarded in the presence of septic arthritis. If septic arthritis is present, thorough debridement of the joint, including the capsule and synovium, is required. Multiple drains should be inserted in the depth of the abscess before closure of the deep structures. Superficial wound closure should be contemplated only if there is no gross contamination or evidence of residual inflammation in the skin or subcutaneous tissue. Wounds that are severely infected (especially with anaerobic organisms) should not be closed. Daily debridement, open packing, and hyperbaric oxygen treatment, if available, are preferable. Vacuum assisted closure (VAC) dressing has been efficacious in management of these difficult wounds.

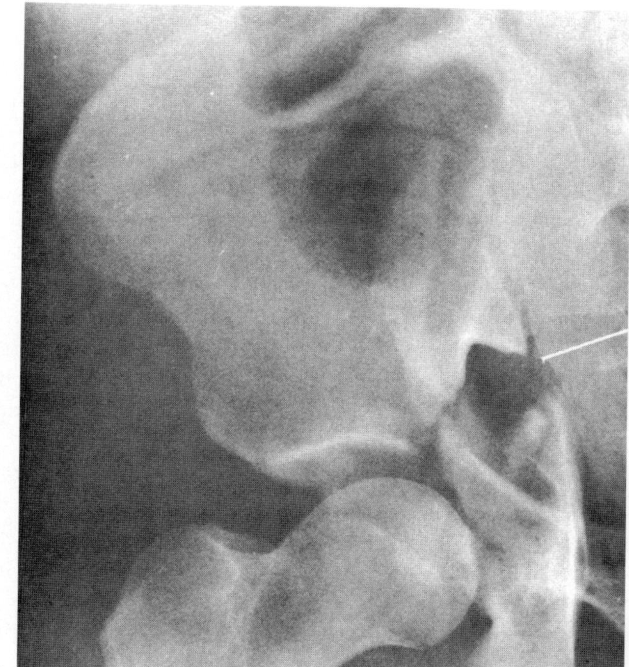

A

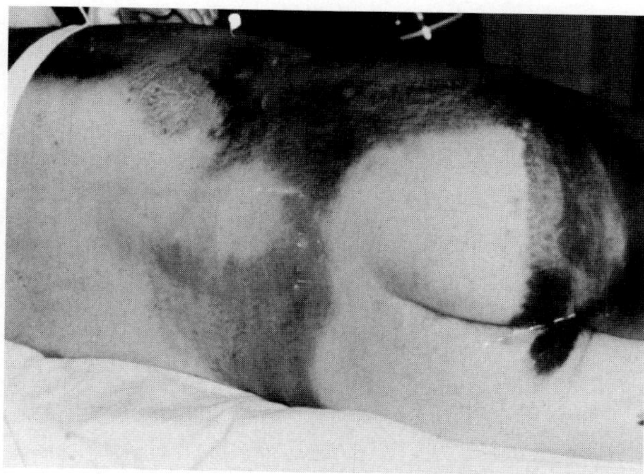

B

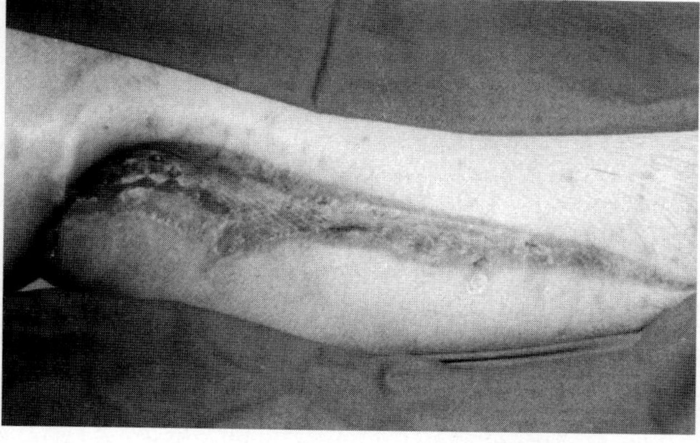

D

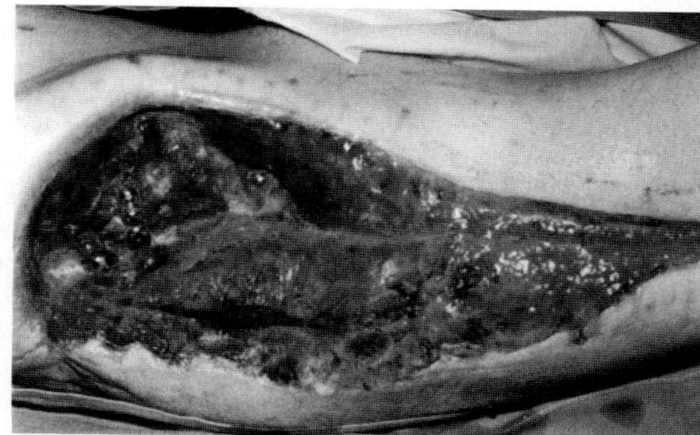

C

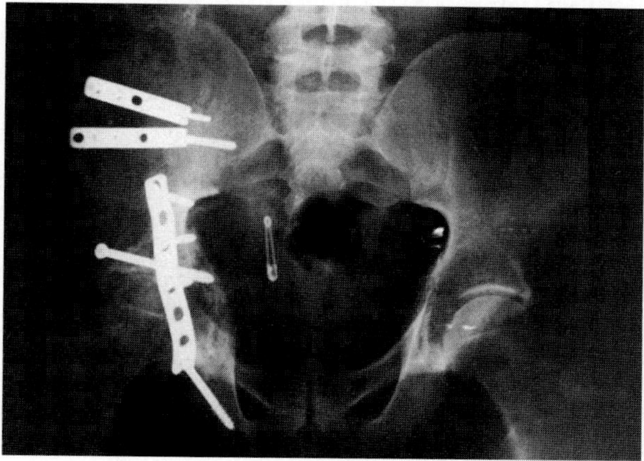

E

FIGURE 39-1. **A:** Anterior-posterior radiograph of a T-type acetabular fracture sustained by a rider thrown from his motorcycle. **B:** Extensive lateral hematoma is visible 10 days following injury (Morel-Lavallée). **C:** An extended iliofemoral approach was performed to effect open reduction and internal fixation. In the postoperative period it became obvious that skin necrosis had developed on the flap as well as in a portion of the gluteus medius. After resection of necrotic muscle and skin it was noted that granulation tissue began to form in the wound. **D:** Healing of this massive wound required a skin flap. **E:** Although the hip joint did not become infected, osteoarthritis was noted 5 years after the injury, in the radiograph.

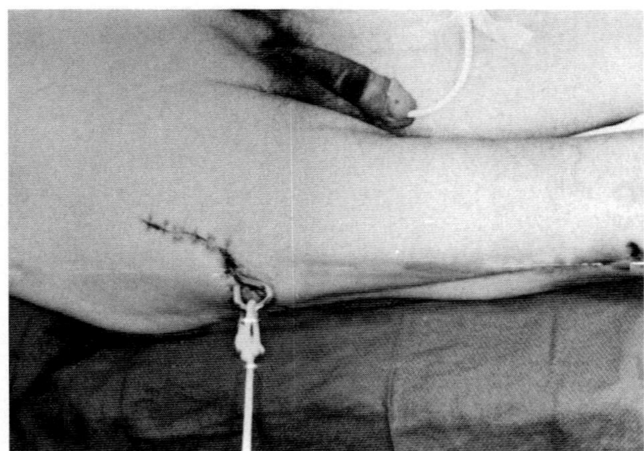
A

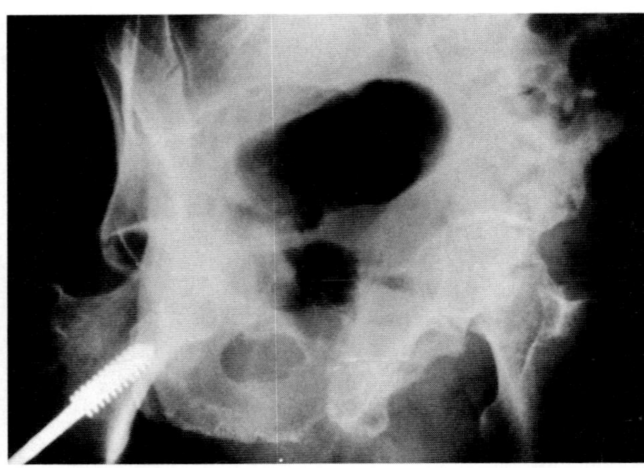
B

FIGURE 39-2. A right transverse posterior wall acetabular fracture in a 75-year-old man was treated with a trochanteric bolt and skeletal distal femoral traction. **A:** Ten days after the injury a clinical photograph demonstrates superficial trochanteric bolt wound problems. **B:** An obturator oblique radiograph demonstrates unacceptable reduction.

NERVE INJURY

Nerve injury is consistently reported as a complication of acetabular fractures and their surgical management (1–6,8–13). Documentation of the extent of such injuries, which can vary from minor sensory paresthesia to complete sensory or motor paralysis, is lacking. This distinction is significant because it represents a functional difference for the patient's outcome. Also, despite reports of the incidence of postoperative nerve involvement, there is little differentiation between those that are the result of the injury (i.e., that were present preoperatively) and those that are a complication of the treatment.

The sciatic (tibial and/or peroneal), femoral, pudendal, obturator, superior gluteal, and lateral femoral cutaneous nerves may be involved, individually or in combination. The most common, and the most significant, is injury to the sciatic nerve or one of its divisions. Two patterns of injury are most common: involvement of both the tibial and peroneal divisions (sciatic) or isolated involvement of the peroneal division.

Sciatic Nerve Injury

The preoperative incidence of sciatic nerve injury varies from 12% to 31% for sciatic nerve injuries (2,4,6,9,33). Letournel and Judet noted a significant association of posterior femoral head dislocation in patients with a sciatic injury (4). The incidence of such injuries was greatest in association with a transverse or posterior wall acetabular fracture and a posterior hip dislocation. In the series presented by Helfet and Schmeling, all the patients with a sciatic nerve injury preoperatively had involvement of the posterior wall or posterior column in their fracture pattern (2).

The reported prevalence of postoperative sciatic nerve injury is 2% to 16% (1–6,8–13,33). Intraoperative measures should be directed toward decreasing the prevalence of postoperative sciatic nerve injury. Letournel and Judet recommended transcondylar femoral traction, holding the knee flexed and hip extended during posterior approaches, and careful use of specially designed sciatic nerve retractors (4). Preoperative neurological evaluation is essential to determine the true prevalence of iatrogenic nerve injuries. Helfet and Schmeling were able to accurately identify posttraumatic nerve injuries with preoperative evaluation by a neurologist (2,34). Helfet and Schmeling reported the intraoperative use of somatosensory-evoked potential (SEP) monitoring, especially when the nerve is injured preoperatively (the high-risk group) or when posterior fracture pattern exists, decreased the rate of iatrogenic sciatic nerve injury to 2% (33,34). Others have also had success with intraoperative SEP monitoring in diminishing postoperative nerve injury (35,36). More recently, spontaneous motor potentials (SMP) have been used to assess intraoperative sciatic nerve function, and subsequently identify impending nerve injury (37). Other authors have confirmed that the methods advocated by Letournel and Judet (4) to decrease postoperative nerve injury are all that is required. In fact, Middlebrooks and colleagues conclude that the use of SEP or SMP are not justified because hip flexion and knee extension and careful retraction can reduce the incidence of postoperative nerve injury to a negligible level (38).

Once injured, the sciatic nerve or the peroneal division has the capacity to recover as long as 3 years after injury. Fassler and coworkers reviewed 14 patients with a sciatic nerve injury, to document carefully the extent of the injury and its recovery (39). Patients with a mild peroneal, mild tibial, or severe tibial nerve injury all had satisfactory nerve recovery. Only one third of those with a severe peroneal division nerve injury had satisfactory nerve recovery. Helfet and Schmeling observed 100% recovery from postoperative severe peroneal division nerve injuries (34). Tile found that 75% of traumatic nerve injuries and 100% of iatrogenic nerve injuries either completely recovered or exhibited partial return of function (40). Letournel and Judet found in their series that 62% of the sciatic nerve injuries had total or significant recovery and an additional 24% had partial recovery (34). Fassler's series had only one patient that did not have satisfactory functional recovery although some required a brace to walk (39). The potential for functional sciatic nerve recovery is good. Observation and prolonged physical therapy are indicated.

Femoral Nerve Injury

Femoral nerve injury is an exceptionally rare sequela of acetabular fractures or their surgery. Helfet and Schmeling reported the prevalence of posttraumatic nerve injury was 2% (2). Both injuries recovered completely. Tile had one patient with a complete laceration of the femoral nerve from a pubic ramus fracture that never recovered and required a tendon transfer (40). Letournel and Judet reported two postoperative cases of femoral nerve injury (4). Both patients recovered. The ilioinguinal approach puts the nerve at risk from traction during fracture manipulation. Care must be taken with lateral traction of the iliopsoas compartment, because the femoral nerve lies on its medial side.

Lateral Femoral Cutaneous Nerve Injury

The lateral femoral cutaneous nerve is at risk from ilioinguinal and extensile approaches. Helfet and Schmeling reported the incidence of postoperative nerve injury to be 18% using the ilioinguinal approach (2). Letournel and Judet reported that 45 of 351 (12%) patients complained of persistent neuralgia after exposures that placed the nerve at risk (4). Most resolve if the nerve is not incised or avulsed. With the extensile approaches, it is very difficult to preserve the integrity of the lateral femoral cutaneous nerve. Injury to the nerve resulting in sensory loss on the lateral side of the thigh seems to be more of an annoyance to the patient than a functional problem.

Pudendal Nerve Injury

Postoperative pudendal nerve injury is usually caused by pressure of the perineal post during posterior approaches with the patient in the prone position. Helfet and Schmeling reported the incidence to be 6% (2). All the patients were males and all recovered spontaneously. This is consistent with Brumback and coworkers, who found a 90% recovery rate for pudendal nerve injuries resulting from traction during femoral nailing at 3-month follow-up (41). In their series, the injury correlated with the magnitude of the pressure on the traction post rather than the duration of the procedure. The traction post must be padded and the duration of the peak traction force observed to help prevent this injury.

Superior Gluteal Nerve Injury

The superior gluteal nerve and superior gluteal vascular bundle exit the pelvis high in the sciatic notch. The neurovascular bundle is at risk in fractures that exit high in the greater sciatic notch and during posterior surgical exposures. Should bleeding be identified in this area, ligation without careful dissection of the neurovascular bundle may place the superior gluteal nerve at significant risk for injury. Letournel and Judet reported 14 injuries to the superior gluteal vascular bundle during 461 Kocher-Langenbeck exposures (4). Four of these patients sustained associated injuries to the superior gluteal nerve. They felt these were not directly related to ligation. If bleeding is identified in the greater sciatic notch, Letournel and Judet recommend packing the area for as long as possible to achieve hemostasis (4). If this is not successful, great care should be used to identify the superior gluteal nerve prior to ligation of the bleeding vessel.

Summary

Perioperative neurologic injury can represent a significant complication of acetabular fractures. The incidence of preoperative sciatic neurologic injury, when actively pursued during a careful preoperative examination, may be much higher than was previously reported (31%) (2). Preoperative neurologic consultation in conjunction with proper positioning and retraction techniques may help decrease the incidence of postoperative sciatic nerve injury in the presence of posterior fracture patterns, or in cases of preoperative identification of neurologic deficit (34,37,38). The role of intraoperative SEP or motor evoked potentials monitoring needs to be better defined.

MALREDUCTON

The aim of surgery must be both anatomic reduction of the weight-bearing surface of the acetabulum and a congruent reduction of the femoral head under the acetabular dome. When this is accomplished, >80% of patients have an excellent or a good result in all series reviewed (1–6,8–13). Similarly, nonanatomic reduction or subluxation of the femoral head results in less favorable outcomes (see Chapter 46) (Fig. 39-3).

Mayo and coworkers reported the success of reoperation in 64 patients with either malreduction or early secondary loss of reduction following ORIF of an acetabular fracture (42). The authors were able to achieve reduction within 2 mm based on plain x-ray in 36 patients (56%). Good to ex-

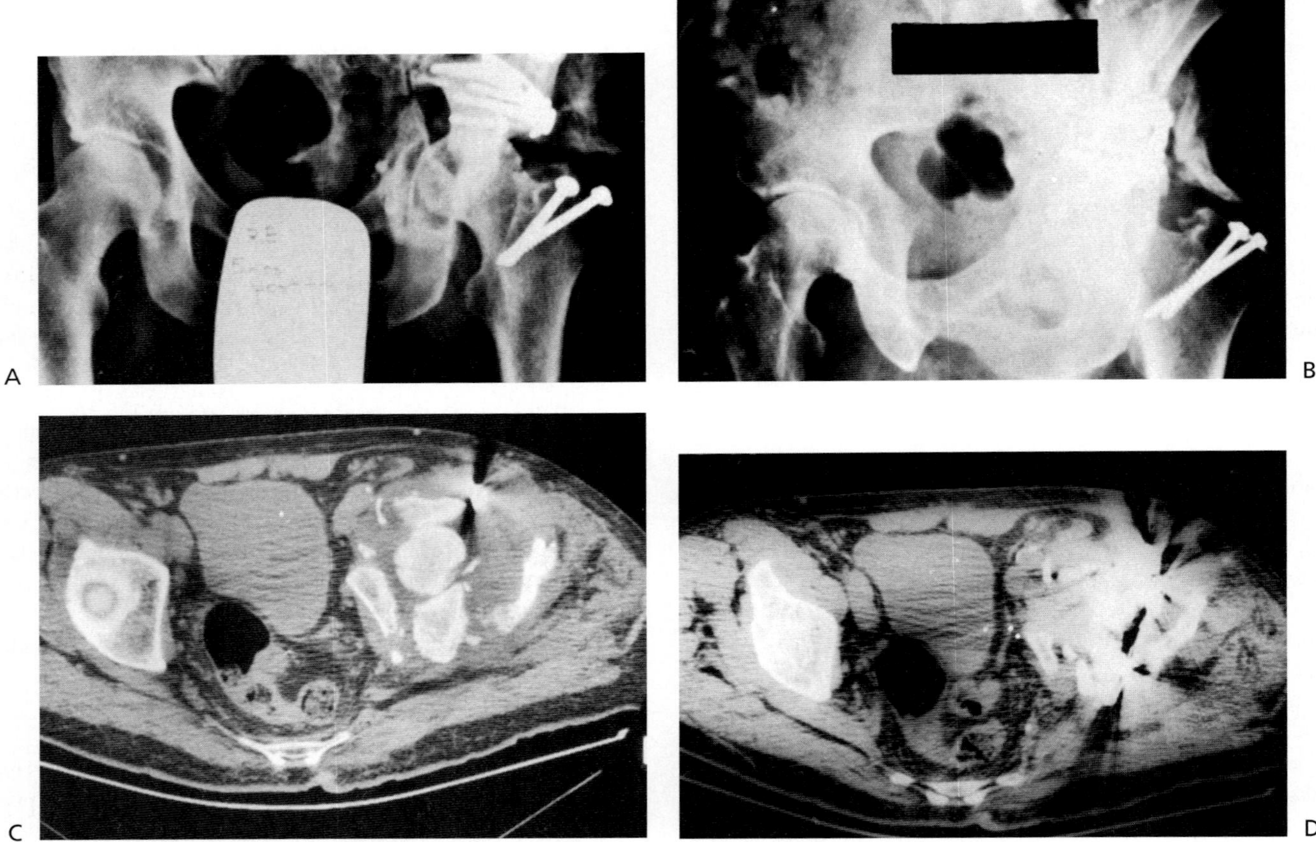

FIGURE 39-3. Five months after surgery for a left associated both-column acetabular fracture, a 65-year-old man had severe pain and limitation of motion owing to inadequate reduction and internal fixation. An anteroposterior pelvis radiograph **(A)**, an obturator oblique radiograph **(B)**, and computed tomography images **(C,D)** demonstrate malreduction of the acetabulum with persistent medial subluxation and deformity of the femoral head and malunion and nonunion of the acetabulum. The only remaining option for salvage for this patient is a difficult total hip arthroplasty.

cellent results were found in 27 patients (42%) at 4-year follow-up. Patients undergoing reoperation within 3 weeks of injury had better results (57% good to excellent) than those whose reoperation was delayed >12 weeks (29% good to excellent). Although results are not nearly as good as primary surgery, early reoperation affords the best chance at successful salvage of malreduction or loss of reduction, as long as the anatomy of the femoral head has been maintained and the articular surface of the acetabulum is reasonable.

Moed and coworkers emphasized the correlation of fracture reduction and favorable clinical outcome (43). The authors evaluated the results in 94 patients with posterior wall acetabular fractures treated with ORIF. Postoperative radiography demonstrated an anatomic reduction (0 to 1 mm) in 92 and an imperfect reduction (2 to 3 mm) in two patients. Postoperative CT scans were obtained in 59 patients. The CT scans revealed step-offs of >2 mm in six patients and fracture gaps of ≥2 mm in 44 patients. Clinical outcomes were excellent in 36%, good in 52%, fair in 2%, and poor in 10%. Risk factors for poor outcomes that were identified included: age >55, delay in hip reduction >24 hours, residual fracture gap >1 cm, intraarticular comminution, and involvement of the weight-bearing portion of the acetabular dome. This study demonstrates that malreduction is not the only factor associated with a poor clinical outcome for posterior wall fractures. It also leads one to question how the assessment of the quality of reduction of the acetabulum is done. CT scans should be used to further define the reduction because plain radiographs alone may not be adequate.

FAILURE OF FIXATION

Letournel and Judet reported six cases of failure of fixation (1%) in their series (4). Helfet and Schmeling had two such patients (2). One was an 81-year-old with a low anterior column-anterior wall fracture with marked comminution of the quadrilateral plate. Anatomic reduction was accomplished through an ilioinguinal approach. Three weeks postoperatively, the patient was found ambulating bearing full weight on her operative extremity. Follow-up radiographs revealed medial subluxation of the femoral head (Fig. 39-4). The other patient, a 67-year-old with a T-type fracture, had an anatomic reduction through a Kocher-Langenbeck approach. Follow-up films revealed progressive subluxation of the femoral head. Both of these patients had marked osteopenia and were noncompliant with their toe-touch weight-bearing restriction.

Failure of fixation also can occur from inadequate fixation. The ideal construct includes both lag screw fixation and buttress plating. Plate fixation alone cannot counteract the tremendous shear forces along these oblique fractures. Lag screws alone often are inadequate, especially in a posterior wall fracture with osteopenia or comminution (Fig. 39-5).

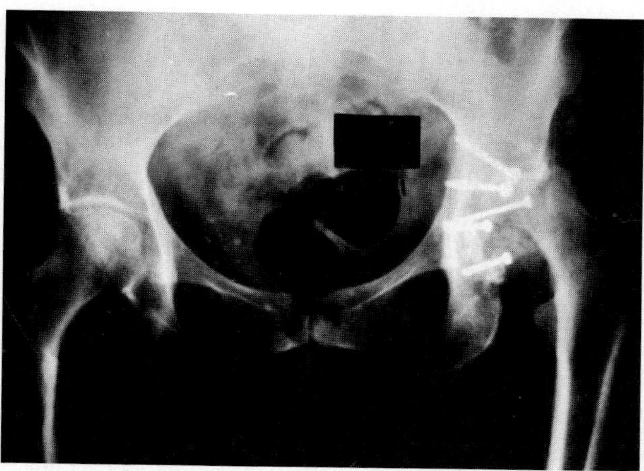

FIGURE 39-5. A 74-year-old woman sustained a left comminuted posterior wall acetabular fracture. An anteroposterior pelvic radiograph 6 weeks after open reduction, and internal fixation with only screws, demonstrates loss of reduction and posterior subluxation of the femoral head.

VASCULAR INJURY

Letournel and Judet found five cases of the superior gluteal vessels being trapped in the fracture at the angle of the greater sciatic notch (4). Care should be taken when bleeding is encountered in this area. Initial attempts at hemostasis should rely on direct pressure and local thrombotic agents. Only if this is unsuccessful should ligatures or vascular clips be used, because of the danger of also compromising the superior gluteal nerve. Injury to the superior gluteal nerve would result in a permanent limp secondary to paralysis of the hip abductors.

Bosse and associates reported on the incidence of superior gluteal artery injuries in complex acetabular fractures with significant fracture displacement into the sciatic notch (29). After angiographic assessment of eight patients, they demonstrated vascular compromise in three. They recommended preoperative angiography for such patients if an extensile exposure and creation of an abductor muscle flap based on the superior gluteal artery is contemplated.

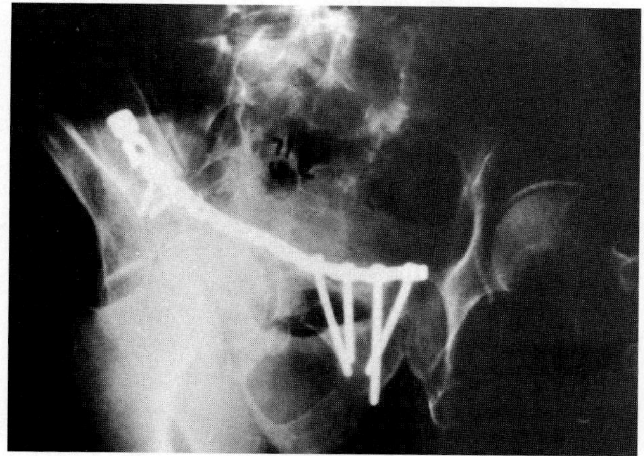

FIGURE 39-4. An 81-year-old man sustained a right anterior column with associated anterior wall acetabular fracture. Following open reduction and internal fixation, an obturator oblique radiograph demonstrates the loss of reduction and anteromedial subluxation of the femoral head.

Reilly and associates (30) looked at the incidence of superior gluteal artery injury following acetabular fracture. The study was designed to look at whether an extended iliofemoral approach associated with superior gluteal artery injury resulted in abductor muscle necrosis. The authors identified 41 of 277 patients with acetabular fractures who were treated with an extended iliofemoral approach. All fractures involved the posterior column. Average displacement of the sciatic notch was 25 mm (6 to 60 mm). Preoperative angiography was not performed. Intraoperative Doppler assessment of the superior gluteal artery was done before and after reduction and fixation of the posterior column. Pulsatile flow was found in 40 of 41 patients. No patients had evidence of complete loss of abductor function, including the patient with superior gluteal artery thrombosis. The authors do not recommend preoperative angiography in patients undergoing acetabular surgery using the extended iliofemoral approach.

Frank and coworkers reported two injuries to the iliofemoral artery in patients with anterior compression pelvic injuries and a displaced high anterior column fracture (44). Intraoperative vascular injuries, even though very rare, have also been reported following acetabular fracture surgery. Johnson and associates had one case of femoral artery injury from lag screw malposition with a posterior approach for a transverse acetabular fracture (45). Helfet and Schmeling reported one case of inadvertent perforation of the femoral vein by a sharp anterior column fracture fragment during attempted fracture reduction (2). Probe and coworkers described thrombosis of the femoral artery as a result of traction during an ilioinguinal exposure (46). Wolinsky and Johnson reported a case of delayed (postinjury day 11, postoperative day 8) rupture of the external iliac artery (47).

Letournel and Judet (4) described an inconsistent connection between the external iliac artery and the deep inferior epigastric artery that they labeled the "corona mortis" or circle of death (Fig. 39-6). They stated that the connection was present in 10% to 15% of exposures. Teague and associates (48) described the retropubic vascular anatomy related to the ilioinguinal exposure. All vessels >2 mm in diameter connecting the obturator system with the external iliac or inferior epigastric system were identified. In 79 ilioinguinal exposures in 40 cadaveric specimens, 59 (73%) had at least one communicating retropubic vascular channel (arterial: 43%, venous: 59%). They found 14 instances of anastomotic connections (37%) in 38 consecutive acetabular fractures treated through the ilioinguinal approach. The incidence of unexpected vascular connections is greater than previously appreciated.

Indirect reduction of the opposite, unexposed column of the acetabulum can be accomplished in complex fractures (2). Fixation of this column is usually completed with a long lag screw. When this screw is placed from posterior to anterior down the anterior column, the femoral vessels are at great risk. The vessel lies just medial to the iliopectineal eminence. The drill bit may exit the bone in this area and perforate the artery or vein, leading to significant blood loss. Immediate exploration and repair are required.

INTRAARTICULAR HARDWARE

Letournel and Judet (4) found five cases of posttraumatic arthrosis that were a direct result of intraarticular hardware (prevalence 0.9%). Routt and coworkers (49) reported one case of inadvertent screw penetration of the hip joint following acetabular fracture surgery that required a second operative procedure for removal. The natural history of intraarticular hardware is progressive articular destruction and arthrosis.

Helfet and Schmeling (2) described the routine use of intraoperative fluoroscopy (Judet views) to determine the position of all hardware as part of their technique for reconstruction of complex acetabular fractures using single, nonextensile exposures.

When intraarticular hardware is suspected, Ebraheim and coworkers (50) recommend intraoperative fluoroscopy or arthrography to verify the position of the hardware. DiPasquale and coworkers demonstrated the value of intraop-

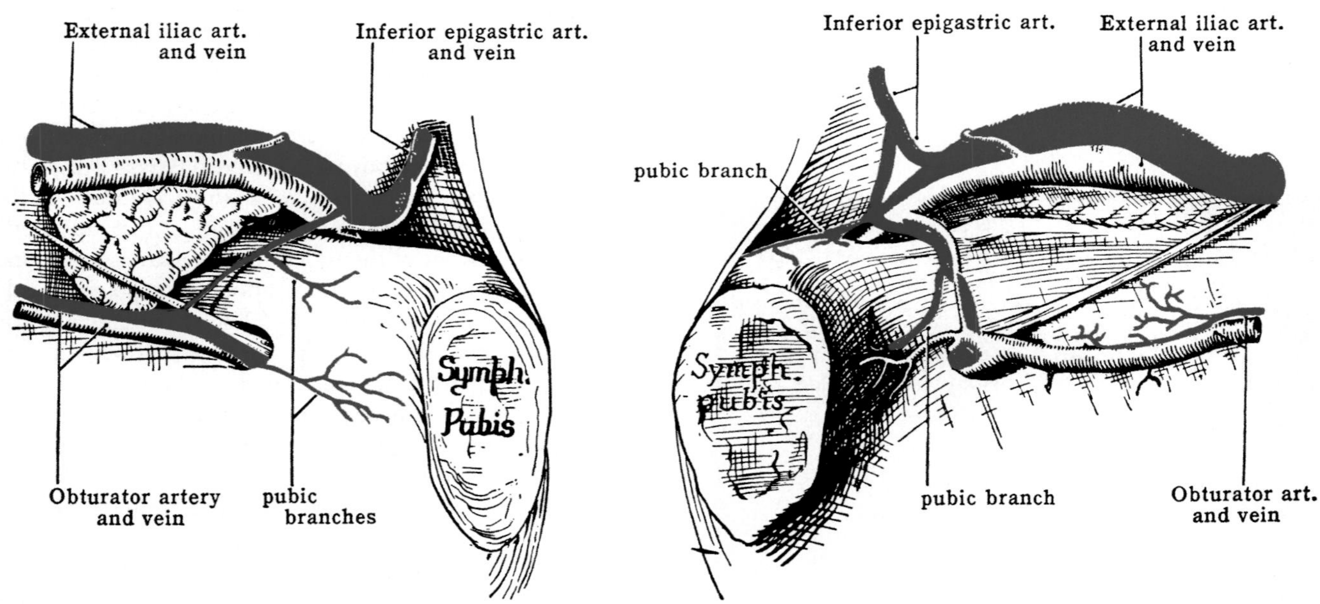

FIGURE 39-6. A: Normal: behind the body of the pubis the pubic branch of the obturator artery forms an anastomosis with the pubic branch of the inferior epigastric artery. **B:** Abnormal (accessory): the obturator artery arises from the inferior epigastric via the pubic anastomosis. In a study of 283 limbs, the obturator artery arose from the internal iliac artery in 70%, from the inferior epigastric in 25.4%, and from both equally in 4.6%. (From: Anderson JE. *Grant's atlas of anatomy,* 8th ed. Baltimore: Williams & Wilkins, 1983, with permission.)

erative auscultation of the periacetabular area with a sterile esophageal stethoscope in helping the surgeon detect intraarticular hardware (51). We suggest that to avoid inadvertent placement of intraarticular hardware the surgeon practice the planned internal fixation on a "saw bone" pelvis preoperatively, use intraoperative fluoroscopy to obtain an anteroposterior view of the pelvis and Judet views to verify the position of the hardware, or auscultate the hip joint intraoperatively with an esophageal stethoscope. Finally, permanent radiographs (anteroposterior pelvis and Judet views) are made in the operating room before the procedure is completed. A postoperative CT scan of the pelvis with 2-mm thin cuts also is recommended to evaluate hardware placement.

TROCHANTERIC OSTEOTOMY

A trochanteric osteotomy is used to extend some surgical exposures (Kocher-Langenbeck) and is part of others (Triradiate). Heck and associates (52) reported the incidence of complications related to a greater trochanteric osteotomy in 55 patients. There was one case of nonunion and two cases of fixation failure (delayed union). Despite the use of indomethacin, the incidence of heterotopic ossification was 44%. Five were Brooker class IV but these five had additional risk factors for heterotopic ossification. Twelve patients had trochanteric bursitis; eight of the 12 required hardware removal. Overall, 11 of 55 patients had an additional procedure related to the osteotomy. Osteotomy of the greater trochanter increases the incidence of complications related to acetabular fracture treatment. The indications for its use should be balanced against this increased complication incidence.

REFERENCES

1. Goulet JA, Bray TJ. Complex acetabular fractures. *Clin Orthop* 1989;240:9–20.
2. Helfet DL, Schmeling GJ. Management of acute, displaced acetabular fractures using indirect reduction techniques and limited approaches. *Orthop Trans* 1991;15:833–834.
3. Kaempffe FA, Bone LA, Border JR, et al. Operative fixation of displaced acetabular fractures: a retrospective review. *Orthop Trans* 1988;12:527.
4. Letournel E, Judet R. *Fractures of the acetabulum,* 2nd ed. Berlin: Springer-Verlag, 1993.
5. Matta JM. *Acetabulum fractures: results of a combined operative and nonoperative protocol.* Presented at the fifty-eighth AAOS annual meeting. Anaheim, CA, 1991.
6. Matta JM. *Preliminary results of a prospective randomized study using prophylactic indomethacin.* Presented at the first International Symposium on Surgical Treatment of Acetabular Fractures. Paris, 1993.
7. Matta JM. Fractures of the acetabulum: accuracy of reduction and clinical results in patients managed operatively within three weeks after injury. *J Bone Joint Surg* 1996;78-A:1632–1645.
8. Matta JM, Letournel E, Browner BD. *Surgical management of acetabular fractures.* Instructional course lectures, 35th ed. St. Louis: CV Mosby, 1986:382–397.
9. Mears DC, Rubash HE. Extensile exposure of the pelvis. *Contemp Orthop* 1983;6:21–31.
10. Ragnarsson B, Mjöberg B. Arthrosis after surgically treated acetabular fractures. *Acta Orthop Scand* 1992;63:511–514.
11. Reinert CM, Bosse MJ, Poka A, et al. A modified extensile exposure for the treatment of complex or malunited acetabular fractures. *J Bone Joint Surg* 1988;70-A:329–337.
12. Salzman EW, McManama GP, Shapiro AH, et al. Effect of optimization of hemodynamics on fibrinolytic activity and antithrombotic efficacy of external pneumatic calf compression. *Ann Surg* 1987;206:636–641.
13. Tile M. *Fractures of the pelvis and acetabulum,* 1st ed. Baltimore: Williams & Wilkins, 1984.
14. Geerts WH, Nanez H, Pagliarello G, et al. Venous thrombosis in trauma: a prospective study. *Orthop Trans* 1990;14:271.
15. Goulet JA, White RH, Daschbach MM, et al. *Deep vein thrombosis following fracture of the pelvis: a prospective study.* Presented at the fourth OTA annual meeting. Dallas, Texas, 1988.
16. Montgomery KD, Potter HG, Helfet DL. The detection and management of proximal deep venous thrombosis in patients with acute acetabular fractures: a follow-up report. *J Orthop Trauma* 1997;11:330–336.
17. Helfet DL, Stickney J. *Deep vein thrombosis prevention in orthopaedic trauma patients.* Presented at the sixth OTA annual meeting. Toronto, Ontario, 1990.
18. Russell JC, Becker DR. The noninvasive venous vascular laboratory. *Arch Surg* 1983;118:1024–1027.
19. Barnes RW, Russell HE, Wu KK, et al. Accuracy of Doppler ultrasound in clinically suspected venous thrombosis of the calf. *Surg Gynecol Obstet* 1976;143:425–428.
20. Flinn WR, Sandager GP, Cerullo LJ, et al. Duplex venous scanning for the prospective surveillance of perioperative venous thrombosis. *Arch Surg* 1989;124:901–905.
21. Foley WD, Middleton WD, Lawson TL, et al. Color Doppler ultrasound imaging of lower-extremity venous disease. *AJR Am J Roentgenol* 1989;152:371–376.
22. Langsfeld M, Hershey FB, Thorpe L, et al. Duplex B-mode imaging for the diagnosis of deep venous thrombosis. *Arch Surg* 1987;122:587–591.
23. Lensing AWA, Prandoni P, Brandjes D, et al. Detection of deep-vein thrombosis by real-time B-mode ultrasonography. *N Engl J Med* 1989;320:342–345.
24. Routt MLC Jr, Winquist RA. *The treatment of 108 consecutive complex acetabular fractures using combined, simultaneous anterior and posterior surgical approaches at the same anesthesia.* Presented at the fifth OTA annual meeting. Philadelphia, October, 1989.
25. Fishmann AJ, Greeno RA, Brooks LR, et al. Prevention of deep vein thrombosis and pulmonary embolism in acetabular and pelvic fracture surgery. *Clin Orthop* 1994;305:133–137.
26. Webb LX, Rush PT, Fuller SB, et al. Greenfield filter prophylaxis of pulmonary embolism in patients undergoing surgery for acetabular fracture. *J Orthop Trauma* 1992;6:139–145.
27. Matta JM. Operative indications and choice of surgical approach for fractures of the acetabulum. *Tech Orthop* 1986;1:13–22.
28. Matta JM, Mehne DK, Roffi R. Fractures of the acetabulum: early results of a prospective study. *Clin Orthop* 1986;205:241–250.
29. Bosse MJ, Poka A, Reinert CM, et al. Preoperative angiographic assessment of the superior gluteal artery in acetabular fractures requiring extensile surgical exposures. *J Orthop Trauma* 1989;2:303–307.
30. Reilly MC, Olson SA, Tornetta P III, et al. Superior gluteal artery in the extended iliofemoral approach. *J Orthop Trauma* 2000;14:259–263.

31. Hak DJ, Olson SA, Matta JM. Diagnosis and management of closed internal degloving injuries associated with pelvic and acetabular fractures: the Morel-Lavallée lesion. *J Trauma-Injury Infect Crit Care* 1997;42:1046–1051.
32. Kellam JF, McMurtry RYH, Paley D, et al. The unstable pelvic fracture: operative treatment. *Orthop Clin North Am* 1987;18:25–41.
33. Helfet DL, Hissa EA, Sergay S, et al. Somatosensory evoked potential monitoring in the surgical management of acute acetabular fractures. *J Orthop Trauma* 1991;5:161–166.
34. Helfet DL, Schmeling GJ. Somatosensory evoked potential monitoring in the surgical treatment of acute, displaced acetabular fractures: results of a prospective study. *Orthop Trans* 1992;16:221.
35. Baumgaertner MR, Wegner D, Book J. SSEP monitoring during pelvic and acetabular fracture surgery. *J Orthop Trauma* 1994;8: 127–133.
36. Trancik T, Mills W, Vinson N. The effect of indomethacin, aspirin, and ibuprofen on bone ingrowth into a porous-coated implant. *Clin Orthop* 1989;249:113–121.
37. Arrington ED, Hochschild DP, Steinagle TJ, et al. Monitoring of somatosensory and motor evoked potentials during open reduction and internal fixation of pelvis and acetabular fractures. *Orthopedics* 2000;23:1081–1083.
38. Middlebrooks ES, Sims SH, Kellam JF, et al. Incidence of sciatic nerve injury in operatively treated acetabular fractures without somatosensory evoked potential monitoring. *J Orthop Trauma* 1997;11:327–329.
39. Fassler PR, Swiontkowski MF, Kilroy AW, et al. Injury of the sciatic nerve associated with acetabular fracture. *J Bone Joint Surg* 1993;75-A:1157–1166.
40. Tile M. Fractures of the acetabulum. *Orthop Clin North Am* 1980;11:481–506.
41. Brumback RJ, Ellison TS, Molligan H, et al. Pudendal nerve palsy complicating intramedullary nailing of the femur. *J Bone Joint Surg* 1992;74-A:1450–1455.
42. Mayo KA, Letournel E, Matta JM, et al. Surgical revision of malreduced acetabular fractures. *Clin Orthop* 1994;305:47–52.
43. Moed BR, Willson Carr SE, Watson JT. Open reduction and internal fixation of posterior wall fractures of the acetabulum. *Clin Orthop* 2000;377:57–67.
44. Frank JL, Reimer BL, Raves JJ. Traumatic iliofemoral arterial injury: An association with high anterior acetabular fractures. *J Vasc Surg* 1989;10:198–201.
45. Johnson EE, Eckardt JJ, Letournel E. Extrinsic femoral artery occlusion following internal fixation of an acetabular fracture. A case report. *Clin Orthop* 1987;217:209–213.
46. Probe R, Reeve R, Lindsey, RW. Femoral artery thrombosis after open reduction of an acetabular fracture. *Clin Orthop* 1992;283: 258–260.
47. Wolinsky PR, Johnson KD. Delayed catastrophic rupture of the external iliac artery after an acetabular fracture. *J Bone Joint Surg* 1995;77-A:1241–1244.
48. Teague DC, Graney DO, Routt MLC Jr. Retropubic vascular hazards of the ilioinguinal exposure: a cadaveric and clinical study. *J Orthop Trauma* 1996;10:156–159.
49. Routt MLC Jr, Swiontkowski MF. Operative treatment of complex acetabular fractures: combined anterior and posterior exposures during the same procedure. *J Bone Joint Surg* 1990;72-A:897–904.
50. Ebraheim NA, Savolaine ER, Hoeflinger MJ, et al. Radiological diagnosis of screw penetration of the hip joint in acetabular fracture reconstruction. *J Orthop Trauma* 1989;3:196–201.
51. DiPasquale TG, Whiteman K, McKirgan C, et al. *The intraoperative detection of intraarticular screws placed during acetabulum fracture fixation: a simple auscultation technique.* Presented at the ninth OTA annual meeting. New Orleans, LA, 1993.
52. Heck BE, Ebraheim NA, Foetisch C. Direct complications of trochanteric osteotomy in open reduction and internal fixation of acetabular fractures. *Am J Orthop* 1997;26:124–128.

40

LATE COMPLICATIONS OF ACETABULAR FRACTURES

GREGORY J. SCHMELING
THOMAS J. PERLEWITZ
DAVID L. HELFET

AVASCULAR NECROSIS

Femoral Head

The reported incidence of femoral head avascular necrosis (F-AVN) is 2% to 10% (1–12). Letournel and Judet reported a 3.8% incidence of femoral head AVN (4). Seventeen of the 22 cases were associated with a posterior dislocation of the femoral head. The prevalence of femoral head F-AVN after a fracture associated with a posterior dislocation was 7.5% (17 of 227); after an anterior dislocation it was 1.5% (one of 63); and after a central dislocation it was 1.6% (four of 243). On further analysis of these cases, Letournel and Judet found no correlation with the time to reduction of the femoral head or the quality of the reduction of the acetabulum (4). They stated, "In fact, the fate of the femoral head appears to be decided from the outset. . . ." However, this may not be true of a pure dislocation, which requires an immediate reduction to avoid AVN.

Helfet and Schmeling reported on four patients who developed significant F-AVN (2). Three had transverse-posterior wall acetabular fractures with an associated posterior femoral head dislocation; one of these three was additionally noted to have a fracture of the femoral head (Fig. 40-1). The fourth case was a patient with a T-type acetabular fracture and significant posterior femoral head subluxation. In all four cases, the initial radiologic diagnosis was made 3 to 6 months postoperatively but before progressive clinical deterioration began. Three of these have been converted to total hip arthroplasties. The remaining patient will likely progress to total hip arthroplasty.

One of the major problems with F-AVN is establishing the diagnosis. The differential diagnosis of progressive destruction of the femoral head includes: AVN, posttraumatic arthrosis (malreduction), and intraarticular hardware. Traditional methods of establishing the diagnosis of F-AVN include plain radiography, technetium scintigraphy, or magnetic resonance imaging. None of these can guarantee the diagnosis postoperatively in patients with acetabular fractures. Posttraumatic arthrosis occurred in 10% of Letournel and Judet's cases, even when anatomic reduction was obtained (4). Letournel and Judet made the diagnosis of femoral head F-AVN in 86% of the cases within the first 18 months (4). If radiographs were normal at 18 months, they believed that F-AVN would not occur.

We recommend that the diagnosis of F-AVN of the femoral head be reserved for cases of progressive destruction of the femoral head following anatomic reduction of the acetabulum with no evidence of intraarticular hardware. The diagnosis should be established within the first 18 months after surgery. Other causes of progressive joint space narrowing must be excluded before establishing the diagnosis of femoral head AVN.

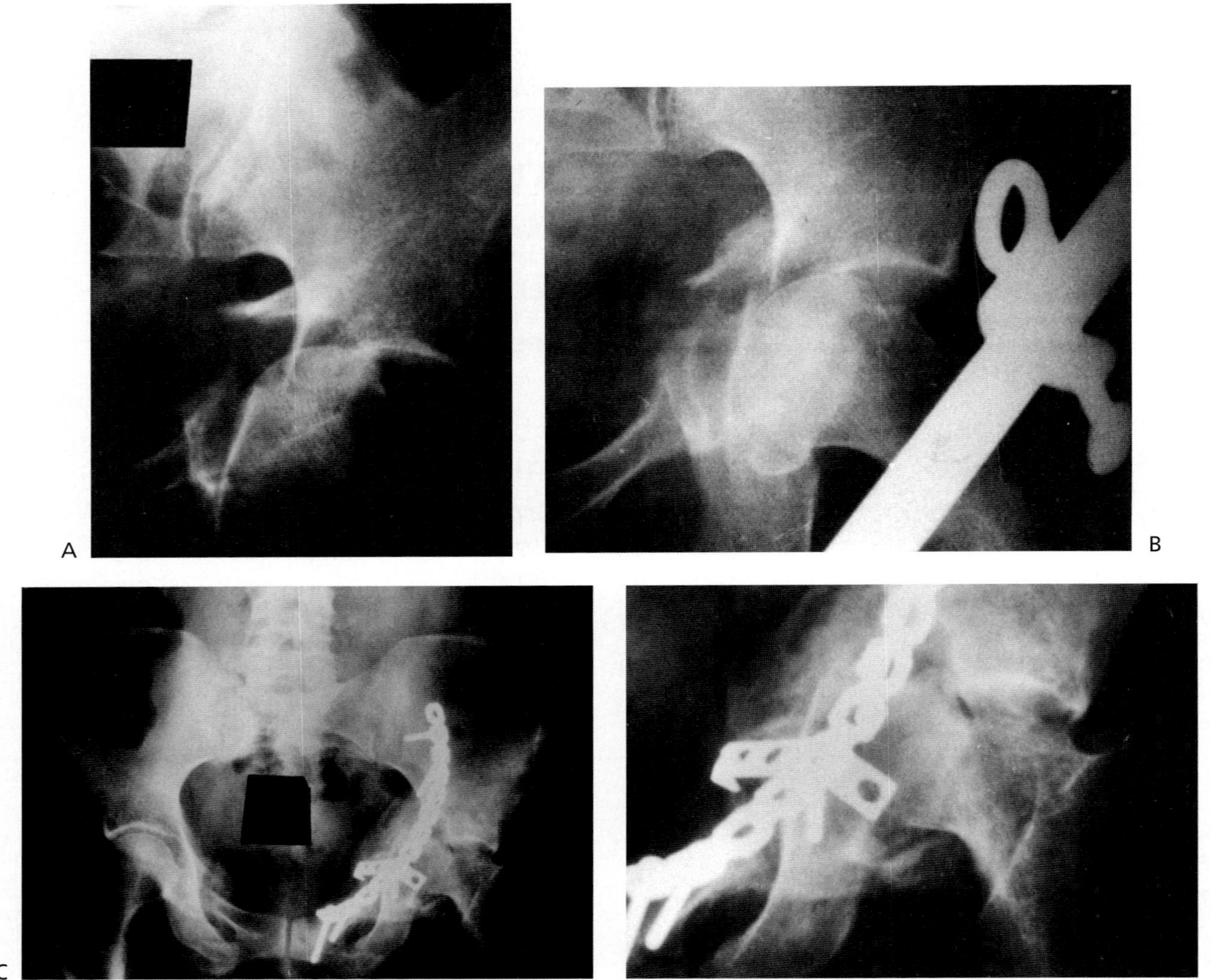

FIGURE 40-1. A left transverse with anterior wall acetabular fracture in a 49-year-old woman. **A,B:** Anterior-posterior pelvis radiographs demonstrate persistent medial subluxation and an impression fracture of the femoral head, despite traction. **C,D:** Anterior-posterior pelvic radiographs at 3 months after open reduction and internal fixation through an ilioinguinal approach demonstrate avascular necrosis of the femoral head and subsequent loss of reduction.

Necrosis of the Acetabulum

The only report in the literature of acetabular avascular necrosis (A-AVN) is by Letournel and Judet (4), who documented three cases of anterior column A-AVN in the first edition of their book. In the second edition after critical reevaluation, two of these cases were found to be the result of intraarticular hardware. The cause of the third case is still in question, but Letournel (4) has labeled this case cartilage necrosis.

Letournel and Judet found three cases of posterior wall AVN associated with F-AVN (4). Intraarticular hardware was found at revision surgery in all three cases. The question they ask is whether the posterior wall crumbled, exposing the hardware, or the F-AVN caused irregular wear of the posterior wall leading to is destruction. They suggested there was no answer to this question. Helfet and Schmeling found no cases that suggested avascular necrosis of the acetabulum (2).

In spite of lack of evidence in the literature, surgeons with a large experience in total hip arthroplasty after acetabular fracture frequently see areas of articular collapse, which in some cases may represent AVN of acetabular fragments.

Devascularization of the iliac wing, especially the anterior column, during extended or combined exposures is certainly a concern. Some of the soft-tissue attachments must be preserved when these types of exposures are used. Soft-tissue stripping of the wing should be done sparingly, as needed, and indirect reduction techniques should be used if possible.

LATE INFECTION

Late infection following acetabular fracture surgery also is a rare complication. Letournel and Judet reported five cases (4). Three cases were diagnosed within a few months of surgery and the other two several years after surgery. Helfet and Schmeling reported only one case (Fig. 40-2) (2). The patient, an immunocompromised man, underwent open reduction and internal fixation of a posterior wall acetabular fracture. The initial postoperative course was benign; however, 4 to 6 months postoperatively the patient began complaining of increasing pain in his hip joint. Radiography showed progressive narrowing of the joint space and, subsequently, some breakdown of the posterior wall. Cultures were obtained from samples obtained through fluoroscopically guided aspiration of the hip joint. *Staphylococcus epidermidis, Enterobacter cloacae,* and *Citrobacter* species were isolated from the culture. The patient required posterior arthrotomy, removal of hardware, drainage, and a prolonged course of antibiotics. Owing to extensive destruction of the hip joint intraarticular and extraarticular hip fusion subsequently were performed. The patient has had no further sequelae.

PSEUDOARTHROSIS

Nonunions are exceedingly rare because of the rich vascularity of the pelvis. Letournel and Judet reported four cases (4) (prevalence 0.7%). Two were both-column fractures, one was a transverse posterior wall fracture, and the fourth was an anterior column posterior hemitransverse fracture. In three cases the transverse component did not heal, and a second operation was undertaken to achieve union. One of the three is doing well. One patient did well for 20 years and then had a total hip arthroplasty. The third result is rated only fair after 1 year. The fourth patient, who did not require a second operation to achieve union, had a total hip arthroplasty at 7 years. Mears and coworkers (8,13) also reported on one case (prevalence 1%) of pseudoarthrosis of the acetabulum following acetabular fracture surgery.

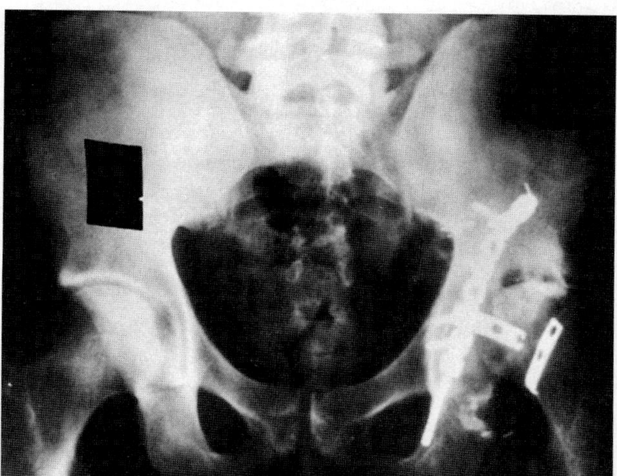

FIGURE 40-2. A left posterior wall acetabular fracture in a 27-year-old man 6 months after open reduction and internal fixation. An anterior-posterior pelvic radiograph demonstrates post-traumatic septic arthritis of the left hip joint.

Nonunions are best managed by revision of the fixation and bone grafting (Fig. 40-3). This is a difficult procedure at best, because of the complex anatomy and previous surgery. Extensive preoperative planning is required. These problems are best managed by surgeons experienced with acetabular fractures.

HETEROTOPIC OSSIFICATION

Heterotopic ossification is a well-recognized complication of acetabular fracture surgery. The reported incidence varies from 3% to 69% (1–12). The lack of consistent use of a single classification scheme makes this rate difficult to interpret. Some authors report only heterotopic ossification that is "significant" (4,14); others report heterotopic ossification only if it resulted in loss of active range of motion >20% of normal (6,15,16). Others use the system developed by Brooker and associates (2,3,6,10,15–18). The Brooker classification is based on a single anterior-posterior radiograph of the involved hip, which is obviously inadequate for this three-dimensional problem. Inclusion in one of the various rating schemes in the preceding seems somewhat arbitrary. In addition, no distinction is made as to whether this is based on a single anterior-posterior view or on additional data obtained from the Judet views or computed tomography (CT).

Heterotopic ossification after an acetabular fracture has been shown to be related to extensile surgical exposures, male sex, associated head injury, significant delays to ORIF, the fracture type, the severity of the injury, and preexisting skeletal conditions (1–7,9,10,14,16,19–25). Heterotopic ossification has also been reported to be a frequent complication of combined anterior and posterior approaches is most common with the extensile exposures; especially those that require greater trochanter osteotomy (Fig. 40-4).

Mears and Rubash (8) reported a 69% prevalence (6% significant) in their series of 100 cases. Ninety-seven of the patients either had a triradiate or extended iliofemoral exposure. Reinert and coworkers (10) reported a prevalence of 25% of Brooker (17) III and IV lesions with the use of their extensile approach and trochanteric osteotomy. Letournel and Judet (4) found an overall rate of 24%; the rate for Brooker III and IV heterotopic ossification (17) was 12%. The incidence varied based on the surgical approach used. The incidence of Brooker III and IV heterotopic ossification for the Kocher-Langenbeck exposure was 10.5%; for the ilioinguinal exposure it was 2%; for the extended iliofemoral it was 35%; and for the combined Kocher-Langenbeck/ilioinguinal exposures it was 27%. Routt and Winquist (26) reported a 54% rate (8% Brooker III and IV) in their 108 cases treated with combined anterior and posterior approaches. Daum and associates (19) described a series where 37 of 38 patients were treated with the Kocher-Langenbeck, triradiate, or combined Kocher-Langenbeck/ilioinguinal surgical exposures. Eighteen of the 38 patients developed some form of heterotopic ossification. Webb and associates (25) reported the results of acetabular fracture reconstruction in head-injured patients. Twenty-two of the 23 patients developed heterotopic ossification. There were seven cases of Brooker III and six cases of Brooker IV heterotopic ossification (17).

Despite aggressive stripping of the iliopsoas muscle from the internal iliac fossa, heterotopic ossification is never significant and almost never is seen inside the pelvis with the ilioinguinal approach. It has been reported in the external iliac fossa with the ilioinguinal approach, probably related to a small extrapelvic extension of the approach for the purpose of applying forceps to the iliac wing for fracture reduction (2,4). In conclusion, from these reports it appears that the amount of heterotopic ossification probably is related directly to trauma to the hip abductor musculature, whether traumatic or iatrogenic-related to intraoperative exposure.

Prophylaxis

Based on the literature for the prevention of heterotopic ossification following total hip arthroplasty, several authors developed series using indomethacin, radiation therapy, or a combination of the two to prevent heterotopic ossification following acetabular fracture surgery. Moed and Maxey (23) reported on their experience using indomethacin, 25 mg p.o. t.i.d., for 6 to 12 weeks beginning on the first postoperative

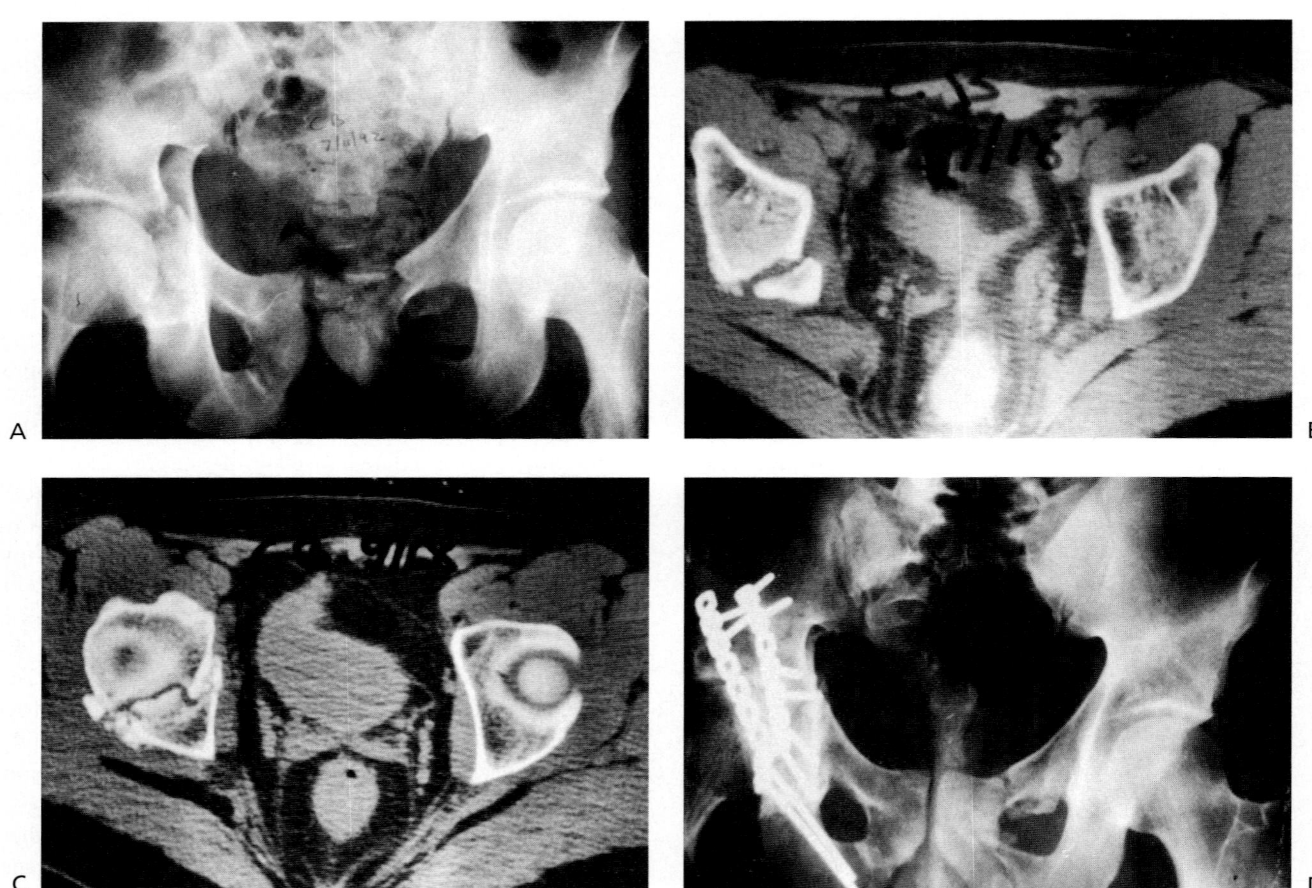

FIGURE 40-3. A right transverse posterior column acetabular fracture in a 22-year-old man resulted in painful nonunion. Because of his multiple injuries, including traumatic thrombosis of the subclavian artery, the fracture was treated conservatively despite persistent displacement of the posterior column with femoral head subluxation. **A:** An anterior-posterior (AP) pelvic radiograph demonstrates nonunion with persistent medial subluxation of the femoral head, whereas computed tomography **(B,C)** of the acetabulum demonstrates the persistent nonunion. **D:** An AP pelvic radiograph 3½ months after surgery indicates healing of the nonunion. At that stage, the patient was bearing full weight and had no pain.

TABLE 40-1. LATE ACETABULAR COMPLICATIONS

Investigator	Cases	Avascular Necrosis (%)	Posttraumatic Osteoarthritis (%)	Heterotopic Ossification (%)	Nonunion (%)
Letournel et al.[a]	569	3.9	17	24.4	0.7
Matta et al.[b]	43	9	NR	NR	NR
Matta[c]	226	NR	NR	11	NR
Matta[d]	259	3	5	18 (9)[m]	0
Mears et al.[e]	100	3	4	69 (6)[n]	1
Goulet et al.[f]	31	3	NR	3	NR
Reinert et al.[g]	20	0 (5)[k]	NR	25[m]	0
Kaempffe et al.[h]	55	10	48	64	NR
Routt et al.[i]	108	2	5	54 (9)[m]	NR
Helfet et al.[j]	84	4	23[l]	2	0

[a] Letournel E, Judet R. *Fractures of the Acetabulum,* 2nd ed. Berlin: Springer-Verlag, 1993.
[b] Matta JM, Anderson LM, Epstein HC, et al. Fractures of the acetabulum: a retrospective analysis. *Clin Orthop* 1986;205:230–240.
[c] Matta JM. *Immediate and long term results of surgical treatment of acetabular fractures.* Presented at the first International Symposium on Surgical Treatment of Acetabular Fractures. Paris, May, 1993.
[d] Matta JM. Fractures of the acetabulum: accuracy of reduction and clinical results in patients managed operatively within three weeks after injury. *J Bone Joint Surg* 1996;78-A:1632–1645.
[e] Mears DC, Rubash HE, Sawaguchi T. Fractures of the acetabulum. The hip. *Proceedings of the thirteenth open scientific meeting of the hip society.* St. Louis: CV Mosby, 1985:95–113.
[f] Goulet JA, Bray TJ. Complex acetabular fractures. *Clin Orthop* 1989;240:9–20.
[g] Reinert CM, Bosse MJ, Poka A. et al. A modified extensile exposure for the treatment of complex or malunited acetabular fractures. *J Bone Joint Surg* 1988;70-A:329–337.
[h] Kaempffe FA, Bone LA, Border JR, et al. Operative fixation of displaced acetabular fractures: a retrospective review. *Orthop Trans* 1988; 12:527.
[i] Routt MLC Jr, Swiontkowski MF. Operative treatment of complex acetabular fractures: combined anterior and posterior exposures during the same procedure. *J Bone Joint Surg* 1990;72-A:897–904.
[j] Helfet DL, Schmeling GJ. Management of acute, displaced acetabular fractures using indirect reduction techniques and limited approaches. *Orthop Trans* 1991;15:833–834.
[k] Acetabular atrioventricular necrosis.
[l] Prevalence with satisfactory reduction, 17%; unsatisfactory reduction, 80%.
[m] Loss of motion >20%.
[n] Significant heterotopic ossification.

day. They found the overall incidence of heterotopic ossification to be similar in both the control and the treated groups; however, the rate of Brooker III and IV heterotopic ossification was significantly reduced in the indomethacin-treated group. They also noted no significant complications related to the use of indomethacin. In a follow-up study, Moed and Karges (27) noted that the maximal extent of heterotopic ossification was evident by 6 weeks postoperatively. These authors also found that, in patients receiving indomethacin, the grade of heterotopic ossification did not progress following discontinuance of the drug. McLaren (14) reported his experience with indomethacin, 25 mg p.o. t.i.d. for 6 weeks beginning postoperatively. The overall rate of heterotopic ossification was 65% in the control group and 50% in the treated group. The incidence of Brooker 13 III/IV in the control group was 38%, whereas in the treated group it was 0%. Only one patient stopped taking the medication because of gastritis. Letournel and Judet (4) in their series, found the overall incidence of heterotopic ossification to be 25% (Brooker III/IV, 11%) when no prophylaxis was used. The overall incidence fell to 10% (Brooker III/IV, 2%) when indomethacin was used for prophylaxis of heterotopic ossification. Matta and Siebenrock (21) used plain radiographs and volumetric CT analysis to determine the extent of the heterotopic ossification following acetabular fracture fixation. Patients were randomized into two groups: indomethacin and no prophylaxis. The surgical exposures in the indomethacin group were: Kocher-Langenbeck, 22; extended iliofemoral, 14. In the control group the exposures were 15 and 16, respectively. The overall incidence of heterotopic ossification on plain radiographs in the indomethacin group was 62% (Brooker II, III or IV, 9%), and in the control group it was 62% (Brooker II, III, IV, 5%). The volumetric CT results for the heterotopic ossification were: indomethacin group 1.7 cm^3 and 3.6 cm^3. These differences were not significant.

Bosse and colleagues (28) reported on their experience using 1,000 rad of radiation therapy (200 rad each day for 5 days beginning on the third postoperative day). They found the overall incidence of heterotopic ossification decreased from 90% in the control group to 50% in the treated group; the incidence of Brooker III and IV heterotopic ossification decreased from 50% in the control group to 11% in the treated group. They reported no complications that could be attributed specifically to the radiation therapy protocol. Daum and associates (19) found Brooker III/IV heterotopic ossification in six of 24 patients who did not receive radiation therapy and in 0 of 14 who had radiation therapy for heterotopic ossification.

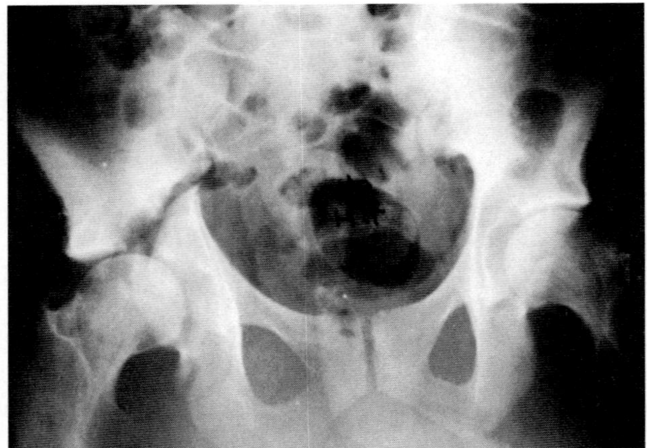
A

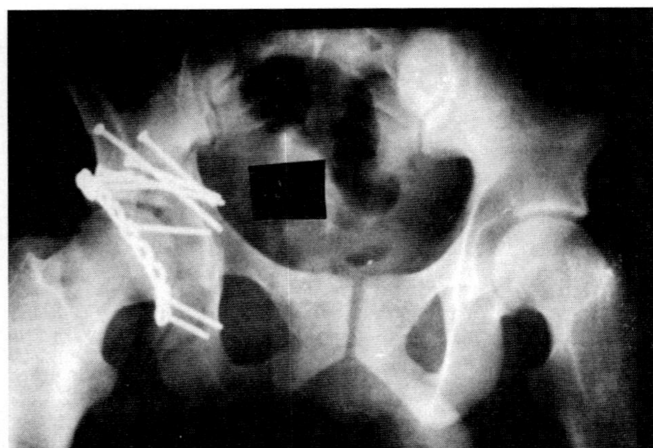
B

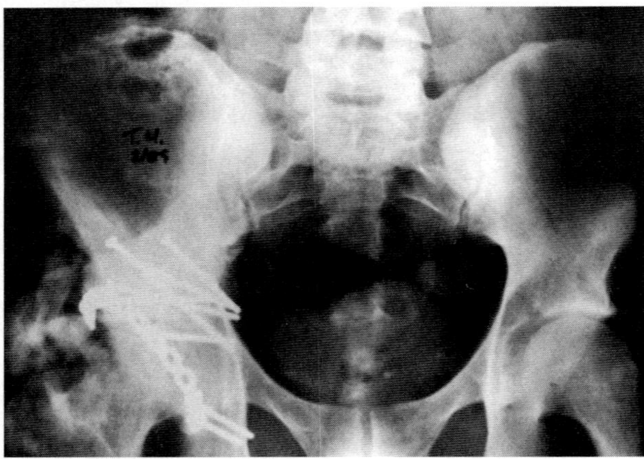
C

FIGURE 40-4. A 32-year-old man sustained a right transverse posterior acetabular fracture plus multiple other orthopedic and visceral injuries. He was transferred late for surgical treatment of the acetabular fracture, necessitating an extensile (extended iliofemoral) approach. **A:** An anterior-posterior (AP) pelvic radiograph demonstrates a transverse posterior wall acetabular fracture. **B:** A postoperative AP pelvis radiograph demonstrates open reduction and internal fixation through an extensile (extended iliofemoral) approach. **C:** An AP pelvic radiograph 5 months after surgery demonstrates Brooker III heterotopic ossification despite indomethacin prophylaxis.

Moed and Letournel (22) reported their experience using both radiation therapy and indomethacin for the prevention of heterotopic ossification. In their series, the overall incidence of heterotopic ossification was 18%. The incidence of Brooker III/IV heterotopic ossification was 0%. The combination of therapies nearly eliminated all heterotopic ossification. The risks involved for both therapies must be weighed carefully against this benefit.

Haas and coworkers (29) reviewed their experience with radiation therapy for heterotopic ossification prophylaxis in acetabular fracture surgery. They compared two protocols: 10 Gy administered in five 2-Gy doses (33 patients) and a single 8-Gy dose (11 patients). An additional three patients received 6 to 7 Gy in a single dose. Forty-four of the 47 patients began or received their treatment <48 hours after surgery. The overall incidence of heterotopic ossification was 51% (24 of 47). There were six cases of Brooker III heterotopic ossification and no cases of Brooker IV. There was no statistical difference between the two protocols. A single fraction of 7 to 8 Gy within 24 to 48 hours of surgery significantly reduced the incidence of clinically significant heterotopic ossification.

Schneider and coworkers (30) looked at heterotopic ossification prophylaxis after total hip arthroplasty in an animal model. They looked at the efficacy of preoperative and postoperative radiation; specifically, at the timing of prophylaxis and a dose–response relationship for single-fraction radiation prophylaxis in a rabbit model. They found that 8 Gy was the minimal effective dose for single-fraction prophylaxis and that postoperative radiation therapy was effective in prevention of heterotopic ossification. They also found that the closer to the time of surgery that preoperative radiation was given the more heterotopic ossification resulted. There was a significant difference between animals dosed at 24 hours preoperative and those dosed at 4 hours preoperative. Preoperative, single dose of radiation therapy may be the future of heterotopic ossification prophylaxis.

Moore and colleagues (31) reported the results of a randomized prospective protocol comparing radiation therapy and indomethacin for the prevention of heterotopic ossification. There were 33 patients in the radiation group and 39 in the indomethacin group. All heterotopic ossification was present by 6 weeks. The incidence of Brooker III heterotopic ossification (17) in the radiation group was 9% and in the indomethacin group it was 13%. The incidence of Brooker IV heterotopic ossification in the radiation group was 0% and in the indomethacin group it was 5%. There was no significant difference between groups. The authors noted that the two patients in the indomethacin group with Brooker heterotopic ossification (17) failed to receive proper doses of the drug and that radiation therapy was 200 times more expensive.

Potential complications of irradiating the pelvis and its contents include radiation-induced malignant degeneration, sterility, and genetic alterations to sperm or ova. Although these possibilities are exceedingly remote, patients must be well informed of the risks. The complications associated with the use of indomethacin and other nonsteroidal antiinflammatory drugs include the well-known side effects of the medications. There can be gastrointestinal disturbances, coagulopathies, or allergic reactions, among others, and the theoretical potential for delayed union of the fracture. Decreased new bone formation, impaired fracture healing, decreased torsional strength of healing bone, and inhibition of haversian bone remodeling in a rabbit model have been reported (23,27,32).

We currently recommend the use of indomethacin, 25-mg tablets three times per day for 6 weeks or a single 75-mg sustained release capsule per day for 6 weeks. If heterotopic ossification appears in the first 6 weeks, then the indomethacin is continued for a total of 12 weeks after surgery. The indomethacin is begun on postoperative day one for all posterior exposures, all extended exposures, and any anterior exposures in which extrapelvic placement of clamps was used.

If indomethacin is not tolerated or is contraindicated or other risk factors are present, radiation therapy is recommended. We currently use 7 to 8 Gy in a single dose or 10 Gy in five divided doses. The radiation therapy is begun within 24 to 72 hours of surgery.

Treatment

Heterotopic ossification requires surgical resection only if it has functional significance (i.e., significant limitation of hip motion or hip ankylosis). Traditionally, surgical resection should be delayed until the heterotopic bone has reached full maturity. This has been assessed clinically, radiographically, by monitoring serum alkaline phosphatase levels, and by technetium bone scintigraphy. Newer information suggests that early resection may be considered. Radiation therapy should be used in conjunction with early resection.

Planning for the surgical resection should include CT to determine the exact location of the heterotopic bone, how much bone is present, and the location of anatomic structures that may be at risk during the surgery (e.g., sciatic nerve, femoral artery). CT also can be used to assess the quality of the remaining articular surface of the hip joint. Surgical resection is recommended for patients with minimal posttraumatic arthrosis. Prophylaxis against recurrence should consist of radiation therapy alone, indomethacin combined with radiation therapy, or perhaps, indomethacin alone. Patients must be cautioned that excision of the heterotopic bone does not guarantee that it will not recur or that a normal range of hip motion can be restored.

CARTILAGE NECROSIS

Cartilage necrosis is defined as painful hip motion with concomitant early (6 to 12 months postoperative) progressive joint space narrowing without alteration in the underlying femoral head or acetabular bone (Fig. 40-5). Intraarticular hardware and infection must be ruled out before progressive joint space narrowing is called "cartilage necrosis." In Letournel and Judet's (4) series, the prevalence was 1% (six of 569). They describe two cases of progressive joint space loss that were labeled cartilage necrosis but later were found to be a result of intraarticular hardware. That is a missed diagnosis rate of 25% (two of eight). Postoperative CT scanning has made this diagnosis much easier.

Treatment for cartilage necrosis is mainly supportive. After the possibility of infection and intraarticular hardware is excluded, physical therapy and antiinflammatory agents may be helpful. The outcome the patient can expect with this complication is fair to poor, with likely progression to total hip arthroplasty (4).

POSTTRAUMATIC OSTEOARTHROSIS

Osteophytes

Letournel and Judet (4) describe a collar of osteophytes that may form around the femoral head and neck following acetabular fracture surgery. The majority of these small, discrete osteophytes were clinically insignificant in the short term. The clinical significance of the collar was unpredictable; however, the appearance of this collar of osteophytes was a negative prognostic sign in the early postoperative period and may be the forerunner of clinical osteoarthritis.

Osteoarthritis

The reported prevalence of osteoarthritis ranges from 4% to 48% (1–12). Letournel and Judet (4) reported an overall rate of posttraumatic osteoarthritis of 17%. The incidence following perfect reduction was 10% and that following imperfect reduction was 36%. Of the 113 cases in which osteoarthritis developed, 16 were a result of infection or AVN and 45 were a result of imperfect reduction. Five were related to intraarticular hardware, two to femoral head injuries noted at the time of surgery, and one owed to failure of fixation. The remaining 45 had no identifiable cause. Some of these patients developed arthritis many years after their injury. The investigators felt that some of these cases may not have been related to the injury or its treatment. Letournel and Judet (4) also found the peak onset of arthritis was 10 years earlier in those patients with an imperfect reduction as

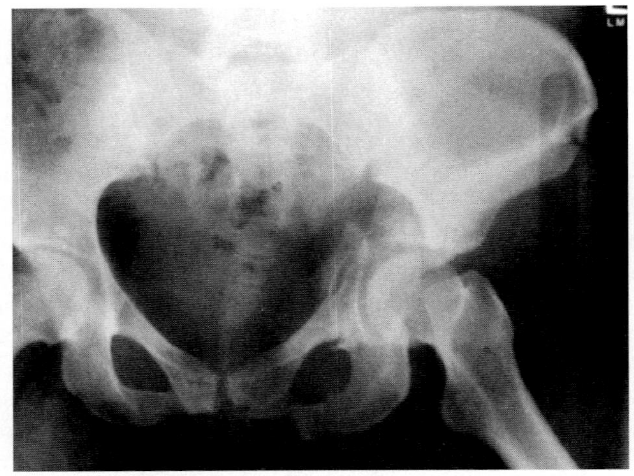

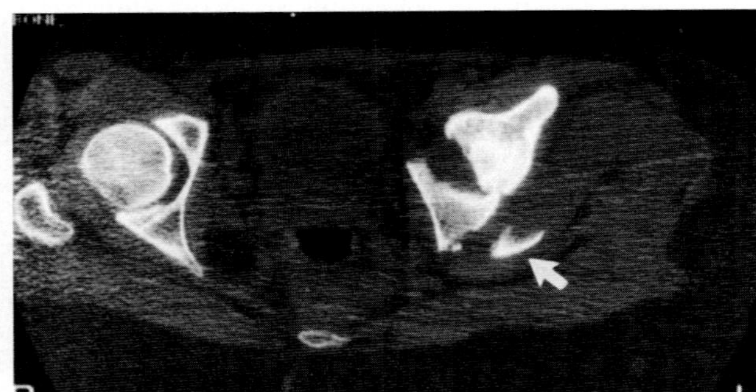

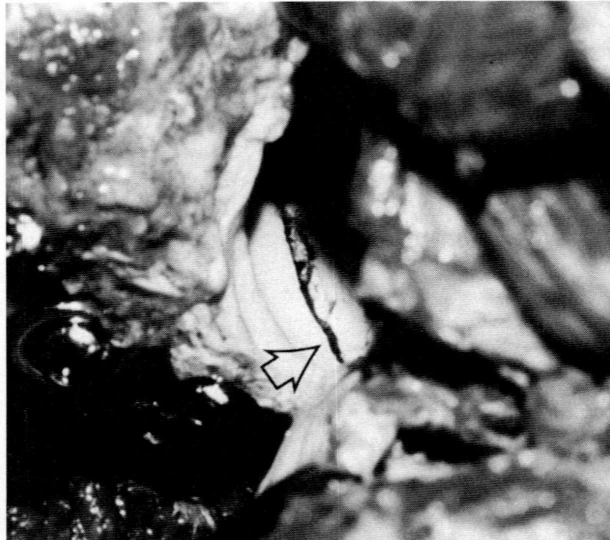

FIGURE 40-5. A: A both-column fracture in a 19-year-old woman injured in a motor vehicle accident. **B:** Computed tomography shows the coronal split characteristic of this pattern and the spur sign *(white arrow)*. **C:** Open reduction and internal fixation was performed through a modified ilioinguinal approach. Note the inspection of the acetabulum, the excellent reduction, and no metal in the joint. **D–F:** Immediate postoperative radiographs show excellent anatomic reduction. The patient did well clinically for 6 months and then developed severe pain.

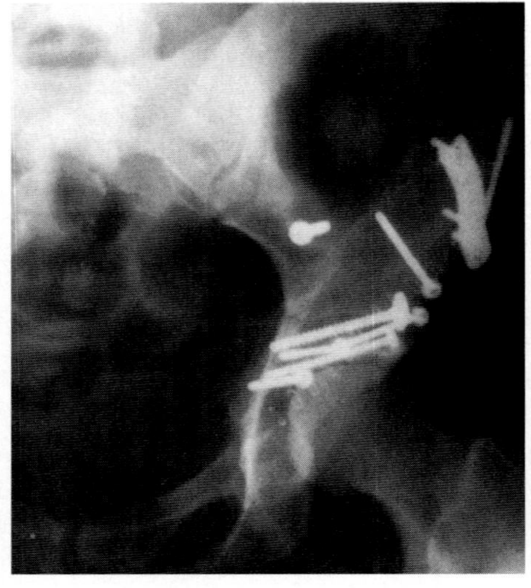

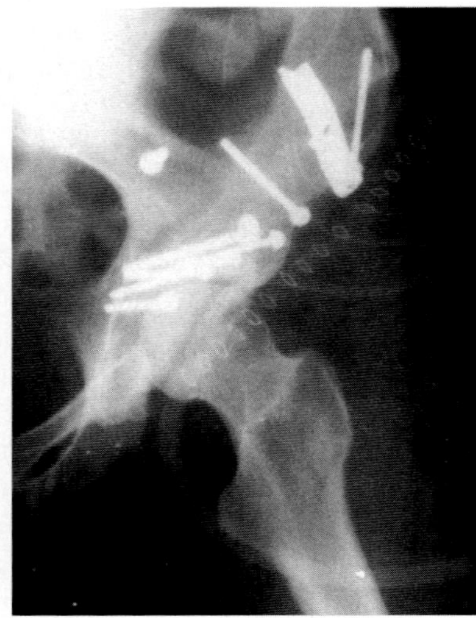

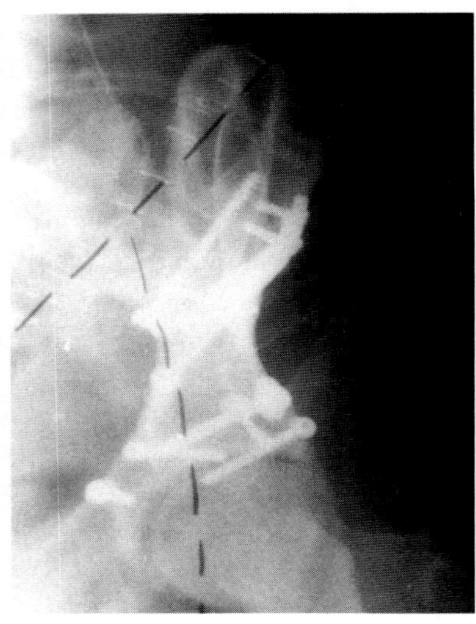

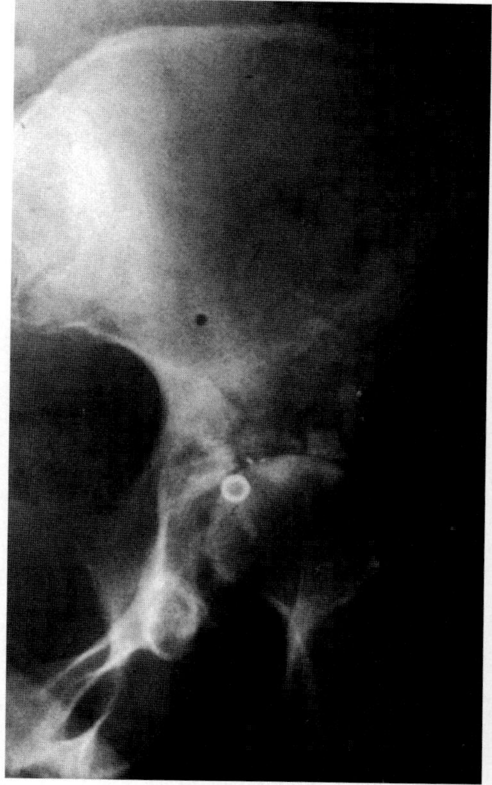

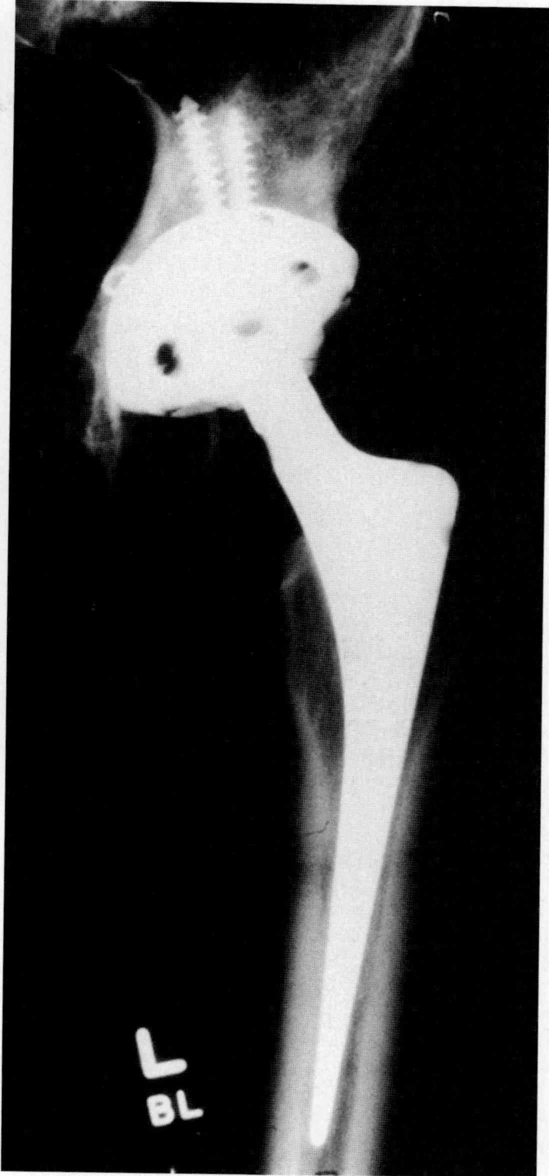

FIGURE 40-5. ***(continued)*** **G:** Cartilage necrosis was diagnosed. When the metal was removed, no metal was found in the joint. **H:** Because of the severe joint destruction, the patient underwent total hip arthroplasty.

compared with those whose reduction was perfect but who nevertheless developed arthritis.

Ragnarsson and Mjöberg (9) retrospectively reviewed the results of surgical reconstruction of acetabular fractures. Arthritis was defined as loss of joint space >50% when compared to the other side. In their series, the prevalence of arthritis with anatomic reduction was 18%. When the fracture was reduced to within 1 to 3 mm, the prevalence of arthritis rose to 58%, and with more than 3 mm of remaining displacement it was 100%. The diagnosis of posttraumatic arthritis was made within 24 months in 88% of the cases and within 32 months in 96%.

To establish the diagnosis of posttraumatic arthritis as a result of an acetabular fracture other possible causes—infection, AVN, intraarticular hardware, or loss of reduction—malunion must be ruled out. The consensus among acetabular fracture surgeons is that restoration of the femoral head under the weight-bearing dome of the acetabulum and restoration of joint congruency is the best prophylaxis against posttraumatic arthritis. Anatomic reduction offers the best chance for a good long-term outcome. As with any osteoarthritis of the hip joint, treatment should be directed to the patient and not the radiograph. Radiographic changes in an asymptomatic patient need not be addressed.

The long-term incidence of osteoarthritis following acetabular fracture is not known at this time, because the insult to the articular surface may not manifest for many years. As with conditions such as Legge-Perthes disease, where the osteoarthritis of the hip may develop after 40-50 years, the same may also be true for the acetabular fracture.

CONCLUSION

High-energy acetabular fractures have the potential for significant morbidity and possible mortality. Many perioperative complications are a consequence of the injury and thereby are unavoidable. However, a number of complications can be influenced by the surgeon with subsequent improved patient outcomes. Acetabular fracture surgery is demanding. Anatomic reduction of the weight-bearing surface of the acetabulum, congruent reduction of the femoral head, timely surgical intervention, and both awareness and avoidance of perioperative complications are the keys to success and acceptable long-term patient outcomes.

REFERENCES

1. Goulet JA, Bray TJ. Complex acetabular fractures. *Clin Orthop* 1989;240:9–20.
2. Helfet DL, Schmeling GJ. Managment of acute, displaced acetabular fractures using indirect reduction techniques and limited approaches. *Orthop Trans* 1991;15:833–834.
3. Kaempffe FA, Bone LA, Border JR, et al. Operative fixation of displaced acetabular fractures: a retrospective review. *Orthop Trans* 1988;12:527.
4. Letournel E, Judet R. *Fractures of the acetabulum,* 2nd ed. Berlin: Springer-Verlag, 1993.
5. Matta JM. Acetabulum fractures: results of a combined operative and nonoperative protocol. Presented at the fifty-eighth AAOS annual meeting. Anaheim, CA, 1991.
6. Matta JM. Preliminary results of a prospective randomized study using prophylactic indomethacin. Presented at the first International Symposium on Surgical Treatment of Acetabular Fractures. Paris, France, 1993.
7. Matta JM, Letournel E, Browner BD. *Surgical management of acetabular fractures.* Instructional course lectures, 35th ed. St. Louis: CV Mosby, 1986:382–397.
8. Mears DC, Rubash HE. Extensile exposure of the pelvis. *Contemp Orthop* 1983;6:21–31.
9. Ragnarsson B, Mjöberg B. Arthrosis after surgically treated acetabular fractures. *Acta Orthop Scand* 1992;63:511–514.
10. Reinert CM, Bosse MJ, Poka A, et al. A modified extensile exposure for the treatment of complex or malunited acetabular fractures. *J Bone Joint Surg* 1988;70-A:329–337.
11. Salzman EW, McManama GP, Shapiro AH, et al. Effect of optimization of hemodynamics on fibrinolytic activity and antithrombotic efficacy of external pneumatic calf compression. *Ann Surg* 1987;206:636–641.
12. Tile M. *Fractures of the pelvis and acetabulum,* 1st ed. Baltimore: Williams & Wilkins, 1984.
13. Mears DC, Rubash HE, Sawaguchi T. *Fractures of the acetabulum. The hip.* Proceedings of the thirteenth open scientific meeting of the Hip Society. St. Louis: CV Mosby, 1985:95–113.
14. McLaren AC. Prophylaxis with indomethacin for heterotopic bone. After open reduction of fractures of the acetabulum. *J Bone Joint Surg* 1990;72-A:245–247.
15. Matta JM. Operative indications and choice of surgical approach for fractures of the acetabulum. *Tech Orthop* 1986;1:13–22.
16. Matta JM, Mehne DK, Roffi R. Fractures of the acetabulum: early results of a prospective study. *Clin Orthop* 1986;205: 241–250.
17. Brooker AF, Bowerman JW, Robinson RA, et al. Ectopic ossification following total hip replacement: Incidence and a method of classification. *J Bone Joint Surg* 1973;55-A:1629–1632.
18. Routt MLC Jr, Swiontkowski MF. Operative treatment of complex acetabular fractures: combined anterior and posterior exposures during the same procedure. *J Bone Joint Surg* 1990;72-A:897–904.
19. Daum WJ, Scarborough MT, Gordon W Jr, et al. Heterotopic ossification and other perioperative complications of acetabular fractures. *J Orthop Trauma* 1992;6:427–432.
20. Ghalambor N, Matta JM, Bernstein L. Heterotopic ossification following operative treatment of acetabular fractures. *Clin Orthop* 1994;305:96–105.
21. Matta JM, Siebenrock KA. Does indomethacin reduce heterotopic bone formation after operations for acetabular fractures? A prospective study. *J Bone Joint Surg* 1997;79-B:959–963.
22. Moed BR, Letournel E. Low-dose irradiation and indomethacin prevent heterotopic ossification after acetabular fracture surgery. *J Bone Joint Surg* 1994;76-B:895–900.
23. Moed BR, Maxey JW. The effect of indomethacin on heterotopic ossification following acetabular fracture surgery. *J Orthop Trauma* 1993;7:33–38.
24. Vrahas M, Gordon RG, Mears DC, et al. Intraoperative somatosensory evoked potential monitoring of pelvic and acetabular fractures. *J Orthop Trauma* 1992;6:50–58.
25. Webb LX, Bosse MJ, Mayo KA, et al. Results in patients with craniocerebral trauma and operatively managed acetabular fracture. *J Orthop Trauma* 1990;4:376–382.
26. Routt MLC Jr, Winquist RA. *The treatment of 108 consecutive complex acetabular fractures using combined, simultaneous anterior and posterior surgical approaches at the same anesthesia.* Presented at the fifth OTA annual meeting. Philadelphia, October, 1989.
27. Moed BR, Karges DE. Prophylactic indomethacin for the prevention of heterotopic ossification following acetabular fracture surgery in high-risk patients. *J Orthop Trauma* 1994;8:34–39.
28. Bosse MJ, Poka A, Reinert CM, et al. Preoperative angiographic assessment of the superior gluteal artery in acetabular fractures requiring extensile surgical exposures. *J Orthop Trauma* 1989;2: 303–307.
29. Haas ML, Kennedy AS, Copeland CC, et al. Utility of radiation in the prevention of heterotopic ossification following repair of traumatic acetabular fracture. *Int J Radiat Oncol Biol Phys* 1999;45:461–466.
30. Schneider DJ, Moulton MJR, Singapuri K, et al. Inhibition of heterotopic ossification with radiation therapy in an animal model. *Clin Orthop* 1998;355:35–46.
31. Moore KD, Goss K, Anglen JO. Indomethacin versus radiation therapy for prophylaxis against heterotopic ossification in acetabular fractures. A randomised, prospective study. *J Bone Joint Surg* 1998;80-B:259–263.
32. Tile M, Joyce M, Kellam JF. Fractures of the acetabulum: classification, management protocol, and early results of treatment. *Orthop Trans* 1984;8:390.

41

SURGICAL MANAGEMENT OF DELAYED ACETABULAR FRACTURES

ERIC E. JOHNSON

Surgical reconstruction of acute displaced acetabular fractures has become the accepted treatment of choice for achieving the best long-term results following injury (1–7). Similarly, surgical reconstruction ranges from stabilization of simple wall fracture to the use of extensile approaches and multiple planes of fixation for the complex fracture types. It is generally accepted that acetabular fracture surgery should be performed relatively early when the patient has stabilized and the potential for surgical complications has been minimized (1–7). The surgeon should have an excellent knowledge of the anatomy and possess the expertise to stabilize these fractures with the minimum amount of operative trauma.

The operative treatment of acetabular fractures may achieve >80% good to excellent results if stabilized within 14 days of injury in most cases (1–4,6–8). As the time from injury to reduction and stabilization increases beyond 21 days definite changes occur in the surrounding soft-tissue envelope, scar tissue formation increases between bony fragments and the absence or resorption of acute fracture lines becomes prevalent. These factors result in a more difficult exposure, reduction, and stabilization and a decrease in good to excellent long-term results (1–5). Fracture surfaces remodel and lose their anatomic fit, fracture gaps fill with maturing fibrous tissue and callus formation and the muscles attached to individual fragments shorten because of loss of position and counterbalancing forces attainable only when the fragments are reduced in their anatomic position (Fig. 41-1).

Letournel divided acetabular fracture surgery into three time periods following injury (4,5). These time periods include from injury to 21 days, from 21 days to 120 days and >120 days following fracture. Fractures stabilized between 21 to 120 days usually possess some recognizable fracture lines that help in final reduction of the bony fragments. After 120 days these fracture lines become indistinguishable and malunion becomes the most difficult problem to correct. With ever-increasing delay in stabilization, the lack of anatomic joint motion may also produce detrimental effects on both acetabular and femoral head cartilage. The major difficulties encountered in treating acetabular fractures beyond 3 weeks from injury are related to these preceding changes. More than one surgical approach may be required for delayed reconstruction as mobilization of malunited or overriding pubic rami fractures or associated fracture dislocations of the sacroiliac joint or fractures of the iliac wing may become necessary for reduction of the acetabular fracture. Simple fracture patterns may require a more extensile approach with less likelihood of anatomic reduction with delayed reconstruction. Whereas an ilioinguinal or Kocher-Langenbeck operative exposure would have provided sufficient access to the corresponding fracture pattern within 2 weeks of injury an extended iliofemoral approach may be required to completely mobilize a similar fracture pattern after 3 or more weeks of delayed surgical intervention. A delay in acetabular reconstruction may also be detrimental to femoral head viability especially if there is persistent dislocation or subluxation (4,5). Recurrent subluxation of the hip erodes cartilage of both the acetabulum and femoral head. There is an increase in both the incidence of chondrolysis as well as femoral head or posterior wall necrosis with delayed reconstruction of acetabular fracture (1–4,9).

The choice of operative approach in delayed reconstruction depends to a great degree on the specific fracture pattern involved. Anterior column and wall fractures may be stabilized through the ilioinguinal approach even after significant delays in operative treatment. The Kocher-Langenbeck approach for isolated posterior column or wall fractures may also provide sufficient exposure even following prolonged delays in treatment. The use of these incisions for more complex associated fracture patterns may compromise the ability to completely mobilize and reduce all fracture lines. It often is required to use the extended iliofemoral to accomplish reduction of these fractures after significant delay in treatment. Double exposures using the Kocher-Langenbeck and ilioinguinal are infrequently used and abandoned after experience

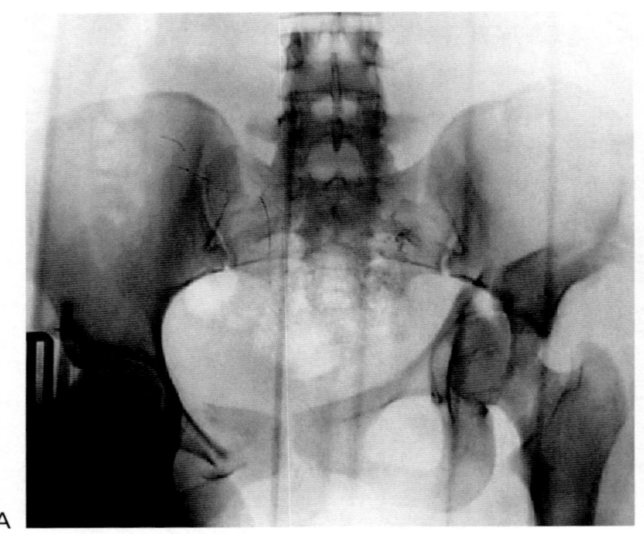

A

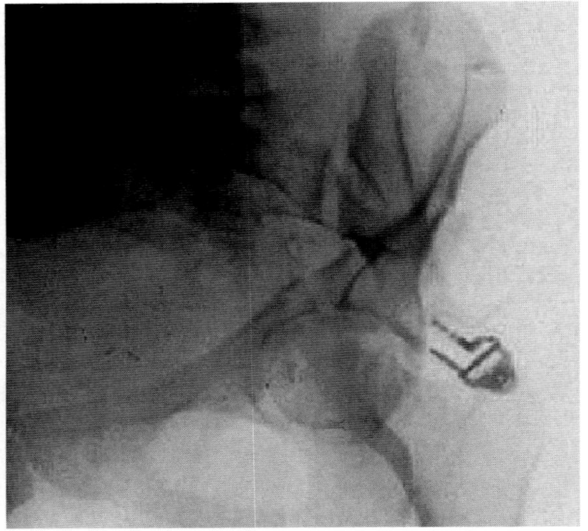

C

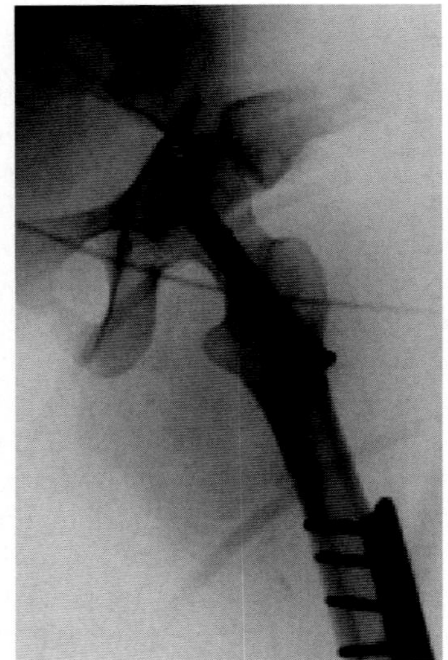

B

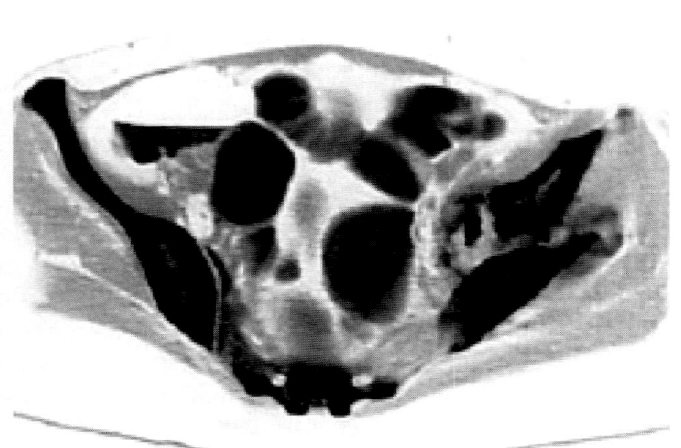

D

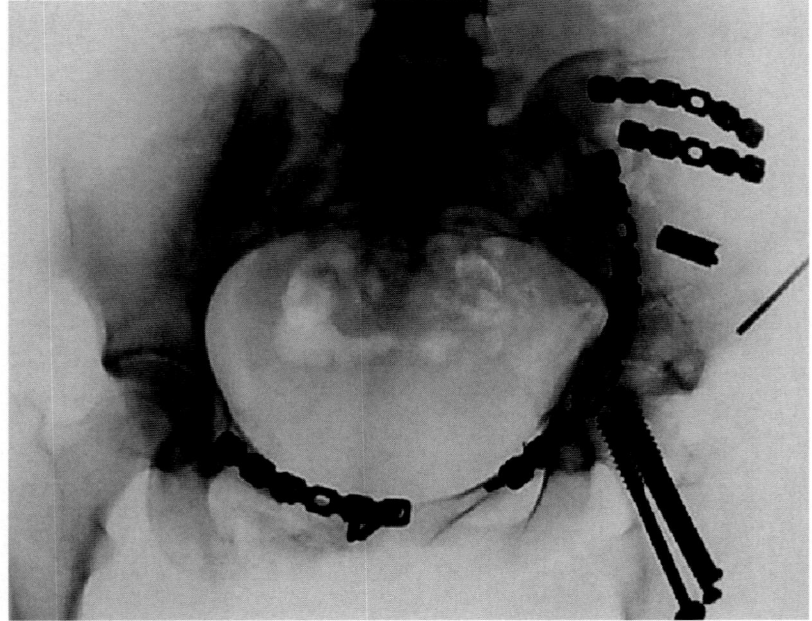

E

FIGURE 41-1. A: Anterior-posterior (AP) radiograph of a left anterior column hemitransverse fracture, open left sacroiliac joint, and ipsilateral femoral neck and shaft fracture at 5 weeks postinjury. The patient suffered severe head injury necessitating delay in operative intervention. **B:** Iliac oblique preoperative radiograph left hip. **C:** Obturator oblique preoperative radiograph. **D:** Computed tomography scan indicating presence of significant callus formation between fragments. **E:** AP radiograph 4 years postoperative management of left acetabular fracture through ilioinguinal approach. A second approach was necessary to mobilize right pubic rami fracture.

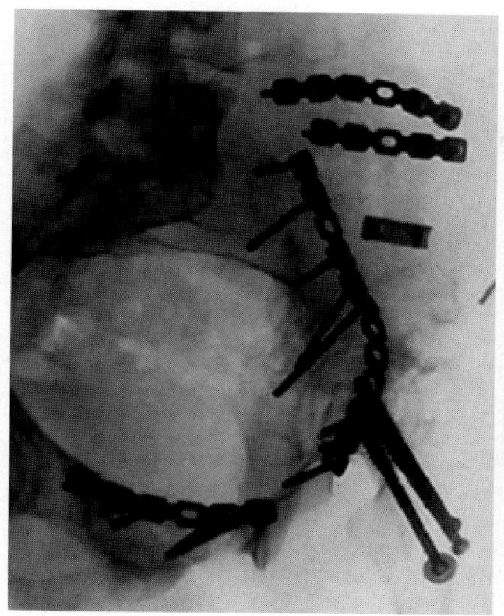
F

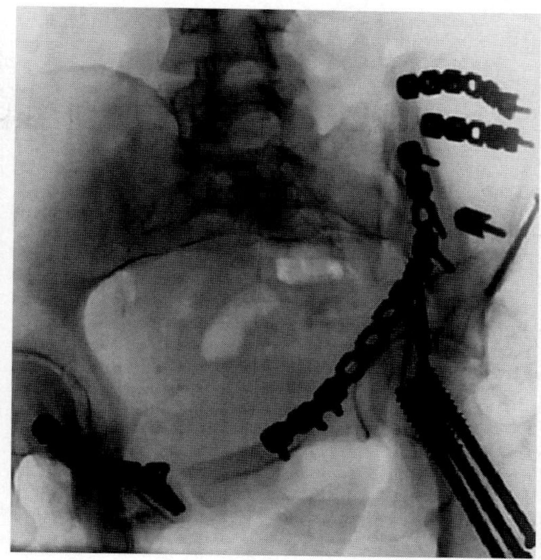
G

FIGURE 41-1. ***(continued)*** **F:** Iliac oblique radiograph at 4 years. **G:** Obturator oblique radiograph at 4 years.

determined that the extended iliofemoral approach offered better access, a higher prevalence of anatomic reduction and stable fixation of the acetabulum. The extended iliofemoral was not described until 1974 by Letournel and Judet (8) and since that time has been used more frequently in delayed surgical reconstruction especially in both-column fractures (4,5). Both the anterior and posterior fracture components of the acetabulum can be controlled using this approach in addition to exposure of both the external and internal aspects of the iliac wing.

If fracture lines are visible and no significant callus formation has occurred the techniques of fragment debridement and reduction with appropriate internal fixation are not significantly different from surgery performed less than 3 weeks from injury. The fragment surfaces are debrided of scar and new callus formation to facilitate anatomic reduction. Care must be used to maintain soft-tissue attachments to small associated wall fragments to avoid devitalization and necrosis of these fragments with loss of reduction and eventual subluxation of the joint. A capsulotomy to gain visualization of the articular surface is helpful in assessing reduction. These cleaned fracture surfaces are irregular and more difficult to anatomically position but once the appropriate reduction is accomplished the standard osteosynthesis is performed.

In the presence of nonunion or malunion, the fibrous tissue is excised or the fragment osteotomized to allow reconstruction. Fractures lines will still be present in the articular cartilage even though they are indistinguishable on the cortical bone surface. An osteotomy through the articular surface followed by resection of the intervening wedge of new bone formation may be necessary to correctly reposition the fracture fragments. Further wedge resections of callus may be necessary to achieve a spherical reconstruction of the acetabulum. Transverse fractures may develop malunion of the anterior fracture line and nonunion of the posterior fragments. A combination of resection of the posterior scar tissue and osteotomy of the anterior malunion is required in this fracture pattern. Multiple trial reductions may be required to align the fragments into their anatomic position. Intraoperative radiography may be necessary to evaluate reduction prior to completion of the osteosynthesis.

Femoral head dislocation or subluxation associated with posterior wall fragments may be especially difficult to mobilize. Isolated posterior wall fracture dislocations also may present difficulty in determining what is malunion bone and where does the wall fragment cortical margin begin. These wall fragments must be separated from new callus formation, freed of associated fibrous tissue and the surgeon must attempt to preserve capsular soft tissue attachments to maintain viability of the wall fragments. Difficulty arises when these fragments are small or multiple in nature and provided no option for stabilization with lag screw fixation. Stabilization of these small wall fragments by multiple lag screws has a high prevalence of intraarticular screw penetration. It may become necessary to stabilize these fragments with "spring plates" reinforced with standard 3.5-mm reconstruction plates (8). Anterior release of contracted capsule or muscle attachments also may be necessary to maintain a concentric reduction and reduce both the tendency for redislocation and the abnormal stress concentration to the femoral head from the posterior wall reconstruction. Preoperative evaluation of all fractures requires the standard Judet radiographic views (anterior-posterior pelvis, 45 degrees internal and external oblique pelvic views). Three-dimensional reconstructed computer axial tomography or coronal and sagittal reconstructed computed tomography (CT) scanning provide the surgeon with additional information crucial to operative decision making. The presence of callus between fracture fragments on CT scan images in-

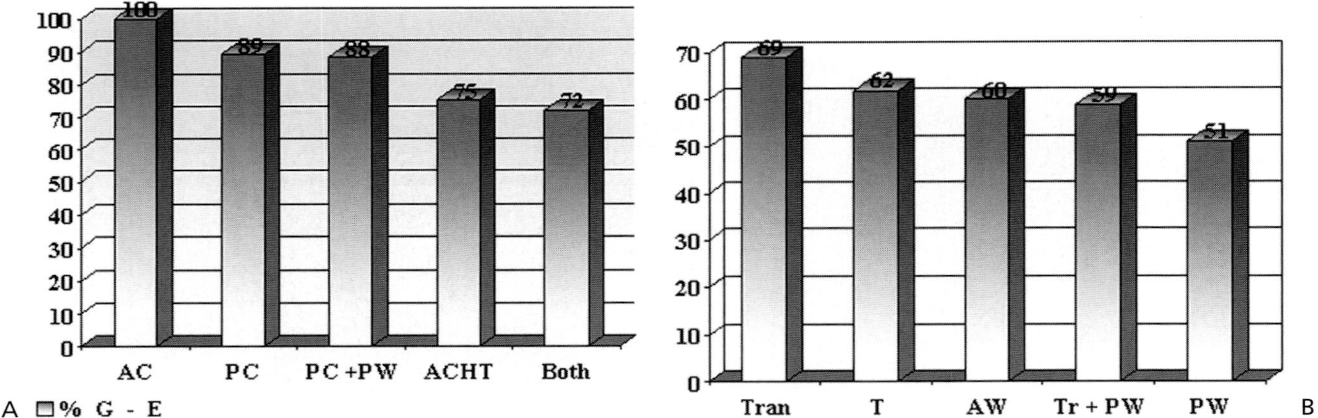

FIGURE 41-2. A: Histogram indicating percentage of good to excellent results in delayed treatment of acetabular fracture in decreasing incidence by diagnosis. **B:** Histogram of decreasing percentage of good to excellent results by fracture diagnosis.

dicate a significant difficulty in operative mobilization of fragments (Fig. 41-1D).

In a reported series of 207 acetabular fractures in 206 patients treated by delayed reconstruction between 21 and 120 days from injury, 187 patients were available for assessment of functional outcome (10). The overall average delay in surgical stabilization from time of injury was 43 days (range: 21 to 120 days). Overall good to excellent results were seen in 65% and fair to poor in 35% (Fig. 41-2). Higher rates of fair to poor results were seen in fracture patterns associated with anterior or posterior wall fractures and T-shaped fractures (Fig. 41-2B). Several authors have reported good to excellent results of early stabilization of acetabular fractures with overall rates averaging ≥80% (1–7,11,12). Within the time interval of 21 to 120 days the patients in this series had a significant decrease in good to excellent results averaging 65%. Other factors including cartilage damage, femoral head erosion and necrosis, and others may be responsible for this decrease in good to excellent results compared to results obtained from early treatment of acetabular fracture.

In this series, there was a surprisingly higher percentage of good to excellent results in the more complex fracture patterns of anterior column posterior hemitransverse (ACHT) and both-column fractures, 75% and 72%, respectively (10). Both-column fractures by definition are serious disruptions of the acetabular anatomy but have a higher success rate after delayed reconstruction than transverse plus posterior wall (59%) and T-shaped fractures (61%). Transverse plus posterior wall fracture may have additional factors that enhance the failure rate, including persistent dislocation of the femoral head, femoral head articular damage, erosion, and avascular necrosis. It can be extremely difficult to obtain an anatomic reduction in T-shaped fractures because of the variable level of anterior column fracture component that may be difficult to access and reduce. Isolated posterior or anterior column fractures gave the best overall rate of very good to excellent results. They usually are easier to approach even with time delays from original injury, and reduction usually is not as difficult as with other fracture patterns. They do not appear to have a significant prevalence of femoral head vascular injury or articular degenerative complications as seen in anterior wall, posterior wall, transverse-posterior wall, or T-shaped fractures.

Complication rates for all major complications are increased in delayed treatment (Fig. 41-3). Postoperative sciatic nerve palsy was a principal complication (10.6%) in this series and the prevalence was high compared to 4.5% (4,6) and 6.5% (8) after early reconstruction of acetabular fractures. This increased prevalence also reflects the difficulty encountered in reconstructing these fractures during

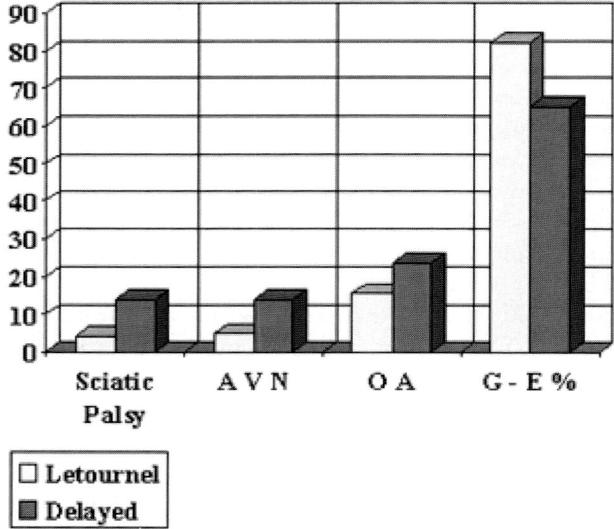

FIGURE 41-3. Histogram of percentage of complication rates of early (Letournel reported series) versus late delayed operative intervention. (From: Johnson EE, Matta JM, Mast JM, et al. Delayed reconstruction of the acetabular fracture: treatment between 21 and 120 days. *Clin Orthop* 1994;305:20–30; and Letournel E. The results of acetabular fractures treated surgically: twenty-one years of experience. In: *The hip: proceedings of the seventh open scientific meeting of the Hip Society.* St. Louis: CV Mosby, 1979, with permission.)

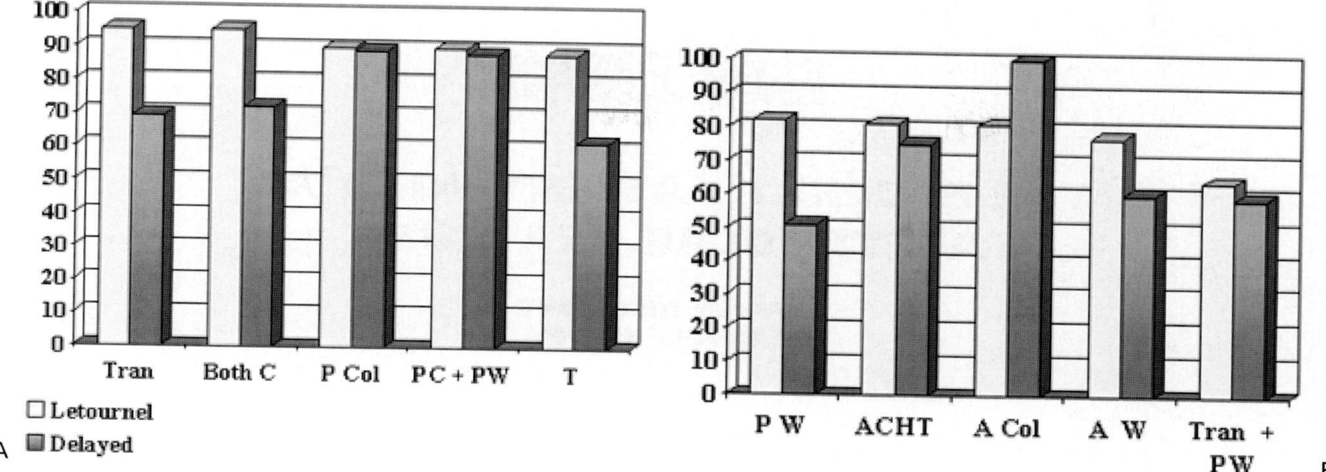

FIGURE 41-4. A: Histograms comparing reported results of early treatment of acetabular fractures compared to results obtained from delayed surgical intervention by diagnosis. **B:** Histograms comparing reported results of early treatment of acetabular fractures compared to results obtained from delayed surgical intervention by diagnosis. (From: Letournel E, Judet R. In: Elson RA, ed. *Fractures of the acetabulum.* New York: Springer-Verlag, 1993; Johnson EE, Matta JM, Mast JM, et al. Delayed reconstruction of the acetabular fracture: treatment between 21 and 120 days. *Clin Orthop* 1994;305:20–30, with permission.)

this delayed time period. Avascular necrosis continues to be one of the most debilitating complications following acetabular reconstruction with a rate in this series of 13.8% as compared to 4.9% reported by Letournel (4). Persistent dislocation of the femoral head or reconstruction of displaced isolated anterior or posterior wall fractures or transverse plus posterior wall fractures have a poor prognosis and a high prevalence of failure following reconstruction. These fracture patterns have the potential to increase femoral head articular damage and erosion through persistent dislocation or subluxation. Remarkably, isolated posterior column and the associated posterior column and posterior wall fracture types had a very acceptable rate of failure of 11% and 13%, respectively. Osteoarthritis in long-term follow-up of patients indicated nearly a twofold increase in incidence (24%), compared to 15% reported by Letournel (4) in early treated fractures. Heterotopic ossification continues to be a serious postoperative complication when using the Kocher-Langenbeck or extended iliofemoral approaches. The ilioinguinal approach had two cases of insignificant heterotopic ossification. Indomethacin appears to reduce both the incidence and severity of heterotopic ossification but did not eliminate it in 11% of cases. The most effective prophylaxis against heterotopic ossification formation was seen in patients treated with both indomethacin and postoperative limited field radiation to the hip. Heterotopic ossification prophylaxis is required for delayed operative treatment of acetabular fractures approached through either the Kocher-Langenbeck or extended iliofemoral exposures. Prophylaxis does not appear to be necessary in the postoperative care when using the ilioinguinal approach.

Operative reconstruction of acetabular fractures within this delayed time period is difficult and requires considerable experience. A decrease in good to excellent results occurs with delayed reconstruction of acetabular fractures during the time period of 21 to 120 days following injury compared to early stabilization of acetabular fracture (Fig. 41-4). There is also an increase in postoperative sciatic palsy, avascular necrosis, and osteoarthritis compared to results reported in early management of comparative fracture patterns.

REFERENCES

1. Letournel E. The treatment of acetabular fractures through the ilioinguinal approach. *Clin Orthop* 1993;292:62.
2. Letournel E. Surgical treatment of hip fractures. *Hip* 1987;157.
3. Letournel E. Acetabular fractures: classification and management. *Clin Orthop* 1980;151:81.
4. Letournel E, Judet R. In: Elson RA, ed. *Fractures of the acetabulum.* New York: Springer-Verlag, 1993.
5. Letournel E, Judet R. In: Elson RA, ed. *Fractures of the acetabulum.* New York: Springer-Verlag, 1981.
6. Matta JM, Anderson L, Epstein H, et al. Fractures of the acetabulum: a retrospective analysis. *Clin Orthop* 1986;205:230.
7. Matta JM, Merritt PO. Displaced acetabular fractures. *Clin Orthop* 1988;230:83.
8. Letournel E, Judet R. *Fractures du Cotyle.* Paris: Mason et Cie, 1974.
9. Letournel E. Les fracture du cotyle. Etude d'une serie de 75 cas. *J Chir (Paris)* 1961;82:47.
10. Johnson EE, Matta JM, Mast JM, et al. Delayed reconstruction of the acetabular fracture: Treatment between 21 and 120 days. *Clin Orthop* 1994;305:20–30.
11. Judet R, Letournel E. Fractures of the acetabulum. Classification and surgical approaches for open reduction. *J Bone Joint Surg* 1964;46A:1615.
12. Letournel E. The results of acetabular fractures treated surgically: twenty-one years of experience. In: *The hip: proceedings of the seventh open scientific meeting of the Hip Society,* pp 42–85. St. Louis: CV Mosby, 1979.

42

THE ELDERLY PATIENT WITH AN ACETABULAR FRACTURE

JEFFREY RICHMOND
DAVID L. HELFET

The elderly represent the fastest growing subset of the population. As such, the frequency of acetabulum fractures in geriatric patients can be expected to increase (1). Given this increase, geriatric patients may represent the largest subset of acetabular fractures by the year 2010 (2). The goals of treatment in this group of patients should be the same as in any other trauma patient: rapid mobilization and restoration of the preinjury level of function. However, the elderly patient poses challenges that are not always seen in the younger acetabulum fracture patient, including the likelihood of significant comorbid medical problems, preexisting degenerative joint disease, osteopenia, and extensive comminution. Treatment of these injuries in this subset of patients warrants special attention.

Although acetabulum fractures in younger patients are typically the result of high-energy trauma, they often result from simple falls in elderly patients owing to the pathologic (osteopenic) nature of the bone. In a high-energy injury, any fracture pattern is possible; however, following a simple fall, anterior column fractures, especially with a fracture of the quadrilateral surface are most common. Regardless of the fracture pattern, significant comminution is often present (Fig. 42-1) along with impaction of the articular surfaces of the acetabulum and the femoral head are also common (2). Associated fractures of the femoral neck or intertrochanteric region are uncommon but should be considered. Careful attention should be directed toward any elderly patient with groin or hip pain because an occult hip or acetabulum fracture may be easily missed (3).

Patients with nondisplaced fractures should be given a trial of nonoperative management consisting of bed to chair transfers with pivoting on the nonfractured side; alternatively, toe-touch weight bearing on the injured side may be allowed if the patient is able to comply with this regimen. Frequent radiographs are necessary in order to insure that there is no displacement of the fracture. Given the excellent vascularity of the pelvis, rapid healing should be expected. Spencer reviewed the results of nonoperative treatment of acetabular fractures in the elderly (4). In this cohort of 25 patients, 68% had no significant displacement initially, and the remainder had an "acceptable" reduction in traction. However, 30% had an "unacceptable functional result." This underscores the need for surgical treatment in all but the cases with minimal displacement out of traction.

Displaced acetabular fractures should be treated surgically according to the same indications used for younger patients. Perhaps a slightly greater tolerance for intraarticular malalignment is appropriate in the setting of an elderly patient who may not be able to tolerate a major operation and has low functional expectations. However, gross subluxation of the joint and significant fracture displacement should not be accepted. Treatment with prolonged bed rest or skeletal traction in an attempt to achieve a concentric reduction has no place in the treatment of these fractures because of the morbidity of prolonged recumbency and the inadequate reductions achieved with traction. There is controversy as to whether these patients should be treated by open reduction and internal fixation, primary total hip arthroplasty, or delayed total hip arthroplasty.

A special situation is the associated both columns acetabular fracture with secondary congruence. In this situation, nonoperative treatment may be successful if articular congruity is maintained without traction and the patient may be mobilized (Fig. 42-2).

Helfet and coworkers (5) reported on the results of open reduction and internal fixation of acetabular fractures in 18 patients over the age of 60, with an average age of 67. Half of these injuries were the result of simple falls, and 16 had complex fracture patterns. All were treated through a single incision (ilioinguinal or Kocher-Langenbeck) within 16 days of the injury. Fixation was with lag screws and buttress plating. A concentric reduction was achieved in all but one case, although a 2- to 3-mm gap owing to comminution was noted in three patients. Seventeen patients were available for

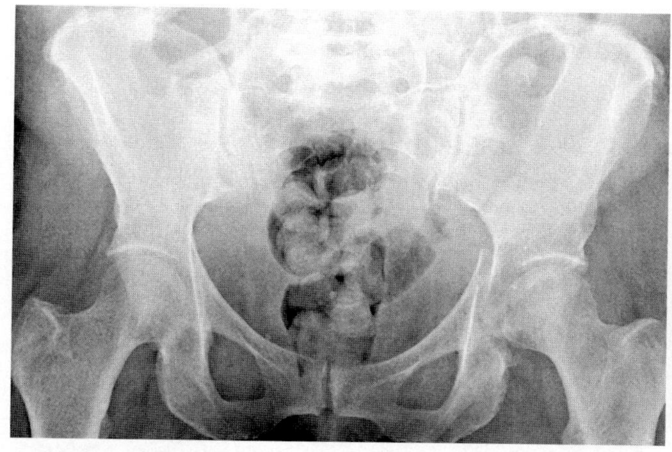

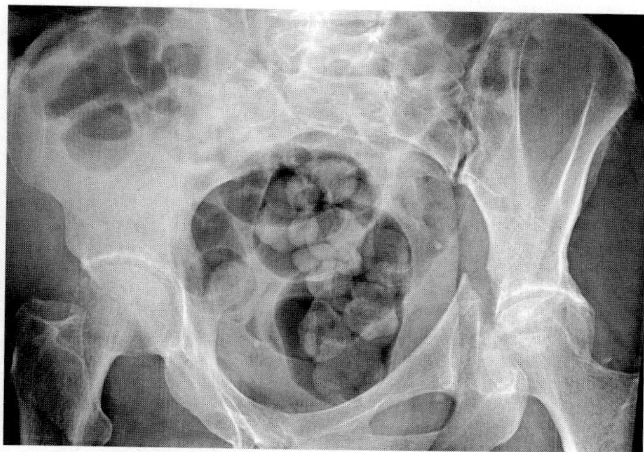

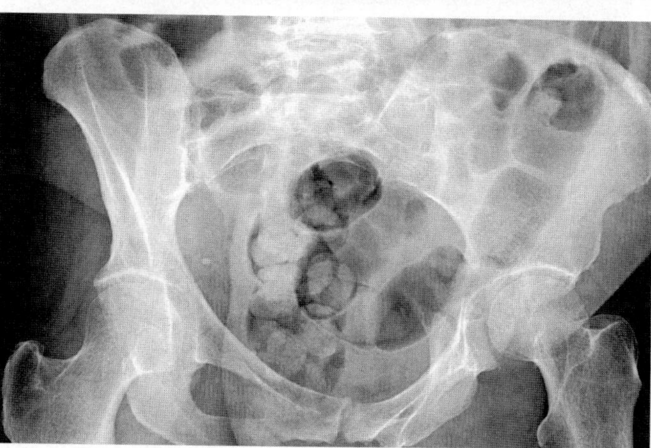

FIGURE 42-1. A–D: A 65-year-old woman was a restrained driver involved in a motor vehicle accident. She was diagnosed with multiple injuries including a left-sided transverse/posterior wall acetabular fracture, a right-sided wrist fracture, and deep vein thrombosis and pulmonary embolus. The patient underwent placement of a Greenfield filter and was then transferred to our institution for definitive management of her orthopedic injuries. She underwent ORIF through a Kocher-Langenbeck approach. Fixation and maintenance of the reduction was accomplished using two 3.5-mm pelvic reconstruction plates along the anterior and posterior wall for the transverse and posterior wall fragments and three one-third tubular buttress plates were also used along the posterior wall owing to the significant comminution and poor bone quality. **E:** The patient returned for follow-up 28 months following her injury with an excellent clinical and radiographic result and preservation of the hip joint space. **F–H:** She has returned to her preinjury activities, including playing golf.

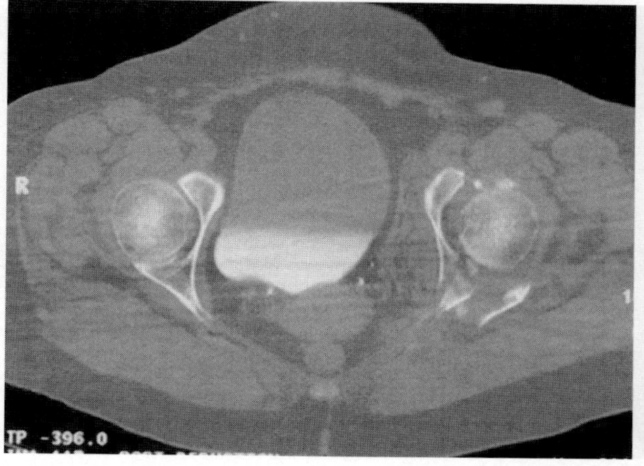

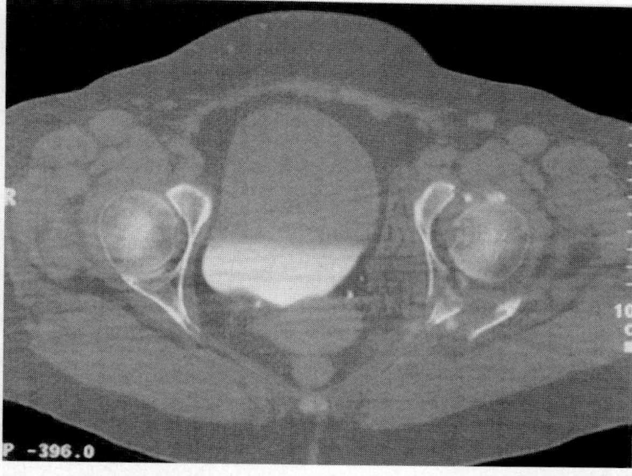

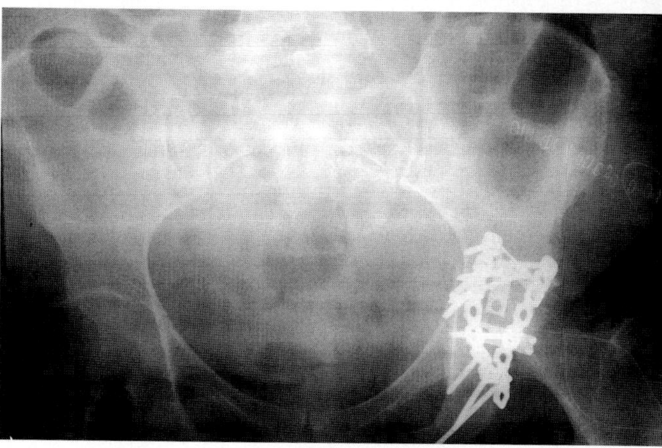

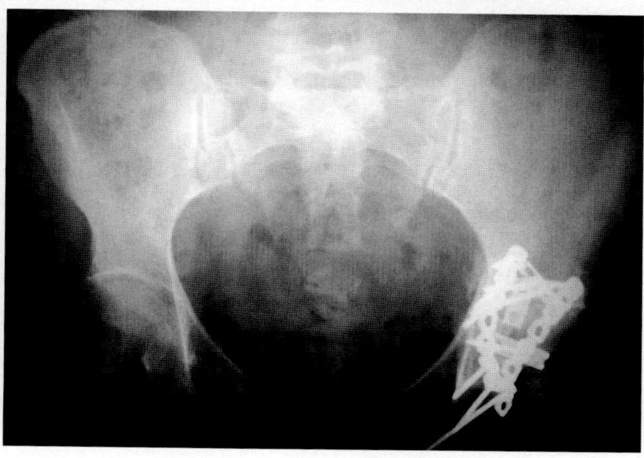

(Figure continues)

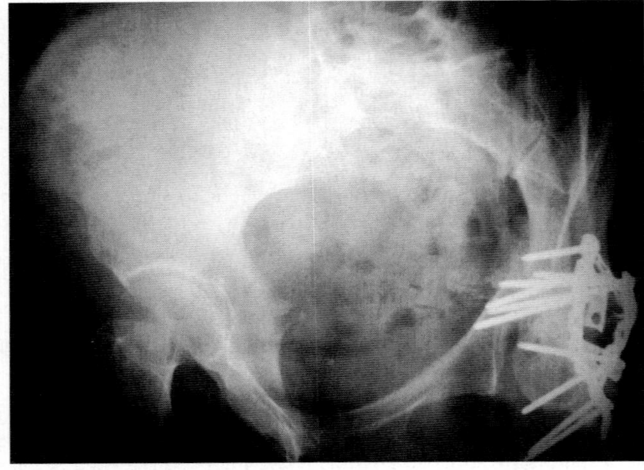
G

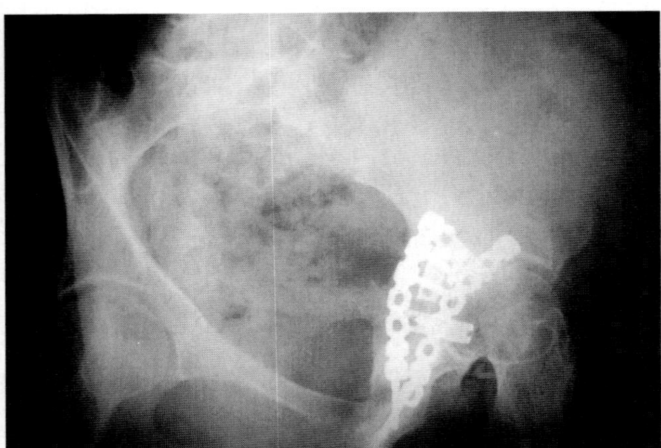
H

FIGURE 42-1. ***(continued)***

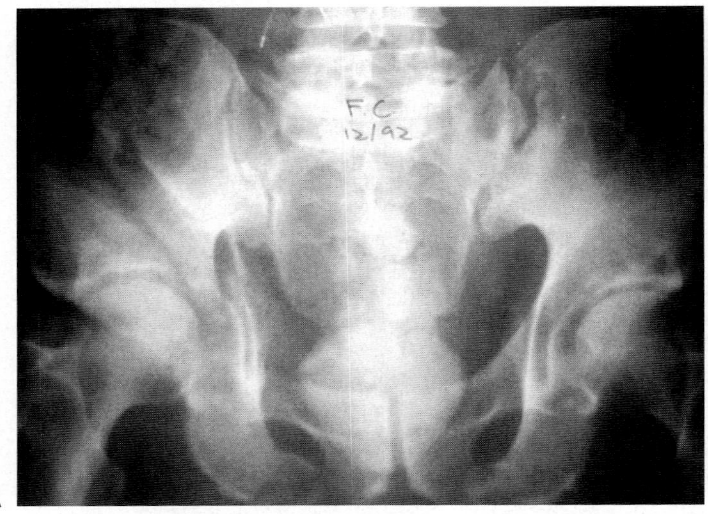

A

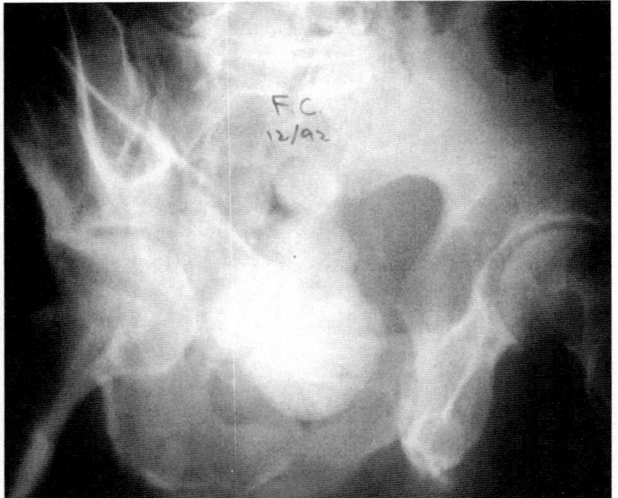

B

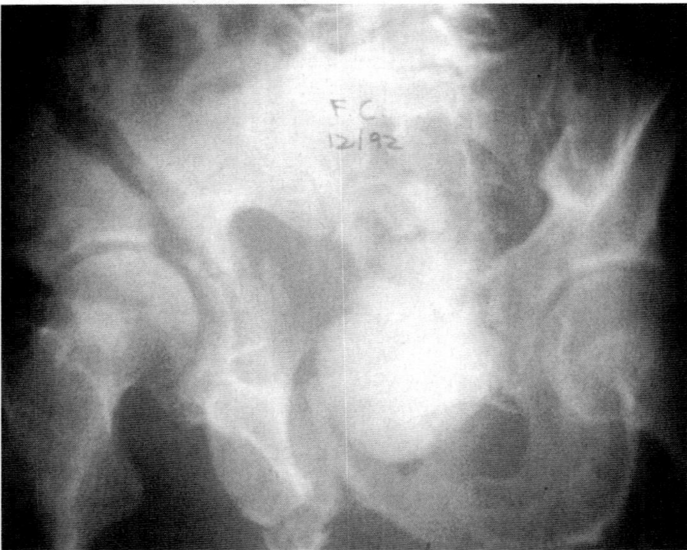

C

FIGURE 42-2. A 60-year-old man was struck by an ambulance while walking in New York City. He sustained a right-sided both-column acetabular fracture. Evaluation at the trauma center revealed an acute myocardial infarction (MI) likely secondary to his injuries. Radiographs provided evidence of secondary congruence of the right hip joint. **A–D:** The setting of an acute MI and secondary congruence of the hip joint mandated nonoperative management of the acetabular fracture. The patient returned for follow-up at 1 year following his injury and radiographs demonstrate a healed both columns acetabular fracture.

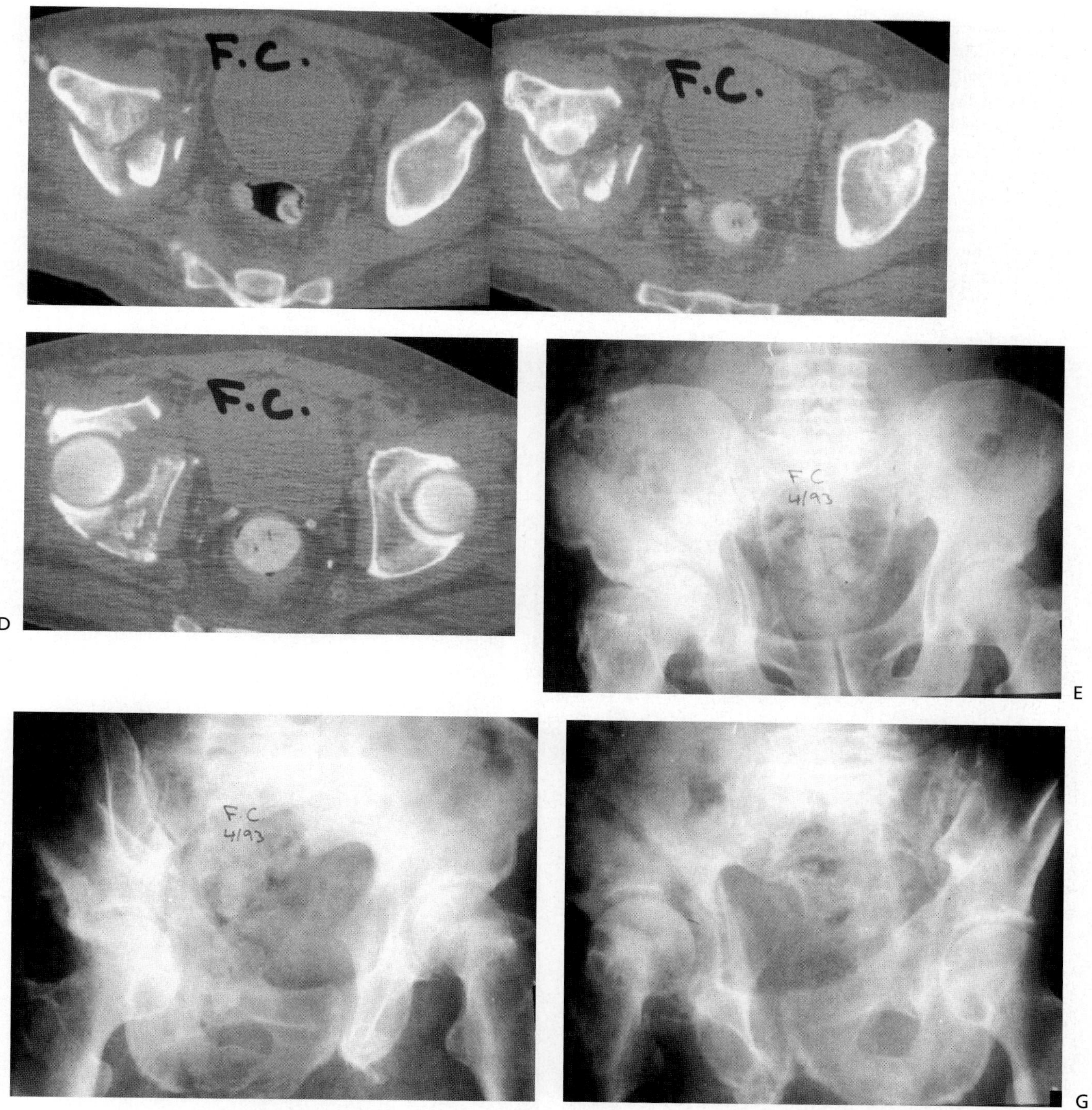

FIGURE 42-2. *(continued)* E–G: The patient noted mild pain at maximum range of motion in his right hip joint.

a minimum follow-up of 2 years (average 31 months). One patient had a partial loss of reduction owing to noncompliance with physical therapy, and one patient required total hip arthroplasty because of posttraumatic arthritis. The average Harris hip score was 90. This study demonstrates that good reductions and a good functional result can be achieved through a single nonextensile operative approach in a majority of elderly patients with acetabular fractures.

In a more recent series, Helfet and Virkus (unpublished data) examined functional outcome in acetabular fracture patients over the age of 55 years. Inclusion criteria included functional ambulators, the ability to tolerate a surgical procedure, and the expectation that an acceptable reduction or restoration of bone stock and stable fixation could be achieved through a single nonextensile exposure with 3 to 4 hours of operative time. Forty-five patients were followed for a minimum of 2 years after surgery. Eleven patients had a femoral head fracture or impaction injury; of these, three were treated with open reduction and internal fixation with acute total hip arthroplasty, and four went on to delayed total hip arthroplasty. An additional four patients required delayed arthroplasty for posttraumatic arthritis. Satisfactory reduction was achieved in 74% of cases. Functional outcome was assessed by the physical component summary of the SF-36 questionnaire. Elderly acetabular fracture patients had relatively high scores after treatment, and this was not significantly less than that for age-matched controls. American Academy of Orthopaedic Surgeons (AAOS) limb scores were also measured. Fracture patients treated by ORIF scored significantly better than patients with primary osteoarthritis. Scores were only marginally lower than for osteoarthritic patients treated with total hip arthroplasty. Overall functional outcome after acetabular fracture treated by open reduction and internal fixation was very good when compared to that of patients with other orthopedic conditions (Fig. 42-3).

Matta reported on a series of 259 patients who underwent operative treatment of an acetabulum fracture (6). Outcome data clearly correlated with the quality of the reduction. Seventy-four percent of patients age 59 years and under had an anatomic reduction compared to 45% of patients ages 60 to

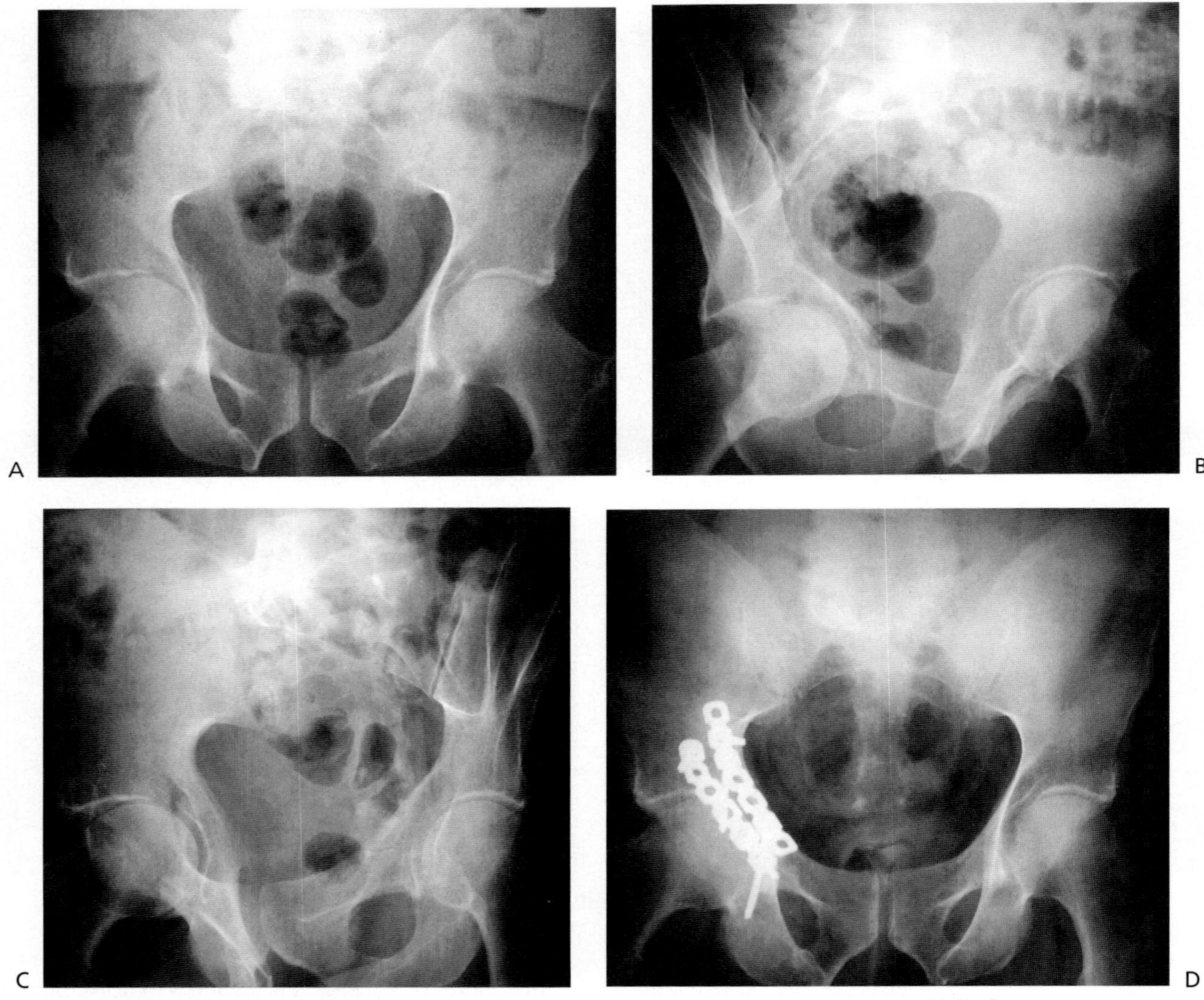

FIGURE 42-3. A–D: A 58-year-old man was riding a bicycle and attempted to stop using only the front brakes and was thrown over the handlebars. He sustained a right-sided anterior wall with an isolated posterior hemitransverse acetabular fracture along with a quadrilateral plate blowout and a protrusio deformity. The patient underwent ORIF of his acetabular fracture through an ilioinguinal approach. Following reduction and placement of two 3.5-mm pelvic reconstruction plates, the first contoured to serve as a buttress plate over the anterior wall fracture and the second contoured to fit along the pelvic brim across the quadrilateral plate. Intraoperative fluoroscopy was obtained and demonstrated anatomic reduction and extraarticular hardware placement.

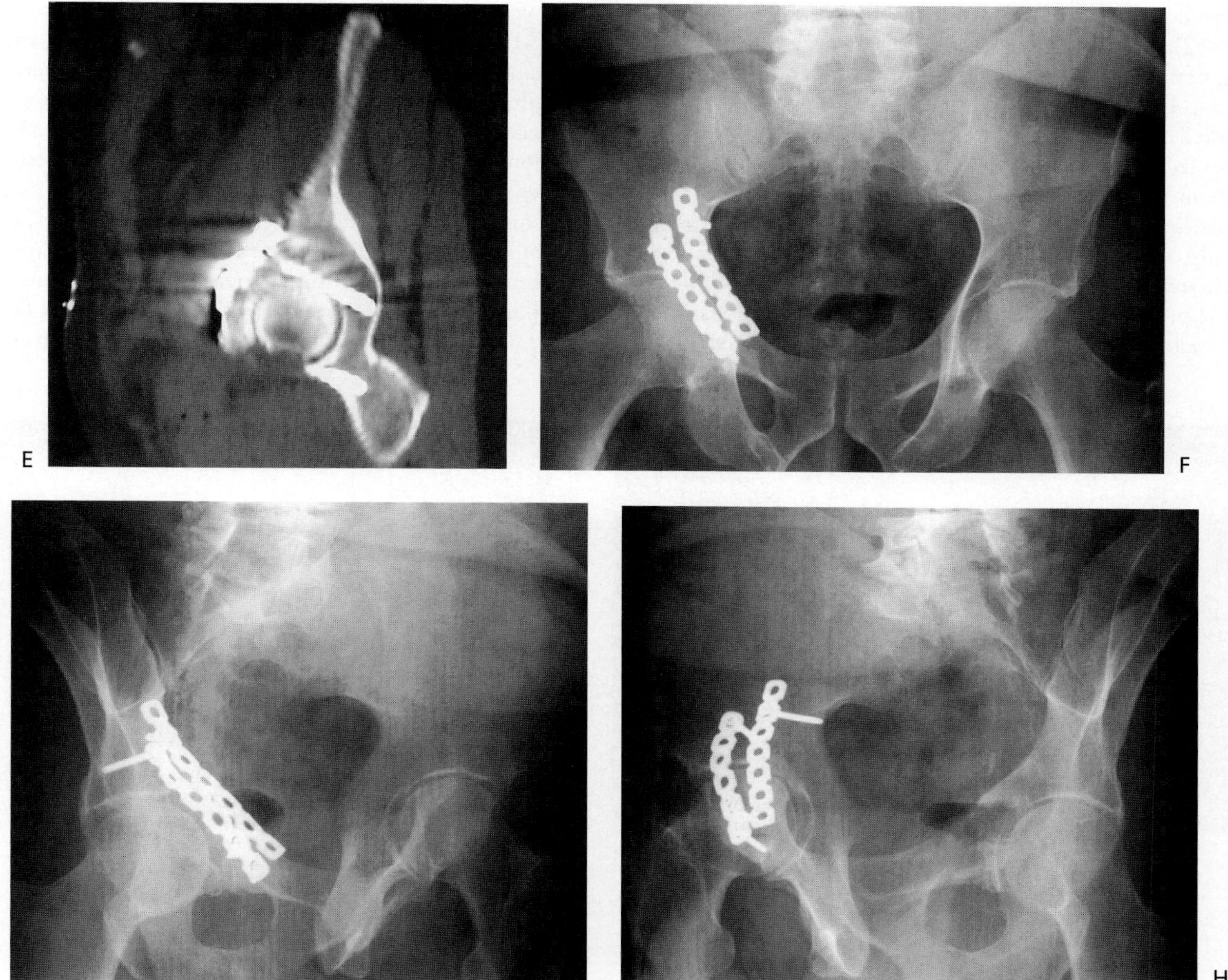

FIGURE 42-3. ***(continued)*** **E:** Routine postoperative computed tomography scan images revealed the presence of screws in the fovea. Therefore, intraarticular screw removal was required/planned for 10 to 12 weeks and then performed. During this interval the patient was kept at toe-touch/20 lbs weight bearing. **F–H:** The patient returned for follow-up at 7 months following his injury and 4 months following removal of intraarticular screws with an excellent clinical and radiographic result. He has returned to his usual activities, including bicycle riding.

90 years. In fact, patients age 40 years and older had considerably worse clinical results than younger patients. However, when fracture reduction was controlled for, the data indicate that it was the quality of the reduction and not the age of the patient that impacted on the clinical outcome. These data show that anatomic reduction is more difficult to achieve in the older patient. Furthermore, impaction of the acetabular surface did not correlate with a poor outcome, whereas the most significant negative prognosticator was a fracture or impaction injury to the femoral head.

Percutaneous methods of stabilization of acetabular fractures are being developed and may be applicable in certain geriatric cases (7,8). This technique involves placement of cannulated screws percutaneously under fluoroscopic guidance in the columns of the acetabulum and as a buttress for the quadrilateral plate. These screws may be placed *in situ* for a minimally displaced fracture, or after specialized clamps are used to achieve a reduction percutaneously. In biomechanical testing, lag screw fixation alone created a very stiff construct in certain fracture patterns. However, load to failure was less than that of traditional plate and screw fixation (9). No specific testing of isolated lag screw constructs have been tested in an osteopenic bone model. Currently there are limited clinical data with regard to this technique; however, it may be applicable in certain patients in order to assist in rapid mobilization and in patients too frail to undergo a standard open reduction and internal fixation.

Given the complexity of acetabular fracture surgery and the difficulty, even in experienced hands, of achieving an anatomic reduction, total hip arthroplasty, either acute or delayed, has been advocated in the elderly population (10–12). Acute arthroplasty is suggested primarily in the setting of an irreparable femoral head injury, but also in cases with preexisting arthritis, significant impaction injuries, marked comminution or the need for extensile approaches in order to achieve an anatomic reduction (Fig. 42-4).

Acute total hip arthroplasty is technically challenging. It is necessary to reduce the gross pelvic deformities sufficiently to provide a bed for the prosthetic acetabular shell, and to achieve stable fixation in order to allow ingrowth into the cup, or a stable, well-fixed cement mantle. Fixation of the fractures may be performed using standard plate and lag-screw techniques, or, alternatively using cables as described by Mears (see Chapter 43) (13). This technique involves passing a braided cable around the ischium and across the quadrilateral surface, exiting the pelvis in the region of the anterior inferior iliac spine and across the supraacetabular region on the outer table of the pelvis. This configuration secures the columns of the acetabulum as well as buttressing the quadrilateral surface. After tensioning the wires, the acetabular shell is impacted into the reamed acetabulum in the standard fashion, with supplemental screw fixation. Mears and Shirahama reported on 19 cases treated in this fashion. All fractures healed, though the cups migrated an average of

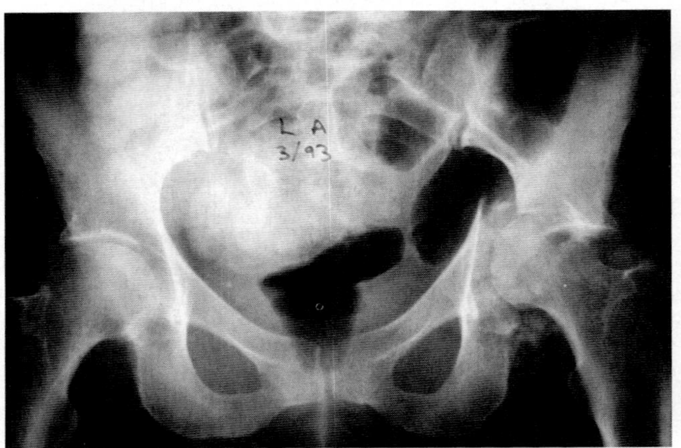

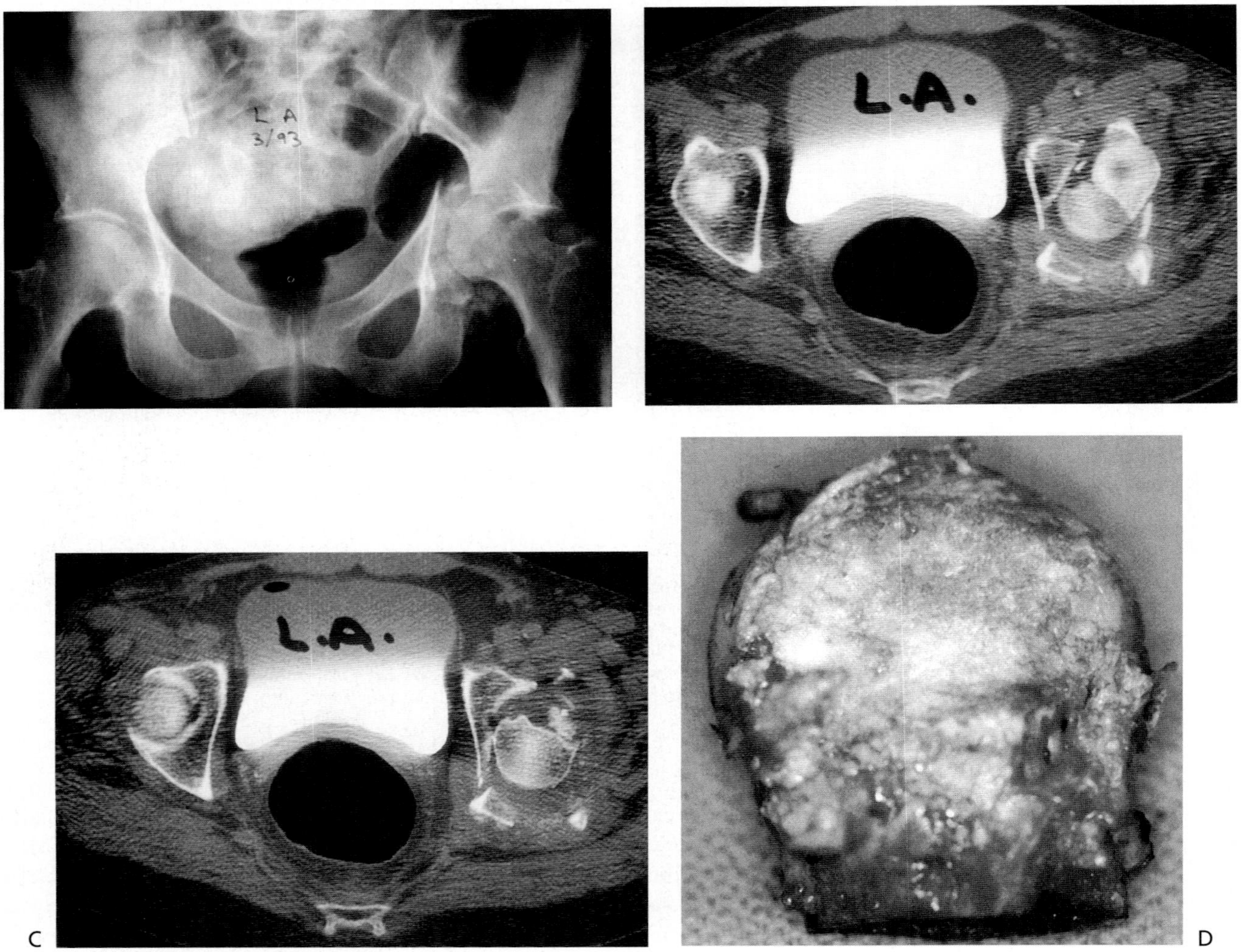

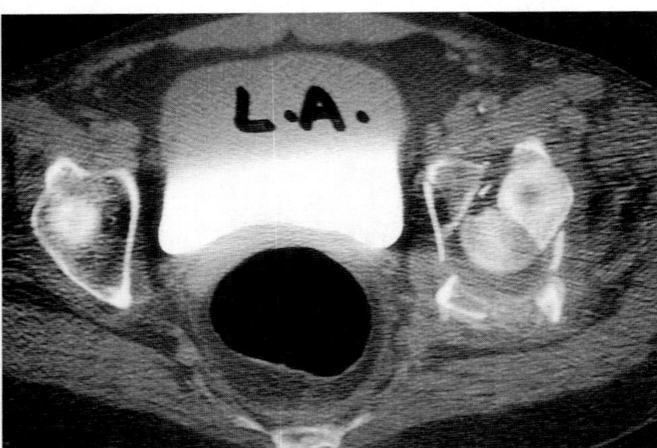

C

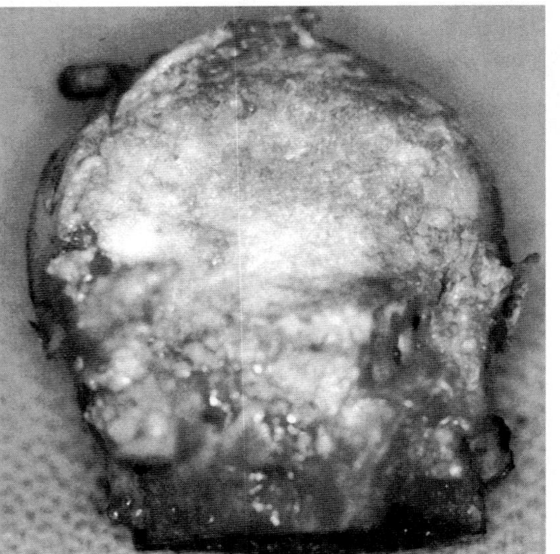

FIGURE 42-4. A 62-year-old woman was an unrestrained driver of an automobile involved in a high-speed motor vehicle accident. She sustained multiple injuries including the chest and also required a splenectomy. She was in the intensive care unit for a prolonged time at another institution. She was also diagnosed with a left-sided transverse/posterior wall acetabular fracture with associated posterior femoral head fracture/dislocation, left-sided distal humerus fracture, and right-sided proximal tibia fracture. The hip was reduced but the femoral head was medially subluxed and abutting on the roof of the acetabulum. **A–C:** After transfer and evaluation of the hip, including computed tomography scan, it was determined the femoral head was unsalvageable. Salvage of the femoral head was determined to not be possible and the patient was taken to the operating room for open reduction internal fixation of her left acetabular fracture **(D)** and immediate total hip arthroplasty

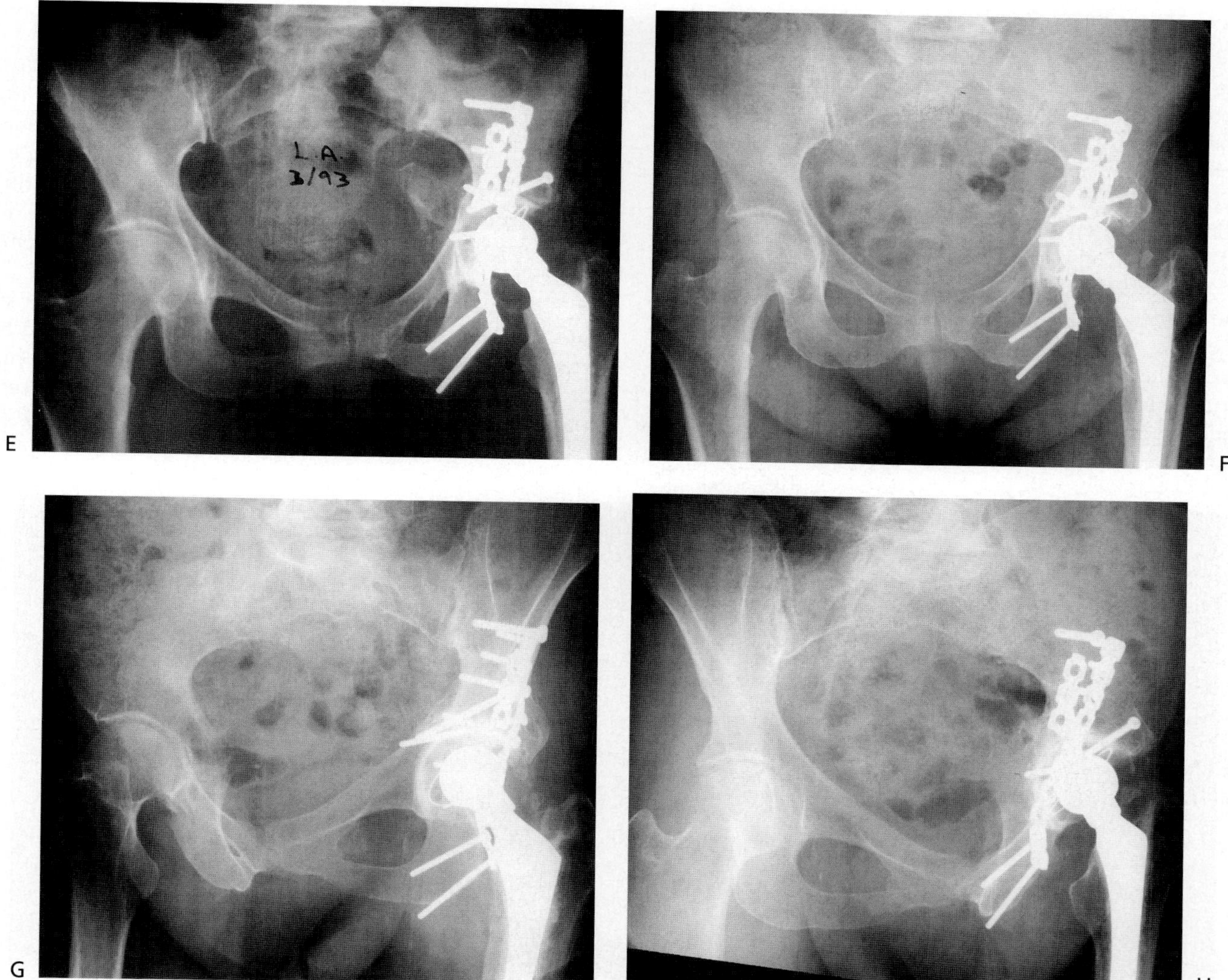

FIGURE 42-4. ***(continued)*** **(E)** and then open reduction internal fixation of her left distal humerus fracture and right tibial plateau fracture. **F–H:** The patient returned for follow-up 8 years following her accident with excellent clinical and radiographic results, a very good hip range of motion, and complete return to preinjury activity level, including swimming at the gym. She has an acceptable functional result of her distal humerus and tibial plateau fractures.

2 to 3 mm. No long-term results were reported for this technique. The initial migration of these acetabular components is a cause for concern, because a stable initial fixation of the component is generally regarded as a prerequisite for bony ingrowth in a noncemented component.

Several authors have examined the results of total hip arthroplasty for posttraumatic arthritis following acetabular fracture (see Chapter 44) (14–16). Romness and Lewallen reported on 55 such arthroplasties, 13 in patients who had undergone operative fixation of their fracture. A variety of prostheses were used. Failure of the acetabular component was noted to be four to five times higher than in cases performed for routine osteoarthritis. Although initial fracture treatment had no demonstrable effect on outcome of the arthroplasty, they attribute the premature failure of the component to loss of acetabular bone stock and suggest that restoration of the bony anatomy may improve results. Weber and colleagues reviewed arthroplasties performed in patients who had undergone internal fixation of their fracture. The procedures were longer when compared to simple arthroplasties, with a higher rate of failure of both the femoral and acetabular component. Failure was associated with age <50 years and, primarily, residual combined segmental and cavitary defects in the acetabular bone stock.

Bellabarba and colleagues reported on exclusively cementless reconstruction after acetabulum fracture and found that survival rates were comparable to procedures performed for primary osteoarthritis. Operative time, blood loss, and transfusion requirements were significantly higher. A single early component failure in this series was in the setting of an acetabular nonunion in which the prosthesis was used as a "hemispherical plate." They conclude that with modern cementless fixation techniques and adequate stability of the acetabular columns, total hip arthroplasty can be a successful salvage procedure after acetabular fracture. A significant limitation of this data is that fracture type and residual displacement was not reported; a significant bias may exist for minimal displacement in patients who had not undergone surgical management of their fracture initially. Therefore, specific conclusions could not be drawn with regard to the value of open reduction and internal fixation for future arthroplasty. However, the fact that patients who had undergone internal fixation required less bone grafting suggests that prosthetic reconstruction was easier in this population because fewer bony defects were present.

Total hip arthroplasty is undoubtedly a useful salvage procedure in all acetabular fracture patients suffering from posttraumatic arthritis. However, several studies demonstrate inferior results when compared to arthroplasties performed for osteoarthritis, and the single study reporting equivalent results, although not controlled for pelvic deformity, suggests that prior restoration of the bony anatomy makes for a simpler reconstruction.

The question that remains controversial is whether or not geriatric patients with acetabulum fractures should be treated by open reduction and internal fixation or total hip arthroplasty, either acute or delayed. Anatomic reconstruction of the acetabulum has been shown conclusively to

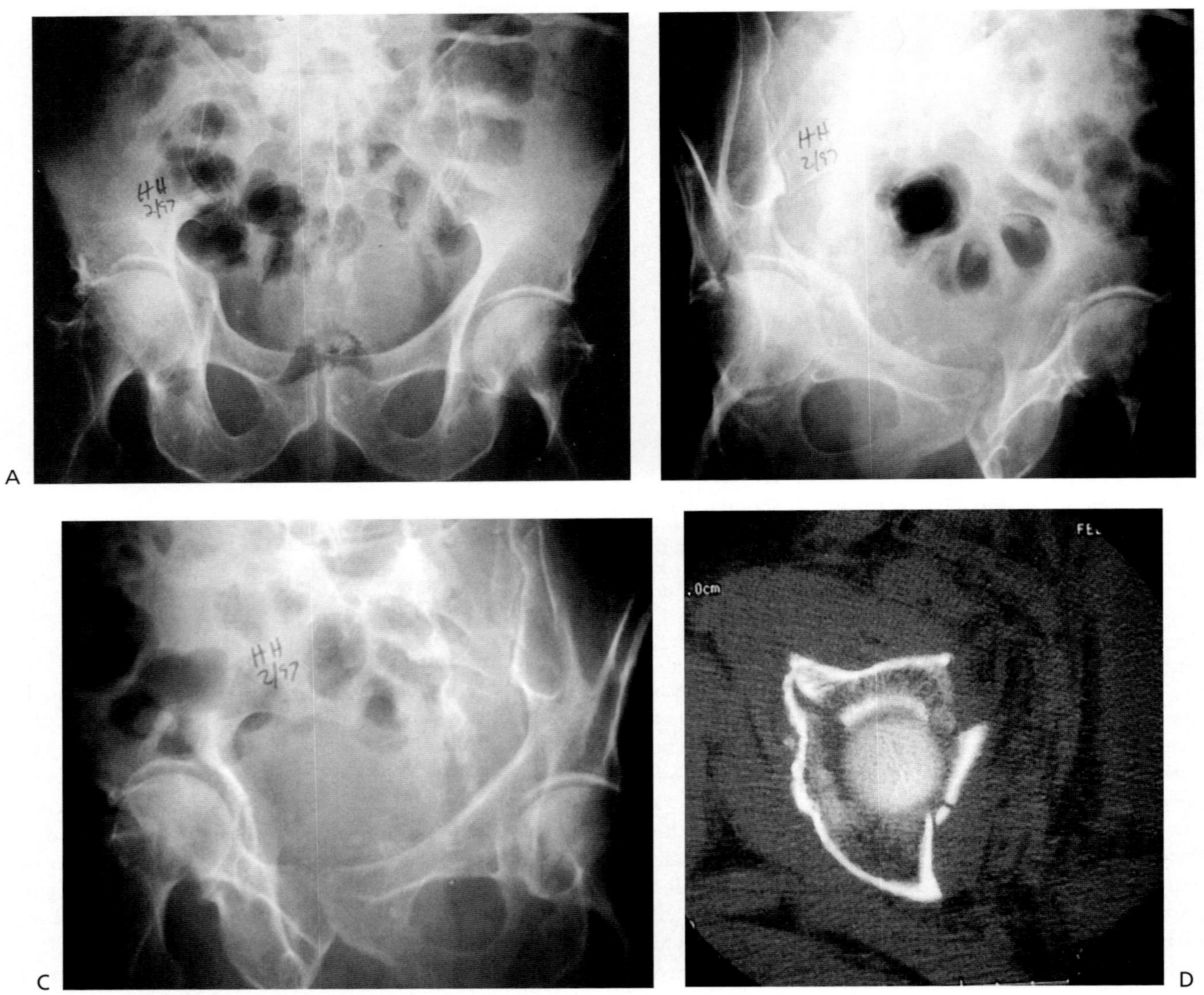

FIGURE 42-5. A–D: A 68-year-old man who fell between a subway car and waiting platform. He was diagnosed with an isolated right-sided extended anterior wall acetabular fracture. He was taken to the operating room where ORIF was performed through an ilioinguinal approach.

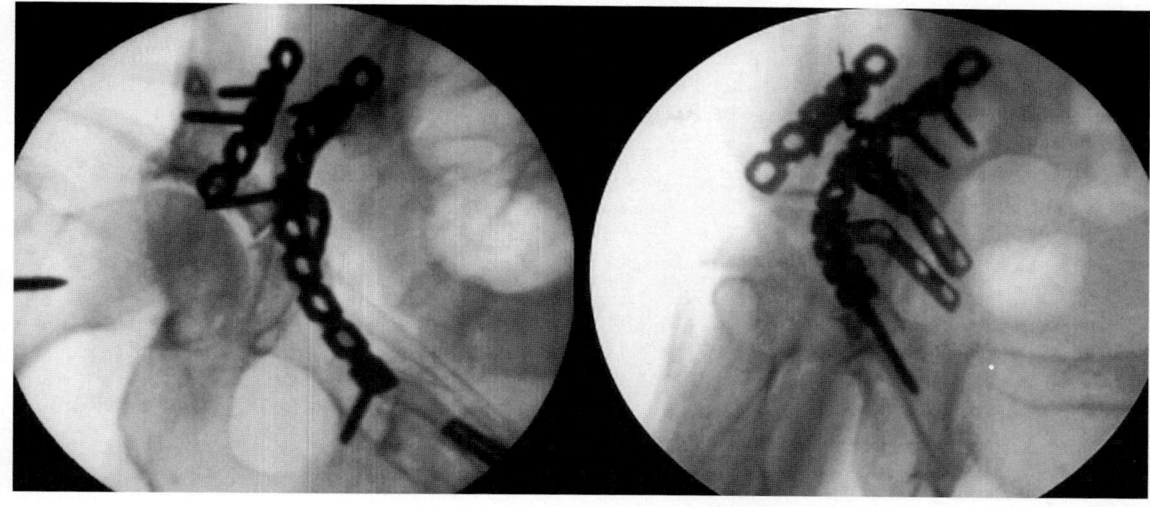
E

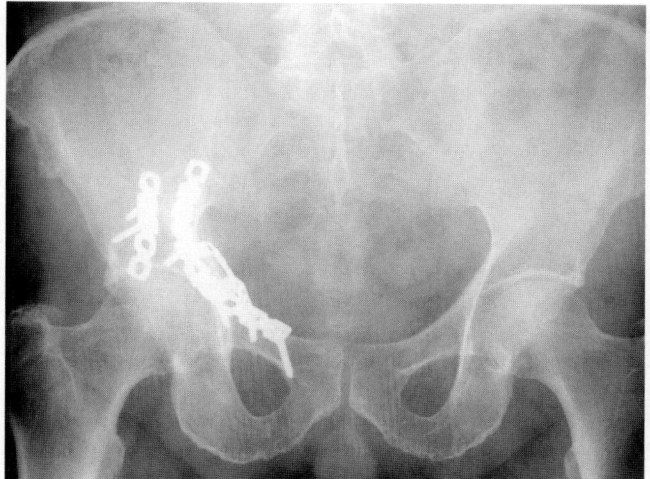
F

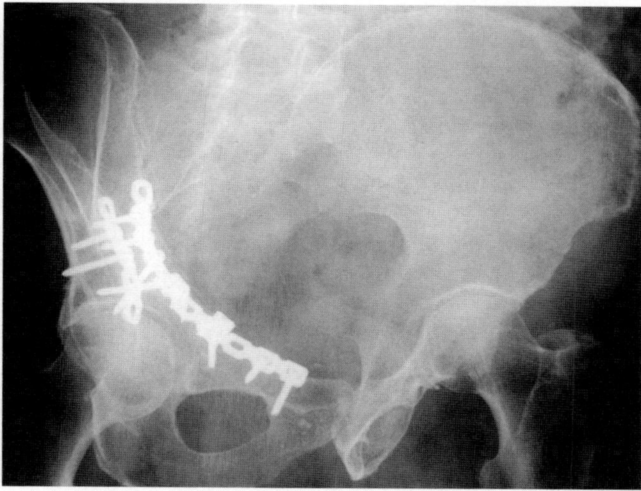
G

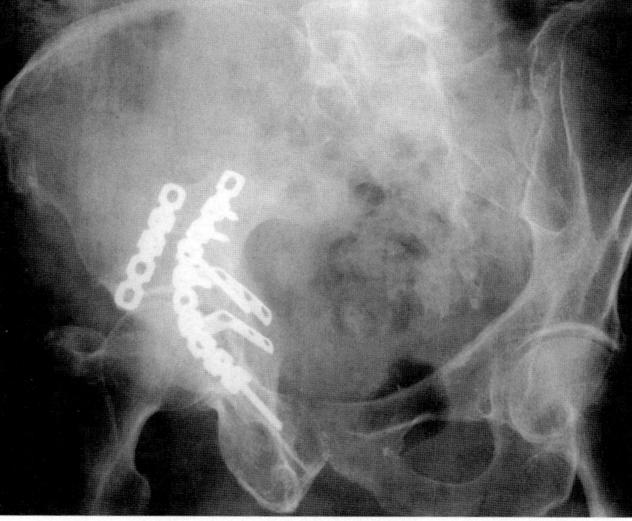
H

FIGURE 42-5. ***(continued)*** **E:** The longer reconstruction plate acts as a buttress plate along the anterior column. Spring plates fashioned from one-third tubular plates were contoured to a 70 degrees angle and placed to maintain the reduction of the quadrilateral plate. **F–H:** At 2 years following surgery the patient returned for follow-up with an excellent clinical/radiographic result and full range of motion.

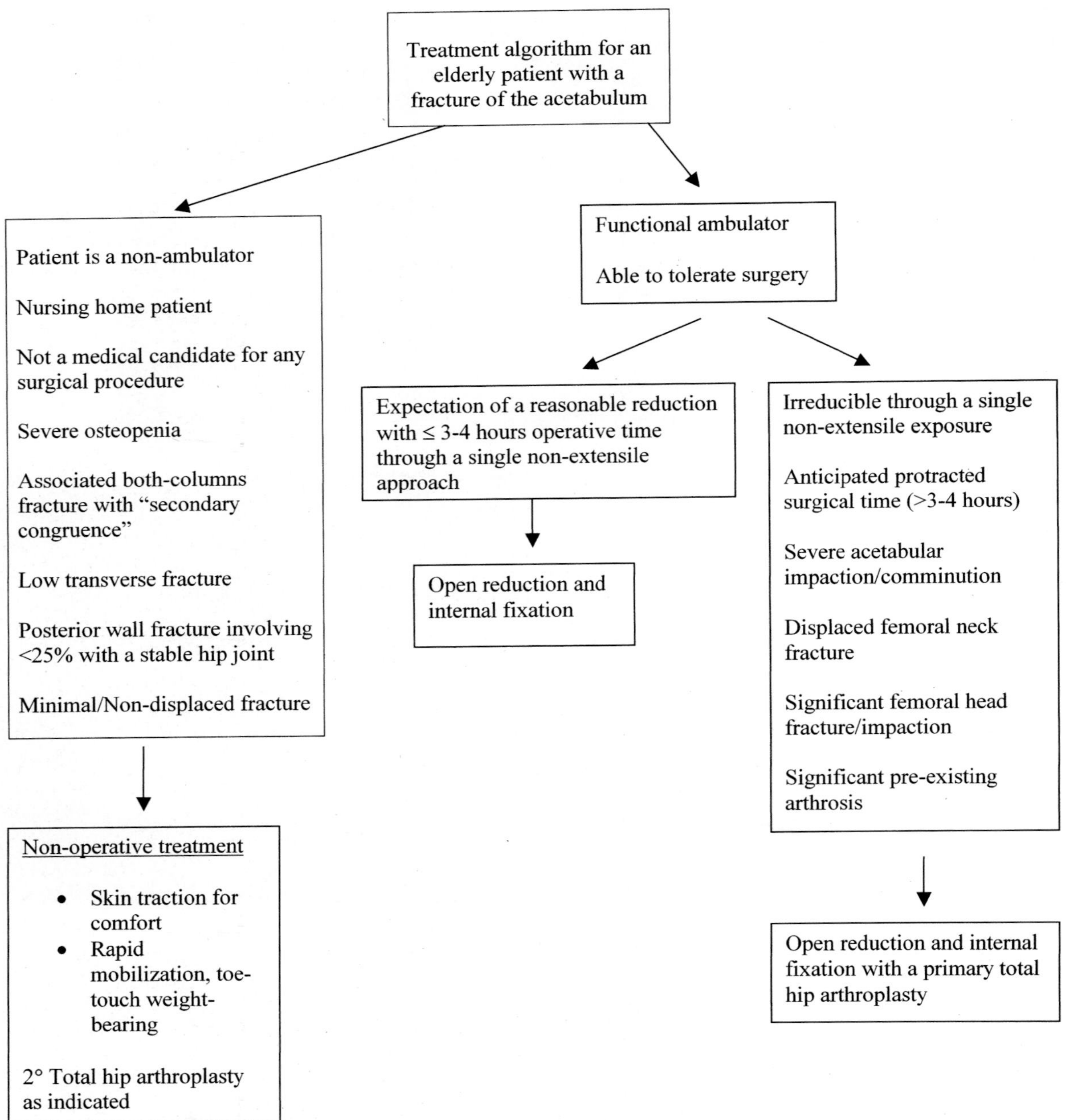

FIGURE 42-6. Treatment algorithm for acetabular fractures in the elderly.

provide excellent long-term outcome; this is clearly preferable to prosthetic reconstruction because it obviates many of the well-known complications of arthroplasty in this setting. This holds true even in the geriatric population, although anatomic reconstruction may be more difficult. In the event that posttraumatic arthritis develops, prior reconstruction of the bony anatomy will provide far better bone-stock for the arthroplasty. Initial nonoperative treatment may be justified if there is no gross pelvic deformity or subluxation of the hip joint without resorting to traction. Minimally invasive stabilization techniques may have a role at some point, but they do not obviate the need to obtain an acceptable reduction.

We recommend open reduction and internal fixation of the medically well elderly patient with an acetabular fracture in the majority of cases (Fig. 42-5). Our indications are based on a fracture pattern amenable to fixation through a single nonextensile exposure without performing a trochanteric osteotomy or disrupting the abductor musculature, with adequate bone quality for fixation, no femoral head injury and a reconstruction that may be performed in a reasonable surgical time (i.e., 3 to 4 hours). Transfer to an appropriate referral center for definitive treatment is to be encouraged.

Other possibilities are nonoperative care for the undisplaced fractures or those with secondary congruence (Fig. 42-2) or acute total hip arthroplasty (Fig. 42-6).

Acute total hip arthroplasty should be reserved for geriatric patients in whom the prognosis for a functional hip joint is hopeless, even in skilled hands at an appropriate referral center (Fig. 42-7). Such cases should be limited to significant lesions of the femoral head, a truly unreconstructable fracture, such as with massive comminution of the quadrilateral surface, or the need for an extensile exposure. Stabilization of the bony anatomy must be achieved in order to achieve a successful prosthetic reconstruction. We caution against the use of the prosthetic shell as a "hemispherical plate" and recommend the use of standard plate and screw fixation, possibly augmented by cable fixation, in this select group of cases.

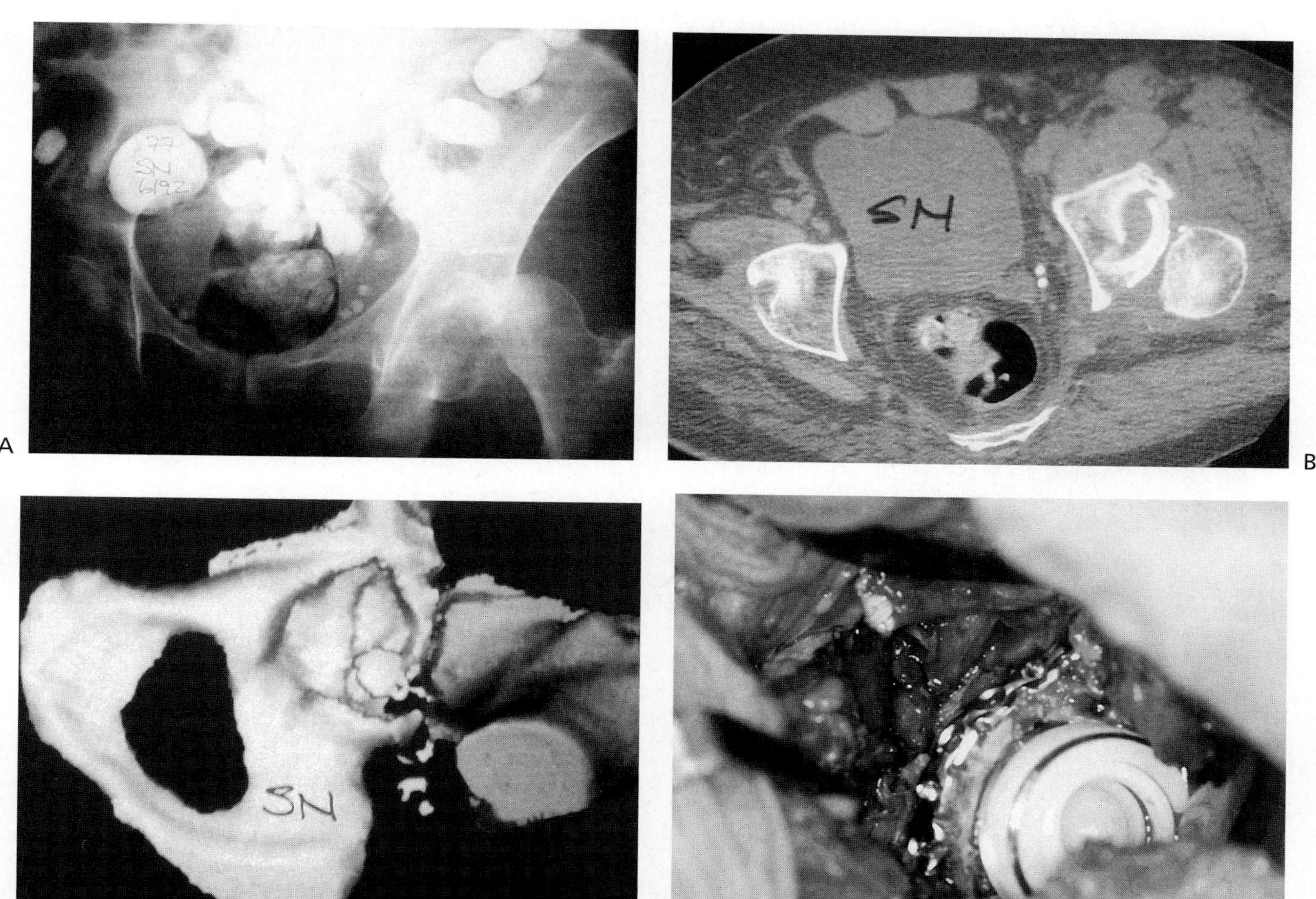

FIGURE 42-7. A 77-year-old man was a restrained driver of an automobile struck by another automobile in a head-on collision. **A:** The patient was transferred from an outlying hospital to our institution and diagnosed with an isolated left-sided posterior wall acetabular fracture with associated posterior dislocation of his left hip. **B,C:** Attempted closed reduction proved unsuccessful and further examination was performed including computed tomography scan that demonstrated extensive impaction of the medial portion of the femoral head. His surgery was further delayed by the fact that he had herpes zoster extending onto his operative site. Preoperatively, the patient had a significant foot drop. **D:** The femoral head was determined to be unsalvageable and the patient was brought to the operating room for emergent open reduction and internal fixation of his acetabular fracture and immediate total hip arthroplasty.

(Figure continues)

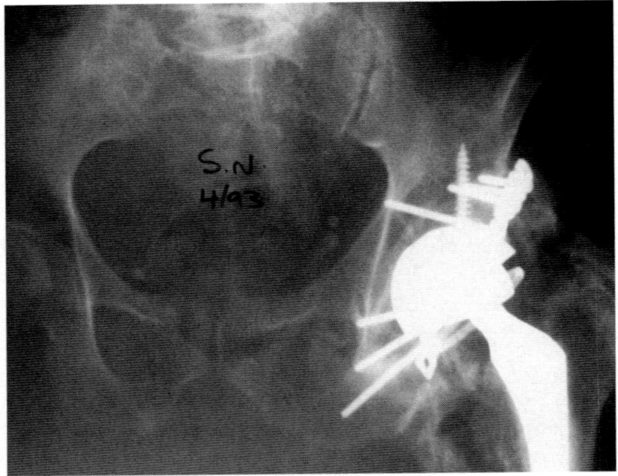

E

F

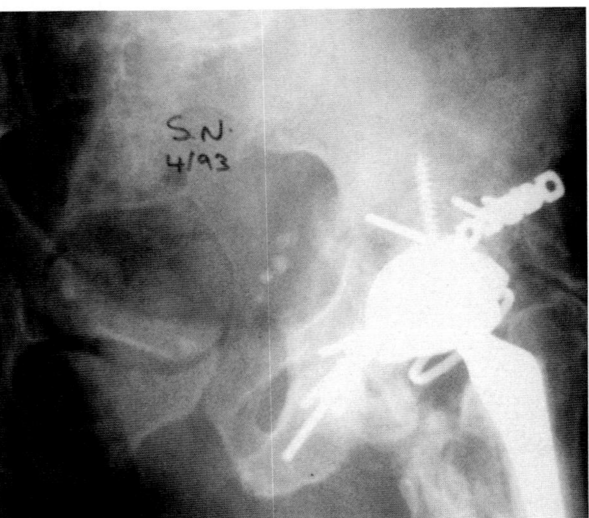

G

FIGURE 42-7. *(continued)* E–G: The patient returned for follow-up evaluation at 8 months following his acetabular fracture with a good clinical and radiographic result and a return to preinjury activity level with the exception of driving an automobile.

REFERENCES

1. Lonner JH, Koval KJ. Polytrauma in the elderly. *Clin Orthop* 1995;318:136–143.
2. Mears DC. Surgical treatment of acetabular fractures in elderly patients with osteoporotic bone. *J Am Acad Ortho Surg* 1999; 7(2):128–141.
3. Tornkvist H, Schatzker J. Acetabular fractures in the elderly: an easily missed diagnosis. *J Orthop Trauma* 1993;7:233–235.
4. Spencer RF. Acetabular fractures in older patients. *J Bone Joint Surg Br* 1989;71(B):774–776.
5. Helfet DL, Borrelli J, DiPasquale T, et al. Stabilization of acetabular fractures in elderly patients. *J Bone Joint Surg Am* 1992; 74(A):753–765.
6. Matta JM. Fractures of the acetabulum: accuracy of reduction and clinical results in patients managed operatively within three weeks after the injury. *J Bone Joint Surg Am* 1996;78(A): 1632–1645.
7. Starr AJ, Reinert CM, Jones AL. Percutaneous fixation of the columns of the acetabulum: a new technique. *J Orthop Trauma* 1998;12(1):51–58.
8. Starr AJ, Jones AL, Reinert CM, et al. Preliminary results and complications following limited open reduction and percutaneous screw fixation of displaced fractures of the acetabulum. *Injury* 2001;32(s1):SA45–50.
9. Chang JK, Gill SS, Zura RD, et al. Comparative strength of three methods of fixation of transverse acetabular fractures. *Clin Orthop Rel Res* 2001;392:433–441.
10. Joly JM, Mears DC. The role of total hip arthroplasty in acetabular fracture management. *Op Tech Orthop* 1993;3:30.
11. Mears DC, Shirahama M. Stabilization of an acetabular fracture with cables for acute total hip arthroplasty. *J Arthroplasty* 1998; 12:104–107.
12. Mears DC. Surgical treatment of acetabular fractures in elderly patients with osteoporotic bone. *J Am Acad Ortho Surg* 1999; 7(2):128–141.

13. Mears DC, Shirahama M. Stabilization of an acetabular fracture with cables for acute total hip arthroplasty. *J Arthoplasty* 1998; 13:104–107.
14. Romness DW, Lewallen DG. Total hip arthroplasty after fracture of the acetabulum: long term results. *J Bone Joint Surg Br* 1990;72(B):761–764.
15. Weber M, Berry DJ, Harmsen WS. Total hip arthroplasty after operative treatment of an acetabular fracture. *J Bone Joint Surg Am* 1998;80:1295–1305.
16. Bellabarba C, Berger RA, Bentley CD, et al. Cementless acetabular reconstruction after acetabular fracture. *J Bone Joint Surg Am* 2001;83A:868–876.

43

PRIMARY TOTAL HIP ARTHROPLASTY FOR AN ACETABULAR FRACTURE

DANA C. MEARS
JOHN H. VELYVIS

INTRODUCTION

Historically, for most displaced acetabular fractures, the preferred method of treatment has been an open reduction and internal fixation (1–8). From the pioneering observations of Judet and Letournel (9), an accurate open reduction was felt to provide the greatest likelihood for a favorable outcome and the best potential for a secondary reconstructive procedure if the initial treatment culminated in an unfavorable outcome. Although this hypothesis has withstood the test of time for the vast majority of acetabular fractures, recently it has been seriously questioned for a sizable and rapidly growing minority of injuries. On a careful examination of the results of Letournel, Judet (10) and Matta (11), even in their highly experienced hands, certain fracture patterns possess a poor likelihood for a favorable outcome after an open reduction. For example, the former authors reported excellent to good results for eight of 17 posterior column-posterior wall fractures (47%), as opposed to 18 of 19 transverse patterns (95%). One explanation of the high incidence of fair and poor results for the former injury pattern was the predilection for elderly individuals to sustain this injury pattern. The clinical results of both Letournel (10) and Matta (11) display a progressive deterioration with aging of the patients. In a more recent series of 424 patients by Mears and coworkers (12), where 25% of the patients were over 60 years of age, the unfavorable impact of aging was even more striking. Admittedly, in a selective group of active elderly individuals, Helfet and coworkers (13) reported highly favorable results after an open reduction. Nevertheless, in many elderly patients, the impact of disuse osteoporosis and of other comorbidities that compromise the structural integrity of bone may culminate in a highly comminuted or impacted acetabular fracture after a minor traumatic insult such as a simple fall (Fig. 43-1). From previous epidemiologic studies by Melton (14), Ragnarsson and Jacobsson (15), and Kannus and coworkers (16), an octogenarian possesses a tenfold increased risk to sustain a pelvic or acetabular fracture versus a 25 year-old. For females of any adult age, the risk is twice that of a male counterpart. With the explosive increase in the numbers of elderly individuals, a trend that is anticipated to continue well into the present century, the numbers of geriatric acetabular fractures are likely to steadily grow (16,17). Meanwhile, with the improved safety of automobiles and the recent favorable response to legislation that addresses driving under the influence of alcohol and drugs, the numbers of young adult acetabular fracture victims, nominally with normal dense bone, has been decreasing (18,19). The impact of these epidemiologic factors is likely to create a progressive increase in

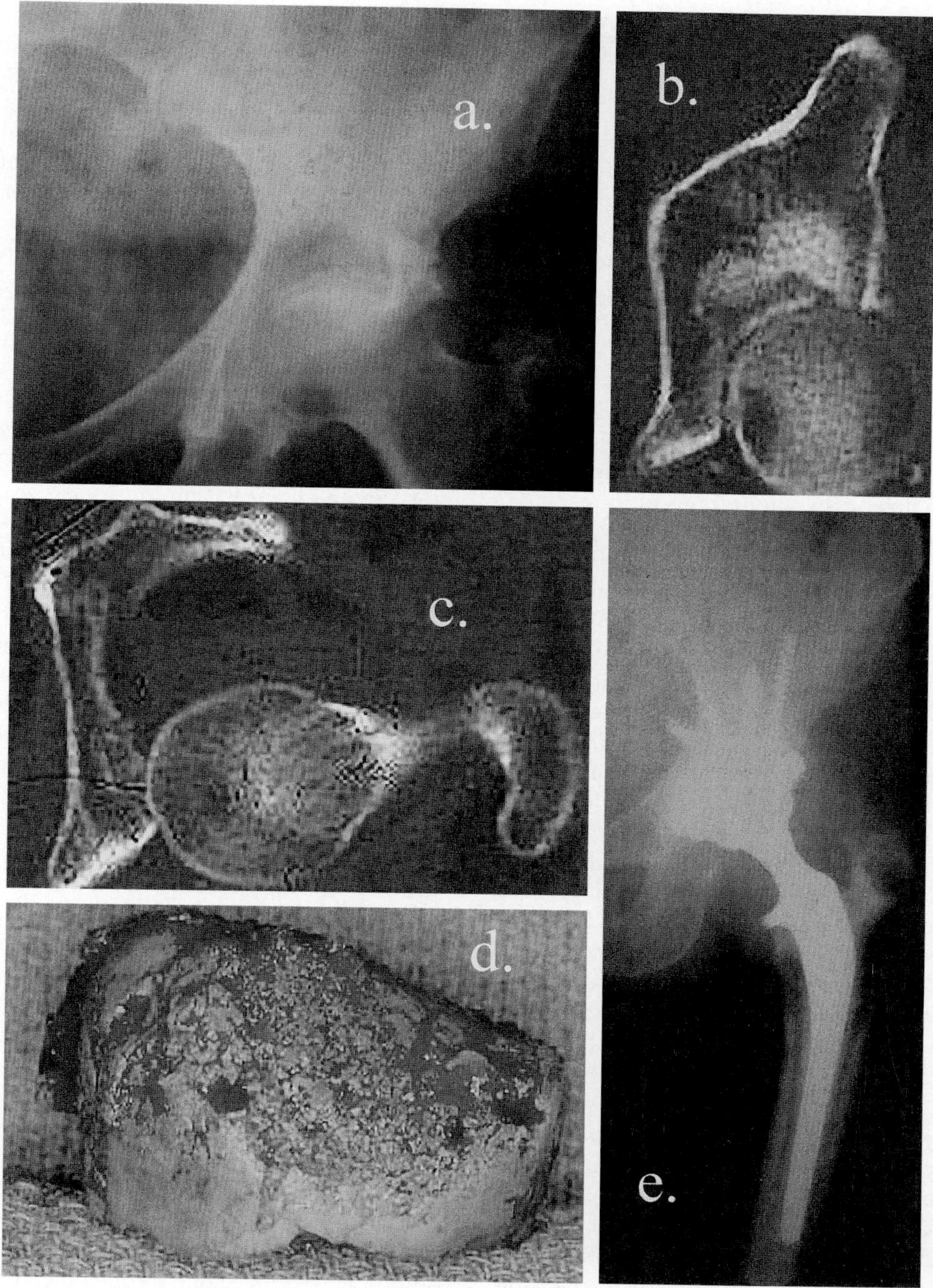

FIGURE 43-1. This 78-year-old woman sustained a simple fall and provoked a posterior wall fracture with marked impaction of the femoral head and acetabulum. The severity of the impaction is poorly evident in the preoperative images but readily apparent in the intraoperative view, and provided the indication for the acute total hip arthroplasty. **a:** Preoperative anterior-posterior (AP) radiograph. **b:** Preoperative computed tomography (CT) scan through impacted dome. **c:** Preoperative CT scan through impacted posterior wall. **d:** Intraoperative photograph. **e:** Postoperative AP view at 2 years.

the numbers of acetabular fractures that are unlikely to achieve favorable outcomes after an open reduction by resorting to the currently available techniques.

The problem is further complicated by the consideration of the young adult who sustains violent trauma to the hip. Despite the presence of dense, normal bone, the forceful impact may provoke marked acetabular comminution or impaction of both the femoral head and the acetabulum. From the series by Mears and Velyvis (20), other complicating factors that compromised the clinical outcome following an open reduction included a late presentation and morbid obesity.

After a patient with an unfavorable prognosis after an open reduction is identified, the question remains as to the optimal therapeutic alternative (21). One possibility is an initial nonoperative course, followed by a total hip arthroplasty after the acetabulum has united (22). Although this strategy avoids the potential complications of an open reduction, previously surgeons have reported an unacceptably high failure rate of late arthroplasties that were attributed to the high incidence of an acetabular nonunion or a large defect (4,23–25). In the largest reported series of 55 arthroplasties in 53 prior acetabular fracture victims, Romness and Lewallen (4) documented a fivefold greater rate of both radiographic and symptomatic loosening of their cemented cups, than for a comparable series of patients who underwent a total hip arthroplasty for degenerative arthritis. The control series was reported by Stauffer (24) with a mean follow-up evaluation of 10 years. In another series by Weber and coworkers (26), which reviewed both cemented and cementless cups, the results of 22 cementless cups were analyzed at a 10-year follow-up evaluation. None of the cups had been revised or displayed radiographic features of loosening.

Another possible strategy is a limited open reduction that eliminates large fracture gaps and restores pelvic stability even though it does not address acetabular comminution and impaction or concomitant damage to the femoral head. This method has the potential for complications without providing a high likelihood for a successful outcome for the acetabulum. A late total hip arthroplasty may be required after the acetabulum is united.

A few other authors have reported the results of late total hip arthroplasty after acetabular fractures that initially were managed with an open reduction (26–29). Such an arthroplasty is liable to the presence of impediments, including heterotopic bone, dense scar tissue, interposed hardware, and potentially an occult infection. The reports of late total hip arthroplasties performed after initial closed or open treatment of an acetabular fracture are notable for significantly higher complication rates than for arthroplasties undertaken for degenerative arthritis.

A third possibility is an acute total hip arthroplasty. At first glance, this treatment option appears to foster many formidable technical challenges, including the means to adequately stabilize the cup and eliminate a potentially large acetabular defect. Historically, acute total hip arthroplasty was preceded by the unsuccessful attempts of Kelly and coworkers (30) and Westerborn (31) to employ a cup arthroplasty. Coventry (32) reported equally unsuccessful results for an acute cemented total hip arthroplasty. Joly and Mears (33) described a successful clinical outcome with a modified technique whereby an uncemented, multiscrewed cup was used as a "hemispherical plate" to draw the fracture fragments into a stable and substantially reduced configuration. Subsequently, while examining diverse methods to achieve stability of the accompanying acetabular fracture, Mears and Shirahama (34) described the use of cerclage cables. Also, techniques of impaction grafting with the use of femoral head autograft and supplementary mesh were evaluated. More recently, Mears and Velyvis (20) reported the late outcome for 57 patients who underwent an acute total hip arthroplasty for an acetabular fracture and were followed for a mean of 8 years and for not less than 2 years. Overall the results were highly favorable, with 45 of the patients (79%) achieving an excellent or good Harris hip score. The principal source of lower scores occurred in the elderly 70- and 80-year-old patients who achieved very good relief of hip pain but who possessed a pretraumatic impairment of ambulation that required the use of a cane. Although these results will be analyzed in more detail, in brief, they have provided a confirmation that the method appears to hold considerable promise, especially for selected elderly patients. The use of an acute total hip arthroplasty in a highly selective young adult is further complicated by the longer life expectancy and the greater likelihood for a premature arthroplastic failure and need for a revision procedure, possibly hampered by extensive lysis of the bone (35). Certain young adults with an acetabular fracture possess a highly self-destructive behavioral pattern that may be accompanied by alcohol and drug abuse. Such a patient is a very poor candidate for an acute or late total hip arthroplasty.

INDICATIONS FOR AN ACUTE TOTAL HIP ARTHROPLASTY

As a general principal, the indication for an acute total hip arthroplasty is irreversible destruction of the acetabulum and/or femoral head that accompanies the fracture (21). The mechanisms for such destruction include extensive impaction, comminution, or full-thickness abrasive loss of the articular cartilage. In elderly patients, profound osteopenia is a major contributing factor. Other considerations include the presence of a nonreconstructible fracture of the femoral head or a concomitant, displaced fracture of the femoral neck that is irreducible by closed or open means. The last situation creates an exceedingly great likelihood for avascular necrosis of the femoral head. A prior history of severe degenerative or inflammatory arthritis is an occasional factor. Rarely, the presence of another antecedent problem such as avascular necrosis of the femoral head is a consideration. Certain fracture patterns possess the greatest predilection for one or more of the traumatically induced problems in a geriatric patient:

1. A posterior wall fracture with extensive impaction of the acetabulum and femoral head (Fig. 43-1). In our experience (12), impaction of either articular surface that compromises more than 20% of the surface area possesses a very poor prognosis, whereas involvement of more than 40% of the surface achieved abysmal results after an open reduction, despite elevation and bone grafting of the lesion.
2. A comminuted anterior column fracture that involves the anterior column, wall, and adjacent quadrilateral surface (Fig. 43-2). This injury pattern often occurs after a simple fall in an elderly person who lands on his or her side, to fracture the weakest part of the acetabulum.
3. An anterior wall, anterior column-posterior hemitransverse, or a both-column injury

Two fracture types that have the greatest predilection for extensive impaction in a young adult who sustains a highly forceful injury.

1. A transverse or T-type fracture, with impaction of the acetabular roof along the transverse fracture line
2. A posterior fracture-dislocation as a transverse-posterior wall or a posterior column-posterior wall fracture. These injuries are vulnerable to extensive impaction of both the posterior wall and the femoral head.

The contraindications to an acute total hip arthroplasty include the following.

1. Any fracture that is suitable for conventional closed treatment or an open reduction and internal fixation
2. A patient, especially a young adult, who possesses self-destructive tendencies for a return to activities or employment that favors a rapid failure of the arthroplasty. Alcohol and drug abuse are included in this category.
3. A neighboring contaminated wound or septic or potentially septic hip. In certain cases, this may be a temporary contraindication where the source of the problem can be eradicated.
4. Other potentially transient contraindications include hemodynamic instability, an unstable cardiac arrhythmia, electrolyte imbalance, or other unstable comorbidity. Usually, such a problem can be brought under control so that ultimately the procedure can be performed.
5. A past history of irradiation therapy to the acetabulum. The presence of a pathologic fracture with markedly impaired healing of bone is beyond the scope of this chapter. The potential for intraoperative problems, such as the inability to effectively anchor the cup in the profoundly osteopenic and avascular bone, and for postoperative complications including a deep wound infection and premature failure of the cup merit special consideration.

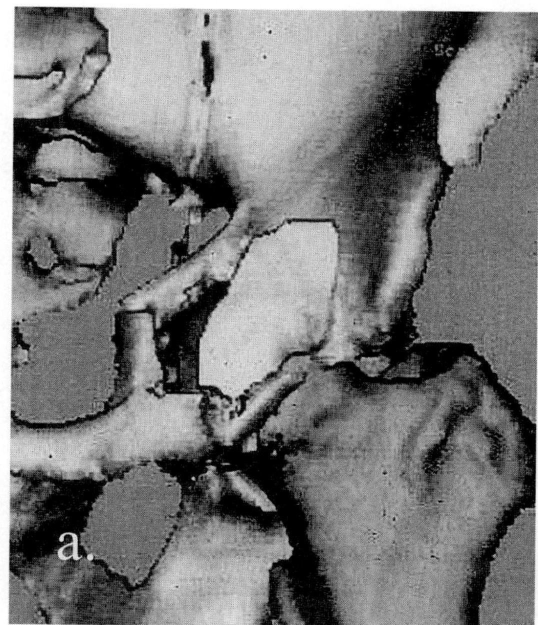

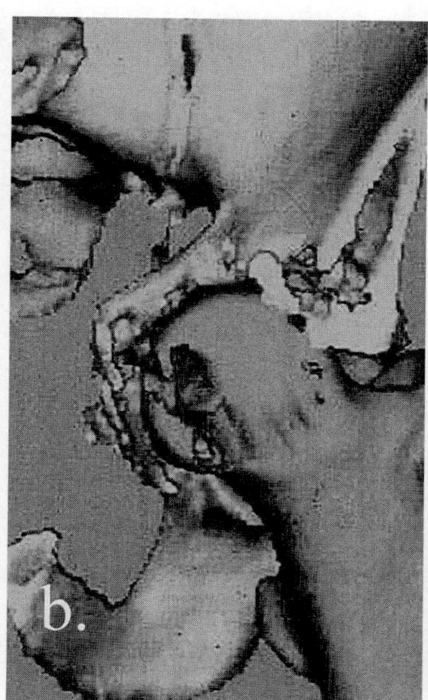

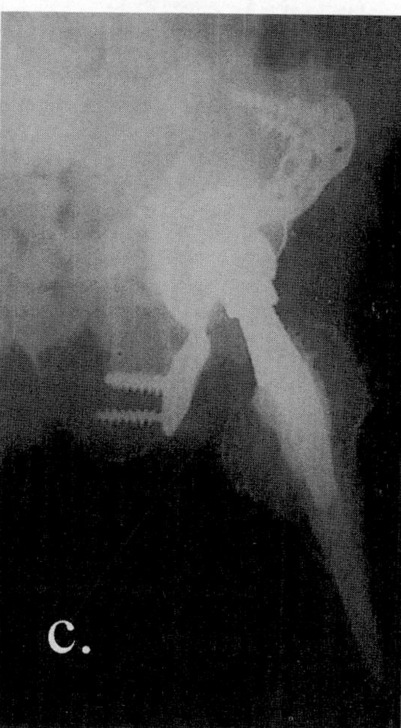

FIGURE 43-2. This 81-year-old man fell from a low stool and provoked a characteristic geriatric fracture pattern with comminution of the anterior column and involvement of the quadrilateral surface. As part of the acute total hip arthroplasty, a Busch-Schneider cage was used to stabilize the fracture. The fracture gap was obliterated with morselized cancellous autograft. **a:** Preoperative three-dimensional computed tomography (3DCT) image. **b:** Preoperative 3DCT sagittal reconstruction to highlight the central comminution. **c:** Postoperative iliac oblique view with residual displacement, 3 years later. The screws in the superior plate have loosened somewhat but radiographically are unchanged from their positions of 2 years earlier.

PREOPERATIVE ASSESSMENT

The force of the provocative blow provides insight into the strength of the bone or the potential presence of osteoporosis. A major traumatic insult is consistent with a motor vehicular accident or a fall from a height. In contrast, a moderate or minor event, such as a fall from a standing position that provokes an acetabular fracture is highly suspicious for the presence of osteoporosis (17). Other contributing factors for osteoporosis such as the chronic use of oral corticosteroids are evaluated. Likewise, a past history of degenerative or inflammatory arthritis of the hip or of avascular necrosis is sought.

Other relevant features of the history include an evaluation for drug and alcohol abuse, and the nature of vocational activities or hobbies that may provide a high likelihood for falls, major accidents, heavy lifting, or other abuse of the hip. For an elderly individual, the presence of posturing of the hip, marked weakness of the hip abductor muscles, or a comorbidity that culminates in recurring falls merits consideration as a contraindication to an acute arthroplasty.

A radiographic evaluation of the hip and pelvis includes the standard anterior-posterior (AP), iliac, and obturator oblique views, along with a computed tomographic (CT) scan (36). The images are assessed carefully for the presence of impaction that is optimally visualized in sagittal and coronal reconstructions (Fig. 43-3). On the standard CT transaxial images, a surprisingly large area of impaction of the femoral head or of the dome may not be visualized. In an osteoporotic individual who sustains a fracture after a

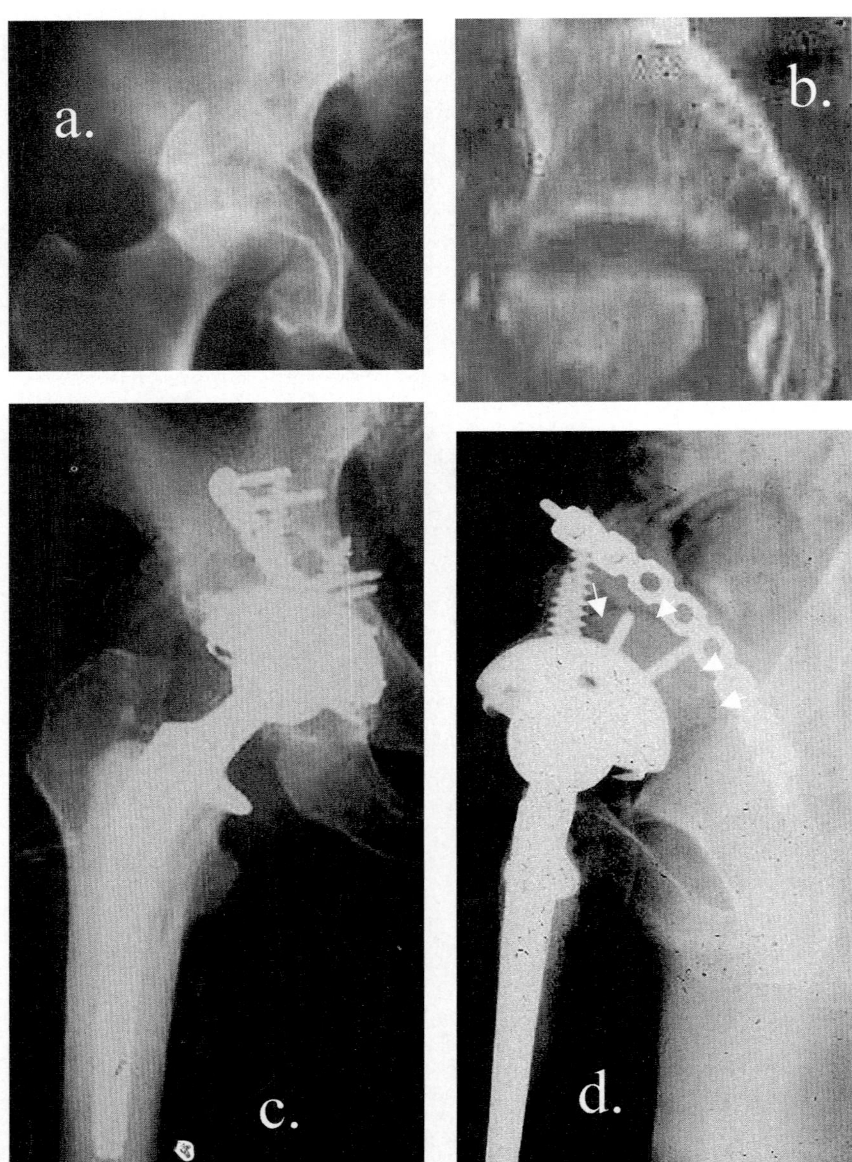

FIGURE 43-3. This 65-year-old man sustained a fall while skiing and provoked a posterior wall fracture. During the acute total hip arthroplasty, a structural autograft of femoral head was used to restore the acetabular defect. **a:** Preoperative anterior-posterior (AP) radiograph. **b:** Preoperative computed tomography sagittal reconstruction displays extensive damage to the femoral head. **c:** Postoperative AP view, 1 year later. **d:** Postoperative iliac oblique view displays the incorporated structural graft in the posterior wall.

simple fall, despite minimal radiographic evidence of impaction, an extraordinarily large area of impaction or of abrasive damage may be encountered at the time of the surgical procedure.

For the surgical consent, in the presence of complicating features that lead to a decision to perform an acute arthroplasty, consent for the acute arthroplasty is obtained. In a patient with a potentially reconstructible hip but who possesses osteopenic bone, we prefer to obtain consent for an open reduction and/or a total hip arthroplasty and to make the decision intraoperatively after the hip joint has been inspected.

THE STANDARD SURGICAL TECHNIQUE

We prefer to use a radiolucent graphite-composite table with the capability for intraoperative image intensification (33). Under a general or a spinal anesthetic, the patient is positioned in lateral decubitus with the use of an inflatable mattress or kidney rests to provide support of the trunk. The ipsilateral lower extremity is freely draped and prepared in the surgical field. Usually, a standard anterolateral or posterolateral approach is made. This decision rests largely on the surgeon's preference. For a posterior fracture-dislocation where the choice of an open reduction or a total hip arthroplasty will be made after the exposure, a posterolateral approach is used. Under special conditions, an extensile approach, such as a triradiate or an extended iliofemoral incision can be made (10,37,38). In either case, the gluteal insertions on the greater trochanter and the greater trochanter itself are preserved. Once a decision to replace the hip is made, the femoral neck is osteotomized with the use of a standard femoral neck guide. The femoral head and neck bone are saved for autograft. The subsequent steps are tailored to the particular fracture pattern.

TECHNIQUES FOR PARTICULAR FRACTURE PATTERNS

Posterior Wall Fracture

Visualization of this injury can be achieved either from a posterolateral or anterolateral incision. In either case, the capsular attachment to the principal wall fragment is carefully preserved to maintain its blood supply. In this way, the fragment serves as a vascularized bone flap for the bulk autograft of femoral head. With standard acetabular reamers, the acetabulum is prepared to achieve a bleeding osseous bed of subchondral bone. The femoral head is prepared with the reverse reamers, akin to previous cup arthroplasty reamers. After appropriate measurements for sizing have been obtained, the femoral head is shaped with a V-shaped cut to facilitate its subsequent impaction on the intact fracture surface of the posterior wall. Then, the bone graft is trimmed to remove the femoral neck. The graft is properly oriented on the fracture surface and gently impacted (Fig. 43-3). Three 2.5-mm drill bits are inserted through the graft into the underlying intact acetabulum. The drill bits are oriented so that they do not obstruct the pathway for the insertion of the acetabular cup. In turn, each drill bit is replaced with a 4-mm fully threaded cancellous screw after enlargement of the corresponding gliding hole in the bone graft. While each screw is inserted, the graft remains anchored by two drill bits or screws. Morselized reamings of bone are packed into any visible gaps along the interface between the graft and the intact acetabulum. Afterward, the acetabulum is re-reamed to the appropriate size. A cementless, multiscrew cup is selected that is oversized by 1 or 2 mm. With the use of a suitable aligning and insertional tool, the cup is positioned in the acetabulum and impacted. Three or four 6.5-mm anchoring screws are inserted into the cup to augment its fixation. One or two screws are directed into the bone graft. A power saw is used to trim any excessive graft that might serve as a source of impingement for the arthroplasty. Then a trial liner is inserted into the cup.

The standard reamers and broaches are used to prepare the femoral canal for the insertion of a cementless or cemented stem. After a suitable trial reduction is performed, the appropriate acetabular liner is inserted into the cup. The selected cementless or cemented stem is introduced into the femur with a standard technique. The femoral head component with the appropriate neck length is impacted on the Morse taper of the stem. The hip joint is reduced for a final assessment of stability and limb length. Then the wound is closed in a conventional fashion.

Transverse or T-Type Fracture

From the perspective of an exchange arthroplasty, a transverse fracture is an example of a dissociation. Compared to the typical complex dissociation that is encountered with an exchange arthroplasty, this traumatically induced variant is simplified by the preservation of the acetabular roof. With the use of a standard multiscrew cup or a cage or ring (39,40), effective anchorage of the component can be readily achieved. The most recent cage designs possess a porous outer surface for bony ingrowth and anchorage. Also, the attachment of the liner is achieved with a mechanical interlock that is similar to a conventional acetabular liner. The technical challenge pertains to the reduction and immobilization of the inferior half of the acetabulum.

Following a standard exposure and removal of the femoral head, the acetabulum is visualized. The intact articular cartilage on the acetabular roof is debrided with the use of curettes and acetabular reamers. For a reduction of the inferior half of the acetabulum, one of several different strategies can be used. One of the large pelvic bone-holding forceps with eccentric tenaculum jaws can be inserted with the longer jaw placed on the inner acetabular surface (41). This jaw can be advanced through the greater sciatic notch to rest upon the quadrilateral surface. Alternatively, it can be positioned next to the anterior inferior iliac spine (AIIS) and slid along the pelvic brim until it advances to the quadrilateral surface. The shorter jaw is positioned on the lateral wall of the pelvis, superior to the acetabulum. The central displacement is corrected by a manipulation of the forceps.

To eliminate an associated rotational component of the deformity, one of several techniques can be used. A Steinmann pin, Schanz screw, or external fixation pin can be inserted into the tubercle of the ischial tuberosity. Manipulation of the pin permits a realignment of the fracture. Alternatively, a Lambotte-Farabeuf forceps (10) can be applied to the heads of two opposing screws that are inserted in the posterior column. Another possibility is to apply a 3.5-mm reconstruction plate across the fracture on the posterior column.

Another method of fixation employs one or two cables or heavy wires that serve both to reduce and stabilize the fracture. A 2.5-mm drill hole is made in the base of the AIIS. A 2-mm cable or a large wire is passed through the hole. The cable has to be of the free-ended variety, without a securing clamp on either end. The free end of the cable on the inner pelvic surface is grasp with a Statinski clamp and passed along the quadrilateral surface to the greater sciatic notch (Fig. 43-4). A finger can be placed in the greater notch to help guide the cable. Alternatively, prior to the reduction of the fracture, the cable can be passed from the drill hole in the AIIS to the anterior fracture surface. In stages, the cable can be advanced to the posterior fracture surface and ultimately out of the greater notch. The critical factor is to keep the cable directly on the inner pelvic table and away from the roof of the greater notch, in proximity to the sciatic nerve and the superior gluteal neurovascular bundle. Now

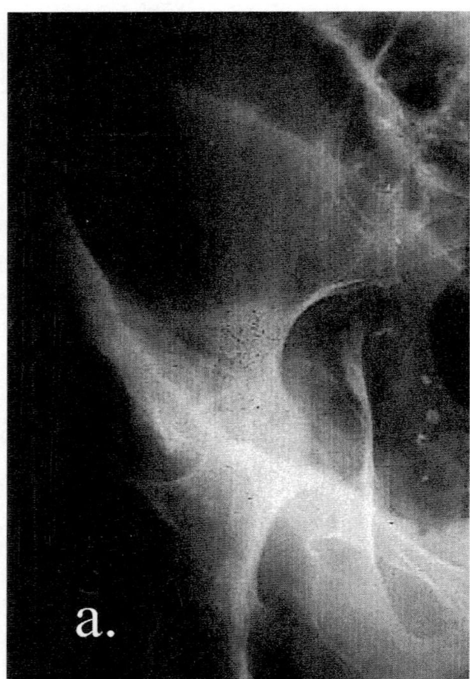

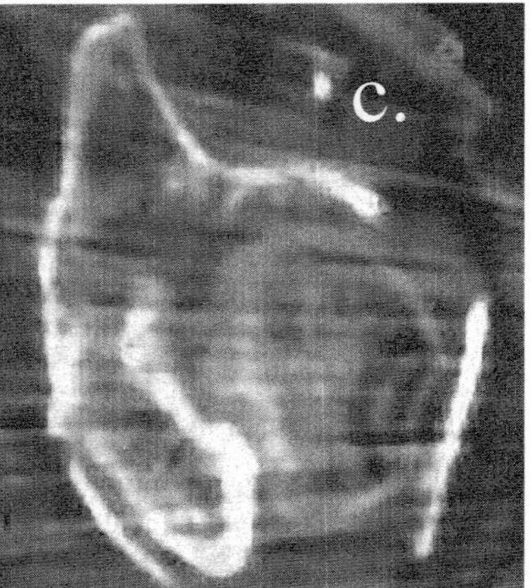

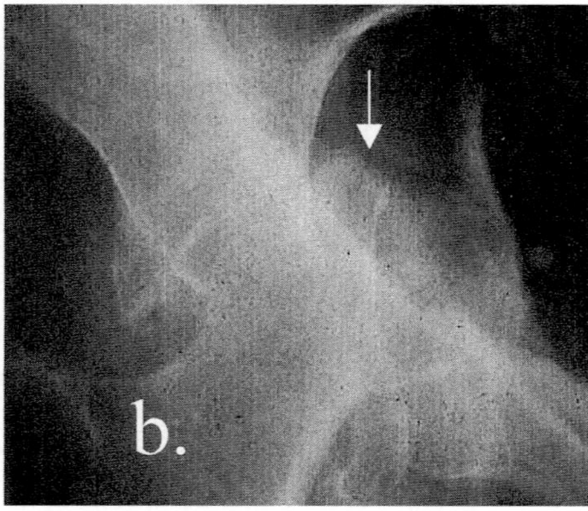

FIGURE 43-4. This 89-year-old woman sustained a simple fall and provoked this T-type posterior wall fracture with marked acetabular impaction. Cable fixation accompanied the acute total hip arthroplasty. **a:** Preoperative iliac oblique view. **b:** Preoperative obturator oblique view. **c:** Preoperative computed tomography scan.

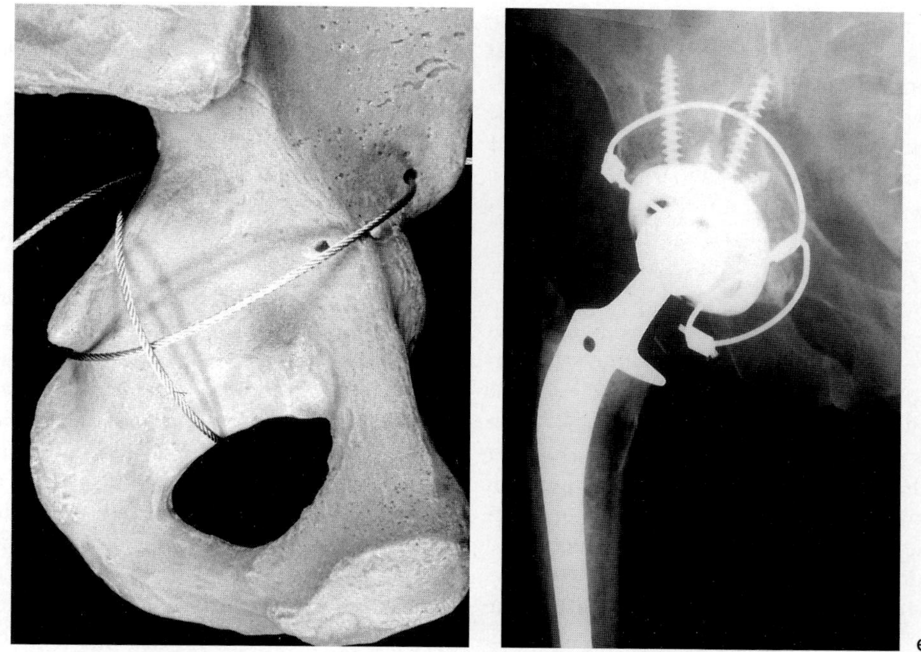

FIGURE 43-4. ***(continued)*** **d:** Model with cable buttressing the quadrilateral surface. **e:** Postoperative anterior-posterior view taken 6 weeks afterward. A free sleeve anchors the two cables on the inner pelvic table.

the passing tool is used to pass the posterior end of the cable from the greater notch to the lesser sciatic notch, where the cable exits from the inner pelvic surface and is directed up the outer surface of the posterior column. The two ends of the cable are connected above the acetabular roof. Where the posterior fracture line extends superior to the greater notch to create a large "beak" of dense bone, the first cable can exit from the greater notch, so that it gains purchase on the beak of the posterior column fragment, rather than exiting from the lesser sciatic notch.

A second cable is passed through another drill hole in the AIIS. The free inner end of the cable is advanced along the outer surface of the anterior wall. The Statinski clamp is passed through the anterior fracture line of the quadrilateral fragment and advanced through the obturator foramen where it exits at the base of the anterior wall. This site is about 3 cm lateral to the obturator vessels. The free end of the cable is grasped and retracted into the acetabulum. In stages, the cable is passed to the posterior fracture line and out through the greater sciatic notch. The two ends of the cable are connected above the acetabular roof. If the standard Dall-Miles tightener and crimping tool are used, the superior acetabular region is the optimal one for the insertion of these bulky tools into a standard incision for a total hip arthroplasty. Alternatively, two of the single-ended tightening tools can be used, with one applied to either end of the cable. After the reduction and prior to the final crimping of the retaining clamps on the cable, imaging is suggested to ascertain the accuracy of the reduction. Then the sleeve is crimped.

Once the transverse fracture is reduced and provisionally stabilized, the acetabulum is reamed progressively to the appropriate size. Morselized reamings are packed into the fracture line. The largest of the previously employed reamers is used in a reverse mode to pack the bone graft. Then the appropriate cup is impacted into the acetabulum, on the aligning tool. Four to six 6.5-mm fixation screws are inserted into the cup to anchor it to the intact acetabulum as well as to the inferior fragment(s). The procedure is completed in a conventional manner.

Anterior Column Fracture

The most frequently encountered variant in a geriatric patient possesses a large fragment of quadrilateral surface as well as separate pieces of anterior column and wall (42). In one of his publications, Letournel (43) recognized this injury pattern as a distinct associated category. The technical challenge has been the development of a method of stabilization that can be undertaken with the use of a standard approach for a total hip arthroplasty. The quadrilateral fragment is extremely thin and thereby unsuitable for fixation with the use of screws. In the exceptional case, the posterior portion of the fragment can be anchored with a screw. Cables have been very effective for these cases (20,34). After the exposure and removal of the femoral head, the quadrilateral fragment is reduced with the use of the eccentric pelvic forceps. Image intensification can be used to confirm the reduction. Then the cabling technique is undertaken. An alternative site where the cables can be connected is the posterior column, although some additional exposure of this region is required, with respect to a standard incision for a total hip arthroplasty (THA).

Both-Column Fracture

This injury pattern usually possesses a high and a low anterior column fragment as well as a posterior column fragment that includes the quadrilateral surface. In contrast to the previously described procedures, the high anterior column fragment requires an initial stabilization. After the exposure and removal of the femoral head, the high anterior fragment is reduced under image intensification with tenaculum forceps. For fixation, two cannulated screws are inserted through a stab wound, superficial to the AIIS. The screws are inserted under image intensification with the use of the obturator and iliac oblique views. The screws are directed into the greater sciatic buttress, above the roof of the greater sciatic notch. With a thickness of more than 3 cm, this site represents a large target zone. Afterward, the two principal inferior fracture fragments are reduced and immobilized in a manner that is comparable to the previous description for a T-type fracture, including the use of cable fixation.

ALTERNATIVE STRATEGIES FOR THE FRACTURE FIXATION AND BUTTRESSING OF BONE GRAFT

Clearly, many other techniques are available to immobilize the fracture and support the bone graft in a bone defect. One method employs mesh to support the morselized bone graft (Fig. 43-5). This technique was popularized by Sloof and coworkers (44), primarily for application to an exchange arthroplasty and in conjunction with the use of cancellous allograft. In that situation, the authors recommend the use of a cemented polyethylene cup. For an acute acetabular fracture, where routinely the femoral head and neck are available as morselized cancellous autograft, the authors prefer to use a multiscrew cementless cup. Either titanium or stainless steel mesh is preferred to one made of cobalt-chromium alloy. The last is too stiff to readily contour and too difficult to cut. A preformed mesh is commercially available that is shaped to fit in the central defect or is applied to the posterior and superior wall. For a central defect, initially, the fracture is reduced under image guidance. Provisional fixation is undertaken with one of the previously described techniques. The central acetabulum is inspected for a persistent full-thickness defect, possibly secondary to marked comminution of osteoporotic bone. Some of the bone graft is placed in the base of the defect. Then a circular mesh of the appropriate size is placed in the defect. The mesh extends across the

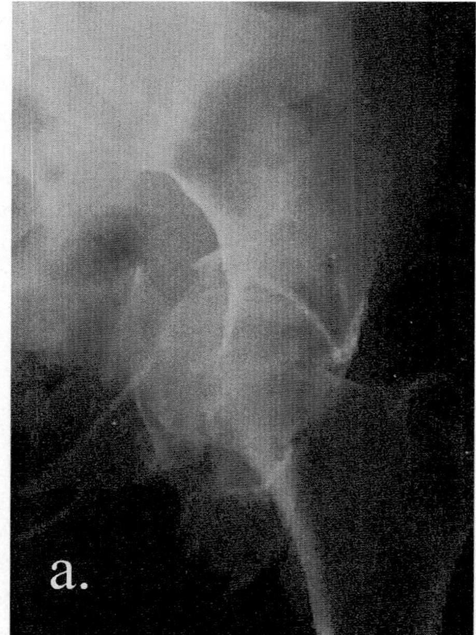

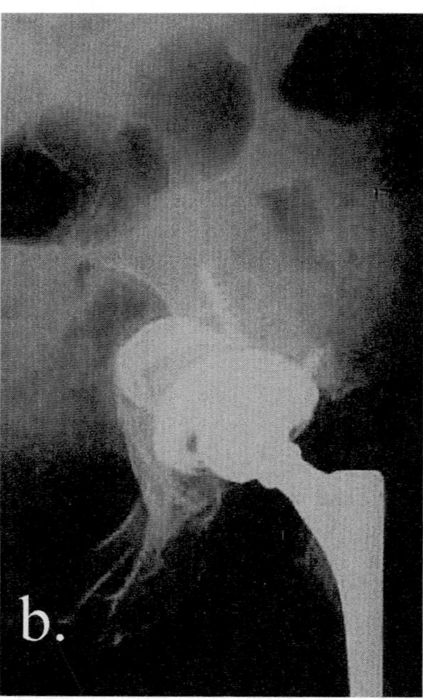

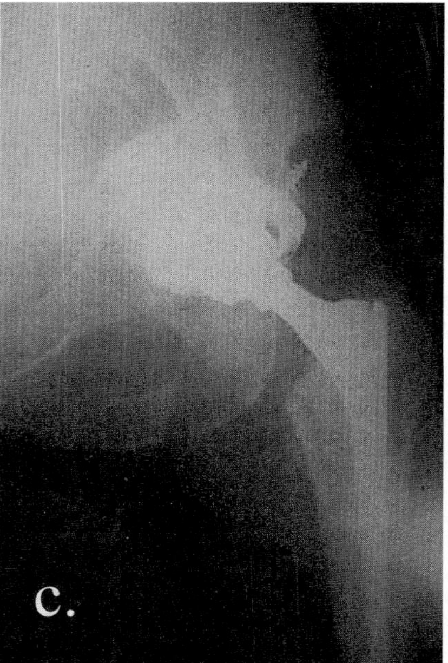

FIGURE 43-5. This 75-year-old woman sustained a simple fall and provoked a comminuted anterior column fracture, including displacement of the quadrilateral surface. A stainless steel mesh was contoured to obliterate the fracture gap and to partly stabilize the fracture. An impaction autografting was performed along with the acute total hip arthroplasty. **a:** Preoperative anterior-posterior view. **b:** Postoperative iliac oblique view, 6 months later. **c:** Postoperative obturator oblique view to display the position of the mesh.

defective zone so that its periphery rests on supportive bone. If the defect is very large, the mesh can be anchored with small screws around its periphery. Additional cancellous graft is placed on the exposed surface of the mesh. An acetabular reamer of the appropriate size is used in reverse mode to impact the graft. This step may be repeated until a complete bony bed is visualized. Then a cup of the corresponding size is impacted into the acetabulum and supplementary screw fixation is undertaken. For a defective posterior wall, a crescentic mesh of appropriate size can be anchored over the defect with multiple screws. Impaction autografting is undertaken followed by the insertion of the cup.

Another technique employs the use of a ring or cage (39). The newest generation of cage possesses an outer ingrowth surface and a mechanical interlock for the attachment of the liner, instead of the use of methylmethacrylate cement. This design is particularly suitable for use in a younger patient with dense bone. With the earlier technique, the cement was liable to a premature failure. Also, in the absence of bone ingrowth, a conventional cage is vulnerable to loosening with backing-out of the screws. In an osteoporotic patient with osteopenic bone, the use of cement may serve to augment the fixation of the cage. The asset of the cage is to facilitate the stabilization of the fracture and to solidly anchor the cup. If the fracture propagates into the posterior column or elsewhere, generally an alternative design of cage such as the Bursch-Schneider design (40) is preferred to optimize the fixation (Fig. 43-2). For a both-column fracture, supplementary lag screw fixation of the high anterior column is necessary. A liability of the Bursch-Schneider design is its inferior plate, which hampers its application to the bone unless a considerable enlargement of the standard incision is made. For the authors, the principal role for a cage is a late presentation where an incomplete reduction may contribute to the anticipated bony defect.

Where the use of a cage is planned, after a careful assessment of the preoperative images, the appropriate type of cage is selected. Prior to its insertion, the optimal reduction of the fracture is achieved and provisionally stabilized with a combination of bone-holding forceps, K-wires, screws, or cables. The acetabulum is debrided of residual articular cartilage with the use of acetabular reamers and curettes or a power burr. If the initial trial fit of the cage is suboptimal, the reduction of the fracture may be adjusted. Once the fit of the cage is improved, a persistent fracture gap or osseous defect is filled with impacted bone graft. Then the cage is inserted and properly oriented. For the conventional cage in which the liner is cemented into place, the orientation of the cage is not critical. With its independent insertion, the orientation of the liner can be directed to optimize the stability of the arthroplastic hip. For the cage with a mechanical attachment of the liner, the orientation of the cage is a critical factor to ensure a stable arthroplastic hip. In the latter instance, the near anatomic realignment of the hemipelvis is essential to ensure that the cage is properly oriented.

RESULTS

Between 1985 and 1997, the clinical and radiographic results after an acute total hip arthroplasty for selective displaced acetabular fractures were evaluated in 57 patients who were followed for a mean duration of 8.1 years (range, 2 to 12 years). The mean age of the patients was 69 years (range, 26 to 89 years), with 30 men and 27 women. The mechanism of injury was minor trauma in 47% (27 cases), indicative of the presence of significant osteoporosis, and major trauma in 53% (30 cases). All of the patients were assessed both clinically and with imaging that included AP and Judet radiographs and a CT scan. Of the 25 (51%) simple fractures, there were 11 posterior wall, three posterior column, 10 transverse, and one anterior column injuries. Of the 32 (49%) associated fractures, there were six posterior column-posterior wall, four transverse-posterior wall, three T-type, four both-column, six anterior column-posterior hemitransverse, and nine comminuted anterior column disruptions with quadrilateral surface involvement. All of the cases possessed complicating features such as extensive comminution with 10 or more articular fragments, impaction, full-thickness abrasive loss of the articular cartilage of the femoral head, or acetabular or femoral head impaction involving more than 40% of the articular surface that included the weight-bearing area. Other occasional indications included severe preexisting degenerative arthrosis or an associated completely displaced femoral neck fracture that was unreduced for more than 1 week. Notable features of osteoporosis included the presence of a minor traumatic event in 27 patients, a previous minor traumatic fracture in 19 patients, including five hip fractures, and a positive Singh index (45) for osteoporosis in 33 patients. One other patient on chronic hemodialysis had severe renal osteodystrophy.

For the surgical procedure, a Harris-Galante I or II cup (Zimmer, Warsaw, IN) was used in all of the cases. For the younger patients with dense bone, an Anatomic or a Multilock uncemented stem (Zimmer, Warsaw, IN) was used. In patients with osteopenic bone, a Harris-Design 2 component (Zimmer, Warsaw, IN) was used in seven earlier cases, along with one Precoat stem. For the last 29 such cases, a collarless, polished, double tapered CPT stem (Zimmer, Warsaw, IN) was used. The cementation technique as described by Bourne and coworkers (46)—using lavage, a brush, a cement plug, and desiccation of the canal—was employed for all of the cemented cases. Following the procedure, the patients were encouraged to undertake a touchdown gait with the use of crutches or a walker. Six weeks later, weight bearing was increased as tolerated with a conversion to a cane at 10 weeks. The patients were routinely anticoagulated with coumadin or low molecular weight heparin for a 3-week period (47). No prophylaxis for heterotopic bone formation was used (48,49). All of the patients were evaluated clinically and radiographically at periods of 6 weeks, 3 months, 6 months, 12 months, and yearly thereafter. The assessment included a Harris hip score (50) and a series of radiographic parameters. A satisfaction index was recorded for each postoperative assessment that evaluated the patient for relief of pain, independence of ambulation based on the preoperative level, restoration of activities of daily living, and of preinjury employment or other activities.

At the latest clinical evaluation, 49 patients (87%) had no or slight and intermittent pain and 18 undertook some degree of laboring activity. Forty-five patients (79%) possessed an excellent or good Harris hip score. When the Harris hip scores were categorized by patient age in decades, a strong correlation was evident, with the highest scores achieved for the youngest patients and a progressive deterioration of the scores with advancing age. This trend was particularly evident for the 70- and 80-year-old patients, with scores of 87 ± 8 for the former and 75 ± 12 for the latter. Whereas 39 patients (68%) displayed normal ambulation or at most a slight limp, 13 others (23%) required a cane for long distances. Of the five patients who were limited ambulators, four were between 70 and 89 years old, whereas the other sustained a complete traumatically induced lumbosacral plexopathy with a footdrop. Of the 13 patients who used a cane, nine were 70 years old or more and had used a cane before their surgery. For the clinical outcome, all of the patients were extremely satisfied or satisfied; none was dissatisfied.

Radiographically, all of the fractures united within 12 weeks, of which six fractures (11%) were healed at 6 weeks. There were no delayed or nonunions. After 12 weeks, two cases of Brooker (51,52) grade I heterotopic bone (3.5%), three cases of grade II (5.2%), and one case of grade IV (1.7%) were documented. In a quantitative assessment for subsidence of the cups using the method of Russotti and Harris (53), the average medial displacement was 3 mm (range, 1 to 4 mm) at 6 weeks and the average vertical displacement was 2 mm (range, 1 to 4 mm). No further displacement was detected in the subsequent radiographs. No angular changes in the cups were documented. No correlation in the magnitude of the displacement and the pattern of the acetabular fractures was identified. There was no late loosening of any cup in the series, by the definition of Russotti and Harris (53). Also, no loose or broken screws were detected, apart from one patient with renal osteodystrophy. In this case, at 12 weeks after the surgery, radiographic halos were present around the screws. One year later, the patient underwent a successful cadaveric renal transplant. Six months later, the halos vanished.

Postoperatively, six cups (10.5%) were medialized secondary to a residual protrusion and a suboptimal reduction of the fracture, all of which involved the anterior column. The obturator oblique view provided the optimal projection of this displacement (Fig. 43-6). The magnitude of the me-

A

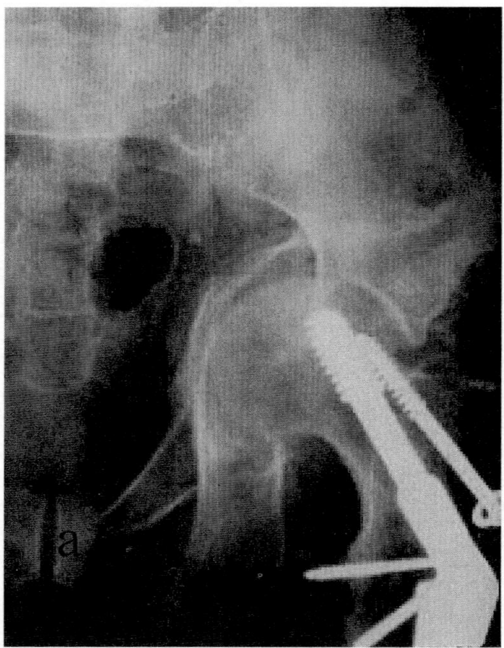

B

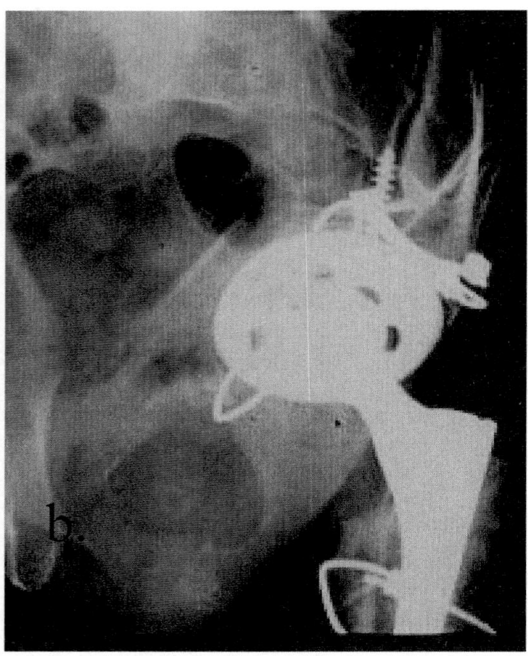

FIGURE 43-6. This 63-year-old man with a history of chronic alcoholism, fell from a 3-foot ladder to sustain a comminuted transverse-posterior wall fracture. Two years earlier, he underwent an ORIF for an ipsilateral intertrochanteric fracture. When the acute total hip arthroplasty was performed, the protrusion was not anatomically corrected. Although he achieved an excellent clinical outcome, the fixation of the cup was suboptimal. **A:** Preoperative anterior-posterior view. **B:** Postoperative obturator oblique view, 6 months afterward.

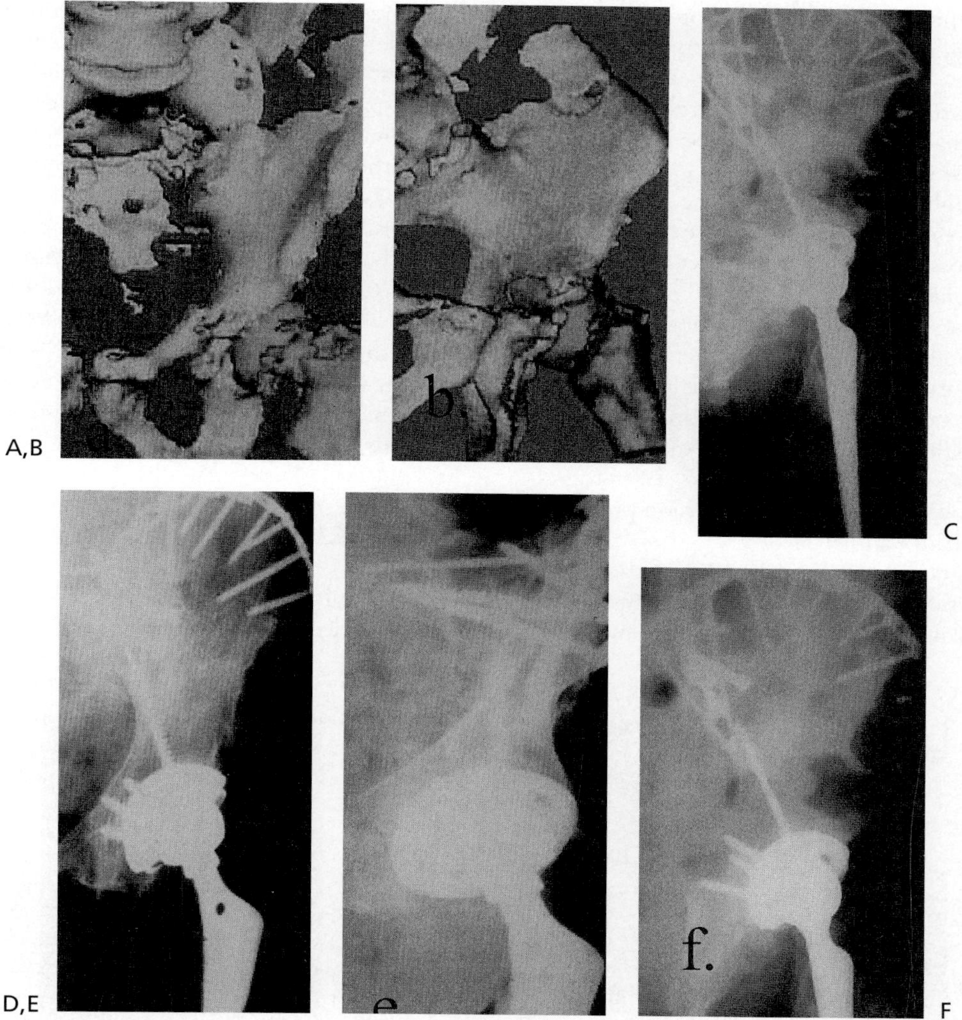

FIGURE 43-7. This 58-year-old woman bus driver sustained a motor vehicle injury when her vehicle plunged over a 100-ft cliff. Her injuries included a left-sided fracture-dislocation of the sacroiliac joint, an anterior column fracture, and an ipsilateral displaced femoral neck fracture. She required an emergency splenectomy and intubation for a bilateral unstable chest injury. Three weeks later, when pelvic surgery became feasible, an ORIF of the pelvic fracture, along with an acute total hip arthroplasty were performed through an extended iliofemoral approach. Although her hip recovered uneventfully, her traumatically induced lumbo-sacral plexopathy and foot-drop did not resolve. A comparison of her immediate postoperative radiograph with views taken four years later illustrates the spontaneous obliteration of gaps in the bone graft within zones I and II. **A:** Preoperative anterior-posterior (AP) view. **B:** Preoperative three-dimensional computed tomography internal iliac oblique view. **C:** Postoperative iliac oblique view, with gap around the superior margin of the cup. **D:** AP view 4 years later. **E:** Four-year obturator oblique view. **F:** Four-year iliac oblique view.

dialization of the six cups ranged from 0.4 to 1.8 cm, with an average of 0.9 cm. None of the malpositioned cups loosened.

Voids between the acetabular bed and the acetabular component were documented on the immediate postoperative radiographs in 36 of the 57 hips (63%). There were 8 hips with gaps in Gruen (54) zone I, 19 with gaps in zone II, and 9 with gaps in zone III. In 27 (75%) of the 36 hips with gaps after surgery, the gaps resolved completely by the one year postoperative evaluation (Fig. 43-7). In four other cases, the gaps disappeared radiographically within 2 years after the procedure. In three other hips, the gaps resolved within some zones but remained unchanged in other zones. In the remaining two hips, the original gaps resolved but new ones formed in different zones. Of the 21 hips with no gaps after surgery, 15 cups displayed no gaps at the time of the last follow-up evaluation. Four hips developed gaps of 0.5 mm or less at the time of the last assessment and two other hips developed gaps of 0.5 to 2.0 mm. None of the hips showed a continuous gap in all three zones to indicate loosening, either immediately after the surgery or at the latest evaluation.

Osteolysis was measured in the acetabular zones with the technique of DeLee and Charnley (55). Localized cavitary acetabular osteolysis occurred in 12 hips (21%). Ten cases were limited to peripheral resorption in zone I, seven cases in zone II, and four cases in zone III. No case of linear osteolysis extending across multiple zones was identified, and no cups were radiographically loose.

Polyethylene wear was documented in nine hips (16%), where the corresponding eccentricity of the femoral head was >2 mm. The earliest time after implantation when wear was detected was at 3 years, whereas most examples were first observed after 5 years. For the few cases with 5- to 12-year follow-up assessments, there was no clear progression of the wear process (Fig. 43-8). No revision procedure was performed to change a liner.

From the radiographic evaluations, four of the 17 cementless stems subsided between 1 and 3 mm within the first year after implantation. No progression of the subsidence was documented with the subsequent evaluations. At the time of the last evaluation, seven of the cases displayed focal resorption adjacent to the uppermost extent of the ingrowth pads on the stems, but none was radiographically or clinically loose.

For the 40 cemented stems, the cementation was characterized as 12 type A, 23 type B, and five type C cement columns. There were no type D examples. None of the 11 Harris Design-2 stems displayed any migration and all were neutrally aligned. On average, the CPT stems displayed 1.5 mm of subsidence during the initial 6-week period after implantation. Subsequently, no further subsidence was evident. At the last evaluation, using the criteria of Harris and McGann (56), none of the cemented stems was possibly or definitely loose.

COMPLICATIONS

During the initial 6-week postoperative period, there were no deaths, deep wound infections, dislocations, sciatic nerve

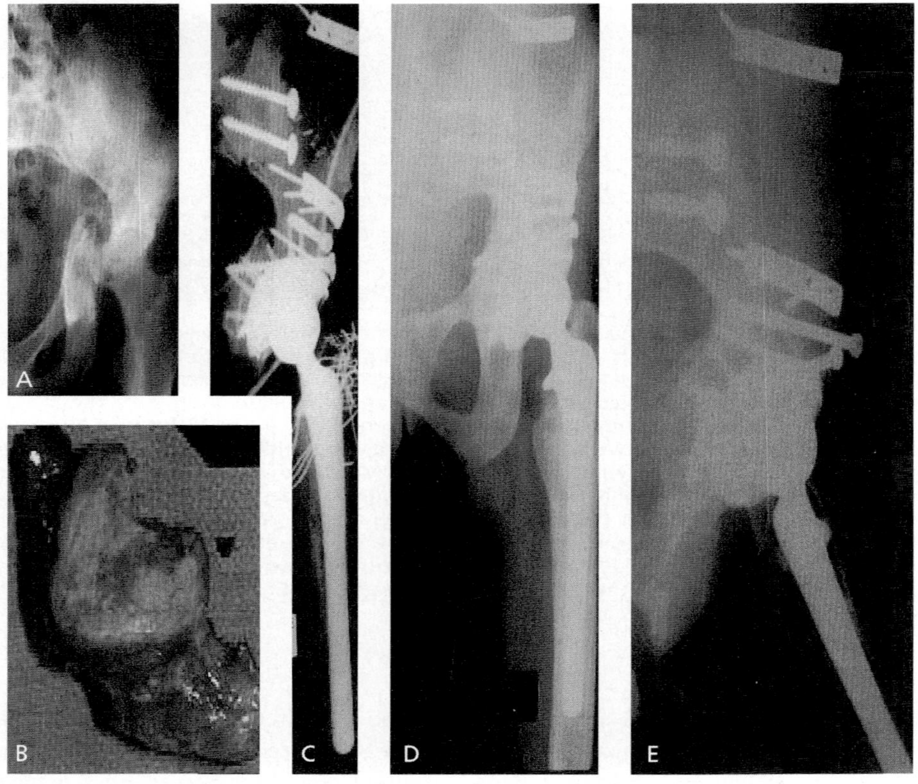

FIGURE 43-8. This 28-year-old woman sustained a both-column fracture with a sacroiliac subluxation in a motor vehicle accident. Her femoral head was markedly impacted. An acute total hip arthroplasty was performed at the time of the ORIF with plates and screws. One year later, symptomatic hardware on the greater trochanter was removed. Otherwise, she achieved an excellent clinical outcome. In the 5-year radiographic study, features of polyethylene wear were evident, although subsequently, no progression was documented in the 12-year assessment. **A:** Preoperative anterior-posterior (AP) view. **B:** Intraoperative view of femoral head. **C:** Initial postoperative AP view. **D:** AP view at 12 years. **E:** Twelve-year iliac oblique view to highlight cup wear.

palsies, or pulmonary emboli. Three cases of symptomatic deep venous thrombosis were managed with short-term heparinization and longer-term coumadinization. During the late postoperative period beyond 6 weeks, there were two dislocations (3.5%). One was successfully managed with a closed reduction, whereas the other progressed to a revision of the cup for a malalignment. One case with a painful trochanteric wire progressed to a localized metal removal, 1 year after the arthroplasty. For the case of grade IV heterotopic bone, a resection was performed 1 year after the arthroplasty. Early postoperative irradiation therapy with 700 cGy units followed. The patient achieved an excellent clinical result, without a recurrence of the heterotopic bone. There were no late deep infections and no other late surgical procedures.

DISCUSSION

Following a review of the recent results of acute total hip arthroplasty, the method appears to hold considerable promise when it is applied to a highly select group of acetabular fractures and particularly for elderly patients. For the purpose of this discussion, the term "elderly" was reserved for an individual of more than 60 years of age. The term does not necessarily indicate physiologic deterioration above and beyond an otherwise healthy individual of that chronological age and sex-dependent degree of postmenopausal osteoporosis. Currently, the elderly population is growing rapidly, a trend that is anticipated to continue for at least a few decades. Nevertheless, certain elderly patients who sustain a displaced acetabular fracture are optimally managed with an open reduction and internal fixation. The wide variability in physiologic age of an elderly individual and the corresponding diversity in the quality of the bone are well recognized. Certainly, an active octogenarian who sustains a simple displaced and incongruent acetabular fracture that is uncomplicated by comminution or impaction is optimally managed by an open reduction and internal fixation. The indications for an acute total hip arthroplasty for a young adult with an acetabular fracture with extensive impaction and concomitant damage to the femoral head is a more complex judgment. With the potential for an active lifestyle and a long life expectancy, in the young adult a total hip arthroplasty is a less satisfactory therapeutic option. Nevertheless, in the authors' opinion, the method also possesses a limited role for carefully selected young adults.

For the current study, the most significant feature of structurally compromising osteoporosis was the provocation of the acetabular fracture by minor trauma, such as a simple fall, in 27 patients (Figs. 43-1 and 43-4). A comparable factor was a past history of a fracture owing to minor trauma in 19 patients, including five with a prior hip fracture. Twenty-one patients had marked osteoporosis according to their Singh index. In this series, 33 patients possessed one or more of these manifestations of osteoporosis. Following a minor traumatic event other significant indicators of markedly osteoporotic bone include acetabular or femoral head impaction involving more than 40% of the surface area or comminution with more than 10 intraarticular fragments.

One unanticipated finding in the current series was the difficulty to accurately determine the degree of damage to the femoral head or the surface area of involvement of the acetabulum with marginal impaction by a review of the preoperative radiographs and CT scan. The typical scenario is a geriatric patient who sustains a posterior fracture-dislocation involving the posterior wall from a minor traumatic event (Fig. 43-1). On the AP and the Judet oblique views, the femoral head may appear to be intact. From the transaxial CT views, a small defect may be evident in the femoral head, which, at the time of surgery actually may involve 30% to 50% of the surface area. Intraoperatively, adequate visualization of such a defect may be further hampered by its typical location on the anterior and superior quadrant of the head where it is difficult to appreciate without the use of an endoscope or dental mirror. For such a case, we routinely obtain surgical consent for either an open reduction and internal fixation or a total hip arthroplasty and make the determination for the preferred treatment based on the operative findings.

For the current series, a notable observation was the common but self-limiting subsidence of the cups by 1 to 4 mm during the first 6 weeks after implantation. Typically, these small voids in the bone at the periphery of the cups resolved within 1 year. This remodeling of the bone adjacent to an impaction grafting that was imperfectly performed was a reassuring observation. Similarly, the absence of any loose cups was encouraging. Clearly, the approximated fracture fragments or autologous cancellous bone graft around the cup tends to culminate in a solid construct of bone that effectively anchors the cementless cup.

A technical concern in six cases was the excessive medialization of the cup by an average of 0.9 cm. The excessive medialization represents an inadequate reduction of central protrusion. This problem is most likely to occur in the presence of a comminuted anterior column fracture that includes the quadrilateral surface, an anterior column-posterior hemitransverse, or a both-column fracture. Intraoperative imaging, especially the obturator oblique view, can be used to minimize the risk of this complication. Although this failure to adequately correct an acetabular protrusion did not lead to associated complications nor to inferior late clinical outcomes, it is undesirable from several perspectives. For an intact acetabulum, the superior anchoring screws are directed along the axis of the ilium, between the inner and outer tables. In a protruded acetabulum, these screws may be directed medial to the ilium and penetrate the thin adjacent inner pelvic wall to compromise the fixation of the cup. The medial screws approximate the hazardous portion of the roof that is adjacent to the overlying anterior iliac vessels (57). Finally, the protruded cup is not well supported by dense superior iliac bone to withstand the normal weight-bearing forces.

Ironically, the functional outcomes for the elderly patients, as determined by the Harris hip scores, were inferior to the scores of the younger patients. Previously, a similar observation for a group of elderly arthroplastic patients with an initial diagnosis of degenerative arthritis was reported by Bourne and coworkers (46). These patients with preexisting osteoarthritis often had a functional impairment prior to the procedure, possibly with the need to use a cane. Frequently, such a situation is unlikely to be improved by the arthroplasty and thereby serves to compromise the hip score. In the current series, in terms of pain relief, whereby 49 patients (86%) had no pain or only slight and intermittent pain, and six others (9.5%) had only occasional pain after ambulation, the results were very good for 96% of the cases. Likewise, in terms of satisfaction of the patients with their outcome, 41 (81%) of the 57 patients were extremely satisfied and 11 others (19%) were satisfied; none were dissatisfied. From these perspectives, acute total hip arthroplasty to manage selective acetabular fractures is a highly successful procedure. Nevertheless, the shortcomings of this technique cannot be underestimated. For an active young adult with a long life expectancy, a total hip arthroplasty is vulnerable to a premature failure, possibly with extensive lysis of bone and a potential for a periprosthetic fracture (58,59). For such an individual who displays a prior history of self-destructive behavior and possibly of alcohol or drug abuse, the outlook for the arthroplastic hip is heavily compromised. In consideration for an acute total hip arthroplasty, the selection of the appropriate patient along with a rigorous assessment of the complicating features of the acetabular fracture represent crucial factors in the preoperative decision-making process to determine the optimal therapeutic protocol.

REFERENCES

1. Goulet JA, Bray TJ. Complex acetabular fractures. *Clin Orthop* 1989;240:9.
2. Pipkin G. Treatment of grade IV fracture-dislocation of the hip. *J Bone Joint Surg* 1957;39-A:1027.
3. Rommens PM, Broos PL, Vanderschot P. Preparation and technique for surgical treatment of 225 acetabular fractures. Two-year results of 175 cases. *Unfallchirurg* 1997;100:338.
4. Romness DW, Lewallen DG. Total hip arthroplasty after fracture of the acetabulum. *J Bone Joint Surg* 1990;72-B:761.
5. Rowe CR, Lowell JD. Prognosis of fractures of the acetabulum. *J Bone Joint Surg* 1961;43-A:30.
6. Ruesch PD, Holdner H, Ciaramitaro M, et al. A prospective study of surgically treated acetabular fractures. *Clin Orthop* 1994;305:38.
7. DeRidder VA, de Lange S, Kingma L, et al. Results of 75 consecutive patients with an acetabular fracture. *Clin Orthop* 1994; 305:53.
8. Mayo KA. Open reduction and internal fixation of fractures of the acetabulum. Results of 163 fractures. *Clin Orthop* 1994; 305:31.
9. Judet R, Judet J, Letournel E. Fractures of the acetabulum: classification and surgical approaches for open reduction: preliminary report. *J Bone Joint Surg* 1964;46-A:1615.
10. Letournel E, Judet R. *Fractures of the acetabulum,* 2nd ed. New York: Springer-Verlag, 1993.
11. Matta JM. Fractures of the acetabulum: accuracy of reduction and clinical results in patients managed operatively within three weeks after the injury. *J Bone Joint Surg* 1996;78-A:1632.
12. Mears DC, Velyvis JH, Chang CP. Is an open reduction and internal fixation the preferred method of treatment for most patients after acute displaced acetabular fractures? 2003;406:261.
13. Helfet DL, Borrelli J Jr, DiPasquale T, et al. Stabilization of acetabular fractures in elderly patients. *J Bone Joint Surg* 1992;74-A:753.
14. Melton LS. Epidemiological features of pelvic fractures. *Clin Orthop* 1981;155:43.
15. Ragnarsson B, Jacobsson B. Epidemiology of pelvic fractures in a Swedish county. *Acta Orthop Scand* 1992;63:297.
16. Kannus P, Palvanen M, Niemi S, et al. Epidemiology of osteoporotic pelvic fractures in elderly people in Finland: sharp increase in 1970–1997 and alarming prospects for the new millennium. *Osteoporosis Int* 2000;11:443.
17. Lonner JH, Koval KJ. Poly-trauma in the elderly. *Clin Orthop* 1995;318:136.
18. Liu S, Siegel PZ, Brewer RD, et al. Prevalence of alcohol impaired driving. *JAMA* 1997;288:122.
19. Reduction in alcohol-related traffic fatalities—United States, 1990–1992. *Morbid Mortal Wkly Rept* 1993;42(47):905.
20. Mears DC, Velyvis JH. Acute total hip arthroplasty for selective acetabular fractures: two to twelve-year results. *J Bone Joint Surg (Am)* 2002; 84A:1–9.
21. Mears DC. Surgical treatment of acetabular fractures in elderly patients with osteoporotic bone. *J Am Acad Orthop Surg* 1999;7: 128.
22. Jimenez ML, Tile M, Schenk RS. Total hip replacement after acetabular fracture. *Orthop Clin North Am* 1997;28:435.
23. Boardman KP, Charnley J. Low-friction arthroplasty after fracture-dislocations of the hip. *J Bone Joint Surg* 1978;60-B:495.
24. Stauffer RN. Ten-year follow-up study of total hip replacement. *J Bone Joint Surg* 1982;64-A:983.
25. Malkin C, Tauber C. Total hip arthroplasty and acetabular bone grafting for unreduced fracture-dislocation of the hip. *Clin Orthop* 1985;201:57.
26. Weber M, Berry DJ, Harmsen S. Total hip arthroplasty after operative treatment of an acetabular fracture. *J Bone Joint Surg* 1998;80-A:1295.
27. Berry DJ. Total hip arthroplasty following acetabular fracture. *Orthopedics* 1999;22(9):837.
28. Pritchett JW, Bortel DT. Total hip replacement after central fracture dislocation of the acetabulum. *Orthop Rev* 1991;20(7):607.
29. Rogan IM, Weber FA, Solomon L. Total hip replacement following fracture-dislocation of the acetabulum. *J Bone Joint Surg* 1979;61-B:252.
30. Kelly PJ, Lipscomb PR. Primary vitallium-mold arthroplasty for posterior dislocation of the hip with fracture of the femoral head. *J Bone Joint Surg* 1958;40-A:675.
31. Westerborn A. Central dislocation of the femoral head treated with mold arthroplasty. *J Bone Joint Surg* 1954;36-A:307.
32. Coventry MB. The treatment of fracture-dislocation of the hip by total hip arthroplasty. *J Bone Joint Surg* 1974;56-A:1128.
33. Joly JM, Mears DC. The role of total hip arthroplasty in acetabular fracture management. *Op Tech Orthop* 1993;3:80.
34. Mears DC, Shirahama M. Stabilization of an acetabular fracture with cables for acute total hip arthroplasty. *J Arthroplast* 1998; 13:10.
35. Dowdy PA, Rorabeck CH, Bourne RB. Uncemented total hip

arthroplasty in patients fifty years of age or younger. *J Arthroplast* 1997;12:853.

36. Mears DC, Ward AJ, Wright MS. The radiological assessment of pelvic and acetabular fractures using three-dimensional computed tomography. *Int J Orthop Trauma* 1992;2:196.
37. Mears DC, MacLeod MD. Surgical approaches: triradiate and modified triradiate. In: Wiss DA, ed. *Master techniques in orthopaedic surgery: fractures.* New York: Lippincott-Raven, 1997:701–728.
38. Mears DC, Rubash HE. *Pelvic and acetabular fractures.* Thorofare, NJ: Slack, 1986.
39. Paprosky WG, Magnus RE. Principles of bone grafting in revision total hip arthroplasty. Acetabular technique. *Clin Orthop* 1994;298:147.
40. Peters CL, Curtain M, Samuelson KM. Acetabular revision with the Bursch-Schneider anti-protrusio cage and cancellous allograft bone. *J Arthroplast* 1995;10:307.
41. Muller ME, Allgower M, Schneider R, et al. *Manual of internal fixation,* 3rd ed. Berlin: Springer-Verlag, 1990.
42. Letournel E. Acetabular fractures: classification and management. *Clin Orthop* 1980;151:82.
43. Letournel E. Classification and evaluation of acetabular fractures. In: O'Brien T, ed. *Techniques in orthopaedics.* Denver: Aspen, 1990:524.
44. Sloof TJ, Scheurs BW, Buma P, et al. Impaction morcellized allografting and cement. In: American Academy of Orthopaedic Surgeons. *Instructional course lectures,* vol. 48. Rosemont, IL: American Academy of Orthopaedic Surgeons, 1999:79–89.
45. Singh N, Nagrath AR, Mairi PS, et al. Changes in trabecular pattern of the upper femur as an index of osteoporosis. *J Bone Joint Surg* 1970;52-A:456.
46. Bourne RB, Rorabeck CH, Skutek M, et al. The Harris design-2 total hip replacement fixed with so-called second-generation cementing techniques. A ten to fifteen-year follow-up. *J Bone Joint Surg* 1998;80-A:1775.
47. Templeman DC, Olson S, Moed BR, et al. Surgical treatment of acetabular fractures. In: *Instructional course lectures,* vol. 48. Park Ridge, IL: American Academy of Orthopaedic Surgeons, 1999:481–496.
48. Matta JM, Siebenrock KA. Does indomethacin reduce heterotopic bone formation after operations for acetabular fractures? A prospective randomized study. *J Bone Joint Surg* 1997;79-B:959.
49. Moed BR, Letournel E. Low-dose irradiation and indomethacin prevent heterotopic ossification after acetabular surgery. *J Bone Joint Surg* 1994;76-B:895.
50. Harris WH. Traumatic arthritis of the hip after dislocation and acetabular fractures: treatment by mold arthroplasty. An end-result study using a new method of result evaluation. *J Bone Joint Surg* 1969;51-A:737.
51. Brooker AF, Bowerman JW, Robinson RA, et al. Ectopic ossification following total hip replacement: incidence and a method of classification. *J Bone Joint Surg* 1973;55-A:1629.
52. Moed BR, Smith ST. Three-view radiographic assessment of heterotopic ossification after acetabular fracture surgery: correlation with hip motion in 100 cases. *J Orthop Trauma* 1996;10:93.
53. Russotti GM, Harris WH. Proximal placement of the acetabular component in total hip arthroplasty. A long-term follow-up study. *J Bone Joint Surg* 1991;73-A:587.
54. Gruen TA, McNiece GM, Amstutz HC. "Modes of failure" of cemented stem-type femoral components: a radiographic analysis of loosening. *Clin Orthop* 1979;141:17.
55. DeLee JG, Charnley J. Ectopic bone formation following low friction arthroplasty of the hip. *Clin Orthop* 1976;121:52.
56. Harris WH, McGann WA. Loosening of the femoral component after use of the medullary-plug cementing technique. Follow-up note with a minimum five-year follow-up. *J Bone Joint Surg* 1988;68-A:1064.
57. Wasielewski RC, Cooperstein LA, Kruger MP, et al. Acetabular anatomy and the trans-acetabular fixation of screws in total hip arthroplasty. *J Bone Joint Surg* 1990;72-A:501.
58. Heekin RD, Callaghan JJ, Hopkinson WJ, et al. The porous-coated anatomic total hip prosthesis, inserted without cement. Results after five to seven years in a prospective study. *J Bone Joint Surg* 1993;75-A:77.
59. Piston RW, Engh CA, DeCarvalho PI, et al. Osteonecrosis of the femoral head treated with total hip arthroplasty without cement. *J Bone Joint Surg* 1994;76-A:202.

44

DELAYED TOTAL HIP ARTHROPLASTY FOLLOWING ACETABULAR FRACTURE

MARVIN TILE
MATTHEW L. JIMENEZ
CORY BORKHOFF

INTRODUCTION

Even in the hands of experts, the results of treatment of acetabular fractures can never be perfect in all patients because of many factors described elsewhere in this book. These include patient factors such as advanced age, medical infirmity, and osteopenia, as well as factors inherent in the fracture itself, such as excessive comminution and bruising of articular cartilage, and avascular necrosis (Fig. 44-1) of the femoral head and/or the acetabulum. Postoperative complications such as sepsis or soft-tissue problems (Fig. 44-2) also can mitigate against a satisfactory result. Therefore, there will always be a role for total hip arthroplasty, both early and late. For biologic and technical reasons, approximately 10% of cases fail within a 2-year period. Beyond that there is a gradual fall off of good to excellent results, depending on the length of follow-up. Most of the literature reports 5–15-year results, with the exception of Letournel, whose series is 3 to 33 years.

Five-, 10-, and even 15-year results may not tell the whole story. The long-term prognosis may be similar to that found in Legge-Perthes disease, where the results beyond 40 years show a major change in the incidence of clinical osteoarthritis, whereas the incidence is relatively low prior to that. The same is true in the posttraumatic acetabular population, where the results may be excellent for 15 years and then show a rapid deterioration (Fig. 44-3). Therefore, the true incidence of osteoarthritis can only be known with results that extend over a 30- to 40-year period.

Outcome of Total Hip Arthroplasty Following Previous Acetabular Fracture

We have recently completed a comprehensive study of the late cases of postacetabular fracture treated by late total hip arthroplasty (1). This was a matched cohort study comparing the group of postacetabular fracture patients with a similarly matched group of patients with primary osteoarthritis.

The literature on this subject (2–7) can be summarized as follows: Most used Harris hip scores, which have now been validated (8). There was no direct comparison between patients with and without a history of previous acetabular fracture undergoing total hip arthroplasty. Although Boardman and Charnley reported results similar to all their other hip population, the other authors indicated much poorer outcomes owing to early acetabular loosening (2). The incidence of acetabular loosening led to an early acetabular revision.

In our study, as well as looking at the cohort, comparing fracture cases to osteoarthritic cases, we also assessed any differences in the outcome of total hip and acetabular fractures in those patients who were treated operatively versus nonoperatively for their original fracture (Table 44-1).

The two groups were almost identically matched with 94 patients in each group. Comparing the patients with previous acetabular fracture treated operatively (67) versus nonoperatively (33), the incidence of male to female predominance was 49 to 18 versus 16 to 17; the higher incidence of nerve injury and hip dislocation in the operatively treated patients was statistically significant.

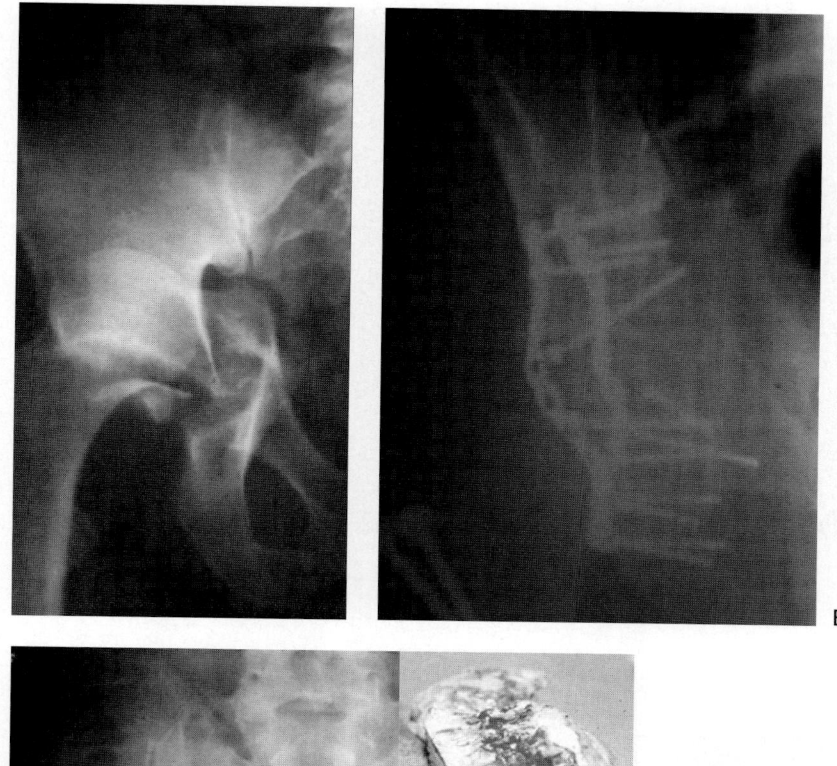

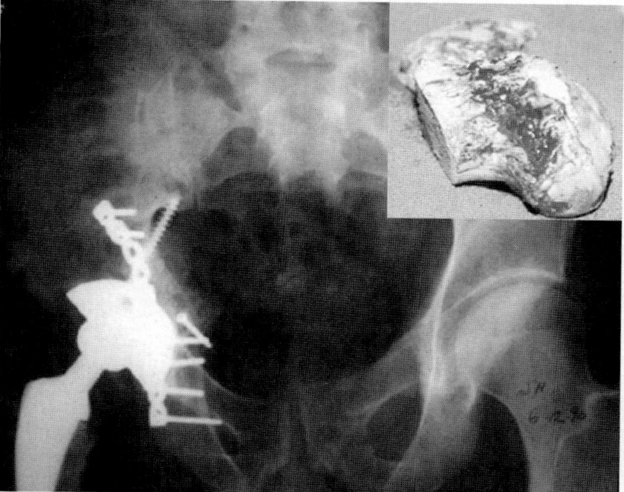

FIGURE 44-1. A: Severe transverse fracture right acetabulum with posterior wall and posterior dislocation of hip and postoperative radiograph **(B).** Within 1 year the femoral head collapsed *(inset),* leading to a total hip arthroplasty **(C).**

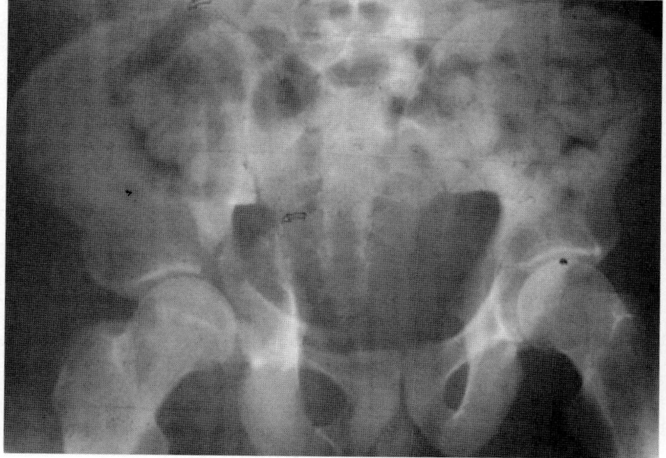

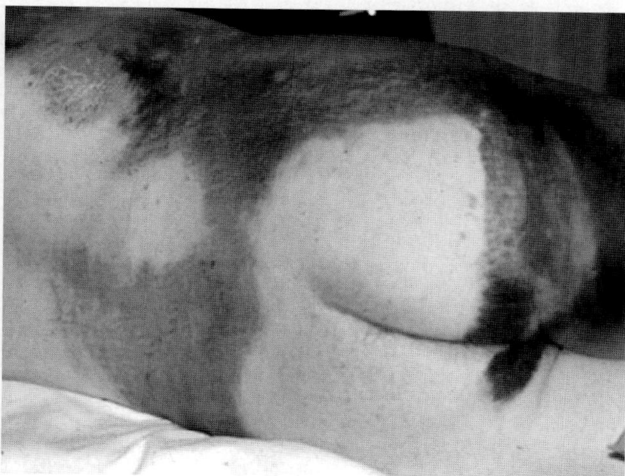

FIGURE 44-2. A: Both-column fracture right acetabulum associated with a severe Morel-Lavelle avulsion type injury of the skin. **B:** Open reduction led to sepsis and then early failure.

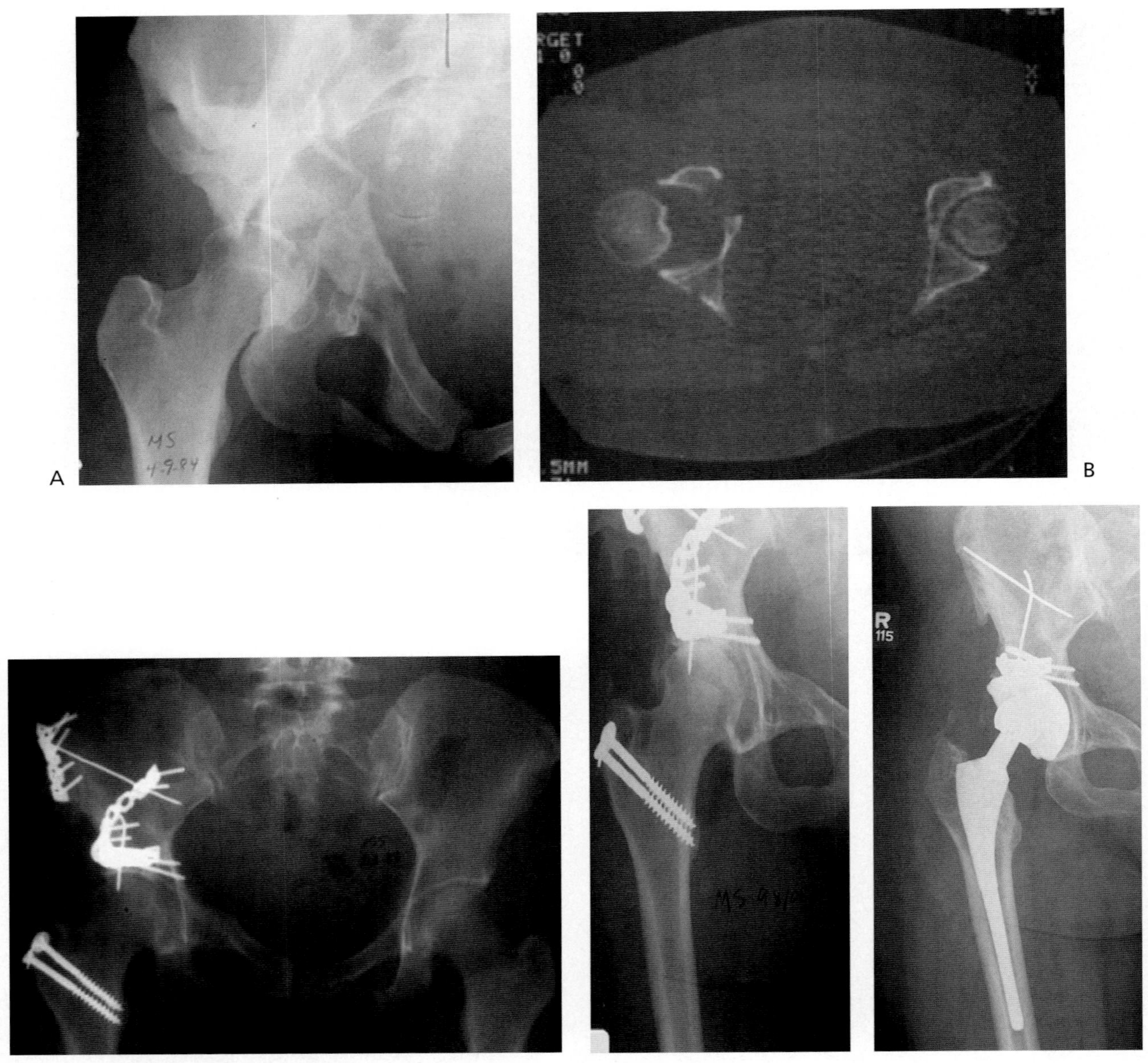

FIGURE 44-3. A: Severely comminuted both-column fracture right acetabulum in a 29-year-old woman. See accompanying computed tomography. **B:** Thirteen years postoperatively, the anatomic reduction looks excellent **(C)** but, at 15 years, severe osteoarthritis has occurred with virtual destruction of articular cartilage **(D),** leading to a total hip arthroplasty **(E).**

TABLE 44-1. DEMOGRAPHIC CHARACTERISTICS OF PATIENTS WITH A PREVIOUS ACETABULAR FRACTURE

	Patients with Previous Acetabular Fracture[a]	
Variable	Operative (n = 67)	Nonoperative[b] (n = 33)
Mean follow-up (years)	6.9	8.5
Male:female	49:18	16:17
Mean age at fracture (years)	44.7	47.2
Polytrauma (%)	58.2	45.5
Nerve injury (%)	26.9	12.1
Hip dislocation (%)	64.2	36.4
Mean time to OR (days)[c]	4.2	NA

[a] One patient (a 70-year-old female) whose posterior wall acetabular fracture was treated acutely with a THA was included in the matched comparison but was not included in the acetabular fracture management comparison.
[b] Two patients (one female and one male) had bilateral acetabular fractures, both of which were managed nonoperatively.
[c] Includes only patients who underwent surgery.

Outcome measures included functional validated measures including the WOMAC, MFA, and SF 36 as well as a clinical and radiographic review. The results of our study indicated that the functional outcome in the fracture group using the WOMAC, MFA, and SF 36 was worse in each group (Fig. 44-4).

The complication rate was significantly higher in the group of ORIF patients versus the nonoperative group (Table 44-2). An important finding was the time to revision, owing to acetabular loosening in most incidences. In the elective total hip arthroplasty group, time to revision was 7.8 ± 3.9, versus 3.5 ± 4.4 years for the fracture groups.

There was a major difference between those fractures treated operatively and nonoperatively. Whereas the nonoperative group approached the elective total hip group for osteoarthritis in time to revision, the operative group had a statistically significant earlier revision.

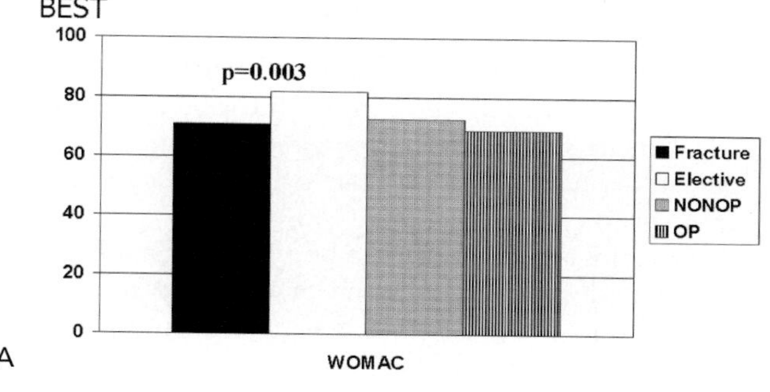

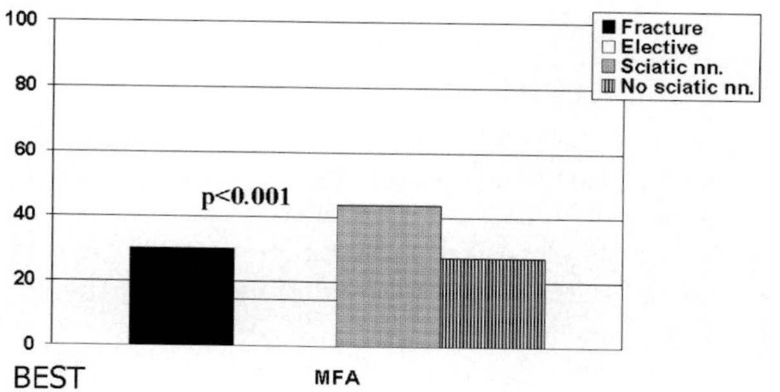

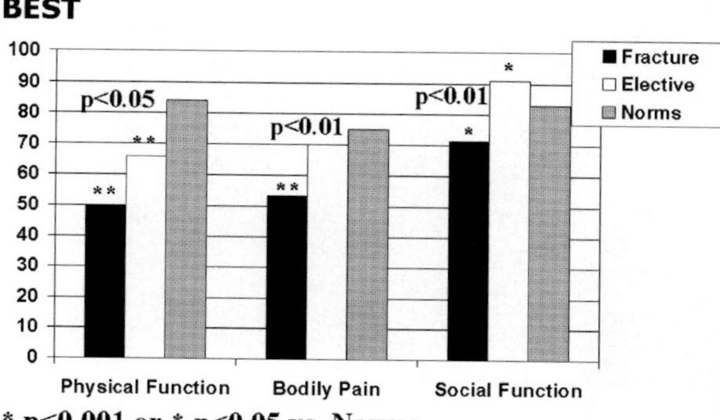

FIGURE 44-4. Using the WOMAC **(A)**, MFA **(B)**, and SF 36 **(C)**, the functional outcome in all show that the fracture group did not fare as well as the osteoarthritis group.

TABLE 44-2. COMPARISON OF COMPLICATIONS POST TOTAL HIP ARTHROPLASTY (THA)

	THA After Previous Acetabular Fracture[a]			Elective THA
Variable	Operative (n = 65)	Nonoperative (n = 29)	Total (n = 94)	Total (n = 94)
Postoperative Complications				
Infection (N)	2	1	3	0[b]
Iatrogenic sciatic nerve Injury (N)	2	1	3	0[b]
Hip dislocation (N)	9	2	11	7

[a]One patient was treated acutely with a THA.
[b]$p < 0.05$ for difference between fracture group and elective THA group.

DISCUSSION

Our findings indicate that arthroplasty function was worse in patients with a previous acetabular fracture compared to an elective total hip, as measured by WOMAC, MFA, and SF 36, irrespective of fracture management. Also, revision occurred earlier, especially in those cases treated by open reduction and internal fixation.

Why Should This Be the Case?

The results are quite logical after assessing preoperative patient factors: namely, a higher incidence of heterotopic ossification, sciatic nerve injury, and lower extremity fracture, and a higher infection rate at the time of ORIF; as well as surgical factors, including increased operating room time and blood loss owing to hardware removal, deep scarring, and infection. The main technical problem, as well as those mentioned, involves fixation of the acetabular component. The femoral component usually is not a problem.

TECHNICAL DETAILS

The problem of fixation of the acetabular component can be considered similar to that found in revision arthroplasty of the hip. In fact, the classification system published by AAOS (9) is valid for postacetabular patients. Defects in the acetabulum may be:

- Contained
- Segmental
- Combined
- Pelvic discontinuity (nonunion)

Therefore, the technical factors include not only the type of defect mentioned in the preceding but also the difference in those patients treated by previous ORIF versus those treated nonoperatively. Additional factors include the surgical approach, metal removal, previous sepsis, and previous nerve injury. Options for the acetabular socket are a roof ring and a cemented cup and a large uncemented cup, usually fixed with screws for a contained defect (Figs. 44-5, 44-6, and 44-7). All avascular tissue should be removed from the acetabulum to bleeding bone; the femoral head should be ground up and packed in as an autogenous bone graft. In cases where a segmental graft is indicated, the femoral head plus or minus an allograft is used (Fig. 44-5).

Decision making is more difficult for operatively treated fractures. First, sepsis must be ruled out in cases that have had a previous open reduction and internal fixation, especially in those cases that deteriorate rapidly within 1 to 2 years of fracture. The usual bone scanning and aspiration techniques are used as well as biopsy at the time of surgery (Fig. 44-6). Second, a decision must be made regarding metal removal and the approach to be used. The approach is dictated by previous incisions, the type of defect, and metal present in the acetabulum. Although all metal does not require removal, the surgeon must be prepared to remove metal should it interfere with insertion of the socket. Metal that has been in for years may be difficult to remove (Fig. 44-3).

Occasionally, the metal can be removed directly from the socket itself, using a diamond or carborundum drill and burr, if one is faced with a situation where removal of a screw that has been stripped would cause more damage and increase the length of the operative procedure unduly. Therefore, in principle, if the metal interferes with the socket, it should be removed, although it does not require

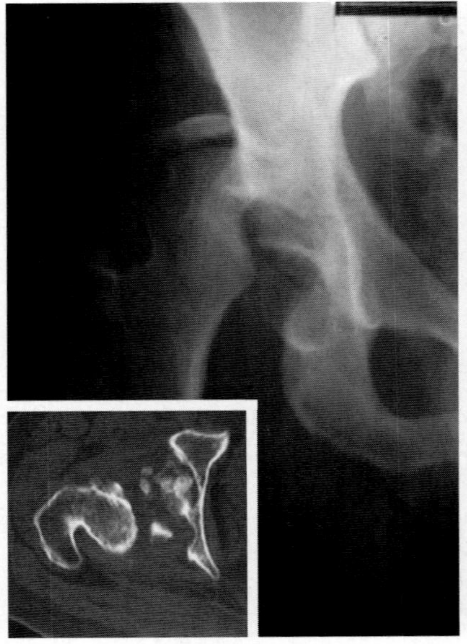

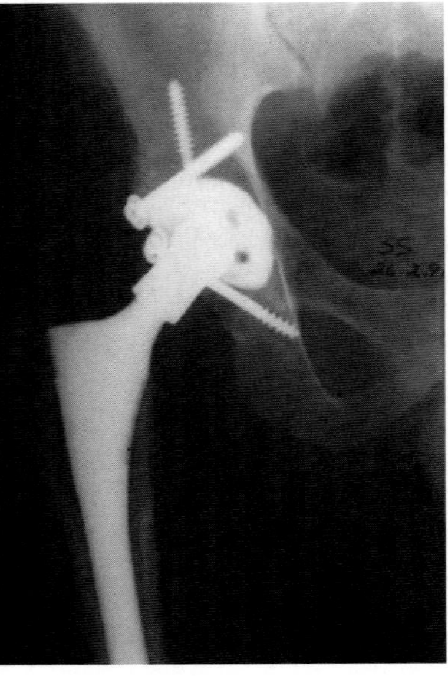

A–C

FIGURE 44-5. Anterior-posterior radiograph of a 38-year-old man who sustained a posterior dislocation of his hip with a large posterior wall fragment. The hip was never reduced and he presented 18 months with this radiograph **(A)** and the computed tomography **(B).** The femoral head was removed and fashioned to create a new posterior wall, and a standard, uncemented total hip arthroplasty using an uncemented acetabular socket with screw fixation was used **(C).** The result was excellent.

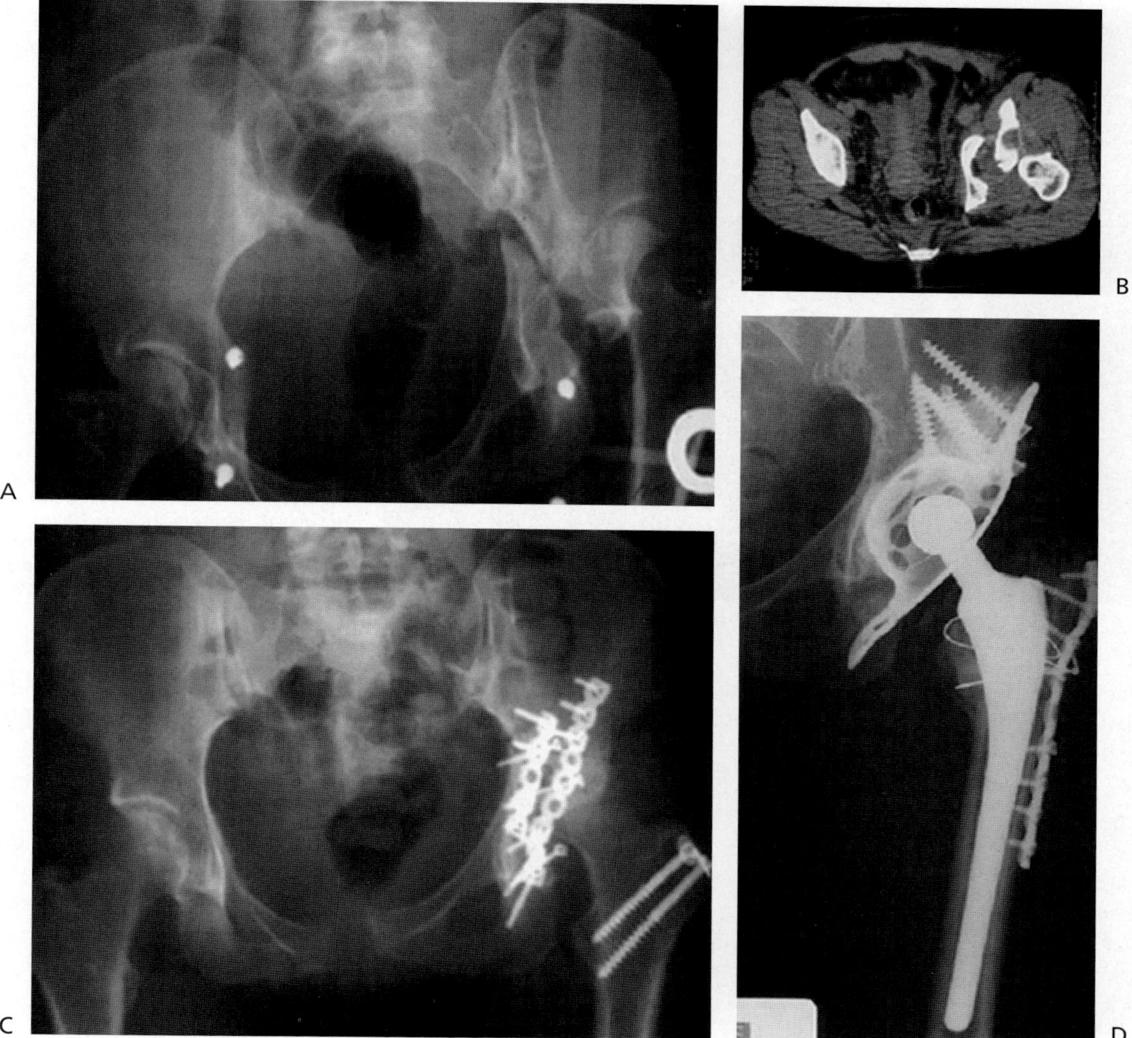

FIGURE 44-6. A: Anterior-posterior radiograph of a 48-year-old woman who sustained a transverse fracture left acetabulum with posterior dislocation, as clearly seen in the computed tomography. **B:** An anatomic reduction was obtained of this difficult fracture but, 8 weeks after open reduction internal fixation the patient complained of severe pain, fever, and a dislocating hip, which is indicative of sepsis **(C)**. The femoral head and all metal was removed. Gram-negative organisms were found. A two-stage procedure was done: first a temporary Prosalac prosthesis with antibiotics; then a permanent prosthesis, including a cemented socket with antibiotics in a roof ring and an uncemented stem, was inserted after the femur was shortened **(D)**. The result was excellent.

routine removal. The surgical approach should be such that the metal can be removed if necessary (Fig. 44-7).

Heterotopic bone also dictates the approach, as well as the presence of metal. Extreme care must be taken because the bone may envelop the sciatic nerve. To obtain reasonable motion, the surgeon must remove adequate amounts of heterotopic bone or the total hip will be extremely stiff.

Postoperatively, the heterotopic bone may reform; therefore, prophylactic medication plus or minus radiation is indicated.

The surgeon must be aware of a past history of sciatic nerve involvement and the present state of the nerve at the time of total hip arthroplasty. Monitoring during surgery is still a controversial issue but the nerve should be inspected if a posterior approach is being used unless a permanent complete sciatic nerve lesion is evident.

Combined defects require both segmental and ground bone grafts, as well as artificial bone graft materials.

Pelvic Discontinuity (Nonunion)

These cases require individual attention. Occasionally one can use a multiple-screw uncemented socket to place screws both proximal and distal to the nonunion. Graft union can be achieved with a large cancellous bone (Fig. 44-8)

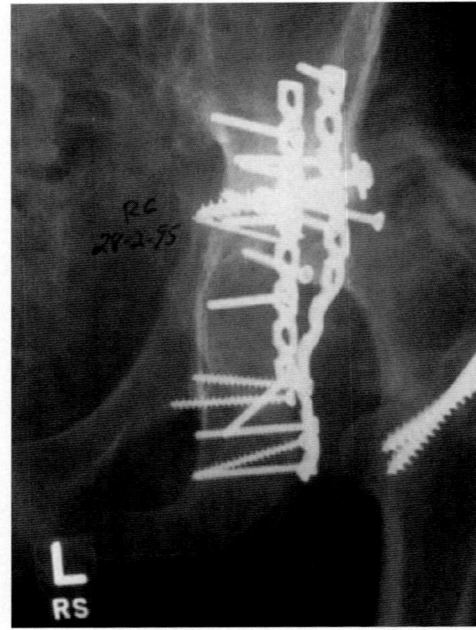

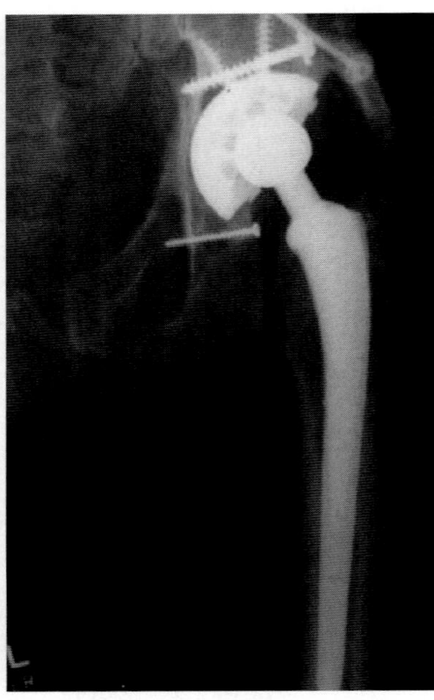

A,B

FIGURE 44-7. A: Anterior-posterior radiograph of left hip showing avascular necrosis after ORIF through a posterior approach. **B:** Most of the metal was removed and an uncemented total hip replacement was inserted.

In extreme cases (e.g., postfusion), nonunion requires very sophisticated techniques and lengthy operative procedures (Fig. 44-9).

CONCLUSION

Total hip arthroplasty remains a viable option in cases with avascular necrosis or osteoarthritis following acetabular trauma. Postseptic cases using modern techniques or eradication of infection may also be salvaged by a total hip arthroplasty.

The patients must be told that the operation may be lengthy, the complication rate higher, and the outcome not as optimal as in other patients whom they may know who have had total hip arthroplasty for osteoarthritis. The major problems are in the acetabular socket, which requires fixation with a roof ring plus a cemented cup or an uncemented cup anchored with screws always accompanied by a large bone graft. The worst patient function in this group is often as a result of associated injuries, previous nerve injuries, and previous sepsis. These patients need to be told that a revision might be necessary at an earlier time.

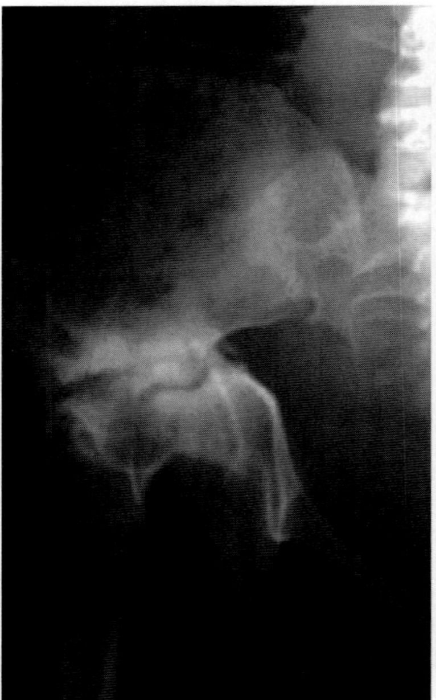

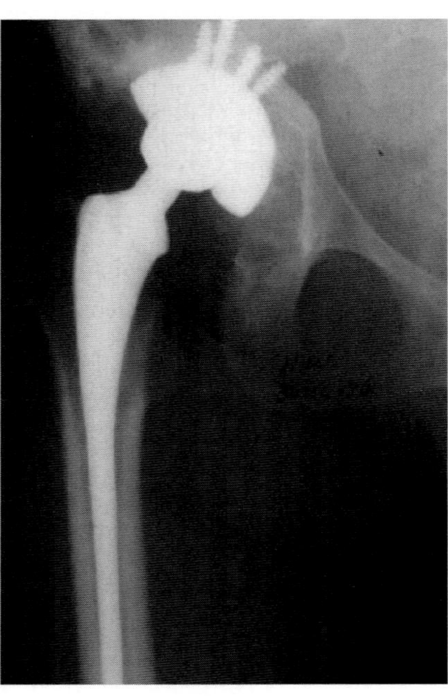

A,B

FIGURE 44-8. A: Anterior-posterior radiograph showing a nonunion of a Chiari osteotomy treated with a primary total hip arthroplasty and bone graft. **B:** The screw fixation extended both proximal and distal to the nonunion, which allowed for this nonunion to heal with the bone graft.

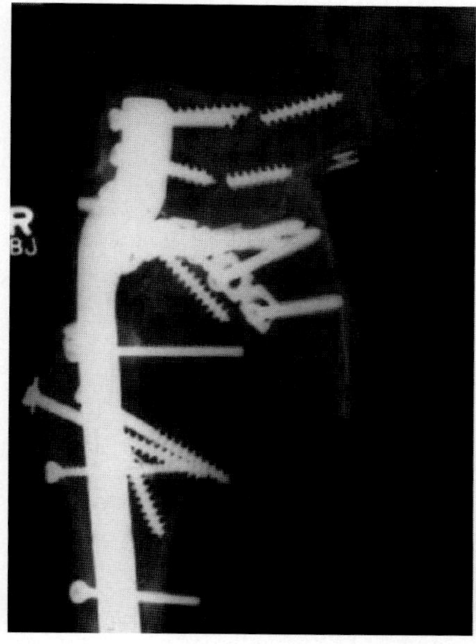

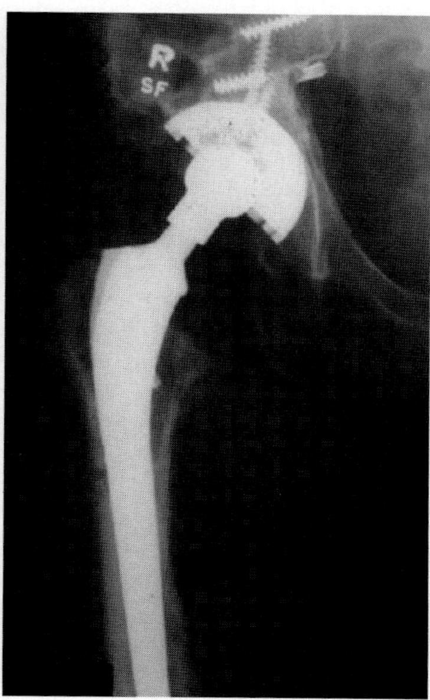

A,B

FIGURE 44-9. A: A patient with five previous attempts at fusion, ending in nonunion, was converted to an uncemented total hip replacement **(B).** Some metal remained. The patient had a good outcome.

This begs the question given the findings of this study group: Could the results of total hip arthroplasty be improved by doing primary total hip arthroplasty in select cases of acetabular fracture? Chapter 43 deals with this, but the final answer is unknown at this time. There is considerable technical difficulty in anchoring the socket in a primary total hip arthroplasty. One such technique is cerclage wiring, as noted in Fig. 44-10.

Therefore, another question one can pose as a result of this study is: Which fractures can be managed nonoperatively with good results over time, especially in the older age group? Certainly, the both-column fracture (Type C) can give results as good or better than those of open reduction in that particular group (11).

These recent studies are defining the role of both early and late total hip arthroplasty in acetabular fracture management.

Given our own results, one would question the old dictum often heard at rounds: We perform an open reduction internal fixation of an acetabular fracture "to improve bone stock." One must question that thesis given the much higher complication rate and poor outcomes.

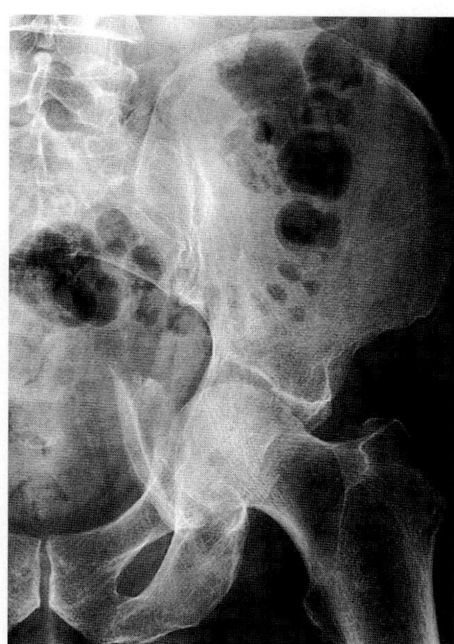

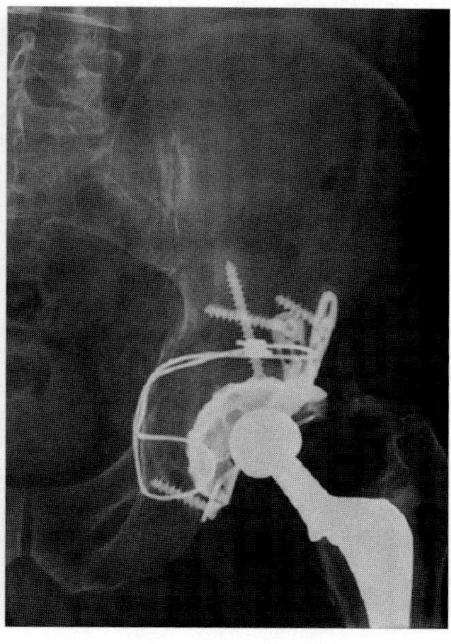

A,B

FIGURE 44-10. A: Anterior-posterior radiograph showing an incongruous anterior column fracture of the left acetabulum in a 78-year-old severely osteoporotic patient. A cemented total hip arthroplasty with bone graft was performed. **B:** Note the cerclage wire fixation of the anterior column.

REFERENCES

1. Borkhoff C, Zaveri G, Kreder H, et al. *Total hip arthroplasty after previous acetabular fracture: a matched cohort study.* Presented at the Canadian Orthopaedic Association Meeting. London, Ontario, June 2001.
2. Boardman KP, Charnley J. Low-friction arthroplasty after fracture-dislocation of the hip. *J Bone Joint Surg* 1978;60(B):495.
3. Rogan IM, Weber FA, Solomon L. Total hip replacement following fracture dislocation of the acetabulum. *J Bone Joint Surg* 1979;61(B):252.
4. Romness DW, Lewallen DG. Total hip arthroplasty after fracture of the acetabulum. *J Bone Joint Surg* 1990;72(B):761.
5. Pritchett JW, Bortel DT. Total hip replacement after central fracture dislocation of the acetabulum. *Orthop Rev* 1991;7:607.
6. Jimenez ML, Tile M, Schenk R. Total hip replacement after acetabular fracture. *Orthop Clin North Am* 1997;28(3):435–445.
7. Weber M, Berry DJ, Scott WS. Total hip arthroplasty after operative treatment of an acetabular fracture. *J Bone Joint Surg* 1998;80(A):1295.
8. Soderman P, Malchau H. Is the Harris Hip Score System useful to study the outcome of total hip replacement? *Clin Orthop Rel Res* 2001;(384):189–197.
9. American Academy of Orthopaedic Surgeons. *Instructional lectures,* vol 48, 1999.
10. Halliwell S, Borkhoff C, Owen PJ, et al. *The associated both-column acetabular fracture: long-term functional outcome of conservative versus surgical management.* Presented at the Canadian Orthopaedic Association Meeting. St. John's, Newfoundland, July, 1999.

PART G. SPECIAL SITUATIONS

45

PATHOLOGIC PELVIS FRACTURES AND ACETABULAR RECONSTRUCTION IN METASTATIC DISEASE

HOLLY K. BROWN
JOHN H. HEALEY

INTRODUCTION

The two primary causes of pathologic fracture of the pelvis are metastatic lesions, and metabolic bone disease. Metastatic lesions can present anywhere within the pelvic ring, and fracture occurs because of resultant bone structural insufficiency. Metastatic lesions also can be associated with a large soft-tissue component that can cause symptoms independent of the bone (i.e., nerve impingement, venous outflow obstruction, traction or impingement on normal soft-tissue structures), and require therapeutic intervention to address these issues. Unlike pelvic pathology owing to trauma, pathologic pelvic fractures do not have the acute soft-tissue disruption associated with high-energy trauma. The majority of pathologic fractures of the pelvis remain undisplaced, and most can be treated nonoperatively. Management of pathologic fractures of the superior or inferior pubic rami, iliac wing, and sacral ala, as well as avulsion fractures involving the anterior superior or inferior iliac spines or ischial tuberosity, includes: pain management, protected weight bearing, and appropriate adjuvant therapy (i.e., radiation and/or chemotherapy) in metastatic situations. However, fractures owing to metastatic disease involving the ischium can continue to be symptomatic despite an appropriate course of conservative management. In these instances, curettage and cementation may be necessary to provide relief (Fig. 45-1).

The acetabulum is the one location that presents a more complex management problem. Pathologic fractures owing to osteoporosis can occur in this area, and management is reflected by the extent of associated bone insufficiency. This factor is discussed further in regard to metastatic disease in this region, and the basic principles can be applied accordingly in osteoporotic lesions. The main difference in dealing with osteoporotic versus metastatic acetabular lesions is that osteoporotic lesions have the potential to heal, whereas in most metastatic cases, healing either does not occur, or occurs in a slow, limited fashion owing to tumor progression and retardation of bone formation by adjuvant therapies such as radiation and chemotherapy (1).

METASTATIC DISEASE OF THE ACETABULUM

Background

Metastatic lesions involving the acetabulum frequently occur in cancer patients. These lesions can progress, leading to pathologic fracture involving the hip joint, or mechanical insufficiency of the acetabulum, causing significant pain and functional compromise. Initial management should incorporate the following modalities, as appropriate: pain management with narcotic analgesics, protected weight bearing, radiation, antineoplastic agents, and bisphosphonates. However, if symptoms continue despite adequate

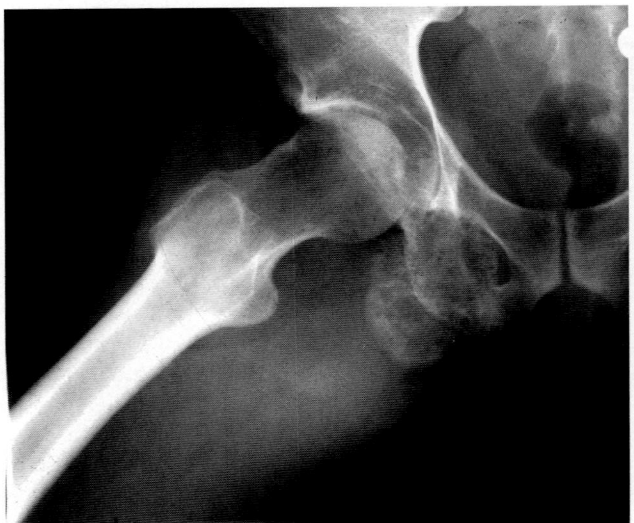

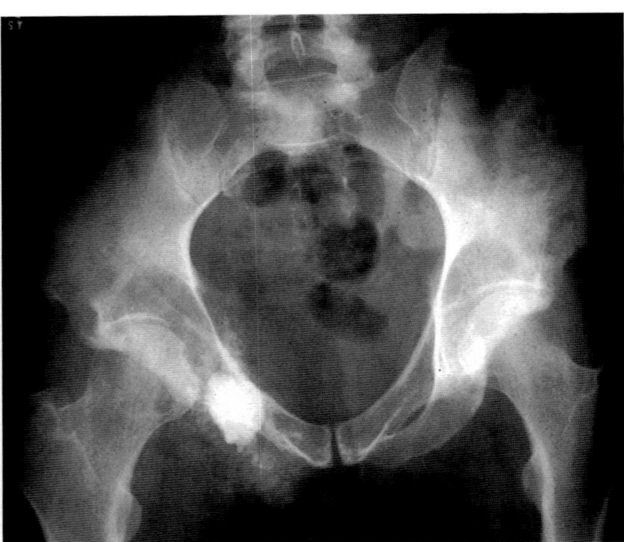

FIGURE 45-1. Metastatic lesion of the right ischium. **A:** Preoperative radiograph demonstrating an expansile mixed lytic/blastic lesion involving the right ischium. This lesion remained symptomatic despite conservative treatment. The patient was unable to sit and had symptoms consistent with sciatic nerve compression. **B:** Postoperative radiograph after the bulk of the extraosseous lesion was excised and the ischial portion curetted and cemented. Symptoms resolved following the procedure.

nonoperative management, surgical intervention may be required to address the problem. Surgery for a metastatic acetabular lesion is a major operative procedure in a patient who often has multiorgan system compromise owing to underlying disease and a reduced life expectancy. Thus, surgery involves significant risks to the patient; however, when performed in the appropriate situation, it can lead to significant and sustained functional improvement and pain relief: 75% of patients maintain satisfactory pain relief, and 60% to 75% maintain the ability to walk and function in the community 6 months postoperatively (2–5).

The general indications for surgical management in patients with metastatic lesions involving the acetabulum take into account patient disability, response to nonsurgical therapy, coincident disease, and longevity. Specifically, surgery is warranted when patients experience: (a) continued acute symptoms despite appropriate nonoperative therapy; (b) continued debilitating pain and poor function 1 to 3 months after radiation of the lesion; (c) pathologic fracture of the ipsilateral femur; (d) impending pathologic fracture of the ipsilateral femur requiring surgery; or (e) coincidental acetabular fracture. To justify surgical intervention, the patient's life expectancy should exceed 1 month, and preferably 3 months (2,6).

The factors found to most directly reflect prognosis in these patients include preoperative performance status, the presence of visceral metastasis, and tumor type. The Eastern Cooperative Oncology Group (ECOG) scale is an effective method for functional evaluation of patients, and has been found to reflect prognosis (Table 45-1) (7–10). In a series of patients presented by Marco and coworkers, the median survival of patients having an ECOG score of ≤ 1 was 15 months, compared to 7 months in those with an ECOG score of >1. Patients without visceral metastasis were found to have a median survival of 12 months, compared to 3 months in those with visceral metastasis ($p < 0.004$). The type of primary tumor also was found to reflect prognosis and survival. Patients with breast cancer bony metastasis survived longer (median 19 months) compared to patients with all other tumor types (median 6 months) (2).

Evaluation and Work-Up

Preoperative evaluation involves a thorough history and physical examination. The patient should undergo a general

TABLE 45-1. PREOPERATIVE PERFORMANCE STATUS BY EASTERN COOPERATIVE ONCOLOGY GROUP SCALE

Value	Description	Number of Patients
0	Normal activity	3
1	Symptoms, but nearly fully ambulatory	12
2	Some bed time, but needs to be in bed <50% of the time	15
3	Bedridden >50% of the day time	16
4	Totally bedridden	9

From: Orr S, Aisner J. Performance status assessment among oncology patients: a review. Cancer Treatment Reps 86 (70):1423–1429, with permission.

medical evaluation, with assessment of ability to tolerate surgery. Laboratory evaluation always should include a serum calcium level, because 5% to 10% of patients with metastatic bone disease can have hypercalcemia of malignancy. This is seen most commonly in patients with the primary diagnoses of myeloma, squamous cell carcinoma of the lung, and breast cancer. Thirty percent of patients with breast cancer metastasis to bone develop hypercalcemia at some point in their course (11). In addition, many of these patients have been bedridden or immobile for a significant period of time preoperatively. Their debilitated condition, in combination with a hypercoagulable state often associated with cancer, can lead to deep vein thrombosis. Preoperative screening with a duplex Doppler ultrasound and prophylactic or therapeutic use of a vena caval filter should be considered in the appropriate patient. Radiographic evaluation is necessary to define the anatomy of the lesion and allow for proper surgical planning, as well as to screen the patient for other sites of skeletal involvement that may impact the clinical situation. For example, a patient with an ipsilateral femoral shaft lesion may require concomitant stabilization with a long-stemmed femoral component to avoid a pathologic periprosthetic fracture below a standard length femoral stem.

Radiographic evaluation of the acetabular lesion should include plain radiographs, as well as a three-dimensional imaging study. An anterior-posterior (AP) pelvis, and AP and lateral views of the full ipsilateral femur to evaluate for additional lesions are basic requirements. Judet views are helpful in further defining the acetabular lesion and the extent of anterior or posterior column involvement. Full-body bone scan screens the rest of the skeleton for metastatic lesions, and can direct further imaging. However, certain types of disease can be cold on bone scan. For example, multiple myeloma or aggressive lytic lesions such as those seen with lung cancer, do not allow for surrounding bone reaction, and therefore do not result in uptake on bone scan. Thus, a negative bone scan does not negate the possibility of other sites of bony disease. Additional skeletal screening by plain radiography also must be guided by the patient's history and physical examination.

Three-dimensional imaging studies include magnetic resonance imaging (MRI) and computed tomography (CT) scan. Each has different capabilities and should be used selectively. Contrast is unnecessary when imaging metastatic disease. MRI of the hip/pelvis has the advantage of showing marrow involvement, and therefore the intramedullary extent of tumor within the pelvis. Unfortunately, the marrow signal abnormality seen on MRI is not diagnostic for tumor, and can result from associated reactive edema. This fact must be taken into account when using MRI for surgical planning. MRI also demonstrates the soft-tissue extent of the tumor, which can be helpful in planning debulking of disease (12,13). In the rare case of a solitary metastasis where curative resection is contemplated, a MRI scan can define the extent of the tumor, allowing for wide resection of all involved tissue. However, MRI is less effective in defining cortical bone involvement, and in assessing the extent of mechanical compromise of the bone. CT scan has the benefit of superior bone imaging over MRI, defining both cortical and cancellous bone involvement, and giving a better indication of mechanical insufficiency. CT also can give information regarding the soft-tissue extent of the lesion, albeit in less detail than that available from MRI. Thus, CT is the study of choice for imaging metastatic acetabular lesions.

Patients with a history of cancer and a solitary bone lesion without a prior diagnosis of bony metastatic disease require a biopsy to confirm the etiology of the bone lesion. Primary bone sarcomas can occur in the same patient population that presents with metastatic disease. For example, Paget's sarcoma, postradiation sarcoma, or chondrosarcoma can all present with a lytic or mixed lytic-blastic lesion, or with a pathologic fracture. Paget's disease also can harbor myeloma or a metastasis that can only be confirmed by biopsy. In addition, the blastic lesions associated with prostate cancer metastasis can mimic pelvic Paget's disease. Metabolic bone disease also occurs within this age group (i.e., brown tumor of hyperparathyroidism or osteomalacia), each of which can present with multiple skeletal lesions mimicking metastasis. Therefore, establishing the diagnosis prior to surgical intervention can avoid potential surgical mismanagement of resectable and curable primary tumors, or overtreatment of metabolic lesions.

Classification

An effective classification system for acetabular lesions should combine the anatomic pathology of the lesion with the surgical intervention required to address it, in a complete, linearly progressive and logical fashion. Harrington originally reported on his experience with reconstruction of metastatic acetabular disease in 1981. At that time he presented a four-class system to define the acetabular lesion, and used to direct the reconstruction. This system divides lesions into four groups.

1. Patients with the lateral cortices, and superior and medial walls structurally intact, reconstructed with a conventional cemented total hip arthroplasty, ± use of medial metallic mesh
2. Patients with a deficient medial wall, but with the superior wall (roof or dome) and lateral cortices intact, reconstructed with a flanged acetabular component
3. Patients with a deficient superior wall, medial wall, and either one or both lateral cortices, reconstructed with threaded Steinmann pins and a flanged acetabular component
4. Patients where resection was required for cure, reconstructed as outlined for Type 3 lesions, or by autoclaving and reimplanting the segment of resected hemipelvis into which an acetabular component is fixed (3).

However, this system does not include all potential lesion anatomic combinations, nor does it flow linearly in regard to extent of disease. Thus it is less intuitive, and difficult to use.

The American Academy of Orthopaedic Surgeons (AAOS) defines an additional classification system for acetabular defects (14). Its primary utility is outlined for definition of lesions associated with osteolysis in total hip arthroplasty. Lesions are divided into five categories based on the type and location of the lesion. The classification incorporates whether the defect is segmental or cavitary, central or peripheral. Type 4 lesions indicate that there is pelvic discontinuity. These lesions were subsequently reclassified/subclassified by Berry and coworkers into groups depending on the cavitary or segmental nature of the lesion, and those associated with radiation (15). This classification focuses on the anatomy of the lesion; however, it does not progress linearly, with segmental defects being present earlier in the classification than cavitary defects. It mixes in other factors, such as prior radiation, not related to the anatomy of the lesion. Also, it does not subclassify or further define combined defects, and this information has a significant impact on the extent and type of reconstruction. Therefore, the AAOS classification system is cumbersome and difficult to use in metastatic disease cases, and it does not define the type of reconstruction required to address a lesion.

A classification system was developed from the Memorial Sloan-Kettering Cancer Center experience with metastatic acetabular disease. This system seeks to combine the strengths of the aforementioned classifications (i.e., the reconstructive focus of the Harrington system), with the completeness and anatomic definition of the AAOS system. The Metastatic Acetabular Classification (MAC) system couples the anatomic definition of the lesion to the reconstructive technique. It divides the acetabulum into four anatomic sections:

1. Dome
2. Medial wall
3. Anterior column
4. Posterior column

Bone in each region is defined as either sufficient or insufficient based on its ability to support an acetabular component. A region is considered insufficient if it contains a fracture, segmental bony defect, or major cavitary defect. This assessment is based on radiographic studies for preoperative planning; however, intraoperative confirmation of bone integrity is necessary before proceeding with the reconstructive plan. If an additional area is found to be incompetent, or an area previously deemed incompetent is found to be structurally sufficient, the reconstruction should be altered accordingly to reflect this change in status (Table 45-2 and Fig. 45-2).

A cavitary defect involving the acetabulum without disruption of the mechanical stability of the subchondral bone can be addressed with a bipolar hemiarthroplasty when a lesion of the proximal femur requires surgical intervention. Direct cementation of the lesion can be performed if a periacetabular lesion is present where the articular congruity of the acetabulum is maintained, but that is symptomatic despite an adequate course of radiation therapy. Pain relief is achieved by supporting the bone in this region, and possibly through the thermal effect of the cement on tumor and cytokine pain pathways. Cementation can be done using ei-

TABLE 45-2. METASTATIC ACETABULAR CLASSIFICATION (MAC) SYSTEM

Lesion Anatomy	Lesion Intervention
Cavitary lesion (dome)	
With intact subchondral bone	Bipolar hemiarthroplasty
With insufficient subchondral bone	Total hip arthroplasty with reinforced cement ± flanged cup/protrusio ring
Medial wall deficiency	
Without a dome deficiency	Total hip arthroplasty with a flanged cup/protrusio ring ± reinforced cement
With a dome deficiency	Total hip arthroplasty with reinforced cement and flanged cup/protrusio ring
Single column deficiency	
Without a dome or medial wall deficiency	Total hip arthroplasty with reinforced cement ± flanged cup/protrusio ring
With a dome and/or medial wall deficiency	Total hip arthroplasty with reinforced cement and flanged cup/protrusio ring
Double column deficiency	
Without a dome or medial wall deficiency	Total hip arthroplasty with reinforced cement and flanged cup/protrusio ring
With a dome and/or medial wall deficiency	Total hip arthroplasty with reinforced cement and flanged cup/protrusio ring, or resection with hemipelvis endoprosthesis or saddle prosthesis.

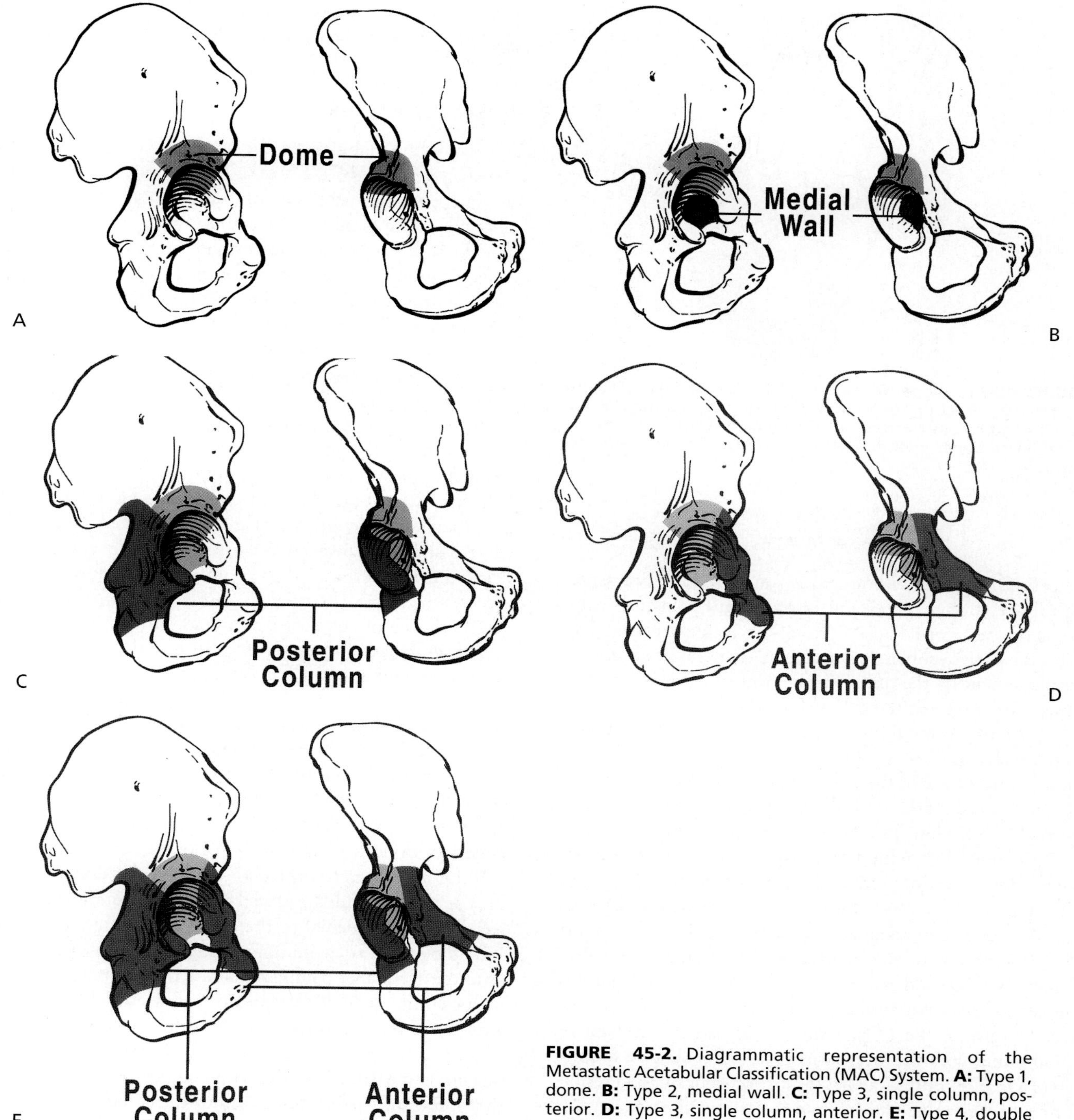

FIGURE 45-2. Diagrammatic representation of the Metastatic Acetabular Classification (MAC) System. **A:** Type 1, dome. **B:** Type 2, medial wall. **C:** Type 3, single column, posterior. **D:** Type 3, single column, anterior. **E:** Type 4, double column.

ther an open technique, where the lesion is curetted and packed with cement, or with radiographically guided percutaneous injection of cement into the lesion. Dangers of the percutaneous technique include cement extravasation into the hip joint with resulting disruption of the articulation and cartilage damage, or outside of the bony confines of the pelvis with potential sciatic nerve or other soft-tissue impingement (16,17).

Lesions resulting in a structurally incompetent acetabulum with adequate bone maintained in the ipsilateral hemipelvis to support internal fixation can be stably reconstructed using a combination of pins or screws and cement with a cemented acetabular component. Lesions involving the medial wall require additional support with a flanged acetabular component or anti protrusio ring. Of note, lesions involving the obturator foramen (region for Type 3 pelvic

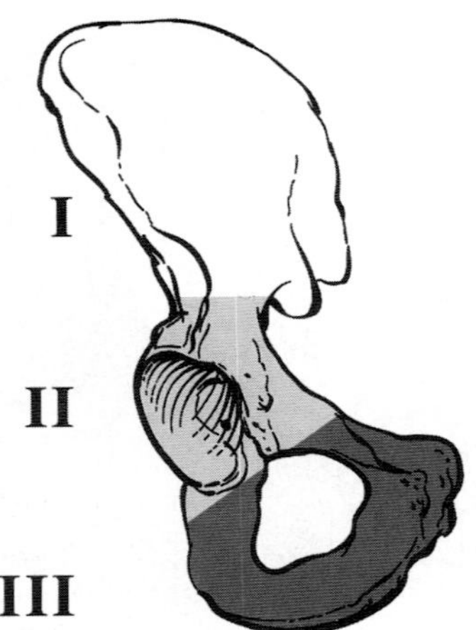

FIGURE 45-3. Basic pelvic resection regions: type I (iliac), II (periacetabular), III (obturator). (From: Enneking W, Dunham W. Resection and reconstruction for primary neoplasms involving the innominate bone. *J Bone Joint Surg* 1978;60:731–746, with permission.)

resection), with or without extension to the inferior aspect of the acetabulum, can result in significant pain and symptoms that are not relieved by total hip reconstruction (18). This is owing to soft-tissue and nerve (femoral or obturator) impingement by the tumor in the confines of this region as these structures exit the pelvis (Fig. 45-3).

When the acetabulum and inferior aspect of the pelvis are extensively involved by tumor (Type 2 ± 3 pelvic resections), this aspect of the pelvis may be excised and the hip reconstructed with a saddle prosthesis (Link America, Denville, NJ). This prosthesis is implanted into the femur using a femoral stem interface. The saddle proximal component allows rotation and articulates with a notch made in the residual ilium (18). This type of reconstruction depends on the presence of adequate proximal iliac bone to support the articulation of the prosthesis, and a stable sacroiliac joint. Aboulafia and associates reported on the results of this procedure in 17 patients, nine with metastatic/systemic disease. Twelve of the 17 patients (71%) had an excellent or good result, with the nine patients still alive at latest follow-up (15 to 62 months), all having an excellent or good result. Three of these nine patients had metastatic disease (19). An additional indication for segmental pelvic resection and saddle reconstruction is a contained solitary lesion (i.e., plasmacytoma or delayed onset renal cell carcinoma metastasis), which is being widely excised for cure (20–23). Large lesions with extensive involvement of the hemipelvis and disruption of the sacroiliac joint may be resected and reconstructed with a pelvic endoprosthesis and total hip arthroplasty. In certain instances, depending on the clinical circumstance, extensive pelvic lesions may best be addressed with a Girdlestone procedure, particularly in bedridden patients with pain at rest and a life expectancy of <3 months (Fig. 45-4).

Basic Principles

The goals of acetabular reconstruction are to: (a) bypass the deficient area(s); (b) establish a line for force transmission across the reconstructed hip joint and through the pelvis; (c) obtain a stable platform for fixation of an acetabular component; and (d) prevent protrusio deformity. Proximal and distal fixation is needed, just as for the treatment of any fracture or discontinuity. Proximal fixation rests on the iliac crest or sacroiliac joint. Distal fixation utilizes periacetabular or ischial bone. Pins or screws span the acetabular defect and are fixed into structurally competent bone. They then act as pilings that help support the acetabular component within the reconstructive construct.

Smooth or threaded ¼-in. Steinmann pins or 6.5-mm cannulated screws are used to reinforce cement. Smooth pins have the advantage of a larger functional pin diameter and increased strength compared to threaded pins of the same diameter. However, threaded pins stably engage both bone and cement, and thus avoid sliding within the construct, which is a potential risk with smooth pins. Pins or screws can be placed either retrograde from within the defect, or antegrade from the iliac crest into the defect, engaging the remaining structurally competent bone of the pelvis. For antegrade fixation, pins or screws are placed from the iliac crest and aimed toward the ischium to reconstruct the posterior column, or aimed toward the pubis to reconstruct the anterior column. Ideally, the screws should be placed along the true medial wall to give a solid medial buttress without excessive lateralization of the cup. Pins or screws placed from both the anterior and posterior iliac crests are used for antegrade reconstruction of superior dome defects. Pins or screws should be placed broadly within the dome defect, above and medial to the acetabular component. Care should be taken to avoid impingement of the pins or screws onto the acetabular component, which can lead to potential malposition. At least two pins or screws should be placed within a defect to avoid rotation of the construct around a single fixation point. Additional fixation can be obtained by placing screws from within the cemented acetabular shell either into intact pelvic bone or into the cement of the construct. A flanged acetabular component gives better fixation to the pelvis than a large cup alone. The flange can be oriented over the region of the remaining intact acetabular rim (if present), whether it is anterior, posterior, inferior, or superior. In addition, the flanged component lateralizes the hip center, establishing a more anatomic hip position, reestablishing muscle tension, and thereby stabilizing the hip joint. This type of component also helps prevent protrusio (Fig. 45-5).

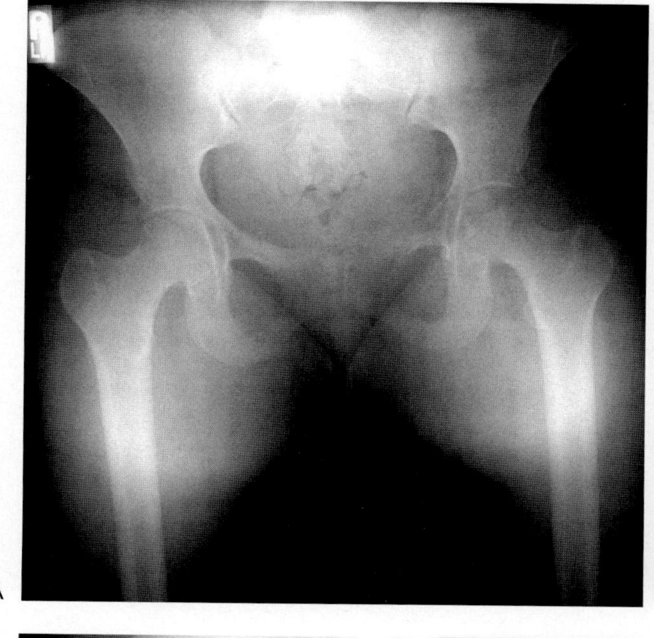
A

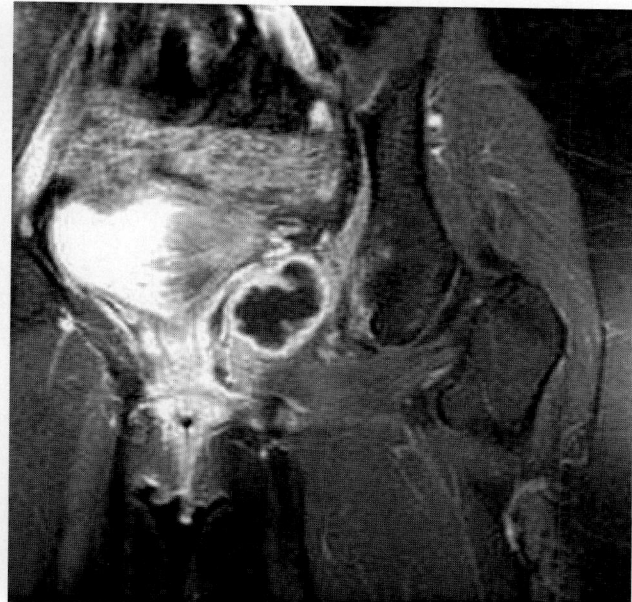
B

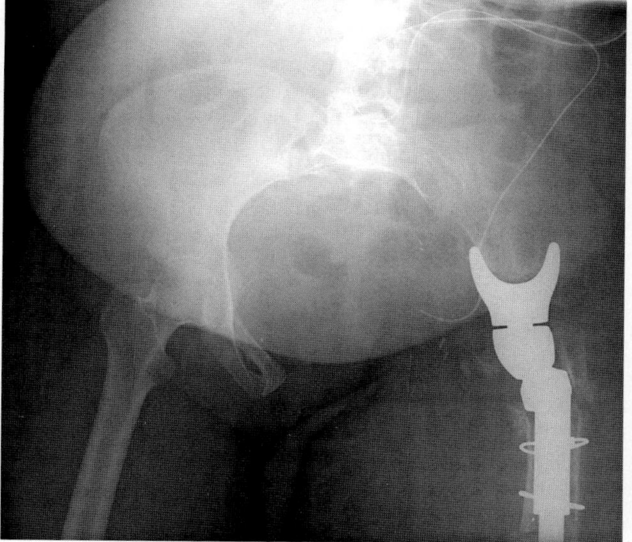
C

FIGURE 45-4. Pelvic lesion requiring a combined type II and III pelvic resection, reconstructed with a saddle prosthesis (Link America, Denville, NJ). **A:** Preoperative radiograph showing a lytic/destructive lesion involving the left superior pubic ramus. **B:** Preoperative magnetic resonance image demonstrating the lesion, with involvement of the medial wall of the acetabulum as well. **C:** After resection and reconstruction with a saddle prosthesis.

When the femur is being surgically reconstructed, it is often prudent to leave pelvic disease alone if it is not symptomatic or mechanically significant. If there is no clear disruption of the subchondral plate, the "thumb test" can help establish whether or not the acetabulum is functionally intact. The thumb test consists of the extended thumb of the surgeon being firmly pressed against the area of the acetabular articular cartilage that appears weakest on inspection and palpation, or that correlates to the region in question radiographically. This creates approximately 100 lb/cm^2 of pressure at the site, and can clinically identify weak regions that require reconstruction. If the acetabular socket can resist this pressure, it is mechanically sound, and these patients can be managed with a bipolar hemiarthroplasty for a femoral metastatic lesion.

Preoperative embolization should be considered in situation where the lesion: (a) is lytic; (b) is of renal, thyroid, or multiple myeloma origin; (c) has a soft-tissue mass; or (d) has not been previously irradiated. General guidelines for embolization are: if all four of the aforementioned factors are present, the lesion should definitely be embolized; if three of four factors are present it should probably be em-

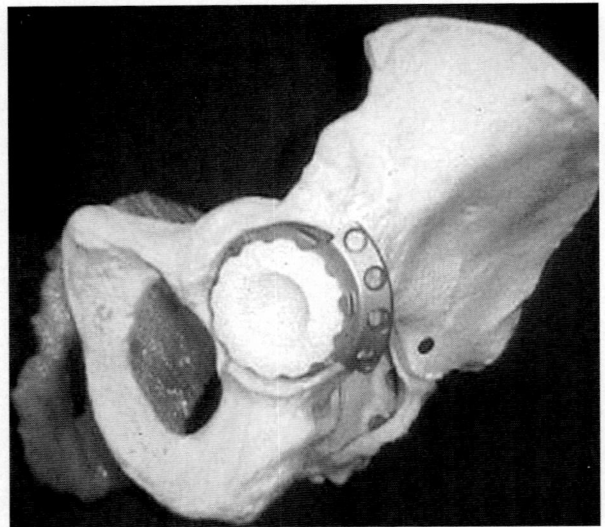

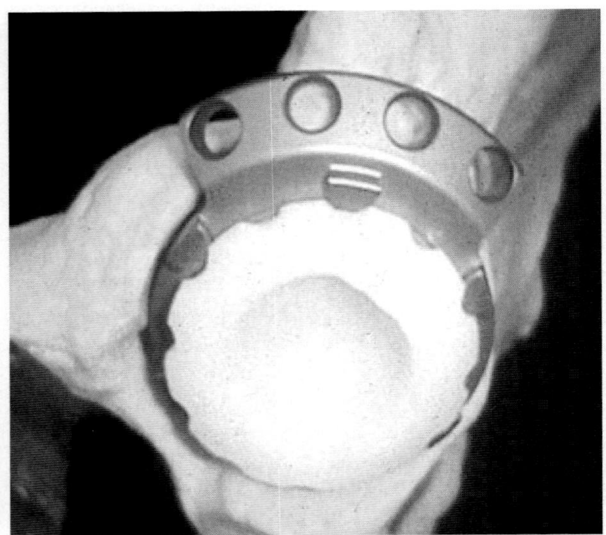

FIGURE 45-5. Flanged acetabular component (Healey Revision Cup; Biomet, Warsaw, IN). **A,B:** The flange may be oriented to contact the region where the remaining cortical bone stock is best.

bolized; if two of four factors are present it should possibly be embolized; and if only one of four factors is present, it should rarely be embolized.

Technique

Marco and coworkers previously described the surgical technique; however, several technical points deserve mention (2):

1. Use an extensive posterolateral approach to optimize acetabular exposure.
2. Remove all gross tumor by curettage. The profuse bleeding associated with this step subsides once the tumor has been fully removed and the defect packed with sponges.
3. Take care to preserve all structurally intact bone to maximize the support of the reconstructive construct. This also maintains anatomic landmarks to guide appropriate positioning of the cup.
4. Place antegrade pins or screws through separate 6- to 8-cm incision(s) made parallel to and directly over the iliac crest.
5. Prepare pin insertion sites prior to performing tumor curettage in patients with highly vascular tumors to minimize the time for bleeding from the cancer and the exposed acetabular tumor bed.
6. Place the pin entry site near the inner one-third of the crest and use a triangulation guide to direct the pins or screws along the iliac wing to maximally engage the bone and prevent penetration of the inner or outer pelvic table.
7. Use either smooth or threaded ¼-in. Steinmann pins or 6.5-mm cannulated screws for fixation.
8. Place pins or screws at least 1 cm apart along the crest, such that they extend into the defect and may be incorporated into the cement used to fill it, but not so far as to impede proper placement of the acetabular component.
9. Insert at least two pins or screws into the defect to adequately stabilize the cement.
10. Countersink pins or screws to prevent pin protrusion and local symptoms related to prominent pins.
11. When placing retrograde pins or screws from within the defect, take care not to penetrate the inner table and cause potential intrapelvic injury, and place them to an adequate depth within the bone to be able to provide stability to the construct.
12. Place a flanged acetabular cup such that the flange resides over the most intact remaining portion of the acetabular rim. In the series reported by Marco and coworkers, 46 of 55 patients (86%) had a flanged acetabular component used in the reconstruction, with the flange oriented over the superolateral rim in most cases (2). Insert the cup in 40 to 55 degrees of vertical inclination.
13. When additional screws are placed in the dome of the cup to obtain added fixation with superior acetabular defects, place the dome screws before the flange screws to prevent the cup from shifting out of position.
14. Cement the construct in two stages for large defects or with medial wall deficiencies. Fill the defect and incorporate the pins or screws in the first stage of cementation, and cement the acetabular component into place in the second stage. Single-stage cementation can lead to incomplete filling of large defects by the cement, and can compromise the accuracy of cup orientation (which is already challenging when reconstructing large de-

fects). Also, where there is a deficient medial wall, pressurization of the cement can lead to a potentially dangerous protrusion of cement into the pelvis (Fig. 45-6).

The femoral side of the reconstruction is performed with use of a cemented femoral stem. A standard stem length or a long stem length (220 to 300 mm) can be used, depending on the clinical situation. Care must be taken with the implantation of long-stemmed cemented femoral components, because there is a significant risk of sudden intraoperative death owing to embolization during this portion of the procedure (24). In light of this, pressurization of the cement in the femoral canal is actively avoided. All long-stemmed prostheses should be cemented after venting the femur distal to the isthmus with a 1/4-in. drill hole. This hole is drilled unicortically in the lateral femoral cortex below the level of the gluteal sling, through a split in the vastus lateralis. A cement restrictor usually is not used in the cementation of long-stemmed implants. After the canal has been prepared and dried, cement is placed into the canal in a more liquid state than is used in traditional third-generation cementation techniques. A finger should be temporarily placed over the vent hole while the cement is injected into the canal. As the component is slowly inserted, the decompression hole is exposed and cement allowed to extrude uninhibited. Tight fascial bands or lateral tissue can act as a fixed diaphragm over the hole, and prevent free egress of cement. The anesthesiologist needs to be actively aware of the progress of the cementation, and maintain blood volume and oxygenation. Routine closure and hip replacement rehabilitation should be started when the patient's condition permits.

Postoperative Adjuvant Therapy

Postoperative adjuvant therapy should be used, depending on the diagnosis and clinical situation. Postoperative radiation, in those patients still eligible, should include the entire operative field, secondary to the possibility of microscopic tumor spread by the dissection or internal fixation. Chemotherapy also should be considered. In the series from Memorial Sloan-Kettering, 78% of patients eligible to receive postoperative radiation did so, with a mean dose of 2,900 $\pm$ 620 cGy, and 75% of the patients received chemotherapy postoperatively. Ninety-eight percent of patients in this series received radiation or chemotherapy either pre or postoperatively (2).

Results

Eighteen of the 55 patients in the Memorial Sloan-Kettering Cancer Center series were nonambulatory preop-

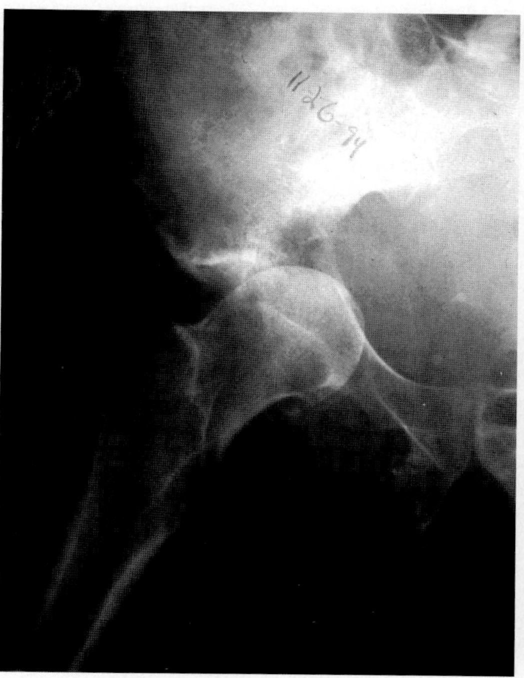

A

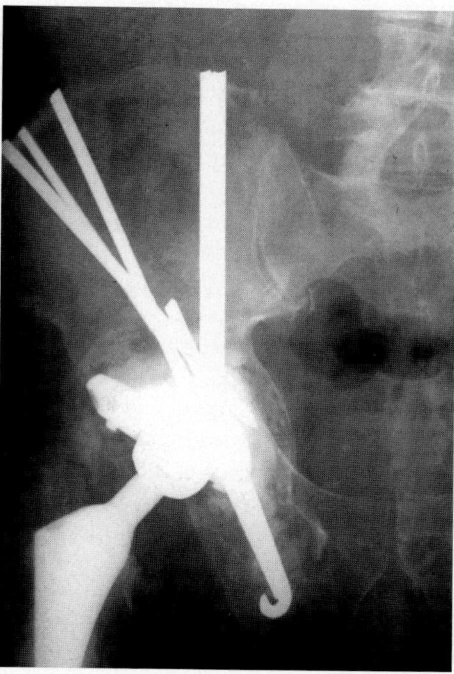

B

FIGURE 45-6. Demonstration of the reconstructive technique using reinforced cement and a flanged acetabular component in a patient with metastatic cancer involving the right acetabulum. **A:** Preoperative radiograph demonstrating a lesion involving the acetabular dome, medial wall, and posterior column. **B:** Postoperative radiograph demonstrating reconstruction using a modified Harrington technique with the use of antegrade pins and rush rods in combination with a total hip arthroplasty.

eratively. Fifty percent of these regained some walking ability postoperatively. At 6-month follow-up, 60% of the patients were still alive, and of these, 76% continued to have pain relief and 58% were able to walk and function in the community. Similar percentages of surviving patients maintained pain relief an ambulatory capacity at 12 and 24 months. Overall mean survival of the patients in this series was 21 months. This was better than the mean survival of 15 months reported in two additional series of patients who underwent acetabular reconstruction for metastatic disease (4,5). Fourteen of the 55 patients showed evidence of local progression of disease. However, late fixation failure occurred in only five patients, and only four of these patients required subsequent surgical intervention to address symptoms (2).

The MAC system is helpful in defining the metastatic acetabular lesions and guiding the operative reconstruction. Mechanically stable and durable acetabular reconstructions for complex acetabular lesions owing to metastatic disease can be performed using basic techniques and implants. Despite the complex nature of management of these lesions, significant and sustained functional improvement and pain relief can be achieved when reconstruction is used in the appropriate patient group.

METABOLIC BONE DISEASE

Pathologic fracture of the pelvis can result from nontumor conditions, including: postirradiation bone insufficiency, osteoporosis, and osteomalacia (often owing to antiseizure medication such as dilantin or phenobarbital, or vitamin D deficiency). Paget's disease as well as brown tumor of hyperparathyroidism also can involve the pelvis and cause pain and symptoms. As discussed, an accurate diagnosis is important to direct therapeutic intervention. Because of the overlap of the clinical pictures of these conditions with metastatic and primary tumors, an index of suspicion, and care in the history and physical examination are important to help direct the diagnostic workup. Often a biopsy is necessary to confirm the diagnosis.

Fortunately, once the diagnosis is made, the bone can be given a chance to recover and heal by addressing the etiology of the problem. In this regard, correcting the metabolic abnormality and managing the patient with pain medication and activity modification can allow for resolution of the symptoms. In some instances, however, the mechanical compromise of a region is extensive enough to require surgical intervention. This usually occurs with lesions involving the acetabulum, where the lesion destroys joint congruity. In these instances, surgical reconstruction of the acetabulum can be conducted as outlined for metastatic lesions. However, in certain metabolic situations (i.e., treatable osteomalacia), bone graft and press fit acetabular components can have utility in reconstruction because these patients do have the capacity to heal and reconstitute their bone stock. In patients with fractures caused by prior irradiation, Paget's disease, and severe osteoporosis, the healing capability of the bone is compromised to such an extent that these lesions are best addressed as in metastatic situations, where the construct stability is not dependent on active bony incorporation.

NONMALIGNANT DISEASE

Fractures caused by osteoporosis and other metabolic disease show patterns similar to those seen in traumatic injuries. Their description and management are dealt with elsewhere in this volume. If a typical fracture, such as a pubic ramus fracture, occurs in a typical patient (i.e., an elderly woman), the diagnosis of osteoporosis should be obvious, and the appropriate metabolic evaluation initiated. A workup also should be considered when there is an atypical fracture pattern, insufficient trauma to account for the fracture, delayed union, or concern regarding a systemic disorder. Evaluation starts with general surveillance tests and then becomes more specific, directed by the study results. Serious medical problems (e.g., renal failure) are clear etiologies of systemic bone compromise. However, to diagnose less obvious causes of metabolic bone disease, first-line tests include complete blood count (CBC), erythrocyte sedimentation rate (ESR), serum protein electrophoresis (SPEP), alkaline phosphatase (Aϕ), serum calcium, serum phosphorus, creatinine, and 24-hour urine collagen crosslinks (i.e., N-telopeptide [NTX]). If the CBC or ESR is abnormal, further evaluation for bone marrow dysplasia or multiple myeloma is necessary. This includes urinary Bence-Jones protein, β2-microglobulin, and iliac bone marrow aspiration/biopsy. If the alkaline phosphatase, serum calcium, or serum phosphorus are abnormal, then intact parathyroid hormone (PTH), 25-OH-vitamin D, and 1,25-(OH)2-vitamin D, need to be evaluated. If the NTX is elevated, then an endocrinopathy should be considered. This includes disruptions in the thyroid, parathyroid, adrenal cortical, or gonadotropin pathways. Bone densitometry (DEXA) is helpful in quantifying or establishing the diagnosis of underlying osteoporosis. However, a specialist in metabolic disease should direct further evaluation and management in cases of endocrine dysfunction (Table 45-3).

Iliac crest bone biopsy is infrequently needed to make the diagnosis or quantitate the degree of underlying osteoporosis. In a series of 100 consecutive cases of women with "osteoporotic" spinal compression fractures, Lane and Healey found occult osteomalacia in 7% (3% with normal blood chemistries), occult endocrinopathy in 10%, and an occult marrow disorder in 4% of patients (two with myeloma, one with lymphoma, and one with myelodysplasia) (Lane and Healey, personal communication). A similar distribution of pathology is likely to be found among patients with pelvic fractures with a diagnosis of osteoporosis.

TABLE 45-3. METABOLIC BONE DISEASE EVALUATION

First-Line Tests	Follow-Up Tests
Hematologic	
Complete blood count	Urinary Bence-Jones protein
Erythrocyte sedimentation rate	B_2-microglobulin
Serum protein electrophoresis	Iliac bone biopsy
Mineral balance	
Alkaline phosphatase	Intact parathyroid hormone
Serum calcium	25-(OH)-vitamin D
Serum phosphorus	24-hour urine calcium
Serum creatinine	24-hour urine creatinine
Endocrinopathy	
24-hour urine *N*-telopeptide (NTX)	Intact parathyroid hormone T4, thyroid stimulating hormone 24-hour urine cortisol

Several specialized situations deserve mention and discussion. Fracture nonunion, particularly when hypertrophic, may result in a central radiolucency surrounded by an "elephant's foot" of bone formation. This radiographic pattern can suggest the diagnosis of malignancy. Biopsy is necessary to rule out an underlying malignant process, but usually shows only callus formation. This type of nonunion is predominantly caused by uncontrolled movement at the fracture site. After an underlying vitamin D deficiency has been ruled out, open reduction with internal fixation is the best resolution for this problem.

Central acetabular fractures are rare, but are recognized sequelae of electroconvulsive treatment, and chronic calcium and vitamin D deficiency. These lesions do not require direct biopsy; however, an iliac crest biopsy for metabolic evaluation of the bone may be helpful. Treatment should include vitamin D and calcium replacement, control of the anticonvulsant medications, and careful mobilization (partial or toe-touch weight bearing). Surgery is warranted only to manage an unreducible central dislocation.

Osteonecrosis is not restricted to the femoral head but may occur within the innominate bone as well. Radiation is the most common cause; however, rarely it develops spontaneously (25,26). Pelvic osteonecrosis often is seen after the treatment of lymphoma, prostate cancer, gynecologic malignancy, or rectal cancer. Surgery should be restricted to situations where clinical symptoms cannot be managed with conservative measures. Infection is a very significant risk in these lesions. Poor osteoblast function delays fracture healing considerably, often doubling the time required to achieve union (27). Remarkably good function can be seen despite bony collapse when the joint remains reasonably congruent. Hip replacement in these situations should be reserved for symptomatic patients (Fig. 45-7).

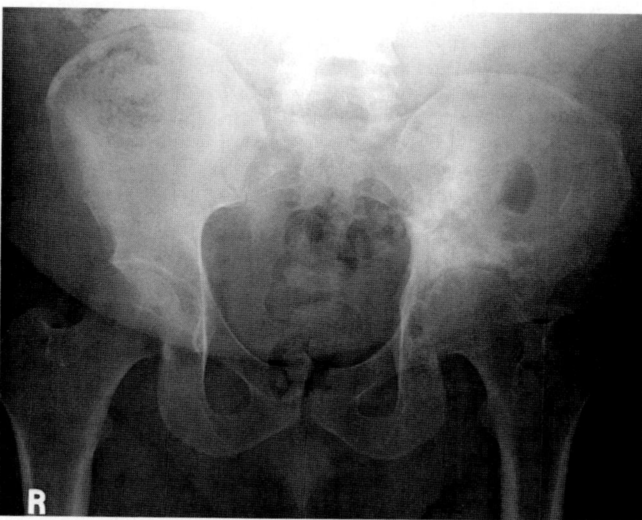

FIGURE 45-7. A 40-year-old man with a history of lymphoma of the left hemipelvis managed with radiation 9 years ago. A sclerotic lesion of the left acetabulum is present with collapse of the bone in the supraacetabular region, and a mild protrusio deformity. However, the joint congruity is maintained. The radiographic appearance of the lesion has remained stable, and the patient does not have hip pain.

Management with uncemented acetabular components is controversial in these situations. All pathologic bone, particularly in the presence of inflammatory arthritis or Paget's disease, is prone to the development of a protrusio deformity. When reconstructing the acetabulum of such patients, the use of a protrusio cup should be considered. Finally, most of these metabolic conditions also have a component of underlying osteoporosis that should be addressed. Second-generation bisphosphonates, such as Fosamax, actually may help accelerate fracture healing. Although this has been established in canine femoral fractures (with the presence of increased callus), it has not been proven to help in humans (28). Other interventions, such as PTH or electrical stimulation, lack experimental or clinical support to recommend their use.

REFERENCES

1. Gainor BJ, Buchert P. Fracture healing in metastatic bone disease. *Clin Orthop* 1983;178:297–302.
2. Marco RAW, Sheth DS, Boland PI, et al. Functional and oncological outcome of acetabular reconstruction for the treatment of metastatic disease. *J Bone Joint Surg* 2000;82A(5):642–651.
3. Harrington KD. The management of acetabular insufficiency secondary to metastatic malignant disease. *J Bone Joint Surg (Am)* 1981;63(4):653–664.
4. Vena VE, et al., Pelvic reconstruction for severe periacetabular metastatic disease. *Clin Orthop Rel Res* 1999;362:171–180.
5. Walker RH. Pelvic reconstruction/total hip arthroplasty for metastatic acetabular insufficiency. *Clin Orthop Rel Res* 1993; 294:170–175.

6. Brown HK, Healey JH. Metastatic cancer to the bone. In: DeVita VT, ed. *Cancer: principles and practice of oncology.* Philadelphia: Lippincott Williams & Wilkins, 1999, pp. 2713–2729.
7. Conill C, Verger E, Salamero M. Performance status assessment in cancer patients. *Cancer* 1990;65:1864–1866.
8. Orr S, Aisner J. Performance status assessment among oncology patients: a review. *Cancer Treat Rept* 1986;70:1423–1429.
9. Roila F, et al., Intra and interobserver variability in cancer patients' performance status assessed according to Karnofsky and ECOG scales. *Ann Oncol* 1991;2:437–439.
10. Verger E, Salamero M, Conill C. Can Karnofsky performance status be transformed to the Eastern Cooperative Oncology Group scoring scale and vice versa? *Eur J Cancer* 1992;28A(8–9): 1328–1330.
11. Galasko CSB, Burn JI. Hypercalcemia in patients with advanced mammary cancer. *Br Med J* 1971;3:573–577.
12. Gosfield E, Alavi A, Kneeland B. Comparison of radionuclide bone scans and magnetic resonance imaging in detecting spinal metastases. *J Nucl Med* 1993;34:2191.
13. Pomeranz SJ, Pretorius HT, Ramsingh PS. Bone scintigraphy and multimodality imaging in bone neoplasia: strategies for imaging in the new health care climate. *Semin Nucl Med* 1994;24:188.
14. D'Antonio JA, et al. Classification and management of acetabular abnormalities in total hip arthroplasty. *Clin Orthop Rel Res* 1989;243:126–137.
15. Berry DJ, et al. Pelvic discontinuity in revision total hip arthroplasty. *J Bone Joint Surg* 1999;81A(12):1692–1702.
16. Weill A, Kobaiter H, Chiras J. Acetabulum malignancies: technique and impact on pain of percutaneous injection of acrylic surgical cement. *Eur J Radiol* 1998;8(1):123–129.
17. Cotten A, et al. Therapeutic percutaneous injections in the treatment of malignant acetabular osteolyses. *Radiographics* 1999; 19(3):647–653.
18. Enneking W, Dunham W. Resection and reconstruction for primary neoplasms involving the innominate bone. *J Bone Joint Surg* 1978;60:731–746.
19. Aboulafia AJ, et al. Reconstruction using the Saddle prosthesis following excision of malignant periacetabular tumors. Complications of limb salvage: prevention, management and outcome. In: Brown, KLB, ed. Montreal: The International Society of Limb-Sparing Surgery, 1991.
20. Saitoh H. Distant metastasis of renal adenocarcinoma. *Cancer* 1981;48:1487.
21. Takashi M, et al., Surgical treatment of renal cell carcinoma metastases: prognostic significance. *Int Urol Nephrol* 1995;27:1.
22. Tongaonkar HB, Kulkarni JN, Kamat MR. Solitary metastases from renal cell carcinoma: a review. *J Surg Oncol* 1992;49:45.
23. Holland J, et al. Plasmacytoma treatment results and conversion to myeloma. *Cancer* 1992;69:1513.
24. Patterson BM, et al. Cardiac arrest during hip arthroplasty with a cemented long-stem component: a report of seven cases. *J Bone Joint Surg* 1991;73A:271–277.
25. Bullough P, et al. Bone infarctions not associated with caisson disease. *J Bone Joint Surg* 1965;47A:477–491.
26. Deleeuw H, Pottenger L. Osteonecrosis of the acetabulum following radiation therapy. A report of two cases. *J Bone Joint Surg (Am)* 1988;70A(2):293–299.
27. Pelker R, Friedlaender G. The Nicolas Andry Award—1995. Fracture healing. Radiation induced alterations. *Clin Orthop* 1997;341:267–282.
28. Peter C, et al. Effect of alendronate on fracture healing and bone remodeling in dogs. *J Orthop Res* 1996;14(1):74–79.

46

RESULTS OF TREATMENT FOR FRACTURES OF THE ACETABULUM

MARTIN D. BIRCHER

> Comparison of a relatively undisplaced crack fracture of the acetabulum with a significantly displaced centrally dislocated bone is like comparing an apple to an orange.

—Marvin Tile, *Fractures of the Pelvis and Acetabulum,* 1st ed, 1983

INTRODUCTION

Professor Emille Letournel's results of 940 operatively managed displaced acetabular fractures is the gold standard: His results may never be bettered. Even in his expert hands only three fourths of patients achieved an excellent or good short-term outcome. He also demonstrated that quality of result diminishes with time (1).

An acetabular fracture is a devastating injury and can seriously influence the quality of a patient's life. In attempting to analyze why one fourth of patients have substandard results, we need to identify factors that point to a good result and more importantly those factors that jeopardize a satisfactory outcome.

In the broadest terms these factors fall under the following headings.

1. The patient. The preinjury level of activities, age, bone quality, and the postinjury requirements and needs. For example, it is hard to imagine a world-class track athlete ever returning to the field after a high-energy transverse acetabular fracture.
2. The fracture type. The degree of displacement and amount of comminution. This reflects the degree of primary bone cartilage and soft-tissue damage.
3. The treatment. The choice of conservative or operative treatment and the factors that lead to this decision making. Timing of this treatment and the expertise of the treating team also have a profound influence on the outcome.
4. Complications (both preoperatively and postoperatively).
5. Length of follow-up.

In the 1950s and 1960s Judet and Letournel demonstrated that it was possible to obtain satisfactory results treating displaced acetabular fractures surgically (2). In the

1970s and 1980s, approaches were modified and refined and instruments developed in an attempt to help the surgeon. It is quite likely that the 21st century will herald improved patient selection. By studying the long-term results of major series, we can begin to identify those patients who need to be treated operatively and which fractures can be treated nonoperatively. A significant subgroup of patients also will be identified where other treatments need to be considered (e.g., acute or delayed total hip replacement). It is now clear that some acetabular fractures are so severe that primary surgical reconstruction is fruitless.

NATURAL HISTORY: WHY OPERATE?

Drawing meaningful conclusions from the orthopedic literature in this area is challenging and occasionally confusing. However, one clear message has appeared over the last 40 years. To obtain a good result following an acetabular fracture it is essential that treatment results in the femoral head being accurately centered beneath the roof of the acetabulum. In a two-dimensional x-ray the relationship between the femoral head and roof of the acetabulum is often referred to as parallelism. When considered in a third dimension, the concept of congruency is introduced. Whether parallelism or congruency is achieved by operative or nonoperative methods seems to be of secondary importance. If operative treatment is undertaken, it is inevitable that a new set of soft-tissue complications may ensue. The outcome then may be jeopardized, even though you may have a centered femoral head.

Some specific fractures (e.g., the associated both-column fracture) demonstrate congruency of the femoral head in the displaced position. These types of fracture have been treated nonoperatively in the past with excellent results (3), although evidence is mainly anecdotal. During the last two decades the assessment of congruity has proved difficult to demonstrate and define. The three classical radiologic views go a considerable way to demonstrating it. The anterior-posterior (AP) x-ray is the most sensitive. If the medial joint space is equal to the superior joint space, it is reasonably safe to assume that there is acceptable congruency. However, x-rays are static pictures and with more unstable injuries medial subluxation of the femoral head may occur when the joint loading is increased.

In a posterior wall fracture the postreduction x-ray may show a congruent relationship between the femoral head and the roof. However, when the hip is flexed (often under anesthetic) it can dislocate. Although in static position we have congruency, recurrent subluxation will again jeopardize an excellent long-term outcome. Therefore, stability and congruity need to be assessed not only statically but using techniques that stress the joint.

The advent of computed tomography (CT) scanning has led to a better understanding of fracture types; but again, congruity is impossible to judge in isolation with these images alone.

If one studies Fig. 46-1, the concept of gaps and steps is introduced. The diagrams are two-dimensional (2D) and the situation with the acetabulum is more complicated because of the three-dimensional (3D) nature of the anatomy. Figure 46-1A demonstrates an acetabulum with a gap. In this situation there is still equal loading of the acetabular articular cartilage. If the cells survive the impact, then this situation is compatible with an acceptable outcome. Figure 46-1B shows an acetabulum with a step. This is an unacceptable situation that will lead to eccentric loading of areas of acetabulum and differential loading on areas of the femoral head. This will lead to abrasion of the articular cartilage on both sides of the joint, cell death, and an early substandard result. This concept has been observed in other joints (e.g., the ankle) (4,5), and the aim of treatment must be to convert steps to gaps and then if possible to close the gaps and produce the ultimate outcome, a perfect reduction.

Another important factor affecting outcome is the retention of loose bodies. In 1960 Epstein (6) showed that following dislocation retained loose fragments will lead to early femoral head abrasion and a poor long-term result. He advocated open inspection and washout of the joint. The presence of loose bodies following an acetabular injury is also an

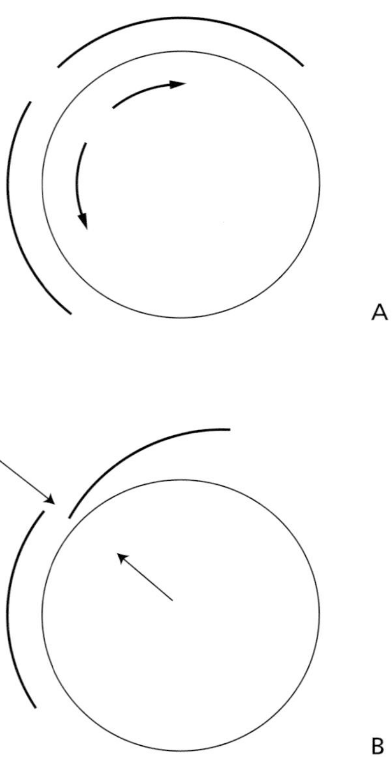

FIGURE 46-1. A: In a gap, the hip may remain congruent because Load A = Load B, thus in C, the load may be evenly distributed. **B:** In a step, the hip is incongruent because Load A > Load B, thus causing point loading.

indicator of significant associated primary articular cartilage damage. What was not appreciated in the 1960s (because CT scans were not available) was that in producing these loose bodies, other areas of articular cartilage suffer impaction ("marginal impaction"). This further contributes to the areas of damaged articular cartilage. This contributes to a substandard result if left malpositioned. CT scans still miss loose bodies in the joint, especially if cuts are >3 mm apart. It is possible for these smaller pieces of articular debris to be retained within the fovea; however, in general terms, any loose fragments that are seen on the scans following dislocation should be removed surgically. During surgery following fracture dislocations, the amount of debris that lies within the joint space is always surprising.

In summary, the hip joint does not tolerate incongruence, instability, or retained loose bodies. If a fracture is minimally displaced, congruent and stable excellent results can be achieved with nonoperative management.

Loose bodies and instability are absolute indications for operative treatment, whereas incongruity is only a relatively strong indicator. This gray area represents the art of acetabular fracture management.

HISTORICAL RESULTS: METHODS OF ASSESSMENT AND OUTCOMES

When studying the historical results, it is essential to ensure that case mix in the studies are comparable and that the method of assessment and quality of the result is not overgenerous. In the past the Harris hip score has been adapted from arthroplasty literature to fracture outcome studies. This is an overgenerous assessment. It is possible to obtain a very high score with an arthrodesed hip. This is because most methods of assessment are strongly biased toward the level of pain. The original D'Aubigne and Postel assessment of 1954 allowed an excellent result, even if a hip had only 90 degrees of flexion. We will only begin to obtain meaningful results from a treatment series when our assessments are accurate and reproducible. Some conclusions drawn from early papers have been inaccurate and have led to significant misconceptions. In 1961 Rowe and Lowell (7) reported 93 acetabular fractures in 90 patients. This paper was used to champion the cause for nonoperative management. The overall results of conservative treatment seem to compare very favorably with those of operative treatment by Judet later in the 1960s. Closer examination of the subgroups within Rowe and Lowell's paper leads to a very different conclusion. As expected, patients with undisplaced cracks do extremely well with nonoperative treatment. The outcome of a subgroup of posterior fracture dislocations paints an entirely different picture. Six of 17 patients with a posterior wall fracture treated by closed reduction and traction had a poor outcome. However, eight of 11 patients with the seemingly comparable posterior wall injury who had an open reduction and internal fixation had a satisfactory outcome. This suggests that operative treatment for a posterior wall fracture is the best choice. Even so, three of the 11 patients who had surgery had a poor result. One also can conclude that the injury itself has a significant influence on the eventual outcome as well as the choice of treatment.

Within the same series, 29 patients with an injury to the quadrilateral plate and/or the anterior column obtained excellent results when congruity was retained between the head and roof by closed methods. Indeed, 90% achieved what is described as "a satisfactory clinical result under these circumstances." However, it was also pointed out that only 83% of the same group had what could be termed a satisfactory radiologic outcome. This was one of the early papers to raise the differences between clinical and radiologic outcome. The conclusions from Rowe and Lowell's paper should *not* be that nonoperative treatment is indicated for all acetabular fractures. It is true that undisplaced crack fractures do not require operative treatment. Likewise, if the femoral head remains under the roof in a stable condition, then surgery again may not be indicated. However, if the hip is unstable or incongruent, then other methods of treatment should be considered. The only way to predictably restore stability and congruity is through operative management.

In 1986 Matta (8) performed a retrospective analysis of 204 acetabular fractures. The follow-up was short (3.7 years). The concept of how much of the acetabular dome or roof was involved in the fracture was introduced. He used these "roof arc angles" in an attempt to assess stability in order to chose between operative and nonoperative treatment. Unfortunately, these angles can only be applied to certain fracture types; for example, they cannot be used in both-column fractures. The paper emphasizes the important relationship between the femoral head and roof of the acetabulum. His conclusions were that closed treatment is only satisfactory for displaced fractures if the weight-bearing dome is intact. Anatomic open reduction in the absence of complications improved the prognosis. This was also one of the first papers to attempt to correlate the clinical result with the quality of fracture reduction.

In 1988 (9) Matta again produced a prospective study of 121 cases. Twenty-three were treated in traction and 98 were managed by open reduction and internal fixation (the large majority through a posterior approach). Radiographic analysis of the quality of reduction deemed a postoperatively displacement of 3 mm or more on x-ray plain films as unsatisfactory. Less than 3 mm was considered satisfactory and less than 1 mm was graded as "anatomic." Using these very generous criteria, 91% of his results were radiographically satisfactory but only 63% were anatomic. Unfortunately, following this paper other workers in the field incorrectly concluded that it was acceptable to reduce an acetabular fracture operatively to within 3 mm. Clearly, this was a mistake. The articular cartilage of the acetabulum is 2.5 mm thick at best. If one accepts a 3-mm step in a reconstruction, then under no circumstances will this produce a satisfactory long-term outcome.

The problem always has been in assessing the amount of postoperative displacement on plain films. It is for this reason that postoperative CT scanning and conventional x-rays should be used in conjunction to assess the quality of reduction.

Other important information that resulted from Matta's 1988 paper related to the experience of the surgeon and the quality of reduction (the learning curve). Figure 46-2 demonstrates a number of unsatisfactory reductions per group of 20 in the first 100 surgically treated cases. This graph demonstrates that as experience increases, the quality of the reduction improves. This point is further underlined in Fig. 46-3. This shows an increasing number of anatomic reductions as experience rises.

Matta's most recent paper in 1996 (10) demonstrates the results in 259 patients. These results mirror Letournel's larger series. Matta's paper included a modified clinical grading system which was much tighter. Matta also evolved a much stricter radiographic assessment. Anatomic reduction was graded between 0 and 1 mm of displacement but imperfect was graded between 2 and 3 mm. A poor reduction was any displacement >3 mm. The fact that his results were almost identical to those of Letournel's, who employed a slightly less rigid scoring system, is intriguing. If one assumes similar surgical capabilities and similar case mix, then it must be that Matta's results are perhaps 5% better than those of Letournel's. This slight improvement of the quality of the results probably reflects 30 to 40 years of worldwide experience with improved techniques, reduced complication rate, and better patient selection.

In summary, the literature in the past has shown that acceptable results following acetabular fracture will be achieved if:

1. The femoral head is centered under the roof and is congruent and parallel and remains there.

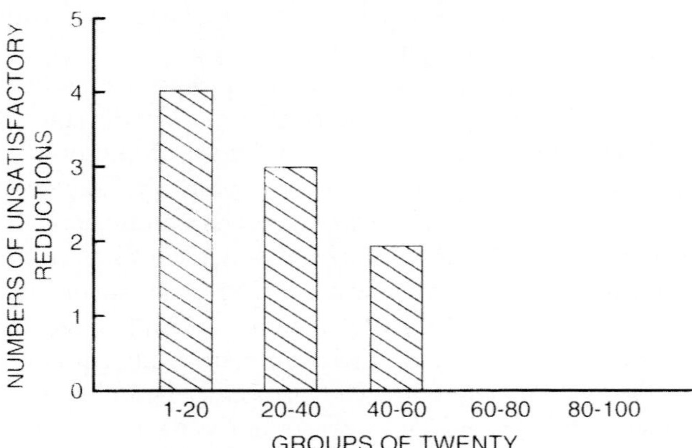

FIGURE 46-2. Number of unsatisfactory reductions per group of 20 for the first 100 surgical cases. (From: Matta JM, Merritt PO. Displaced acetabular fractures. *Clin Orthop* 1988;230:83, with permission.)

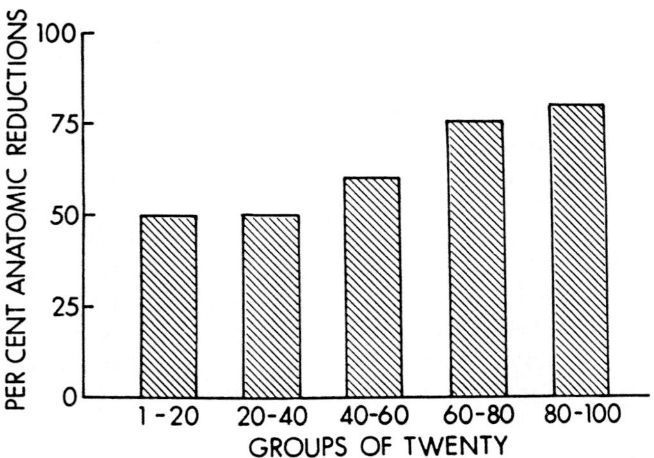

FIGURE 46-3. Percentage of anatomic reductions per group of 20 for the first 100 surgical cases. (From: Matta JM, Merritt PO. Displaces acetabular fractures. *Clin Orthop* 1988;230:83, with permission.)

2. The hip is stable and there are no entrapped loose bodies.
3. Complications are avoided.

Whether these criteria are met by open and closed methods depends more on the type of fracture and the degree of displacement.

LETOURNEL'S RESULTS: THE GOLD STANDARD

The results of operative treatment published by Letournel (1) in 1993 are presented in such a way that already recognizes certain important factors that influence the outcome. The three main factors are the quality of reduction, interval between injury and surgery, and length of follow-up. Time intervals are easy to measure and are accurate. The major problem is measuring outcome in relation to assessment of the quality of reduction. A perfect reduction has always been relatively simple to assess. Letournel defined it as the perfect restoration of the articular congruence and the reestablishment of all radiologic landmarks on three standard radiographic views. It was only his later cases where postoperative CT scans were available. The problem has always lain in the assessment of imperfect reduction. Letournel defined imperfect reductions as those in which one or more of all the acetabular landmarks were not anatomically restored on the three plain radiologic views. The consequence of this was usually some form of postsurgical articular incongruence. The difficulty that arose was how to evaluate the degree of postsurgical incongruence. It was hoped that 3DCT scanning would have made this task easier, but as yet this has not been the case. To date there seems to be no precise method of assessing the amount of postoperative incongruity. Letournel in his last two reviews (1978 to 1980 and 1987 to 1990) decided to assess imperfection by evaluating the posi-

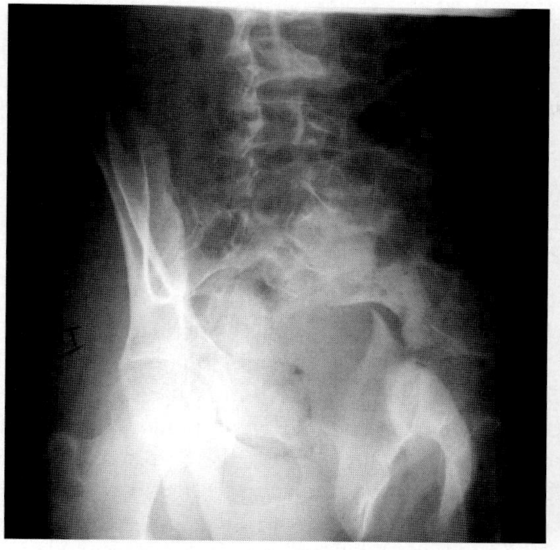
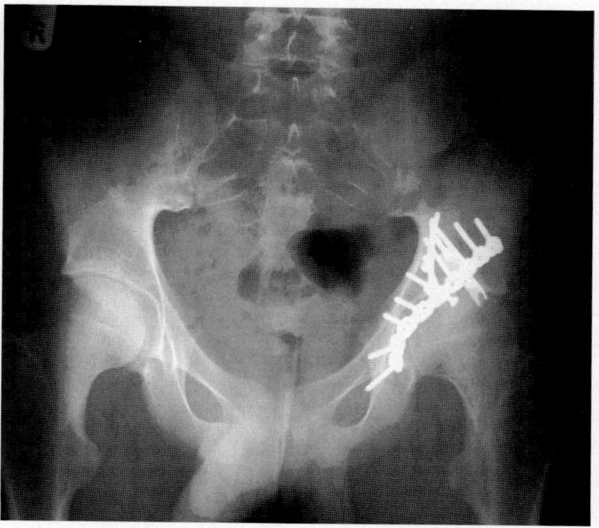

A B

FIGURE 46-4. Anterior-posterior pelvis. Note excellent reduction but apparent loss of parallelism with opening of lateral joint space. However, the hip is in fact normal compared to the other side.

tion of the femoral head with respect to the undisturbed or restored anatomic roof of the acetabulum. Thus, four types of imperfect reductions were described.

1. Reductions where the head/roof congruency is correctly restored but with a malreduction of the acetabulum visible on one of the three views. These malreductions were usually low in the anterior or posterior columns.
2. Cases where there is obvious loss of parallelism of the upper joint space. This would have been invariably related to some form of malreduction higher in the anterior or posterior part of the acetabulum. Letournel, however, drew our attention to the important fact that some "normal hips" do appear to demonstrate a lack of parallelism. Comparison must always be made with the uninjured side if possible. Figure 46-4 demonstrates such a case where all views of the injured side demonstrate an anatomic reduction but there seems to be a loss of parallelism between the head and roof. However, if this is compared to the other side, it can be seen that this normal hip demonstrates this phenomenon of anatomic "loss of parallelism."
3. Imperfect reductions where it is clear that the femoral head is centrally protruded. In these cases, the AP x-ray usually demonstrates the femoral head to be nearer or medial to the ilioischial line with an associated loss of parallelism of the upper joint space.
4. Secondary surgical congruency (Fig. 46-5). In essence these cases represent the end result of surgery where all the fragments of the shattered acetabular articular cartilage are reassembled around a centrally displaced femoral head in a

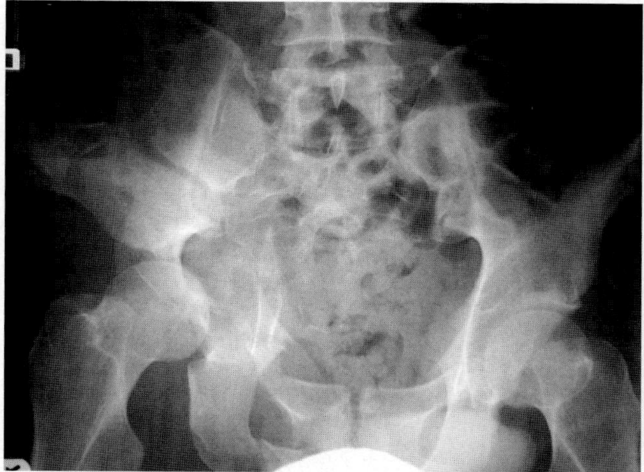
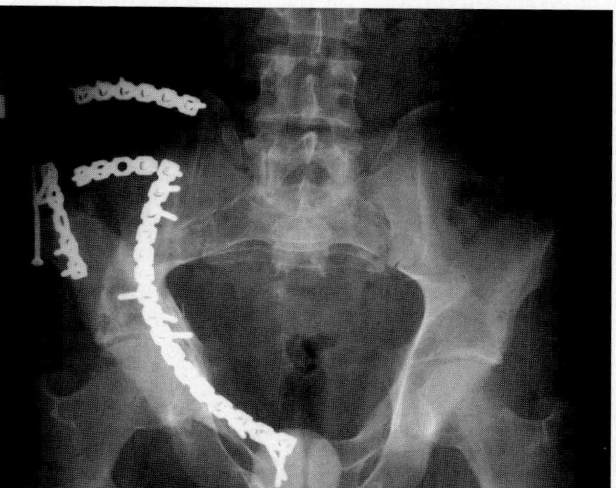

A B

FIGURE 46-5. A: Anterior-posterior (AP) x-ray of complex both-column acetabular fracture. **B:** Postoperative AP x-ray. Secondary surgical congruency with good parallelism between roof and head. The whole hip is still medialized. The ilioischial and iliopectineal lines are not anatomic.

fully congruent manner (the situation often seen in both-column fractures preoperatively). In these cases, congruency has been restored but there are clearly gaps in the joint surface.

It must be noted that it is possible to perfectly restore the ilioischial and iliopectineal lines and still have a significant malreduction. This situation is seen in the elderly or high-energy injuries where there is bone impaction. If an indirect reduction is being made, then a false sense of achievement will ensue. A perfect reduction can be achieved only with the elevation of depressed fragments and internal bone grafting.

Clinical Results of Operations Performed Within 3 Weeks of Injury

Of five hundred sixty-nine patients with an acetabular fracture operated within 3 weeks of injury, 544 had a minimum follow-up period of 1 year. A significant number of patients were lost to follow-up; indeed, only 492 patients were available, of which over 100 had incomplete follow-up. The assessment of their last examination prior to being lost to follow-up was included.

The overall clinical results were assessed on pain, mobility, and gait, according to the slightly modified d'Aubigne Postel system. This is an unduly kind assessment where the maximum score for range of motion is achieved if you only have 90 degrees hip flexion. Using these assessments, the overall accumulation of results was 62.4% excellent, 11% very good, 7.3% good, 6.7% intermediate, and 13.2% poor. This represented over three fourths of the patients having a good or excellent result. These are impressive results but the follow-up is short. There was a strong correlation between good and excellent results and the quality of reduction and it also appeared that certain fracture types seemed to do better than others. For example, only 48.5% of transverse and posterior wall fractures had an excellent result. This must be a reflection on not only the difficulties of reduction but also the presence of primary articular cartilage damage.

Clinical Results of Patients Treated Operatively Between 3 Weeks and 4 Months After Injury

Using the same criteria of 138 patients from 155, only 54.3% achieved a very good or excellent result. Again, there was a correlation between quality of reduction and outcome. It is clear that it is much more difficult to achieve a satisfactory reduction in neglected cases and the chances of a satisfactory outcome are significantly diminished.

Clinical Results of Patients Treated Beyond 4 Months Following Injury

A meaningful conclusion cannot be drawn from this subgroup of patients. Other procedures (e.g., total hip replacements and arthrodesis) are included and the numbers are relatively small. What can be said is that various treatment modalities need to be available to manage this group of patients and anatomic reconstruction usually is not achievable.

Radiologic Results of Operative Treatment in Cases Operated Within 21 Days After Injury

There are 567 cases in this subseries. Four hundred eighteen (73.72%) cases were assessed as perfect reductions.

The best reductions were in the posterior wall and posterior wall/posterior column group (nine out of 10 cases being perfect). It is not clear in what percentage of patients CT scanning was used in assessing the result. The most challenging subgroups according to fracture type are the both-column, the transverse, the T type, and transverse and posterior wall groups. Perfect reductions range here between 60% and 70%. The more comminuted and complex fractures were more difficult to obtain a perfect reduction.

Radiologic Results in Cases Operated Between 3 Weeks and 4 Months

Letournel stressed the diversity of this particular subgroup of cases. Of the 150 surgeries that he carried out between 3 weeks and 4 months after injury, 19 patients were lost to follow-up. However, he achieved an incredible 97 perfect reductions in this group. These sorts of cases should not be seen nowadays, as referral should not be delayed. It is clear that it is still possible to achieve acceptable radiologic results in neglected cases but the difficulty of surgery escalates and the complication rate rises steeply.

Radiologic Outcome in Cases Treated Beyond 4 Months

In 123 cases, 49 cases were deemed as impossible to reconstruct. Of the remaining 74 late-presenting cases, 16 were instances of delayed removal of missed incarcerated fragments and there were three cases of unreduced posterior dislocation. However, a number of these posterior dislocations were not reconstructed and whether or not anatomic reconstruction was achieved seems rather irrelevant because bone grafts and supplementary surgical techniques were used to reinforce the skeleton in many surgeries. It is almost impossible to achieve a perfect reduction of an acetabular fracture if reconstructed 4 months or more after injury. Other options should be considered, such as total hip replacement in the older age group and arthrodesis in the young.

SUMMARY OF LETOURNEL'S RESULTS

Letournel's results demonstrate that acutely performed surgery with minimal primary articular cartilage damage with associated accurate reduction and avoidance of complications will result in an excellent outcome. Any factors that reduce the chances of an anatomic reduction or accelerate primary or secondary articular cartilage damage will jeopardize a satisfactory long-term outcome.

Length of Follow-Up

Letournel expressed this phenomenon in two ways. He regularly reviewed his series of patients over the 33 years and presented his results as an evolution of outcome. For example, in 1966, 111 patients with follow-up of more than 1 year were evaluated. In this group, 63 were rated as excellent. Of the same group, in 1971, only 44 patients of the 63 group had an excellent result. This had become 33 by 1978, and 20 by 1990. This clearly showed that with time, the quality of the result has deteriorated. The most important figure in Letournel's book correlates outcome, length of follow-up, and the quality of reduction. It can be seen from Fig. 46-6 that patients who have imperfect reductions fail at an early stage and are highly unlikely to achieve a long-lasting satisfactory result. The only exceptions to this rule are those patients who have undergone a surgical procedure and ended up with secondary surgical congruency. The best chance of achieving an excellent long-term outcome is with a perfect reduction. However, at the 10- to 15-year mark there are a significant number of failures within the perfect reduction group that develop posttraumatic osteoarthritis. I believe this is more a reflection of the primary chondral damage of injury rather than treatment. Most other series in the literature from experienced surgeons mirror these results, albeit with smaller numbers, and come to similar conclusions (11–14).

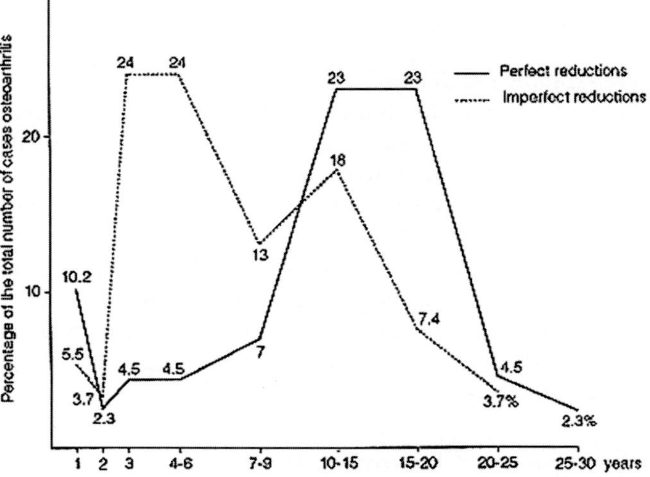

FIGURE 46-6. All injured hips are at risk to the development of osteoarthritis. This risk is much lessened and pushed back further in time with a perfect reduction. (From: Letournel E, Judet R. *Fractures of the acetabulum,* 2nd ed. New York, Springer-Verlag, 1993, with permission.)

Results of Treatment: Conclusions

Preinjury Status

A.E. Nicol introduced the concept of patient and fracture personality. The make-up of the patient along with her or his overall reaction to the injury can strongly influence the end result.

Age

In his 1996 series of 262 displaced acetabular fractures, Matta said that there was a statistical difference in outcome of patients <40 years old compared with those >40 years old. In 160 patients under 40, 81% had an excellent or good result, compared to only 68% of the 96 patients in the 40+ age group. This was not a strong difference but indicates that the age of the patient does have an influence. This relates to the patient's preoperative activities, the quality of both the articular cartilage and bone at the time of the injury, and compliance postoperatively. In elderly patients, much less force is required to fracture the bones and certain fracture patterns occur commonly, for example, the anterior column and associated both-column fractures. The fact that less energy is required is a plus factor but the bone tends to impact and makes surgical management much more challenging. Screw hold is much less reliable than in young hard bones. This, combined with the fact that elderly patients find it very difficult to partial weight bear leads to an increased risk of loss of fixation in the elderly skeleton. Age itself, however, should not be a contraindication to operative treatment. If an acetabulum is unstable (usually posteriorly), then surgical treatment is usually required no matter the age of the patient. However, it may be decided to perform a reconstruction and then proceed to hip replacement at the same sitting (see Chapter 43). Loss of fixation is often blamed on patients by surgical teams but I believe this is more often than not related to an underestimation of the injury associated with poor reduction and inadequate fixation. In Matta's series, eight patients had partial loss of fracture reduction with only one patient achieving an excellent result. Therefore, one must conclude that loss of fixation strongly correlates with a poor outcome.

Patient Personality

If patients are totally noncompliant (e.g., psychiatric patients), then treatment is more challenging and the outcome is often jeopardized by the patients themselves. It may be that minimally displaced fractures become displaced because of inappropriate weight bearing. It could be argued that undisplaced fractures should be stabilized in such noncompliant patients, possibly percutaneously, to prevent this complication. Displaced fractures in a noncompliant group usually require operative treatment, but a poor outcome is often the end result because of loss of fixation. If fixation is undertaken in this particular group of patients, then it is wiser to use double-plating techniques in an attempt to prevent loss of position. In an attempt to overstabilize the fracture, some areas of bone may become devascularized and avascular changes may ensue. This may produce a poor outcome in a different way.

Fracture Type

Certain fracture types are associated with severe chondral damage, which is either primary or secondary. *Severe posterior wall fractures, transverse fractures,* and *T fractures* with or without posterior wall involvement, are always associated with a significant amount of primary articular cartilage damage. If left in an unreduced position with no traction, secondary abrasion of the femoral head also may occur (secondary cartilage loss). The loss of articular cartilage is permanent and even if an anatomic reduction is achieved, a durable long-term outcome will not be achievable.

Certain fracture types are very difficult to reduce anatomically. This is usually owing to the strong forces of the muscles attached to the pelvis or to delay with callus formation. Because the quality of reduction correlates strongly with the outcome, it follows that fracture type also influences the end result. The best example of this is a transtectal transverse fracture. Anatomic reduction is mandatory. This is extremely difficult to achieve through a single approach. Bone often bends in young patients prior to fracture. This can mislead the surgeon if an indirect external approach is made. If a posterior approach is used, then anatomic reduction at the back is achieved quite often. Unfortunately, because of the length of the fracture line and the forces of the attached muscles, there is often significant anterior malposition. It is for this reason that two approaches are advisable for this type of fracture.

The best indicator of the influence of a fracture type on outcome can be gleaned from Matta's 1996 paper. He had 14 T fractures associated with posterior wall injuries. These had the highest incidence of poor results. Only eight cases were excellent or good, whereas six were fair or poor. This represents a 42% failure rate at an average time of 6 years following surgery. This particular subgroup of patients combines the formidable combination of severe primary articular cartilage damage and the most challenging reconstructive procedure.

The both-column fracture is a very common injury, usually representing over one fourth of the cases in a series. Unfortunately, it has been impossible to complete a randomized trial of the management of this injury. Operative treatment stands the greatest chance of having the best long-term result, but surgical reconstructions of both-column fractures are challenging and the complication rate can be high. Selective nonoperative treatment has produced acceptable results in many centers. The biggest mistake within this group of patients is to operate and turn a congruent both-column subluxation into an incongruent fixation.

The Soft Tissues

Postoperative Nerve Injury

The influence of a postoperative sciatic palsy following posterior acetabular surgery has diminished rapidly over the last four decades. Some authors claim this is because of nerve monitoring. I think this is just a reflection of surgical experience and the identification of surgical maneuvers to relax the sciatic nerve (e.g., keeping the hips flexed through surgery). Matta's 1996 paper suggested that an excellent or good result could still be achieved with a foot drop. However, a more sophisticated functional analysis of outcome (see SF 30 results of Kreda) will demonstrate less than a satisfactory outcome. In these patients the radiographic appearance of the skeleton is often excellent but function is compromised because of the neurologic deficit.

Other nerve palsies do not seem to influence outcome (e.g., damage to the lateral cutaneous nerve of the thigh during an anterior approach). Femoral nerve palsy is rare and does have a capacity for recovery. However, permanent femoral nerve palsy following reconstruction is a disaster and will lead to a poor result. Damage to the obturator nerve is not fully documented but can occur with a complex injury entering the obturator foramen. It can also result during the reduction of a quadrilateral plate fracture through the ilioinguinal approach.

Infection

Deep infection following an acetabular reconstruction correlates very strongly with a poor result. The only exceptions to this are those infections that follow the ilioinguinal approach, which are usually retropubic. If a satisfactory joint seal is achieved, then it is possible to obtain an acceptable outcome even with such an infection. Deep infection is a catastrophe in all other external approaches and will influence not only the short-term result but also jeopardize long-term reconstructive procedures (e.g., total hip replacement).

Heterotopic Ossification

Direct trauma to the abductors following injury or surgery will result in the increased risk of the development of heterotopic ossification. Meticulous excision of dead muscle combined with Indocid ± DXT will reduce the incidence and severity of bone formation. Although Brooker's grading is far from satisfactory, grades 3 and 4 will result in a decrease in motion. In the past, because of generous grading systems this has not strongly influenced the reported outcome. With stricter, more modern assessments, the effect on the end result becomes more apparent.

The Timing of Treatment Producing Avascular Necrosis

Early Management

All dislocated hips should be reduced as soon as possible. It has been shown quite clearly that in pure dislocations, time to relocation correlated strongly with avascular necrosis rates (15). If there is an associated fracture it is still important to reduce the hip as soon as possible. Traction should also be applied to prevent secondary abrasion.

The Reconstructive Surgery

Letournel's results show a statistically significant deterioration in the quality of the result if surgery is delayed beyond 3 weeks. Again this message must not be misunderstood. Acetabular reconstructive surgery should be performed as soon as practically possible. Massive reconstruction should not be carried out on polytraumatized patients during the first week. Surgery can be undertaken as an emergency when indicated, but if carried out too soon following injury the "second hit phenomenon" may ensue. This may compromise the patient's safety. Other complications (e.g., infection) may also be increased because of a compromised immune system. However, surgery should not be unduly delayed, and other factors (e.g., theater time) may influence the timing of operation.

The Quality of Reduction

Letournel's and Matta's series all clearly demonstrate that an excellent outcome correlates strongly with acceptable reduction of the fracture. If surgery is performed with the appropriate approach, at the appropriate time, by an experienced team, then it is much more likely that an excellent reduction will follow and this will improve the chances of a good outcome.

HOW DO WE IMPROVE OUTCOME IN THE 21ST CENTURY?

It seems that to improve outcome we must achieve a balance between quality of reduction and the complications that may occur by performing large approaches in an attempt to achieve a perfect reduction. It is clear that these fractures need to be managed by experienced teams and surgery needs to be performed at the appropriate time.

The Timing of Surgery

All dislocations should be as promptly reduced as possible. I believe traction should be applied, particularly in the transverse fracture types to prevent secondary femoral head abrasion. Acetabular reconstruction is rarely indicated in the first 24 hours following injury. The absolute indication for early surgery is irreducible fracture dislocations. This is demanding surgery and consideration should be made for urgent transfer to a specialist unit. All other surgery should be performed in a planned environment after correct assessment and imaging. Children's fractures should be operated on promptly because they heal very rapidly.

Improved Imaging

With the advent of 3DCT and MRI scanning it is now possible to visualize these fractures very accurately. However, the skill of the interpretation of the plain films must not be lost and plain AP and Judet x-rays still must be taken.

Better Equipment

The use of modified clamps and computer-assisted surgery may aid the acetabular surgeon to obtain better reductions.

Prompt Referral

The prompt referral of patients has lessened the need for extensile approaches. It is now possible to reduce parts of the acetabulum directly combined with lesser indirect reductions.

Patient Selection

Within large units it is now recognized that some fracture configurations are not worthy of reconstruction. Arthroplasty may provide better outcomes in an aging population. The real problem still lies with the young patient with high-energy comminuted fractures.

Nerve Repair

It is hoped during the course of the next two to three decades that methods of repairing such nerves may improve with the overall outcome. It is still frustrating for the patient and surgeon to have an excellent radiographic result but poor clinical outcome because of nerve palsy.

REFERENCES

1. Letournel E, Judet R. *Fractures of the acetabulum,* 2nd ed. New York: Springer-Verlag, 1993.
2. Judet R, Judet J, Letournel E. Fractures of the acetabulum: classification and surgical approaches for open reduction. *J Bone Joint Surg* 1964;46A:1615.
3. Tile M. *Fractures of the acetabulum.* Presented at the Canadian Orthopaedic Association annual meeting. Saint John, Newfoundland, Canada, 1992.
4. Hamilton R. Changes in tibiotalar areas of contact. *J Bone Joint Surg* 1976;58A:356–357.
5. Vrahas M, Vennis N. Intra-articular contact stress with simulated ankle malunions. *Orthop Trans* 1990;14:265.
6. Thompson VP, Epstein HA. Traumatic dislocation of the hip: a survey of 204 cases covering a period of 21 years. *J Bone Joint Surg* 1951;33A:746.
7. Rowe CR, Lowell JD. Prognosis of fracture of the acetabulum. *J Bone Joint Surg* 1961;43A:30.
8. Matta JM, Mehne DK, Roffi R. Fracture of the acetabulum. Early results of the prospective study. *Clin Orthop* 1986;205:241.
9. Matta JM, Merritt PO. Displaced acetabular fracture. *Clin Orthop* 1988;230:83.

10. Matta JM. Fracture of the acetabulum: accuracy of reduction and clinical results. *J Bone Joint Surg* 1996;78-A:1632–1645.
11. Moed BR, Carr SE, Watson T. Open reduction and internal fixation of posterior wall fractures of the acetabulum. *Clin Orthop Rel Res* 2000;377:57–67.
12. Chiu F-Y, Chen C-M, Lo W-H. Surgical treatment of displaced acetabular fractures: 72 cases followed for 10 (6–14) years. *Int J Care Injured* 2000;31:181–185.
13. Plaisier BR, Meldon SW, Super DM, Malangoni MA. Improved outcome after early fixation of acetabular fractures injury. *Int J Care Injured* 2000;31:81–84.
14. Liebergall M, Mosheiff R, Low J, et al. Acetabular fractures. Clinical outcome of surgical treatment. *Clin Orthop Rel Res* 1999; 366:205–216.
15. Upadhyay SS, Moulton A. The long-term results of traumatic posterior dislocation of the hip. *J Bone Joint Surg* 1981;63B:548.

SUBJECT INDEX

Page numbers followed by *f* refer to figures; page numbers followed by *t* refet to tables.

B

T